**BMA**

brary

dge, better care

ofession     king for ve

an

*Hamilton Bailey's*

# Demonstrations of Physical Signs in Clinical Surgery

D1141805

1000695

# *Hamilton Bailey's*
# Demonstrations of Physical Signs in Clinical Surgery

## *19th Edition*

**Edited by**

**John S P Lumley**, Emeritus Professor of Vascular Surgery, University of London; Past Council Member and Chairman of Primary Fellowship Examinations, Royal College of Surgeons of England, UK

**Anil K D'Cruz**, Director, Tata Memorial Hospital, Professor & Surgeon, Department of Head & Neck Surgery, Mumbai, India

**Jamal J Hoballah**, Professor & Chairman, Department of Surgery, American University of Beirut Medical Center, Lebanon; Emeritus Professor of Surgery, Vascular Surgery Division, University of Iowa Hospitals and Clinics, Iowa City, USA

**Carol E H Scott-Conner**, Emeritus Professor, Division of Surgical Oncology and Endocrine Surgery, Department of Surgery, University of Iowa Carver College of Medicine, Iowa City, USA

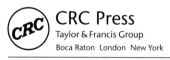
**CRC Press**
Taylor & Francis Group
Boca Raton  London  New York

CRC Press is an imprint of the
Taylor & Francis Group, an **informa** business

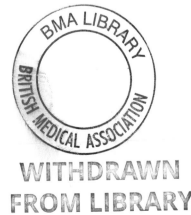
BMA LIBRARY
BRITISH MEDICAL ASSOCIATION

WITHDRAWN
FROM LIBRARY

CRC Press
Taylor & Francis Group
6000 Broken Sound Parkway NW, Suite 300
Boca Raton, FL 33487-2742

© 2016 by Taylor & Francis Group, LLC
CRC Press is an imprint of Taylor & Francis Group, an Informa business

No claim to original U.S. Government works

Printed on acid-free paper
Version Date: 20151109

Printed and bound in India by Replika Press Pvt. Ltd.

International Standard Book Number-13: 978-1-4441-6918-8 (Pack - Book and Ebook) 978-1-4441-6920-1 (Paperback)
International Standard Book Number-13: 978-1-4441-6920-1 (International Students' Edition, restricted territorial availability)

This book contains information obtained from authentic and highly regarded sources. While all reasonable efforts have been made to publish reliable data and information, neither the author[s] nor the publisher can accept any legal responsibility or liability for any errors or omissions that may be made. The publishers wish to make clear that any views or opinions expressed in this book by individual editors, authors or contributors are personal to them and do not necessarily reflect the views/opinions of the publishers. The information or guidance contained in this book is intended for use by medical, scientific or health-care professionals and is provided strictly as a supplement to the medical or other professional's own judgement, their knowledge of the patient's medical history, relevant manufacturer's instructions and the appropriate best practice guidelines. Because of the rapid advances in medical science, any information or advice on dosages, procedures or diagnoses should be independently verified. The reader is strongly urged to consult the relevant national drug formulary and the drug companies' and device or material manufacturers' printed instructions, and their websites, before administering or utilizing any of the drugs, devices or materials mentioned in this book. This book does not indicate whether a particular treatment is appropriate or suitable for a particular individual. Ultimately it is the sole responsibility of the medical professional to make his or her own professional judgements, so as to advise and treat patients appropriately. The authors and publishers have also attempted to trace the copyright holders of all material reproduced in this publication and apologize to copyright holders if permission to publish in this form has not been obtained. If any copyright material has not been acknowledged please write and let us know so we may rectify in any future reprint.

Except as permitted under U.S. Copyright Law, no part of this book may be reprinted, reproduced, transmitted, or utilized in any form by any electronic, mechanical, or other means, now known or hereafter invented, including photocopying, microfilming, and recording, or in any information storage or retrieval system, without written permission from the publishers.

For permission to photocopy or use material electronically from this work, please access www.copyright.com (http://www.copyright.com/) or contact the Copyright Clearance Center, Inc. (CCC), 222 Rosewood Drive, Danvers, MA 01923, 978-750-8400. CCC is a not-for-profit organization that provides licenses and registration for a variety of users. For organizations that have been granted a photocopy license by the CCC, a separate system of payment has been arranged.

**Trademark Notice:** Product or corporate names may be trademarks or registered trademarks, and are used only for identification and explanation without intent to infringe.

**Visit the Taylor & Francis Web site at**
**http://www.taylorandfrancis.com**

**and the CRC Press Web site at**
**http://www.crcpress.com**

# Contents

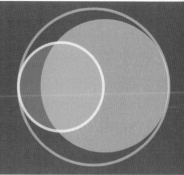

# Hamilton Bailey
# 1894–1961

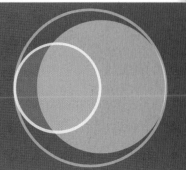

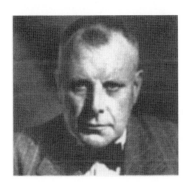

Born in Bishopstoke, Hampshire, where his father was a general practitioner, Henry Hamilton Bailey grew up in Southport, Eastbourne, and Brighton, England, where his father was successfully in practice. His mother was a nurse, so not surprisingly he became a medical student at the London Hospital at the early age of sixteen years, after schooling at St. Lawrence College, Ramsgate.

At the outbreak of the First World War he was a fourth-year medical student, and volunteered for the Red Cross, being dispatched with the British Expeditionary Force to Belgium. Almost inevitably he was taken prisoner-of-war and set to work on the German railways. A troop train was wrecked and Bailey, with two Frenchmen, was held on suspicion of sabotage. One of the latter was actually executed but Bailey was reprieved (apparently by the good offices of the American Ambassador in Berlin) and repatriated via Denmark, where he continued his medical studies temporarily.

In 1916 he joined the Royal Navy as a Surgeon-Probationer, serving in HMS Iron Duke at the Battle of Jutland. During the battle he helped with casualties in near darkness, the electricity supply being damaged for most of the action. While in the Navy he qualified, and later returned to the London Hospital, where he gained the FRCS (Eng) in 1920. During his period as surgical registrar at the London Hospital he pricked his left index finger, and tendon-sheath infection, a common sequel in those days, ensued. The end result was an amputation of the stiff finger, but he soon overcame the disability.

Appointments as Assistant Surgeon at Liverpool Royal Infirmary, Surgeon to Dudley Road Hospital, Birmingham (1925), and finally as Surgeon to the Royal Northern Hospital, London (1931) followed.

In a quarter of a century Bailey produced this work, his *Emergency Surgery*, and *Short Practice of Surgery* [jointly with R.J. McNeill Love (1891–1974), contemporary as a surgical registrar at the London Hospital and as a Surgeon at the Royal Northern Hospital], edited *Surgery of Modern Warfare* during the Second World War, and revitalized *Pye's Surgical Handicraft*. These were his most successful works; all rapidly attained a wide circulation with many editions, and it has been said "... it will readily be conceded that the present excellence of illustrations in medical textbooks owes much to his inspiration and striving for perfection". In addition to these major contributions, he wrote over 130 original papers and nine other books.

All this, together with a busy practice, particularly in surgical emergencies, was too much, even for Hamilton Bailey's massive frame, and in 1948 he suffered a breakdown in health, aggravated, no doubt, by the death of his only child, a son, in a railway accident in 1943. He retired to Deal, Kent, and later to Malaga, Spain, but continued his literary work. He died of carcinoma of the colon, and is buried in the peaceful little English cemetery in Malaga. His missionary zeal for teaching medical students has been perpetuated by the use of the royalties from his books to expand medical libraries in developing countries.

# Contributors

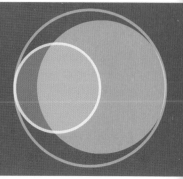

**Dr Ghassan S. Abu-Sittah** MBchB FRCS (Plast), Assistant Professor of Surgery, Head of Division of Plastic & Reconstructive Surgery, American University of Beirut Medical Center, Beirut, Lebanon; Honorary Senior Clinical Lecturer, Queen Mary University of London, UK

**Badih Adada** MD FRCS, Cleveland Clinic Florida, FL, USA

**Muhyeddine Al-Taki** MD FACS, Assistant Professor of Clinical Surgery, American University of Beirut Medical Center, Beirut, Lebanon

**Parth Amin** MD, Clinical Assistant Professor, Western Michigan University School of Medicine, Kalamazoo, MI, USA

**Evgeny V. Arshava** MD FACS, Clinical Assistant Professor, Division Acute Care Surgery, Department of Surgery, University of Iowa Hospitals and Clinics, Iowa City, IA, USA

**Andrea Badillo** MD, Assistant Professor of Surgery, Attending Pediatric Surgeon, Children's National Healthcare System, George Washington University, Washington DC, USA

**Jamil Borgi** MD, Cardiothoracic Surgery Senior Staff, Division of Cardiac Surgery, Henry Ford Hospital, Detroit, MI, USA

**John Byrn** MD, Department of Surgery, University of Michigan, Ann Arbor, MI, USA

**Devendra Chaukar** MS (General Surgery) DNB, Professor and Head, Division of Head and Neck, Tata Memorial Hospital, Mumbai, India

**William Cross** BMed Sci BM BS FRCS (Urol) PhD, Consultant Urological Surgeon, St James's University Hospital, Leeds, UK

**Anil K. D'Cruz** MS DNB FRCS (Hon), Director, Tata Memorial Hospital, Professor and Surgeon, Head and Neck Services, Tata Memorial Hospital, Mumbai, India

**Mitali Dandekar** MS DNB, Clinical Fellow, Department of Head Neck Surgery, Tata Memorial Centre, Mumbai, India

**Anuja D. Deshmukh** MS (ENT) DLO DORL, Associate Professor and Associate Surgeon, Department of Head and Neck Surgical Oncology, Tata Memorial Centre, Mumbai, India

**Shraddha Deshmukh** MS DNB, Assistant Professor, Department of Otorhinolaryngology, Government Medical College, Nagpur, India

**Mandar S. Deshpande** MS (General Surgery) DNB, Consultant Head and Neck Surgeon, Kokilaben Dhirubhai Ambani Hospital, Mumbai, India

**Parul Deshpande** MS (Ophthalmology) DNB, Fellowship (Cornea and Anterior segment) Ophthalmologist and Cornea Specialist, Sarvodaya Eye Hospital, Mumbai, India

**Jesse Dirksen** MD, Surgical Director, Edith Sanford Breast Center, Sioux Falls, SD, USA

**Celia M. Divino** MD FACS, Department of Surgery, Mount Sinai School of Medicine, New York, NY, USA

**Abdel Kader El Tal** MD, Procedural Dermatology, Dermatology Associates Inc. Perrysburg, OH, USA

**Rachid Haidar** MD FACS, Head of Division of Orthopedic Surgery, Professor of Clinical Orthopaedic Surgery, Department of Surgery, American University of Beirut Medical Center, Beirut, Lebanon

**Ali Hallal** MD FRCS (Ed), Assistant Professor of Clinical Surgery, General and Upper Gastro-Intestinal Surgery, Trauma Surgery and Intensive Care, Program Director, Trauma and Surgical Critical Care Fellowship, Department of Surgery, American University of Beirut Medical Center, Beirut, Lebanon

**Natalie Anne Hirst** BSc MBBS MRCS, Clinical Research Fellow, St James's University Hospital, Leeds, UK

**Jamal J. Hoballah** Professor & Chairman, Department of Surgery, American University of Beirut Medical Center, Beirut, Lebanon; Emeritus Professor of Surgery, Vascular Surgery Division, University of Iowa Hospitals and Clinics, Iowa City, IA, USA

**Maen Aboul Hosn** MD FEBS, Division of Vascular Surgery, University of Iowa Hospitals and Clinics, Iowa City, IA, USA

**Hamed Janom** MD, Surgical Resident, PGY5, Division of Plastic and Reconstructive Surgery, American University of Beirut Medical Center, Beirut, Lebanon

**Subbiah Kannan** MS (ENT), Fellow (Head and Neck Onco-surgery), Consultant Head and Neck Onco-surgeon, Apollo Speciality Hospital, Chennai, India

**Firas Kawtharani** MD, Chief Resident, Orthopaedic Surgery, American University of Beirut Medical Center, Beirut, Lebanon

**Murad Lala** MS (General Surgery), MCh (Surgical Oncology) FICS, Consultant Surgical Oncologist, Department of Surgical Oncology, P. D. Hinduja National Hospital and Research Centre, Mumbai, India

**Ingrid Lizarraga** MBBS, Clinical Assistant Professor of Surgery, Division of Surgical Oncology and Endocrine Surgery, University of Iowa Carver College of Medicine, IA, USA

**John S. P. Lumley** Emeritus Professor of Vascular Surgery, University of London; Past Council Member and Chairman of Primary Fellowship Examinations, Royal College of Surgeons of England, UK

**Karim Masrouha** MD, Orthopaedic Surgery Resident, American University of Beirut Medical Center, Beirut, Lebanon

**Mira Merashli** MD, NIHR Leeds Musculoskeletal Biomedical Research Unit, Leeds Teaching Hospitals NHS Trust, University of Leeds, Leeds, UK

**Basant K. Misra** MBBS MS (General Surgery) MCh (Neurosurgery) Diplomate National Board (Neurosurgery), Consultant Neurosurgeon and Head, Department of Neurosurgery and Gamma Knife Radiosurgery, P. D. Hinduja National Hospital and Medical Research Centre, Mumbai, India

**Ahmad Moukalled** MD, General Surgery Resident, American University of Beirut Medical Center, Beirut, Lebanon

**Kelly Morris** MB, Northamptonshire Healthcare NHS Foundation Trust, Kettering, UK

**Maurice Murphy** MRCPI, Consultant Physician, Barts Health NHS Trust, London, UK

**Imad S. Nahle** MD, Chief Resident, Orthopaedic Surgery, American University of Beirut Medical Center, Beirut, Lebanon

**Sudhir V. Nair** MS (General Surgery) MCh (Head and Neck Oncology), Associate Professor, Head and Neck Service, Tata Memorial Centre, Mumbai, India

**Deepa Nair** MS DNB DORL, Associate Professor, Head and Neck Surgical Oncology, Tata Memorial Centre, Mumbai, India

**Rabih Nayfe** MD, Department of Internal Medicine, Akron General Medical Center, Cleveland Clinic Affiliate, Akron, OH, USA

**Gouri Pantvaidya** MS DNB MRCS, Associate Professor, Department of Head Neck Surgery, Tata Memorial Hospital, Mumbai, India

**Elie P. Ramly** MD, Surgery Resident, Department of Surgery, Oregon Health and Science University, Portland, OR, USA

**S. Girish Rao** MDS FDSRCS (Eng) FFDRCSI (Ire), Professor & Head, Department of Maxillofacial Surgery, RV Dental College Bangalore, India

**Lynn Riddell** FRCP, Clinical Director and Consultant Physician, Integrated Sexual Health Services, Northamptonshire Healthcare NHS Foundation Trust, Northampton, UK

**Bernard H. Sagherian** MD, Instructor of Clinical Surgery, American University of Beirut Medical Center, Division of Orthopedic Surgery, Department of Surgery, Beirut, Lebanon

**Carol E. H. Scott-Conner** MD PhD, Emeritus Professor of Surgery, Division of Surgical Oncology and Endocrine Surgery, University of Iowa Carver College of Medicine, IA, USA

**Pierre M. Sfeir** MD FACS, Associate Professor of Clinical Surgery, Head, Division of Cardio-Thoracic Surgery, Director, Residency Program Department of Surgery American University of Beirut Medical Center, Beirut, Lebanon

**Arpit Sharma** MS DNB DORL, Assistant Professor, Department of Otorhinolaryngology, Seth G. S. Medical College and K. E. M Hospital, Mumbai, India

**Fawwaz R. Shaw** MD, Congenital Cardiac Surgery Fellow, University of Washington, Seattle Children's Hospital, Seattle, WA, USA

**Malini D. Sur** MD, Department of Surgery, Mount Sinai School of Medicine, New York, NY, USA

**Shivakumar Thiagarajan** MS (ENT) DNB MS (ENT) DNB, Fellowship in Head and Neck Surgical Oncology, Assistant Professor, Department of Surgical Oncology, Malabar Cancer Centre, Kerala, India

**Imad Uthman** MD MPH FRCP, Professor of Clinical Medicine, Head, Division of Rheumatology, American University of Beirut Medical Center, Beirut, Lebanon

**Abhishek Vaidya** MS DNB, Assistant Professor, Head Neck Surgical Oncology, DMIMS, Wardha, India

**Richa Vaish** MS, Senior Resident, Head and Neck Surgical Oncology, Tata Memorial Centre, Mumbai, India

**Sagar S. Vaishampayan** MDS (Oral & Maxillofacial Surgery), Fellowship in Head & Neck Oncosurgery, Associate Professor, Department of Maxillofacial Surgery, MGM Medical University, Navi Mumbai, Maharashtra, India

# Preface to the 19th edition

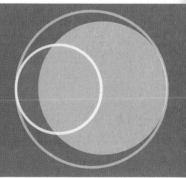

A complete history and full clinical examination are the foundation of excellence in clinical practice. It is therefore essential that these modalities are retained at the core of undergraduate and postgraduate training, irrespective of enormous technical and scientific advances and the competing demands from other disciplines.

These clinical principles have been the key elements of *Hamilton Bailey's Demonstrations of Physical Signs* since its first publication in 1927. The ease of world travel has facilitated the rapid spread of infection, while chronic conditions such as obesity, diabetes, cardiovascular conditions and many cancers are increasingly prevalent internationally, and clinicians have to be aware of this in their differential diagnoses. The current edition reflects this global nature of disease in its choice of editors and contributors from across the world.

Although Hamilton Bailey and his wife Vita would not recognise the current edition, they would appreciate its aims for clarity of text and full colour illustration. Its system-based organization mirrors the structure of the current edition of *Bailey & Love's Short Practice of Surgery*, re-establishing the link between these two seminal surgical textbooks. We hope that the nineteenth edition will continue to provide an invaluable source of clinical information for students worldwide.

John Lumley on behalf of the editorial team
London, 2015

# PART
# 1

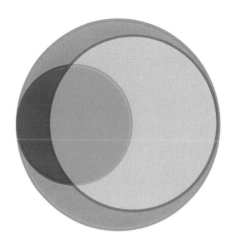

# Principles

# History-taking and General Examination

John S. P. Lumley and Natalie Anne Hirst

## LEARNING OBJECTIVES

- To be able to take a concise, structured patient history
- To understand the basis for a systematic general examination of the patient
- To know the methods for taking a manual blood pressure reading

- To be able to undertake a focused examination of systems and a formulation of initial working diagnoses
- To be aware of the specific requirements of the neonate and child in the surgical examination

## HISTORY-TAKING

A patient usually comes to see a doctor with a specific problem (a symptom) and the doctor's aim is to make the patient better. To do this, the doctor tries to work out what is causing the problem (the diagnosis), determine its severity (assessment) and then institute appropriate treatment. The total process of assessment and treatment is termed 'management'.

Disease may be due to social and psychological as well as physical abnormalities – the surgeon must be aware of, and sensitive to, all of these factors. To diagnose and assess a patient's problems, the doctor can obtain information from three sources:

- taking a history;
- carrying out a physical examination;
- requesting appropriate investigations.

The history is the single most important factor in making a diagnosis. Although this textbook is primarily concerned with eliciting abnormal physical signs, these are not always present at the time a patient presents. The history directs the clinician to search for the physical abnormalities and find them at the earliest possible stage of the disease, thus facilitating further management.

The skilled clinician becomes an expert on the pattern of diseases, but their greatest skill is to listen to what the patient volunteers. This is the key to the diagnosis and the clinician must not shape, elaborate, flavour or direct a history into a particular category just so that it fits a classical package. Such prompting may result in misdiagnosis.

Sometimes it is not possible to make a diagnosis. However, the process of assessment serves to exclude serious abnormalities, allowing the clinician to reassure the patient and advise symptomatic treatment. This strategy is based on the nature and duration of the symptoms. It allays the patient's fears and avoids an overinvestigation of trivial and self-limiting disease.

A decision must be made, however, on whether the patient needs to be seen again for further assessment. Continual explanation to the patient and good patient rapport are of vital importance and will translate into a more accurate diagnosis and increased patient knowledge. Management occasionally has to be initiated before a definitive diagnosis has been made, such as in the control of severe pain or haemorrhage.

The following scheme for history-taking is intended as an introduction to the subject and outlines the prime headings that need to be considered when interviewing each patient.

## SCHEME FOR HISTORY-TAKING

First record the **date and time** of the examination. Note the patient's **name, age, sex, occupation** (past and present) and **who they live with at home** (including any dependants). The history emerges from the patient's description of the problem, directed by your planned questioning. It is conveniently recorded under the following six headings.

### Present Illness

#### Presenting Complaint(s)

'Can you tell me why you've attended the hospital today?' This must be put in a short statement, preferably using the patient's own words, for example 'c/o [complaining of] abdominal pain and vomiting for the last 24 hours' or 'increasing breathlessness for 2 weeks'. If there is more than one complaint, these are listed and then taken in turn through the following two sections.

### History of Presenting Complaint(s)

This should record the details of each problem, using mainly the patient's own words. Record as accurately as possible how long the complaint has been present and include the sequence of events in chronological order with dates (e.g. 1 year ago, 1 month ago, yesterday). Let the patient begin by telling the story in their own words without interruption. Afterwards, ask specific questions using terms readily understood by the patient, either enlarging upon or clarifying their symptoms.

The presenting disorder is usually related to one system, and questions referable to this – and any other system involved in the presenting complaint – are delivered at this stage. Pain is one of the most common symptoms; appropriate questions are given below. Many of these questions can also be applied to other symptoms.

If the patient is a poor historian or is unable to give a history, or you suspect them of giving unreliable information, it may be helpful to talk to relatives or witnesses. Record the source of this and all aspects of the history that are not obtained directly from the patient.

### Previous History of Presenting Complaint(s)

If the patient has had similar symptoms in the past, obtain detailed information in chronological order, including any treatment received and the results of any investigations (if known). Report any past event with a clear bearing on the present condition, such as operations, trauma, weight loss, medication, contact with others with disease or any recent travel abroad.

## Past Medical History

Note all other previous non-trivial illnesses, operations, accidents and periods of admission to hospital for non-related illnesses, together with their dates. For children, note illnesses, investigations and immunizations. In adults, note relevant childhood problems, for example chronic respiratory disease, cardiac problems and rheumatic fever.

## Drugs and Allergies

Note all drugs being taken, their doses and for how long they have been taken. Ask what drugs have been taken in the past and for what conditions. Ensure that non-prescription medications, for example St John's Wort, and any other drugs the patient may not consider as medication, such as the oral contraceptive pill, are also documented. Record drug allergies and any allergic symptoms. Ask what is meant by any admitted allergy or sensitivity.

## Social and Personal History

Note any current smoking habit, the number of years smoked and any changes over this time. Note the usual alcohol consumption in units per day or per week and what is drunk. Sensitively question whether the subject has ever been a heavy drinker. Ask whether any recreational drugs are used, which drugs, when and in what quantities.

Record details of the patient's work and, where relevant, any difficulties with their job, family or finances. Note any recent mental stress or problems with their sleeping pattern. Does the patient live alone? Which floor? Are there lifts? Is the lavatory on a different floor? Are friends and/or relatives nearby? Do they receive or need home help or meals on wheels? Will the patient be able to return to their previous residence and/or employment?

## Family History

Enquire into the state of health or cause of death of the patient's parents, siblings, other close relatives and partner. Ask whether any members of the family are suffering, or have suffered, from the presenting condition(s). It often helps to draw a family tree.

## Review of Systems

The history of the presenting complaint encompasses a detailed enquiry into at least one of the body's systems; this part of the history reviews the remaining systems for unsuspected abnormalities. It is carried out using specific questioning pertinent to each system, and this is then considered alongside the examination of the relevant system. Important non-specific symptoms may also be present such as fever, lassitude, malaise and weight change.

### PAIN

Pain is an indicator of disease and is frequently the presenting symptom for every body system. It varies with the disease process and the tissue involved and may be characteristic and diagnostic. Pain may be present at the time of interview but – although this allows a first-hand experience of the patient's problem – it can also interfere with the assessment.

Pain is very subjective and can be influenced by what the patient thinks or suspects its cause to be and by its implications. Patients may have worries about the seriousness of a certain condition and because relatives or friends have been disabled by or died from similar problems. They may want to impress or convince the doctor, or may underplay the symptom in order not to interfere with their own plans and needs. Responses to pain also vary with age, sex, ethnic origin, education and personality. A doctor should guard against categorizing and interpreting a pain to suit a chosen diagnosis and – even if leading questions are needed – there must be a free choice of answers.

Although friends and relatives can provide a good indication of how the pain is interfering with the patient's everyday activities, they cannot describe the features of the pain. In this respect, the use of interpreters can be difficult since the words used to describe the nature and severity of pain may have different meanings in different languages – the interpreter may be giving their own opinion rather than the patient's. In addition, patients may be unwilling to admit their fears or disclose the precipitating causes of a pain via an interpreter.

Each doctor must therefore develop an efficient and reliable method of questioning a patient about their pain, using clear, understandable language. The following section outlines the areas that need to be covered. It is worth studying these questions and reshuffling them into a form that you can easily remember, perhaps converting them into an acronym or an anagram – SOCRATES is a well-known example:

- S: Site;
- O: Onset;
- C: Character;
- R: Radiation;
- A: Associations;
- T: Timing;
- E: Exacerbating/relieving factors;
- S: Severity.

## Site

The site of the pain is a good indicator of its origin. Ask the patient where the pain is, and get them to point to the area of maximum intensity. This may be **focal** and indicated with one finger, such as an infected maxillary air sinus or a fractured lateral malleolus. Injuries in particular can usually be localized by the site of the pain and tenderness – pain is what is experienced by the patient, while tenderness is elicited by the examining doctor.

Pain arising from the skin and subcutaneous tissues is better localized than that from deeper structures as pain in the latter may be **diffuse**. Headache from an intracranial lesion may be indicated by the patient placing a whole hand placed over the side or top of the head. Similarly, cardiac pain may be demonstrated by a hand over the central chest wall, and abdominal pain by a hand over a quadrant of the abdomen. Severe limb ischaemia is another example of diffuse pain, with the rest pain involving the forefoot or sometimes the whole foot and lower leg.

Pain may **radiate** from the site of origin to another region of the body; for example, protrusion of an intervertebral disc may trap a nerve, giving local back pain, but may also produce pain down the back of the thigh and possibly into the calf or foot. Pain from posterior abdominal wall structures – such as the pancreas and abdominal aorta – may radiate through to the back. Renal colic may radiate from the loin around to the iliac fossa and into the groin. Gallbladder pain may be felt between the shoulder blades, while the pain of a myocardial infarction may radiate from the chest into the neck and down the left arm. The radiated pain may have different features from the local pain and may occur independently of it.

**Referred** pain implies pain occurring at a site far removed from the originating disease. It is due to visceral nerve impulses stimulating the somatic afferent pathways of the same dermatome. A classic example is pain over the tip of the shoulder from disease under the diaphragm, the visceral nerve involved being the phrenic, and the somatic dermatome the fourth cervical.

## Timing

When asking about the timing of a pain, include its onset, progress and offset. The **onset** may be sudden or gradual. Sudden pain is typical of pain associated with an injury or with the blockage or rupture of an artery (as in myocardial infarction or a ruptured abdominal aorta) or the rupture of a viscus (such as a spontaneous pneumothorax or a perforated peptic ulcer). Most patients are be able to describe the precise time of onset in these examples.

With a gradual onset, the timing may vary greatly. Acute inflammatory lesions may progress during a day or overnight, while claudication from degenerative arterial disease or the pain of an osteoarthritic knee may build up over many years before the patient realizes that a vague ache is a specific problem and seeks medical advice. 'Gradual' in these examples implies a gradual awareness of the pain; it also indicates a gradual increase in the severity of the pain.

Note the **progress** of the current attack, whether it is changing and whether there is any **pattern** to the pain. Pain may gradually increase or decrease or become continuous or persistent. It may also fluctuate. There may be total relief from the pain between bouts. The latter is characteristic of **colic**, which is due to waves of contraction down an obstructed hollow viscus, such as with adhesions obstructing the small bowel, a cancer obstructing the large bowel or a stone blocking the ureter. Note how often these attacks occur and their duration. The pain may be continuous with exacerbations producing peaks of pain. Factors exacerbating or precipitating the pain are considered below (see 'Modification', below).

Enquire carefully about **previous** bouts of pain or anything similar in the past. Record the patterns of previous attacks, their frequency, how many there have been in all and their duration. Note whether they are changing in character. The terms 'exacerbation' and 'recurrence' are used to denote changes in a disease as well as in its symptoms.

Like the onset, the **offset** of pain may be gradual or sudden, and this may be characteristic of the condition. Relief of the pain usually indicates an improvement in the disease or a removal of the precipitating cause. Improvement may be obtained by treating the patient with analgesics, surgically or with other therapies. Very occasionally, a reduction of pain is a bad sign, for example with the rupture of a tense abscess into the cerebral ventricles or the peritoneal cavity. The previous history and a knowledge of any underlying disease can provide guidelines on the likelihood of a further recurrence of the pain.

## Severity

The quantity of pain is generally related to the severity of the underlying disease. However, individuals vary extensively in their pain tolerance, and this is further influenced by anxiety and a fear of the possible implications of the pain. Sometimes there may be a desire to impress the doctor over the extent of the problem or conversely to play down the symptoms for some personal reason.

A useful indicator is the influence of the pain on the patient's lifestyle. Ask whether they have had to stop work or go to bed and whether they are losing sleep because of the pain. If they have pain at the time of the interview, their response to it can be directly assessed. However, by this time they may already have had some appropriate analgesia.

A rough quantitative measure can be obtained using a pain scale of 0 to 10. The patient is asked to grade their pain on this scale, with 0 being no pain at all and 10 being the worst possible pain imaginable. Although this is still very subjective and dependent on the individual's response, it can be of value in assessing change within the individual.

## Character

The character or quality of the pain is another subjective assessment; it may have specific characteristics but these may be difficult to categorize. The terms used can be linked to previous experiences – common descriptions are sharp, stabbing or knife-like. Such terms are associated with most wounds.

Inflammation and pain from deeper organs are often described in less precise terms, such as aching, bruising, burning, gripping, crushing, twisting and breaking. Colic has already been referred to above for gut obstruction, when the patient may also complain of a distended or bloated feeling; this may also occur in childbirth and urinary retention.

A throbbing pain implies a tense, sensitive area with an increase in tension with each heart beat. Such situations can occur with vascular tumours, acute inflammation with or without an abscess, and raised intracranial pressure and vascular lesions such as an expanding aneurysm or a complicated arteriovenous malformation or fistula.

## Modification

Some of the factors that precipitate and influence a pain may have already been elicited by this stage in the history. Now ask the patient specifically what makes the pain worse or better, and what they do in an attack.

**Aggravating/exacerbating** factors include eating spicy foods (for peptic ulcers) and fatty foods (with biliary disease), movement such as coughing (for pleuritic pain and pain due to peritonitis) or walking (with lower limb injuries or ischaemia), and certain postures such as sitting and standing (with lumbar disc protrusions) and raising the leg (in severe foot ischaemia or sacral nerve root compression).

**Relieving** factors include analgesics and specific medications such as antacids. Eating may relieve the pain of duodenal ulcers, and resting a limb may ease the inflammatory pain and pain caused by an injury. The severe pain of lower limb ischaemia may be helped by hanging the leg out of bed.

The application of heat from a hot flannel, a fire or a hot water bottle is often used, and specific aids such as transcutaneous electrical nerve stimulation can help. The repeated use of heat such as a fire to the shins or a hot water bottle on the abdomen may produce a characteristic mottled brown skin pigmentation (erythema ab igne), providing an important physical sign.

Remember that denervation may render an area insensitive and therefore subject to repeated trauma and inflammatory changes without the protective benefit of pain sensation. Such examples are seen in diabetic neuropathy, where perforating ulcers are commonly seen over the pressure areas of the sole. Extreme examples are seen in leprosy, where there can be a progressive loss of digits and limbs.

## Associated Symptoms

The systemic effects of pain may be primary or secondary. Primary effects are specific events such as the vomiting that is seen with peptic ulcers and the diarrhoea of inflammatory bowel disease. However, these same symptoms can be seen as non-specific effects in severe pain originating outside the alimentary tract. Similarly, nausea, malaise, sweating, loss of sleep and restricted fluid and food intake are frequently encountered. It is of paramount importance to ascertain any weight loss due to its frequent correlation with malignancy. Attempts should be made to quantify this, either by a change in the patient's weight on measuring scales or in terms of whether the patient has noticed their clothing getting looser.

## Cause of Pain

It is important to ask the patient's opinion on the cause of their pain as they may know or think they know what this is. They may be afraid or unwilling to tell you the cause as there may be a guilt complex, such as with current or previous self-abuse, but there may still be some hints on the underlying cause of the pain. Such clues must be carefully noted. The patient may well have given a lot of thought to the potential causes of their pain, and it is important to identify areas of anxiety, which can often be treated by immediate reassurance.

### GENERAL PHYSICAL EXAMINATION

When undertaking a physical examination, aim to keep the patient comfortable, relaxed and reassured. Talk through what is going to happen – if this is not obvious – and ensure there is minimal discomfort and inconvenience. A warm environment is essential and, similarly, the examiner's hands must be warm. The privacy of a small room or a curtained area is desirable, with optimal, preferably natural, lighting.

The patient should undress down to their underclothes and put on a dressing gown. They will then lie supine on a couch with an adjustable back to provide head support, covered with a sheet or blanket. Each area must be adequately exposed as needed without embarrassing the patient. A cardinal principle is to expose both sides when examining paired structures in order to compare the diseased with the normal, for example a limb or breast. A chaperone may be appropriate when examining members of the opposite sex. Relatives are usually best excluded, except when examining children.

The examiner stands on the right side of the patient. The order of examination is **regional** rather than by system, although the central nervous system is often examined as an entity, together with various parts of the locomotor system, at the end of the procedure.

It is usual to start the examination with the patient's hands and then to proceed methodically from head to toe, surveying all the systems and later integrating these findings, as subsequent verbal presentations and recordings in the notes are usually by system. Thoroughness is important – efficiency and speed develop with practice. The examination time should not be prolonged for ill or frail patients, and in emergencies it may be appropriate to concentrate on diseased areas, completing the routine examination at a later time.

## General Impression

Throughout the history-taking, the clinician is gaining an impression of the patient's physical and mental status and the severity of their disability, as well as attempting to make a diagnosis. The physical examination continues these observations, giving information on the patient's general state of health, shape, posture, state of hygiene and mental and physical activity. The patient must be considered as a whole but initially the doctor should observe the exposed parts, particularly the hands, skin, head and neck.

The patient may be fit and well, but problems with diet and disease can lead to an alteration in nutrition and hydration such as obesity, weight loss, cachexia, loss of skin turgor or skin laxity. In the clinic, it is important to weigh the patient; other factors that should be routinely charted are the pulse rate, blood pressure and urine test results. A subject can usually state their height, but an accurate assessment, together with measurements of segments and spans, may be important when considering endocrine abnormalities. Admission to hospital usually indicates more severe disease states, and additional monitoring then includes temperature, respiratory rate, bowel habit and the examination of the sputum and faeces.

### Mental Status

A patient's behaviour may be influenced by the unaccustomed situation of being a patient or by the effect of the disease, particularly if there is pain. This may be manifest by the patient's facial expression, the degree of eye contact, restlessness, sweating, anxiety, apathy, depression, lack of cooperation or aggression. Stress may be indicated by rapid respiration, a rapid pulse rate and sweating. Note whether the patient's comprehension and acuity equate to what one would expect from the history, or whether this could have changed in relation to the disease.

Drugs, head injuries and other diseases of the central nervous system can affect the level of consciousness, varying through alert, slow and confused, lacking concentration and a reduced level of response to spoken and physical stimuli. The patient's orientation in time, place and person should be noted: the Glasgow Coma Scale (see p. 140, *Table 6.2*) is a valuable way of documenting the level of consciousness for serial measurement. A patient's speech may be impaired by diseases of the central nervous system, producing dysphasia or dysarthria, and there may be voice changes such as hoarseness in laryngeal infection or myxoedema. Impairment of motor function can produce weakness or spasticity, and this may affect the speech.

The posture and gait should be noted, as should the ability to perform other activities such as undressing. There may be added movements such as the fine tremors of age, thyrotoxicosis, parkinsonism and alcoholism, the flapping tremors of hepatic, respiratory, renal and cardiac failure, or more specific neurological abnormalities producing a lack of coordination and involuntary movements.

Psychiatric assessment is not usually part of a surgical examination, but if abnormalities are present or suspected, note the general behaviour and any disturbances of consciousness and orientation. Record the patient's emotional state, insight, thought processes and content, as well as any hallucinations, delusions and compulsive phenomena, and include an assessment of cognitive and intellectual function.

## Abnormal Facies and Body Configuration

A number of congenital and endocrine diseases have characteristic general features amenable to a spot diagnosis. However, one needs experience to differentiate between minor changes and the extremes of normality so be aware of the danger of jumping to false conclusions. Congenital examples are Down, Turner's and Marfan's syndromes, achondroplasia and hereditary telangiectasia. Endocrine abnormalities include acromegaly, Cushing's disease, myxoedema and thyrotoxicosis. Other spot diagnoses included are Paget's disease, parkinsonism and myopathies (see Chapters 2 and 18). Some general disease states can be found in Chapter 2 and include weight loss, dehydration, oedema and pyrexia of unknown origin, as well as examples from the above list. Other examples included elsewhere are the features of hepatic and renal failure.

## The Hands

The general examination starts with the patient's hands: sweating or abnormal soft tissue may have been noted during the introductory handshake. The hand may be unusually large, as in acromegaly (**Figure 1.1**), or small or deformed, perhaps relating to a previous injury or to systemic disease. Skin abnormalities of the palm and dorsum of the hand may be easier to see in a white-skinned individual but are usually visible in all races and should be carefully noted. They include pallor, cyanosis, polycythaemia, pigmentation (**Figure 1.2**), bruises, rashes (**Figures 1.3** and **1.4**) and nicotine stains (**Figure 1.5**). Many of these features are more easily seen in the head and neck, and are further considered in the next section.

### Nails

The nails can be an indicator of local and systemic disease. There can be stunted growth, and they may be brittle and deformed. Nail-biters can be identified from the loss of the projecting

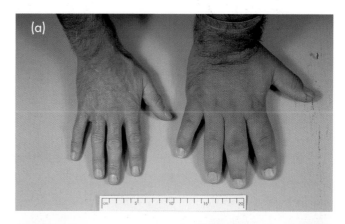
Figure 1.1 The acromegalic hand is large with wide long fingers.

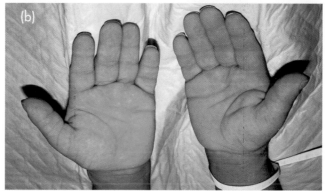
Figure 1.2 Skin pigmentation of the dorsum of the hand in a white patient with Nelson's syndrome.

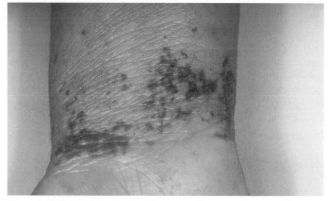
Figure 1.3 Hyperpigmentation of an area of atopic eczema on the wrist of a patient with Addison's disease.

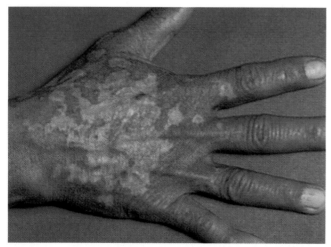

Figure 1.4 The rash of discoid lupus erythematosus of the dorsum of the hand.

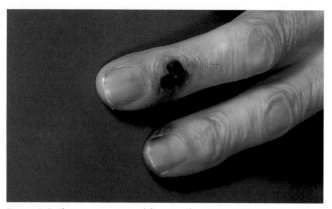

Figure 1.5 The nicotine-stained fingers of a chain smoker.

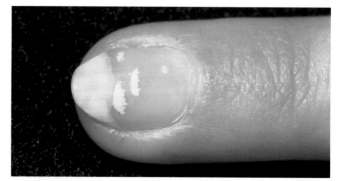

Figure 1.6 White spots within the nails indicating previous trauma.

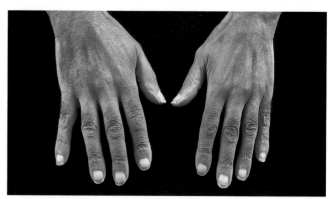

Figure 1.7 The colour of the nails in an anaemic patient.

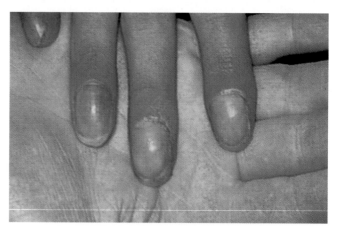

Figure 1.8 Marked cyanosis of the nails in a patient with Fallot's tetralogy.

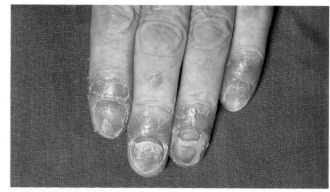

Figure 1.9 The pitted nails of psoriasis.

nail on all the digits of both hands. Whitish spots (**Figure 1.6**) under the nail (leukonychia punctata) are associated with minor trauma. The pallor of anaemia (**Figure 1.7**) and hypoalbuminaemia, and the colour of jaundice and cyanosis (**Figure 1.8**), are usually well shown, and pitting of the nails is common in psoriasis (**Figure 1.9**). Splinter haemorrhages are longitudinal brown strips along the length of the middle of the nail that are seen in subacute bacterial endocarditis and vasculitic disorders. A spoon-shaped depression of the nail is seen in iron deficiency anaemia and is termed koilonychia (**Figure 1.10**).

Transverse grooves at a similar level in a number of nails (Beau's lines; **Figure 1.11**) can denote growth abnormalities related to the onset of a severe systemic disease. The arch over the base of the nail may become brown (Mei's lines) in renal insufficiency, poisoning and some inflammatory disorders. Infections around the nail (paronychia; **Figure 1.12**) are common, but a diabetic aetiology must always be excluded.

## Clubbing

In clubbing of the fingers, the tissues at the base of the nail are thickened and the angle between the nail base and the adjacent skin of the finger, which should measure approximately 160°, becomes obliterated. The application of light pressure at the base of the nail is associated with excessive movement of the nail bed. In clubbing, the nail loses its longitudinal ridge and becomes convex from above downwards as well as from side to side.

In the later stages, there may be associated swelling of the tips of the fingers. Hypertrophic pulmonary osteoarthropathy may be associated with clubbing in bronchial carcinoma (**Figure 1.13**); involvement of the wrist joint can be looked for at this stage.

Clubbing, particularly the congenital variety, may also involve the feet (**Figure 1.14**). Common causes of clubbing are carcinoma and purulent conditions of the lung (bronchiectasis, lung abscess, empyema), congenital heart disease and infective endocarditis. Less common conditions are pulmonary fibrosis, fibrosing alveolitis, pulmonary tuberculosis, pleural mesothelioma, cystic fibrosis, coeliac and inflammatory bowel disease, cirrhosis (**Figure 1.15**), malabsorption, thyrotoxicosis and bronchial arteriovenous malformations.

## Skin

Examination of the skin of the palm of the hand gives some indication of the type of work the patient does. Stretch the skin of the palm to examine the colour of the skin creases – these provide a better indication than the more exposed areas. Erythema of the palmar skin is most marked over the thenar and hypothenar eminences (**Figure 1.16**). It is an important finding in liver disease but may also occur in pregnancy, thyrotoxicosis, polycythaemia, leukaemia, chronic febrile illnesses and rheumatoid arthritis. Liver disease may also give rise to spider naevi on the skin as well as yellow discoloration of the conjunctivae (**Figure 1.17**). The skin on the back of the hand is a useful site to assess skin turgidity and to look for generalized pigmentation (**Figures 1.18–1.20**) and bruising (**Figure 1.21**). Other cutaneous abnormalities (**Figures 1.22–1.24**) are considered on (see Table 18.1, p. 291). Laxity (**Figure 1.25**) is seen in older subjects but may indicate extensive dehydration at all ages. Similarly, areas of bruising and senile keratosis (**Figure 1.26**) are normal features of ageing but may also indicate disease or anticoagulant therapy. Skin nodules and moles are common (see p. 312).

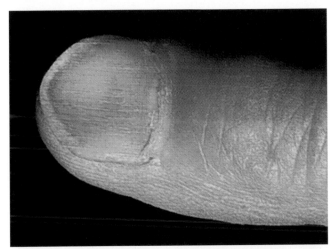

Figure 1.10 **The spoon-shaped depressions of koilonychia.**

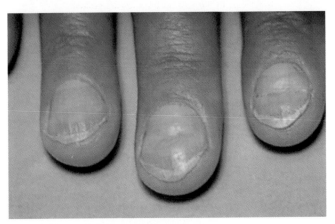

Figure 1.11 **Beau's lines.**

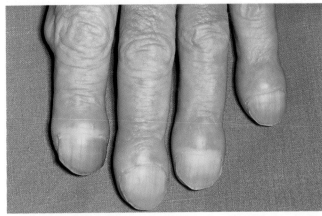

Figure 1.13 Clubbing associated with bronchial carcinoma.

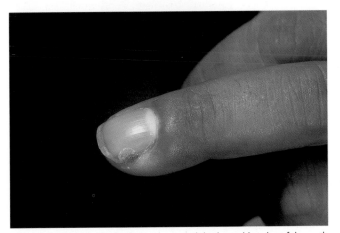

Figure 1.12 **Paronychial infections around the lateral border of the nail.**

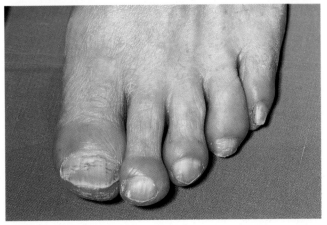

Figure 1.14 **Congenital clubbing of the feet.**

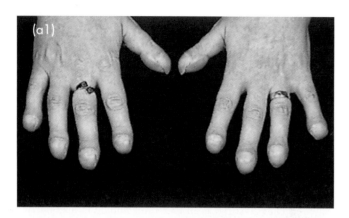

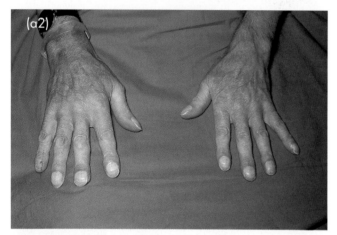

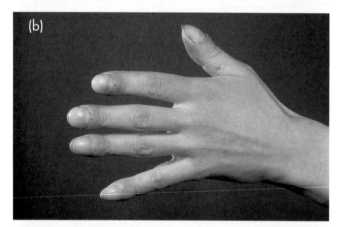

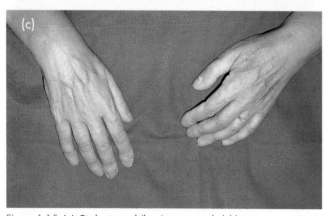

Figure 1.15 (a) Cirrhotic and (b, c) congenital clubbing.

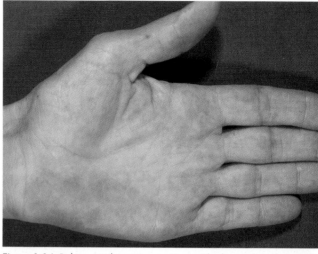

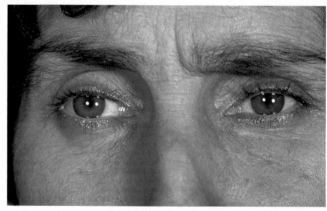

Figure 1.16 Palmar erythema in a patient with chronic liver failure.

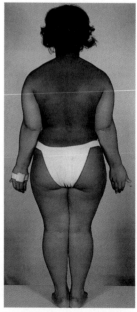

Figure 1.17 Primary biliary cirrhosis – yellow discoloration of the conjunctivae from jaundice.

Figure 1.18 Acanthosis nigricans – cutaneous pigmentation and thickening associated with an underlying malignancy. It is common in older individuals, associated with itching and commonly seen in the groin, hands and face. It may also affect the oral mucosa.

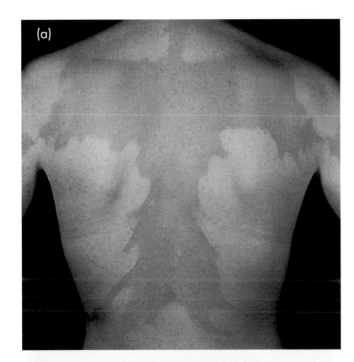

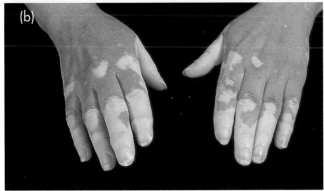

Figure 1.19 Vitiligo of (a) the back and (b) the hands. Vitiligo involves an autoimmune destruction of melanocytes often associated with other autoimmune diseases. The condition may be familial, lesions occasionally developing with changes in melanoma.

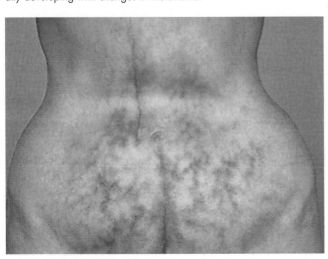

Figure 1.20 Erythema ab igne – reticular pigmentation following repeated application of a heat source, in this case a hot water bottle to soothe local pain.

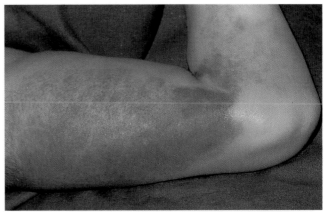

Figure 1.21 Bruising. Individuals vary in their ease of bruising, but spontaneous or major bruising requires investigation.

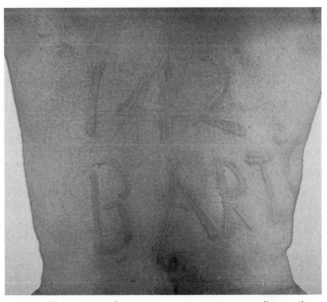

Figure 1.22 Dermography. Urticaria is a transient swelling with or without flushing, produced by physical and chemical agents. The demographia shown is a hypersensitive response to scratching.

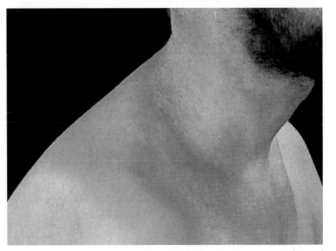

Figure 1.23 Light-sensitive dermatitis. Sunburn occurs a number of hours after exposure but light sensitivity as demonstrated occurs immediately, particularly over infrequently exposed areas.

PART 1 I PRINCIPLES

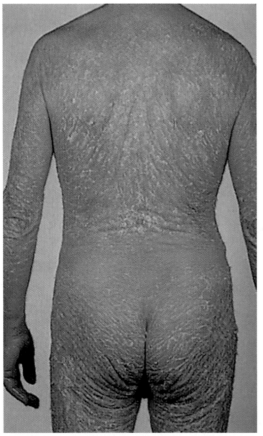

Figure 1.24 Exfoliative dermatitis, or erythroderma. Dermatitis is inflammation of the skin and may occur in response to an allergen, although the cause is often unknown.

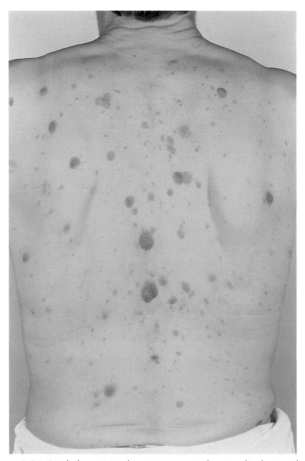

Figure 1.26 Senile keratosis – benign pigmented warty skin lesions that occur with age.

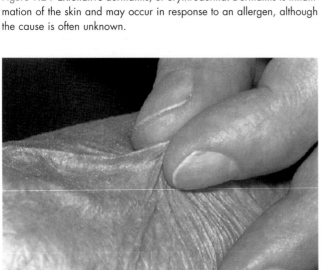

Figure 1.25 Laxity. With ageing, skin becomes thinner and loses its elasticity, as demonstrated by laxity.

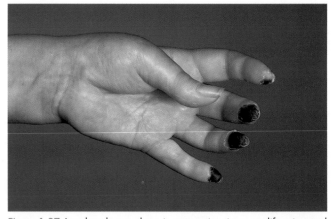

Figure 1.27 In scleroderma, there is connective tissue proliferation and inflammatory cell infiltration. It usually affects the skin layer, also producing necrosis or other tissue abnormalities.

Note the nutrition of the fingertips in scleroderma (Figure 1.27), rheumatoid arthritis (Figure 1.28), other collagen diseases and ischaemic conditions. There may be a loss of pulp and small areas of ulceration around the fingertips. Painful nodules around the fingertips are seen in infective endocarditis (Osler's nodes). Thickening of the palmar fascia – Dupuytren's contracture (Figure 1.29) – may be idiopathic, hereditary or associated with cirrhosis and various gut and pulmonary disorders.

## Muscles and Joints

The small muscles of the hand provide an early indication of general and muscular wasting as well as peripheral nerve injury. Note particularly the dorsum of the hand, the loss of substance of the interossei of the thumb and index finger (Figure 1.30), and the loss of muscle bulk deep to the long extensor tendons. Local causes of muscle wasting include carpal tunnel syndrome, proximal lesions of the median and ulnar nerves and their roots (Figure 1.31), motor neurone disease, poliomyelitis, syringomyelia, peripheral neuropathy and rheumatoid arthritis.

The joints of the hands are commonly affected in rheumatoid arthritis (see p. 168), and the terminal interphalangeal joint is occasionally involved in osteoarthritic changes. There may be

palpable osteophytes in this area, for example Heberden's nodes in osteoarthritis (Figure 1.32).

Examination of the pulse is considered in more detail under the vascular system (see p. 458), but at this stage in the general examination it is counted for at least half a minute and abnormalities of volume, character and rhythm are noted. The pulse rate at birth is approximately 135 beats per minute, falling to 100 at 5 years of age, 80 in the teens and 72 in the adult. This is also a useful point at which to note the blood pressure as it may be inadvertently omitted if not routinely positioned in the examination.

## Blood Pressure

The upper limb is fully exposed while the patient sits or lies on a couch. An appropriately sized blood pressure cuff must be used: in adults this is 12.5 cm. It should not impinge on the axilla or the cubital fossa and should be wrapped closely and evenly around the upper arm. Smaller cuffs are available for children. Too small a cuff can give a falsely high reading, while too large a cuff prevents access to the brachial artery. The manometer should be at the observer's eye level.

The radial pulse is palpated as the cuff is inflated. The pressure is raised to approximately 30 mmHg above the level at which the pulse disappears. A stethoscope is then lightly applied over the brachial artery on the medial aspect of the cubital fossa and the

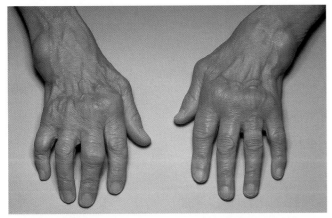

Figure 1.28 Rheumatoid arthritis. The chronic inflammatory changes in rheumatoid arthritis mostly affect the joints, producing deformity and disability.

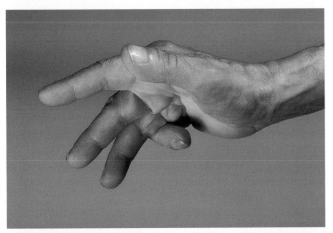

Figure 1.29 Dupuytren's contracture.

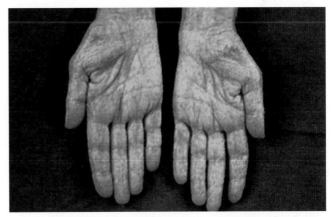

Figure 1.31 Leprosy. The muscle wasting is due to peripheral nerve damage.

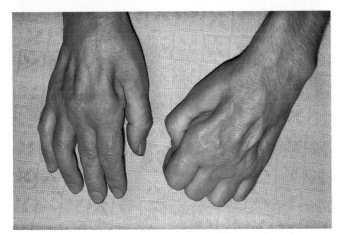

Figure 1.30 Small muscle wasting. Wasting of the small muscles in the hand may be part of general weight loss or specific abnormalities of muscle innervation.

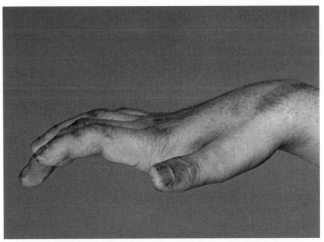

Figure 1.32 Heberden's nodes – inflammatory nodules of the skin overlying the joints in osteoarthritis.

cuff pressure is lowered 5 mmHg at a time. The systolic blood pressure is the level at which the sound is first heard. The diastolic pressure is the point at which the sound becomes suddenly faint or inaudible (Korotkoff sounds: I – appearance; IV – muffling; V – disappearance).

In cardiovascular disease, the blood pressure is taken in both arms and – in patients with treated or untreated hypertension – in the lying and standing positions. If a patient is anxious, a falsely high reading may be obtained together with an increased pulse rate. When abnormal readings are obtained, the recording should be repeated, the pressure in the cuff being allowed to drop to zero between measurements.

In peripheral vascular disease, the blood pressure may also be measured in the lower limbs. A wider cuff is required for thigh compression, and a Doppler probe is used to detect the presence or absence of a distal pulse. The systolic blood pressure is the point at which audible pulsation reappears when the cuff is deflated.

## The Face

Generalized weight loss may be apparent in changing facial and cervical contours. Excess tissue fluid – oedema (Figure 1.33) – is subject to the effect of gravity, and although mostly observed in the lower limbs towards the end of the day it may also be obvious in the face, particularly the eyelids, after a night's sleep. Regional oedema of the head, neck and upper limbs is seen in superior vena caval obstruction, and the oedema of myxoedema may be particularly obvious in the eyelids, associated with skin and hair changes (Figures 1.34 and 1.35).

Whereas pallor and cyanosis of the hands may be due to the cold or to local arterial disease, these signs in the warm, central areas of the lips and tongue have a more generalized significance. The pallor of anaemia is most noticeable in the mucous

membranes, although the sign lacks specificity. The inner surface of the lower lid is an important area to demonstrate this, as well as pallor being seen in the mucous membranes and the palmar creases.

Cyanosis is the blue discoloration given to the skin by deoxygenated blood. However, a minimum of 5 g/dL is required to produce visible cyanosis; it is thus not detectable in severe anaemia. Cyanosis is best observed in areas with a rich blood supply, such as the lips and tongue. It may also be noted in the ear lobes and fingernails, but these areas can react to cold by vasoconstriction, producing peripheral cyanosis in the presence of a normal oxygen saturation.

Central cyanosis is usually due to cardiorespiratory abnormalities (Figures 1.36 and 1.37) but may also occur at high altitudes and with methaemoglobinaemia and sulphhaemaglobinaemia. Cardiac conditions include a number of congenital abnormalities with a right-to-left shunt, while cyanosis may be

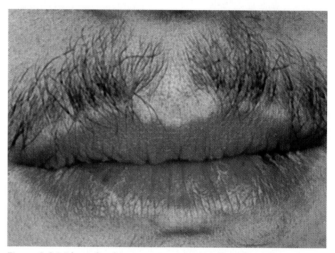

Figure 1.34 Idiopathic hirsuties. 'Hirsute' usually refers to a male pattern of hair growth in a female patient. Female hair growth varies in different races but is increased in a number of endocrine disorders.

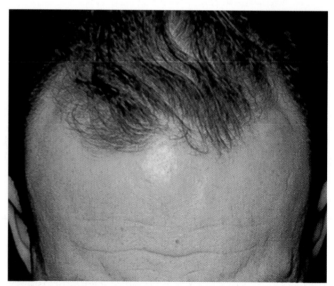

Figure 1.35 Alopecia. Frontal recession and thinning of scalp hair is age- and sex-related. Alopecia also occurs in a number of conditions, particularly with the use of cytotoxic drugs.

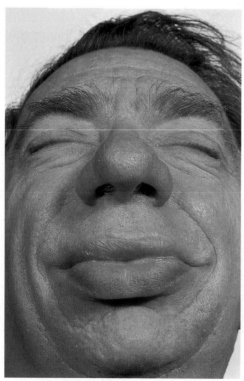

Figure 1.33 Facial oedema.

related to hypoventilation (head injuries, drug overdosage), chronic obstructive pulmonary disease and mismatched arterial ventilation and perfusion (pulmonary embolism, pulmonary shunts, arteriovenous fistulas). Cyanosis is difficult to elicit in dark-skinned people with anaemia. Polycythaemia is an excess of circulating red cells and may produce a purple–blue skin discoloration, mimicking cyanosis. However, it is also prominent in the cheeks and the backs of the hands (**Figure 1.38**).

Jaundice is a yellow discoloration caused by excess circulating bile pigments. Mild degrees of jaundice are easily picked up by staining of the sclerae (see Figure 1.17). Be careful not to confuse the uniform yellow colour of jaundice with the yellowish peripheral discoloration of the sclera that can be seen in normal individuals. As the jaundice becomes more pronounced, there is yellow discoloration of the skin and this may progress to yellow/orange or even dark brown with high levels of plasma pigment. Other generalized changes in skin pigmentation are considered on p. 312.

## The Mouth

The mouth is a valuable indicator of systemic illness as well as of local pathology. The mouth has a complex embryological origin, being the site of the junction of the ectoderm and endoderm, and receiving contributions from the pharyngeal arch mesoderm. The tongue muscles are derived from suboccipital somites that have migrated forwards around the pharynx, bringing their nerve supply with them. This origin is also reflected in the variety of diseases. These include skin and gut mucosal abnormalities together with other lesions that encompass a number of medical and surgical disciplines.

The breath must be examined for halitosis (unpleasant or abnormal – fetor oris); this may be an indicator of respiratory, upper alimentary or systemic disease. Purulent oral infection producing halitosis most commonly involves the gums in association with poor dentition (**Figure 1.39**). Oral candidiasis (**Figure 1.40**) – a white coating with fungus – may occur in relation to debilitating disease, prolonged antibiotics or steroid therapy, immunological diseases (such as sarcoidosis), immunodeficiency disorders (such as HIV infection) and immunosuppressive drugs. Certain drugs – such as paraldehyde – have a specific fetor.

Nasal and sinus infections and degenerative tumours in these areas may give offensive odours, as does the infection of bronchiectasis.

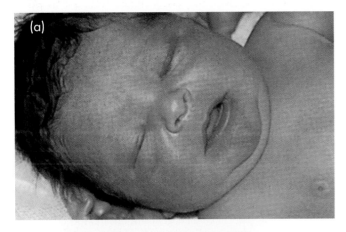

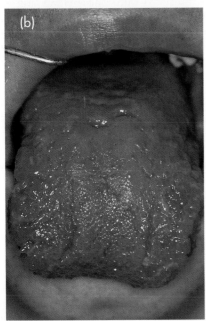

Figure 1.36 (a) A blue baby with cyanotic heart disease. (b) Cyanosis secondary to tetralogy of Fallot.

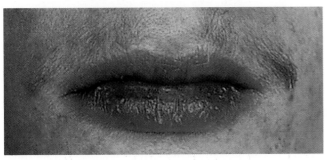

Figure 1.37 Cyanosis in a teenager with a single ventricle.

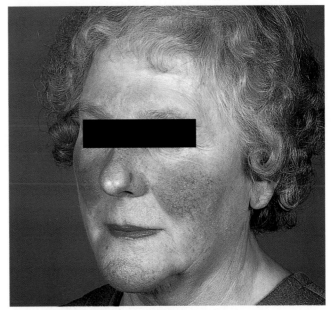

Figure 1.38 A malar flush. Facial flushing occurs in individuals who are regularly exposed to the elements and is a feature of mitral and pulmonary stenosis. It is found in Cushing's and carcinoid syndromes and some collagen diseases.

Alimentary odours may be related to gastroenteritis, obstruction of the pylorus and small or large gut, and overindulgence in food or alcohol. The latter aroma depends on the timing and the quantity imbibed.

Systemic diseases producing characteristic odours are diabetic ketosis and renal and hepatic failure. The sweet smell of ketotic breath may be related to insulin deficiency but also to an increased metabolic rate – such as with a fever and fasting – particularly in childhood disorders. In renal and hepatic disease, there may also be systemic manifestations of the conditions. The ammoniacal smell of hepatic coma has been likened to musty old eggs.

## Examination of the Mouth

Examination of the mouth requires a good light. This may be provided by daylight, but a torch or lamp is usually necessary. A spatula allows movement of the lips, cheeks and tongue to observe all areas; this may be aided by a dental mirror. Palpation is with a gloved finger, the second hand being used for bimanual exploration of the floor of the mouth and the cheeks. The tongue may be pulled forwards by holding it with a swab to examine its sides and the adjacent structures.

Specific disorders of the tongue – such as congenital abnormalities – and benign and malignant tumours are considered on

p. 371–375 but the tongue is often a good indicator of systemic disease. There is a good deal of variation in ethnic pigmentation and papillary patterns, such as 'geographic tongue'. The pallor of anaemia, central cyanosis and the yellow tingeing of jaundice may be recognized in all races.

Many tongue coatings have no clinical significance or may reflect a recent meal. Roughage in the diet can serve to remove particulate matter and therefore coatings do relate to dietary habit. Dietary deficiencies such as of vitamins C and D may produce an abnormally smooth tongue. The coating is increased in heavy smokers and mouth breathers. Mouth breathing may also dehydrate the surface of the tongue. However, this, together with the loss of skin turgor and sunken eyes, is a valuable indicator of the general state of dehydration postoperatively, in fevers and with reduced fluid intake. There may be tongue atrophy in Plummer–Vinson syndrome, associated with angular stomatitis (**Figure 1. 41**) and abnormalities of the gastric mucous membrane.

## Ulcerated Tongue

Ulceration of the tongue is common and is usually due to dental trauma or aphthous ulcers. In the former, there may be sharp teeth or poorly fitting dentures, and the gums must be carefully checked for any associated damage. Falls, fits and sports or other injuries may be associated with tongue-biting, and fish bones may lodge anywhere in the tongue or alimentary tract, producing trauma and infection.

Aphthous ulcers (**Figure 1.42**) may be associated with generalized disease but are usually of unknown aetiology. Ulcers may also be associated with inflammatory changes of the tongue and this glossitis may be due to generalized disease. Examples are drug reactions such as the Stevens–Johnson and MAGIC syndromes. Sexually transmitted diseases causing glossitis and inflammation include HIV, syphilis and gonorrhoea, and may be part of Reiter's syndrome. Autoimmune and connective tissue disorders and occasionally gut abnormalities – such as ulcerative colitis and Crohn's disease (**Figure 1. 43**) – may have associated mouth ulceration.

A coating of candida has already been considered in the mouth. White patches also include lichen planus, a disorder of unknown aetiology. It has a number of characteristic patterns, usually involving the edges of the tongue, associated with mucosal atrophy and erosion. An important differential

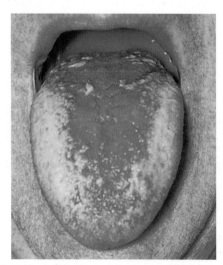

Figure 1.39 **Poor dentition.**

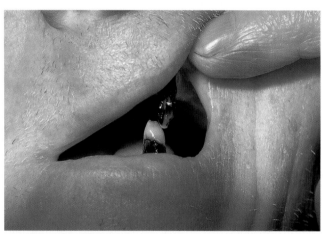

Figure 1.40 **Oral candidiasis.**

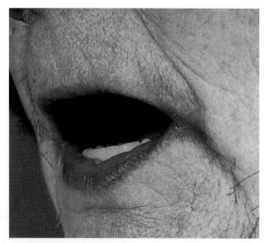

Figure 1.41 Angular stomatitis with cracking and fissuring of the lips, a feature of vitamin deficiency.

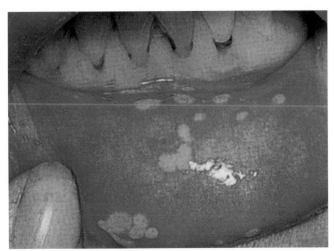

Figure 1.42 Aphthous ulcers are common and usually of unknown aetiology. They are frequently a complication of autoimmune deficiency.

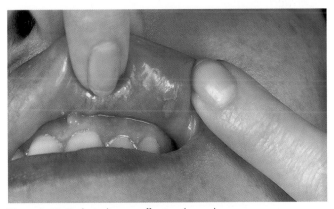

Figure 1.43 Crohn's disease affecting the oral mucosa.

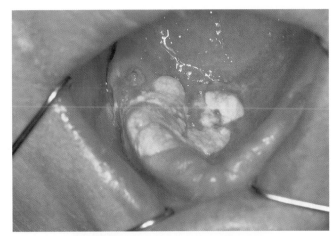

Figure 1.44 Leukoplakia.

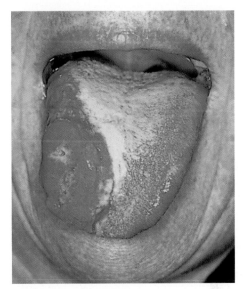

Figure 1.45 Carcinoma of the tongue.

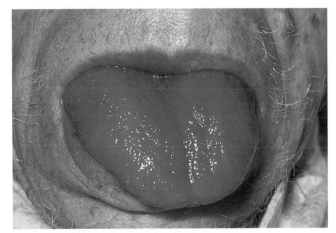

Figure 1.46 Macroglossia of acromegaly.

diagnosis of a white coating is leukoplakia, a premalignant condition (Figures 1.44 and 1.45). An important finding is that it cannot be removed by scratching the mucosal surface.

Large tongues are seen in hypothyroidism and acromegaly (Figure 1.46), in developmental abnormalities and associated with some congenital syndromes such as Down syndrome.

The tongue receives bilateral cortical innervation so wasting only occurs with bilateral upper motor neurone lesions (pseudobulbar palsy). However, the XIIth nerve nucleus may be affected by motor neurone disease and the nerve damaged in surgical or other trauma. With a lower motor neurone paralysis, the tongue deviates towards the side of the lesion (Figure 1.47). Tongue weakness and difficulty swallowing may be present in myasthenia gravis and the tremor of Parkinson's disease. Thus, disease can often be well demonstrated by asking the patient to stick their tongue out.

Many of the features described for examination of the mouth and tongue apply equally to the mucous membrane of the oropharynx.

## SYSTEMIC EXAMINATION

After completing the general examination – as outlined above – the examination takes a regional approach as indicated in subsequent chapters. Some specific clinical syndromes that need to be identified and understood are covered in Chapter 2.

The skin of each area provides further information on the state of nutrition and hydration, colour changes and scratch marks. Venous and arterial pulsation can be observed in the neck, and respiratory movements in the chest and abdomen.

PART 1  |  PRINCIPLES

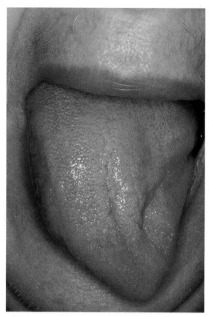

Figure 1.47 **XIIth nerve palsy (hypoglossal).**

Table 1.1 **Aids to diagnosis**

| System | Anatomy | Pathology |
| --- | --- | --- |
| Cardiovascular | Skin | Congenital |
| Respiratory | Subcutaneous tissues, fat, | Inflammatory |
| Gastrointestinal | vessels, nerves | Traumatic |
| Genitourinary | Muscles | Neoplastic |
| Musculoskeletal | Bones | Degenerative |
| Neurogenic | Joints | Metabolic |
| Haemopoietic | Related viscera | Hormonal |
| | | Haematological |
| | | Poisons |
| | | Chemicals |
| | | Psychiatric |
| | | Idiopathic |
| | | Iatrogenic |

Abnormal movements such as those caused by neurological abnormalities (see p. 170) and hiccups may become more obvious, as may an abnormal posture in relation to pain and deformity.

When the examination of each region and system has been completed, cover the patient and make sure they are comfortable. Examine all excreta available and request the collection of these when appropriate. The excreta include sputum, vomit, faeces, the contents of surgical drainage bottles and any discharges. Discharges may be from ulcers, wounds or other sites, and smaller amounts can also be observed on dressings.

## FORMULATING A DIAGNOSIS

Having completed the history and examination, the clinician has usually come to a working diagnosis. This is supported or not by further investigations and the subsequent progress of the disease.

It is sometimes difficult to diagnose a patient's problem. This may be linked to inexperience, the condition may already be resolving or difficulty of diagnosis may be encountered in the very early stages of presentation. Table 1.1 is intended to generate ideas for possible diagnoses and differential diagnoses in these circumstances.

First try to identify the system involved. Backache, for example, may be musculoskeletal but consider neurological causes or referred pain from the cardiovascular system (e.g. a ruptured abdominal aortic aneurysm) or alimentary system (e.g. pancreatic or biliary disease). The anatomy of the region of interest should be considered when there is pain or a lump. This may be sited superficially in the skin, subcutaneously or more deeply in muscle or viscera. The pathology list – 'diagnostic sieve' – is of particular value when assessing a lump but is equally applicable to any symptom.

The original 'surgical sieve' included the five headings: congenital, infection, traumatic, neoplastic and degenerative. Inflammation is 'the body's response to injury' and is a wider title than infection. The injury includes not only infection from a virus or bacterium, but also infection with other organisms, antigen responses and inflammation surrounding a traumatic wound or infiltrating neoplasm. It is a useful heading under which autoimmune diseases can be placed.

Neoplasia should be divided into benign and malignant, and the latter into primary and secondary lesions. Degenerative disease is a useful heading under which to place atheromatous disease, dementia and other diseases of the aged.

## COMMUNICATION

Taking a detailed history and performing a thorough examination establishes a unique doctor–patient relationship. This privileged relationship must be reinforced by a frank explanation of the findings to the patient in terms that they fully understand, together with the proposed course of action. The degree of empathy that a clinician achieves with different patients is dependent on both their personalities. However, with all patients, the clinician must aim to establish a mutual respect of the relationship based on trust and honesty. In the case of children or mentally disabled patients, these discussions should be with the appropriate guardian.

In the case of a specialist referral, the letter must ensure that the referring clinician is kept fully informed of all actions taken. This is similarly true when a patient is discharged from hospital, when the general practitioner should receive an immediate discharge letter followed as soon as possible by a summary of the admission.

Accurate records are essential to document progress and to ensure effective continuity of care; they also have important medicolegal significance.

## SURGICAL EXAMINATION OF THE CHILD

Many relatively common surgical conditions occur exclusively during childhood. In addition, each stage of childhood has specific problems. Childhood is characterized by growth, which can lead to its own disorders, while other conditions can adversely affect the growth and development of the child. Children also pose difficulties in terms of examination, especially in infancy and early childhood.

This section deals with the approach to the child as a whole during the different stages of growth and development, referring the reader to other parts of the text when disorders are discussed with related adult conditions.

## Examination of the Neonate

The growth and development of the individual begins at conception and even at this stage disease may become evident. Most genetic disorders and genetically damaged blastocysts or embryos do not implant or are miscarried before the mother is even aware that she is pregnant. Previous pregnancies or the parents' family histories may point to the possibility of genetically determined disorders, and genetic population screening will in future lead to an increased awareness of these problems.

*In vitro* fertilization techniques provide a means by which abnormal embryos may be diagnosed and excluded from implantation. Genetic information can also be obtained by taking a sample of the covering membranes of the fetus (chorionic villus sampling) or fetal cells in the amniotic fluid (amniocentesis). Further assessment of the growth and development of the fetus is by ultrasound examination of the fetus *in utero*. In particular, defects affecting the spine and the neurological and cardiovascular systems may become apparent.

Apart from predetermined genetic disease, the growing and developing fetus is in danger from infective agents that can cross the placenta, such as rubella virus, cytomegalovirus or *Toxoplasma* – these organisms can lead to disorders of organ growth and development. Maternal health and adequate nutrition also determine the health of the fetus, as do the mother's ingestion of alcohol and drugs and her inhalation of tobacco.

The general health of the growing fetus can to a large extent be assessed by examining the mother. The growth (by fundal height), heart rate (by auscultation) and fetal movement are useful markers. The amount of amniotic fluid is a guide to the function of the gastrointestinal tract and urogenital systems. Excess amniotic fluid – polyhydramnios – may be a sign of a high gastrointestinal defect or diabetes mellitus, and a reduced volume may be a sign of a problem of renal failure or expulsion of urine, or intrauterine growth retardation.

Finally, the baby may undergo harm or injury during birth. Anoxia during birth may lead to neurological impairment, and the baby can suffer serious nerve (in particular brachial plexus) and musculoskeletal injury (including fractures) during obstructed or otherwise complicated deliveries, for example with shoulder dystocia; these injuries may be iatrogenic, although they are occasionally unavoidable. Forceps- or suction-assisted deliveries have characteristic injury patterns, and the baby may be injured during a caesarean section. Examination of the newborn infant should therefore take into account the health and medical history of the mother and any previous siblings, the health of the mother during pregnancy, the progress of the pregnancy and the mode of delivery.

All parents are keen to know that their newborn child is normal so a brief but important examination is always carried out immediately. The baby is first inspected for signs of life such as adequate spontaneous respiration and adequate circulation, leading to a healthy skin coloration and the spontaneous activity of all the limbs, the eyes and the head. If these are not present, the baby requires immediate resuscitation. These initial physical signs are grouped together and scored to give the 'Apgar' score – this is an index of the immediate physical state of the neonate, usually recorded at 1 and 5 minutes after delivery (Table 1.2).

The baby can then be examined more carefully, first by inspection. Low scores indicate the need for immediate resuscitative measures; however, they do not relate to the long-term outcome. Particular attention is paid to the head and spine. Meningomyelocele and anencephaly are usually obvious but other types of spinal dysraphism may not be immediately apparent. They may be evident from a degree of abnormal curvature of the spine or a patch of hair over the spine. The eyes are inspected. Pronounced canthal folds together with a large tongue and the distinctive continuous single 'simian' crease in the palm lead to a suspicion of Down syndrome. The syndrome is associated with other abnormalities, notably congenital heart defects and duodenal atresia.

The mouth should be inspected – cleaned out if necessary – to exclude a cleft lip or palate. The chest wall and abdominal wall are examined to exclude defects such as bladder extrophy; the umbilical cord is examined to ensure that it contains the usual configuration of three vessels – abnormalities are suggestive of renal deformities. Failure of the intestine to return to the abdominal cavity *in utero* leads to exomphalos. The anus is examined to exclude a very low obstruction of the intestinal tract. The genitalia, having been examined carefully by one and all to determine the sex of the baby, are examined more carefully to ensure that there is no abnormality.

The limbs are examined, confirming the normal configuration and the correct number of digits. Fractures and dislocations caused during difficult labours are usually obvious, as is talipes – club foot – from its characteristic equinovarus deformity. The baby's skin is examined for the presence of rashes, discolorations and accessory skin tags. The chest is ausculated to ensure that the lungs have expanded and that there are no cardiac murmurs.

Finally the baby is weighed. A low birth weight may be due to prematurity, intrauterine growth retardation, congenital abnormalities, intrauterine infection or maternal poor health. Large babies – macrosomia – can be due to maternal diabetes, and these infants are in danger of birth injury, hypoglycaemia, neonatal jaundice and respiratory distress.

When all is deemed to be well, the child is returned to the mother and feeding is started. Failure to feed – in particular cyanosis during attempted feeding – together with the presence of frothy saliva around the mouth in between feeds leads to the suspicion of oesophageal atresia and a tracheo-oesophageal fistula.

Table 1.2 **Apgar score chart**

| | Apgar score | | |
|---|---|---|---|
| | 0.00 | 1.00 | 2.00 |
| Response to stimulation | None | Facial grimace | Cry |
| Respiration | Absent | Gasping | Regular |
| Heart rate (bpm) | 0.00 | <100 | 100+ |
| Colour of trunk | White | Blue | Pink |
| Muscle tone | Flaccid | Some flexion | Normal with movement |

Vomiting soon after feeding may be due to a more distal obstruction. If bile is present, this is likely to be distal to the second part of the duodenum. Intestinal obstruction may be due to atresia, obstructing bands, intestinal organs compressing the intestine, notably an annular pancreas, or inspissated meconium. The latter suggests a diagnosis of cystic fibrosis.

Failure to pass urine may suggest urethral obstruction or problems of renal function. Failure to pass stool can be due to obstruction of the distal colon, rectum or anus by agenesis, the presence of bands or the absence of a functioning myenteric plexus – Hirschsprung's disease.

The baby is re-examined carefully and methodically at 48 hours, care being taken to exclude congenital dislocation of the hips and, in boys, absent testes. A more detailed examination of the cardiovascular system is carried out to exclude murmurs and to assess the presence or absence of the femoral arteries. The character of the peripheral pulses may also be significant – if full they may signify a patent ductus arteriosus, if weak a major defect compromising cardiac output.

A number of abnormalities are commonly found that are benign and either resolve independently or require minor treatment for removal. These include the following:

- *Mongolian blue spots* are areas of blue or black pigmentation that are usually found on the buttocks or at the base of the spine, and are more common in dark-skinned babies. They usually resolve spontaneously.
- *Capillary or macular haemangiomas*, which are very common, are usually found around the eyes or on the neck at the nape. They usually disappear, especially if they are around the eyes.
- *Breast enlargement* is common in both boys and girls due to the presence of maternal hormones. Milk –'witch's milk' – can also be secreted for a short period of time. Both the enlargement and the section resolve spontaneously.
- *Milia* are white spots caused by blocked sebaceous glands, usually on the nose and cheeks. They clear spontaneously.
- *Mouth cysts* can occur in the midline of the palate (Epstein's pearls), on the gums (epulis) and on the floor of the mouth. Most of these cysts disappear spontaneously.
- *Accessory skin tags* are common on the face and around the ears.
- *Dimples* may occur over the sacrum and should be gently palpated to exclude underlying cysts.

## Examination of the Infant and Child

This varies little from the examination of the adult, but one has to be flexible as each part of the examination often has to be carried out when a suitable opportunity arises. The clinician must be sympathetic to the needs of the child and to recognize that he or she may be frightened, especially if in pain.

A number of gambits exist to calm the anxious child, including the use of dolls or the parents to show what will happen and that nothing harmful is to be undergone. For instance, the child's hand can be guided over their abdomen where tenderness is suspected. Each individual finds the best techniques to suit not only themselves, but also the individual child in terms of their mental and social development. During these examinations, always bear in mind the relative growth and development of a child, and if necessary chart these over time.

### Key Points

- The assessment of a patient's symptoms should consist of a history, an examination and any relevant adjunctive investigations as necessary.
- A thorough history is the single most important factor in making a diagnosis. This should follow a structured, systematic scheme that can then be focused on for each patient on an individual basis depending on the nature of the patient's symptoms.
- After a history has been taken, the patient should be adequately exposed before undertaking a methodical general examination from head to toe, with the results of a full examination of all the systems being interpreted to make an initial diagnosis.
- The general examination of a patient should include their hands, skin, face and mouth.
- Frank, honest communication with the patient is key in establishing and maintaining the doctor–patient relationship. Thorough, accurate documentation in the patient's case notes and when referring to or informing other doctors is essential for continuity of care and for medicolegal purposes.
- The surgical assessment of the child and neonate requires a special consideration of the anatomy and specific childhood surgical conditions, as well as an awareness of issues of compliance related to the history and examination.

## QUESTIONS

### SBAs

**1. Which nail sign is most characteristic of iron deficiency anaemia?:**
 a  Koilonychia
 b  Clubbing
 c  Splinter haemorrhage
 d  Leukonychia punctata
 e  Beau's lines

**Answer**

*a Koilonychia. Koilonychia is a spoon-shaped depression of the nail seen in iron deficiency anaemia.*

**2. Which of the following disorders involving the mouth is a premalignant condition?:**
 a  Lichen planus
 b  Candida
 c  Aphthous ulcer
 d  Glossitis
 e  Leukoplakia

**Answer**

*e Leukoplakia. Leukoplakia is a white coating seen in the mouth and is a premalignant condition. It is differentiated from conditions such as candidiasis by the inability to remove it by scratching its surface.*

**3. Over which artery are the Korotkoff sounds heard when taking a regular manual blood pressure reading?:**
 a  Radial
 b  Brachial
 c  Subclavian
 d  Ulnar
 e  Femoral

**Answer**

*b Brachial. When using a stethoscope to take a manual blood pressure reading, Korotkoff sounds are heard over the brachial artery. The radial pulse may be palpated first when inflating the cuff to ascertain an approximate systolic reading before making a true assessment.*

### EMQS

**1. For each of the following descriptions, select the most likely cause of the pain from the list below. Each option may be used once, more than once or not at all:**
 1  Biliary colic
 2  Pancreatitis
 3  Myocardial infarction
 4  Acute limb ischaemia
 5  Chronic limb ischaemia
 6  Renal colic
 7  Pleuritic chest pain
 8  Peptic ulcer
 9  Duodenal ulcer
 a  A central crushing chest pain radiating down the left arm and into the neck
 b  A burning epigastric pain radiating up into the throat. It is aggravated by spicy foods and is not relieved by eating
 c  A right upper quadrant pain lasting several hours after the consumption of fatty foods and alcohol, but with complete resolution
 d  A crampy calf pain on walking that is rapidly relieved by resting
 e  A right loin pain radiating to the groin that comes in waves. The patient moves around unable to get comfortable

**Answers**

*a 3 Myocardial infarction. This is a classic description of myocardial infarction. Pleuritic chest pain is, in contrast, typically aggravated on deep inspiration.*

*b 8 Peptic ulcer. The symptoms given suggest gastrointestinal ulcer disease, more likely to be a peptic than a duodenal ulcer as duodenal ulcer pain may be relieved by eating.*

*c 1 Biliary colic. Biliary colic is commonly associated with fatty foods and/or alcohol consumption, with attacks lasting several hours. It is differentiated from pancreatitis, which typically presents as an epigastric pain radiating through to the back and is severe.*

*d 5 Chronic limb ischaemia. The symptoms are typical of a chronic limb ischaemia in which there is intermittent claudication when increased blood flow to the limb is needed. On resting, there is a rapid resolution of symptoms. Acute ischaemia is in contrast commonly described by the 'six Ps': pale, pulseless, painful, perishing cold, paraesthetic and paralysed.*

*e 6 Renal colic. Pain described as coming in waves is typical of colic, with renal colic usually being sited in the loin to groin area. In contrast to the pain of peritoneal irritation, in which the patient lies still, patients with renal colic move around unable to settle or get comfortable.*

**2.** For each of the following descriptions, select the most relevant answer in neonatal examination from the list below. Each option may be used once, more than once or not at all:

1 Fundal height
2 Mother's weight
3 Amniocentesis
4 Glasgow Coma Scale
5 Cytomegalovirus
6 Rubella
7 Apgar score
8 Capillary haemangioma
9 Chorionic villus sampling
10 AVPU score
11 Mongolian blue spots

a A method of sampling the covering membranes of the fetus for genetic testing
b An infective agent that can cross the placenta and lead to development disorders that is currently screened for in the UK
c A marker of growth of the fetus
d An index used for the immediate physical state of the neonate, usually recorded at 1 and 5 minutes after delivery
e Areas of black pigmented areas on the buttocks or base of the spine

Answers

a **9 Chorionic villus sampling.** *This involves the covering membranes of the fetus being sampled and tested. In contrast, amniocentesis is the sampling of cells in the amniotic fluid.*

b **6 Rubella.** *Both rubella and cytomegalovirus are agents that are able to cross the placenta and lead to development disorders of the fetus, but cytomegalovirus is currently not routinely screened for in the UK.*

c **1 Fundal height.** *The fundus is measured and used as a marker of fetal growth.*

d **7 Apgar score.** *The Apgar score is used for the initial physical assessment of the neonate.*

e **11 Mongolian blue spots.** *The description here given is classic of these lesions. They usually resolve spontaneously.*

# Distinctive Clinical Syndromes

John S. P. Lumley and Natalie Anne Hirst

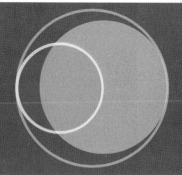

## LEARNING OBJECTIVES

To understand and be able to manage a number of important clinical conditions with surgical relevance including:
- Fluid balance/oedema
- Shock
- Bleeding and coagulation disorders
- Anaemia
- Pyrexia
- Weight loss/gain
- Acromegaly
- Thyrotoxicosis/myoxedema

- Cretinism
- Cushing's syndrome
- Addison's disease
- Myasthenia gravis
- Ehlers–Danlos syndrome
- Marfan's syndrome
- Genetic disorders
- Dwarfism
- Paget's disease
- Parkinson's disease
- Congenital syphilis

## INTRODUCTION

Many diseases have characteristic and diagnostic physical signs. This text aims to include all those of surgical relevance. The current chapter brings together a number of clinical states in which a disease presents with multiple – often unique – signs. They are important to recognize as methods of treatment and problems of management are well documented.

Some of the conditions require operative procedures to treat or prevent complications, while others have abnormalities that may produce anaesthetic difficulties and require skilled postoperative care. Once the condition has been diagnosed, patients can benefit from previous experience and their prognosis can be clearly defined.

The importance of these conditions to the examination candidate is disproportionately high. The patients have chronic diseases and are frequently available for clinical examinations. The examiners also expect candidates to recognize the signs and to know many details of the diseases and their management.

The clinical states included are of mixed aetiology. The reason for inclusion at this point is the generalized nature of the conditions, affecting more than one region of the body and involving more than one system. They include shock, bleeding disorders, anaemia, pyrexia of unknown origin (PUO), weight disturbances, endocrine abnormalities and some inherited disorders. Other conditions – such as hepatic and renal failure – and skeletal abnormalities, although producing widespread signs, have fitted more appropriately into the relevant section in the subsequent text.

## ABNORMALITIES OF FLUID BALANCE

Water makes up approximately 55 per cent of the body weight in men, but less in women because of their higher fat content. About two-thirds of this fluid is intracellular, with potassium being the main ion contributing to the osmolality; 98 per cent of the body's potassium resides within the cells. Sodium is the main extracellular ion, and Na/KATPase is the source of energy required to keep the sodium and potassium in the extra- and intracellular compartments, respectively. This ionic balance is influenced by pH, aldosterone, insulin and the adrenogenic nervous system.

The volume of the extracellular fluid is regulated mainly by the kidney, through a number of mechanisms, the most important of which is antidiuretic hormone (ADH; also known as vasopressin). Lowered sodium levels and reduced blood volume stimulate hypothalamic receptors, leading to the release of ADH; they also stimulate thirst. There are similar osmoreceptors in the aortic arch and probably in the gut and portal circulation. ADH increases permeability in the terminal distal tubule and collecting ducts of the kidney to allow more water reabsorption.

Other factors influencing renal tubular function include the renin–angiotensin–aldosterone axis, neurogenic reflexes – such as from the baroreceptors – prostaglandins and atrial natriuretic peptide/factor. Atrial natriuretic peptide is a peptide stored in granules in the walls of the atria and released in response to excess atrial filling. It increases renal perfusion and salt excretion to reduce the circulating volume.

PART 1 | PRINCIPLES

Plasma comprises about one-quarter of the extracellular fluid. A delicate balance is maintained between the colloid osmotic – oncotic – pressure of the plasma and the capillary hydrostatic pressure, forcing fluid through the capillary wall. This is influenced by the arteriolar and venous pressures, the permeability of the capillary membrane and the lymphatic drainage of the interstitial fluid.

A normal fluid intake is approximately 2.5 L per day, drink providing 1.8 L and food the remainder. The equivalent loss is mainly from urine, at 1.5 L. Exhaled gases and insensible loss, for example sweating, make up 0.9 L, and faeces 0.1 L.

## Oedema

Increased fluid intake is usually compensated for by an increase in urine output. The kidney is capable of increasing this to 750 mL/h, and fluid overload is well compensated for in the healthy individual. Some generalized or focal diseases can give rise to an excess of interstitial fluid. When this excess is clinically detectable by subcutaneous pitting on digital pressure, it is termed oedema. The common causes of oedema are listed in Table 2.1. Generalized causes include cardiac, renal and liver failure, and hypoproteinaemia.

Although it is tempting to think of cardiac oedema as being the result of an increase in venous pressure due to poor emptying of the right atrium, the capillary hydrostatic pressure in this condition is not markedly raised and the prime cause is reduced renal perfusion and reduced sodium excretion, with a resultant rise in blood volume and pressure in the interstitial fluid. The oedema of renal failure can be due to a failure of salt and water excretion or be secondary to hypoproteinaemia, as in nephrotic syndrome. The oedema of liver failure relates to a low plasma albumin level and also to interference with the metabolism of enzymes such as aldosterone. Hypoproteinaemia reduces plasma oncotic pressure, altering the balance between the plasma and interstitial fluid pressure measurements. The majority of causes of hypoproteinaemia originate in the gut. They include starvation, malnutrition and malabsorption, together with protein-losing enteropathies; vomiting, diarrhoea and intestinal fistulas are other causes.

Fluid retention occurs premenstrually and in pregnancy, and ADH hormone-secreting tumours reduce water and sodium excretion. Inappropriate ADH secretion may also be present in some malignancies. Certain drugs – particularly steroids – promote sodium retention and similar problems are encountered with an excessive sodium intake. This can be a problem in infants if sodium is added to a milk diet. Fluid retention in myxoedema is partly in the interstitial fluid and may pit. Idiopathic oedema in women is an unusual condition, usually diagnosed by exclusion.

Excessive intravenous hypotonic solutions, such as 5 per cent dextrose and the use of water for bladder or peritoneal washouts, may give rise to water retention. Similar effects may be obtained if a careful fluid balance is not maintained during haemo- and peritoneal dialysis.

Increased capillary permeability can present as an acute, even fatal, event. There is leakage of proteins, markedly influencing the plasma–intercellular pressure gradient; fibrinogen is one of the plasma proteins that readily leaks in these circumstances and can produce additional problems from fibrin deposition blocking the lymphatic drainage. Such allergic reactions (Figure 2.1) can occur with certain foodstuffs – particularly nuts and shellfish – as well as drugs and chemicals. A snake bite or bee sting can have rapid and serious consequences via this mechanism.

Focal oedema may be related to inflammation associated with infection or collagen diseases, or around traumatized tissue and neoplasms. Venous and lymphatic oedema are considered on p. 511.

## History and Examination in Oedema

The history and examination of the patient with oedema are directed at establishing its cause. In cardiorespiratory causes, there may be a history of valvular heart disease, myocardial

Table 2.1  **Causes of oedema**

| Condition | Cause |
|---|---|
| Systemic disease | Cardiac failure |
| | Renal failure |
| | Hepatic failure |
| | Hypoproteinaemia (nephrotic syndrome, liver failure, malnutrition, malabsorption, protein-losing enteropathy) |
| Fluid retention | Premenstrual |
| | Pregnancy |
| | Tumours secreting ADH |
| | Inappropriate ADH secretion |
| | Sodium-retaining drugs/steroids |
| | Added salt in milk diet (infants) |
| | Myxoedema |
| | Idiopathic oedema (in women) |
| Water intoxication | Excess intravenous hypotonic solution |
| | Bladder/peritoneal washout with water or hypotonic solutions |
| | Overload during haemo-/peritoneal dialysis |
| Abnormal capillary permeability | Angioneurotic oedema |
| | Allergy (food, drugs, chemical, toxins) |
| | Snake bites |
| | Bee stings |
| Local oedema | Inflammation |
| | Venous hypertension |
| | Impaired lymphatic drainage |
| | Prolonged dependency |
| | Tight bandaging |
| | Fictitious |

ADH, antidiuretic hormone.

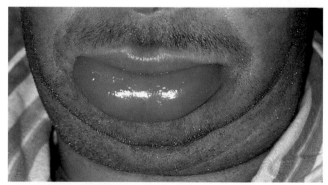

Figure 2.1  **Angio-oedema.**

infarction or angina. Dyspnoea is common, and in more severe cardiac and respiratory problems there is orthopnoea, paroxysmal nocturnal dyspnoea and a chronic history of cough and sputum. Signs may include cardiomegaly, heart murmurs and added respiratory sounds. The signs of congestive cardiac failure include a raised jugular venous pressure (JVP; **Figure 2.2**), ascites, pleural effusion, hepatomegaly, basal crepitations and central (**Figure 2.3**) and peripheral oedema.

In renal disease, the symptoms and signs may be few. There is anaemia with malaise, pallor and renal angle tenderness; palpable renal and pelvic masses should be excluded. Hepatic failure is usually obvious, with jaundice (**Figure 2.4**) and malaise. There may be – at least initially – hepatomegaly (**Figure 2.5**) and the signs of liver flap, palmar flushing (**Figure 2.6**), cutaneous telangiectasia (**Figure 2.7**) and purpura. Ascites may be present (**Figure 2.8**).

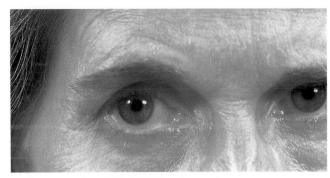

Figure 2.4 Jaundiced conjunctiva.

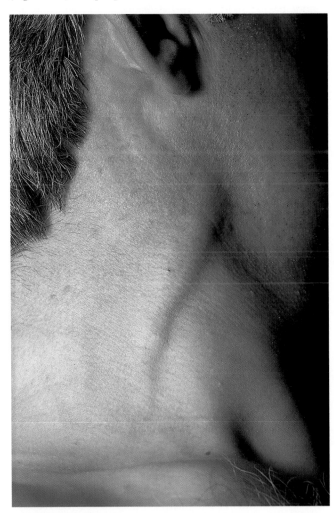

Figure 2.2 Raised jugular venous pressure.

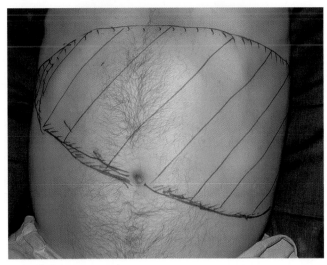

Figure 2.5 Hepatomegaly.

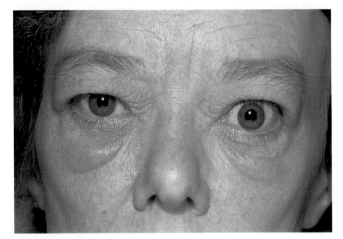

Figure 2.3 Eyelid oedema.

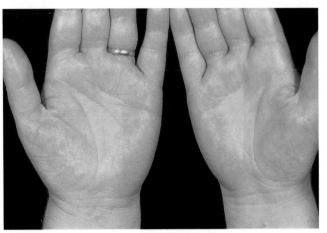

Figure 2.6 Palmar flushing.

PART 1 | PRINCIPLES

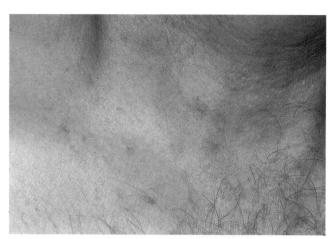

Figure 2.7  Spider naevi.

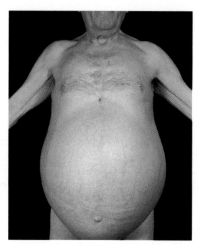

Figure 2.8  Ascitic liver disease.

Table 2.2  Reduced body fluid

| Reason | Cause |
| --- | --- |
| Reduced intake | Debilitation |
| | Oral pathology |
| | Dysphagia |
| | Coma (trauma, metabolic, intracranial lesions/surgery) |
| Fluid loss | Fever |
| | Exercise |
| | Hot, dry climates |
| | Vomiting |
| | Gut fistulas |
| | Diarrhoea |
| | Intestinal obstruction |
| | Paralytic ileus |
| | Small bowel infarction |
| | Peritonitis |
| | Acute pancreatitis |
| | Drained ascites |
| | Severe haemorrhage (multiple trauma, ruptured abdominal aortic aneurysm) |
| | Burns |
| | Extensive weeping eczema |
| | Increased metabolism |
| | Respiratory loss (hyperventilation, unhumidified tracheostomy, metabolic acidosis) |
| | Diabetes insipidus (hypothalamic disease, idiopathic) |
| | Renal diuresis |
| | Diuretic drugs |

In the alimentary system, note any weight loss in the history and examination and ask about dietary habits, indigestion, abdominal pain and bowel habits, particularly noting changes and the number, form and colour of the stools. Examine the hands, mucous membranes and mouth and the root of the neck for nodes. In the abdomen and pelvis, look for tenderness, enlarged organs and abdominal masses.

In questioning for the miscellaneous other groups causing oedema, discuss all the patient's current symptoms and previous illnesses, particularly rashes or vague symptoms following any particular food and any recent, unusual diets such as shellfish. Check the salt and fluid intake, drug history, whether on prescription or over the counter, and any recreational drugs, as well as exposure to toxins or chemicals at work or in other environments. In all forms of oedema, note weight changes and keep careful records of the weight and fluid intake and output.

## Reduced Body Water

Inadequate body fluids may be due to a reduced intake, increased needs or an increased loss of water. This is usually accompanied by a low body sodium level. Common causes of a reduced body water content are listed in **Table 2.2.**

A reduced intake may be due to a lack of available water or a lack of the desire to drink. There may be an inability to drink, such as with oral pathology, dysphagia or coma. Increased

needs include fever, where every degree rise in body temperature equates to an increased fluid requirement of 10 per cent. An increased basal metabolic rate – as in thyrotoxicosis – carries with it an increased water requirement. With raised external temperatures, especially with high humidity, an additional 250 mL of fluid is required for every degree above 29°C.

Fluid loss is commonly related to diseases of the alimentary tract. This loss may be externally – through diarrhoea, vomiting or fistulas – or due to a sequestration of fluids within the gut (as in paralytic ileus) or within the peritoneal cavity (e.g. acute pancreatitis and ascites), particularly if the latter is being continually drained. Fluid loss may be through the skin, such as in widespread burns or extensive weeping eczema. The loss may be through haemorrhage, as with major trauma or a ruptured aortic aneurysm.

An increased loss from the lungs may be caused by a lack of humidification of a recently fashioned tracheostomy or by hyperventilation. Renal loss can occur in the diuretic phase of the recovery from renal failure, with the overuse of diuretic drugs and in diabetes insipidus.

The clinical features of an abnormally low body water content usually relate to the underlying disease. There is also at first lethargy, malaise, drowsiness and muscle twitching, eventually leading to coma. With a few exceptions – for example, diabetes insipidus – there is oliguria, together with the signs of dehydration including tachycardia and hypotension. The skin is dry, with a loss of elasticity that can be noted when picking it up between the thumb and finger. The eyes are sunken, the mouth is dry and the tongue is usually furred.

## Shock

In extreme cases of fluid depletion – when the circulating volume does not match the circulating capacity – there is an accompanying failure of tissue perfusion. This failure of perfusion to meet the metabolic requirements of the tissues is termed shock. The syndrome incorporates a number of entities such as extremes of cardiac failure and abnormal capillary permeability. The conditions grouped within the syndrome of shock are listed in Table 2.3.

The low tissue perfusion produces a profound lactic acidosis, and the low pH gives rise to dyspnoea. Initial vasoconstriction is present although dilatation may occur as a terminal event. There is low cerebral perfusion, producing confusion, agitation and finally coma. Low renal perfusion gives rise to renal failure and possibly acute tubular necrosis, while lowered gut perfusion can allow the absorption of bacterial vasodilator toxins, accentuating the existing hypotension.

As has already been emphasized, shock is a syndrome encompassing a number of different causes of altered tissue perfusion. The presenting signs and symptoms differ, and it is important to identify the cause since the treatment is specific and appropriate treatment for one group may be harmful for another. Two main varieties of shock exist: those accompanied by **high systemic vascular resistance** and those with **low systemic vascular resistance**.

Table 2.3 Causes of shock

| Condition | Type of shock |
|---|---|
| With high systemic vascular resistance | Cardiogenic Pulmonary embolism Cardiac tamponade Hypovolaemic (fluid loss, haemorrhage) |
| With low systemic vascular resistance | Septic Anaphylactic Amniotic embolism |

High systemic vascular resistance is seen in cardiogenic shock, pulmonary embolism, cardiac tamponade and hypovolaemic shock. **Cardiogenic shock** occurs as a result of pump failure, commonly due to myocardial infarction. The heart failure is accompanied by low blood pressure and a tachycardia with a low-volume pulse. There may be a gallop rhythm and audible third or fourth heart sounds. Failure of the left ventricle gives rise to acute pulmonary oedema, and failure of the right ventricle to a raised JVP. These features – and the high peripheral resistance – produce a cold, clammy periphery and marked dyspnoea. There may be slight cyanosis with added chest sounds and possibly a pleural effusion.

In massive **pulmonary embolism**, the signs are similar to those of cardiogenic shock but the symptoms are of very sudden onset, usually 2–10 days after an operative procedure. There is acute chest pain and breathlessness, and a vagal reflex may produce a desire to defecate. The ECG may show the typical picture of S1 Q3 T3 (an S-wave in lead I, and a Q-wave and an inverted T-wave in lead III) but may only show right axis deviation or a right bundle branch block, or may even be normal.

**Cardiac tamponade** – due to fluid within the pericardial cavity compressing the heart – is seen in aortic dissection, after cardiac surgery and with acute pericarditis and thoracic malignancy. There is decreased ventricular filling producing signs similar to those of cardiogenic shock, but there may also be pulsus paradoxus, the pulse volume falling with inspiration rather than showing the usual rise, and similarly the JVP rising rather than falling in inspiration (Kussmaul's sign).

**Hypovolaemic shock** is due to a marked loss of tissue fluid. Of particular note are acute pancreatitis, severe burns and acute massive haemorrhage. Hypovolaemia leads to reduced cardiac output and low blood pressure; there is a tachycardia and the intense peripheral vascular constriction is due to reflex sympathetic stimulation. The patient is cold and clammy with dyspnoea and cyanosis. This pattern is similar to that of cardiogenic shock but does not show a raised JVP, pulmonary oedema or added heart sounds. Hypovolaemic shock may be considered in four stages (Table 2.4). A useful memory aid to represent the percentage volume of blood loss at each stage is to consider the scores in a game of tennis: 15 per cent, 15–30 per cent, 30–40 per cent, >40 per cent. Stage 1 is by definition compensated, and there must be an awareness of the relatively normal measured parameters to prompt early management, preventing further deterioration.

Table 2.4 Classes of haemorrhagic shock

| | I | II | III | IV |
|---|---|---|---|---|
| Blood loss (mL) | <750 | 750–1500 | 1500–2000 | >2000 |
| Blood loss (% blood volume) | <15 | 15–30 | 30–40 | >40 |
| Pluse rate (/min) | <100 | 100–120 | 120–140 | >140 |
| Blood pressure | Normal | Normal | Decreased | Decreased |
| Pulse pressure (mmHg) | Normal/increased | Decreased | Decreased | Decreased |
| Respiratory rate (/min) | 14–20 | 20–30 | 30–40 | >35 |
| Urinary output (mL/hour) | >30 | 20–30 | 5–15 | Negligible |
| Central nervous system – mental status | Slight anxiety | Mild anxiety | Anxiety, confusion | Confusion, lethargy |

In low systemic vascular resistance **septic shock**, the septicaemia is usually due to gram-negative organisms originating from infection in the gastrointestinal or genitourinary system. Other important sources are infected intravenous lines and large burns. Trivial infections of the nasopharynx or skin occasionally provide the source and at times almost every bacterium has been implicated. There is an increased incidence in those who are elderly or malnourished and in alcohol and drug abusers. The toxins produced from the infection give rise to massive arteriolar and peripheral venous dilatation, accompanied by hypotension and a low central venous pressure. The clinical picture differs markedly from the cold, clammy state of cardiogenic and hypovolaemic shock. The sympathetic drive produces a positive inotropic action and there is a full, bounding pulse with a tachycardia, warm extremities and no rise in JVP. However, the gut and kidney are shut down, the poor gut perfusion gives rise to the absorption of further exacerbating toxins and there is early acute renal failure. Symptomatically, there is fever, rigor, headache, lethargy and decreasing mental function.

In **anaphylactic shock**, the allergic reaction produces a massive histamine response, altering the capillary permeability and producing peripheral vascular dilatation. There is an increased cardiac output and tachycardia, producing a warm periphery, as with septic shock, but in addition there is marked pulmonary oedema with bronchospasm and mucosal airway obstruction, giving rise to marked dyspnoea.

**Amniotic fluid embolism** is a rare condition caused by amniotic fluid or other material of fetal origin entering the maternal circulation. There is a resulting deposition of fibrin and platelets, giving rise to disseminated intravascular coagulation (DIC). The circulatory response is rapid and profound, with hypotension and a cold, clammy periphery and cyanosis. If the patient survives the initial reaction, they are subject to adult respiratory distress syndrome.

## BLEEDING DISORDERS

Homeostasis is dependent on free-flowing blood within the vessels and on effective mechanisms for haemostasis should a vessel wall be damaged. The failure of this delicate balance can result in death from intravascular thrombosis or haemorrhage. Control of the system is therefore complex, incorporating many inhibitors and feedback loops. The degree of control can be appreciated when one considers that there is enough thrombin in 10 mL of blood to clot the whole of the vascular system if left unopposed. Bleeding abnormalities may give rise to increased natural loss (e.g. as in menorrhagia), spontaneous haemorrhage (e.g. purpura), haemarthrosis and bleeding from the nose and alimentary tract. It is of particular relevance to the surgeon in managing trauma and surgical wounds. **Haemostasis** is achieved by three mechanisms:

- coagulation of the blood;
- platelet adhesion and aggregation;
- vessel wall contraction.

**Abnormalities** of coagulation, platelets and the vessel wall – although uncommon – encompass a large number of congenital and acquired defects. The more important of these are listed in Tables 2.5–2.7. Those of surgical relevance are considered below, after a general discussion of the history and examination of patients with bleeding disorders.

Table 2.5 Disorders of coagulation

| Congenital/acquired | Disorder |
| --- | --- |
| Congenital | Haemophilia A and B |
| | Von Willebrand's disease |
| | Abnormalities of other clotting factors |
| Acquired | Vitamin K deficiency |
| | Acquired anticoagulants |
| | Disseminated intravascular coagulation |
| | Haemolytic–uraemic syndrome |
| | Thrombotic thrombocytopenic purpura |
| | Anticoagulant medication |
| | Snake bites |

Table 2.6 Platelet abnormalities

| Congenital/acquired | Disorder |
| --- | --- |
| Congenital | Hereditary thrombocytopenic purpura |
| | Bernard–Soulier syndrome |
| | Fanconi syndrome |
| | Storage pool failure |
| Acquired | Reduced platelet production (marrow and megakaryocyte abnormalities) |
| | Increased destruction (idiopathic thrombocytopenia, drug induced, infection, autoimmune) |
| | Abnormal consumption (disseminated intravascular coagulation, thrombotic thrombocytopenic purpura, infection, haemangioma: Kasabach–Merritt syndrome; pump oxygenation) |
| | Splenic sequestration |

Table 2.7 Vessel wall abnormalities

| Congenital/acquired | Disorder |
| --- | --- |
| Congenital | Hereditary haemorrhagic telangiectasia |
| | Connective tissue disorders |
| Acquired | Endothelial damage (anoxia, chemical, immunological) |
| | Abnormal vessel wall (senile purpura, protein abnormalities, scurvy, steroids, amyloid) |

## History

The history and examination aim to determine whether there is a potential problem with bleeding, which of the three mechanisms it involves, whether it is a congenital or an acquired abnormality, and if it is the latter, the underlying cause.

A previous history of serious or prolonged bleeding is the most likely way in which a bleeding problem comes to light. Enquire about bleeding after dental extraction, trauma, venepuncture and any surgical operation. Spontaneous bleeding commonly comes from the nose, from the mouth on tooth-brushing and from the gastrointestinal tract, although the latter may go unnoticed. There may be a tendency to bruise easily and purpuric patches may be present. Haemarthroses cause severe pain and must be differentiated from a septic arthritis. Bleeding into the psoas is a common muscular complication and may produce a flank mass and paralysis of the femoral nerve. Bleeding into the central nervous system is the most common cause of death in abnormalities of bleeding.

Congenital problems often first present at 2.5–3 years of age when a child starts to run and sustain heavier falls. A family history may be present but many congenital lesions occur spontaneously. It is important to determine the mode of transmission – congenital lesions are usually of a recessive nature, haemophilia being sex-linked. A history of previous infection may be present, such as a febrile illness 2–3 weeks previously. A full drug history is essential as drugs influence all three haemostatic mechanisms and around 100 preparations contain aspirin. Most of these problems resolve within a few weeks of stopping the drug but some preparations – for example, gold – are bound to the tissues so take longer to return to normal levels.

In adults, a large number of diseases give rise to problems with bleeding and should be sought for in the history. These include malabsorption, collagen diseases, liver and renal failure and malignancy, particularly of haematological origin or with bony secondaries.

## Examination

The examination must be full in view of the large number of potentially related diseases. The whole body must be examined for subcutaneous haemorrhage. Small bleeding points are termed petechiae (Figure 2.9); these differ from telangiectases (Figure 2.10) in that they do not blanch under pressure. They can occur along scratch lines and at pressure points, such as where the clothes rub, and may occur around the lower legs and ankles due to increased hydrostatic pressure.

Blowing up an arm cuff to 80 mmHg can produce underlying and distal petechiae. In the Hess test, a positive result in this manoeuvre is present if more than 15 petechiae are produced within a 5 cm cutaneous circle under the cuffed area after 10 minutes of inflation, indicating capillary fragility. Larger bruises are termed ecchymoses. Purpura is a spontaneous subcutaneous haemorrhage that can be produced by coagulation and platelet and vessel wall abnormalities. The site of purpuric patches may provide some indication of the underlying disease. Senile purpura and that due to excess steroids usually occur over the backs of the hands and arms, Henoch–Schönlein purpura is seen over the buttocks and thighs, and secondary thrombocytopenic purpura commonly occurs around the ankles secondary to hydrostatic

pressure. Fictitious purpura – and that seen in psychiatric patients – is commonly found over the front and sides of the thighs and legs, sparing the back of the legs and trunk. In general, purpura is the hallmark of platelet abnormalities, and haematomas that of clotting defects.

Examination of the mouth may show ulceration and haemorrhagic gums in cases of neutropenia, leukaemia and thrombocytic purpura, while congenital haemorrhagic telangiectasia can produce numerous buccal lesions. The joints of haemophiliac patients often undergo progressive degeneration and ankylosis due to recurrent haemarthrosis, whereas they are hyperextensible in patients with Ehlers–Danlos syndrome or pseudoxanthoma elasticum. There may be widespread general features of collagen disease and of liver and renal failure (see pp. 561 and 640); splenomegaly (Figure 2.11) may be present. Examine the retina for fundal haemorrhages – these suggest severe thrombocytopenia.

In general, platelet abnormalities produce a prolonged bleeding time, whereas coagulation defects prolong the clotting time. Routine blood tests include the prothrombin time as an assessment of the extrinsic pathway, and the activated partial thromboplastin time as a measure of the intrinsic pathway. More detailed studies include those of platelet morphology and assay for individual clotting factors.

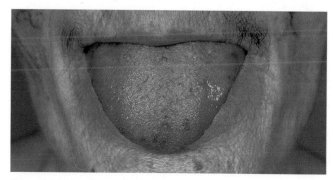

Figure 2.10 Hereditary telangiectasia.

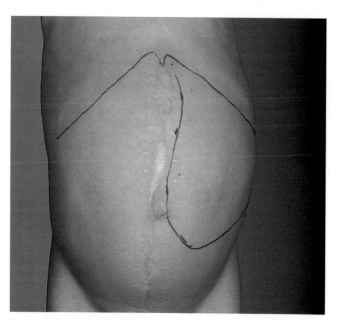

Figure 2.11 Splenomegaly.

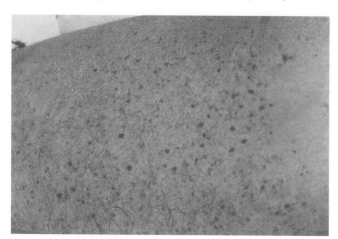

Figure 2.9 Petechial rash.

## Disorders of Coagulation

Congenital abnormalities of coagulation include haemophilia A (factor VIII deficiency), haemophilia B (factor IX deficiency – Christmas disease) and von Willebrand's disease. Haemophilia occurs in 30–120 cases per million of the population, affects all races and is widely distributed geographically. It is a sex-linked, recessive transmission but occurs sporadically in one-third of cases. It produces a drastic slowing of thrombin generation via the intrinsic pathway. Haemarthroses are common; in the late stage, fibrosis and ankylosis develop. Spontaneous muscle haemorrhage particularly involves the psoas, with associated femoral nerve palsy and a loin mass (Figure 2.12). Haematuria and gastrointestinal haemorrhage are common, as is continuous bleeding after dental extraction. Serious consequences include bleeding into the central nervous system and around the sublingual or pharyngeal regions, giving rise to suffocation.

Von Willebrand's disease exhibits autosomal dominant transmission. It is a deficiency of von Willebrand factor, a protein that promotes platelet adhesion and protects factor VIII against premature destruction. Other deficiencies occasionally encountered include those of factors II, VII, XI and XII, afibrinogenaemia and abnormalities of fibrinogen.

Acquired coagulation defects include vitamin K deficiency. They interfere with hepatic prothrombin metabolism. They may be due to a reduced intake of vitamin K – as in starvation (Figure 2.13) – or poor dietary habits, malabsorption and primary liver disease. Circulating anticoagulants are probably autoimmune in nature and can occur in collagen diseases, drug reactions and postpartum.

Disseminated intravascular coagulation interferes with both coagulation and platelet function. The condition is one of a consumptive coagulopathy, laying down fibrin throughout the microcirculation. The resultant necrosis can lead to damage to essential organs such as the brain, liver and heart. In fulminating cases, this is followed by fibrinolysis, depletion of clotting factors and complete thrombocytopenia, the patient paradoxically presenting with widespread haemorrhage. DIC is associated with a number of clinical conditions including malignancy – adenocarcinoma of the gut, prostate and ovary, and promyelocytic leukaemia - gram-negative septicaemia (Figure 2.14), fat embolism and severe injuries. It occurs in obstetric practice in antepartum haemorrhage, amniotic fluid embolism and, in the more chronic state, with a retained dead fetus and in pre-eclampsia.

Haemolytic–uraemic syndrome (HUS) and thrombotic thrombocytopenic purpura, like DIC, show widespread microvascular coagulation but the clotting mechanism is different. They usually follow infection of the respiratory and gastrointestinal tracts. The former predominantly affects the renal vasculature and usually presents in childhood. The latter is most common in young women.

A detailed anticoagulant history is important as the patient may not have mentioned treatment for prosthetic valves, atrial fibrillation or previous thrombotic episodes. Snake bites need the appropriate anti-venom; if the snake has not been identified, an informed guess is made based on the locality.

## Platelet Abnormalities

Platelets contribute to haemostasis in that they adhere to damaged endothelium. They aggregate in response to thrombin, ADP, serotonin and other clotting factors and their presence

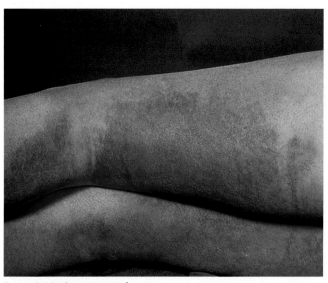

Figure 2.13 The purpura of scurvy.

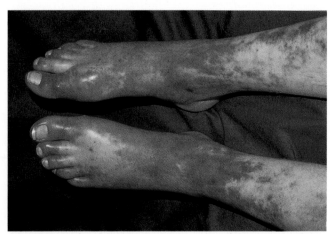

Figure 2.14 Septic coagulopathy.

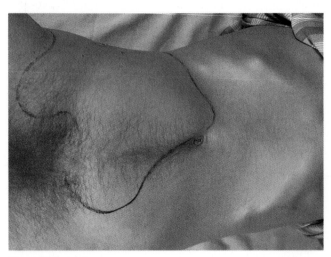

Figure 2.12 A loin mass.

can accelerate thrombin generation by as much as 1000 times. Congenital disorders of platelet function are rare. Platelets can be reduced in number, such as in hereditary thrombocytopenic purpura and Fanconi's anaemia. There may be reduced platelet adhesion, as in Bernard–Soulier syndrome, and there may be failure of the platelets to release ADP – with abnormal platelet aggregation – as in storage pool diseases.

There are a large number of acquired disorders of platelet activity, including reduced production, increased destruction, consumptive loss and sequestration. Reduced production occurs in marrow disease – such as bone marrow infiltration with metastases, myeloproliferative disorders and leukaemia – and defective thrombopoeisis, as in vitamin $B_{12}$ and folate deficiency, uraemia and alcohol abuse, and with some drugs, particularly thiazide diuretics.

An increased destruction of platelets by immune mechanisms – such as idiopathic thrombocytopenic purpura – occurs in children 2 or 3 weeks after viral infections (e.g. mumps, infective mononucleosis or rubella, or post-immunization). It can occur as a complication of a large number of drugs – of particular note are chloramphenicol, septrin, sulphonamides, quinine, quinidine, anti-tuberculous drugs, phenylbutazone, aspirin, gold, heparin, high-dosage penicillin and non-steroidal anti-inflammatory drugs. Destruction can also accompany a number of diseases, particularly collagen diseases and infective conditions.

A massive consumption of platelets may be seen in DIC, HUS and thrombotic thrombocytopenic purpura (see above). It can also occur with prosthetic heart valves and giant haemangiomas, in extracorporeal circulations and with massive blood loss. Abnormal sequestration of platelets can occur in hypersplenism.

## Vessel Wall Abnormalities

Congenital vessel wall abnormalities are seen in hereditary telangiectasia, most commonly in adults, and in connective tissue disorders such as Ehlers–Danlos syndrome and pseudoxanthoma elasticum. The latter are both associated with lax skin and hyperextensible joints; patients bruise easily. Acquired vessel wall abnormalities may be limited to the endothelium or represent an abnormality of the whole wall. The former occurs in anoxia, with poisons and with immunological disorders, such as Henoch–Schönlein purpura.

More extensive wall abnormalities are seen in senile purpura, disproteinaemias, scurvy, steroids (Cushing's disease and therapeutic administration) and amyloid. Most of these conditions present with varying degrees of purpura, particularly over pressure areas, and with easy bruising and bleeding from the mucous membranes.

## ANAEMIA

The prime function of red blood cells is to deliver oxygen to the tissues. Anaemia is the reduction of the haemoglobin concentration, the red cell count or the packed cell volume to below normal levels. This has the effect of reducing the oxygen-carrying capacity of the red cell mass. Anaemia is one of the most common conditions encountered and affects around 15–20 per cent of the population worldwide. It may be due to abnormalities of erythropoiesis – red blood cell production – or to an increased loss of red blood cells. It should be considered to be a symptom rather than a disorder in its own right, and there are a large variety of causes (**Tables 2.8–2.12**).

Table 2.8 Anaemia due to defective erythropoiesis

| Type of defect | Disorder |
|---|---|
| Abnormalities of erythropoietin | Renal disease |
| | Reduced oxygen requirements (hypopituitarism, hypothyroidism) |
| | Reduced oxygen affinity of haemoglobin |
| | Erythropoietin autoantibodies |
| Defective proliferation | Iron deficiency |
| | Marrow failure: |
| | – aplastic anaemia (primary, secondary – radiotherapy, chemicals, toxins, drugs) |
| | – tumour invasion (leukaemia, lymphoma, myelofibrosis, secondary carcinoma) |
| | Chronic diseases (infection, collagen disease, malignancy) |
| Defective maturation | Nuclear abnormalities (vitamin $B_{12}$ and folate deficiencies) |
| | Globin abnormalities: |
| | – genetic (thalassaemia, sickle cell disease) |
| | – acquired (met-, carboxy- and sulphaemoglobinaemia) |
| | Sideroblastic anaemia: |
| | – genetic |
| | – idiopathic |
| | – secondary (alcohol abuse, anti-tuberculosis drugs, collagen, infection, lead poisoning, malignancy) |

Table 2.9 Haemolytic anaemias

| Genetic/acquired abnormalities | Reason |
|---|---|
| Genetic (intrinsic) | Haemoglobin (thalassaemia, sickle cell disease) |
| | Membrane (hereditary spherocytosis) |
| | Enzyme (glucose 6-phosphate dehydrogenase deficiency) |
| Acquired (extrinsic) | Trauma (burns, heart valves) |
| | Drugs (phenacetin) |
| | Immune (incompatible blood, haemolytic disease of the newborn) |
| | Autoimmune (leukaemia, lymphoma, systemic lupus erythematosus) |
| | Toxins (lead, copper) |
| | Hypersplenism |
| | Malaria |
| | Snake and insect bites |
| | Disseminated intravascular necrosis |
| | Haemolytic–uraemic syndrome |

Table 2.10 Blood loss through acute haemorrhage

| System | Condition |
| --- | --- |
| Gastrointestinal | Haemorrhoids |
| | Salicylate ingestion |
| | Non-steroidal anti-inflammatory drugs |
| | Peptic ulcer |
| | Hiatus hernia |
| | Large bowel tumour |
| | Hookworm |
| | Telangiectasia |
| Genitourinary | Kidney (autoimmune nephritis, carcinoma) |
| Uterine | Bladder (polyps, schistosomiasis, carcinoma) |

Table 2.11 Reasons for vitamin $B_{12}$ and folate deficiencies

| Vitamin $B_{12}$/folate | Source of deficiency |
| --- | --- |
| Vitamin $B_{12}$ | Nutritional (vegan, neglect) |
| | Malabsorption: |
| | – gastritis |
| | – gastric atrophy/carcinoma/resection |
| | – abnormalities of intrinsic factor |
| | – blind loop syndrome |
| | – tropical sprue |
| | – fish tapeworm |
| | – drugs (neomycin, colchicine, metformin, anticonvulsants, alcohol) |
| Folate | Excess requirements (pregnancy, infection, malignancy) |

Table 2.12 Anaemia classified by red blood cell morphology

| Morphology | Condition |
| --- | --- |
| Microcytic | Iron deficiency |
| | Thalassaemia |
| | Sideroblastic |
| Macrocytic | Vitamin $B_{12}$ and folate deficiency |
| | Haemolysis |
| | Alcohol abuse |
| Normocytic | Primary disease of the bone marrow (aplastic anaemia) |
| | Renal failure |
| | Hypopituitary/hypothyroidism |
| | Chronic diseases (infection, collagen, malignancy, scurvy) |
| Leukoerythroblastic | Leukaemia |
| | Myelosclerosis |
| | Metastatic carcinoma |

In the following paragraphs, erythropoiesis is considered first – to identify where disorders may occur – and this is followed by comments on classification. Subsequent sections discuss the presenting history and examination of the anaemic patient. Consideration is given to the types of anaemia encountered transglobally.

**Erythropoiesis** is stimulated by the release of the hormone erythropoietin. In the adult, this is stored predominantly in the kidneys and is released in response to lowered tissue oxygenation. Maturation of the red blood cell in the marrow from its precursors takes 7 days. During this time, the nucleus shrinks and gradually disappears, and haemoglobin is synthesized within the cell. The cell becomes enucleate by the seventh day but still contains residual RNA and organelles. In this stage of maturation, the cell is termed a reticulocyte, and red blood cells are released into the circulation in this form. The nuclear remnants are detectable for a further 24 hours. The life cycle of the mature red blood cell is about 120 days. About 1 per cent of the circulating red cell mass is destroyed daily, being replaced by an equivalent number of reticulocytes.

Initial abnormalities of maturation are due to a failure of release of erythropoietin due to renal damage, to altered sensitivity to oxygen, to reduced oxygen requirements – such as in endocrine abnormalities – and to the autoimmune destruction of erythropoietin. Factors affecting maturation within the bone marrow can be divided into those inhibiting cell proliferation and those affecting the development of the mature cell. Some factors can affect both these aspects of red blood cell development.

**Iron deficiency** is the most common factor inhibiting red cell proliferation. Similar effects can occur with primary or secondary marrow failure and with infiltration of the marrow in malignant disease. Chronic debilitating diseases – such as infection, collagen abnormalities and malignancy – also inhibit proliferation.

**Vitamin $B_{12}$** and folate deficiencies inhibit early maturation of the precursor cell membrane. Globin abnormalities include genetic variants – especially **thalassaemia** and **sickle cell disease** – and the rare acquired abnormalities of methaemoglobin, carboxyhaemoglobin and sulphaemoglobin. Abnormalities of haem maturation are due to altered iron metabolism, giving rise to iron loading of the red cell, a condition termed **sideroblastic anaemia**; this can present as a mild genetic form. Acquired sideroblastic anaemia may be idiopathic or secondary to a number of causes, including alcohol abuse and drugs used in the treatment of tuberculosis.

The second group of factors giving rise to anaemia comprise increased red blood cell loss and haemolysis. Blood loss may be due to **acute haemorrhage** but is more commonly due to **chronic loss**, particularly from the gastrointestinal tract, the uterus and the genitourinary tract; malignancy should always be a consideration. The causes of gastrointestinal haemorrhage vary with age and locality. In Western civilization, aspirin ingestion makes up approximately 10 per cent of cases, and there is also a high incidence in piles, peptic ulceration and hiatus hernia. In developing countries, hookworm is the most common cause, another potent cause being schistosomiasis.

**Haemolysis** may be congenital or acquired. It may be due to abnormal haemoglobin (thalassaemia or sickle cell disease), an alteration in the cell membrane (hereditary spherocytosis) or abnormalities of the enzyme systems of the red blood cell (glucose 6-phosphate dehydrogenase [G6PD] deficiency). A variety of extrinsic factors make up the acquired group. Haemolysis may be an immune abnormality such as with incompatible blood transfusions or haemolytic disease of the newborn. Blood can be damaged by the trauma of an artificial heart valve or in burns, and an abnormal destruction of red blood cells occurs in hypersplenism. The most common form of acquired haemolytic anaemia is due to the malarial parasite.

## Classification of Anaemia by Red Cell Morphology

Whereas the division of anaemias into abnormalities of erythropoiesis and blood loss helps with understanding and memorizing the large number of causes, a useful clinical classification is by the microscopic study of a simple blood film. In this way, anaemias can be divided into **microcytic**, **macrocytic** and **normocytic**. These divisions have direct clinical relevance to both the diagnosis and the presenting symptoms and signs.

A **microcytic anaemia** (Figure 2.15) is one in which the red blood cells are reduced in size. It is commonly encountered with reduced circulating or stored iron, and this is usually accompanied by hypochromia, that is, reduced staining with haematoxylin and eosin due to a decreased amount of cellular haemoglobin. The most useful of the indices in this type of anaemia is a reduction in the mean corpuscular volume. The mean corpuscular haemoglobin and mean corpuscular haemoglobin concentration are also abnormal.

Microcytosis may also occur in thalassaemia, sideroblastic anaemia and occasionally the anaemia of chronic disorders. Further measurements of body iron include serum iron, total iron-binding capacity, serum ferritin and the iron stores present in the marrow. In the clinical assessment, include questions on menstruation, postmenopausal bleeding and frank bleeding from the gastrointestinal or urinary tracts. Examine the faeces for occult blood, cysts, ova and parasites. As appropriate, undertake endoscopy and barium studies of the oesophagus, stomach and duodenum, and examine the anus, rectum and colon. Undertake urinalysis to exclude haematuria.

Megaloblastic red blood cells – **macrocytic anaemia** – in the peripheral circulation or the marrow commonly occur in relation to vitamin $B_{12}$ and folate deficiency. There is also an increase in mean corpuscular volume. Megaloblastic circulating red blood cells also occur in myelodysplasia, anaemia related to alcohol abuse and occasionally haemolytic anaemias. A megaloblastic pattern always warrants further investigation.

**Normocytic anaemias** occur in a wide variety of disorders. They are usually normochromic and have normal red blood cell indices. They include primary diseases of the bone marrow and aplastic anaemias. White blood cell and red blood cell precursors (Figure 2.16), including enucleate red cells, myelocytes and metamyelocytes, may be present in the peripheral field. There may be hypoplasia of all cell groups and also dysplasia. Examination of the marrow may show the underlying cause of disease. The majority of anaemias encountered in chronic disease fall into this category. They include the anaemias of renal failure, hypopituitarism, hypothyroidism, inflammation, collagen diseases and malignancy.

Examination of a peripheral blood film may show associated abnormalities of the red and white blood cells; such anaemias are termed leukoerythroblastic. They include the anaemias of leukaemia, myelosclerosis and metastatic marrow carcinoma. The film may show the primitive blast cells of leukaemia. White blood cell abnormalities are also seen with iron deficiency anaemia (parasites, especially hookworm, allergic conditions, enteritides and Hodgkin's disease). In vitamin $B_{12}$ and folate deficiency, there may be hypersegmented polymorphs and platelet abnormalities, producing a bleeding diathesis (see p. 30).

Examination of the peripheral blood film may identify other classical red and white cell abnormalities that may be of diagnostic importance:

- Anisocytes and poikilocytes are abnormally shaped red blood cells that are useful cell markers of iron deficiency anaemia.
- An increased number of circulating reticulocytes is characteristic of haemolytic anaemia and chronic blood loss. Fragmented cells can be seen in cases of haemolysis and microangiopathies.
- Spherocytes are abnormal, spherically shaped red blood cells encountered in hereditary spherocytosis and malaria.
- Target cells have a characteristic darker centre, providing the multiple ringed appearance. They occur in thalassaemia and liver disease, and after splenectomy.
- Punctate basophilia of the red blood cells is an abnormality of erythropoiesis seen in lead poisoning.
- Heinz bodies are abnormal subunits of globin or precipitated haemoglobin that are particularly seen in G6PD deficiency.
- Howell–Jolly bodies are nuclear fragments, particularly seen after splenectomy. Sideroblasts are red blood cells with iron granular inclusions that are seen in sideroblastic anaemias and post-splenectomy.

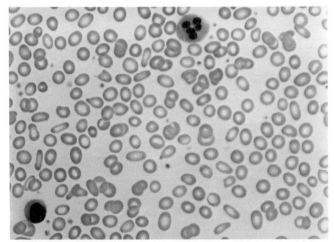

Figure 2.15 A blood film from a patient with microcytic anaemia. Note the hypochromic small red blood cells (also the lymphocyte, polymorph and platelets).

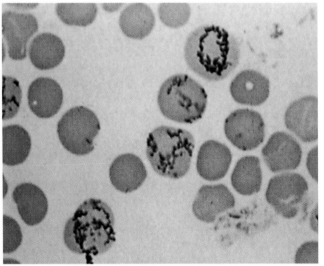

Figure 2.16 Reticulocytes in a blood film.

- Rouleaux formation – the stacking of red blood cells in columns – occurs in multiple myelomatosis and dysproteinaemia.

Haemoglobin abnormalities – such as those of thalassaemia and sickle cell disease – are identified by electrophoresis. More sophisticated tests are becoming available and are used to study milder and rarer forms of haemoglobin abnormality and their mode of inheritance. Different forms of anaemia may coexist, such as iron deficiency in thalassaemia.

## CLINICAL ASSESSMENT OF THE ANAEMIC PATIENT

### History

The anaemic patient may present with the symptoms of anaemia or its underlying cause. Occasionally, a blood test undertaken for a routine health screen or prior to an operative procedure brings the anaemia to light. The symptoms depend on the rate of onset and severity; for example, in chronic, unrecognized bleeding from the stomach, bowel, kidneys or bladder, the haemoglobin can fall to less than 5 g/dL without noticeable symptoms. Similarly, with chronic menorrhagia or hookworm infestation, a haemoglobin of 10 g/dL may well be the norm.

The lowered oxygen tension defining anaemia has widespread effects on all the tissues: the symptoms are often diffuse. The aim of the history and examination should be to identify the existence of anaemia and to search for any underlying cause. Subsequent investigations help to define the particular type and severity of the anaemia and provide further diagnostic clues, as discussed earlier.

The general symptoms of chronic anaemia are tiredness, weakness and lassitude. There may be a reduced appetite and weight loss. Mental changes of headache and dizziness are common and to these can be added confusion, particularly in the elderly. Exertional dyspnoea is an early symptom.

More severe symptoms of anaemia usually relate to the effects on cardiac function since the cardiac output has to be increased to deliver adequate tissue oxygen in the presence of an inadequate transport medium. If the disease progresses, a high-output cardiac failure occurs. Tachycardia and a high output give rise to palpitations, increased headache and dizziness. Breathlessness becomes more severe, with orthopnoea and paroxysmal nocturnal dyspnoea. Anaemia accentuates angina and claudication from underlying coronary and lower limb arterial disease. Cardiac failure is accompanied by ankle and sacral oedema and a cough with frothy white sputum.

Having found anaemia, explore the possible causes, particularly in the gastrointestinal, urological and menstrual history. Fresh alimentary bleeding may be noted from the gums and piles. A painful mouth and tongue may be related to the anaemia and produce eating difficulties. Note any low dietary intake due to neglect or starvation, as well as dietary habits, food fads and psychiatric disorders. A total absence of meat and dairy products can give rise to vitamin $B_{12}$ deficiency. Note dysphagia, indigestion, abdominal pain and distension, and changes in bowel habit. The symptoms may suggest malignancy, other gut disease or sickle cell crises. The locality or overseas trips may suggest specific parasitic problems of the gut or elsewhere, such as hookworm and malaria. Pruritus can occur in iron deficiency anaemia.

In the menstrual history, assess the degree of loss, such as the number of pads and tampons used and any recent change in loss.

Bleeding problems may become apparent through easy bruising after minor trauma, spontaneous purpura or bleeding after tooth extraction, cuts and surgery. Associated diseases may be obvious, such as acute haemorrhage and the symptoms of shock and collapse, severe infections and widespread malignancy. Bone pain may indicate local pathology.

A detailed drug history is essential as the ingestion of non-steroidal anti-inflammatory agents is common and patients may be taking anticoagulants. Drug reactions are diverse and – once the list is complete – may require reference to the appropriate literature.

Alcohol abuse can produce a number of haematological effects through liver disease as well as specific haemolysis and its effects on the bone marrow. Adhesives, lead and some other chemicals linked with occupations or hobbies must be identified. The racial origin of the subject may suggest the possibility of thalassaemia or sickle cell disease, and a detailed family history of bleeding problems should be questioned and a family tree constructed.

### Examination

Anaemia is characterized by pallor, although clinical assessment of the degree of pallor is unreliable. It is most easily observed in the mucous membranes of the mouth or the conjunctiva, and peripherally in the nail beds and palmar creases. Examination of the skin and subcutaneous tissues may reveal bruising, purpura or other manifestations of bleeding diatheses, such as petechiae and telangiectasia. There may be extensive bruising around any venepuncture sites. Fundal haemorrhages may also be noted on retinoscopy.

Cardiac signs include tachycardia, a large pulse volume and a hyperdynamic flow murmur. The hyperdynamic state might give rise to cardiac failure, the signs including peripheral oedema, a raised JVP, basal crepitations, hepatomegaly and fluid collections in the pleural and peritoneal cavities.

In patients with iron deficiency anaemia, there may be weight loss due to a deficient intake from neglect, starvation, food fads or psychiatric problems, or malabsorption and losses through fistulas. The tongue is smooth and shiny (**Figure 2.17**) and there may be angular stomatitis. The nails characteristically show koilonychia, that is, spooning and widening of the nails, which are brittle and fragile (as shown in Figure 1.10).

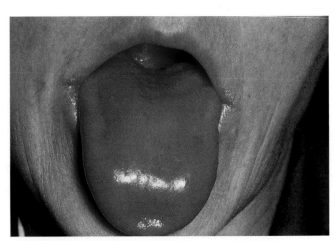

Figure 2.17 Plummer–Vinson syndrome – a smooth tongue.

Patients with vitamin $B_{12}$ and folate deficiencies often have a pronounced pallor but also a lemon yellow tinge to their skin. They may have angular stomatitis and glossitis, together with mouth ulceration. A specific feature of pernicious anaemia is the presence of subacute combined degeneration of the spinal cord. In this condition, the peripheral neuropathy is more pronounced in the lower limbs, especially involving the lateral columns, affecting vibration and position sense; the knee jerks are lost, and there may be an extensor plantar response, a positive Rhomberg sign and optic atrophy. Megaloblastic changes may be accompanied by thrombocytopenia, with splenomegaly, hepatomegaly and purpura. Other signs may be related to an underlying carcinoma of the stomach, with weight loss, an abdominal mass, hepatomegaly and supraclavicular nodes.

In haemolytic anaemia, there may be a mild jaundice and – if a haemoglobinopathy is present – there may be gallstones, secondary splenomegaly and chronic leg ulceration. Areas of bone necrosis may occur in sickle cell disease. Autoimmune anaemias may occur in chronic lymphatic leukaemia, lymphoma and systemic lupus erythematosis; there may be signs of these diseases and associated splenomegaly.

Malignancy can give rise to other abnormal physical signs. These include an abdominal mass, liver secondaries, hepatosplenomegaly and widespread lymphadenopathy; the latter may be primary or secondary malignant involvement. Endocrine anaemias may be accompanied by pituitary, adrenal or thyroid insufficiency.

## Geographical Distribution of Anaemias

The prominence of anaemia as a worldwide problem has already been emphasized. However, this high incidence has a marked geographical variation: anaemia is particularly frequency in parts of Africa, Asia and China. The large populations of these areas are dependent on local agriculture, and this in turn is subject to many natural and man-made disasters, especially drought, flood, earthquake and war. The ultimate effect is starvation, mass migration and refugee problems. The associated poverty diminishes the potential for alternative food and fresh water supplies. These conditions give rise to deficiency anaemias and anaemias due to infection. The third problem is the genetic haemoglobin abnormalities that already exist in some of these areas.

Starvation gives rise to anaemia through deficiencies of iron, vitamin $B_{12}$, folate, vitamin C and protein. Dietary habits in different continents influence the pattern of endemic anaemias. Common diets are based on rice, wheat and maize, all of which are low in vitamin $B_{12}$, and this can become a problem if the diet is also low in meat and devoid of dairy products. Worldwide, however, folate deficiency is more common. Folates are destroyed by the prolonged boiling of vegetables, and in this respect folate deficiency is seen less in China, where vegetables are lightly boiled, than in India, where spicy foods are heated for longer periods. Pregnant women and children are particularly prone to folate deficiency because of their high physiological requirement. Fresh fruit is a valuable source of folate.

Acute infections commonly follow disasters, and the establishment of a clean water supply and adequate sanitation are of prime concern in the management of these events. Many infections, however, are endemic and give rise to widespread, chronic anaemias. Hookworm is a prime offender, it being estimated that 450 million people harbour this parasite, which not only sucks blood through the mucous membrane of the alimentary tract, but also secretes an anticoagulant. Although the body is very

effective in using ingested iron, it cannot necessarily keep up with the loss produced by such parasites. There is also an increased requirement in children and adolescence, menstruation and pregnancy. Schistosomiasis is another serious cause of anaemia and affects 50 million people worldwide.

According to the World Health Organization, there were an estimated 207 million cases of malaria in 2012, with approximately 627 000 deaths. Mortality rates from malaria have reduced by 42 per cent worldwide since 2000. The majority of deaths from malaria are in children living in Africa. Mortality from malaria in African children has, however, also decreased, by an estimated 54 per cent since 2000. In malarial regions, a number of varieties of haemoglobin have developed that provide partial protection against the haemolytic effects of the parasite. Well over 100 genetic varieties have so far been identified. Many are produced by changes in a single amino acid in the haemoglobin chain, and the majority have no clinical relevance. However, a few, such as those which cause thalassaemia and sickle cell disease, have serious haematological consequences.

Thalassaemia is the most common inherited single-gene disorder in the world and is the most common inherited haematological abnormality. It is thought that approximately 5 per cent of adults worldwide are carriers of a haemoglobinopathy, these being approximately equally divided between thalassaemia (2.9 per cent) and sickle cell disease (2.3 per cent). With the improvement in health care in endemic areas leading to increased survival, the prevalence of these disorders is increasing.

The thalassaemias are widely encountered, predominantly in Asia but also in the southern Mediterranean and North Africa. Thalassaemia in its most severe form gives rise to fetal deaths so it is less commonly encountered in adults. Typical clinical features of α, β and other varieties of thalassaemia include failure to thrive, fever, poor feeding and reduced resistance to infection; there is also splenomegaly. Late problems include iron overload from repeated transfusion, folate deficiency, weight loss and terminal infections.

Patients with sickle cell disease originate predominantly from North Africa. They have a mild icterus, splenomegaly and a high incidence of leg ulcers. They are also prone to systemic infections. Major problems arise if there are bouts of anoxia, from example from respiratory infections or anaesthesia. These produce acute haemolysis, giving rise to vascular occlusion and focal infarction, which present with areas of aseptic bone necrosis and gut and cerebral infarction.

G6PD deficiency is a red cell enzyme deficiency widely distributed through Africa and the Middle and Far East. There are more than 400 variants, and it has been estimated that 400 million people are affected. It usually produces mild chronic haemolysis but acute haemolysis may be precipitated by intercurrent illnesses and exposure to oxidant drugs, including antimalarials.

Urgent treatment is often required for severe anaemia. This may include blood transfusion. However, it is important to take blood for all the appropriate tests prior to the commencement of any therapy as the latter may alter the haematological picture and obscure an accurate diagnosis.

## PYREXIA

The body temperature can be raised after exercise and is subject to physiological variation, for example at the time of ovulation. The temperature is also raised in response to disease, the condition being known as pyrexia or fever. The mechanism is uncertain but is probably related to the release of endogenous pyrogens from damaged tissue. The highest and most constant fevers occur in infectious diseases but they are also associated with collagen disease and some neoplasms, thrombosis, ischaemia and drug reactions.

The cause of a pyrexia is usually obvious. Most acute infections have run their course within 3 weeks and the fever commonly has a characteristic pattern of onset, duration and lysis (see p. 35). A few viruses – such as infective mononucleosis, hepatitis and cytomegalovirus – may have a prolonged course, as do chronic granuloma-producing organisms such as those giving rise to tuberculosis, actinomycosis, toxoplasmosis, histoplasmosis and candidiasis. A number of endemic infectious diseases – for example, malaria, schistosomiasis, amoebiasis and trypanosomiasis – must be considered in their chosen habitat and in visitors from these areas (see Chapter 4).

The inflammatory response produces pyrexia in non-infective disorders, particularly immunological conditions including the collagen diseases, rheumatoid arthritis, systemic lupus erythematosus, polyarteritis nodosa, temporal arteritis and polymyalgia. Some tumours characteristically have a fever, including hypernephroma, leukaemia, lymphoma and occasionally pancreatic carcinoma, liver metastases and sarcomas. Other less common causes include venous thrombosis, pulmonary embolism, cirrhosis and sarcoidosis.

Intracranial disease and associated surgery can interfere with the hypothalamic control of temperature, producing marked pyrexia that may be difficult to control. Almost any drug can produce a febrile reaction but of note are sulphonamides, penicillin and barbiturates.

A fictitious pyrexia is occasionally encountered, the patient placing a thermometer in a cup of tea or exchanging thermometers. Watching the patient during a sublingual measurement provides an accurate result. Suspicion is raised if the pyrexia is not accompanied by an equivalent rise in pulse rate.

## Pyrexia of Unknown Origin

Patients may present with a pyrexia with no obvious cause. The title of pyrexia of unknown or uncertain origin (PUO) is usually applied when this pyrexia persists for more than 3 weeks or if the diagnosis has not been made after 1 week of inpatient investigation. A limit of 38.4°C can be added to provide uniformity for comparative studies. In view of the serious nature of many underlying causes, the patient should be fully investigated, with PUO as a diagnosis of exclusion. A diagnosis is eventually made in 90 per cent of these cases through a careful and repeated history, examination and investigation. About 40 per cent of patients turn out to have an infective source, 20 per cent collagen disease and 20 per cent neoplasia. The diagnosis is usually one of a common condition presenting in an unusual fashion, rather than a rare disease.

## History

A patient with a PUO will already have had their history taken on a number of occasions. This means that each subsequent history must be taken in even more detail to capture any subtle change in symptoms. Great skill is required and the condition provides a great diagnostic challenge. Every system must be questioned in detail and even trivial symptoms or slight nuances in the history must be fully assessed. A PUO may be accompanied by anorexia, malaise, lassitude, weight loss and non-specific symptoms of associated anaemia. Skin abnormalities include rashes, eruptions and irritation. Enquire whether the patient has had previous illnesses, accidents, transfusions or surgery. For the alimentary tract, question for changes in appetite, dental problems, dysphagia, abdominal discomfort or distension, changes in bowel habit, the presence of mild diarrhoea, changes in stool colour, perianal pain, pruritus or discharge. Enquire for dyspareunia and urethral or vaginal discharge.

For the head, neck and respiratory system, ask about eye discomfort, redness or discharge, earache or discharge, nasal discharge, pain or tenderness over the sinuses, sore throats, cough or dyspnoea. There may be aches or swelling of the muscle, bones and joints, or abnormal sensation or motor function. Question for contacts with sick individuals, whether these are family, friends or at work. Animal contacts produce a large number of potential pyrexial diseases.

Foreign travel is of prime importance. Visits to malarial zones without appropriate prophylaxis raises the question of malarial infection. Other potential infective diseases from tropical and other zones worldwide include typhoid, paratyphoid, hepatitis, amoebiasis, brucellosis, schistosomiasis, trypanosomiasis, filariasis, leishmaniasis, Rocky Mountain spotted fever, typhus, Lassa fever and rabies. Incubation periods vary in these diseases and require reference to appropriate texts (see also Chapter 4).

In the drug history, consider prescribed medications and non-prescription drugs, which may have been bought over the counter for minor ailments. Also ask about recreational drugs and any injections the patient has received.

The family history may identify chronic infective diseases such as tuberculosis, collagen diseases or unusual anaemias.

## Examination

In the examination, note the pulse, blood pressure and respiratory rate. Check the temperature, watching that the patient is not interfering with the reading. A temperature chart indicates the level and characteristics of the fever. A swinging record implies the presence of pus, while night fever may be associated with tuberculosis.

The patient's general appearance indicates whether they look unwell and are pyrexial, whether they are pale or jaundiced and whether there is obvious weight loss; also measure the patient's weight. The hands may show clubbing, suggesting respiratory or gut disorders, or the splinter haemorrhages of endocarditis. Examine the skin over the whole body for infective lesions, rashes, scratch marks, petechiae, purpura, ulceration and staining, such as in the flanks from pancreatitis, over a hernia due to dead bowel or over superficial venous thromboses.

In the head and neck, examine for eye abnormalities and tenderness over the mastoid air cells, nasal sinuses, teeth and temporal arteries. Examine the mouth for bad teeth and an inflamed throat. Generalized lymphadenopathy often presents in the neck. Examine all the node groups, particularly nodes that are not usually palpable such as the occipital and external and anterior jugular nodes. Supraclavicular examination behind a lax sternomastoid muscle may reveal a palpable scalene node. Examine the axillae and groins, as well as the epitrochlear nodes.

The heart valves may be the site of infective carditis. Listen for soft murmurs or established valvular abnormalities, as well as for pericardial and pleural rubs and focal lung disease. Percuss the lung bases to establish whether the diaphragm is moving or could be splinted by subdiaphragmatic disease. This is a common site, as evidenced by the aphorism 'pus somewhere, pus nowhere, pus under the diaphragm'.

Hidden and unsuspected causes of PUO are commonly found in the abdomen. Examine for superficial, deep and rebound tenderness and for tenderness in the renal angles. Palpate for masses and viscera, especially for hepatosplenomegaly and perinephric masses. Abnormalities along the large bowel – such as malignancy or pericolic abscesses – may be palpable. Check the hernial orifices to ensure that they do not contain ischaemic bowel or omentum. Listen for peritoneal rubs and hepatic bruits. Pelvic examination, including rectal and gynaecological digital and instrumental examination, is a very important assessment. Pus or tumour may be present in the pouch of Douglas, and tubo-ovarian disease may be detected.

During the remainder of the examination, note any tenderness and swelling of the muscles, bones and joints; look for pain on movement of the joints and of the back and for any neck stiffness. There may be deep tenderness over areas of venous thrombosis.

In a seriously ill patient with a non-specific abnormal white blood count or raised erythrocyte sedimentation rate, there is occasionally an indication for laparoscopy or even laparotomy. In addition, if certain illnesses are suspected, there may be an indication for prescribing antibiotics, steroids or anti-inflammatory, anti-tuberculous or antimalarial therapy.

## WEIGHT LOSS

Weight loss in the absence of dieting is usually a symptom of underlying disease and a greater than 5 per cent weight reduction must be fully investigated. A very sudden loss of weight is usually due to fluid loss from dehydration or the operative removal of fluid, the correction of fluid overload in renal, cardiac and liver disease, being post-partum and to a lesser extent being postmenstrual or having been catheterized.

If a patient presents with increased appetite and loss of weight, it is important to exclude thyrotoxicosis, diabetes mellitus and malabsorption. This group of patients may also include those with unrecognized psychiatric problems (see below) or an early malignancy with a high metabolic rate.

Weight loss is usually due to a decreased intake of food and fluid (dieting, or anorexia due to systemic or psychiatric disease), increased loss (diarrhoea, vomiting or fistulas) or increased metabolism (fever and malignancy). In the assessment, it is important to establish the patient's normal weight and usual pattern of intake and output, and to document changes in these patterns.

Weight loss may be evident in any alteration of features or form and lax skin folds over the arms, trunk and buttocks. The patient's clothes may be too large. Weight reduction can be due to fluid loss as well as tissue reduction. Signs of dehydration include dry, inelastic skin, sunken eyes and dry mucous membranes.

Table 2.13 indicates the large number of causes of weight loss. General examination must include an assessment of the hands

Table 2.13 Causes of weight loss

| Malabsorption | Low intake | Systemic disorders |
|---|---|---|
| Chronic diarrhoea | Starvation | Subacute and chronic infection |
| Laxative abuse | Dieting | |
| Coeliac disease | Senility | Malignancy |
| Colitis | Neglect/disability | Cardiorespiratory disease |
| Crohn's disease | Oral pathology | |
| Acute/chronic gut infection | Dysphagia | Uraemia |
| | Obstruction of the upper alimentary tract | Collagen disease |
| Abnormal gut flora | | Alcohol abuse |
| Liver/biliary/pancreatic disease | Vomiting | Recreational drugs Poisons |
| Gut resection | Anorexia nervosa | |
| Endocrine (diabetes mellitus, thyrotoxicosis, panhypopituitarism, hypoadrenalism) | Food fads | |
| | Psychoses | |

and skin for pallor, pigmentation, rashes, clubbing, splinter haemorrhages and spider naevi. Examine for a goitre, eye changes, skin signs, tremor, sweating and tachycardia to identify thyrotoxicosis. Look for occult malignancy in the abdomen, pelvis, breasts and lymph nodes, and identify fluid collections in the pleural and peritoneal cavities. Measure the patient's temperature and undertake urinalysis for evidence of glycosuria and proteinuria. After establishing baselines, it is necessary to follow up with precise measurements of intake and output, weight and skin thickness.

Starvation affects all ages but weight loss at other times is markedly influenced by the patient's age. In children, severe gastroenteritis and malabsorption are frequent causes; the latter may also present in later life. In young adults, common causes are tuberculosis, reticuloses and psychiatric problems. In middle-aged patients, consider endocrine disease and malignancy. In older age groups, the cause is usually related to more than one factor. The tissues of old people tend to shrink and there is a loss of stature. Although this may be associated with a reduction of appetite, it is important to exclude other causes, particularly neglect and senility. Cancer is common and cardiorespiratory as well as alimentary diseases are accompanied by weight loss.

**Anorexia nervosa** is a psychiatric disorder that occurs in young adults, particularly women. There is a total preoccupation with weight, obsession with a thin figure, fear of weight gain and altered body perception. There is rigorous dieting with ritualized eating patterns that can be accompanied by vigorous exercise programmes – the weight loss can be considerable (Figure 2.18). Associated endocrine abnormalities include depression of the pituitary–gonadal axis and hypothyroidism, with an accompanying loss of libido and potency, and amenorrhoea. In extreme cases of emaciation, there may be bradycardia and hypothermia. The condition carries a 5 per cent mortality, usually from a cardiomyopathy induced by nutritional changes in the heart.

**Bulimia nervosa** is also a psychiatric problem noted in young adults that relates to a fixation with weight. In this case, the patient develops a cycle of excessive eating followed by vomiting,

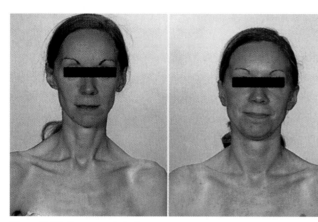

Figure 2.18 An anorexic twin.

these habits taking up much of the day. There may be associated laxative abuse. The weight loss does not equate to that of anorexia nervosa patients, the patients usually maintaining their weight near normal despite a high volume of intake.

## OVERWEIGHT

In the adult, the quantity of most tissues is fixed but the amount of fat can vary dramatically. Fat is contained both in the superficial adipose layer and in other tissues such as liver, muscle and bone. In normal adult men, fat makes up 12 per cent of the body weight, and in women it accounts for 26 per cent. An individual is termed 'fat' when there is a 20 per cent increase in body weight, and 'obese' after 30 per cent. Obesity is the most common nutritional disorder in the developed world. Average values are based on height–weight tables, and follow-up studies use weight change and measurement of skin fold thickness.

Obesity may also be classified in relation to the body mass index (BMI). This is calculated by dividing the weight in kilograms by the square of the height in metres. A BMI greater than 30 kg/m$^2$ is classified as obesity, morbid obesity being denoted by a figure greater than 40. An ideal body weight in kilograms is the height in centimetres minus 100 in men and minus 105 in women.

Obesity is usually due to overeating and too little exercise, but it is important to identify a weight increase due to focal or generalized fluid retention and that due to pregnancy. Focal fluid collections include ascites and ovarian cysts. Generalized fluid retention may be secondary to cardiac, renal or liver failure.

Obese people eat more but the basis of the hyperphagia can be metabolic or hypothalamic in origin, an example of the latter being a hypothalamic tumour. Genetic causes are usually due to hypogonadism; hormonal causes include hypothyroidism, Cushing's syndrome and abnormal sex hormone metabolism. Drugs include the contraceptive pill and some psychotherapeutic medications.

Eating is also influenced by cultural and environmental factors, the variety of food available and its nutritional value; some individuals are habitual or compulsive overeaters.

The distribution of fat is particularly noticeable around the face, abdomen and buttocks but it may be more focally sited, such as the 'buffalo hump' of Cushing's syndrome. Rapid weight gain may be accompanied by skin stretching with paper-thin striae.

A number of diseases are closely linked with obesity, including atherosclerosis, hypertension, hiatus hernia, gallbladder disease, diabetes, respiratory dysfunction, joint diseases, deep venous thrombosis and endometrial carcinoma. The dangers of obesity are also seen during anaesthesia and may be associated with psychiatric problems. Respiratory problems are due to an increased oxygen consumption and increased carbon dioxide production. A reduced functional residual capacity results in airway closure during normal tidal breathing, promoting anoxia. In severe cases, there will be sleep apnoea, cyanosis, polycythaemia and eventually right ventricular hypertrophy and heart failure.

Anaesthetic problems include respiratory depression, cardiac disease and hypertension. Intubation may be difficult in a bull neck, and there is an increased risk of aspiration of the gastric contents due to hiatus hernia and delayed gastric emptying. There is an altered distribution of anaesthetic drugs due to lipid binding, and mild liver abnormalities from fatty infiltration. Postoperative drugs must be chosen with care to prevent respiratory depression, and measures must be taken to reduce the incidence of deep venous thrombosis.

Reducing weight is predominantly a dietary problem but pathological causes of obesity must be identified and treated appropriately. Regular exercise should be encouraged. Increasing the metabolic rate by other means can reduce weight, but as this is usually dependent on thyroid hormones, smoking or amphetamine-like drugs, such treatment is usually inappropriate.

## ACROMEGALY

Acromegaly is produced by growth hormone secretion from a pituitary acidophilic adenoma, starting after the completion of normal growth; hyperactivity before this time results in gigantism. The clinical features of acromegaly are due to overgrowth of the bony and soft tissues.

The skin is thickened and greasy due to increased sebum production, and there may be hirsutism and hyperpigmentation. In the hands, the bones, especially the distal phalanges, are longer and broader, producing a long hand with wide fingers (**Figure 2.19**). The feet are larger, especially in width, and patients may have noticed increasing glove and shoe sizes.

The skull is enlarged, particularly the prognathic jaw (**Figures 2.20 and 2.21**) and nasal air sinuses. A skull radiograph usually shows an enlarged pituitary fossa. An increase in the soft tissues of the face includes a prominent lips, nose and tongue. Most patients present or are recognized because of these changes in their features.

There is not usually marked growth of the long bones of the arms and legs but there are exuberant osteoarthritic changes. The spine is subject to spondylitic changes, and a dorsal kyphosis can make the arms look longer. There is visceromegaly, including of the liver, spleen, kidneys and lungs.

The overgrowth of bone and soft tissue can induce nerve entrapment problems, particularly carpal tunnel syndrome, spinal nerve compression with sciatica and brachial neuropathy. There may be a proximal myopathy. Nerve pain, visual disturbances due to compression of the optic chiasm and headache may bring the patient to a doctor.

Associated conditions – due to an increase in basal metabolic rate – include intolerance to heat, with excess sweating. There may be diabetes mellitus, hypercalcaemia and hypophosphataemia. Hypopituitarism may give rise to a goitre and sometimes myxoedema. The condition may be part of a multiple endocrine syndrome. The patients are subject to cardiomyopathy and obesity, and there is an increase in cerebrovascular disease.

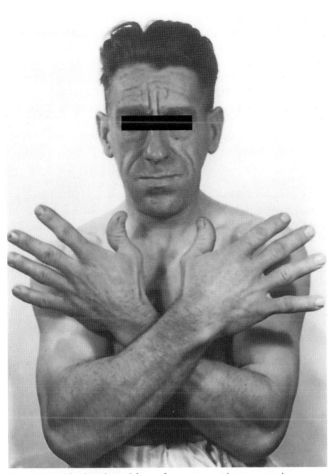

Figure 2.19 The hands and face of a patient with acromegaly.

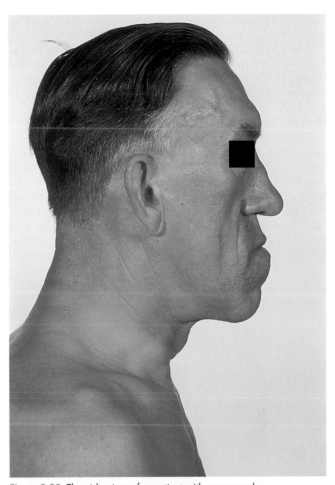

Figure 2.20 The side view of a patient with acromegaly.

In the respiratory system, soft tissue abnormalities can produce an increased lung volume and voice changes. There is an increase in malignancy in males.

## THYROTOXICOSIS

Thyrotoxicosis is due to excess circulating thyroid hormone in the form of thyroxine or tri-iodothyronine. Its effects are an increased basal metabolic rate, increased sensitivity of β-adrenergic responses and – if it occurs before the end of the growth phase – early maturation and a slight increase in growth rate. Primary thyrotoxicosis (see p. 409) is associated with thyroid-stimulating antibodies and may occur in conjunction with autoimmune conditions such as vitiligo, myasthenia gravis and pernicious anaemia. A few rare cases may be due to drugs such as thyroxine and iodine, an increased release of thyroid-stimulating hormone (TSH) from the pituitary, or a well-differentiated thyroid carcinoma. Secondary thyrotoxicosis (see p. 409) describes the development of thyrotoxicosis in a patient with a pre-existing goitre. It is seen in areas where endemic goitres occur due to a deficient iodine intake.

The effects of thyrotoxicosis are seen in all systems but are most marked in the cardiovascular and neuropsychiatric responses. The onset may be precipitated by sepsis or stress but may also appear at puberty or during pregnancy. The onset is usually gradual but occasionally explosive. The metabolic effects of an increased metabolic rate include a marked increase in

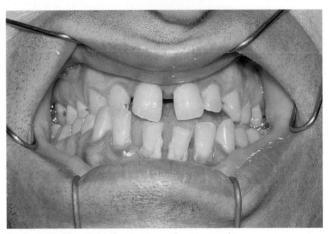

Figure 2.21 The teeth of a patient with acromegaly.

appetite yet a loss in weight. Occasionally, there is nausea and vomiting and usually a mild diarrhoea.

The excess heat production gives rise to sweating and a dislike of hot weather. Palmar erythema and spider naevi may be present. Skin changes also include pretibial myxoedema, alopecia and onycholysis.

Cardiovascular symptoms may dominate the clinical features and patients may present with the dyspnoea of cardiac failure. There is a tachycardia – which persists through sleep – palpitations, extrasystoles and commonly atrial fibrillation. These factors may lead to a high-output congestive cardiac failure with extreme dyspnoea and debilitation.

The neurological features are those of agitation, nervousness, restlessness, irritability and insomnia. There is marked emotional lability, rapidly changing from an excited and manic state to anxiety, depression and melancholia, with frequent bouts of crying. Patients are often short–tempered and occasionally an overt psychosis may occur.

Muscle wasting is common – accompanying the weight loss – and may be severely disabling. It particularly affects the facial muscles of the cheek, giving rise to hollow cheeks, the small muscles of the hands and the shoulder muscles (**Figure 2.22**). Fatigue is common and may mimic myasthenic symptoms. Movements are jerky and a fine tremor is usually present, particularly seen in the outstretched hand and tongue. There may be hyperaesthesia but – in spite of the motor problems – there is no sensory loss.

Eye signs are the most noticeable clinical features of thyrotoxicosis (**Figures 2.23** and **2.24**) but care must be taken in their diagnosis since some of the signs are occasionally seen in normal individuals. There is lid retraction, exposing the sclera above and below the iris and giving a wide-eyed, staring look, and proptosis from retro-ocular fatty infiltration.

In other systems, there may be oligomenorrhoea or amenorrhoea and loss of libido. The thyroid gland, as well as being enlarged from diffuse, single or multiple nodules, usually has a soft systolic bruit over it.

## MYXOEDEMA

Myxoedema is a hormonal disease resulting from a reduction in circulating thyroid hormone levels. In primary myxoedema, the abnormality is in the thyroid gland. Examples include agenesis, atrophy, destruction by autoimmune disease, thyroiditis, malignancy, radioactive iodine, surgical excision, iodine deficiency and drug suppression. Secondary myxoedema is due to reduced levels of TSH as a result of tumours or infarction involving the hypothalamic–pituitary axis.

The disease can occur at any age but peaks between 56 and 60 years; it is more common in women, by a ratio of 5:1. The symptoms are due to a reduction in the basal metabolic rate and are initially insidious. They include fatigue and lethargy, tiredness

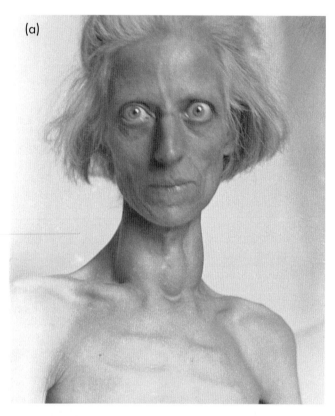

(a)

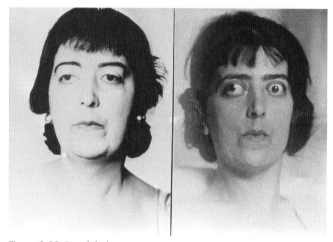

Figure 2.23 Exophthalmos.

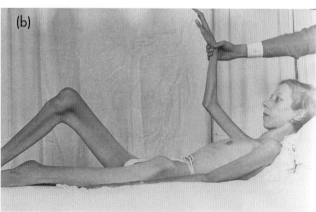

(b)

Figure 2.22 Muscle wasting in thyrotoxicosis: (a) facial and (b) general.

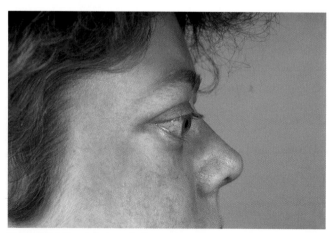

Figure 2.24 Exophthalmos (side view).

and weakness. They are vague and can bring the patient to many different clinics, and are thus easily missed. There may be aches and pains, cramps and stiffness, with feeling the cold and a dislike for cold weather. Constipation and menorrhagia are common.

There is usually a reduction in mental activity, with slowness of thought, speech and action. Rare complications include myxoedema psychosis and myxoedema coma, the latter being precipitated by cold, exposure, narcotics and analgesics. It is often seen in the aged patient living alone. It is a serious complication with a 50 per cent mortality, as it is very difficult to warm the patient without precipitating cardiac abnormalities and failure. The temperature may drop to 24°C, the patient being cold, dry and cadaveric with no shivering.

On examination, the patient is slow in communication and actions. The deposition of mucinous substance within the skin and subcutaneous tissue produces a thickening in these layers. The non-pitting, fatty tissue is prominent over the supraclavicular region, the back of the neck, the shoulders and the face, the latter producing puffy eyelids and gross features. The tongue may be enlarged. The voice is deep, gruff and weak with some hoarseness.

The skin is cold, dry, scaly, thickened and pale. A malar flush, together with the pale skin colour, produces a 'strawberries and cream' complexion and there may also be a tinge of yellow. This has also been described as a 'peaches and cream' picture (**Figure 2.25**). The hair is dry, coarse, lacklustre, inelastic and brittle, and falls out, producing baldness and commonly loss of the outer aspects of the eyebrows (**Figure 2.26**). The hands are cold and puffy (spade-like) with cyanosed tips.

The thyroid gland may be felt but this depends on the underlying pathology (see p. 409). The cardiac deposition of mucinoid material can produce cardiac failure, the signs being accentuated by a coexistent pericardial effusion, there being a weak pulse, peripheral oedema, a raised JVP, dyspnoea and basal crepitations.

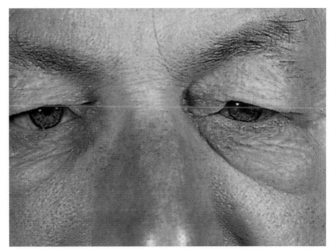

Figure 2.26 Loss of the eyebrow in myxoedema.

The ECG shows a low voltage with flattening and inversion of the T-waves.

In the nervous system, there may be mental changes as commented on in the history, slurring of speech, ataxia, weakness, myopathy, polyneuritis and sluggish reflexes with a characteristically delayed relaxation phase of the ankle jerks.

## CRETINISM

Although myxoedema can occur in children, hypothyroidism in the newborn produces cretinism (**Figure 2.27**); older children may have a mixture of myxoedema and cretinism (**Figure 2.28**). In the syndrome, there is a reduction of growth, poor bone maturation and abnormal mental development. The clinical picture may not appear for a number of weeks and can be difficult to detect. This has important clinical implications since irreversible damage usually commences after 6 weeks, the full picture of mental and physical retardation taking some months to develop.

The initial symptoms are feeding problems, respiratory difficulties, constipation and jaundice. The established syndrome is dwarf-like stature with a wide skull, short limbs and trunk, and spade-like hands. There is hypertelorism and macroglossia, the skin is dry, the abdomen is protruberant and there may be an umbilical hernia. Mental retardation may be marked.

Most hypothyroid infants are picked up by routine screening at birth. Causes may be agenesis and ectopic thyroid. A goitre is present in a third of patients.

## CUSHING'S SYNDROME

Cushing's syndrome is due to excess circulating corticosteroids. This is most commonly due to adrenal stimulation by a pituitary tumour, but it may be related to a primary adrenal tumour, steroid medication or an ectopic steroid source, such as a small cell carcinoma (oat cell carcinoma) of the bronchus. Other tumours of the lung, pancreas or thymus may also secrete corticosteroids, as can a medullary carcinoma of the thyroid. Hypersecretion in children may be accompanied by arrested growth.

The skin in Cushing's syndrome is thin with atrophy of the elastic lamina. Stretching occurs, with paper-thin scars that may be pale but are usually light purplish in colour. Healing

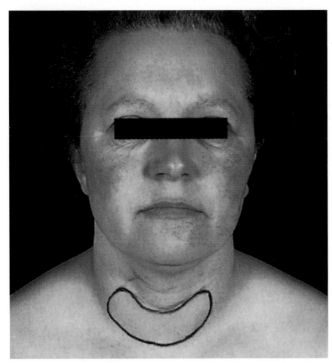

Figure 2.25 Myxoedema of the face.

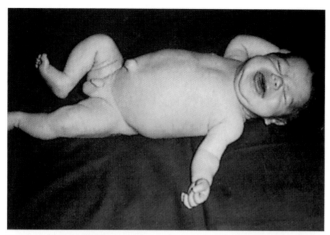

Figure 2.27 Neonatal cretinism.

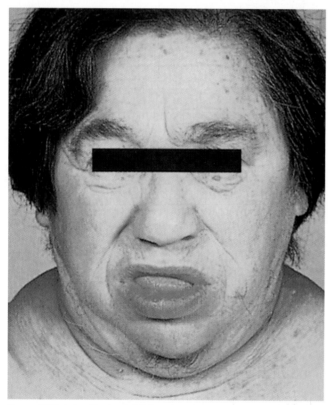

Figure 2.28 Late effects of childhood cretinism.

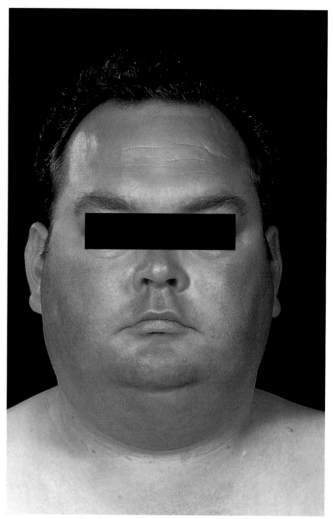

Figure 2.29 The moon face of Cushing's syndrome.

is poor. The superficial capillary network may be easily seen through the skin, giving rise to plethora, which is most marked on the face. Capillary fragility is accompanied by spontaneous purpura. Acne is common. Pigmentation may accompany excess circulating adrenocorticotropic hormone as with pituitary tumours, particularly if adrenalectomy is undertaken. There is an increase of lanugo hair and facial hirsutism. The scalp hair is often lost.

There is characteristically an increase in weight, this being due both to oedema from fluid retention and to obesity. The obesity mostly occurs around the face (moon face; Figure 2.29), the trunk and the back of the neck (buffalo hump; Figure 2.30). The limbs remain thin. The appearance has been likened to a central lemon with projecting matchsticks.

Associated conditions are hypertension, diabetes mellitus (30 per cent), myopathy with proximal wasting, oligomenorrhoea, impotence and infertility. Osteoporosis – particularly of the axial skeleton – is present, with occasional fractures of the ribs and vertebrae. Mood lability is common and about 20 per cent of patients suffer from depression.

Due to the frequent associated conditions, important differential diagnoses include hypertension, diabetes, psychoses and obesity. A sudden weight gain, as for example in pregnancy, may give rise to cutaneous striae (Figures 2.31–2.33).

## ADDISON'S DISEASE

Addison's disease is the clinical manifestation of adrenal failure. A variety of abnormalities can produce bilateral adrenal lesions, including tuberculosis, metastases, granulomatous lesions, autoimmune conditions, amyloid and infection. Pigmentation is a common finding, most marked in the skin creases, particularly of the palm, in scars, inside the lips and cheeks and on exposed areas (Figures 2.34–2.36). Depigmentation is very occasionally present, interspersed with pigmentation or normal skin. Skin changes may be absent in autoimmune-induced disease.

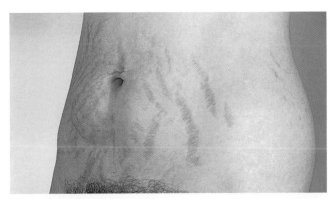

Figure 2.32 Striae post-gravidarum.

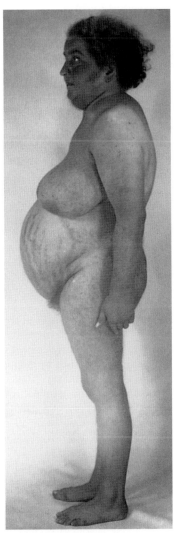

Figure 2.30 Cushing's stature.

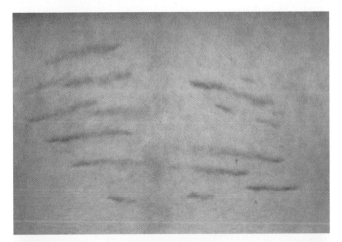

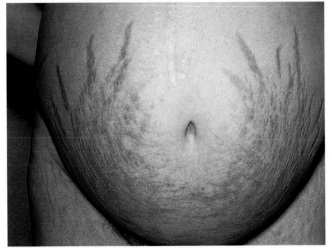

Figure 2.31 Striae in Cushing's syndrome.

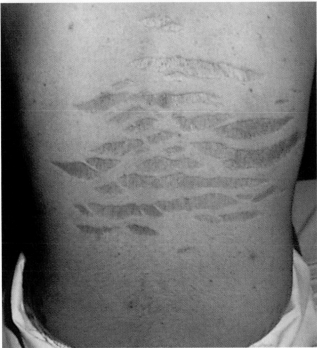

Figure 2.33 Striae post-pancreatitis.

Weight loss, diarrhoea and vomiting are commonly present, together with non-specific abdominal pain, colic, malaise, loss of energy, postural hypotension, muscle cramps and unexplained pyrexia. In extreme cases, hypovolaemic shock may be present accompanied by hyponatraemia, hypertension and hyperglycaemia.

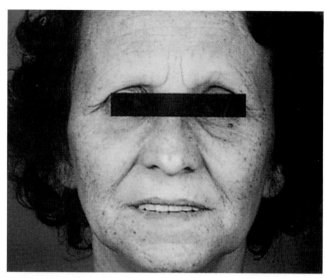

Figure 2.34 Addison's pigmentation of the face.

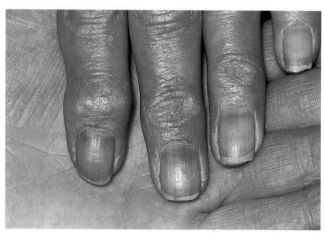

Figure 2.35 Addison's pigmentation of the nails.

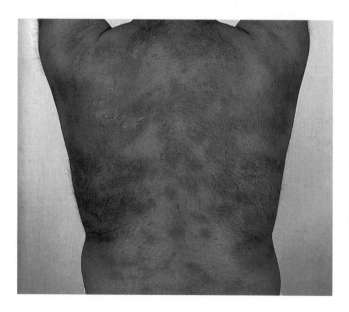

Figure 2.36 Addison's pigmentation of the back.

## MYASTHENIA GRAVIS

Myasthenia gravis is an autoimmune muscular disorder producing abnormal fatigue on exercise. Movement and power return after resting but repeated testing produces a more rapid decline. Wasting and permanent weakness are a late feature of the disorder but tendon reflexes are preserved. In the initial stages, the abnormality is confined to or predominantly in a single muscle group. The disorder is particularly marked in the extraocular and bulbar muscles but extends in the later stages to involve the neck, the shoulder girdle and, later still, respiratory, trunk and proximal lower limb movements.

The early symptoms are ptosis and a weakness of facial and jaw movements. The ptosis may initially be uni- or bilateral (Figure 2.37) and is accentuated by an upward gaze. The pupillary size and responses are not affected. The orbicularis oculi are rarely spared, and weakness of these muscles and difficulty of retraction of the angles of the mouth means that a 'smile' produces more of a 'snarl'.

Weakness of the palate, pharynx, larynx and tongue produces difficulty in swallowing and chewing as a meal progresses, with fluid regurgitation up the nose. Difficulties of articulation occur with prolonged speech, there being progressively less distinct articulation and a nasal tone. In the later stages of the disease, neck muscle weakness is accompanied by dropping of the head onto the trunk, limb weakness producing difficulty in bringing the hands to the mouth and often terminal respiratory failure due to weakness of the respiratory movements. An injection of anticholinesterase drugs can temporarily alleviate the symptoms and is diagnostic. The condition is occasionally helped by thymectomy.

## EHLERS–DANLOS SYNDROME

Ehlers–Danlos syndrome is a heterogeneous group of inherited connective tissue disorders, largely characterized by defects in collagen. It can be inherited by both dominant and recessive transmission. Patients are of short stature, their skin is smooth and velvety, demonstrating poor healing, and vascular fragility can lead to prolonged bleeding and spontaneous haemorrhage. The ligaments are lax and produce extensible joints, making them susceptible to recurrent dislocation. In certain forms of the disease, there may be ocular abnormalities.

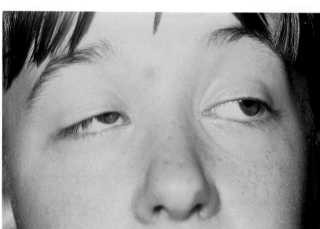

Figure 2.37 Myasthenic ptosis.

## MARFAN'S SYNDROME

Marfan's syndrome is a dominantly inherited disorder of connective tissue. The abnormal collagen synthesis affects the basal cement layer, particularly in the musculoskeletal, vascular and ocular systems. In the latter, there is a tendency to lens dislocation with resultant blindness. Individuals are tall and thin, the span being greater than the height, and the lower segment being greater than the upper. There is arachnodactyly (spidery fingers and toes; Figure 2.38). The sternum may be depressed and twisted, with an associated scoliosis.

Weakness of the joint capsules and aponeuroses can lead to joint dislocation and hernia formation. This also influences physical tests of stretch, for example passing the thumb across the ulnar edge of the palm and overlapping the fingers when gripping around the opposite wrist.

Other features are a high-arched palate, dissecting aneurysms, aortic valve incompetence and mitral valve prolapse.

## KLINEFELTER'S SYNDROME

Klinefelter's syndrome denotes a male patient with usually an XXY chromosomal pattern, but many karyotypic variations also exist. Patients are often tall and there is subnormal testosterone production. The testes are small and soft, and there may be maldescent. There is no spermatogenesis so individuals are infertile.

The body hair is masculine in distribution but the body fat has a female distribution around the breasts and pelvis and there may be mental retardation.

## TURNER'S SYNDROME

Turner's syndrome denotes a female patient with an XO chromosomal pattern resulting in mild skeletal and soft tissue abnormalities, amenorrhoea and occasionally associated coarctation of the aorta, horseshoe kidney and lymphoedema. Skeletal abnormalities include a masculine build, short stature, wide shoulders, cubitus valgus, a short fourth metacarpal, a high-arched palate, a wide (shield) chest with separation of the nipples, and a narrow pelvis.

The breasts are underdeveloped and there is scanty axillary and pubic hair. The neck is wide and there is classically webbing of the skin from the neck to each shoulder (Figure 2.39).

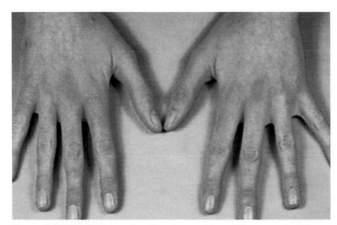

Figure 2.38 Marfan's arachnodactyly.

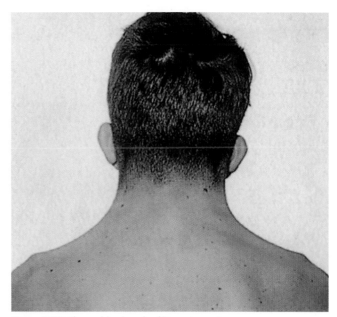

Figure 2.39 The webbed neck of Turner's syndrome.

## DOWN SYNDROME

Down syndrome is the single most frequent cause of mental retardation, accounting for 20–30 per cent of these patients. The condition is a genetic abnormality caused by an extra chromosome 21 (trisomy 21). The condition occurs in all races and is equally frequent in males and females. There is a marked increase in the incidence of Down syndrome with advancing maternal age – whereas the usual incidence is 1 in 1000, this rises to 1 in 20 with a maternal age of 46.

The syndrome comprises a number of congenital anomalies some of which are fatal. About two-thirds of fetuses do not reach term. Affected babies are floppy and hypotonic and already demonstrate recognizable adult features of the syndrome.

The outer angles of the eyes are raised, the sloping appearance, prominent epicanthic folds and hypertelorism giving a Mongoloid appearance (Figure 2.40), hence the earlier name for the condition. There may be a squint, nystagmus and myopia, keratoconus is found in adults, and there are pigment (Brushfield) spots (Figure 2.41) on the iris.

The head is bradycephalic with flattening of the face, and a prominent fold of redundant skin is present over the nape of the neck. The tongue is large and fissured, and the ears hypoplastic. The skin and hair are smooth and fine.

The stature, especially the limbs, is short and the hands are small. There is characteristic shortening of the middle phalanx of the fifth finger and typical palmar crease markings. Mental retardation is a constant finding but extremely variable in severity. Individuals are practical and personable, with a sense of humour and a preservation of musical appreciation, but with poorly developed numeracy and abstract thought. Their speech is dysarthric and hoarse. Walking is delayed and remains broad-based throughout life. Epilepsy occurs in over 5 per cent of cases.

A congenital cardiac anomaly is present in 40 per cent of individuals. This is usually an atrial or ventricular septal defect,

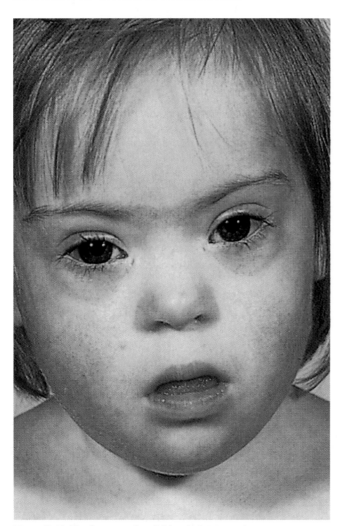

Figure 2.40 The features of a child with Down syndrome.

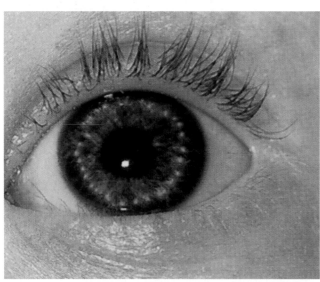

Figure 2.41 Brushfield spots.

but patent ductus arteriosus and tetralogy of Fallot also occur. Other congenital anomalies include duodenal atresia and imperforate anus. There is male sterility.

## DWARFISM

Dwarfism can be classified into proportionate and disproportionate forms.

The **proportionate** group includes some genetic abnormalities – such as Turner's syndrome – and mucopolysaccharide deficiency. The majority of this group are related to systemic abnormalities. Examples include renal and hepatic disorders, congenital heart disease, hypothyroidism, low growth hormone production and increased corticosteroid secretion.

Nutritional disturbances giving rise to dwarfism include starvation and coeliac and fibrocystic disease. The vitamin D deficiency produced by these gut abnormalities gives rise to the abnormality of rickets (Figure 2.42). This is characterized by lateral bowing of the long bones, especially the femur and tibia, scoliosis and prominent costochondral junctions. The lumps produced by the latter have been termed the 'rickety rosary'. Another chest wall abnormality is the transverse groove around the attachments of the diaphragm – Harrison's sulcus.

The **disproportionate** group comprises a disparate set of genetic abnormalities. The most common is achondroplasia, but there are also a number of rare abnormalities resembling achondroplasia. They have a different genetic profile but express a variety of achondroplasia-like symptoms. Severe osteogenesis imperfecta can also present with a disproportionate loss of stature.

Achondroplasia is the most common form of dwarfism. It most often occurs as a result of a spontaneous mutation associated with

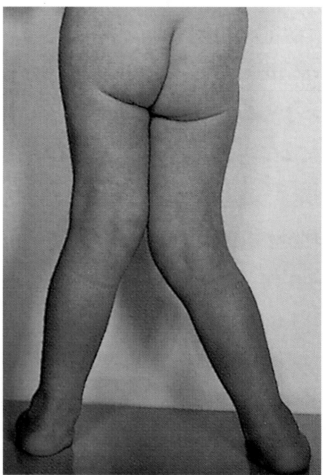

Figure 2.42 Rickets.

advanced paternal age, or it may be inherited as an autosomal dominant gene. The abnormalities are due to growth failure of the epiphyseal cartilage; periosteal bone development is normal. There is a marked shortening and deformity of the long bones, the umbilicus being below the midpoint of the vertical height. The hands are trident-like with short fingers and may only reach the iliac crest, thus giving difficulties in toiletry. The trunk is shortened, and there may be increased lumbar lordosis, wedging of the upper vertebrae and scoliosis. The gait is waddling. Late complications include spinal stenosis and osteoarthritic changes.

The head is relatively large, with bulging of the vault. The face is short, with flattening of the bridge of the nose. Intelligence is normal.

## PAGET'S DISEASE (OSTEODYSTROPHIA DEFORMANS)

Paget's disease is a bony disorder of unknown aetiology in which there is active osteoclastic bony reabsorption. Although there is an equivalent replacement by osteoblastic activity, the bone so formed is soft, deformed and lacking in normal mineralization. There is a marked increase in the blood supply of the affected area,

which is warm, and – if there is widespread bony involvement – it may lead to high-output cardiac failure.

The involved bones may be painful and in about 1 per cent of patients there is a sarcomatous malignant change. Although very thick, the bone may be fragile and brittle, and pathological fractures may occur, the most common being the classical transverse fracture of the femur just below the lesser trochanter. Any bone may be involved in the process but typically the skull, spine, pelvis and long bones are affected. The skull vault is enlarged (Figure 2.43) with overgrowth above the eyes and the ears. Enlargement of the skull base may produce compression of the cranial nerves, particularly producing deafness, dysphagia and dysarthria. There may be associated raised intracranial pressure. The long bones are thickened and may be bowed forwards and outwards (Figure 2.44).

## PARKINSON'S DISEASE

Parkinson's disease is a disorder of movement due to dopamine deficiency in the substantia nigra of the midbrain. The abnormalities are rigidity, tremor, akinesia and postural changes. They are often insidious in origin.

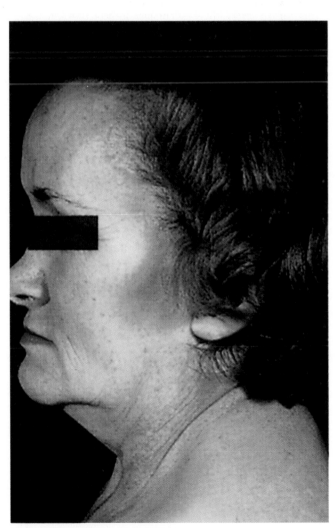

Figure 2.43 The skull in Paget's disease.

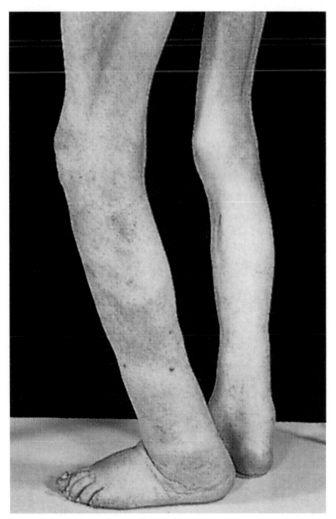

Figure 2.44 Tibial deformity in Paget's disease.

Rigidity is most marked in the head, trunk and proximal limbs. The movements are slow and stiff. There is an absence of facial expression with an unblinking, blank, mask-like stare. The volume of the voice is reduced, with a loss of modulation producing a soft, monotonous tone. Eye movements are usually preserved. There is slight 'plastic' resistance to passive movement, this being constant through the full range of movement. However, when tremor coexists, the resistance may show some 'cog-wheel' features.

Tremor may involve the hands, head, jaw or limbs. It is most common in the hands where it is of a pill-rolling form produced by wrist rotation. It is increased with emotional stress but absent in sleep. It may be unilateral.

Akinesia presents with poverty of movement. Postural changes include flexion of limbs, neck and trunk. This produces an alteration of the centre of gravity and instability when standing and walking, with a tendency to fall forwards. Although akinesia produces difficulty in initiating walking, there is also difficulty in stopping, the short, shuffling steps taking the subject forwards until a suitable obstruction is reached.

Sitting is in a flexed, motionless position, and getting out of a chair or out of bed may be impossible. Eating and swallowing become increasingly difficult as the disease progresses, there being some drooling and similar difficulties in washing and toileting. The handwriting becomes tremulous, small and untidy. Somatic and cranial nerve sensation remain intact, but abnormal sensations of pain, hot and cold may be experienced in the feet. Constipation is universal and there may be a lack of urinary control. The mental state remains intact, but the symptoms may give rise to depression and there is a higher risk of dementia than occurs in the normal population.

## CONGENITAL SYPHILIS

Syphilitic disease is very rare in the newborn and if present is a fulminating infection with a poor prognosis.

**Infantile syphilis** appears at 10–12 months and rarely before 7 months. The symptoms are of a cutaneous rash and destructive granulomatous lesions of the nasal cavities, mouth and anus. The rash is symmetrical and bullous, the bulli containing highly infectious fluid. The rash does not persist but healing produces linear scars. On the face, the scars are prominent and radiate from the lateral angles of the mouth and eyes – termed rhagades (**Figure 2.45**) – producing the wrinkled 'old man' look.

Nasal granulomas produce an active rhinitis; the symptoms are termed 'snuffles'. The subsequent destruction of the nasal septum produces flattening and widening of the bridge of the nose and a typical saddle nose (**Figure 2.46**). The disease of the oral and anal mucosa produces condylomas at these sites.

Congenital syphilis in **children and young adults** occurs after the age of 2 years. It has been summarized as producing a blind, deaf and lame subject. The blindness is due to interstitial keratitis and optic atrophy, and the deafness to atrophy of the vestibulocochlear nerves. The entire skeleton is underdeveloped, producing a small stature. A symmetrical, painless synovitis particularly involves the knees and produces swelling – Clutton's joints. The bones are thickened but the tibia is also bowed anteriorly (sabre tibia).

Rhagades, saddle nose and nasal perforation may again be present, with prominent parietal and frontal bulging – Parrot's nodes. The permanent incisors have a characteristic central notching along their margins. These have been termed Hutchinson's teeth. Hutchinson's triad is interstitial keratitis, nerve deafness and the tooth abnormalities.

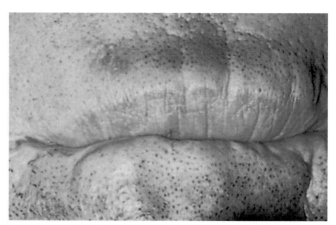

Figure 2.45 Rhagades in congenital syphilis.

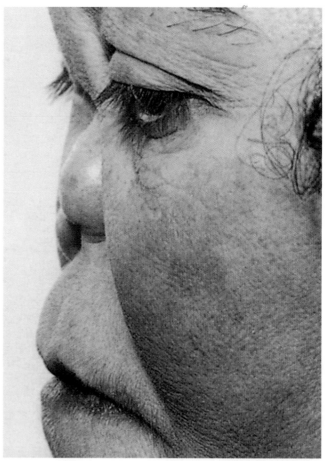

Figure 2.46 Saddle nose.

## Key Points

- Fluid balance is of prime importance in the surgical patient. It is primarily regulated by the kidney through a number of mechanisms, the most influential of which is ADH.
- Oedema is an excess of interstitial fluid and is caused by a number of generalized and focal disease processes including cardiac, renal and liver failure. Important surgical considerations are hypoproteinuria from malnutrition, malabsorption and protein-losing enteropathies such as fistulas. An excessive use of hypotonic intravenous fluid may also cause oedema.
- Reduced body water commonly arises in the surgical patient from alimentary tract loss both externally due to diarrhoea, vomiting, fistulas and a high stoma output, and internally in 'third space losses' such as with paralytic ileus or pancreatitis.
- The failure of perfusion to meet the metabolic requirements of the tissues is termed shock. Types of shock include cardiogenic, pulmonary embolic, cardiac tamponade, hypovolaemic, septic and anaphylactic. The characteristic differences must be identified to make a diagnosis as the management varies for each cause.
- Abnormalities of coagulation, platelets and the blood vessel wall comprise a large number of congenital and acquired defects. Anaemia is an important surgical consideration as blood may be lost from the gastrointestinal tract, uterus or genitourinary tract, and a malignant cause should always be considered.
- Weight loss and weight gain require an assessment and elucidation of the cause if they cannot be fully explained by a change in dietary intake. Weight loss may indicate malignancy, increased losses through diarrhoea/vomiting, thyrotoxicosis, diabetes or psychiatric disorders. Obesity presents a challenge in the surgical patient, with increased risks during anaesthesia and in the postoperative period.
- A number of endocrine and genetic disorders have surgical relevance in terms of both operative management and specialist requirements during the pre-, intra- and postoperative periods.

## QUESTIONS

### SBAs

**1. Which of the following hormones does not lead to increased fluid resorption in the body?:**
 a  ADH
 b  Aldosterone
 c  ANP
 d  Angiotensin
 e  Renin

**Answer**

**c ANP.** *ANP (atrial natriuretic peptide) is released in response to excess atrial filling. It acts to increase renal perfusion and salt excretion in order to reduce fluid reabsorption and circulating blood volume. In this way, it has the opposite function to ADH and the renin–angiotensin–aldosterone systems, which act directly and indirectly to resorb fluid.*

**2. Which of the following disorders is a sex-linked recessive condition that is characterized by a lack of functional clotting factor IX?:**
 a  Haemophillia A
 b  Haemophillia B
 c  Von Willebrand's disease
 d  Disseminated intravascular coagulopathy
 e  Thrombotic thrombocytopenic purpura

**Answer**

**b Haemophilia B.** *Haemophilia B, also known as Christmas disease, is a recessive sex-linked genetic disorder in which there is a lack of functional clotting factor IX. It accounts for approximately 20 per cent of all cases of haemophilia.*

**3. Which of the following symptoms is least likely to be seen in thyrotoxicosis?:**
 a  Sweating
 b  Irritability
 c  Baldness
 d  Weight loss
 e  Palpitations

**Answer**

**c Baldness.** *Dry, brittle hair that falls out leaving baldness is more likely to be seen in myxoedema, a disorder resulting from hypothyroidism. Hair loss can, however, occur in thyrotoxicosis, particularly at the outer third of the eyebrows.*

### EMQS

**1. For each of the following patients, select the most likely type of shock from the list below. Each option may be used once, more than once or not at all:**
 1  Cardiogenic
 2  Pulmonary embolism
 3  Cardiac tamponade
 4  Hypovolaemic
 5  Septic
 6  Anaphylactic
 7  Amniotic fluid embolism
 a  A 52-year-old man who underwent coronary artery bypass grafting 3 days ago. He denies any chest pain but appears breathless at rest. Observations reveal temperature 37.0°C, pulse 120 bpm and BP 75/45 mmHg. He has a raised JVP and pulsus paradoxus
 b  A 65-year-old man in A&E with a 1 day history of chest/epigastric pain. His past medical history includes angina, osteoarthritis and gallstones. He is clammy and has cool peripheries. Observations reveal temperature 37.5°C, pulse 110 bpm, BP 90/75 mmHg, RR 20/minute and saturation 99 per cent on room air. A cardiovascular examination is normal with no raised JVP or added heart sounds. His ECG appears synormal

**Answers**

**a  3 Cardiac tamponade.** *The recent history of cardiac surgery with specific signs of a raised JVP and pulsus paradoxus (pulse pressure falling with inspiration) make this the most likely diagnosis.*

**b  4 Hypovolaemic shock.** *In the absence of any cardiovascular signs and with a normal ECG, this patient is likely to have acute pancreatitis caused by his gallstones, leading to huge third space fluid losses and hypovolaemic shock.*

**c  2 Pulmonary embolism.** *The recent long-haul air travel and classic description of pleuritic chest pain and deep vein thrombosis mean that pulmonary embolism is the most likely diagnosis.*

**d  5 Septic shock.** *The common history of confusion, pyrexia, a bounding pulse and warm peripheries as a consequence of the gross vasodilatation seen means that this patient is likely to have septic shock. His indwelling suprapubic catheter is the probable source of the infection.*

c A 70-year-old man who returned home from Australia 2 days ago. He has a 1 day history of sharp, right-sided chest pain, worse on deep inspiration. Observations reveal a pulse of 115 bpm and BP of 95/50 mmHg but are otherwise normal. His left leg appears erythematous, swollen and hot to the touch. His ECG shows a right bundle branch block

d A 90-year-old man from a nursing home with ischaemic heart disease and an indwelling suprapubic catheter. He denies any chest pain or shortness of breath but appears confused, which staff say is new. Observations reveal a temperature of 38°C, a bounding pulse of 130 bpm, BP 90/60 mmHg, RR 12/minute and saturation of 98 per cent on room air. His peripheries are warm to the touch. His ECG shows a right bundle branch block

e A 55-year-old lawyer in A&E who collapsed at work. He gives a history of chest pain over the last hour that extends across his chest in a tight band, into his neck and down his left arm. Observations reveal a pulse of 100 bpm and BP 110/75 mmHg. and he appears grey and clammy. An ECG shows deep Q waves with ST elevation in leads V1–V4

e **1 Cardiogenic shock.** *The description and ECG changes are indicative of an anterior myocardial infarction causing cardiogenic shock in this patient.*

2. **For each of the following patients, select the most likely reason for weight loss from the list below. Each option may be used once, more than once or not at all:**
   1 Thyrotoxicosis
   2 Anorexia nervosa
   3 Malignancy
   4 Diabetes mellitus
   5 Malabsorption
   6 Dieting
   7 Gastroenteritis

   a A 21-year-old woman with a 5 week history of weight loss. She also complains of lethargy and urinary frequency

   b A 65-year-old man with a 6 month history of weight loss. He has been more constipated over the last 2 months and has noticed occasional dark red rectal bleeding. He is found on a full blood count to be anaemic

   c A 35-year-old woman with Crohn's disease who underwent a small bowel resection with loop ileostomy 6 weeks ago and is awaiting a reversal. She has lost weight since her operation. She changes her stoma bag up to ten times a day and notices the contents are very watery.

   d A 45-year-old woman who presents with diarrhoea and weight loss over the last 4 months. She also has symptoms of increased sweating and insomnia. On examination, she has a tremor and is tachycardic

   e A 17-year-old girl who presents with amenorrhoea. Her mother states that she has lost a lot of weight, has been avoiding eating with the family at home and spends a lot of time in her room exercising

Answers

a **4 Diabetes mellitus.** *The age of the patient and the symptoms of weight loss with lethargy and urinary frequency make the likely diagnosis type 1 diabetes mellitus.*

b **3 Malignancy.** *Weight loss with a change in bowel habit, dark rectal bleeding and anaemia is most likely to represent a gastrointestinal malignancy in this patient.*

c **5 Malabsorption.** *This patient with weight loss and a recent ileostomy with a high output is likely to have malabsorption.*

d **1 Thyrotoxicosis.** *Symptoms of weight loss with diarrhoea, sweating and insomnia with signs of a tremor and tachycardia are most likely to represent thyrotoxicosis.*

e **2 Anorexia nervosa.** *This presentation of a young girl with features of weight loss, loss of periods and behavioural changes may indicate anorexia nervosa.*

# Lumps, Ulcers, Sinuses and Fistulas

John S. P. Lumley and Natalie Anne Hirst

## LEARNING OBJECTIVES

- To be able to take a history, examine and systematically describe a patient presenting with a lump
- To be able to undertake a history of and examine an ulcer, with an understanding of

the aetiological types and their subsequent management
- To understand the differences between a sinus and a fistula and the pathophysiology and types of each

## LUMPS

### History

In the history, determine as precisely as possible when the patient **first noticed** the lump and what brought it to their attention. A common history is one of minor trauma, but the trauma often merely draws attention to the lump rather than causes it. The lump may be observed or felt when washing or may be observed by another person, as with a thyroid swelling; alternatively, it may become apparent because of pain. Ask about any changes in the lump. Rapid enlargement may imply inflammation, particularly if it is painful, whereas progressive enlargement may signify neoplasia.

It is common for patients to report a variation in size of a lump. This may be a genuine **change** but can also be due to its prominence in certain movements or positions. Note whether it has ever disappeared completely. True examples of variation are the obstructed parotid gland enlarging on eating and the reduction of a hernia. Blood-filled lumps – for example, varicose veins and some fluid-filled lumps such as communicating bursae – can be emptied by positional changes or direct pressure. Ask whether there is anything the patient can do to make the lump get bigger or smaller, such as tensing the abdominal wall or performing a Valsalva manoeuvre. Some lumps may discharge, in which case ask about the quantity, colour, consistency and smell of the contents.

**Painful** lumps are commonly caused by trauma and inflammation, but malignant lumps may also be painful when rapidly expanding, breaking down or invading nervous tissue. A **previous history** of the lump or other similar lumps may help in the diagnosis. Congenital lumps may be associated with multiple abnormalities.

Note the systemic effects that can be produced by infection, trauma or neoplastic changes. Ask the patient what they think the lump is as they might know or suspect a cause.

The word **deformity** is frequently used by both patient and doctor but not necessarily with the same meaning. Although it can be applied to any marked deviation from the normal size or shape of the whole or part of the body, and as such is applicable to any disease, it is usually used in relation to musculoskeletal abnormalities, particularly contractures of soft tissue, fixation of joints and bony angulation.

Lumps are commonly presented to the student, who is expected to communicate with the patient before palpating the lesion. The most important question is whether the lump is tender, but also ask **how long** it has been present and whether it is **changing** in size. To these questions add 'Where is it?' if a lump you have been asked to examine is not immediately obvious (Table 3.1).

### Examination

The clinical examination of a lump provides important clues to its diagnosis as many lumps have characteristic features. The following description is of the features that must be considered with every lump. Although all the features are not applicable in every situation, considering them in an organized fashion will mean that important steps will not be omitted.

It has previously been emphasized that the student and trainee must be able to describe accurately the clinical features elicited. This will ensure that they will remember to look for each sign and will be able to give an opinion on its presence or absence. The description may have to be given to a senior colleague over the telephone. As the recipient may be basing the diagnosis and management plans on this description, it must be full and reliable.

Table 3.1 Features to consider in the description of lumps and ulcers

| Feature | Definition/aetiology |
|---|---|
| Pathogenesis | Tissue of origin, single/multiple, classification<br>Incidence, age, sex, familial, ethnic, occupational, environmental |
| Symptoms | Appearance, progress, disappearance<br>Precipitating, exacerbating and/or relieving factors<br>Course of symptoms, pain, discharge<br>Systemic effects, social history |
| Signs* | Site: anatomy, depth, relations<br>External: colour, temperature, tenderness, shape, size, surface, edge, mobility<br>(Edge: sloping, punched-out, undercut, raised, everted)<br>Internal: consistency, fluctuation, transillumination, compression, reducibility, cough impulse, thrill, pulsation, resonance, bruit<br>(Base: slough, granulation, deep tissues, fixation, discharge)<br>Surroundings: induration, spread, fixation, penetration, perforation, lymphangitis, nodes, veins, arteries, nerves, muscle, bones, joints |

*Substitute 'edge' and 'base' for 'external' and 'internal' to describe ulcers.

Useful descriptive features are highlighted in bold in the following text. A later attempt is made to make these signs more memorable (see p. 68), but at this stage remember that the examination covers four aspects: the site, the external and internal features of the lump, and its effect on the surrounding tissues (remember the mnemonic 'SEIS').

## Site

The position of a lump has important implications for its likely aetiology, so details of both its surface markings and its depth must be recorded. The **site** (Figure 3.1) is measured from fixed bony prominences such as the manubriosternal angle, olecranon or tibial tubercle. The **relations** of the lump define its anatomical **origin**, its anatomical plane and the structures covering the surfaces of the lump. It may arise from the skin, subcutaneous tissues, bones, joints or muscles, or lie within one of the body cavities. The abnormality may be due to a **deformity** (Figure 3.2) of one or more tissues, perhaps of congenital or post-traumatic origin. When a lump is rapidly changing in size, for example with a haematoma or an abscess, its progress can be monitored by outlining the circumference with a skin marker (see Figure 2.12).

## Exterior of a Lump

### Size

First, measure the size (Figure 3.3) of the lesion. This should be carried out quantitatively, with a tape measure for example, as an inaccurate estimate can lead to a false interpretation of the change of size at the next visit. Lumps are three-dimensional so three measurements should be written down. It may not be possible to measure deeply placed lumps with a tape measure so learn how to estimate these sizes to within 0.5–1 cm. As the hand is always available for comparison, measure the width of your

thumb nail, the length of your thumb from the interphalangeal joint to its tip, your index finger from the metacarpophalangeal joint to the tip and your digital span. These measures can serve as a reference. Oranges and grapefruit, while useful for describing the shape of a lump, are, like walnuts and even golf balls, subject to variations in size.

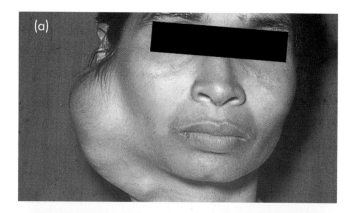

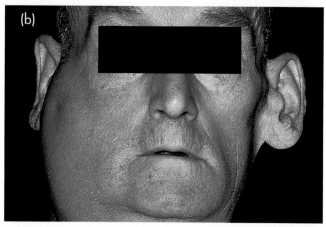

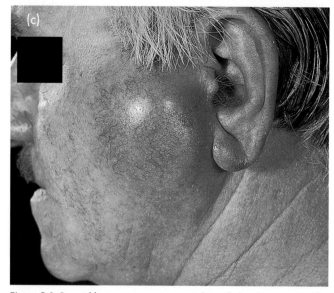

Figure 3.1 Parotid lumps: as you progress through the chapter, consider how you would describe these three lesions (a), (b) and (c) over the telephone.

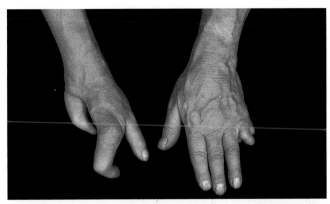

Figure 3.2 Lobster claw deformity of the hand.

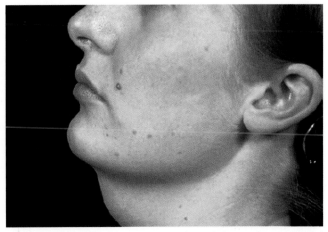

Figure 3.4 The smooth, regular, hemispherical shape of a suprahyoid thyroglossal cyst.

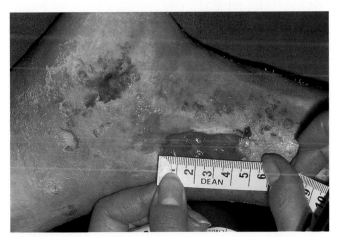

Figure 3.3 Clinical measurement starts with a tape measure.

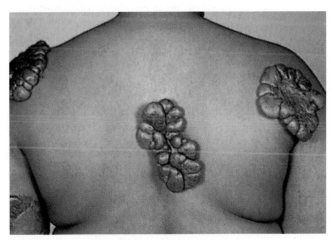

Figure 3.5 The irregular surface of a keloid scar.

## Shape, Surface and Edge

The **shape** of a lump is, like its size, three-dimensional so descriptive terms should take this into account. Common terms – round (**Figure 3.4**), oval, flattened, triangular, rectangular, square, irregular (**Figure 3.5**) – should be used for each plane being described. Likening the lump to common objects can be helpful, and the shape may be characteristic of the organ of origin, such as an enlarged kidney, gallbladder or thyroid gland. Many lumps are poorly defined (**Figure 3.6**) and all these features should be noted. Cutaneous lumps may be raised above the skin surface and the base may be narrowed, producing a polypoid lesion.

The **surface** of a lump can provide an indication of its aetiology. The surface is described in terms such as smooth and regular (**Figure 3.7**), rough and irregular (**Figure 3.8**) or any mixture of these. Lesions arising in the epidermis may exhibit a surface abnormality, such as the irregularity of a wart, and there may be a pit or punctum when the lump arises from a dermal appendage, such as a sebaceous cyst. Deeper lesions are usually covered with normal skin. There may be a specific pattern to an irregular surface, such as small or large nodules; the terms 'lobulated', 'cobblestone' and 'bossellated' are sometimes used to describe these features.

The **edge** of a flattened or projecting lump may be clearly (**Figure 3.9**) or poorly defined (**Figure 3.10**), and may be sharp, rounded, regular or irregular. The use of simple, well-known terms ensures that the description is fully understood.

## Colour, Temperature and Tenderness

The **colour** of a lump, in the case of a cutaneous lesion, may be that of the lesion itself, but when the lump is more deeply placed, its colour can be due to normal skin or changes in the overlying skin. Pigmentation (**Figure 3.11**) is an important characteristic as it may be the brown melanin of a malignant melanoma. Basal cell carcinomas (rodent ulcers) and squamous cell carcinomas can also contain melanin, as can a number of benign moles. Xanthelasmas are the yellowish colour of their fatty content, while gouty tophi are the white of their calcific content. Vascular lesions may be stained from iron pigments or may be discoloured because of the excess circulating blood in surface vessels.

Inflammatory and necrotic tissue changes from infiltration of the overlying skin produce colour changes varying from the pink or red of hyperaemia to black dead tissue. The latter is further considered with the features of the base of an ulcer. The overlying skin may be pale due to tissue oedema or cyanosed due to the reduction in oxygenated haemoglobin.

Increased blood flow in the superficial tissues increases their **temperature**; this is seen in inflammatory changes (**Figure 3.12**), tumours with a rich blood supply and tumours of vascular tissue.

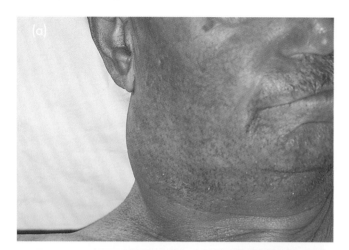

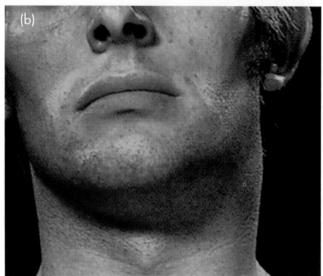

Figure 3.6 A poorly defined submandibular mass.

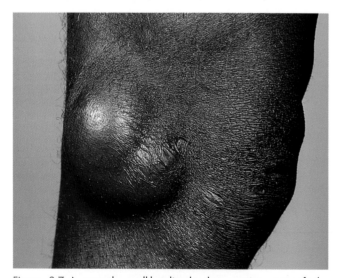

Figure 3.7 A smooth, well-localized, degenerative cyst of the lateral meniscus.

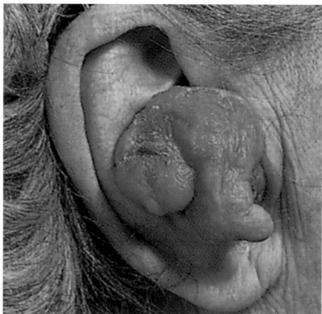

Figure 3.8 An irregular papilliferous lesion growing out of the auricular canal.

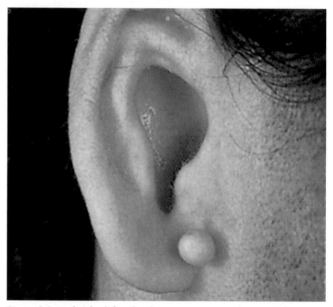

Figure 3.9 A clearly defined right accessory auricular appendage.

Large masses may reduce the temperature of the overlying skin or more distal areas. In temperature assessment, compare the local temperature with that of the adjacent skin and an equivalent site on the other side of the body. The examining hand is a sensitive indicator of temperature – the dorsum has the advantage over the palm in that it has fewer sweat glands and is dryer, making assessment easier. Gently draw the back of the fingers over the area being assessed and then over the area being used for comparison.

**Tenderness** may accompany trauma, inflammation and malignant lumps that are expanding rapidly, degenerating or

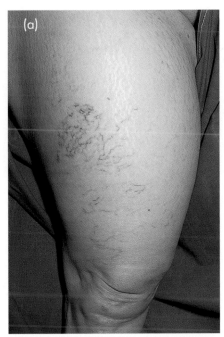

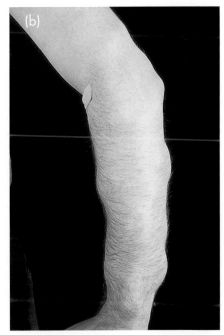

Figure 3.10 (a) A poorly defined thigh mass that proved to be a large subfascial lipoma. (b) Multiple lipomata in the forearm.

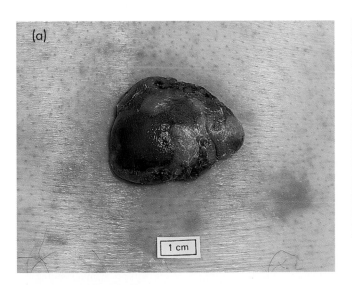

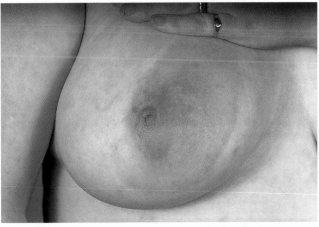

Figure 3.12 A red, inflamed oedematous, tender breast abscess.

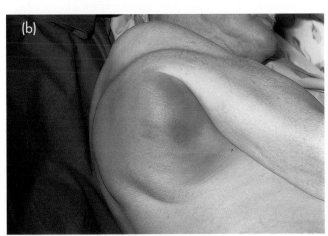

Figure 3.11 (a) Dark pigmentation in a malignant melanoma of the back. (b) A sarcoma of the right shoulder.

invading nervous tissue. It has already been emphasized that a patient must be asked before any lump is examined whether there is any tenderness. With this information, the appropriate degree of pressure can then be applied during palpation. If in doubt, always watch the patient's face when carrying out these manoeuvres.

## Mobility of the Lump

The mobility of a lump depends to a large extent on its tethering and fixation to the surrounding tissue (this is considered in a later section). However, the local features of the lump and its site of origin can also produce characteristic signs of mobility. A lipoma, for example, is one of the more common subcutaneous lumps, and if its edge is pressed the swelling slips from under the finger, producing a characteristic 'slip sign'.

Tension in the underlying muscles and fascia makes all subcutaneous lumps more easily palpable. If, however, a lump is more deeply situated, for example within a muscle compartment, muscle contraction tenses the deep fascia and often renders the lump impalpable. Similarly, a lump beneath the deep investing fascia of the neck can become impalpable when the patient presses their chin towards the opposite side of the neck against the examiner's hand. Lipomas and other lumps within the muscle may become more prominent on muscle contraction. The muscle is still mobile from side to side and is more prominent at the site of the lump. In addition, muscle bulges through splits in the deep fascia; such protrusions become more prominent on muscle contraction, the patient being asked to tense the relevant muscle group to show this.

Certain postures can make some lumps more palpable. Standing with an extended knee, for example, brings into prominence some masses in the popliteal fossa – such as a Baker's cyst – while flexion of the knee can accentuate infra- and prepatellar bursae. Flexion of the wrist can bring a ganglion of the dorsum of the hand into prominence.

Movement may also produce characteristic crepitus when moving inflamed tendons, for example in de Quervain's disease of the wrist or osteoarthritic joints. In joints, the crepitus may be a fine, 'squeaky' sensation (from subacute or chronic infections), coarse (e.g. from contact of the irregular surface of the femur, patella and tibia in osteoarthritis) or a click from a loose body or torn cartilage. In fractures, the broken ends produce a grating sensation on testing the movement. Demonstrating crepitus in this situation is, however, likely to be extremely painful and diagnosis should be by other means (see p. 147). Clicking of a tendon may be seen and felt, as in a trigger finger, when the tendon nodule is pulled through a narrow area of sheath.

Abdominal masses have a characteristic mobility. The kidney, gallbladder and liver typically descend longitudinally on deep inspiration. It may be possible to 'bounce' mobile abdominal lumps anteroposteriorly or from side to side – this is termed ballottement. In the supine position, a renal mass can be pushed forwards with short, sharp finger movements from a hand placed under the loin and felt anteriorly by the palm of the other hand. An enlarged spleen, untethered by adhesions, may also be ballottable.

An ovarian mass and other mobile abdominal swellings, such as a mass of secondaries in the greater omentum, can be ballotted from side to side, or backwards onto the posterior abdominal wall. The sign is more prominent when ascites is also present. A pregnant uterus and a large bladder can be felt bimanually by a hand placed suprapubically when pressure is applied on the mass by a digit inserted into the pelvis through the rectum or vagina.

If an abdominal viscus is dilated with fluid and air, a splashing noise can be elicited by holding the trunk and shaking it from side to side. This is a succussion splash.

## Interior of a Lump
### Contents

The contents of a lump can be composed of cells, fluid or gas (Figure 3.13); the cells may be normal or abnormal. Normal cells may increase in number, as with the overgrowth of a congenital anomaly, in hyperplasia or with a benign tumour. Abnormal cells may arise from an alteration in the local tissues, such as a malignant change, or from invasion by other cells, such as inflammation and secondary malignant deposits.

Fluid is usually extracellular, as in the swelling of oedema due to inflammation and venous or lymphatic obstruction.

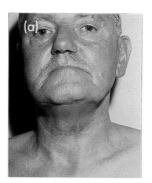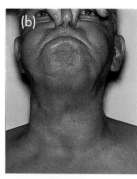

Figure 3.13 (a) A laryngocele. (b) The laryngocele becoming apparent when the patient exhales against closed lips and palate (the Valsalva manoeuvre).

Focal collections include encapsulated secretions, abscesses or intravascular blood retained within abnormal vessels, such as arteriovenous malformations, and some scrotal swellings.

Gas is usually within the gut, such as within an inguinal hernia, but can be within an abnormal segment of lung or within the tissues, for example after an incision, trauma or dental extraction damaging a nasal sinus, infection with a gas-forming organism, lung damage in rib fractures, tension pneumothorax, trauma to the larynx and tracheotomy, and as a complication of a ruptured oesophagus. Gas in the tissues – termed subcutaneous or surgical emphysema – has a characteristic crepitus on palpation.

This 'crackling' sensation is also audible if a stethoscope is pressed on the tissues.

### Consistency

Lumps range from stony hard to very soft. The simplest classification of consistency is the bony hardness of the forehead, the firmness of the nasal cartilages and the softness of the lip. Another useful classification is bony (stony hard), rubbery (hard but can be indented slightly), spongy (i.e. squeezable) and soft with (e.g. jelly) or without (e.g. butter) resilience.

### Compressibility and Reducibility

Lumps are termed **compressible** when they can be emptied by squeezing but reappear on release. These features are characteristic of blood-filled lesions, such as a cavernous haemangioma, but may also be seen with a lymphangioma or narrow-necked meningocele. This sign of emptying in cavernous haemangiomas may be accompanied by blanching as blood is expressed from the lesion. Blanching may also be seen by pressing a glass slide on a telangiectasia or other superficial vascular lesion such as a capillary naevus. Refilling of vascular lesions is due to arterial pressure, and in some instances this can be demonstrated by pressure on the feeding artery and filling being delayed.

**Reducibility** indicates that a lump can be emptied by squeezing but does not return spontaneously – this requires an additional force, such as a cough or the effect of gravity. A classic example is an inguinal hernia. A hernia may also demonstrate two other important signs – a cough impulse and, by pressing on the neck of the sac, possibly an ability to control the impulse, preventing refilling.

There is some overlap between the features of a lump that is 'compressible' or 'reducible' and in some instances both terms can be applied. An example is that of a saphena varix that can be compressed digitally and controlled by appropriate digital pressure. It can also be reduced by elevating the limb and will then refill under the influence of gravity. In this lesion, a cough impulse can usually be palpated as, with increased abdominal pressure, blood is expelled from the inferior vena cava and iliac vessels proximally into the heart and distally down to the first competent valve. Incompetence of the saphenofemoral junction means that blood is expelled into the great saphenous vein and a fluid thrill can be palpated.

### Indentation and Fluctuation

If the contents of a lump are solid or semi-solid and not too tense, they can be **indented** by pressure. This can be well demonstrated by compressing the faeces in the palpable sigmoid colon in the left iliac fossa. It may also be possible to demonstrate this sign in a lax sebaceous cyst and in large dermoid cysts.

If pressure is applied to one side of a fluid-filled lump, the fluid tends to protrude in all other directions, and provided it cannot escape into another compartment, this bulging of the rest of the wall can be demonstrated, this being termed **fluctuation** (Figure 3.14). The cyst is held between thumb and finger (the watching digits) of one hand, and pressure is then applied downwards between them with a digit from the other hand (the displacing digit); the watching digits can feel the expansion.

This same expansion can be felt if a bundle of muscle fibres is held transversely, but the sign is not present if an attempt is made to hold the muscle longitudinally. Therefore, when testing for fluctuation, it is important to examine in two planes at right angles to one another. With a small cyst, it may not be possible to apply three digits at the same time and in two planes, but downward digital pressure may still demonstrate the bulging if the lesion is over a firm surface. When lumps of less than 2 cm in diameter are situated over soft tissues, pressure displaces the lump and gives a false impression of fluctuation in solid masses; the test is therefore unreliable in this group.

Examples of cystic lesions are hydroceles, spermatoceles, abscesses – do not try to demonstrate the sign on these if there is excessive tenderness – and branchial cysts. At body temperature, fat is semi-fluid and fluctuation can be demonstrated in superficial lipomas provided they are not too tense.

### Expression and Discharge

When the skin over a cystic lesion breaks down, the contents may be **discharged** (Figure 3.15) onto the surface; this is a common feature of sebaceous cysts and abscesses. In the former, the contents are putty-like and granular and on **expression** are expelled in spurts as large particles intermittently block the punctum. The smell of these contents can be bad, as is common when dead cutaneous elements are retained and degraded; a putrid smell is also present with necrotic, degenerating, malignant skin lesions.

Abscesses are variable in their smell, depending on the organisms involved. Faecal organisms in particular are foul-smelling, and this can be a useful sign when a perianal abscess is released as a foul-smelling discharge usually indicates a fistulous connection with the anal canal.

### Pulsation

If a lump lies adjacent to an artery, it can be felt to pulsate (Figure 3.16). This transmitted pulsation may be demonstrable in a pancreatic mass situated in front of the abdominal aorta. Other masses, for example an abdominal aortic aneurysm, are expansile as well as pulsatile. This can be demonstrated by gently

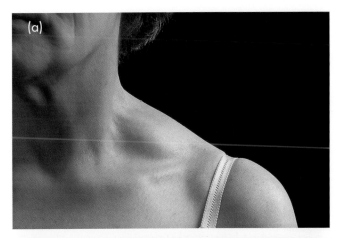

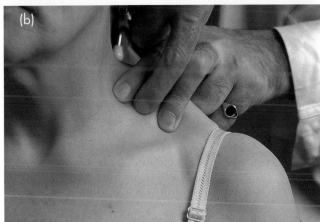

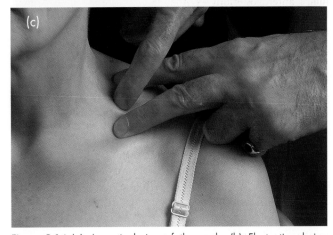

Figure 3.14 (a) A cystic lesion of the neck. (b) Fluctuation being demonstrated in one plane. (c) Fluctuation being demonstrated in a plane at a right angle to that in (b).

pressing a finger of each hand on either side of the mass, the fingers then being moved outwards away from each other, whereas in transmitted pulsation they both move in the same direction. The size of an aneurysm can be assessed by measuring the horizontal distance between a finger pressed onto each side of it.

Vascular malformations and the veins of arteriovenous fistulas may also be expansile. Compression of a feeding artery may reduce the size and pulsation of a focal vascular malformation. A carotid body tumour situated in the carotid bifurcation usually has a rich blood supply and is expansile as well as transmitting

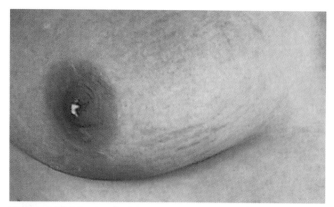

Figure 3.15 Nipple discharge in a patient with a galactocele prolactinoma.

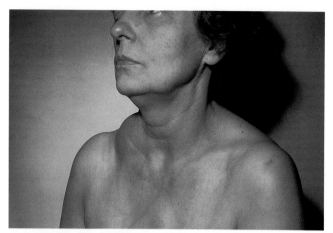

Figure 3.16 A pulsatile right supraclavicular mass caused by a subclavian aneurysm.

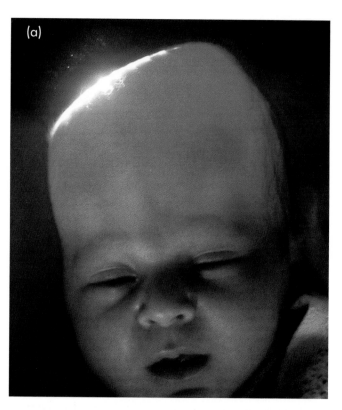

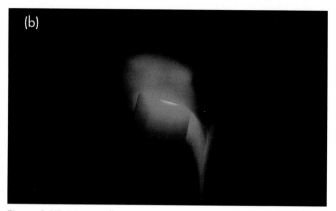

Figure 3.17 (a) Transillumination across the skull demonstrating fluid in an anencephalic infant. (b) Transillumination of the supraclavicular cystic mass shown in Figure 3.14.

pulses from the external and internal carotid arteries within which it is embedded. This is an important sign since a biopsy or removal of this tumour requires an experienced surgeon and, if the preoperative diagnosis is not made, serious complications can ensue. Some other tumours, usually sarcomas, have a large enough blood supply to make them expansile.

## Transillumination

Clear fluid transmits light. This transillumination (Figure 3.17) is a valuable diagnostic sign – a lump containing such fluid glows when the beam from a pen torch is shone across it. There are, however, a number of precautions to take when demonstrating this sign. Fat transilluminates, as can be demonstrated when placing a thumb or finger over the end of the torch. Thus, pressing the end of the torch onto the skin produces a surrounding glow, which can be misinterpreted as the transillumination of an underlying lump.

'Trans' means through, and the lump must be big enough to shine the beam across it for transillumination to be confirmed. A bright torch with a unidirectional beam is essential, and it may also be necessary to cut out surrounding light or demonstrate the sign in a dark room. A fine cardboard tube placed over the skin opposite the torch excludes outside light and helps to demonstrate the sign.

Vaginal hydroceles and epididymal cysts are brilliantly transluminant, spermatoceles less so. Hydroceles with thick walls or those containing blood may not transilluminate. Cystic hygromas, ganglia and to a lesser extent branchial cysts and bursae transilluminate, as does cerebrospinal fluid in a meningocele and a hydrocele of the canal of Nuck. Non-cystic lesions that can transilluminate include lipomas and, in a baby or young child, an inguinal hernia containing small intestine.

## Percussion

Percussion is used routinely on the chest and abdomen to demonstrate the resonance of gas-filled organs such as the lung and gut, and the dullness of solid structures such as the heart and liver; it is also useful over some masses. An enlarged bladder, a pregnant uterus and an ovarian cyst are dull to percussion, whereas gas-distended loops of gut, such as the stomach or an obstructed intestine, are resonant. An enlarged thyroid gland may extend deep to the sternum, and this retrosternal portion may be detected by dullness to percussion over the manubrium sterni.

Ascites is dull to percussion, the fluid level being demonstrated by percussing towards each side from the central, resonant, gas-filled intestine. If these levels are marked on the skin and percussion is repeated after turning the patient through 45°, the line of dullness changes since the fluid level of the ascites remains horizontal. This is a useful diagnostic sign termed **shifting dullness**.

Tapping fluid produces a ripple through it; this **fluid thrill** may be demonstrable, for example with ascites. With the patient lying supine, place one hand on one side of the abdomen and flick a finger against the opposite side. As the flick will produce an impulse through the fat over the centre of the abdomen, the patient or a third person is asked to place the side of a hand along the midline to block out such additional movement.

### Auscultation

Listening to a mass can reveal a number of characteristic diagnostic signs. Examples include bowel sounds in a hernia, bruits over vascular lesions, crepitus over a joint and **friction rubs** over pleuritic and pericardial surfaces. The **bruits** of vascular lesions include the machinery murmurs of an arteriovenous fistula and also masses, such as an enlarged toxic thyroid gland, that may have an audible blood supply.

## Surrounding Tissues

A lump can produce characteristic signs in the surrounding tissues, one of which is **induration**. Whereas most terms used to describe a lump are drawn from everyday language, induration is a specific medical term implying thickening and firmness of the surrounding tissues due to oedema or infiltrating neoplasia. If there is the former, it is often due to an inflammatory response. The hardness and indentability vary with the amount of fluid. To confirm oedema, sustained digital pressure must be exerted for 10–15 seconds. A positive sign is a residual, temporary denting at the pressure point that can be seen, or for minor degrees, felt by passing a finger over it. The amount of pressure needed depends on the amount and type of oedema. Venous and lymphatic obstruction and the oedema of systemic disease are initially soft, pitting with gentle finger pressure. Inflammatory oedema requires increased pressure, usually with the thumb. As there may also be tenderness, watch the patient's face during this test and increase pressure very slowly.

The indurated area may also be tender, and bleeding within the tissues may produce bruising and pigmentation. Measure the size of the indurated area and record its shape so that its progress can be mapped. If the induration is due to neoplastic invasion, there may be irregularity of the surface from tumour nodules, or the tumour may spread through tissue planes or along veins and may produce satellite or distant metastatic lesions.

The **mobility** features of a lump have already received some consideration, but the lump can also become tethered or fixed to the surrounding tissues, for example by inflammation or neoplastic involvement. The latter carries important prognostic implications. In the early stages, tethering to the skin and adjacent fascia may be difficult to demonstrate.

To and fro movement or gentle squeezing of the skin over the lump in at least two directions at right angles to one another is necessary to exclude early signs of **pitting**, wrinkling or pulling on the skin. Gentle squeezing of the skin over a sebaceous cyst accentuates the central depression at the site of the blocked duct if this punctum is not already obvious. This sign demonstrates that the lesion is of dermal rather than subcutaneous origin.

When looking for **tethering** to deeper structures, grip the lump between finger and thumb, and move it in two planes at right angles to one another. Repeat the movement once the underlying fascia has been tensed by appropriate muscle contraction, for example by asking the patient with a breast lump to place their hands on their hips and apply downward pressure. An untethered lump moves equally in both planes whether the underlying tissues are tensed or relaxed.

As the attachment to the adjacent tissues progresses, there is less independent movement of the lump and, as fixation may be to adjacent bone or other organs, further signs may develop, such as **peau d'orange** of the skin in a malignant breast lesion (see p. 421). In this case, oedema stretches the skin between the dermal pegs, giving the surface a pitted, orange-peel appearance. A lesion may also perforate the surrounding skin and adjacent viscera, discharging its contents, or erode into a blood vessel, causing haemorrhage.

The draining **lymph nodes** must always be palpated as part of the examination of a lump – this usually means the axillary, groin and cervical nodes (Figures 3.18–3.20). Remember that the lymphatic drainage of the testis is to the para-aortic lymph nodes so the abdomen must be palpated in this instance. Inflammation may occur along the line of the superficial lymphatics, producing **lymphangitis**, which is characterized by pain, redness and swelling.

The **blood vessels** supplying or draining a lump may undergo change. The enlarged feeding arteries of vascular malformations have already been referred to under 'Compressibility and reducibility'. The veins may become more prominent in association with a lump, and there may be local thrombosis, accompanied by pain and oedema.

Large masses in the thoracic inlet, such as a retrosternal goitre or matted malignant nodes, can compress the superior vena cava; similarly, pelvic masses can cause inferior vena caval obstruction (Figure 3.21). In these instances, the veins over the trunk dilate to provide alternative channels for venous return to the heart. The direction of flow in these abdominal wall varices can be demonstrated by compressing a point in the vein with the index finger of the left hand and using the right index finger to empty a segment of the vein by milking it away from the compressed point. By releasing the pressure from the right index finger, the emptied segment fills rapidly if the obstruction is in the direction of milking. Repeat the test milking a segment of vein in the opposite direction; this will show slow refilling towards the non-obstructed direction.

Involvement of the adjacent **nerves** by the disease process may give rise to pain or motor and sensory abnormalities (Figure 3.22). This usually indicates infiltration from neoplastic disease. Examine for sensory loss around and distal to the lump, and for the power of the related muscles.

Having completed the examination of the external and internal features of a lump, and their effects on the surrounding tissues,

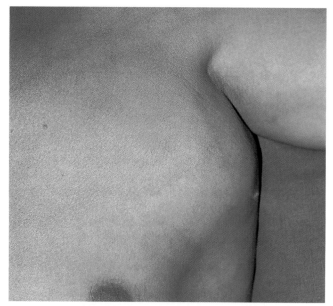

Figure 3.18 A malignant axillary mass.

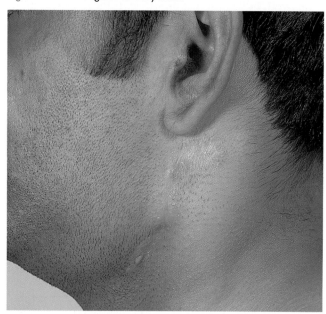

Figure 3.19 Tuberculous lymphadenitis.

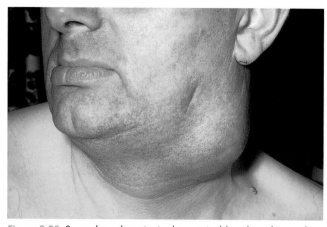

Figure 3.20 Secondary deposits in the cervical lymph nodes resulting from a primary nasopharyngeal carcinoma.

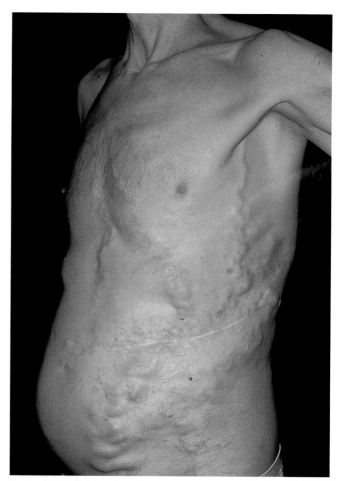

Figure 3.21 Abdominal wall varicosities secondary to inferior vena caval obstruction.

it is usually possible to formulate a diagnosis or a differential diagnosis of possible causes. Information also has to be gained from the history and full general examination of the patient. The latter should be routine to exclude systemic disease related or unrelated to the lump. Signs may include weight loss, malaise and increased pulse rate and temperature.

The process of formulating a differential diagnosis when there is still doubt is considered in Table 1.1 and uses additional anatomical, aetiological and systemic clues. The diagnosis may be further confirmed by specific investigations such as imaging or needle biopsy. A lump may need to be excised to obtain a definitive diagnosis, for example with persistently large cervical lymph nodes, but a warning has already been given (see p. 59) to exclude a possible carotid body tumour before such an exploration.

Most lumps are easily diagnosed, and undergraduate and postgraduate candidates are expected to recognize lipomas, sebaceous cysts, benign and malignant skin lesions, vascular abnormalities, enlarged thyroid and salivary glands, breast lumps, hernias, scrotal swellings, abdominal masses and lymph nodes. All of these are more readily diagnosed if they have been seen before. Hence clinical experience is an essential part of medical training, but never disregard the stages of examination referred to above as a 'spot' diagnosis should not preclude the careful palpation of a lump and an assessment of its mobility, as well as an examination for regional node enlargement.

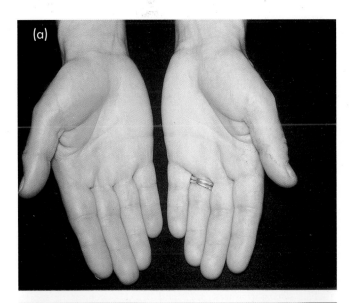

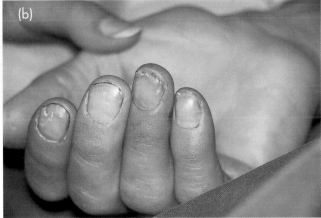

Figure 3.22 A cervical rib causing (a) pallor on elevation and (b) digital ischaemia.

# ULCERS

## History

An ulcer is a persistent discontinuity of an epithelial surface that can occur in the skin or in the mucosa of the alimentary and respiratory passages.

Ulcers differ from the defects of acute surgical or other trauma in their persistence, this being due to recurrent minor physical or chemical injury, ischaemia, neoplastic change and a poor healing response, as in patients with malnutrition or other systemic disease.

Features to look for in the history and examination of an ulcer are similar to those described for a lump, and the reader is referred for more detail to the previous section. In the history, ask when the patient first noticed the ulcer and what brought it to their attention. This latter may have been due to symptoms such as pain, discharge, bleeding or smell. Neuropathic ulcers may be painless and often out of sight, for example on the sole of the foot. In individuals with diabetes, this may become compounded by visual impairment. These patients must be taught how to regularly examine their feet with a mirror, by palpation or with the help of a carer to identify early lesions and initiate therapeutic and preventive measures.

Annual checks at the diabetic clinic also aim to detect changes early on.

The progress of the ulcer should be determined, particularly with reference to its size, shape, depth, base, discharge and response to any treatment. As with lumps, enquire about previous local or similar lesions, any systemic symptoms and what the patient thinks the lesion is.

## Examination

Note the **site**, **edge**, **base** and **surrounding** tissues ('SEBS' – compare this with the SEIS mnemonic for a lump and note how many of the terms used are equally applicable).

## Site

The site of the ulcer is usually characteristic. The three lower limb ulcers that a student can expect to see in qualifying examinations are venous, arterial and diabetic neuropathic ulcers.

**Venous ulcers** (Figure 3.23) (see p. 509) are sited just above the malleolus. They are usually medial but in the more florid states can become circumferential.

**Arterial ulcers** (Figure 3.24) (see p. 478) occur when occlusive arterial disease reduces the arterial pressure in the foot to critically low levels. They are situated distally, that is, over the tips of the toes and between the toes, where the pressure is lowest, and over the malleoli and heels where minor pressure

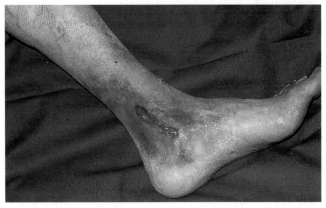

Figure 3.23 A venous ulcer. Healing has reduced the size of the ulcer to a linear defect. Note the typical pigmentation and residual varicosities.

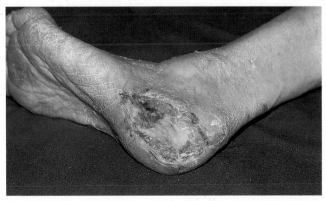

Figure 3.24 An arterial ulcer caused by ischaemic pressure on the heel.

PART 1 | PRINCIPLES

such as lying in bed is sufficient to abolish capillary flow and produce ischaemic skin necrosis. A bandage can have similar effects over the Achilles tendon and the tibialis anterior tendon across the ankle.

Diabetic ulcers (Figure 3.25) (see p. 479) are of multiple aetiology. Arterial disease occurs in these patients about 10 years earlier than in the rest of the population. They are also subject to microvascular disease, are more susceptible to infection and are subject to neuropathic changes, including motor, sensory and autonomic abnormalities. Diabetic arterial ulcers are similar to those already described. With peripheral neuropathy, the small muscles of the foot may be paralysed, allowing unopposed action of the powerful long flexor tendons. The shortening of the longitudinal arches means that the heads of the metatarsals are subject to an additional load during walking. The loss of the protective sensation of pain places an area such as the sole at particular risk from repetitive excessive trauma or unnoticed damage by sharp objects. The most common site for a diabetic neuropathic ulcer is therefore over the heads of the first and second metatarsals.

The shin is particularly susceptible to direct trauma. The tibia is subcutaneous and the lack of underlying muscle means that the skin's blood supply is reduced, with poor healing potential. Skin and bony injuries at this site can give rise to long-standing ulceration.

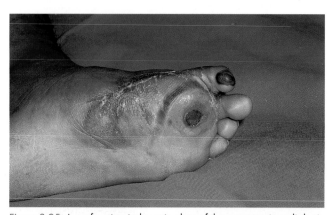

Figure 3.25 A perforating ischaemic ulcer of the great toe in a diabetic patient. Note also the swelling of the proximal sole associated with this foot abscess.

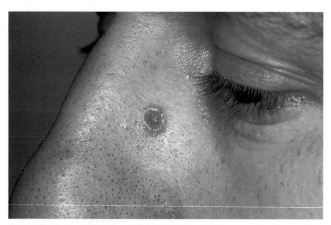

Figure 3.26 A rodent ulcer of the nose.

Peptic ulcers are usually sited in the distal stomach and proximal duodenum, while malignant ulcers are common in the oesophagus, stomach, colon and rectum.

Malignant ulcers can also occur in typical locations; for example, rodent ulcers (basal cell carcinomas) occur on the upper part of the face (Figure 3.26).

## Edge

The edge of an ulcer must be accurately drawn in the patient's record, noting the shape and measuring the size in at least two directions. As one does not wish to rest a tape measure on the surface of the ulcer, the size may have to be gauged by the measure being held taut just above the surface. More accurate records can be made by resting a gauze on the surface and then measuring the imprint, or by placing a sheet of cellophane over the surface and tracing the edge. The cellophane can be retained, cut out or reproduced in the patient's notes. The edge may be characteristic of the underlying pathology:

- *Flat sloping* (Figures 3.27 and 3.28) – venous or septic, often with a transparent healing edge along part of its circumference.
- *Punched-out* – syphilitic, trophic, diabetic, ischaemic (Figure 3.29), leprosy.
- *Undermined* – tuberculosis, pressure necrosis (Figure 3.30); particularly over the buttocks, carbuncles.
- *Raised* – rodent ulcer (Figure 3.31), often with a slightly rolled appearance.
- *Raised and everted* – carcinoma (Figure 3.32).

The colour of the edge may be red from inflammation, or pale or cyanosed from ischaemia, although in the later stages of ischaemia the skin has a permanent staining of blue, purple or black. Pigmentation may be present around venous ulcers and also malignant melanomas. A basal cell carcinoma has a characteristic pearly edge, while keratinization of the edge is common in neuropathic ulcers of the sole.

Ulcers may be very tender, particularly when inflamed, when the local temperature may also be raised. Arterial ulceration is usually painful, the pain also being due to ischaemia of the surrounding tissues. Neuropathic ulcers are by definition associated with far less pain than one would expect, while venous ulcers are not usually very painful. Vasculitic ulcers (see p. 491) can be very painful and the pain may precede the appearance of the ulcer.

## Base

In the base, note the **depth**, the **covering** (the floor) and any **discharge**. The depth can be described in millimetres and in terms of the tissue the ulcer has **penetrated**. With venous ulcers, there may be full or partial thickness skin loss, but the ulcer does not usually extend deeper than the subcutaneous tissues. With ischaemic ulcers, it is not uncommon to see fascia, tendons, bones and joints in their base. Inflammatory ulcers usually extend only into the subcutaneous tissue but they may communicate with a deep abscess cavity. Skin cancers initially spread circumferentially, but as their bulk increases there is a progressive deepening through the subcutaneous tissue to deeper structures, with fixation to fascia, muscles and bone. Penetration of the wall of a viscus may lead to **perforation** into a body cavity or **fistulation** into another organ.

The base provides an indication of the ulcer's progress; a wound may expose normal tissues. Primary healing indicates

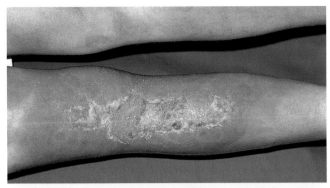

Figure 3.27 Flat, sloping ulcers in a burn lesion of the leg.

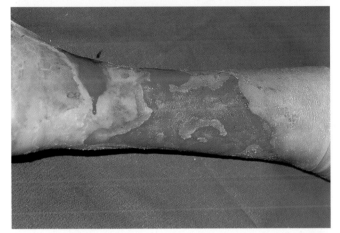

Figure 3.28 A healing, granulating ulcer with skin islands. Epithelialization can extend from these islands as well as from the surrounding skin edge.

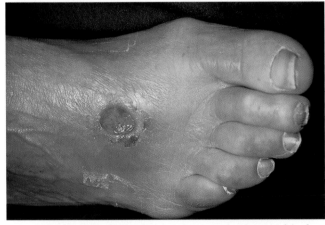

Figure 3.29 A punched-out ischaemic ulcer over the dorsum of the foot.

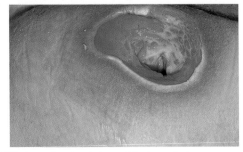

Figure 3.30 An undermined ulcer of the buttock due to pressure.

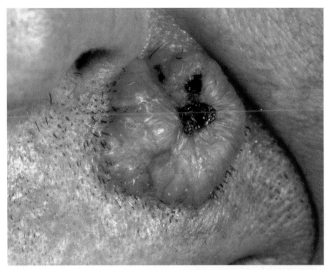

Figure 3.31 A rodent ulcer of the face. The typical pearly, rolled edge is present at some points on its circumference.

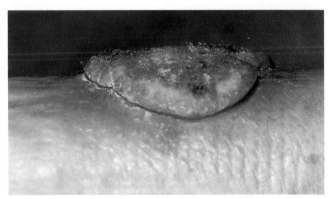

Figure 3.32 The raised and inverted edge of a carcinoma of the forearm.

the apposition of cut edges and the establishment of continuity through the ingrowth of fibroblasts and blood vessels, with minimal inflammatory change. In secondary healing, there is no initial skin cover, and capillary loops and fibroblasts grow towards the surface. Initially, there is an inflammatory response with the production of **slough** (**Figure 3.33**), a yellowish, adherent surface made up of dead tissue and inflammatory cells stimulated by trauma and subsequent infection.

Signs of a healing in an ulcer occur when the slough is replaced by granulation tissue (**Figure 3.34**) and the skin creeps in over the granulating surface. Granulation is usually pink with red dots at the site of the capillary loops, but it may have other characteristic appearances, such as the bluish granulation in tuberculosis and the wash-leather appearance of a syphilitic ulcer. With ischaemic ulcers, there may be no evidence of any healing or granulation formation, the underlying tissues being exposed, for example tendons crossing the ulcer and deep fascia, or bone and joint surfaces.

Slough and small amounts of discharge may dry to become a scab, and a layer of dead tissue may become dehydrated and form a dark brown or black eschar (**Figure 3.35**), for example after a burn or ischaemic necrosis. The base may be formed of malignant

PART 1 | PRINCIPLES

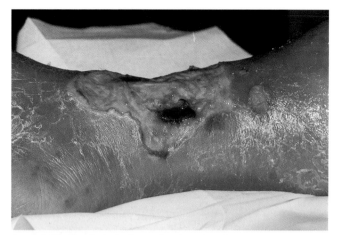

Figure 3.33 Slough in the base of a deep leg ulcer.

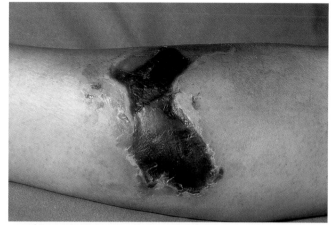

Figure 3.35 Eschar following shin trauma.

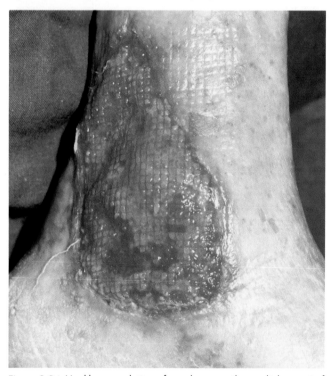

Figure 3.34 Healthy granulation of an ulcer over the medial aspect of the ankle: the surface should accept a skin graft and, in view of the size, this may the best option.

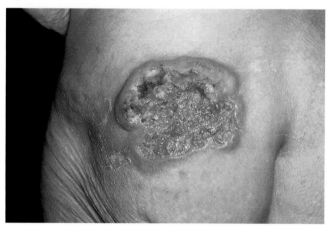

Figure 3.36 A malignant ulcer. Note the dead tissue over its base, with no evidence of granulation formation.

Dead tissue, such as that associated with a malignant ulcer, and wet gangrene may also be foul-smelling. An ulcer may bleed from the initial or subsequent trauma. A healing granulating surface bleeds with minimal abrasion. Bleeding may also indicate the erosion of adjacent vessels, particularly in malignant disease.

## Surrounding Tissue

As with lumps, the effect of ulcers on the surrounding tissues is largely dependent on their aetiology. The depth of penetration and possible perforation has already been referred to. Induration of the surrounding tissues is seen particularly in the inflammatory response to infection, trauma and malignancy, or it may be from direct invasion in a malignant process. Blood vessels may be prominent, with an increase in blood supply and venous drainage in an inflammatory response. Pigmentation is common around a venous ulcer, and the surrounding skin may be scarred from previous ulceration.

If the prime aetiology of the ulcer is neuropathic, there is sensory loss over the adjacent skin, and reduced sweating in an autonomic neuropathy. Neuropathy may also be related to damage to the adjacent nerves by the ulcer. The mobility of the ulcer depends on the degree of penetration and the effects of induration on the surrounding tissues. The skin may show adherence to the underlying fascia or muscle, tethering or subsequent fixation. As with lumps, it is essential

tissue (Figure 3.36), which does not produce normal granulation tissue or allow skin ingrowth.

Any discharge may be serous, serosanguinous or purulent. Serous discharge is of normal tissue fluid as other discharges imply superadded infection. Pus requires culture to determine the causative organism, although in a few cases the colour provides preliminary clues: staphylococci produce yellow, creamy pus; that from streptococci is watery and opalescent; pus from *Pseudomonas* is blue/green; an amoebic liver abscess produces purplish-brown pus; and actinomycosis gives yellow granules. The discharge may be more copious when associated with oedema, whether from venous or lymphatic obstruction, or generalized oedema such as in cardiac, liver and renal failure.

The smell of the discharge may provide a clue to the infecting organism, faecal organisms being particularly offensive.

to examine for local and more distant nodal involvement by the disease process.

## SINUSES AND FISTULAS

A **sinus** is a tract lined with granulation tissue that connects an abnormal cavity to an epithelial surface (Figure 3.37). The cavity usually commences as an abscess in which the normal healing process is impaired. The granulations may be exuberant and protrude through the opening. A number of factors can lead to delayed healing and sinus formation. These include the following:

- There may be inadequate drainage of an abscess.
- Chronic inflammation may be occurring. The tuberculous, syphilitic and leprosy bacteria, the fungal infection actinomycosis and some diseases such as Crohn's disease stimulate a chronic inflammatory granulomatous response from the body from which there is a slow resolution. Typical examples of sinus formation in this group are a collar stud tuberculous abscess in the neck, the multiple sinuses of actinomycosis (Figure 3.38) and Crohn's sinuses along the alimentary tract.
- A foreign body in an abscess cavity stimulates a prolonged inflammatory response and recurrent infection. A foreign body may gain access through injury, as with clothing material, or at operation, such as with a non-absorbable suture or an orthopaedic or vascular prosthesis. The latter have particularly serious consequences since it may only be possible to eradicate the sinus by removing the prosthesis. Hair or the bony sequestrum of osteomyelitis may act as a foreign body, preventing healing and promoting sinus formation. A pilonidal sinus (see p. 618) is an example of the former.
- Epithelium in the cavity wall prevents the resolution of an abscess. This can result from congenital or acquired lesions. Examples of the former are congenital epithelial rests, such as dermoid cysts, along the embryological lines of facial fusion. The abscess may become infected and start to discharge its contents onto the surface. Penetrating injuries to the pulp of the finger can bury surface epithelium in the subcutaneous tissue, producing an implantation dermoid and leading to sinus formation.

- Malignant disease in a cavity wall can prevent healing and precipitate sinus formation. The opening of a sinus can be onto the skin or a mucous membrane, and this can be sited some way from the cavity. A sinus probe may be passed, gently negotiating the lumen of the tract, to enter the cavity and establish its depth and position.

A sinus can give symptoms through recurrent discharge and recurrent bouts of acute infection of the abscess cavity. These are likely to persist until removal of the causative factors listed above.

A **fistula** is an abnormal tract between two epithelial surfaces (Figure 3.39). It is usually produced when an abscess cavity breaks into two adjacent epithelial surfaces; the aetiological factors that prevent closure of the tract and normal healing include those listed under sinus formation. An additional factor, however, is that the epithelial surfaces may be of adjacent organs, and the contents of these organs may pass through the fistulous tract and prevent healing. Examples are fistulas between adjacent

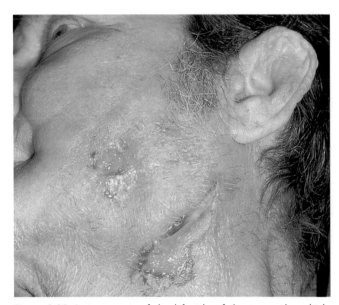

Figure 3.38 Actinomycosis of the left side of the jaw with multiple sinus formation.

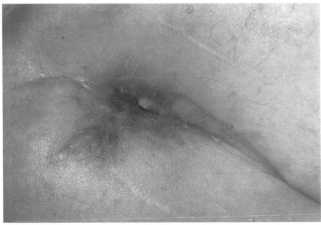

Figure 3.37 A sinus caused by septic arthritis of the shoulder due to actinomycosis.

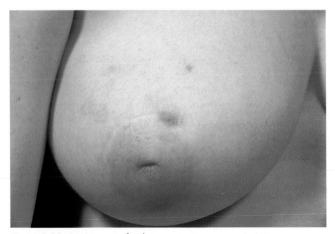

Figure 3.39 A mammary fistula.

loops of gut (entero-enteric fistulas) in Crohn's disease, and between the gut and the bladder (entero-vesicular fistulas) in diverticulitis or malignant disease of either organ.

Perianal abscesses may communicate with the rectum and the anal canal, and in these cases surgical drainage produces a fistula that may persist with continued discharge. Foul-smelling pus suggests faecal organisms and the likely presence of a fistulous connection. Treatment is by a seton suture placed through the tract to allow it to remain open and drain so that healing can commence. Diseased gut may perforate and discharge its contents onto the abdominal wall. Again there may be foul-smelling discharge, and the presence of gas bubbles is confirmation of the alimentary connection. Tracheobronchial fistulas are usually congenital anomalies, presenting soon after birth, but may follow malignant invasion of the adjacent organs in later life.

## CHECKLIST FOR LUMPS AND ULCERS (**bold** type relates to **both** abnormalities)

| ▼ Site | ▼ Lumps | ▼ Ulcers |
|---|---|---|
| ▶ Site | ▶ **Tissue of origin** | |
| | ▶ **Relations** | |
| ▶ Exterior | ▶ **Size** | ▼ Edge: |
| | ▶ **Shape** | ▶ flat sloping |
| | ▶ **Surface** | ▶ punched-out |
| | ▶ **Colour** | ▶ undermined |
| | ▶ **Temperature** | ▶ raised |
| | ▶ **Tenderness** | ▶ everted |
| | ▶ **Mobility** | |
| ▶ Interior | ▶ Consistency | ▼ Floor: |
| | ▶ Compressibility | ▶ depth |
| | ▶ Reducibility | ▶ covering |
| | ▶ Cough impulse | ▶ discharge |
| | ▶ Fluid thrill | ▼ Base: |
| | ▶ Indentation | ▶ penetration |
| | ▶ Fluctuation | ▶ fistulation |
| | ▶ Discharge | |
| | ▶ Pulsation | |
| | ▶ Expansion | |
| | ▶ Transillumination | |
| | ▶ Bruit | |
| ▶ Surroundings | ▶ **Induration** | |
| | ▶ **Tethering/ fixation** | |
| | ▼ **Invasion:** | |
| | ▶ **nerves** | |
| | ▶ **vessels** | |
| | ▶ **other tissue** | |
| | ▶ **Nodes** | |
| | ▶ **Related disease** | |

## Key Points

- A lump may arise in any part of the body. Important points to elucidate from the history are its tenderness, duration and any change in size.
- The examination of a lump should be carried out in an organized fashion comprising its site, its external and internal features, and its effect on the surrounding tissues (SEIS). Adjunct techniques to assist with diagnosis include transillumination.
- An ulcer is a persistent discontinuity of an epithelial surface. The structured examination of an ulcer may be considered using the headings of site, edge, base and surrounding tissues (SEBS).
- Common lower limb ulcers are venous, arterial and diabetic neuropathic ulcers, each with specific sites and characteristics.
- A sinus is defined as a tract lined with granulation tissue that connects an abnormal cavity, frequently an abscess, to an epithelial surface. A common example is a pilonidal sinus. Symptoms of recurrent infection of the cavity and discharge are likely to persist unless the causative factors, such as presence of a foreign body or inadequate drainage, are resolved.
- A fistula is the abnormal communication between two epithelialized surfaces. Important examples to note are those arising from perianal disease, for which the treatment may be complex and require a consideration of sphincter preservation, and enteric, enterovesicular and enterovaginal fistulas, which may be caused by malignancy or inflammatory disease.

## QUESTIONS

### SBAs

**1.** 'Empties on being pressed or squeezed, but may reappear on release or on the patient coughing.' Which of the following best describes this feature of a lump?:
  **a** Compressibility
  **b** Fluctuation
  **c** Ballottement
  **d** Crepitus
  **e** Reducibility

**Answer**

**e** *Reducibility. This classically described feature of a lump is termed reducibility. Common examples of lumps that demonstrate reducibility are inguinal hernias.*

**2.** Which of the following is **not** usually transilluminable?:
  **a** Lipoma
  **b** Hydrocele
  **c** Inguinal hernia in a neonate
  **d** Saphena varix
  **e** Epididymal cyst
  **f** Cystic hygroma

**Answer**

**d** *A saphena varix. This is a dilatation of the saphenous vein at its junction with the femoral vein in the groin. In common with an inguinal hernia, it may demonstrate a cough impulse, but it is not known to transilluminate as the other options shown do. Inguinal hernias in neonates and young children can transilluminate if they contain small intestine.*

**3.** Which of the following is **not** a feature of ascites?:
  **a** Resonance to percussion
  **b** Shifting dullness
  **c** Fluid thrill
  **d** Dullness to percussion
  **e** Flank bulging

**Answer**

**a** *Resonance to percussion. Ascites is dull to percussion. Gas-filled structures such as the intestine are resonant to percussion, and this feature can be used to demarcate the fluid level of ascites.*

### EMQs

**1.** For each of the following descriptions, select the most likely type of lump from the list below. Each option may be used once, more than once or not at all:
  **1** Malignant melanoma
  **2** Lipoma
  **3** Inguinal/inguino-scrotal hernia
  **4** Haemangioma
  **5** Sebaceous cyst
  **6** Arteriovenous fistula
  **7** Baker's cyst
  **8** Hydrocele
  **9** Renal mass
  **10** Saphena varix
  **a** A painless scrotal lump present for 3 years and slowly increasing in size. It is possible to 'get above' the lump, and it is brilliantly transilluminable
  **b** A painless lump over the scapular region. On examination, it is subcutaneous, soft, large in size and fluctuant, and demonstrates a 'slip sign'
  **c** A smooth swelling on the neck. On examination, it is attached to the skin and a punctum may be seen
  **d** A lump on the leg of a 25-year-old woman. On examination, it is pigmented with an irregular edge and it bleeds easily
  **e** A mass seen in the popliteal fossa on asking the patient to stand up with an extended knee

**Answers**

**a** *8 Hydrocele. This is differentiated from an inguino-scrotal hernia by the ability to 'get above' it and by its ability to transilluminate.*

**b** *2 Lipoma. The signs given are those of a lipoma, with the specific 'slip sign' confirming the likely diagnosis.*

**c** *5 Sebaceous cyst. The feature of a punctum, although not always present, is usually specific to a sebaceous cyst.*

**d** *1 Malignant melanoma. A pigmented lesion with an irregular edge should raise a suspicion of malignant melanoma. The age and gender of the patient and site of the lesion seen here are common presentations.*

**e** *7 Baker's cyst. This is a description of a Baker's cyst. Asking the patient to adopt certain postures to make a lump more palpable is of great importance.*

PART 1 | PRINCIPLES

**2.** For each of the following descriptions, select the most likely type of lesion from the list below. Each option may be used once, more than once or not at all:

    **1**  Arterial ulcer
    **2**  Venous ulcer
    **3**  Basal cell carcinoma
    **4**  Neuropathic ulcer

**a**  A painless 2 cm lesion over the head of the right second metatarsal. It has a regular, clean outline following the contour of the skin, and is deep to bone. The surrounding skin is normal, the skin temperature is normal and the peripheral pulses are present

**b**  A 3 mm lesion on the tip of the left second toe in a patient with atherosclerosis. The edge is punched-out, with a sloughy base appearing to extend deeply down to bone. Peripheral pulses are absent and the limb is cold

**c**  A large lesion just above the right medial malleolus. It has an irregular margin with a sloping edge. The base consists of pink granulation tissue, with lipodermato-sclerosis seen in the surrounding skin. Peripheral pulses are present

**d**  A nodular lesion on the arm of a 75-year-old man. On examination, it has a well-defined rolled, pearly edge that is fixed deep to the skin

**Answers**

**a**  **4 Neuropathic ulcer.** *The painless lesion over a load-bearing area with no associated features is classic of a diabetic neuropathic ulcer.*

**b**  **1 Arterial ulcer.** *The features of an arteriopathic patient with a punched-out, deep ulcer, absent pulses and a cold limb indicative of poor perfusion make the likely diagnosis an arterial ulcer.*

**c**  **2 Venous ulcer.** *The site and description, with lipodermatosclerosis in the surrounding skin and normal pulses, most likely indicate a venous ulcer.*

**d**  **3 Basal cell carcinoma.** *A pearly lesion with a nodular, rolled edge seen on a sun-exposed site in an elderly person is most likely to be a basal cell carcinoma.*

# Inflammation

Natalie Anne Hirst and John S. P. Lumley

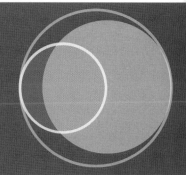

---

## LEARNING OBJECTIVES

- To understand the pathophysiology and characteristic features of, and the relationship between, acute and chronic inflammation
- To be aware of the criteria and described stages of the systemic inflammatory response syndrome and compensatory mechanisms
- To be able to describe types of infection, including those caused by common bacterial pathogens, and categorize them accordingly

- To understand the pathogenesis of abscess formation, its presentation and its sequelae
- To gain knowledge of viral, fungal, worm and parasitic disease processes
- To be aware of specific infections arising in the hand and foot
- To understand the classification and pathophysiology of surgical wounds, complications arising from wound healing and the principles of wound repair

---

## INTRODUCTION

Inflammation may be defined as the body's physiological response to tissue injury. Its main purpose is an attempt to eliminate or minimize the harmful effect of the injury, although it may also be counterproductive, with inappropriate exacerbation by innocuous stimuli, as in allergy.

Inflammation may be classified by its time course and according to the different types of cell involved in the inflammatory response as:

- acute inflammation: the preliminary response to injury;
- chronic inflammation: the persistent tissue responses subsequent to the initial damage.

## Acute Inflammation

Acute inflammation is characterized by its time course, usually lasting from hours to days. The most common injuring agents are microorganisms such as bacteria and viruses; the condition is then termed infection. Other causes include hypersensitivity reactions, for example to parasites, physical agents such as burns, chemical agents such as acids, and invading tumours giving rise to tissue hypoxia and necrosis.

The first four cardinal signs of inflammation – redness (rubor), swelling (tumour), heat (calor) and pain (dolor) – were described by Celsus in the first century AD. Loss of function was added by Galen a century later. In dark-skinned individuals, the redness is masked, but the stretching of the skin by oedema produces a characteristic shiny surface.

The initial stage of acute inflammation involves the local vasculature, the immune system and the clotting system. An initial vasodilatation of vessels allows a transient increased blood flow to the injured area. This change is offset by an increase in vascular permeability caused by the release of mediators such as histamine, allowing plasma and inflammatory cells to escape into the tissues at the site of damage. Consequently, more fluid leaves the vessels than is returned to them, giving rise to a net escape of protein-rich fluid named the **fluid exudate**, which is responsible for the **oedema** seen.

As the blood cells remain in the circulation, there is a relative blood stasis in which leukocytes may adhere to the vessel endothelial wall and begin to migrate into the tissues. This process involves initial margination before adhesion, 'pavementing' and migration through the venule walls, facilitated by both the complement and cytokine systems. The hallmark histological feature of acute inflammation is the presence of neutrophil polymorphs within the extracellular space.

Other mediators of inflammation released from the cells include prostaglandins, which potentiate vessel permeability and platelet aggregation, leukotrienes, which have vasoactive properties, and chemokines, which attract specific leukocytes to the site of tissue damage. The specific enzymatic cascade systems present in the plasma that are implicated in acute inflammation consist of complement, the kinins, the coagulation cascade and the fibrinolytic system, all of which interrelate and have a variety of roles in neutrophil chemotaxis, increasing vascular permeability and activating the various clotting components of the inflammatory exudate.

The lymphatic capillaries also dilate, and inflammatory fluid, bacteria and other cellular debris pass to, and are filtered by, the local lymph nodes. The associated lymph node enlargement is termed **lymphadenopathy** (see pp. 399 and 521).

As well as local tissue effects, inflammation produces systemic responses. The effects include pyrexia as endogenous pyrogens from neutrophils and macrophages have a direct effect on hypothalamic thermoregulation. General symptoms include anorexia, malaise and weight loss. Splenomegaly may occur with intracellular organisms such as the malarial parasite, while haematological changes include a normochromic, normocytic anaemia due to blood loss in exudates, haemolysis from bacterial toxins and/or the depression of the bone marrow seen in prolonged inflammation.

The outcome of acute inflammation may be the following:

* *Resolution:* The phagocytosis of bacteria and cellular debris by neutrophils and macrophages, and their removal by efficient drainage, bringing about a return to the normal architecture and function of the tissue, for example in acute pneumonia.
* *Organization:* The replacement of damaged tissue by the proliferation of fibroblasts and new capillaries, covered by an ingrowth of epithelial tissue, giving rise to a fibrotic scar. This commonly occurs after gross damage or in tissues that are unable to regenerate.
* *Abscess formation:* A localized collection of **pus** formed from unresolved dead tissue and cells surrounded by granulation tissue due to a persistent infective agent, usually a pyogenic bacterium. The terms 'purulent organisms' and 'process of suppuration' are often applied in this instance.
* *Chronic inflammation* (see below).

## Chronic Inflammation

When an inflammatory response lasts for a number of weeks or longer, it is termed chronic. Chronic inflammation may follow acute inflammation or be a primary event. It is characterized by differences in the cohort of cells and systems activated. The key mechanism is an immune response to a persistent damaging agent, and this may be seen in a variety of conditions:

* The presence of exogenous or endogenous indigestible substances. The former include suture material, prostheses, asbestos and silica. The latter irritants include fragments of hair (pilonidal sinus), keratin (ruptured epidermoid cyst) and uric acid crystals (gout).
* Organisms with a persistent but low toxicity that incite a cell-mediated immune response. Of particular note are tuberculosis, leprosy, syphilis and fungal and parasitic infections.
* Autoimmune disease – in which the body reacts against its own proteins – is characterized by a chronic inflammatory response. Examples include rheumatoid arthritis, chronic hepatitis and Hashimoto's thyroiditis.
* Some chronic inflammatory diseases are of unknown aetiology, such as Crohn's disease, sarcoidosis and Wegener's granulomatosis.

An essential feature of all chronic inflammation is that it occurs simultaneously with tissue repair. This is in contrast to acute inflammation, where inflammation and healing are sequential. Another important feature of healing in chronic inflammation is an intense fibrous reaction; this can damage the adjacent normal tissue, as seen in pulmonary fibrosis or silicosis.

The predominant cell types infiltrating the tissues in chronic inflammation are lymphocytes and macrophages. Activated B lymphocytes undergo transformation to plasma cells with a subsequent production of antibodies as part of the humoral immune system. Cell-mediated immunity is principally controlled by T lymphocytes, which release cytokines to recruit macrophages and other lymphocytes to the site. The main role of macrophages is to phagocytose, or ingest, pathogens and cellular debris.

**Granulomatous** inflammation is a specific form of chronic inflammation that occurs particularly with *Mycobacterium tuberculosis* but also with fungi and parasites, and in a foreign body granuloma. In the case of tuberculosis, the cheesy content of degenerating granulomas is termed **caseous** rather than purulent pus. Macrophages undergo a transformation to epithelioid histiocytes and often fuse to produce multinucleated giant cells.

## Systemic Inflammatory Response Syndrome

As described above, the inflammatory response is a physiological protective response by the body that is under the tight control of a variety of systems. A loss of this control or an overly activated response results in an excessive uncontrolled inflammation, which is clinically defined as the systemic inflammatory response syndrome (SIRS). Causes include both sepsis – defined as SIRS with an infective origin – and non-infective causes, such as major surgery, trauma, burns and pancreatitis.

Criteria for SIRS were established in 1992 as part of the American College of Chest Physicians/Society of Critical Care Medicine Consensus Conference. SIRS may be diagnosed when two or more of the following criteria are present:

* Temperature $<36°C$ or $>38°C$.
* Heart rate $>90$ beats per minute.
* Respiratory rate $>20$ breaths per minute or an arterial partial pressure of carbon dioxide $<4.3$ kPa (32 mmHg).
* White blood cell count $<4 \times 10^9$ cells/L or $> 12 \times 10^9$ cells/L or the presence of $>10$ per cent immature (bands) forms.

The pathophysiology of SIRS has been described as occurring in three stages. Stage I is the initial insult giving rise to local inflammation. In stage II, there is a systemic 'spilling over' of inflammatory mediators but with few clinical signs or symptoms. Stage III describes the overt systemic reaction as manifest by multiorgan dysfunction due to the dysregulation of inflammatory systems.

The systemic reaction may have the features of an excess of inflammatory or anti-inflammatory mediators, or may show a mixed picture. An excessive inflammatory response (SIRS) may lead to shock and organ dysfunction (see pp. 27 and 72). An excessive anti-inflammatory response – the compensated anti-inflammatory response syndrome (CARS) – normally a system of balance to maintain homeostasis in the resolution of inflammation, suppresses the immune system and confers increased susceptibility to further infection. The mixed inflammatory response syndrome describes a mixed picture involving the cells and activated systems of both the pro- and anti-inflammatory components. The spectrum of these three responses has been termed CHAOS (**c**ardiovascular shock, **h**omeostasis, **a**poptosis, **o**rgan dysfunction, immune **s**uppression). The clinical value of these classifications lies in directing therapeutic agents in a targeted way, although, currently, this has met with little success.

## INFECTION

The human body is covered with many bacteria and other organisms. These are particularly common on the skin of the axillae and perineum, and the mucosa of the nose, mouth, pharynx and large bowel. Many of these harmless commensals have the potential to become harmful pathogens if they breach the body surface and multiply. The portal of entry may be an abrasion or trauma, or may be 'deliberate' such as with surgical incisions and instrumentation.

Surgical and traumatic wounds are at particular risk. A patient's general resistance to infection may be lowered by trauma, a prolonged surgical illness, malignancy, poor nutrition, immunosuppressive drugs or steroids. Such states allow a minor inoculation with pathogens to produce infection. The problem is compounded in immunocompromised patients (see p. 104) when the inoculation of otherwise non-pathogenic organisms can give rise to serious infective states, a condition called **opportunistic infection**, the organisms then being termed opportunists.

Infection from commensal organisms is termed **endogenous** and that from elsewhere **exogenous**. Most exogenous infections derive from a community source such as other humans, animals and the environment, but hospital-acquired infection is termed **nosocomial** and may be more harmful because of associated drug resistance.

Methicillin-resistant *Staphylococcus aureus* (MRSA) is an example that is a particular problem in current hospital practice. As with ordinary strains of S. aureus, some patients harbour MRSA on their skin or nose without harm (such patients being said to be 'colonized'). However, patients may develop infections if the MRSA then spreads to other parts of the body or cross-infects other patients and colonizes staff. Scrupulous cleaning and hand-washing, the use of isolation procedures and screening using swabs from patients and staff suspected of carrying MRSA are all important in reducing the incidence of infection.

In general, the size of an inflammatory response is related to the number of bacteria involved and their ability to multiply. Several million organisms are required to produce an inflammatory response and many millions for abscess formation. The virulence of an organism is therefore related to its ability to cross resistant surfaces and overcome non-specific tissue defences and specific immune responses. To combat these body defences, bacteria produce various enzymes and a number of toxins. Such toxins may be **exotoxins**, which are secreted by the organism, or **endotoxins**, which are released on the death of the organism. Harmful mechanisms include the enzymes hyaluronidase and streptokinase promoting tissue invasion, leukocidins inhibiting phagocytosis, haemolysins destroying blood cells and neurotoxins such as those of polio, diphtheria and tetanus.

Gram-positive organisms produce peptidoglycan and teichoic acid, giving rise to fever and general malaise. They do not usually have the lethal consequences of the endotoxin of gram-negative organisms, which in high doses can induce the marked abnormalities of tissue permeability and disseminated intravascular coagulopathies that are seen with endotoxic shock (see p. 27). The importance of the number of bacteria present, rather than their physical and chemical properties and pathogenicity, is further demonstrated in immunologically compromised patients in whom acute and chronic infective conditions often do not have organ-specific signs or symptoms, the diagnosis being made by bacteriological culture.

The terms 'bacteraemia' and 'septicaemia' are often used interchangeably; however, **bacteraemia** implies the culture of bacteria from the blood of an asymptomatic patient and does not necessarily carry any serious clinical significance. **Septicaemia** denotes a systemic disturbance due to organisms or their toxins being disseminated throughout the bloodstream, as in septicaemic shock. The term 'pyaemia' is best avoided.

## CELLULITIS

Inflammation of the cellular tissue can be superficial or deep. Superficial – that is, cutaneous and subcutaneous – is more common type and is easier to diagnose. The affected part is swollen, tense and tender. Later it becomes red, shiny and boggy. From the point of view of the differential diagnosis, superficial cellulitis may be said to have no edge, no fluctuation, no pus and no limit.

Cellulitis frequently commences in an infected wound (**Figure 4.1**). If no wound is obvious, a small puncture, blister or abrasion where organisms could have gained entrance should be sought. In the absence of a breach in continuity of the skin, a common site of origin for cellulitis is an infected anatomical bursa, for example olecranon or prepatellar, or an adventitious bursa, for example the bunion over a hallux valgus.

In children in whom no obvious abrasion is found, bear in mind Morison's aphorism: 'Cellulitis occurring in children is never primarily in the cellular tissues but secondary to an underlying bone infection.'

Cellulitis is commonly accompanied by pyrexia and general malaise. Examine for regional lymph node enlargement; inflamed superficial lymphatic vessels (**acute lymphangitis**; **Figure 4.2**) may be seen coursing from the site of infection to the regional lymph node. The telltale red lines are principally

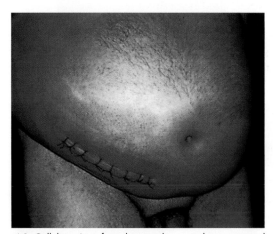

Figure 4.1 Cellulitis. An infected appendix wound is a potential complication in any patient undergoing surgery for suppurative appendicitis.

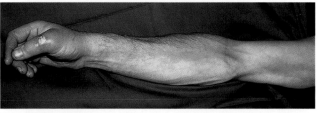

Figure 4.2 Lymphangitis on the arm and forearm following an infection of the thumb.

seen on the arm or leg. The initiating lesion is occasionally difficult to find.

## Erysipelas

Streptococcal cellulitis has a characteristic rosy or crimson colour. It is peculiarly smooth and has a characteristically shiny appearance.

The face is the most common site of origin in cellulitis (Figure 4.3), and oedema is prominent and may completely close the eyelids. The cellulitis has a distinct, raised surrounding edge. The regional lymph nodes are usually moderately enlarged. The eruption reaches its peak on the fifth day; the brilliant erythema then changes to a livid hue after which it turns to brown and later yellow. An exudate sometimes occurs beneath the cutis to form vesicles, later turning to pustules. Other sites involved include the hands, genitalia, the umbilicus in young infants and the lower limb, particularly associated with lymphoedema.

Milian's ear sign differentiates non-specific cellulitis from erysipelas in that the latter involves the pinna because it is a cuticular lymphangitis. On the other hand, subcutaneous inflammation stops short of the pinna because of the close adherence of the skin to the cartilage.

## Orbital Cellulitis

Orbital cellulitis (see also p. 351) may arise from hair follicles and other facial infections or from penetrating orbital wounds. It most commonly follows infection of the nasal sinuses, especially the ethmoidal and frontal. It is not surprising that ethmoiditis is the most common cause of orbital cellulitis as the paper-like lamina papyracea of the ethmoid bone forms the major part of the medial wall of the orbit. In infants, the infection may follow infection of the gums and teeth.

The condition is accompanied by prominent swelling of the eyelids, and on parting the lids the proptosis and frequent chemosis become apparent. Because of pressure on or involvement of the optic nerve, acuity of vision is often reduced. The condition carries two dangerous complications – cavernous sinus thrombosis and infection of the globe of the eye (see p. 360).

## Ludwig's Angina

Ludwig's angina is cellulitis involving the sublingual and submandibular spaces beneath the deep cervical fascia; it is almost invariably due to dental sepsis. In many instances, the floor of the mouth becomes oedematous, and in severe cases there is stridor and difficulty breathing.

Other examples of superficial and deep cellulitis occur in:

- the layers of the abdominal wall;
- the scrotum;
- spreading subcutaneous gangrene in the diabetic patient;
- pelvic cellulitis, for example parametritis, occurring in the connective tissue around the uterus.

These conditions result from infection with a mixture of aerobic and anaerobic organisms, and are termed **synergistic**. The spread is along the tissue planes and is accompanied by a high degree of oedema, tissue necrosis and gangrene. Gas-forming organisms are frequently also present.

## Meleney's Synergistic Gangrene or Ulceration

The condition is usually of the abdominal or chest wall following surgery for septic conditions. An area of cellulitis progresses rapidly, with the formation of a central purplish zone surrounded by angry, red inflammation. The whole area is exquisitely tender, with gross oedema of the surrounding skin. The purplish zone soon becomes gangrenous, and if unchecked the gangrene spreads widely. At first, the general signs are mild unless the patient is already debilitated from underlying disease. The gangrene and skin slough, producing an ulcer with an undermined edge.

## Pyoderma Gangrenosum

Pyoderma gangrenosum (Figure 4.4) has a similar acute pathology to synergistic gangrene but is related to recent wounds. Tender blue nodules progress to skin necrosis with multiple sinuses and exuberant granulation. Half of the patients affected have a depression of their immune system; associated diseases include Crohn's disease, ulcerative colitis, rheumatoid arthritis, plasma cell dyscrasia and leukaemia.

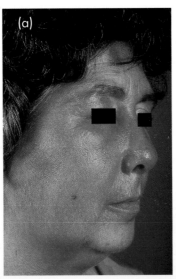

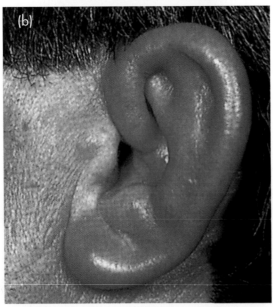

Figure 4.3 (a) Erysipelas of the face. (b) Erysipelas of the left ear.

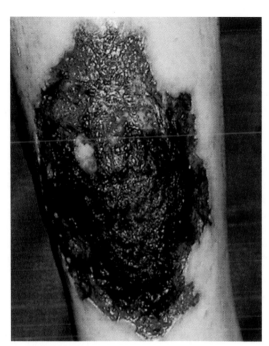

Figure 4.4 Pyoderma gangrenosum.

## Fournier's Gangrene of the Scrotum

This rare condition is notable for its rapidity of onset and absence of precipitating causes. It starts as an acute inflammatory oedema of the scrotum followed, in a matter of hours or days, by sloughing gangrene. Diabetes should be excluded and a search made for perianal sepsis.

## NECROTIZING FASCIITIS

This life-threatening condition may follow minor abrasions or innocuous surgical procedures. Risk factors include an immunocompromised state and diabetes, although it can occur in those who are otherwise healthy.

Necrotizing fasciitis is the spread of infection along the fascial planes, leading to extensive necrosis. The skin may appear normal in the early stages, with rapid progression to painful, red areas and finally necrosis due to compromise of the underlying blood supply. Patients are severely ill with systemic fever, toxaemia and septic shock, and mortality is high despite aggressive treatment including the extensive surgical excision of affected areas.

## ABSCESSES

An abscess (Figure 4.5) is an end product of unresolved inflammation. It consists of a collection of pus surrounded by an inflammatory zone and a lining of granulation tissue (historically known as the 'pyogenic membrane' although it is neither a true membrane nor itself pyogenic). The production of pus is termed suppuration. Pus is a fluid composed of living and dead bacteria, dead fixed and free cells (the latter representing the body's phagocytic response) and foreign material such as sutures, implants and splinters. The granulation tissue seals off the cavity from the surrounding structures. The natural progression of an abscess is to discharge through an epithelial covering or into a body cavity. The fibroblasts and capillary ingrowth of the wall then proceed to heal the cavity.

If the contents cannot discharge, they may become a sterile collection that is gradually reabsorbed, particularly if antibiotics have sterilized the pus. In this case, the residual collection is termed an **antibioma**. The organisms may continue to proliferate, with expansion and further destruction of the abscess wall. This may be seen, for example, in a deep breast abscess. Abscess formation is particularly common with staphylococcal infections and to a lesser extent pneumococcal and streptococcal. Abscesses of the large bowel commonly contain coliforms and *Bacteroides*.

Superficial abscesses are often associated with hair follicles, nail beds and wounds. Intra-abdominal abscesses are commonly associated with the appendix, the colon and tubo-ovarian disease, producing paracolic, subphrenic and pelvic abscesses. Less frequently, intra-abdominal abscesses are located around the kidney (perinephric) and liver (related to biliary and portal infection, and amoebic and hydatid organisms). Perianal abscesses are relatively common.

Infection related to bone (Figure 4.6) and joints is difficult to eradicate, as evidenced by the subperiosteal sequestration

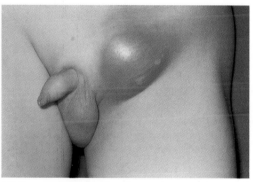

Figure 4.5 Suppurative inguinal nodes may be secondary to infection in the leg, abdominal wall, penis, scrotum or perineum.

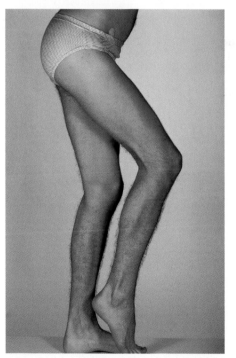

Figure 4.6 Pus from a vertebral infection, particularly tuberculosis, can track within the psoas sheath, and a psoas abscess may therefore present as a lump in the groin. Associated spasm causes hip flexion.

(Figure 4.7) of bone and prolonged infection in joint prostheses. Abscesses of the head and neck include styes, those of the teeth (Figure 4.8), tonsil, mastoid and retropharyngeal space and those of the intracranial cavity.

The local symptoms and signs of an abscess are those of inflammation, with redness, swelling, heat and tenderness as well as regional node involvement. At this stage, the lesion may be effectively combated by the body's own defences or by the addition of antibiotics. If the infection progresses, the swelling becomes soft centrally and the abscess cavity spherical. If the abscess is large enough, fluctuation may be demonstrated. The pain becomes more intense and throbs. The entry of bacteria and toxic products into the bloodstream gives rise to pyrexia, which is characteristically swinging in variety. The pyrexia and raised white blood count may be the only signs of a deep-seated abscess, and the aphorism 'pus somewhere, pus nowhere, pus under the diaphragm' should always be heeded.

Septicaemia may subsequently develop and may be accompanied by the complications of septic shock. The natural discharge of an abscess, for example through the skin, gut or bronchus or by surgical drainage, is accompanied by a rapid resolution of the pain and pyrexia. The abscess **points** after the destruction of a pathway to the surface; this pathway is termed a **sinus** (Figure 4.9). If discharge is complete, the cavity fibroses and the sinus opening heals as a scar. If discharge is incomplete, recurrent symptoms and recurrent, multiple sinuses can be expected. Chronic abscesses of this form and sterile collections as described above only resolve after adequate drainage and debridement. This healing does not occur if foreign bodies such as prostheses, mesh, bone sequestra or necrotic tendon remain.

The physical characteristics of a purulent discharge are of limited value in suggesting the causal organism, with bacteriological examination always being required. Various gross characteristic descriptions may, however, be given. Streptococcal pus from newly infected tissues is watery and slightly opalescent. It is sometimes also bloodstained. Staphylococcal pus is yellow and of a creamy consistency. Blue or bluish-green pus is typical of *Pseudomonas* infection. The purplish-brown coloured pus from an amoebic abscess of the liver is very characteristic.

Pus resulting from the activity of certain microorganisms emits a characteristic odour. This is particularly true of coliform bacteria, producing abdominal abscesses or sinuses and perianal abscesses that are in communication with the anal canal. *Bacteroides*, also common in intra-abdominal suppuration and infections of the abdominal wall, gives rise to an odour similar to that of over-ripe Camembert cheese. The smell of the gas gangrene infection caused by *Clostridium perfringens* emits a peculiar, sickly-sweet odour like decaying apples.

## Chronic Abscesses

Chronic abscesses as well as being caused by foreign bodies and inadequate drainage, may also be due to a communication with a hollow viscus. If the abscess cavity communicates with a second epithelial surface such as another loop of gut or the surface, a **fistula** develops. Other causes of chronic abscess that must be excluded are an associated malignancy and the presence of epithelium in the wall of the abscess cavity, such as a sebaceous cyst, which prevents healing.

Certain types of infection, such as tuberculosis (Figure 4.10), leprosy and syphilis, produce a granulomatous response. The

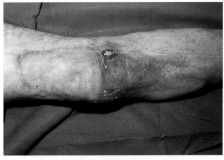

Figure 4.7 Sequestrum of the right tibia.

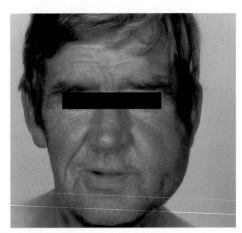

Figure 4.8 A dental abscess.

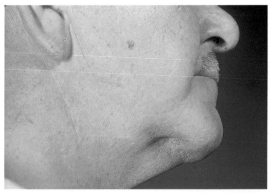

Figure 4.9 A sinus from a tooth abscess.

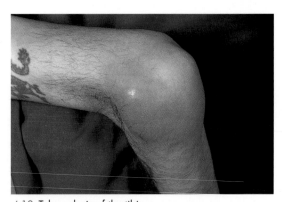

Figure 4.10 Tuberculosis of the tibia.

liquefaction of caseous material produces a thin, creamy, as opposed to purulent, discharge. Tuberculous abscesses are termed cold abscesses since they do not produce local heat and redness and do not have an associated, marked pyrexia. The neck is a common site due to degenerative nodes, and this is termed **scrofula (Figure 4.11)**. These may be collections both superficial and deep to the deep fascia, producing a **collar stud abscess**. The reactions associated with specific bacteria are included in Table 4.1.

## Boils and Carbuncles

Boils **(Figure 4.12)** – folliculitis, furuncles – and carbuncles **(Figure 4.13)** are staphylococcal skin infections commencing in hair follicles. They are common in those with diabetes, and this must always be considered and excluded. Initial inflammation progresses to a pustule, and with carbuncles this infection spreads subcutaneously due to coagulase activity. The subcutaneous

tissue dies, with the production of a core of hard, adherent slough with multiple overlying, discharging sinuses. The lesions are very painful and may be accompanied by systemic symptoms of malaise and pyrexia.

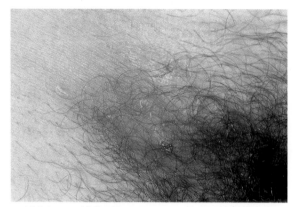

Figure 4.12 Inguinal folliculitis.

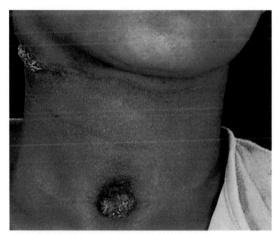

Figure 4.11 Cervical tuberculosis.

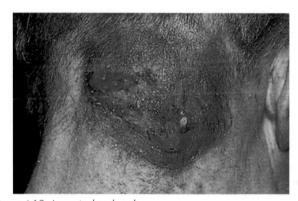

Figure 4.13 A cervical carbuncle.

Table 4.1 Surgical bacterial infections

| Organism | Clinical features |
| --- | --- |
| **Cocci** | |
| ***Gram-positive aerobic*** | |
| *Staphylococcus* (in bunches) *aureus* | Common commensal of the skin, nose and perineum. Resistant to dehydration; therefore viable in dust. Boils, carbuncles, wound infections, deep and superficial abscesses, osteomyelitis. Produces coagulase that clots plasma and limits access of neutrophils. Problem of antibiotic resistance, particularly in hospitals, because of methicillin-resistant *S. aureus*. Danger in intensive care units and surgical and neonatal wards |
| *epidermidis* (*albus*) | Usual skin commensal; increasing awareness of infections of intravascular lines and prosthetic implants |
| *Streptococcus* (in chains) *pyogenes* | Common nasal commensal in children. Throat infections, cellulitis, erysipelas, wound infections, lymphangitis, lymphadenitis, septicaemia |
| *viridans* | Oral commensal but potential for endocarditis after dentistry in susceptible individuals |
| *pneumoniae* | Pneumonia, meningitis, peritonitis in susceptible and occasionally fit individuals |
| *faecalis* | Gut commensal. Pathogen in urogenital and biliary tracts and endocarditis |
| Anaerobic staphylococci and streptococci | Commensals in the gut. Commonly found in the mixed growth of intra-abdominal abscesses. Can be gas-forming and therefore an important differential diagnosis of *Clostridium perfringens* |

*contd...*

PART 1 | PRINCIPLES

Table 4.1 Surgical bacterial infections (*contd...*)

| Organism | Clinical features |
| --- | --- |
| **Gram-negative** | |
| *Neisseria* | Aerobic intracellular diplococci |
| *gonorrhoeae* | One of the most common sexually transmitted diseases |
| *meningitidis* | May be a commensal. Epidemic meningitis in children and young adults; endemic in infants. The endotoxin is capable of producing fulminating septicaemia and meningitis |
| **Bacilli** | |
| **Gram-positive** | |
| *Clostridium* | Anaerobes, gut commensal, resistant spores proliferate in devitalized tissue |
| *tetani* | In soil, particularly horse droppings. Powerful exotoxin producing neuromuscular excitation |
| *perfringens (welchii)* | Powerful lethal exotoxin, producing myositis and gas gangrene |
| *difficile* | Endotoxin may give rise to pseudomembranous colitis |
| *botulinum* | Powerful exotoxin from contaminated foodstuffs. Mild gastroenteric symptoms followed by progressive symmetrical paralysis of the cranial and spinal nerves. Autonomic dysfunction but no sensory loss |
| Actinomycosis | Branching mycelial network spreading infection, abscess formation, yellow granules in pus |
| Anthrax | Spore-forming, highly resistant. Animal carriers, in wool, hides, bones. Cutaneous lesions, boil-like but no pus, and coal-black centre. Pulmonary and intestinal manifestations |
| *Mycobacterium tuberculosis* | Primary lymphadenopathy, meningeal infection, secondary and tertiary pulmonary, urinary tract infection (see pp. 79 and 643). |
| *leprae* | 'Tuberculoid' variety localized to skin and peripheral nerves<br>'Lepromatous' generalized bacteraemia, lesions also involving many systems |
| **Gram-negative** | |
| Enterobacteria (coliform) | Normal gut flora, non-spore-bearing, both anaerobic and aerobic. Capable of gut infection and opportunistic infection of the host. Produce gram-negative septicaemia, especially in immunocompromised patients and neonates |
| *Escherichia coli* | Gut and urinary tract infection |
| *Salmonella* | Typhoid and paratyphoid fevers commencing as gut infection but becoming widespread, potentially lethal infections affecting many organs |
| *enteritidis/typhimurium* | Salmonella food poisoning producing 2–3 days of acute diarrhoea, tenesmus, bloody stool, malaise, fever and abdominal pain. Patient continues to secrete organisms for 4–8 weeks. One of the leading causes of intestinal perforation in Africa and Asia |
| *Shigella* | Bacillary dysentery, ranging from mild to fulminating infection, fever, malaise, headache, diarrhoea |
| *Yersinia* | Mesenteric adenitis with or without terminal ileitis. Also produces plague, 'bubonic' from rats via flea vector, massive discharging lymphadenopathy. 'Pneumonic' human cross-infection from pulmonary involvement |
| Enterobacter | Gut infections and common organism in post-infective malabsorption (also *Escherichia coli* and *Klebsiella*) |
| *Klebsiella* | Gut infection and common opportunistic pneumonia |
| *Proteus* | Common urinary tract infection |
| *Pseudomonas aeruginosa* | Common, hospital-acquired infection, resistant to many chemical disinfectants, antiseptics and antibiotics. Important pathogen in burns, producing blue–green discharge. Problems in ophthalmic surgery and potential fatal septicaemia as is an opportunistic organism |
| *Haemophilus* | Common upper respiratory tract commensal. Acute epiglottitis, pneumonia, meningitis |
| **Coccobacilli** | |
| *Brucella* | Primarily an animal parasite, infection from close contact with cattle and carcasses. High, swinging fevers, dramatic sweating, severe, generalized aches and pains |
| *Bacteroides* | Common synergistic organism in bowel infections and intra-abdominal abscesses |

*contd...*

Table 4.1 Surgical bacterial infections (*contd...*)

| Organism | Clinical features |
| --- | --- |
| **Curved bacilli** | |
| *Vibro cholerae* | Epidemic in the Indian subcontinent. Colonizes small bowel. Enterotoxin impairs reabsorption from the gut, producing severe, extracellular fluid depletion. Characteristic 'rice water stool' |
| *Campylobacter* | Acute, self-limiting infectious diarrhoea |
| **Spiral bacteria** | |
| *Treponema pallidum* | Syphilis, venereal disease, demonstrated by dark field illumination as their size is on the limits of light microscopy. Worldwide distribution, no geographical or racial barriers. Profoundly influenced by the discovery of penicillin. Capable of congenital transmission |

## Hidradenitis Suppurativa

Suppurative hidradenitis (**Figure 4.14**) is an infection of the sweat glands that usually occurs in the axillae, often bilaterally. The condition may also involve the groins, the back of the neck and the perineum; in the last site, it must be differentiated from perianal fistulas. The infection is usually recurrent and persistent, with multiple abscess and sinus formation occurring over many years. It can be very disabling due to the associated pain.

## CAT-SCRATCH DISEASE

Cat-scratch disease (**Figure 4.15**) is a benign infectious disease resulting from a cat bite or scratch. The intercellular bacterium *Bartonella henselae* is responsible. The disease occurs about 10 days after inoculation, by which time a minor breach in the skin has usually healed. Although one should search for a primary lesion, the initial sign is considerable lymphadenitis without visible intervening lymphangitis, the axillary and inguinal nodes being almost exclusively affected. The constitutional symptoms are often considerable.

## PHLEBITIS

This is thrombosis of a superficial vein accompanied by marked pain and an inflammatory response in the overlying tissues. The thrombus is palpable as a tender, hard cord following the line of the varicose or superficial vein; propagation can be mapped by the cord and by the inflammatory response.

## TUBERCULOSIS

*Mycobacterium tuberculosis* infections occur in three stages: the primary complex, secondary dissemination and tertiary focal disease.

The primary lesion is usually a Ghon focus sited in the lungs and spreading to the hilar lymph nodes, but the portal of entry may be through the skin or alimentary tract. The infection is usually subclinical, residual evidence being a pulmonary scar, calcified lymph nodes and a positive skin test.

Secondary dissemination may occur months or many years later, commonly activated by immune suppression, and causes widespread haematogenous spread with multiple lesions. Any organ but commonly the lungs, bones and kidneys may be

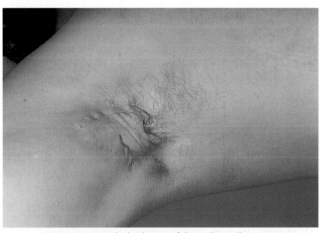

Figure 4.14 **Suppurative hidradenitis of the right axilla.**

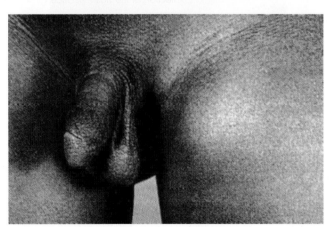

Figure 4.15 **Left inguinal lymph adenopathy from unsuspected cat-scratch disease.**

involved. Tuberculous meningitis is common in some localities, particularly across Asia. Systemic resistance develops or the condition is treated.

Tertiary lesions are usually focal and granulomatous, with extensive cellular destruction and possible abscess formation. Again the lungs, bones and kidneys are the common target organs. The cutaneous manifestation of tuberculosis is lupus vulgaris (**Figure 4.16**), which commences as a hyperaemic nodule and proceeds to a spreading, undermined ulcer (**Figure 4.17**), healing with extensive, pale scarring.

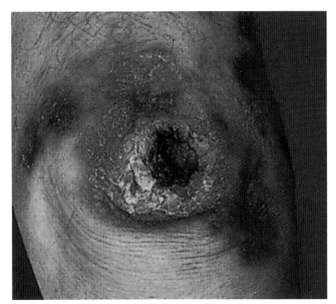

Figure 4.16 Lupus vulgaris.

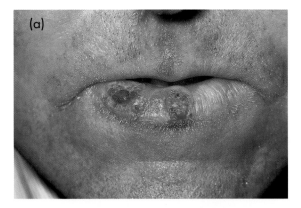

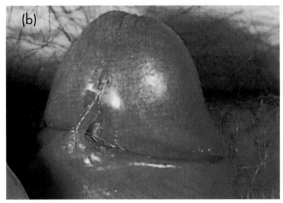

Figure 4.18 (a) Primary chancre of the lower lip. (b) Chancroid of the penis.

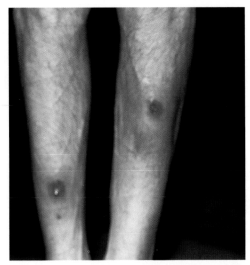

Figure 4.17 A tuberculous ulcer of the shin.

## SYPHILIS

This, usually sexually transmitted, infection caused by the spirochaete *Treponema pallidum* follows a similar pathological course to tuberculosis: a primary lesion, secondary haematogenous spread and tertiary local tissue destruction.

The primary lesion is a solitary, painless, erythematous nodule occurring 9–90 days, usually about 21, after exposure (see p. 645). The lesion breaks down to form a hard ulcer, a chancre, usually of the penis but it may occur on the lips, anus, nipples or fingers (**Figure 4.18a, b**). It has a sloping edge and a bloodstained discharge. The ulcer is accompanied by regional non-suppurative lymphadenopathy. Inguinal nodes from a penile lesion are hard and shotty, but the nodes are usually much larger when associated with extragenital lesions.

A penile lesion (see p. 651) must be differentiated from carcinoma of the penis and **chancroid** (**Figure 4.18b**) – the latter

is a softer, less indurated, painful lesion that may be multiple. It is due to the gram-negative bacillus *Haemophilus ducreyi* and is also sexually transmitted. Regional lymph node involvement may suppurate.

Secondary syphilis occurs 4–10 weeks after the primary infection and is a generalized disease accompanied by fever, malaise, a skin rash and generalized lymphadenopathy. There may be glossitis and pharyngitis, as well as oedematous papules of the mouth, penis, anus and vulva.

The tertiary focal granulomatous stage of syphilis is the gummatous ulcer. The lesion never reaches a large size. At first it is firm, but soon the centre softens and the overlying skin becomes infiltrated and reddish-purple. Finally, there is central necrosis with ulcer formation. It is punched out and painless. The base is covered with a characteristic wash-leather ('chamois leather') slough, which contains one or more 'islands' of normal tissue that have escaped the necrosis. The healed gumma is seen as a circular, characteristic, paper-thin scar with surrounding pigmentation; although the scar of yaws is a similar lesion, there are usually other manifestations of a previous syphilitic infection.

Tertiary syphilis may occur approximately 3–15 years after the initial infection, although patients are no longer able to transmit the infection to others. Any organ may be affected by tertiary syphilis, hence its name of the 'great imitator'. Classic gummatous lesions are found in the skull (**Figure 4.19a**). The syphilitic lesions of the ascending aorta may produce superior mediastinal aneurysms. Neurosyphilis comprises general paresis, tabes dorsalis (**Figure 4.19b**) and meningovascular disease.

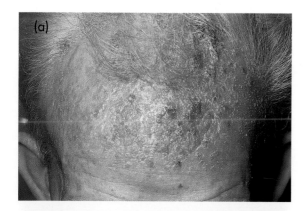

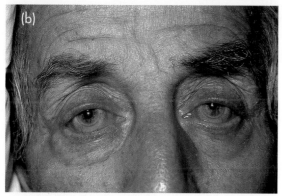

Figure 4.19 (a) A gummatous syphilitic lesion of the skull. (b) Tabes dorsalis – tertiary syphilis.

## ACTINOMYCOSIS

*Actinomyces* is a branching, filamentous, gram-positive bacterium. It gives rise to a chronic, spreading infection with indurated, woody lesions. The subcutaneous involvement gives the overlying skin a dusky appearance (see p. 336). Abscess formation is common, with multiple discharging sinuses, the pus containing characteristic 'sulphur-like' granules. Spread is directly through the bloodstream without lymph node involvement. Common sites involved are the jaw (from dental infection), neck, lungs, caecum and liver.

## TETANUS

Tetanus is a lethal condition produced by the powerful neurotoxic exotoxin of the gram-positive, anaerobic, spore-bearing bacillus *Clostridium tetani*. The bacillus is a commensal of the gut found in human and animal faeces and in soil. It is therefore a common contaminant of dirty wounds and can multiply in dead and ischaemic tissue.

Widespread programmes of anti-tetanus prophylaxis have rendered tetanus an uncommon disease in Western civilization. However, tetanus is still a major health problem in the developing world, neonatal tetanus being a particularly lethal condition. The incubation period ranges from a few days to a few weeks but usually 10–14 days. The initial symptoms are of lassitude, irritability, dysphagia and muscle spasm. Spasm of the facial muscles – trismus – produces the characteristic painful smile, risus sardonicus. This is followed by rigidity – lockjaw – and generalized tonic and clonic spasm. The prognosis is worst when

there is a short incubation period and a short interval between the onset of the symptoms and the first convulsions.

## GAS GANGRENE

A number of anaerobic infections can produce gas and crepitus within the tissues; examples of gas-producing synergistic gangrene have already been discussed. However, the term 'gas gangrene' usually refers to infection with *Clostridium perfringens* (*welchii*), the condition being a toxic myositis with myonecrosis produced by an exotoxin. The organism is a commensal of the alimentary tract and a potential infective agent in gangrenous bowel. Gas gangrene can also follow elective gastrointestinal surgery or vascular surgery for an ischaemic limb, with ischaemic muscle injuries at particular risk (Figure 4.20).

The diagnosis may be based on clinical grounds as *Clostridium* spp. may be contaminants of wounds, producing mild cellulitis or more lethal myositis depending on the local conditions. Pain is frequently the first symptom. A rising pulse out of proportion to the temperature increases suspicion and requires inspection of the wound. The characteristic odour is a sickly-sweet smell suggestive of decaying apples, and the wound shows a surrounding area of red, brawny swelling with a distended limb due to gas spreading along the muscle planes. Crepitus may be elicited at some distance from the wound.

Later, general signs suggestive of clostridial septicaemia include hypersensitivity and irritability, dyspnoea and tachycardia out of proportion to the pyrexia. Profound systemic symptoms of shock, obvious crepitus, a bluish-brown skin discoloration and the formation of bullae with a watery discharge and pronounced odour are present. The fluid from the bullae provides a heavy growth of the causative organism.

## VIRAL DISEASES

Viral diseases are common worldwide and affect every system. Although they require less surgical involvement than the pus-forming bacteria, surgical patients are susceptible to viral infection, and viral diseases may require surgical intervention, often because of secondary bacterial infection. The surgeon is also at risk of contracting certain viral infections such as hepatitis and HIV (see p. 105) from patients.

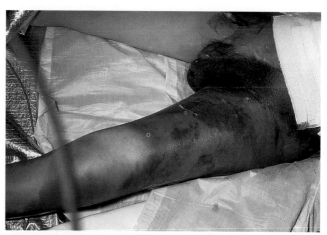

Figure 4.20 Gas gangrene of the upper thigh with skin staining from muscle destruction.

The classification of viral disease can be based on the physical properties, protein coat or nucleic acid core of the viruses but a more practical division is based on the prime organ of involvement. Systemic effects are also common and the incidence of multiorgan pathology is increased in immunocompromised patients, a specific example being **cytomegalovirus**, which gives rise to serious consequences after organ transplantation. Some viruses are endemic, such as **plague**, which is transmitted via wild animals, and many are tropical in their distribution, such as the mosquito-borne **alphaviruses**. Other groups may become epidemic, such as the influenza viruses, while plague and **typhus** are prevalent in malnourished refugee populations.

In the respiratory tract, the common cold is produced by **rhinoviruses**, while specific virus groups also affect the lungs, for example influenza viruses. Other organs commonly involved include the central nervous system, for example in **poliomyelitis** and **rabies**, and the gut, as in **hepatitis** and **yellow fever**. Many viral infections have cutaneous manifestations, examples being **herpes simplex** (Figure 4.21), **herpes zoster** (see pp. 109 and 369), **measles**, **mumps** and **chickenpox** (Figure 4.22). A few viruses are largely restricted to cutaneous manifestations, such as warts on the hands and the plantar aspects of the feet, and the lesions of molluscum contagiosum (see p. 110; see Figures 5.22 and 5.23).

## FUNGAL INFECTIONS (MYCOSES)

Fungi affect humans in a number of ways. They can destroy crops, thereby promoting starvation in tropical areas; some fungi, such as certain mushrooms, are poisonous; they can act as allergens, producing asthma and hypersensitivity pneumonitis; and some fungi are invasive. The latter may be subdivided into those invading the skin, the subcutaneous tissues and the deep tissues.

Superficial infections of the skin include thrush (*Candida albicans*; Figure 4.23) and ringworm (tinea cruris and tinea capitis; Figure 4.24). Subcutaneous fungal infections are usually tropical in distribution, the prime example being mycetoma (see p. 93). Deep visceral fungal infections are often opportunistic, occurring in immunocompromised individuals; an example is cryptococcosis, which affects the lungs and produces meningitis.

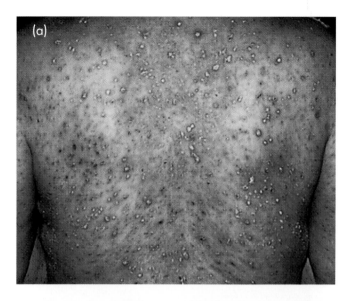
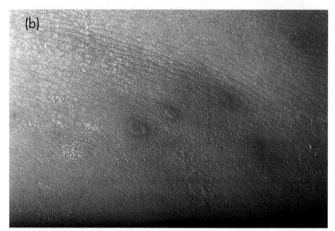
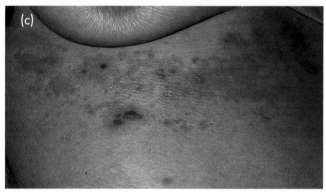

Figure 4.22 (a) The cutaneous lesions of chickenpox. (b) Close-up of a chickepox rash on the back. (c) Submammary shingles.

## PROTOZOA AND WORMS

Parasitic infections are common in the tropics (see pp. 82–87), but are also widely distributed in temperate zones. The majority pass their life cycle in more than one host, producing millions of eggs to ensure survival and reaching humans by way of a vector. Many of these diseases, particularly those affecting the alimentary tract, involve surgical management.

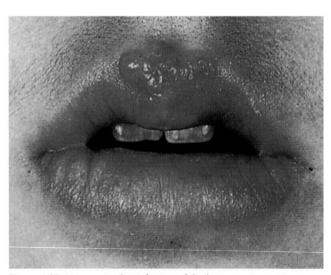

Figure 4.21 Herpes simplex infection of the lip.

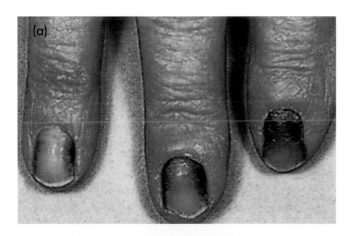

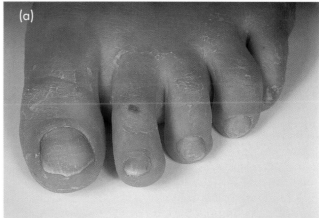

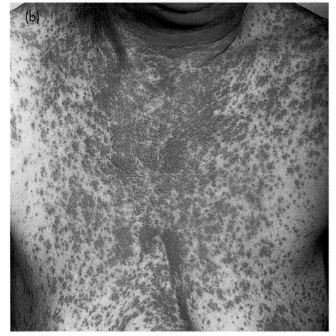

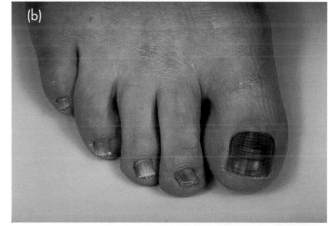

Figure 4.23 (a) Candidial infection of the nails. (b) Systemic candidiasis secondary to hairy cell leukaemia.

Protozoal infections include amoebiasis, malaria (the mosquito being the vector), trypanosomiasis (carried by the tsetse fly in Africa), toxoplasmosis (usually contracted from household pets) and leishmaniasis (carried by the sandfly) (see pp. 82–87).

## Amoebiasis

Amoebiasis is a gastrointestinal infection producing inflammatory dysentery that is caused by **Entamoeba histolytica**. Occasionally, there is systemic involvement, which usually takes the form of inflammatory amoebomas of the large bowel – this mass most commonly occurs in the caecum. Portal venous invasion can lead to a liver abscess, which is usually solitary; rupture through the diaphragm into the bronchial tree produces the characteristic purplish-brown sputum from red–brown necrotic liver tissue. The disease is endemic and sometimes epidemic in the tropics, but sporadic cases occur elsewhere. Cysts are excreted in the stool, the disease being contracted through poor hygiene or insect transfer.

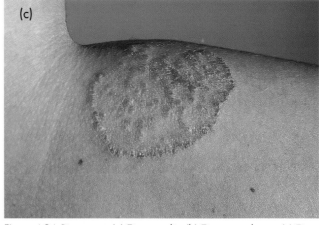

Figure 4.24 Ringworm. (a) Tinea pedis. (b) Tinea ungulatum. (c) Tinea corporis.

## Malaria (*Plasmodium falciparum, P. vivax, P. ovale* and *P. malariae*)

Malaria (Figure 4.25) is the pre-eminent tropical disease, with 200 000 000 sufferers and probably an annual mortality of 1 000 000. It is transmitted by the blood-sucking female *Anopheles* mosquito. Parasites are trapped by the liver within 30 minutes of infection, and the symptoms then usually occur within 1 month but may appear within 5 days or rarely after 1 year. The diagnosis

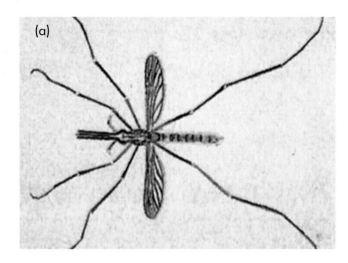

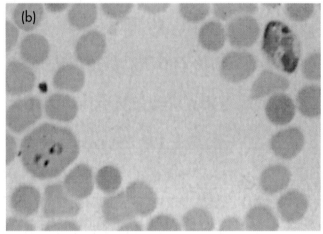

Figure 4.25 (a) The female *Anopheles* mosquito. (b) Intracellular *Plasmodium falciparum* in a blood film.

is suspected on clinical grounds and confirmed by the presence of parasites within red blood cells viewed on a thick blood film.

The importance of malaria to the surgeon lies mainly in its differential diagnosis. Fever, headache, nausea and myalgia occur in many tropical conditions but the rigors may be diagnostic in their timing (see p. 35). Anaemia, abdominal pain, jaundice and diarrhoea are also common, together with splenomegaly, particularly with *P. malariae*. The large spleen is fragile, rupturing with minor trauma and having a high mortality. Most deaths are from *P. falciparum*, with patients usually suffering from cerebral malaria accompanied by shock, hypoglycaemia and renal failure.

## Trypanosomiasis

In **African trypanosomiasis**, the first sign is the nodule at the site of the tsetse fly bite. This is followed by fever and lymphadenopathy. Central nervous system involvement, with the onset of the characteristic mental changes of sleeping sickness, may take a month or over a year to appear.

**American trypanosomiasis** is located in North and South America and is transmitted by the house bug. The disease was initially described by, and is now named after, Chagas. There is local swelling at the site of the bite, but the chronic symptoms may take many decades to appear. These involve chronic

inflammation of the cardiac muscle producing a cardiomyopathy, and involvement of the smooth muscle and nerve plexuses of the gut producing a mega-oesophagus and megacolon, and causing dysphagia and constipation.

## Toxoplasmosis

Toxoplasmosis is a worldwide infection, usually carried from infected mice by household cats. The majority of infections go unnoticed but patients may present with painless lymphadenopathy. The disease, however, has serious implications in immunocompromised patients, in whom fatal encephalitis can develop. Neonatal infections may also be accompanied by fatal cerebral involvement and/or necrotizing retinochoroiditis (**Figure 4.26**).

## Worms

Worms include **roundworms** (nematodes), **tapeworms** (cestodes) and **flukes** (trematodes); a common finding is an eosinophilic response to their foreign protein. Among the roundworms, **hookworm** is one of the most prevalent diseases in the world (**Figure 4.27**). The larvae migrate to the top of blades of grass and enter humans through skin abrasions. They pass through the lungs and then to the small intestine. The head becomes firmly attached to the intestinal wall and, although each worm is small – less than 2 cm long – a chronic, debilitating anaemia results as the worms are present in their thousands.

The *Ascaris* worm (**Figure 4.28**) is the common roundworm that resembles the earthworm in shape but may be 20–30 cm

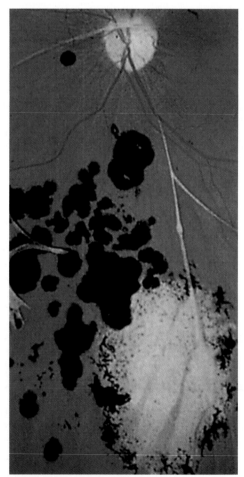

Figure 4.26 Choroid retinitis following toxoplasmosis infection.

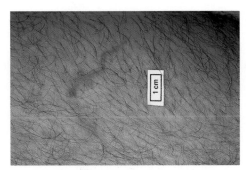

Figure 4.27 Hookworm of the right leg.

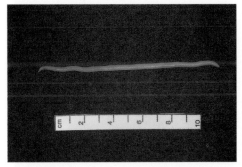

Figure 4.28 The common roundworm – *Ascaris*.

long. Large collections of these worms can produce intestinal obstruction, especially in children. They also produce systemic disturbances as larvae that have been ingested penetrate the gut wall and pass to the lungs via the circulation. They then break into the bronchi, migrate to the epiglottis and are again swallowed; they mature in the small intestine. Very occasionally, and usually after irritation by drugs or manipulation during surgery, a worm may migrate into the appendix or the common bile or pancreatic ducts, giving rise to obstruction and secondary infection.

**Filarial** infections (*Wuchereria bancrofti*) are also produced by roundworms of 6–8 cm that are transported in their larval form by the mosquito. The adult worms migrate into the human lymphatics, producing gross secondary lymphoedema of the legs and scrotum (Figure 4.29) that is termed elephantiasis. Obstruction of the thoracic duct may give rise to chylous ascites, and subcutaneous nodules may be produced by an inflammatory response surrounding a local worm. **Pinworms** or **threadworms** are up to 1 cm long and are common in children. Their presence in the perianal area produces intractable itching.

## Guinea Worm and Larvae Migrans

The guinea worm, *Dracunculus medinensis* (Figure 4.30), is extensively distributed across central Africa and Asia. The secondary host is the water flea and transfer to humans is in contaminated water. The worm migrates from the gut to the surface. The male worm usually dies after mating but the adult female can grow

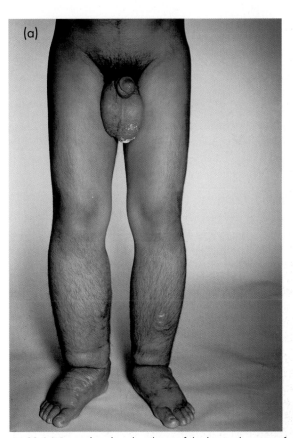

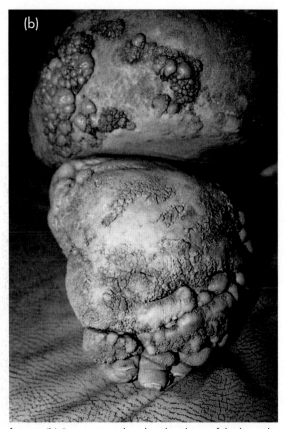

Figure 4.29 (a) Secondary lymphoedema of the leg and scrotum from filarial infection. (b) Severe secondary lymphoedema of the lower leg due to filarial infection.

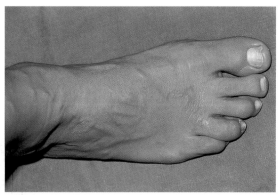

Figure 4.30 Guinea worm infection of the right foot.

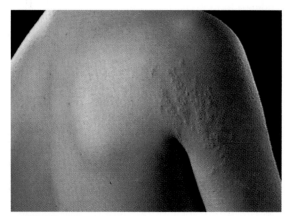

Figure 4.31 Cutaneous larvae migrans.

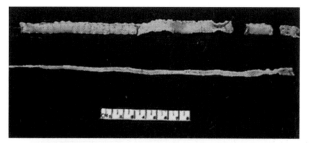

Figure 4.32 Tapeworm – *Taenia saginatum*.

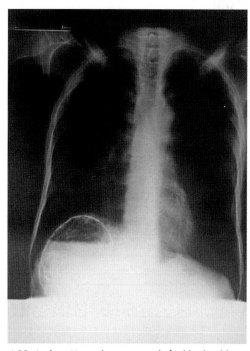

Figure 4.33 A chest X-ray showing a calcified hydatid lung abscess.

to 70–120 cm in length and 2 mm wide. The local inflammatory response may be intense. It is sometimes possible to extract the full length of the worm once it has surfaced.

Cutaneous larvae migrans, **Strongyloides stercoralis** (Figure 4.31), occurs in the West Indies and central Asia. The worm is about 3 mm long and is atypical in that it can produce several generations within the same human host, leading to heavy infestation and prolonged symptoms. Its cutaneous migration is accompanied by a marked inflammatory response.

## Flat Tapeworms

The flat tapeworms have a wide distribution. In those whose secondary host is cattle (*Taenia saginatum*) (Figure 4.32), pigs (*Taenia solium*) or fish (*Diphyllobothrium latum*), the adult tapeworm is found in the alimentary tract of the human. Some grow to many metres in length. The symptoms are usually mild, although a severe anaemia occasionally occurs in the Chinese fish tapeworm and rarely bile duct adenocarcinoma can develop. If the eggs of *Taenia solium* are transferred directly from one human to another, the cysticercus stage may occur in man. The symptoms of cysticercosis are usually severe neurological problems due to invasion of the central nervous system.

The **hydatid tapeworm** *Echinococcus granulosus* differs from the others in that the cystic stage occurs in man, the other hosts being the dog and the sheep. The ingested eggs penetrate the bowel wall and are carried by the portal vein to the liver and thence around the body; cysts develop mainly in the liver, lung (Figure 4.33), kidneys and brain. The cysts cause pressure as well as toxic effects in many systems.

## Liver Flukes

Liver flukes are prevalent parasites in China, and **lung flukes** are common parasites in Japan and China. The most important disease caused by flukes is, however, **schistosomiasis** (bilharzia; Figure 4.34). The *Schistosoma* organism produces granulomas, particularly of the bladder and liver, and causes bladder dysfunction, recurrent infections (Figure 4.35) and in the late stages transitional cell carcinoma. The intermediate host of the flukes is the water snail (Figure 4.36) – larvae enter the human through skin abrasions and mature in the liver.

## External Parasites

Common external parasites include scabies (Figure 4.37), lice (Figure 4.38) and fleas (Figure 4.39); these belong to the jointed arthropods. Their bites may be painful and cause hypersensitivity and itching. They may also carry diseases, particularly epidemic typhus and relapsing fever. The reactions to insect bites vary from mild hyperaemia to acute allergic local or systemic effects (Figure 4.40).

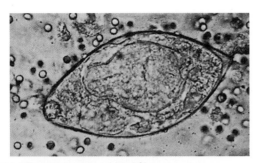

Figure 4.34 Bilharzia eggs in a blood film.

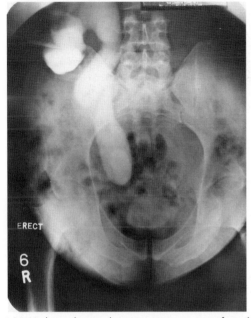

Figure 4.35 Hydronephrosis due to ureteric stenosis from bilharzial infection.

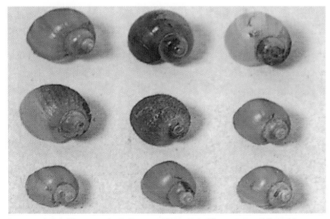

Figure 4.36 The snail *Bulinus physopsis*. The intermediate host in bilharzia infection.

## HAND INFECTIONS

Hand infections have become less common in the UK in recent decades. This is due to the mandatory wearing of protective apparel including gloves in the workplace and to the automation of many industries, with a consequent reduction in manual labour. Nevertheless, hand infections still make up 0.7 per cent

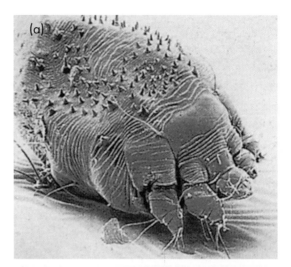

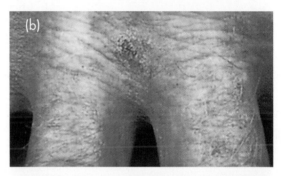

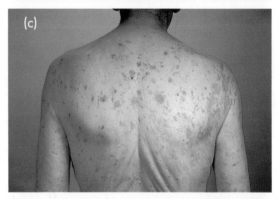

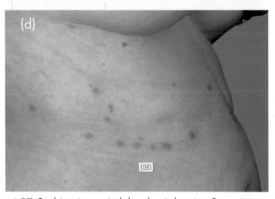

Figure 4.37 Scabies is carried by the itch mite *Sarcoptes scabiei*. (a) The female burrows into the skin to lay her eggs, producing a papule, the site of the lesion commonly being on the dorsum of the web space. (b) This produces intense itching. (c) A scabies rash on the back. (d) Post-scabetic nodules.

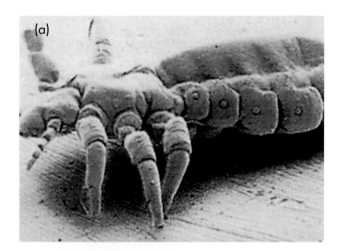

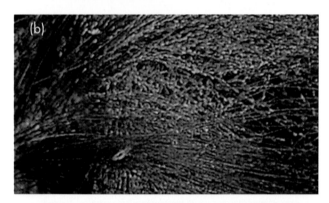

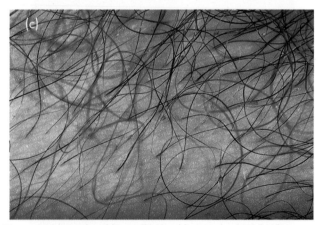

Figure 4.38 (a) A head louse. (b) Head lice *in situ*. (c) Pubic lice.

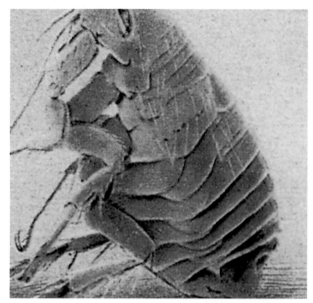

Figure 4.39 There are more than 20 species of flea that attack humans, the most common variety in the UK being *Pulex irritans*. The bites can cause irritation and erythema. These effects vary remarkably between individuals.

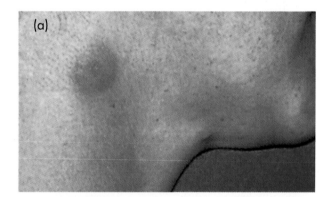

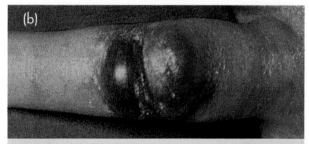

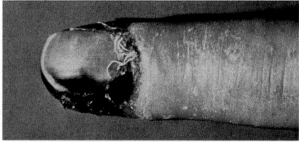

Figure 4.40 (a) An insect bite. (b) An acute allergic response secondary to an insect bite.

of accident and emergency attendances in the UK, and the early recognition and treatment of these lesions are important to prevent prolonged loss of work and hand deformity. Those particularly at risk include manual workers, patients with diabetes and those who are immunosuppressed. Patients with ischaemia, whether from large or small vessel disease, such as scleroderma, are subject to recurrent infection with necrosis and tissue loss.

When describing hand conditions, it is important to document the digits as the thumb and the index, middle, ring and little fingers. Numbering the digits leads to confusion, with disastrous results if an amputation is being undertaken. The infected hand is held in the position of rest, this being with all joints flexed to 5–25° and a flexed elbow.

Oedema is usually prominent, being most evident on the dorsum of the hand irrespective of the site of the lesion; this is due to the greater laxity of the skin and fascia over the dorsal aspect of the hand. Cellulitis is common with superficial lesions. Lymphangitis may present as red streaks along the arm and is accompanied by axillary lymphadenopathy, the supratrochlear node being enlarged with infection of the medial aspect of the forearm and hand. Focal tenderness is the cardinal sign of pus, and demonstration of this tenderness is a very important diagnostic tool, particularly when searching for deep infection such as in a tendon sheath. There may be an associated pyrexia and general malaise.

Streptococci (50 per cent) and staphylococci are the most common infecting organisms, but wounds may become infected with coliforms (19 per cent) and *Bacteroides* and other anaerobes. Viral infections, for example herpes simplex, can occur, and opportunistic organisms should be considered in immunosuppressed individuals.

## Paronychia

Paronychia (**Figure 4.41a, b**) is the most common hand infection (30 per cent), encountered in every walk of life and affecting both sexes in all age groups. The infection arises underneath torn nails or damaged cuticles, with subeponychial suppuration spreading around the nail fold, often to the collateral side. In 60 per cent of cases, pus burrows beneath the nail (a subungual abscess; **Figure 4.41c**). In this case, pressure on the nail evokes exquisite pain.

The infection may persist as a chronic inflammation around the nail fold (**Figure 4.42**). Chronic lesions may also be secondary to fungal infections such as candidiasis.

## Apical Abscess

An apical abscess (**Figure 4.43**) lies beneath the free edge of the nail following a sharp injury, such as from a splinter. Pus may burst through the subungual epithelium to lie in the distal nail bed.

## Pulp Space Infection

Pulp space infection (**Figure 4.44**) is a common (14 per cent) and potentially serious infection following penetrating injury, the index finger and thumb being the most susceptible. The space is filled with compact fat, partly partitioned by septa and separated from the rest of the finger by a distinct transverse septum at the level of the epiphyseal line of the terminal phalanx.

A dull ache and swelling are initially present, with cellulitis. With pus formation, there is a severe nocturnal exacerbation of throbbing pain interfering with sleep and marked local tenderness. The subcutaneous abscess may break through and spread under the dermis or may extend deeply to involve the bone (**Figure 4.45**). In the former (collar stud abscess), the deeper component may only be recognized after deroofing the subcuticular abscess.

## Infection over the Middle and Proximal Phalanges

These infections have a similar aetiology and clinical course to terminal pulp space infections, but the oedema is more marked due to greater skin laxity. Infection over the middle phalanx is localized by proximal and distal septa, but over the proximal

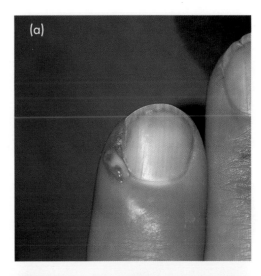

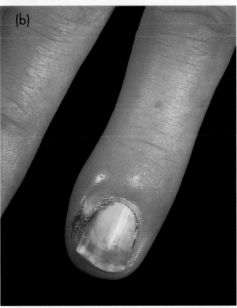

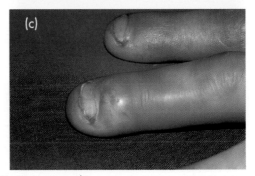

Figure 4.41 **Acute paronychia.**

phalanx (**Figure 4.46**) pus can communicate freely with the adjacent web space of the hand.

**Web space infections** produce gross oedema of the web space and extend over the dorsum of the hand. The infection may be poorly localized, with marked systemic symptoms. The differential diagnosis of tendon sheath infection is difficult until pus forms locally, when the redness becomes more focal. Pus may

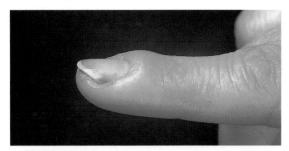

Figure 4.42 Chronic paronychia.

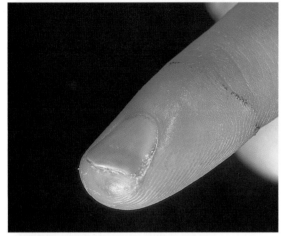

Figure 4.43 An apical abscess.

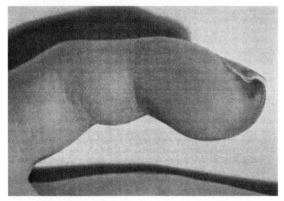

Figure 4.44 Pulp space infection.

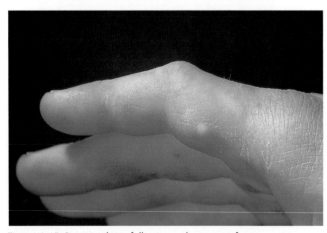

Figure 4.45 Septic arthritis following pulp space infection.

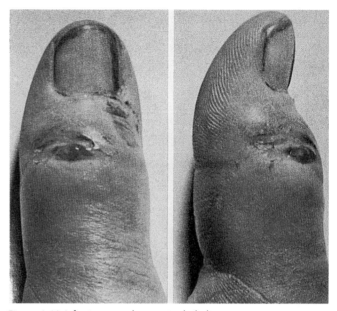

Figure 4.46 Infection over the proximal phalanx.

track across the palmar surface of the base of the fingers from one web space to the next and into the proximal digital compartment of the adjacent fingers.

## Thenar Space Infection

The thenar compartment encloses the short thenar muscles and long tendons to the thumb. There is marked ballooning of the thenar eminence with thenar space infection. Flexion of the distal phalanx may be pronounced but it lacks the resistance to extension that is present in infection of the sheath of flexor pollicis longus. The **hypothenar space** may be similarly affected, but this is less common.

## Mid-palmar Space Infection

Infection of the mid-palmar space containing the long digital flexor tendons deep to the palmar fascia (Figures 4.47 and 4.48) usually follows penetrating injuries but can follow the rupture of an infected tendon sheath. There is obliteration of the concavity of the palm with bulging and extreme swelling of the dorsum, giving the characteristic 'frog hand' appearance (Figure 4.49).

## Infection of the Tendon Sheaths

Infection of the tendon sheaths usually follows penetration by a sharp pointed object such as a needle or thorn, particularly over the digital flexor creases where the sheath is near the surface. Very occasionally, the infection may spread from more superficial abscesses. The whole sheath is rapidly involved and within a few hours of the injury throbbing pain is felt in the affected digit, with an accompanying pyrexia. The involved finger is held in a flexed position and as the infection proceeds there is symmetrical swelling of the whole finger, with puffy swelling on the dorsum of the hand. Although the finger can be moved back and forth by lumbrical action, active finger flexion is absent. Passive extension produces extreme pain. There is marked tenderness along the tendon sheath, this being extreme at the proximal and distal limits of the sheath where it extrudes outside the fibrous containing bands.

The little finger communicates with the ulnar bursa, and the thenar flexor sheath with the radial bursa. The proximal limit of tenderness with bursal involvement extends proximal to the flexor retinaculum. As there is usually a communication between the radial and ulnar bursae, it may be difficult to distinguish the

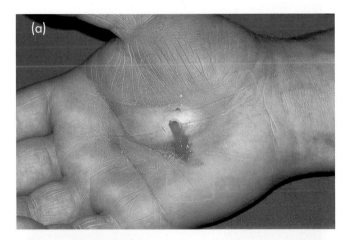

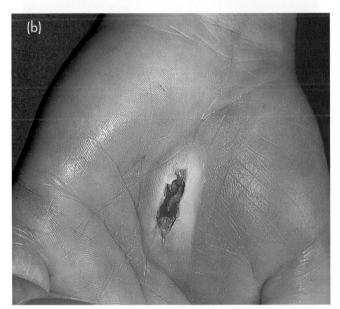

Figure 4.47 (a) Palmar infection. (b) On excision. The superficial component proved to be a collar stud abscess involving the mid-palmar space.

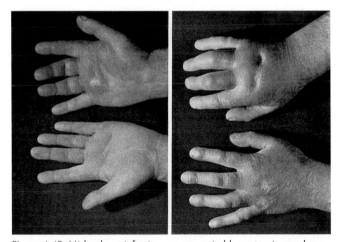

Figure 4.48 Mid-palmar infection accompanied by extensive oedema.

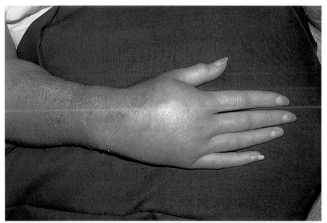

Figure 4.49 A 'frog hand' showing extensive oedema over the dorsum of the hand. The prime focus may be situated on the palmar aspect.

infection of one bursa from that of the other. Associated palmar and dorsal swelling can make the differential diagnosis from other palmar infections difficult, but the absence of extension and the extreme pain on movement are usually diagnostic.

Other infections of the palm include barber's pilonidal sinus (see p. 622) and penetrating injuries from spray guns dispensing oils, solvents and paints (grease gun injuries). These are serious injuries, and the damage can be underestimated in the early stages due to small entry wounds, lack of bleeding, numbness masking the pain and the area being cold on palpation rather than demonstrating the classical signs of inflammation. Debridement can thus be delayed, with subsequent extensive subcutaneous necrosis that may involve the tendons and tendon sheaths.

## Infection of the Dorsal Space

This is unusual but may accompany boils and carbuncles, and extensions of these lesions can involve the extensor tendon sheaths. Focal tenderness over the infected area differentiates it from dorsal swelling associated with palmar lesions.

Animal and human bites may also cause a variety of superficial and deep infections from a range of pathogenic organisms. The healing of penetrating injuries may be followed by implantation dermoid cysts, most commonly seen in the pulps of the fingers.

For **warts** and *Candida* infection of the nail, see p. 83; Figure 4.23.

## Uncommon Hand Infections

In addition to the infections described above, the hand is subject to a number of other characteristic lesions. **Cutaneous erysipeloid** (Figure 4.50) is due to infection with *Erysipelothrix rhusiopathiae* bacteria, which contaminate meat, game and fish; it is seen particularly in butchers.

### Orf and Anthrax

Orf and anthrax are acquired by animal contact. Orf (Figure 4.51) is a poxvirus carried by sheep, cattle and goats, and occurs in shepherds, farmers, abattoir workers and veterinary surgeons. The vesicular macular lesions break down and are usually painless until secondary infection occurs. Generalized disease is very rare.

Anthrax (Figure 4.52) is a gram-positive bacterium whose resistant spores can be transported in animal hides, wool, hair and bone. The latter is ground down in the preparation of gelatin and

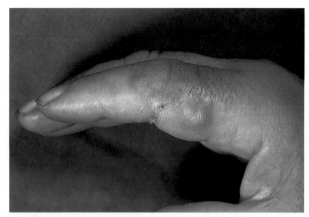

Figure 4.50 Erysipeloid infection.

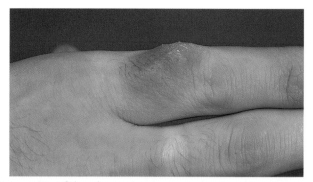

Figure 4.53 A fish tank granuloma.

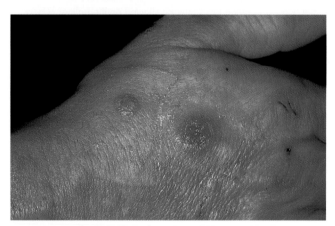

Figure 4.51 Orf infection.

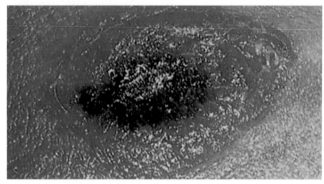

Figure 4.52 Anthrax infection.

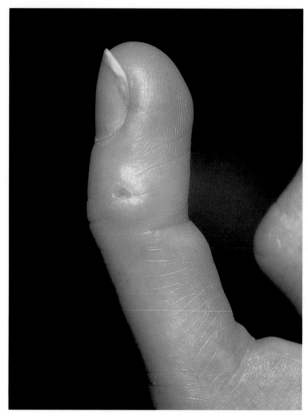

Figure 4.54 A herpetic whitlow.

glue. The lesions are found in those coming into direct contact with infected animals or animal products. The lesions consist of a black, firmly adherent scab surrounded by oedematous, purplish vesicles. These aggressive-looking lesions cause surprisingly little pain. Systemic infection may follow, typically affecting the lungs, intestine and more rarely the meninges.

## Fish Tank Granuloma

Fish tank granuloma (Figure 4.53) is acquired in an abrasion from a fish tank that is infected with atypical mycobacteria. A soft, subcutaneous nodular lesion is produced, which becomes secondarily infected. There is often associated tracking lymphangitis.

## Herpetic Whitlows

Herpetic whitlows (Figure 4.54) are caused by the herpes simplex virus and occur in medical and other health professionals in contact with infected patients. The digital lesions are painful blisters, initially containing clear fluid but later exuding pus and debris. The lesions take a number of weeks to heal.

## Systemic Infection

Cutaneous infection may be secondary to systemic disease such as meningococcal meningitis Figure 4.55. The dissemination of septic emboli may produce deep or superficial lesions such as the septic lesion on the thumb shown in Figure 4.56.

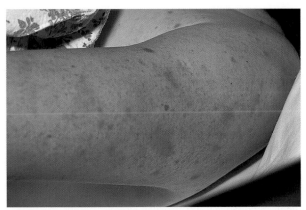

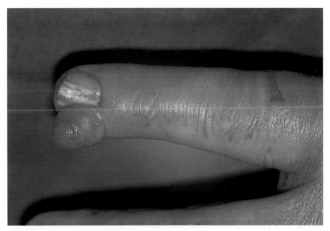

Figure 4.55 Cutaneous infection may be secondary to systemic disease such as meningococcal meningitis.

Figure 4.57 A foreign body granuloma.

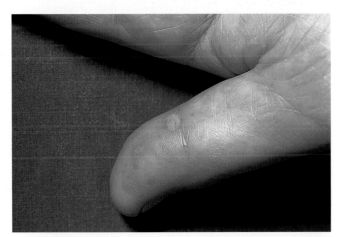

Figure 4.56 The dissemination of septic emboli may produce deep or superficial lesions such as this septic lesion on the thumb.

*Foreign Body Granulomas*

Foreign body granulomas (**Figure 4.57**) are produced by the subcutaneous implantation of external debris and bacteria.

Tropical infections are considered on pp. 82–87.

## FOOT INFECTIONS

Infection of the sole of the foot is common among those who walk barefoot so is seen mostly in the tropics. Tight, rigid footwear can produce blisters over the heel and prominent joints, and pressure on the great toenail can precipitate the problem of an ingrowing toenail. Neuropathic feet are prone to unnoticed injury, with secondary infection; this is particularly common in diabetic patients (see p. 479).

The dense fascial layers of the foot and their various septa tend to localize any infection, due to spread from one compartment to another being slow. Pus within a compartment produces extreme local tenderness and throbbing pain that may interfere with sleep. As in the hand, associated oedema may appear over the dorsum or lateral aspects of the foot rather than over the sole. If the infection is in the **heel space**, the patient dare not put the foot to the ground. Infection of the **deep fascial spaces**

of the sole may track along neurovascular bundles or into tendon sheaths. Penetrating injuries may allow **subcutaneous** infection to produce collar stud abscesses, and **web space** infection to spread through the tissue planes and track into the plantar or dorsal aspects of the foot.

## Mycetoma (Madura Foot)

This fungal infection is endemic in tropical Africa, India and South and Central America. It is almost exclusively confined to individuals who walk barefoot and are liable to the contamination of mild abrasions with road dust.

The first manifestation is a firm, painless, rather pale nodule, usually on the foot. This increases in size and others appear. In the early stages, especially if the sole is involved, a malignant melanoma may be suspected. In approximately a week, vesicles appear on the surface of the nodules, and these soon burst to reveal the mouth of a sinus, which discharges purulent, mucoid fluid. The fluid contains black, red or yellow granules depending on the species. The black variety spreads mainly subcutaneously, but the red and yellow varieties spread early to the muscles and underlying bone. Nerves and tendons are resistant, and neurological signs are conspicuously absent; there is no associated lymphadenitis or blood-borne dissemination.

Sooner or later, secondary infection supervenes, producing gross swelling of the foot with obliteration of the concavity of the instep (**Figure 4.58**).

## Differential Diagnosis of Multiple Sinuses in the Foot

A large number of tropical infections may cause foot ulceration and sinus formation. The diagnosis depends on a knowledge of the local endemic infections and on isolating the causative organisms. Tuberculosis is common in the tropics and often goes long untreated. Kaposi's sarcoma (see p. 109; Figure 5.21), in which soft nodules often become infected, can resemble Madura foot (above). Tropical ulcer (see p. 409) may also occur in the foot.

## Ingrowing Toenail (Onychocryptosis)

An ingrowing toenail usually affects the great toe (**Figure 4.59**), particularly on the lateral side. It develops when there is excessive

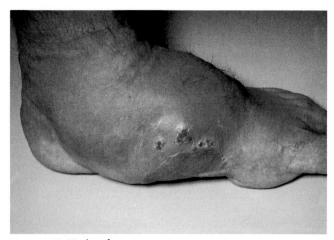

Figure 4.58 **Madura foot.**

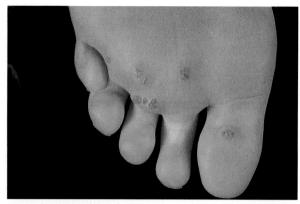

Figure 4.60 **A plantar wart.**

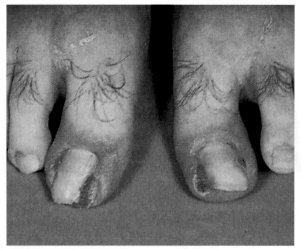

Figure 4.59 **An ingrowing toenail.**

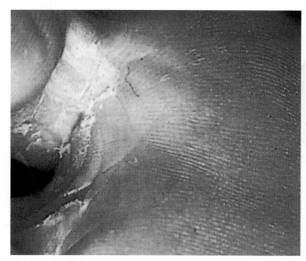

Figure 4.61 **Tinea pedis.**

outward growth of the nail into the nail fold. It may be precipitated by tight shoes or by cutting the corner off the nail; the sharp residual edge then penetrates the nail fold as it grows forwards rather than growing clear of the skin.

The laceration produced allows the entry of bacteria and a painful infection. In chronic cases, there can be protuberant granulation tissue. The lesion is very tender and the patient wears capacious shoes or sandals to prevent a painful limp.

## Plantar Wart

Plantar warts or verrucas (Figure 4.60) are produced by infection with the human papillomavirus. They occur on the weight-bearing areas of the ball of the foot or the heel. The pressure of walking inverts the warty lesion so that it is surrounded by a rim of cornified skin with a central red or black pitted area. There may be adjacent satellite lesions. Verrucas are usually found in children and can be exquisitely tender.

## Tinea Pedis

Tinea pedis or athlete's foot is a fungal infection that produces maceration between the toes, usually the fourth interspace, and itching (Figure 4.61). In its more aggressive form, it produces purplish-red, raised skin around the web, which may blister. Interdigital infection with the fungus *Candida albicans* can mimic these symptoms. It can also infect the nail fold and nail, producing chronic paronychia and a ridged and brown pigmented nail.

## WOUNDS

Injuries may be open or closed, the former implying a break in the epithelial covering and thus having a potential to undergo bacterial invasion. The terms 'open' and 'closed' are not synonymous with 'major' and 'minor' since a lethal injury, for example cardiac or cerebral trauma, may occur in either group.

The term 'wound' usually implies a break in the skin, irrespective of its aetiology, for example surgery or accidental injury, or of the amount of underlying tissue damage. There are a number of different classifications of wounds related to their position, their depth and the amount of tissue damage, for example incision, laceration and contusion. A common classification of surgical wounds is by their potential for infection:

- *Clean* wounds are those related to elective operations performed under sterile conditions with access through non-infected or non-contaminated skin. There is no breach of the gastrointestinal, genitourinary, biliary or respiratory tract. Direct primary closure (see below) can usually be achieved. Examples of clean operations include hernia repair.

- *Clean-contaminated* wounds are those in which urgent or emergency surgery is undertaken that would otherwise be described as clean. The operation is therefore under sterile conditions but there is elective opening of the respiratory, gastrointestinal, biliary or genitourinary tract with minimal spillage. No infected fluids, for example infected urine or bile, are encountered. Appendicectomy and cholecystectomy are examples.
- *Contaminated* surgery is that in which non-purulent inflammation is encountered. There may be gross spillage from the gastrointestinal tract, or entry into the biliary or genitourinary tract in the presence of infected bile or urine. Open fractures, penetrating trauma less than 4 hours old and bite injuries are contaminated wounds.
- *Dirty* wounds occur when an operation is carried out in the presence of pus such as an abscess, with preoperative perforation of the respiratory, biliary, gastrointestinal or genitourinary tract, or when there is penetrating trauma over 4 hours old. The risk of wound infection is considerably increased in these cases, which must be closely monitored for and promptly treated if it occurs.

Although such classifications are of practical value, each wound must be assessed independently for associated problems since even a small insect bite may result in a lethal anaphylactic response or be followed by marked cellulitis. The body responds to all injuries with an inflammatory response, this being capillary dilatation and the production of an inflammatory exudate incorporating both cellular and humoral responses to the damaged tissue.

Surgical incisions are placed along tension lines (Langer's lines) or skin creases and aim to avoid the underlying vessels, nerves and organs. In a wound closed with sutures, the apposed edges are sealed with the exudate and fibrin clot, and there is a firm union in 3–4 days. This is the first phase of **primary repair**.

In the second phase, there is capillary proliferation with an outgrowth of capillary buds and fibroblast migration, collagen deposition and epithelial ingrowth from each edge. This stage lasts from 4 to 15 days, during which there is increasing strength across the wound such that in the absence of tension, for example on the face and neck, the stitches can be removed in 3–4 days. In the abdomen, where there can be tension – coughing, straining and distension – stitches are left in for 10–14 days.

In the third phase of healing, there is contraction and maturation of the scar, with normal strength returning by approximately 3 months.

**Delayed primary repair** may be desired if a wound is initially contaminated; in this the wound is cleaned and left unapproximated before surgical closure 3 or 4 days later.

In non-apposed wounds, healing is by **secondary intention**, the inflammatory response producing a slough of damaged and dead tissue, foreign material and organisms. The capillary growth and fibroblast activity occur towards the surface and gradually replace the green slough with pink granulating tissue, with epithelial ingrowth from the surrounding edge. This type of wound healing is therefore described as healing 'from the bottom up'.

**Drains** may be placed in wounds to remove existing or anticipated blood, pus or body fluids, or to drain dead spaces where such collections may occur. They are removed when they stop draining, usually after 24–48 hours post-injury.

## Complications

Postoperative healing is promoted by the delicate handling of the tissues, minimizing tissue damage and bleeding, removing foreign or dead material, obliterating any dead space and ensuring the meticulous alignment of the skin edges, apposing the tissues without tension. Conversely, delayed healing occurs when there is residual dead, damaged or ischaemic tissue or foreign material, or when undrained dead space or a haematoma prevents tissue apposition. Foreign material, such as synthetic vascular grafts and joint prostheses, delays tissue ingrowth.

**Infection** is one of the most common complications of wound healing. There is variability in the reported rate but it is approximately 1–2 per cent in clean wounds and up to 8 per cent in those classified as dirty. Infection rates have drastically reduced with the use of routine prophylactic antibiotics – dirty wounds previously carried infection rates of up to 40 per cent. Signs of cellulitis are redness and discharge, which may become purulent. Staphylococci and streptococci are the usual organisms but gut flora may be involved or opportunistic infection in immunocompromised patients.

The majority of patients experience trivial discomfort and delayed healing. However, infection in a haematoma and collections with abscess formation carry a more serious prognosis. Persistent dead tissue or foreign bodies can result in sinus formation, and leaks from gut anastomoses may result in a **fistula**.

A number of factors have been implicated in delayed healing. These include malignancy, old age, hormonal abnormalities, steroid therapy, anaemia, diabetes and obesity. However, controlled studies of these factors are not well documented. Malnutrition, particularly hypoproteinaemia and vitamin C deficiency, does produce fragile wounds and poor healing but the degree of deficiency necessary to delay healing is unusual in Western society.

Vertical abdominal wounds are liable to stretch due to the tension from abdominal distension, trunk movements and coughing. Such wounds are prone to the late development of **incisional hernias** (Figure 4.62), particularly if multiple incisions are present.

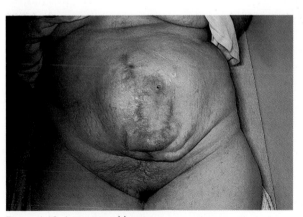

Figure 4.62 An incisional hernia.

PART 1 | PRINCIPLES

The powerful forces of coughing, vomiting and distension, linked with inadequate incorporation of the layers of the rectus sheath or early removal of the sutures, can give rise to a **burst abdomen**. This generally preventable complication is a major cause of morbidity following surgery. The burst may be heralded by a pink discharge of serous peritoneal fluid, indicating disruption of the deeper layers, before the skin gives way. The wound should be immediately covered with sterile gauze soaked in saline and a sterile occlusive dressing before taking the patient back to theatre as a matter of urgency. In theatre, the wound is usually reopened to remove the suture material and wash the wound out before resuturing, often with tension sutures.

## Hypertrophic Scars and Keloids

Some wounds are accompanied by a fibrous overgrowth and enlargement of the scar. In a **hypertrophic scar** (Figure 4.63), this fibrous reaction is limited to the margins of the scar, which is pink, may be tender and may itch. The scar can continue to enlarge for about 6 months but it regresses after a year to pale, thin, stretched scar tissue.

The heaping-up and overgrowth of the scar in **keloid** formation (Figure 4.64) is composed of hyperplastic vascular collagen fibres, which can extend in a claw-like fashion into the adjacent tissues. The process can continue for a number of years. It is common in individuals with pigmented skin, in children and in pregnancy, and it may be familial. Keloid is distributed more commonly in the midline over the face and the neck, the sternum and the anterior abdominal wall. It can be copious after burns, radiotherapy, scarification and puncture wounds, such as BCG (bacille Calmette–Guérin) inoculation sites and pierced ears.

Hypertrophic tissue in a wound may be due to a foreign body response to a suture or other foreign material (Figure 4.65).

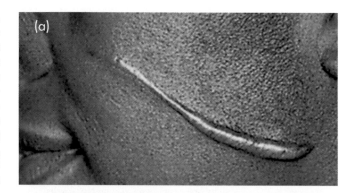

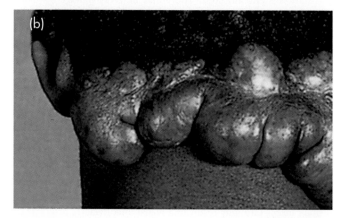

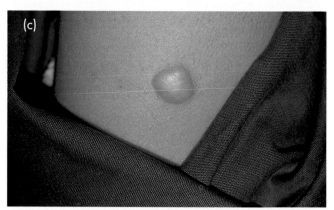

Figure 4.64 (a) Facial keloid. (b) Cervical keloid. (c) Keloid at a vaccination site.

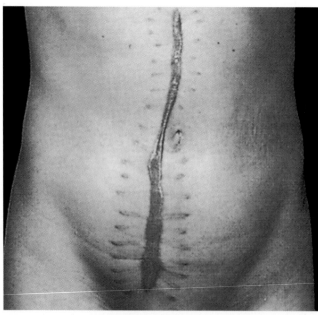

Figure 4.63 A hypertrophic abdominal scar.

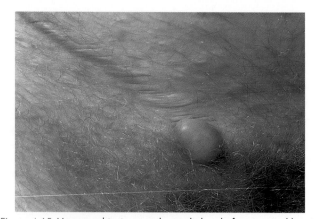

Figure 4.65 Hypertrophic tissue at the medial end of an inguinal hernia wound due to a foreign body response to a suture.

## Key Points

- Inflammation may be defined as the body's physiological response to tissue injury. It is usually classified into acute and chronic based on its time course and characteristic pathophysiological features.
- Acute inflammation constitutes a range of local (redness, swelling, heat, pain, loss of function) and systemic (pyrexia, weight loss) signs and symptoms.
- Chronic inflammation is a sequela of acute inflammation in which the key mechanism is an immune response to a persisting damaging agent.
- The SIRS is an excessive, uncontrolled inflammatory state defined by criteria including temperature, the heart and respiratory rates and the white cell count. Compensatory mechanisms such as CARS are described, with the balance of each leading to the patient's clinical presentation and outcomes.
- Infections commonly arise from regular skin commensals becoming pathogens by breaching the body surface and multiplying. Immunocompromised patients are susceptible to opportunisitic infections in which non-pathogenic organisms may cause infective states. Common skin infections include cellulitis. Necrotizing fasciitis is a life-threatening spread of infection along the fascial planes that requires urgent surgical excision.
- An abscess is a collection of pus resulting from unresolved inflammation, usually requiring drainage. Chronic abscesses may arise from infections such as tuberculosis leading to a granulomatous response.
- Common viral, fungal, worm and parasitic diseases such as malaria impact upon the surgical presentation as a differential diagnosis or for management, as do characteristic infections of the hand and foot.
- The surgical classification of wounds into clean, clean-contaminated, contaminated and dirty serves to pre-empt the likelihood of infection and the requirement for antibiotics.
- Wound healing is by primary repair (sutures), delayed primary repair (sutured after the initial procedure) or secondary intention by allowing granulation. Complications include infection, fistulas, wound dehiscence, incisional hernias and hypertrophic and keloid scar formation.

## SBAs

**1. Which of the following is not a diagnostic criterion for the systemic inflammatory response syndrome?:**

a Heart rate >80 bpm
b Respiratory rate >20 breaths per minute
c Temperature <36°C
d Temperature >38°C
e White cell count < 4 × 109 cells/L or >12 × 109 cells/L

**Answer**

*a* **Heart rate >80 bpm.** *The criteria for systemic inflammatory response syndrome state a heart rate of >90 bpm.*

**2. Which of the following mediators of inflammation is primarily involved in chronic inflammation?:**

a Neutrophils
b Prostaglandins
c Macrophages
d Chemokines
e Leukotrienes

**Answer**

*c* **Macrophages.** *The predominant cell type mediating chronic inflammation is macrophages, to phagocytose, or ingest, pathogens and cellular debris.*

**3. Which of the following would be classified as a 'clean-contaminated' surgical wound?:**

a Appendicectomy
b Hartmann's procedure for perforated diverticular disease
c Incision and drainage of a perianal abscess
d Open inguinal hernia repair
e External fixation of an open tibial fracture

**Answer**

*a* **Appendicectomy.** *Appendicectomy is an example of a clean-contaminated procedure, which describes an urgent or emergency case undertaken that would otherwise be described as clean. The operation is carried out under sterile conditions, but there is elective opening of the respiratory, gastrointestinal, biliary or genitourinary tract with minimal spillage. No infected fluids, for example infected urine or bile, are encountered.*

## EMQs

**1. For each of the following descriptions, select the most likely type of infection from the list below. Each option may be used once, more than once or not at all:**

1 Cellulitis
2 Syphilis
3 Meleney's synergistic gangrene or ulceration
4 Pyoderma gangrenosum
5 Fournier's gangrene
6 Tetanus
7 Necrotizing fasciitis
8 Hidradenitis suppurativa
9 Tuberculosis
10 Actinomycosis

a A diabetic patient with a painful, erythematous leg after an insect bite. The pain initially appears disproportionately high compared with the clinical signs, but the patient rapidly becomes unwell with pyrexia and tachycardia 24 hours later, with the skin becoming grey and necrotic

b A 35-year-old woman with an abscess in her left axilla. On examination, she has extensive scarring and sinus formation in both axillae

**Answers**

*a* **7 Necrotizing fasciitis.** *Risk factors for necrotizing fasciitis include diabetes, and it may follow innocuous insect bites or surgical wounds. There must be a high index of suspicion as the skin changes are initially few, but the pain the patient experiences is disproportionately high. Patients rapidly progress to systemic septic shock and mortality is high.*

*b* **8 Hidradenitis suppurativa.** *This is a description of hidradenitis suppurativa, in which abscesses develop in the sweat glands, commonly in the axillae. The progression is that of persistent abscess formation requiring incision and drainage, leaving chronic scarring and sinus formation.*

*c* **4 Pyoderma gangrenosum.** *This is a description of pyoderma gangrenosum, which typically occurs on the legs. It is associated with diseases such as inflammatory bowel disease, as well as with arthritides and haematological disorders such as leukaemias.*

*d* **2 Syphilis.** *The description is of sexually transmitted syphilis caused by Treponema pallidum.*

**c** A patient with Crohn's disease found to have a lesion on the leg that appears as tender blue nodules progressing over time to skin necrosis. Multiple sinuses and exuberant granulation are seen

**d** A patient presenting with a penile lesion 25 days after an unprotected sexual encounter. The lesion appears to be ulcerative, with a sloping edge and a bloodstained discharge. There is associated regional non-suppurative lymphadenopathy

**e** A patient arriving from Africa 1 week ago presenting with dysphagia, irritability and trismus. He has a wound on the sole of his left foot made by stepping on a rusty nail 8 days ago

2. **From each of the following descriptions, select the most likely type of hand infection from the list below. Each option may be used once, more than once or not at all:**
   1 Herpetic whitlow
   2 Tendon sheath infection
   3 Paronychia
   4 Orf
   5 Thenar space infection
   6 Apical abscess
   7 Pulp space infection

**a** A sheep farmer presenting with a painless, vesicular macular lesion on the tip of his left index finger. He is otherwise fit and well

**b** A painful, erythematous swelling at the side of the right middle finger nail fold in a kitchen porter

**c** A seamstress presenting hours after a penetrating injury from a needle to the left index finger flexor crease with a throbbing pain in the area. On examination, she is found to be pyrexial and is holding the finger in a flexed position. Active finger flexion is absent, and passive extension elicits severe pain

**d** A nurse presenting with a painful blister over the left thumb found to contain herpes simplex virus

*Important differential diagnoses are carcinoma of the penis and chancroid.*

**e 6 Tetanus.** *Tetanus is still seen in the developing world and is associated with rust harbouring the Clostridium tetani bacterium in a puncture wound. Trismus – spasm of the facial muscles – is an early sign.*

*Answers*

**a 4 Orf.** *Orf is a poxvirus primarily carried by sheep and goats as well as other animals. It presents as a painless lesion with no systemic symptoms.*

**b 3 Paronychia.** *This is a tender, erythematous infection seen after direct or indirect damage to the nails or cuticles, such as that sustained from heavy kitchen work.*

**c 2 Tendon sheath infection.** *The description of a penetrating injury with a rapid progression to systemic features and the hand signs given is typical of a tendon sheath infection. Tenderness along the tendon sheath is also a feature.*

**d 1 Herpetic whitlow.** *These occur commonly in healthcare workers in contact with infected patients. They present as painful blisters initially containing clear fluid but later with pus and debris expelled.*

# HIV and AIDS

Kelly Morris, Maurice Murphy and Lynn Riddell

## LEARNING OBJECTIVES

- To be able to describe the nature of HIV infection and its clinical progression
- To recognize pointers to HIV infection and develop an index of suspicion for the disease
- To indicate the important surgical manifestations of HIV
- To be able to specify principles of HIV testing

- To explain preventive measures for occupational exposure
- To be able to discuss issues surrounding HIV-positive surgeons
- To summarize the general principles of perioperative care in HIV-positive patients

## INTRODUCTION

Human immunodeficiency virus (HIV) and conditions related to HIV infection have had a significant impact on surgical practice. Acquired immunodeficiency syndrome (AIDS) was reported in 1981, and the causal agent (Figure 5.1) was identified in 1984. The latest global figures show that almost 37 million people are living with HIV, with 2.3 million new infections and 1.5 million AIDS-related deaths having occurred in 2013.

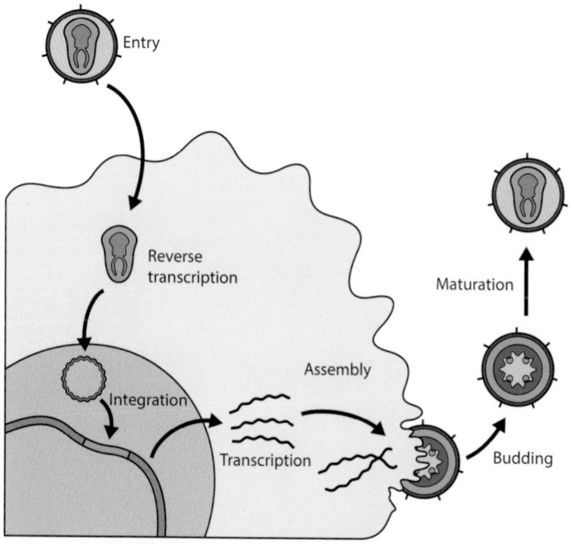

Figure 5.1 The HIV life cycle. Virions enter and bud from the cells. (Redrawn from SIB/ViralZone.)

The spectrum of surgical pathology related to HIV often depends on the geographical location of the surgical practice and whether the area has a high, low or rising prevalence of HIV. Patients with HIV and AIDS also develop the same surgical conditions as an age-, sex- and race-matched population without HIV. However, with advancing immunodeficiency their presentation may differ due to the relative lack of an inflammatory response. Conditions related to treatment of HIV disease are now presenting to surgical practice.

## THE PANDEMIC

HIV is a **blood-borne infection** that is mainly transmitted by:

- sexual intercourse;
- mother-to-child transmission during the birth process or breastfeeding;
- exposure to infected blood, bloodstained fluids or blood products.

The HIV pandemic has evolved and changed as a result of public health responses and the availability of antiretroviral treatment (Figure 5.2 and Table 5.1). Globally, around 50 per cent of people who are infected are thought to be unaware of their status.

Local epidemics vary between different geographical areas, showing three basic patterns of:

- high-prevalence areas, where there are high levels of heterosexual transmission and mother-to-child transmission;
- low-prevalence areas, where infections occur mainly in men who have sex with men (MSM), intravenous drug users, commercial sex workers, immigrants from high-prevalence countries, the recipients of inadequately screened blood and

# Adults and children estimated to be living with HIV|2013

**North America and Western and Central Europe**
**2.3 million**
(2.0 million – 3.0 million)

**Eastern Europe &
Central Asia
1.1 million**
(980 000 – 1.3 million)

**Caribbean
250 000**
(230 000 – 280 000)

**Middle East & North Africa
230 000**
(160 000 – 330 000)

**Asia and the Pacific
4.8 million**
(4.1 million – 5.5 million)

**Latin America
1.6 million**
(1.4 million – 2.1 million)

**Sub-Saharan Africa
24.7 million**
(23.5 million – 26.1 million)

## Total: 35.0 million (33.2 million – 37.2 million)

Figure 5.2 The state of the HIV pandemic, 2013.

Table 5.1 Features of the HIV pandemic in early 2015

The number of new infections and AIDS-related deaths has fallen to the lowest level since the peak of the pandemic

People living with HIV in richer countries experience normal lifespans owing to effective treatment

Large numbers of those eligible for treatment in low- and middle-income countries can access antiretroviral drugs. However, 19 000 000 of those estimated to be infected do not know their status

Measures to reduce transmission have had an enormous impact in many African countries, the Caribbean, South and South-East Asia and India

Epidemics are emerging in Eastern and Central Europe, Central Asia, the Middle-East, North Africa and Oceania

concern in this group is late presentation with advanced immunodeficiency, which carries a substantially increased risk of AIDS-defining illnesses and death. European estimates suggest that 15–38 per cent of individuals with HIV have advanced immunosuppression at the time of their first positive test. Thus, an index of suspicion for HIV disease and a knowledge of the characteristics of the local epidemic are necessary in current surgical practice in order to diagnose the condition (Figures 5.3 and 5.4).

blood products, marginalized groups including indigenous communities and the sexual partners of these groups;
• areas of rising prevalence, where infections are spreading from high-risk groups to the general population.

HIV-positive patients might present to the surgeon:

• declaring their HIV status;
• aware of their HIV status but withholding disclosure;
• unaware of their HIV status.

In the UK, it is estimated that around one-third of HIV-positive individuals are unaware of their diagnosis. Of great

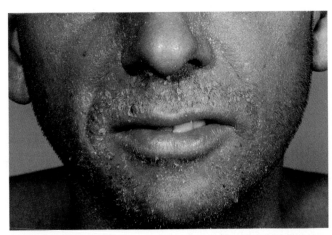

Figure 5.3 Extensive and severe seborrhoeic dermatitis in a gay man from the UK.

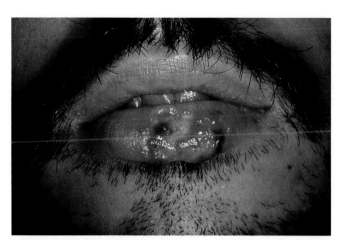

Figure 5.4 Chronic and severe labial herpes simplex. (Courtesy of CDC/Sol Silverman.)

## NATURAL HISTORY

Without treatment, clinical HIV infection invariably progresses to symptomatic disease, AIDS and death. The recognized clinical features of the disease are described below.

## Aetiology and Pathogenesis

HIV is a retrovirus that infects many cell types but shows a propensity for immune cells. Human cellular mechanisms are hijacked to produce further viral particles, and the ongoing viral replication disrupts both cell-mediated and humoral immunity. The primary immune deficit is the loss of CD4-positive T lymphocytes (T helper or CD4 cells). Progressive clinical disease is accompanied by characteristic changes in the levels of both CD4 cells and HIV RNA (Figure 5.5). Progressive immunodeficiency develops and uncommon (opportunist) infections and neoplastic processes occur.

## Primary/Acute HIV Infection

After infection, HIV establishes reservoirs of infection in many tissues. The virus replicates in activated CD4 cells that then migrate to lymphoid tissue. Viral particles appear in the blood from around 4–11 days after infection. Once infection with HIV has occurred, it may take several weeks for the body to mount an immune response. Standard HIV tests detect the presence of antibodies to the virus, so in this early period of infection – the 'window period' – routine HIV testing will be negative (Figures 5.5 and 5.6).

**Seroconversion** occurs once the body has mounted an immune response to the virus and antibodies have been produced. In a minority of patients, an **acute retroviral syndrome** may be reported, often retrospectively. This consists of:

- glandular fever-like symptoms;
- lymphadenopathy;
- a sore throat;
- a maculopapular rash.

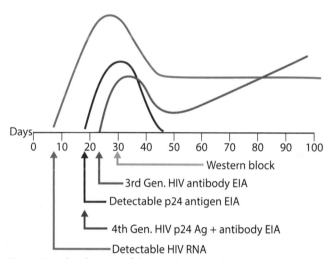

Figure 5.6 The duration of the window period depends on the type of test in use. RNA testing can detect HIV infection in days, whereas other tests become positive later (e.g. fourth-generation tests that detect antigen and antibody usually become positive in 18–42 days). EIA: enzyme immunoassay.

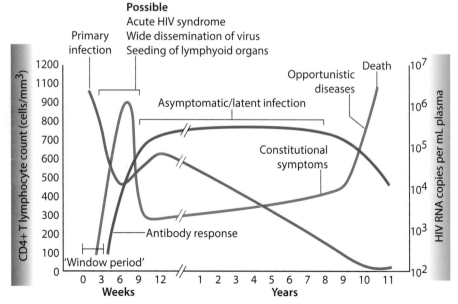

Figure 5.5 A timeline of changes in CD4 count and viral load over time in untreated HIV infection with an antibody response. The initial sharp decline (up to 30 per cent) of the total CD4 cell population is usually rapidly restored once the developing antibodies have mounted a partial response to the virus. HIV tests that rely on detecting antibodies only become positive after the window period (seroconversion).

PART 1 | PRINCIPLES

The identification of **primary infection**, where possible, is extremely important in guiding clinical management and prevent ongoing transmission.

## Latent Infection

After seroconversion, most individuals enter a **clinically latent phase** during which they are relatively asymptomatic despite rapid viral multiplication in the tissues and lymph nodes. Without treatment, the duration of clinical latency varies widely among individuals and may last for 2–8 years.

During this period, CD4 cells – the 'conductors of the immune system' – decline in number and function, by about 60 cells/μL per year. Progressive CD4 cell loss impairs the orchestration of an effective immune response. Individuals with low CD4 counts are particularly susceptible to infection with viruses, fungi and intracellular pathogens such as *Salmonella* and *Mycobacterium tuberculosis*, the cause of tuberculosis (TB). The CD4 count is strongly correlated to the degree of clinical immunosuppression.

Dysfunction of the humoral (antibody) response has many manifestations including:

- a global increase in antibodies (hypergammaglobulinaemia);
- a failure of the function and formation of antibodies (e.g. a failure of immunization and infection with encapsulated organisms, including *Streptococcus pneumoniae* and *Haemophilus influenzae*);
- excessive IgE production causing, for example, eczema, seborrhoeic dermatitis (see Figure 5.3) and urticaria;
- adverse drug reactions (Figures 5.7 and 5.8), which may occur to previously tolerated antibiotics and other medications;
- vasculitis (Figure 5.9).

The **early stigmata** of HIV infection, such as oral candidiasis (Figure 5.10), thrombocytopenia, seborrhoeic dermatitis and hairy oral leukoplakia (HOL) (Figure 5.11), gradually become apparent. Patients may repeatedly present to the healthcare services over a protracted period of time with apparently unlinked physical complaints.

As the CD4 cell count declines, patients become increasingly susceptible to commensal organisms and opportunist infections that would rarely cause pathological disease in healthy individuals. Multiple infectious agents may coexist, so that the isolation of one organism does not exclude the presence of other opportunists, which should be actively excluded. Multiple specimens for microbiology, virology, cytology and histopathology are of paramount importance.

## Symptomatic HIV Disease and AIDS

Untreated patients eventually develop one or more of the designated unusual infections or malignancies that define them as having AIDS. The prognosis of untreated HIV infection is very poor, with death occurring on average 8–10 years after infection and 2 years after a diagnosis of AIDS. However, individual progression varies widely.

Bacterial infections, oral candida, tuberculosis, Kaposi's sarcoma and non-CNS lymphoma occur at a wide range of CD4 counts. However, some AIDS-defining illnesses usually occur once the CD4 count (cells/μL) has fallen below certain thresholds, for example:

- below 200 cells/μL – *Pneumocystis* pneumonia, cryptosporidiosis, microsporidiosis, oesophageal candida;

PART 1  |  PRINCIPLES

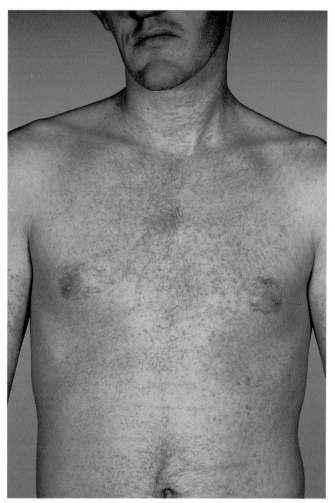

Figure 5.7 **An acute drug reaction. A non-specific maculopapular rash.**

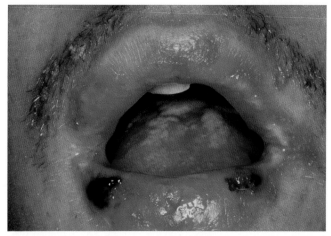

Figure 5.8 Stevens–Johnson syndrome. There may be severe mucosal involvement of the whole gastrointestinal tract as well as of the conjunctiva.

- below 100 cells/μL – toxoplasmosis, cryptococcosis, histoplasmosis, systemic cytomegalovirus (CMV) infection;
- below 50 cells/μL – CMV retinitis, *Mycobacterium avium* complex, CNS lymphoma, progressive multifocal leukoencephalopathy.

However, these thresholds are given for guidance and are not absolute.

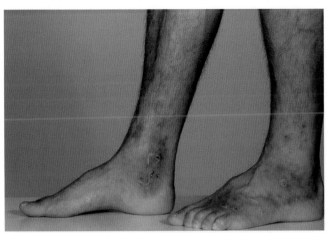

Figure 5.9 A vasculitic rash. Classically seen on the lower limbs, residual pigmentation develops as healing occurs.

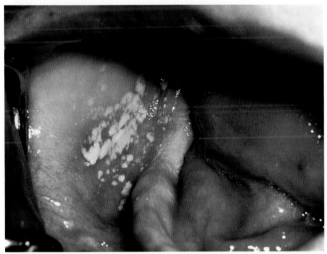

Figure 5.10 Candidiasis affecting the buccal mucosa. (Courtesy of CDC/Sol Silverman.)

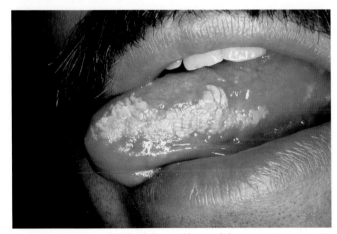

Figure 5.11 Hairy oral leukoplakia. Unlike candidiasis (see Figure 5.10), this cannot be scraped off. (Courtesy of CDC/Sol Silverman.)

The pattern of HIV-related and AIDS-defining illnesses depends upon the population. For example, in developed nations AIDS tends to present with commensal organisms such as *Candida albicans* and *Pneumocystis jirovecii* pneumonia (formerly *Pneumocystis carinii* pneumonia or PCP); MSM are more likely to develop CMV disease, as well as Kaposi's sarcoma (KS) caused by co-infection with human herpes virus 8. Hepatitis B and C co-infections and abscesses are common in intravenous drug users, while TB and severe and recurrent bacterial infections are extremely common in developing countries. Worldwide, epidemics of TB and HIV are acting synergistically to increase both morbidity and mortality.

## TREATMENT

Effective **antiretroviral therapy** (ART), consisting of combination drug treatments taken on an ongoing basis, has had the most impact on the prognosis of HIV. Since the introduction of ART, mortality from HIV disease has fallen by over 90 per cent in industrialized countries, and for at least 5 years after seroconversion remains similar to the mortality in the general population. Effective regimens of antiretroviral agents are now available in most countries. Access to treatment and the availability of newer medications remain limited in some countries.

ART often results in substantial immune restoration. However, patients whose immune systems fail to reconstitute effectively and who have persistently low CD4 counts remain at high risk of opportunist infections. The risk and progression of certain conditions, for example anal cancer, are not, however, affected by ART.

## Complications of Antiretroviral Therapy

**Immune restoration inflammatory syndrome** (Figure 5.12) is a well-recognized complication of ART initiation. Extensive inflammatory reactions, usually to existing pathogens (viable or non-viable), are the most common cause. However, a worsening of some neoplasms and autoimmune phenomena also occur. Patients may present to surgeons, usually 4–8 weeks after starting ART, with rapidly enlarging, painful lymph node(s). Underlying infections, especially viral, fungal and mycobacterial, need to be sought, and discussion with HIV clinicians is helpful to guide diagnostic procedures, such as biopsies, and the use of steroids.

ART can cause significant long-term side-effects, including pancreatitis, renal calculi, accelerated atherosclerosis, bone disease and metabolic syndrome, which may necessitate surgical intervention. HIV-positive individuals now have a longer life expectancy and clinicians are faced with a new spectrum of pathology. As this patient population ages, the need for surgical interventions, such as coronary revascularization, is likely to rise.

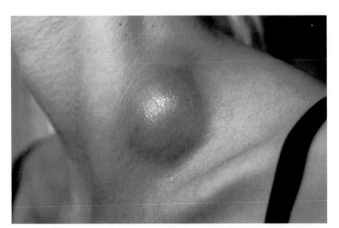

Figure 5.12 Enlarged, inflamed and tender lymph node due to immune restoration inflammatory syndrome. (Courtesy of Professor R. Colebunders.)

## POINTERS TO POSSIBLE HIV INFECTION

When an HIV-positive patient presents to an on-call surgeon with no knowledge of their status, the attending surgeon is in a position to make the diagnosis of HIV. A high index of suspicion facilitates testing and diagnosis, and a positive result can radically alter the management and prognosis of HIV disease. Careful history-taking and examination is key. Certain pointers on examination or the presence of indicator diseases (Table 5.2) should increase the index of suspicion and prompt more detailed questioning on lifestyle factors and a discussion of HIV testing.

## High-risk Behaviour

Questions about high-risk behaviour might be appropriate during history-taking or if pointers to HIV infection are noted on the general examination. With tactful, non-judgemental enquiry, patients may reveal that they have engaged in high-risk activities such as:

- the use of injected drugs and crack cocaine (Figure 5.13);
- unprotected male sex with other men;
- commercial sex work;
- unprotected sex with individuals from countries with a high prevalence of HIV;

Table 5.2 Clinical indicator diseases for adult HIV infection (UK)

| | AIDS-defining conditions | Other conditions for which HIV testing should be offered |
|---|---|---|
| Respiratory | Tuberculosis | Bacterial pneumonia |
| | *Pneumocystis* | Aspergillosis |
| Neurology | Cerebral toxoplasmosis | Aseptic meningitis/encephalitis |
| | Primary cerebral lymphoma | Cerebral abscess |
| | Cryptococcal meningitis | Space-occupying lesion of unknown cause |
| | Progressive multifocal leukoencephalopathy | Guillain–Barré syndrome |
| | | Transverse myelitis |
| | | Peripheral neuropathy |
| | | Dementia |
| | | Leukoencephalopathy |
| Dermatology | Kaposi's sarcoma | Severe or recalcitrant seborrhoeic dermatitis |
| | | Severe or recalcitrant psoriasis |
| | | Multidermatomal or recurrent herpes zoster |
| Gastroenterology | Persistent cryptosporidiosis | Oral candidiasis |
| | | Oral hairy leukoplakia |
| | | Chronic diarrhoea of unknown cause |
| | | Weight loss of unknown cause |
| | | *Salmonella*, *Shigella* or *Campylobacter* |
| | | Hepatitis B infection |
| | | Hepatitis C infection |
| Oncology | Non-Hodgkin's lymphoma | Anal cancer or anal intraepithelial dysplasia |
| | | Lung cancer |
| | | Seminoma |
| | | Head and neck cancer |
| | | Hodgkin's lymphoma |
| | | Castleman's disease |
| Gynaecology | Cervical cancer | Vaginal intraepithelial neoplasia |
| | | Cervical intraepithelial neoplasia Grade 2 or above |
| Haematology | | Any unexplained blood dyscrasia including: |
| | | – Thrombocytopenia |
| | | – Neutropenia |
| | | – Lymphopenia |
| Ophthalmology | Cytomegalovirus retinitis | Infective retinal diseases including |
| | | Herpes viruses and *Toxoplasma* |
| | | Any unexplained retinopathy |
| Ear, nose and throat | | Lymphadenopathy of unknown cause |
| | | Chronic parotitis |
| | | Lymphoepithelial parotid cysts |
| Other | | Mononucleosis-like syndrome (primary HIV infection) |
| | | Pyrexia of unknown origin |
| | | Any lymphadenopathy of unknown cause |
| | | Any sexually transmitted infection |

UK National Guidelines for HIV Testing 2008 (http://www.bhiva.org/documents/Guidelines/Testing/GlinesHIVTest08_Tables1-2.pdf).

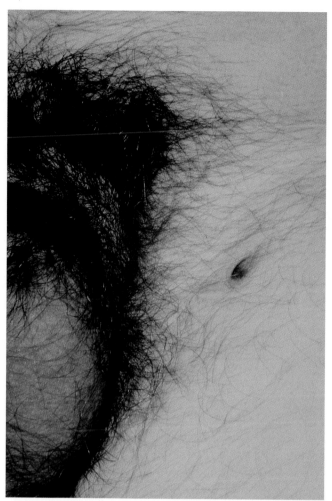

Figure 5.13 Intravenous mainline scarring. Repeated femoral stabs have caused a large single scar. 'Track marks' or small scars along the course of veins and arteries may also commonly be seen on the forearms or feet.

- the receipt of blood transfusions or blood products where screening was not available;
- unprotected sex with individuals that would fit a description in the list above.

## PHYSICAL SIGNS OF HIV INFECTION

This section reviews the signs of HIV disease that a surgeon might encounter and discusses the notable causes within each system. The key principles are as follows:

- a single pathology can present in several systems. For example, common presentations of CMV infection are retinitis and colitis.
- different pathologies can underlie a single presentation. For example, the symptoms of dysphagia (difficulty swallowing) and odynophagia (painful swallowing) could occur with fungal, viral or neoplastic lesions, and all these need to be excluded.
- multiple pathologies often coexist and 'opportunists hunt in packs'. For instance, gastrointestinal endoscopic sampling might concurrently identify mycobacteria, viruses and fungi, while a patient with lymphadenopathy, fever and wasting might have both lymphoma and TB.

Any patient in whom HIV infection is a possibility should, where possible, be discussed with colleagues who are experienced in the management of HIV infection. The following descriptions include the physical manifestations that a surgical practice is most likely to encounter.

## General Examination

### Constitutional Symptoms

Unexplained fever or weight loss accompanied by signs of prolonged ill-health, including wasting, are common in HIV-positive individuals presenting as an emergency.

### Generalized Lymphadenopathy

**Peripheral generalized lymphadenopathy** (PGL) is characterized by lymph nodes of less than 2 cm in diameter that are bilaterally symmetrical, smooth, rubbery, mobile and non-tender (Figure 5.14). By definition, the syndrome requires that the lymph nodes be present at two or more extrainguinal sites for a minimum of 3–6 months with no other diagnosis or explanation for their presence. The most frequently involved node groups are the posterior and anterior cervical, occipital, axillary and submandibular. PGL is a highly sensitive marker for HIV so its presence should prompt an evaluation of HIV status.

Histology of the lymph nodes reveals follicular hyperplasia. The differential diagnosis includes:

- lymphoma, usually of the non-Hodgkin's type;
- TB;
- *Mycobacterium avium* complex (MAC);
- secondary syphilis;
- infectious mononucleosis;
- KS;
- a primary head and neck malignancy.

In endemic areas, TB accounts for the majority of presentations with lymphadenopathy and lymphadenitis. Fine needle aspiration is often the initial diagnostic procedure of choice. However, open biopsy is indicated in a patient with systemic symptoms if the cytology of an aspirate is negative. Where there is a clinical suspicion of lymphoma (often asymmetrical, large or rapidly enlarging nodes), an open biopsy remains the procedure of choice.

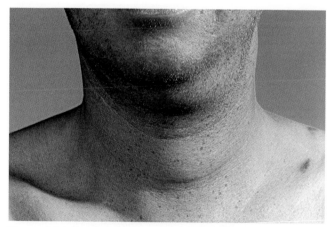

Figure 5.14 Peripheral generalized lymphadenopathy. Enlarged submandibular, submental and cervical lymph nodes – note the two Kaposi's sarcoma lesions on the left shoulder.

### Isolated Lymphadenopathy

Isolated, tender, rapidly expanding or thoracic lymphadenopathies are more suggestive of underlying malignancy or infection (Figure 5.15). Fine needle aspiration or preferably an open biopsy of the nodes is required to exclude conditions such as lymphoma, TB, MAC and KS. Immune restoration inflammatory syndrome needs to be considered in any patient who has recently started on ART, and advice should be sought from HIV specialists.

## Skin

### Evidence of Lifestyle

Careful examination of the skin may provide evidence of 'high-risk' behaviours. Abscess formation and 'track marks' at injection sites, which can occur in numerous body areas, suggest intravenous drug use. Prison tattoos and tattoos undertaken where needle-sharing or reuse is possible increase the risk of blood-borne acquisition of the virus. Evidence of other sexually transmitted infections (STIs) may be significant and their presence increases the risk of HIV.

### Rashes

**Seborrhoeic dermatitis** is evident in about 60–80 per cent of HIV-positive individuals. Although it also occurs with moderate frequency in HIV-negative individuals, it is often extensive and erythematous in the presence of HIV, and may be psoriaform in nature (Figure 5.16; see also Figure 5.3). It is commonly the first clinical manifestation of HIV disease. Patients often complain of 'burning' of the skin in the affected areas, particularly if there is contact with sweat.

**Psoriasis** can be the initial manifestation of HIV disease. It occurs at a prevalence similar to or greater than that seen in the general population, but its onset is often sudden. Involvement of the palms, soles and skin folds, including the groin, is especially common in advanced immunodeficiency.

**Herpes virus infections** occur with increasing frequency as the immune system deteriorates. In patients with a normal immune system, herpes simplex virus (HSV) infection is self-limiting and generally resolves in 4–5 days. Chronic recurrent HSV eruptions (Figure 5.17; see also Figure 5.4) and/or non-healing, ulcerating lesions commonly seen in the genital area may be the first indicator

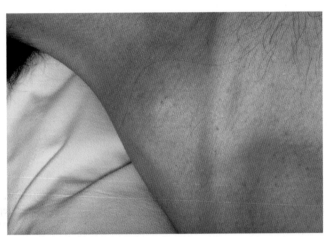

Figure 5.15 Isolated axillary lymphadenopathy. The diagnosis in this case was follicular hyperplasia.

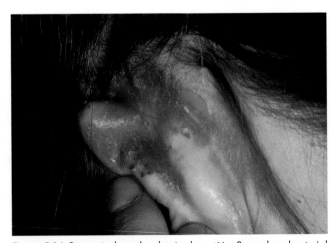

Figure 5.16 Postauricular seborrhoeic dermatitis. Secondary bacterial infection is common.

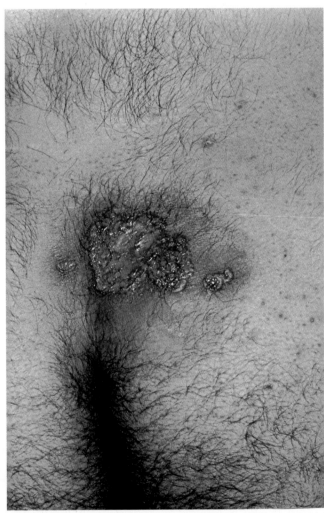

Figure 5.17 Sacral herpes simplex infection. These lesions are painful and, as shown here, commonly secondarily infected with bacteria. The typical blisters are often absent, leaving a widely sloughed ulcerated appearance.

of immunosuppression. Varicella-zoster virus causing shingles may leave characteristic dermatomal scarring (**Figure 5.18**), particularly on dark skin. The typical unidermatomal, vesicular lesion on an erythematous base seen in an otherwise healthy individual may, in HIV, be replaced with multidermatomal, and sometimes haemorrhagic or necrotic lesions (**Figure 5.19**).

## Discrete Lesions

**Cutaneous KS** is not pathognomonic of HIV infection. However, in the presence of HIV, cutaneous lesions are more widely distributed over the skin and occur in younger individuals than with the endemic form. These subcutaneous tumours are painless and non-pruritic, and vary in colour from brownish-red to dark purple (**Figures 5.20** and **5.21**). They occur as solitary or multiple plaques or nodules, and range from a few millimetres to several centimeters in diameter. In HIV infection, KS is not confined to the skin.

The clinical diagnosis of cutaneous KS is usually straightforward, although biopsy may occasionally be required to differentiate KS from other lesions, for example bacillary angiomatosis. Massive lymphoedema (seemingly out of proportion to the extent of the cutaneous KS) and overlying skin breakdown are two common complications that necessitate surgical intervention. In recent years, human herpes virus 8 has been identified as the causative agent.

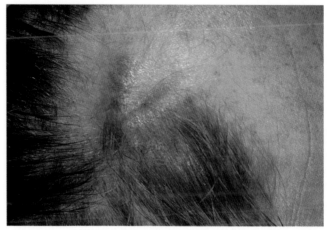

Figure 5.20 Kaposi's sarcoma. This scalp lesion is typically raised and not painful.

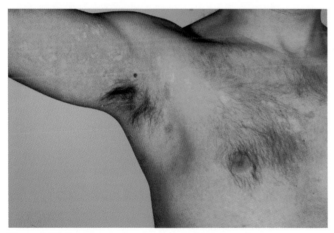

Figure 5.18 Depigmented scars of varicella-zoster infection.

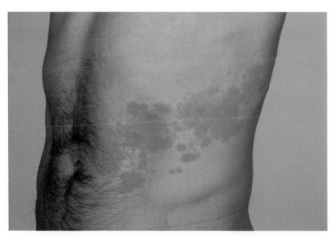

Figure 5.19 Multidermatomal shingles can be an indicator of HIV infection.

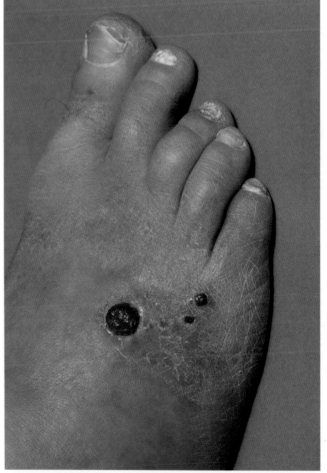

Figure 5.21 Kaposi's sarcoma. The raised lesions are surrounded by less obvious subcutaneous lesions that cause lymphoedema by lymphatic obstruction.

PART 1 | PRINCIPLES

**Molluscum contagiosum** is a benign condition caused by an as yet unidentified poxvirus. It is not confined to immunocompromised individuals. The characteristic small, pearly, firm, umbilicated papules are found on epithelial surfaces. In HIV-positive individuals, they have a predilection for the face (unlike in other adults), where they tend to increase in size, number and severity with advancing immunosuppression (Figures 5.22 and 5.23). Large and/or traumatized lesions may become secondarily infected.

## Head and Neck

Numerous manifestations of HIV infection occur in the head and neck. Oral lesions are especially common and are often the first manifestations of HIV infection. Common causes of lymphadenopathy have already been described, while HIV-associated eye disease is discussed below.

### Oral Cavity Lesions

Up to 90 per cent of people with AIDS have at least one kind of oral lesion. None of these are pathognomonic of infection with HIV, and their presentation and natural course vary considerably. Ominous lesions such as lymphomas may present in diverse forms, such as ulcers, masses and plaques. Biopsies for diagnostic purposes are frequently indicated to exclude a sinister lesion.

Oral and dental lesions strongly associated with HIV infection include:

- candidal infection;
- HOL;
- linear gingival erythema;
- necrotizing ulcerative gingivitis, periodontitis and stomatitis;
- KS;
- non-Hodgkin's lymphoma.

**KS** of the oral cavity, particularly the palate (**Figure 5.24**), may occur in isolation but more commonly indicates that systemic KS is also present. The lesions may be flat or raised – in the latter case they may interfere with normal oral function (**Figures 5.25** and **5.26**). Unlike cutaneous KS, it is not always easy to make a definitive clinical diagnosis from lesions of the oral cavity. Biopsy may be required to exclude lymphoma or infections such as fungal or mycobacterial lesions or syphilitic gummata.

**HOL** is not pathognomonic of HIV infection. However, it is a marker of symptomatic HIV disease and a poor prognostic indicator for progression to AIDS. The lesion is painless, white, raised and striated. Unlike candidiasis, HOL cannot be scraped off easily with a spatula. It occurs most commonly on the lateral borders of the tongue (**Figure 5.27**; see also Figure 5.11) but may also be seen on the tongue's surface, in the buccal mucosa

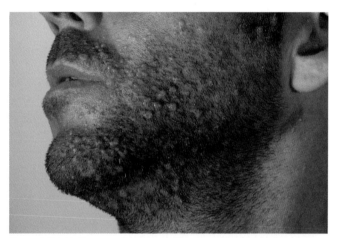

Figure 5.23 Molluscum contagiosum. Trauma from shaving exacerbates the spread of molluscum across the beard area. In adults with no immunodeficiency, such large extensive lesions in this distribution would be highly unusual.

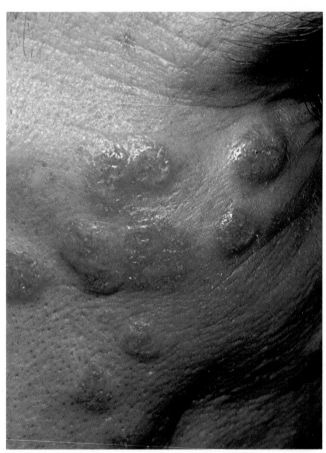

Figure 5.22 Molluscum contagiosum. Umbilication is seen on these large coalescing lesions.

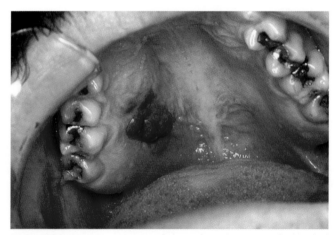

Figure 5.24 Kaposi's sarcoma of the palate. (Courtesy of CDC/Sol Silverman.)

or in the oesophagus (commonly the middle third), where the lesion may have a more plaque-like appearance. HOL is related to uncontrolled replication of the Epstein–Barr virus but is not a premalignant lesion.

**Oral candidiasis** is most commonly seen as an erythematous base from which white curd may be easily scraped (the pseudomembranous form; Figures 5.28 and 5.29; see also Figure 5.10). However, candidal infection may also form flat,

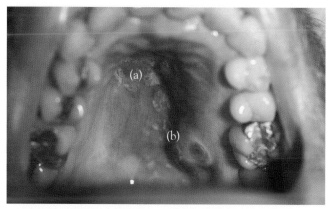

Figure 5.25 (a) Palatal Kaposi's sarcoma (KS). (b) KS lesions may ulcerate. Trauma from eating with subsequent secondary infection may result in severe pain and weight loss.

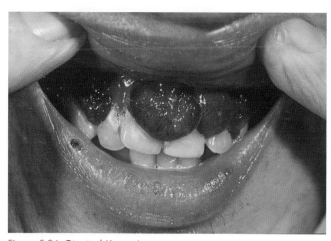

Figure 5.26 Gingival Kaposi's sarcoma.

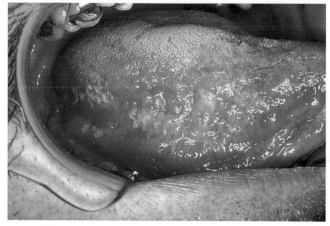

Figure 5.27 Early signs of hairy oral leukoplakia. (Courtesy of CDC/ Sol Silverman.)

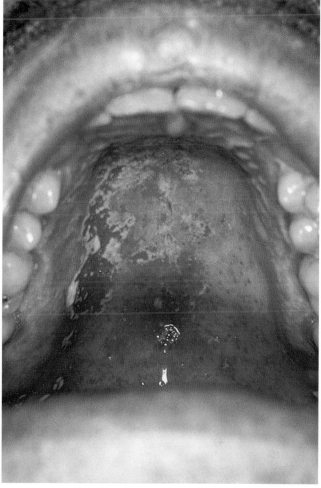

Figure 5.28 Oral candidiasis. The typical erythematous base from which the white plaques have sloughed off is often painful. This is the form most often seen in the oral cavity.

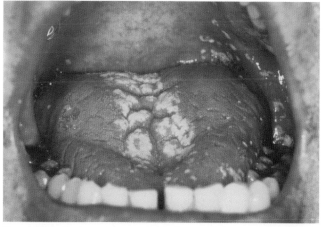

Figure 5.29 Oral candidiasis on the dorsum of the tongue and in the tonsillar bed.

PART 1 | PRINCIPLES

erythematous plaques. Since this atrophic form does not have the classic white exudate, it is often not recognized by clinicians, so an important pointer to an immunocompromised state of health is missed.

Oral candidiasis may exist in a hypertrophic form that manifests as a lesion similar to the plaque form of HOL (**Figure 5.30**). In this form, it may be distributed in similar locations to HOL, for example the lateral margin of the tongue, and may not be easily scraped off. The lesions of angular cheilitis (**Figure 5.31**) are often caused by candidal infection and/or bacterial infection and is a common indicator of iron deficiency.

## Oral Ulceration

Oral ulcers (**Figures 5.32–5.35**) are most commonly caused by HSV. Recurrent severe aphthous ulceration and CMV-induced ulceration may both cause significant pain and should also be included in the differential diagnosis. Polymerase chain reaction (PCR) testing should assist with diagnosis.

Difficulties with swallowing and speech may occur, and significant weight loss is a serious complication. A failure of medical treatment necessitates biopsy to exclude lymphoma and guide further therapy. Some medications and neutropenia may also cause ulceration.

### Tonsillar Lesions

Tonsillar swelling can be unilateral or bilateral. Recurrent tonsillitis can occur in symptomatic HIV infection. In the absence of signs of acute tonsillar infection, the differential diagnosis includes lymphoma, TB and non-neoplastic lymphoid tissue proliferation, including PGL. Unilateral tonsillar swelling raises concerns of a neoplastic cause and biopsy is usually indicated.

## Cardiovascular System

HIV infection is associated with several vascular manifestations, including vasculitis (see Figure 5.9), aneurysms and atherosclerosis. The incidence of cardiovascular disease, particularly coronary artery disease but also peripheral arterial compromise, is likely to be increased in the HIV-infected population compared with age-matched controls. Endothelial dysfunction is possibly the most plausible link between HIV infection and accelerated atherosclerosis, while various forms of frank vasculitis also occur. Antiretroviral agents, in particularly protease inhibitors, are

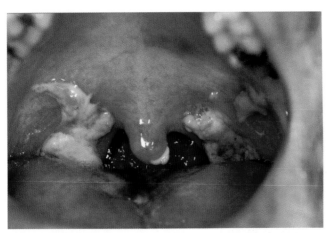

Figure 5.30 Hypertrophic oral candidiasis.

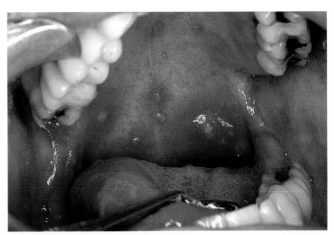

Figure 5.32 Aphthous ulceration. The typical presentation is multiple, small painful ulcers with surrounding erythema. (Courtesy of CDC/Sol Silverman.)

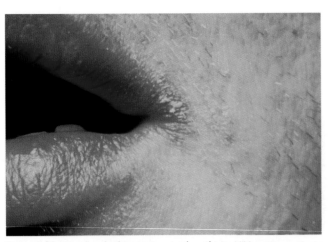

Figure 5.31 Angular cheilitis. Lesions such as this in HIV-positive patients are often due to candidal infection. (Courtesy of Dr M. Nathan.)

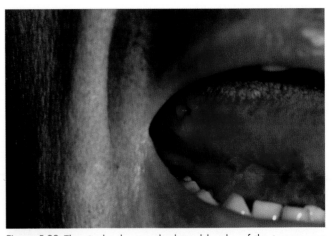

Figure 5.33 The single ulcer on the lateral border of the tongue was due to CMV infection. This diagnosis was made following a biopsy, undertaken after a failure of antiherpetic medication.

linked with a metabolic syndrome – dyslipidaemia, lipodystrophy and insulin resistance – that increases cardiovascular risk.

Pericardial effusion in patients from TB-endemic areas is rarely non-tuberculous. Surgical complications of a pericardial effusion in TB include tamponade and constrictive pericarditis. Aneurysms are reported especially in sub-Saharan Africa and can be atypically located and multiple. Syphilis and TB need to be excluded.

## Respiratory System

Respiratory symptoms with or without pulmonary infiltrates are common in patients with HIV. Often several coexisting organisms are isolated, including bacteria, mycobacteria and fungi. The need to take multiple specimens cannot be overemphasized. Such specimens are usefully obtained by bronchial lavage and transbronchial biopsy (**Figure 5.36**). Specimens should be sent for virological, bacterial, mycobacterial, fungal and histopathological studies.

***Pneumocystis jirovecii* pneumonia** is one of the most common causes of breathlessness in a patient with immunodeficiency (usually with CD4 count <200 cells/μL). It often presents with a normal chest radiograph and few, if any, signs on examination (**Figures 5.37** and **5.38**). A key clinical marker is desaturation on minimal exertion. The presence of signs and lobular or multilobular X-ray changes (**Figure 5.39**) often indicates bacterial infection, which is common. Focal signs raise the

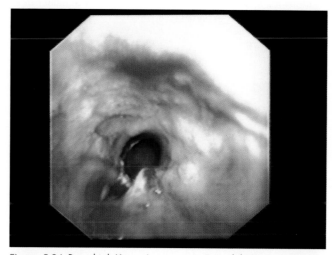

Figure 5.36 Bronchial Kaposi's sarcoma. Raised lesions may cause obstruction with wheezing, cough and recurrent bacterial infections. Sputum, if produced, often resembles marmalade rather than frank blood.

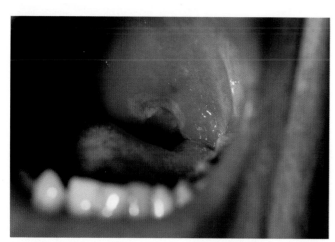

Figure 5.34 **Severe aphthous ulceration. This is a diagnosis of exclusion.**

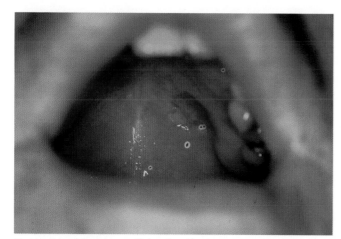

Figure 5.35 Ulceration of the hard palate. A high-grade B-cell lymphoma was identified on histology.

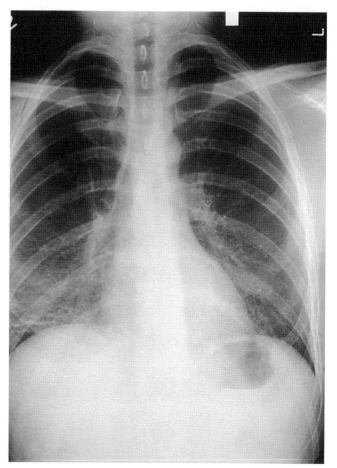

Figure 5.37 Chest radiograph of *Pneumocystis jirovecii* pneumonia. (Courtesy of CDC/Jonathan W M Gold.)

PART 1 | PRINCIPLES

suspicion of alternative pathologies such as tumours, mycobacteria, fungi, CMV and aggressive bacterial infection (**Figures 5.40** and **5.41**). It is common for several pathogens to coexist, and failure to respond to first-line therapy necessitates further investigations for other pathogens and pathologies. The incidence of lung cancer is raised in patients with HIV.

**Surgical complications** of thoracic infections (**Figure 5.42**) include empyema, which is often tuberculous, pneumothorax and bronchopleural fistulas, notably due to *Pneumocystis jirovecii* pneumonia. Pneumothorax secondary to *P. jirovecii* pneumonia has a high mortality rate.

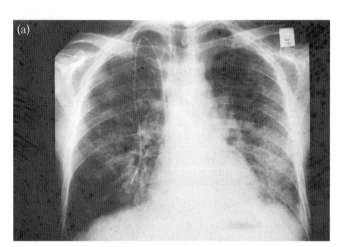 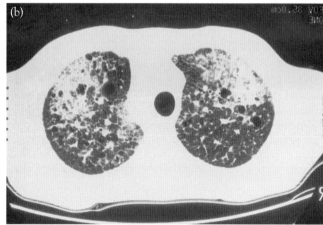

Figure 5.38 Interstitial process typical of *Pneumocystis jirovecii* pneumonia. (a) Chest radiograph. (b) High-resolution CT scan. Both show an extensive mid- and lower zone perihilar interstitial process typical of *P. jirovecii* pneumonia.

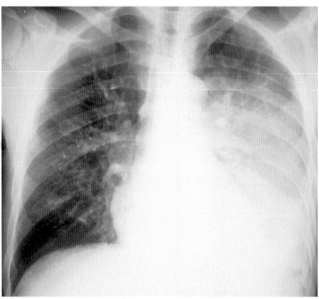

Figure 5.39 Pneumococcal pneumonia. (Courtesy of Professor R. Colebunders.)

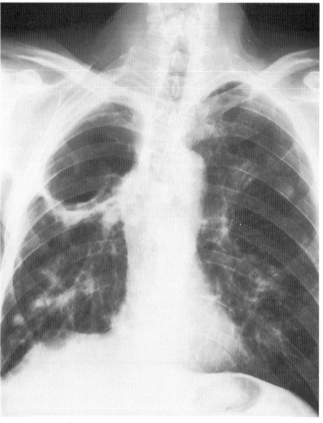

Figure 5.40 Tuberculosis. In a patient with multi-drug-resistant TB. (Courtesy of Professor R. Colebunders.)

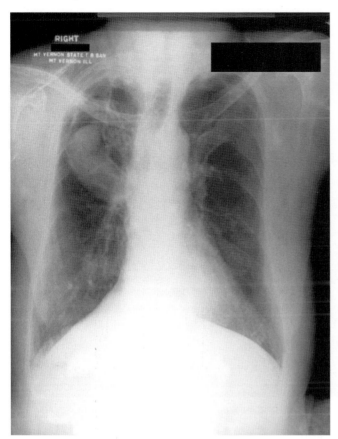

Figure 5.41 A 'ball' formed by fungal infection (right upper lobe), in this case aspergillosis (an aspergilloma). (Courtesy of CDC/M. Renz.)

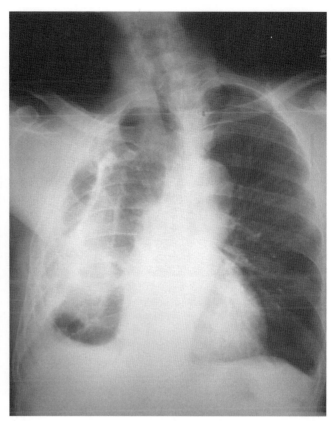

Figure 5.42 A right fibrothorax, thought to be due to a previous empyema. (Courtesy of CDC/Thomas Hooten.)

## Gastrointestinal System

### Oesophagus

Up to 90 per cent of patients with AIDS complain of odynophagia, dysphagia or retrosternal chest pain at some point in their illness. Oesophageal candidiasis is the most common cause. A trial of therapy is considered to be appropriate initial management. Failure to respond warrants further investigation to exclude other pathologies. Oesophagoscopy is the procedure of choice as a definitive diagnosis (or diagnoses) may be obtained by biopsies and brushings. As 10 per cent of patients have multiple pathologies, specimens must be sent for mycobacterial, viral, fungal and histological testing.

The differential diagnosis of dysphagia/odynophagia includes:

- oesophageal candidiasis;
- CMV and other herpetic viruses;
- idiopathic/apthous ulceration;
- KS and lymphoma.

**Oesophageal candidiasis (Figure 5.43)** may occasionally cause no symptoms, but it invariably presents with dysphagia. Nausea and epigastric pain commonly accompany the dysphagia but may occur independently. The upper half of the oesophagus is the most common site of involvement. In up to 30 per cent of cases, there is no concomitant oral candidiasis. Oesophageal stricture and rupture are uncommon.

In terms of **viral infections**, CMV infection tends to involve the lower third of the oesophagus and typically causes large, single, deep, linear ulcers. HSV forms multiple small, shallow ulcers. Ulceration due to Epstein–Barr virus is relatively uncommon and predominantly occurs in the mid-oesophageal region.

Any of the lesions described above may exhibit bacterial superinfection. Although uncommon in the oesophagus, MAC and TB may be isolated.

### Stomach and Bowel

HIV-related disease manifests throughout the gastrointestinal system. It is important to remember that HIV-positive individuals still present with the same routine surgical (and medical) conditions of the abdomen as HIV-negative individuals. The diagnosis of HIV-related gastrointestinal conditions, as with other systems, is based on the predominant symptom(s), the clinical signs, an assessment of immunodeficiency and multiple samples.

Important presentations of HIV-related gastrointestinal disease are:

- abdominal pain;
- diarrhoea;
- gastrointestinal bleeding;
- an abdominal mass;
- obstruction;
- perforation;

PART 1 | PRINCIPLES

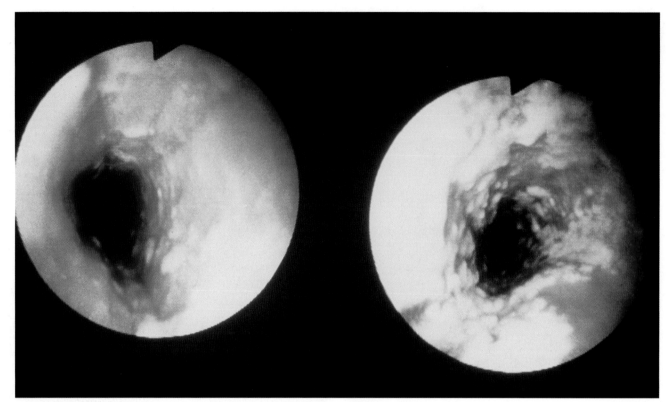

Figure 5.43 Oesophagoscopy macroscopically demonstrating moderately severe oesophageal candidiasis. Histological specimens confirmed the diagnosis and further identified CMV inclusion bodies.

- peritonitis;
- toxic megacolon.

Presentation with an 'acute abdomen' is more common in individuals with HIV than in the general population. The physical signs expected to accompany these conditions can be absent or altered because of the reduced inflammatory response in advancing HIV disease.

### Abdominal Pain

Pain commonly presents as: (1) epigastric pain with or without oesophageal symptoms, (2) right upper quadrant pain with or without jaundice, (3) left or right iliac fossa pain, or (4) diffuse abdominal pain.

The common HIV-related causes of acute pain are:

- CMV;
- MAC or other atypical mycobacterial infections;
- lymphoma;
- visceral KS;
- TB;
- acalculous cholecystitis;
- a combination of the above.

**KS and lymphoma** cause abdominal pain and may present with obstruction, intussusception, bleeding and perforation (**Figures 5.44–5.46**). Both may be seen on endoscopy. Lymphomas, typically of the non-Hodgkin's type, often present while the patient still has a relatively preserved CD4 count. Concurrent TB must be excluded. KS tends to cause problems in later disease. Lymphomas can also present as abdominal masses or with organomegaly. Abdominal KS is usually accompanied by KS lesions of the palate.

Abdominal pain may be caused by mesenteric and retroperitoneal lymphadenopathy (**Figure 5.47**) as well as other abdominal mass lesions, including organomegaly. Extrapulmonary TB is a common differential diagnosis. It tends to occurs in individuals with some degree of immunodeficiency, while MAC is seen in very advanced immunodeficiency. Biopsy is usually required to differentiate between MAC, TB, lymphoma and KS, each of which is potentially treatable but fatal if left to progress. A combination of pathologies also needs to be considered.

### Colitis

Colitis is the second most common presentation of CMV (after retinitis), and is characterized by pain, rebound tenderness in the left iliac fossa, bleeding and diarrhoea. As inflammation and ulceration of the colon progresses, acute ischaemic colitis may occur. This can result in severe pain, massive haemorrhage, toxic megacolon and perforation. CMV infection or reactivation typically occurs with advanced immunodeficiency and affects the gastrointestinal tract from mouth to anus. It also may affect the solid organs. CMV can affect the caecum and terminal ileum and mimic Crohn's disease. Other organisms that cause colitis and gastroenteritis in the presence of HIV infection include HSV, *Shigella, Salmonella, Campylobacter* and *Clostridium difficile*.

### Gastrointestinal Bleeding

Substantial gastrointestinal bleeding occurs in less than 1 per cent of patients with AIDS but is associated with diagnostic challenges. Non-HIV-related causes are almost as common as HIV-related ones. Acute upper gastrointestinal bleeds are associated with reduced survival and are often related to lymphoma, KS, or CMV. Lower gastrointestinal bleeding can occur with or without

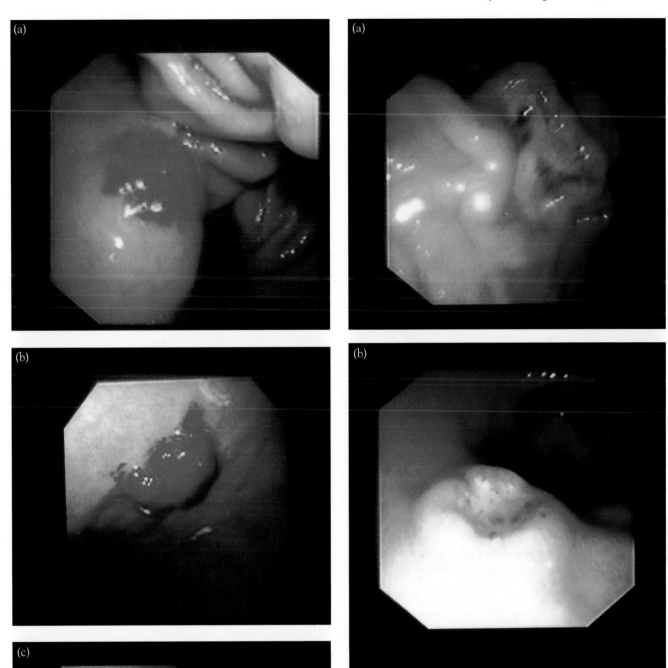

Figure 5.45 Gastric lymphoma. (a, b) Both depict biopsy-proven, Epstein–Barr virus-driven B-cell lymphomas.

Figure 5.44 Gastric Kaposi's sarcoma. (a–c) These three lesions caused early fullness and epigastric pain consistent with moderately severe gastritis.

signs of obstruction and/or perforation, and is usually due to infectious agents, particularly CMV, HSV, C. *difficile* and rarely *Histoplasma*. Idiopathic ulceration, KS and lymphoma are other important causes.

## Diarrhoea

Chronic diarrhoea (lasting for more than 1 month) is extremely common and affects at least 40 per cent of patients with advanced immunodeficiency. It is a cause of marked morbidity and mortality. Spore-forming protozoa, especially cryptosporidia, microsporidia and less commonly isospora and cyclospora, can cause severe and prolonged gastroenteritis. Multiple stool samples for

PART 1 | PRINCIPLES

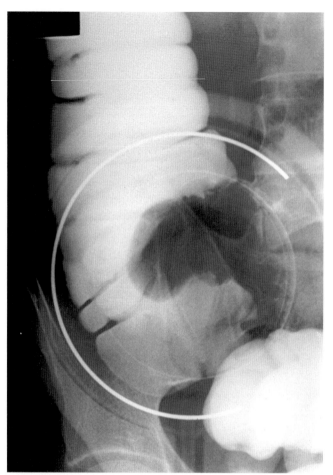

Figure 5.46 Ileocaecal intussusception secondary to lymphoma. A barium enema study shows a filling defect in the caecum. Kaposi's sarcoma may also cause intussusception, particularly if the lesions are raised.

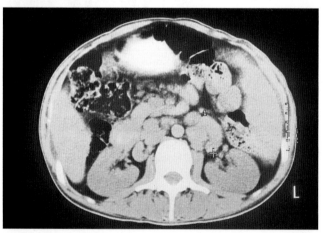

Figure 5.47 An abdominal CT scan showing marked retroperitoneal lymphadenopathy secondary to biopsy-proved MAC infection.

bacteria, *C. difficile* toxin, mycobacteria and ova, cysts, and parasites are indicated. Blood cultures to assess bacteria and MAC should be taken if the patient is febrile. Flexible sigmoidoscopy and biopsy are key investigations in a stool-negative patient. However, many cases of diarrhoea in advanced HIV disease remain pathogen-negative.

## Hepatobiliary System

Hepatic and biliary tract disease often manifests as right upper quadrant pain with an elevated alkaline phosphatase level. It may be accompanied by fever and jaundice but this is not invariable.

### Hepatic Disease

Hepatitis B and C infections are usually the most significant causes of liver disease in HIV-positive patients. Co-infection must be excluded as it substantially increases mortality. While treatment is available, end-stage liver failure and hepatocellular carcinoma are increasingly seen due to the late diagnosis of co-infection. Liver infection with MAC, TB or CMV often occurs in the context of systemic illness.

### Biliary Disease

Small bowel and biliary tract disease caused by opportunist infections is common and debilitating. Endoscopic retrograde cholangiopancreatography, biopsies and duodenal aspirates provide an essential definitive diagnosis where pathogens have invaded the mucosa. When pathogens are found, *Cryptosporidium*, enteric bacteria, CMV and MAC are common isolates.

**Acalculous cholecystitis** is now a frequently diagnosed condition, causing symptoms indistinguishable from those of gallstone disease. Acalculous cholecystitis is thought to be a result of CMV, *Cryptosporidium* or *Campylobacter* infection. Severe colicky abdominal pain in the right upper quadrant, nausea, vomiting, pyrexia and a thickened gallbladder wall, but no gallstones on ultrasound study, are the hallmarks of this condition (**Figure 5.48**). Emergency cholecystectomy is often required to prevent fatal peritonitis following gallbladder rupture.

The term 'HIV cholangiopathy' includes acalculous cholecystitis but also encompasses the conditions of sclerosing cholangitis and papillary stenosis, which also cause debilitating pain. Ultrasound scans may show dilatation and thickening of the bile duct walls. Confirmation is by endoscopic retrograde cholangiopancreatography, which shows beading of the bile ducts and/or an oedematous and swollen ampulla. Sphincterotomy may allow biliary drainage and pain relief, while biopsy is required to isolate the causative agent(s) if possible.

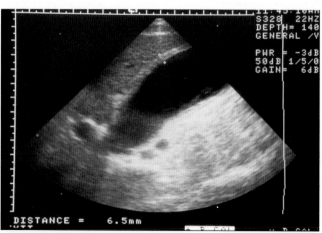

Figure 5.48 Acalculous cholecystitis. Ultrasound showing a dilated gallbladder with intramural oedema.

## Pancreatitis

Pancreatitis is a common cause of abdominal pain in HIV-positive individuals, who are more likely to develop pancreatitis and have higher rates of morbidity and mortality than non-infected individuals. It is commonly caused by alcohol abuse, gallstones, high lipid levels and medications, especially the antiretroviral agent didanosine. Other opportunists and malignancies that cause ampullary mass lesions need to be excluded.

## Anal and Perianal Region

Anorectal pathology is a leading cause of surgical intervention in HIV-positive populations and causes considerable morbidity. The spectrum of anorectal and perineal disease is diverse, including condylomas, tumours, fissures, fistulas, abscesses, ulceration and haemorrhoids (Figures 5.49–5.59). Perianal abscesses may not demonstrate the typical features of fluctuance so a high degree of suspicion is needed. Inadequate management of perianal abscesses can readily lead to the development of fistulas and might be complicated by septicaemia, especially in resource-poor settings.

The differential diagnosis of infective lesions includes:

- human papillomavirus (HPV);
- HSV;
- CMV;
- syphilis;
- gonorrhoea;
- other STIs.

**Perianal HPV** infection is very common. Visible warts can be extensive and frequently fail to clear with conventional therapies. In these instances, they may require surgical intervention (see Figure 5.49). Infection with oncogenic forms of HPV can cause anal intraepithelial neoplasia (AIN) and squamous cell carcinoma (see Figure 5.58). The incidence of AIN (Figure 5.59) is increasing in HIV-positive individuals, particularly in MSM and others who have engaged in repeated high-risk anal intercourse. Up to half of the anal warts that merit surgery in HIV-positive MSM harbour high-grade AIN or squamous cell carcinoma. Digital rectal examination and proctoscopy are indicated. Anal cytology and high-resolution anoscopy are available in some areas, and screening for AIN has been proposed but is currently not routine practice.

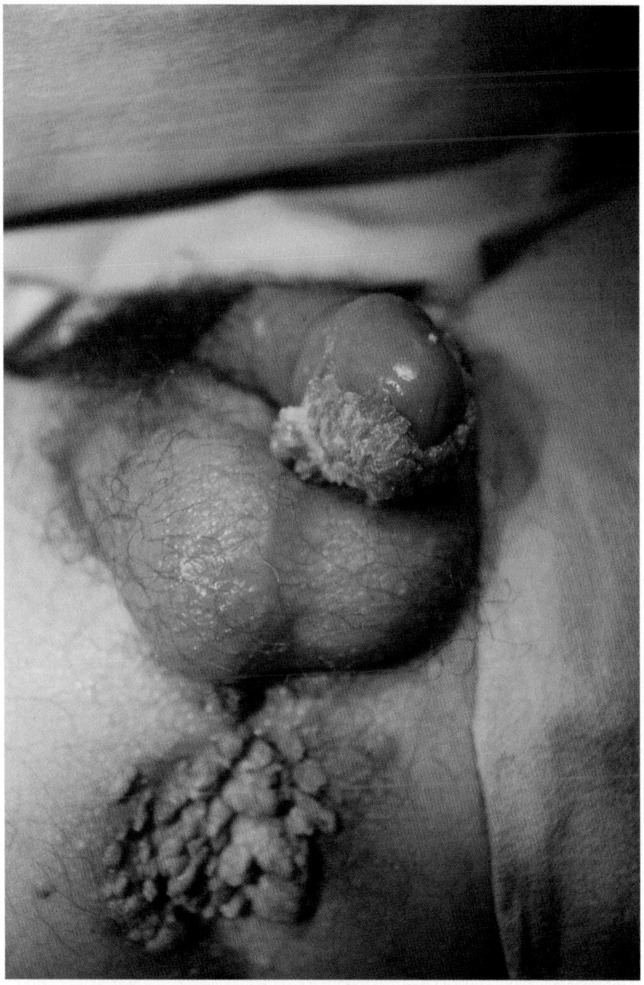

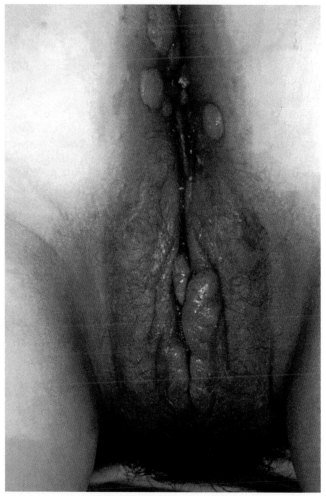

Figure 5.49 Extensive penile and perianal warts. (Courtesy of Mr A. Tanner.)

Figure 5.50 Condylomata lata in a patient with secondary syphilis. (Courtesy of CDC/Robert Sumpter.)

PART 1 | PRINCIPLES

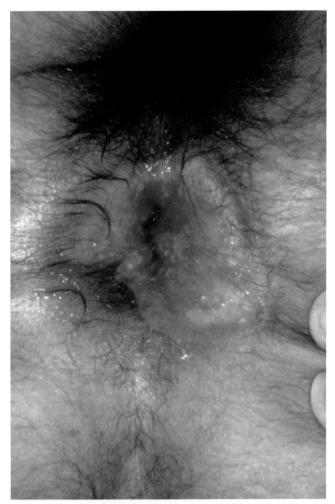

Figure 5.51 Perineal ulceration due to herpes simplex, a sexually transmitted infection. (Courtesy of CDC.)

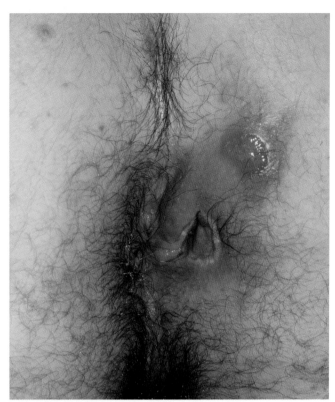

Figure 5.53 Perianal abscess with several underlying fistula tracts and superficial ulceration. Specimens from the superficial ulcers grew herpes simplex virus, but biopsy specimens from the tracts were CMV-positive. *Staphylococcus aureus* and *Enterococcus faecalis* were isolated from the abscess swabs. MRI of the pelvis delineated the multiple fistula tracts and defined a further ischiorectal abscess.

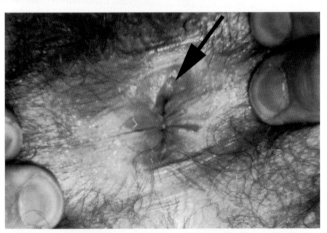

Figure 5.52 Perianal chancre (arrow) of primary syphilis. (Courtesy of CDC/Susan Lindsley.)

Figure 5.54 Deep perianal ulceration. Recurrent non-healing ulcers require biopsy to exclude pathology such as lymphoma (as shown here), squamous cell carcinoma or infections, for example CMV. (Courtesy of Mr A. Tanner.)

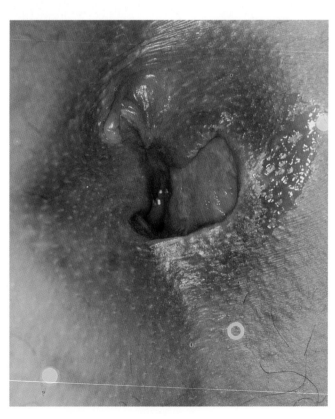

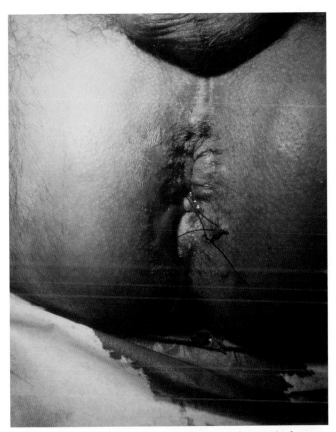

Figure 5.55 High fistula *in ano* secondary to mycobacterial infection.

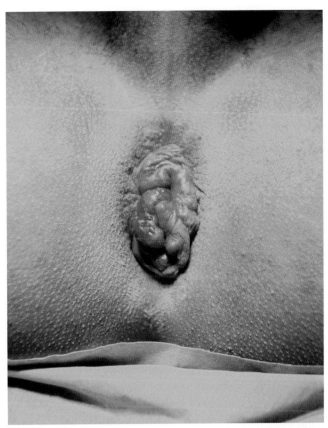

Figure 5.57 Rectal mucosal prolapse secondary to HIV-related perineal neuropathy. (Courtesy of Mr A. Tanner.)

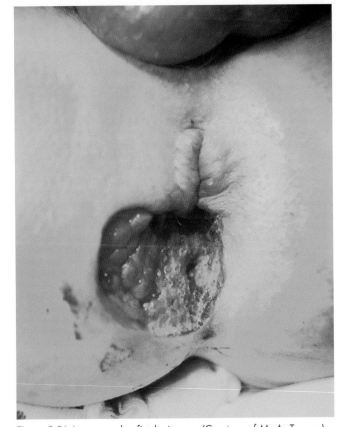

Figure 5.56 Low, complex fistula *in ano*. (Courtesy of Mr A. Tanner.)

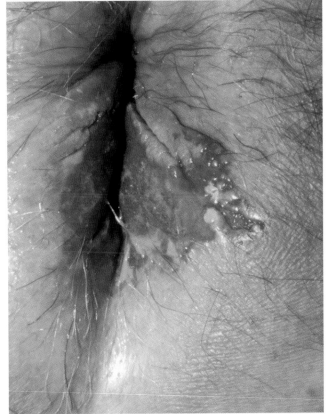

Figure 5.58 Anal squamous cell carcinoma.

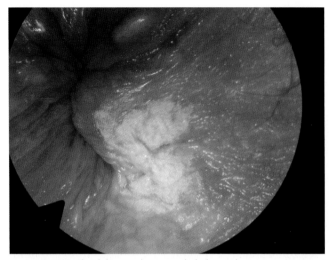

Figure 5.59 Leukoplakic anal intraepithelial neoplasia seen on anoscopy. (Courtesy of Paul Fox.)

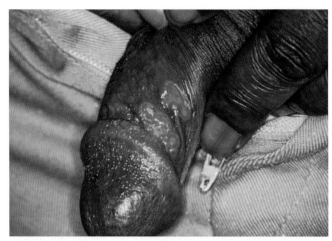

Figure 5.60 Penile ulceration due to primary syphilis (chancres). The differential diagnosis includes herpes simplex virus and lymphogranuloma venereum. (Courtesy of CDC/M. Rein.)

## Urogenital System

**STIs** occur more frequently in people with HIV infection than in the general population, they are often more severe and may be atypical in their presentation. Any STI is an indicator for HIV testing (Figure 5.60). Multiple and atypical organisms can present as persistent or recurrent urinary tract infections, persistent/recurrent urethritis, acute and chronic prostatitis and pelvic inflammatory disease. **Circumcision** reduces the rate of HIV acquisition in certain populations.

Common surgical manifestations of renal disease presenting to urologists are **renal abscess** and **renal calculi**. Renal calculi have been related to the antiretroviral agents indinavir and atazanavir. An analysis of stone composition and/or urine for crystals is warranted. Acute and chronic **urinary retention** can be due to HIV subacute encephalitis and dementia.

**Neoplasms** can affect the kidney, bladder and genitourinary tract. The risk of germ cell and non-germ cell tumours of the testis is markedly raised in HIV patients relative to the general population. Rarely, penile intraepithelial neoplasia and frank penile carcinoma (Figure 5.61) present to the urologist.

**HIV-associated nephropathy** (some cases of which are reversible with ART) and **renal disease** due to hypertension, diabetes and so on are not uncommon and are important perioperative considerations. Continuous ambulatory peritoneal dialysis might be preferred over haemodialysis in some patients with end-stage renal disease, including intravenous drug users and those with hepatitis B/C co-infection. With the improved prognosis due to HIV treatment, renal transplantation is an option in selected patients.

## Gynaecological System

**Invasive cervical carcinoma** is an indicator of AIDS and should prompt HIV testing. Frank cancer and high-grades of cervical intraepithelial neoplasia are much more frequent in HIV-positive women than in the general population and are not always related to clinical immunodeficiency (Figure 5.62). HIV-positive women need to undergo yearly cervical screening, with an accompanying low threshold for colposcopy. Women with intraepithelial

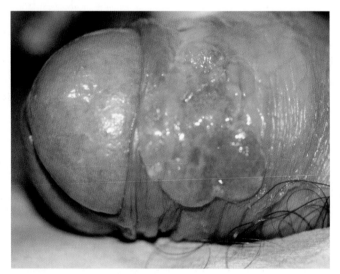

Figure 5.61 Penile squamous cell carcinoma.

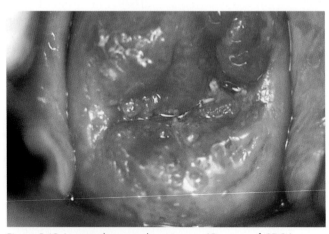

Figure 5.62 Low-grade cervical carcinoma. (Courtesy of CDC.)

neoplasia or carcinoma at one site (cervical, vulval, anal or vaginal) are at increased risk of disease at another site (Figure 5.63). Mortality from cervical carcinoma is high in populations where there is inadequate screening.

## Musculoskeletal System

HIV infection changes the spectrum and presentation of several musculoskeletal disorders. Treponemal disease, especially syphilis, needs to be considered as a cause of bone lesions in areas of high prevalence. An increasing number of patients present with TB of the bones and joints. Muscle and joint infections, such as pyomyositis, psoas abscess and septic arthritis, also occur, as does gangrene secondary to arteritis.

**Haematogenous osteomyelitis (Figure 5.64)** occurs in adults with HIV and is typically subacute. There is a predilection for the upper tibial and lower femoral metaphyses bilaterally. Tenderness, localized swelling and heat are the most common findings. Fluctuant subfascial abscesses may be present. *Staphyloccocus aureus*, non-typhoid *Salmonella* species and other gram-negative organisms have all been isolated from aspiration or incision specimens. Blood cultures are usually sterile.

**Pyomyositis** is now one of the most common and serious consequences of advanced HIV disease in developing countries and tends to affect young men. Lesions are often multiple and recurrent and can be found at unusual sites. Enteric organisms are isolated in up to 10 per cent of affected patients, but the most common cause remains *Staphylococcus aureus*.

## Orthopaedic Complications

The risk of **bone disease** is increased in HIV-positive individuals and with antiretroviral treatments, notably causing osteopenia, osteoporosis and osteonecrosis. The increased prevalence of these conditions is thought to be multifactorial and includes long-term continuous ART, wasting and hypogonadism. The risk of pathological fracture is increased especially among postmenopausal women and men over 50 years.

**Orthopaedic complications** occur in relation to fractures and the insertion of surgical prostheses. Closed fractures usually heal normally, but open fractures have a high incidence of non-union and sepsis. External fixation carries an increased risk of sepsis, and late sepsis of implants has been reported. However, the risk of infection is likely to be lower in those well managed on ART.

## Central Nervous System

Almost all HIV-positive individuals develop some degree of neurological dysfunction during their illness. Conditions that present to neurosurgeons tend to occur later in the disease.

### Intracranial Mass Lesions

The discovery of one or more space-occupying lesions on brain imaging is a common finding in patients who present with focal neurological symptoms or signs. The most common pathologies are:

- toxoplasmosis;
- primary cerebral lymphoma;
- brain abscess.

Neoplastic conditions and opportunist infections cannot always be adequately differentiated on CT and MRI. Tests for pathogens including *Toxoplasma gondii*, *Cryptococcus neoformans*, TB, MAC and *Treponema pallidum* can aid the diagnosis and might prevent the need for a brain biopsy. However, a brain biopsy should be considered where there is any doubt about the diagnosis or where dual pathology is suspected.

A key differential diagnosis of neurological dysfunction is **progressive multifocal leukoencephalopathy (Figure 5.65)**. This demyelinating condition caused by the polyoma JC virus can be distinguished by experienced radiologists on MRI scans. However, a brain biopsy is often required for definitive diagnosis.

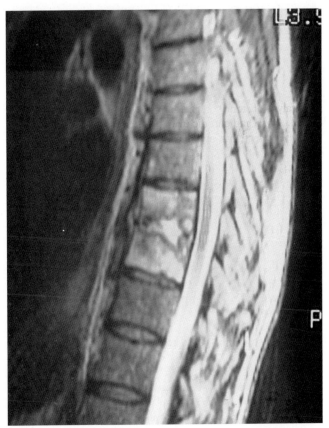

Figure 5.64 Sagittal MRI showing discitis and abscess formation in the T9 and T10 vertebral bodies. Biopsy proved candidal infection.

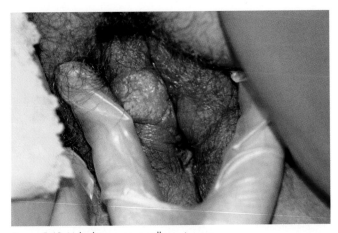

Figure 5.63 Vulval squamous cell carcinoma.

PART 1 | PRINCIPLES

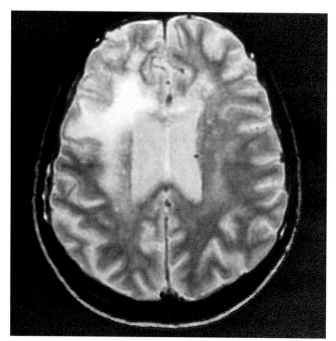

Figure 5.65 Progressive multifocal leukoencephalopathy. MRI shows focal increased signal in the left frontal white matter and to a lesser extent on the right side. Note that progressive multifocal leukoencephalopathy can be focal or diffuse, but in the latter it is usually asymmetrically distributed.

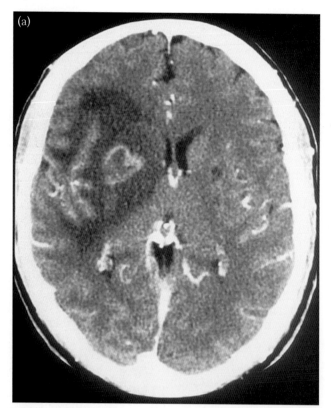

Figure 5.66 (a) MRI showing cerebral toxoplasmosis lesion, on the right side, with surrounding oedema (Courtesy of Professor R. Colebunders). (b, c) Cerebral toxoplasmosis often presents with multiple ring-enhanced lesions, which are more visible on MRI (c) than CT (b), making contrast MRI the investigation of choice where available (Courtesy of HIV Web Study [www.HIVwebstudy.org] at the University of Washington).

**Cerebral toxoplasmosis** is the most common brain mass lesion in patients with advanced HIV disease. It is usually the result of a reactivation of latent infection. It classically presents with rapid-onset headaches, low-grade pyrexia and focal neurological signs. Single or multiple ring-enhancing lesions may be seen on contrast CT scans and MRI (Figure 5.66). The most common

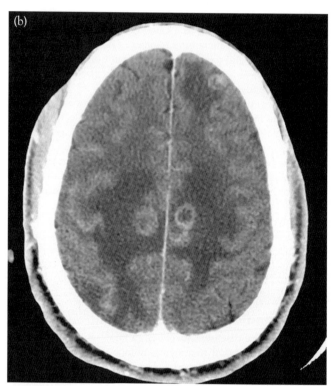

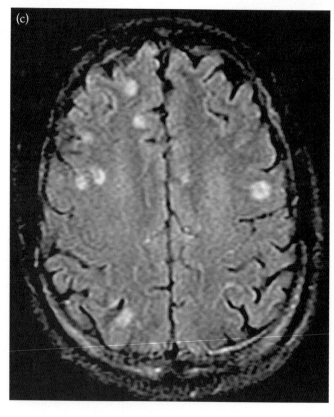

site is in the posterior fossa. The radiographic signs are characteristic enough that a trial of therapy should be commenced in the presence of positive *Toxoplasma* serology. If *Toxoplasma* serology is negative, a brain biopsy becomes mandatory.

**Primary cerebral lymphoma** (Figure 5.67) in an adult under 60 years of age is pathognomonic of HIV infection and AIDS. Patients tend to present with signs of late-stage HIV disease and B symptoms (night sweats, an unexplained fever of more than 38°C and more than 10 per cent weight loss in 6 months). Cerebral lymphomas can be difficult to differentiate from toxoplasmosis both clinically and radiologically. Toxoplasmosis usually involves multiple lesions while cerebral lymphomas are single lesions, but this is not invariable. If any doubt exists about

the diagnosis or if a 2-week course of empirical toxoplasmosis treatment has failed, a rapid definitive diagnosis can be made by a stereotactic brain biopsy.

### Brain Abscesses

The differential diagnosis of an intracranial mass lesion includes infection with:

* TB (a tuberculoma);
* *Cryptococcus neoformans* (a cryptococcoma);
* pyogenic organisms;
* *Candida*, notably in intravenous drug users;
* other fungal species.

**Cerebral TB** may cause meningitis, abscesses or isolated cranial nerve palsies. Infection tends to occur with a higher CD4 count than with other opportunist pathogens of the brain. Neurological complications are more frequent in HIV infection and high swinging fevers are normally found. Respiratory symptoms and abnormal chest radiographs provide important clues to the diagnosis, but their absence or the lack of a positive diagnostic test (e.g. a tuberculin skin test or interferon-gamma-releasing assays) does not exclude the diagnosis of cerebral TB.

Various other **brain abscesses** occur, depending on the geographical location and population involved. They are typically seen as single or multiple ring-enhancing lesions on cerebral CT and MRI (Figure 5.68).

### Raised Intracranial Pressure

Several pathologies that cause meningitis, encephalitis and intracranial mass lesions can result in raised intracranial pressure and hydrocephalus. These include cryptococcosis, toxoplasmosis and cerebral TB. Acute lumbar drainage and the long-term

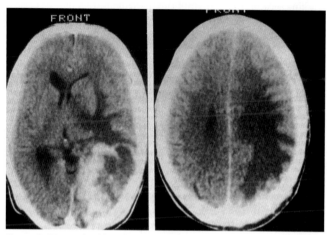

Figure 5.67 Cerebral lymphoma. A contrast-enhanced CT scan shows a large enhancing mass with prominent vasogenic oedema.

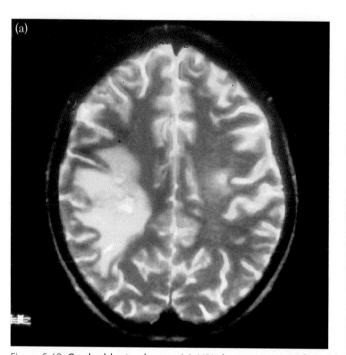
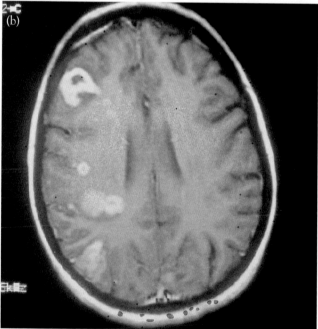

Figure 5.68 Cerebral brain abscess. (a) MRI shows a posterior frontal lobe abscess surrounded by prominent vasogenic oedema. (b) MRI with enhancement shows multiple, predominantly ring-enhancing, abscesses, due to candidal infection in an intravenous drug user. Brain biopsy is essential to exclude other pathogens, such as bacteria, mycobacteria, *Toxoplasma*, *Cysticercus* (particularly in African patients) and *Nocardia*.

PART 1 | PRINCIPLES

placement of a lumboperitoneal or ventriculoperitoneal shunt lead to improved outcomes without substantially increasing the risk of secondary infection.

## Ophthalmic Complications

The ophthalmic manifestations of HIV may be classified as microvasculopathy, infections, neoplasms and neuro-ophthalmic manifestations. Ophthalmic surgeons are involved in the management of visual symptoms as well as in routine screening for CMV retinitis in at-risk patients.

**Retinal microvasculopathy** is the most common ophthalmological manifestation of HIV infection. It is usually a self-limiting condition but may occasionally precede the development of CMV retinitis in the same location.

**CMV retinitis** (Figure 5.69) is the most common ocular infection in people with AIDS and is the leading cause of blindness in this population. Complaints of visual blurring or distortion, visual field loss or an increased number of floaters necessitate urgent retinal examination by an ophthalmologist. The sclerae are white, without pain or photophobia.

Clinical CMV retinitis affects 15–45 per cent of adult patients with AIDS but is rare in children. It occurs in advanced HIV disease, and in the absence of ART treatment implies a low life expectancy. Untreated CMV retinitis progresses in all cases, with involvement of the optic disc or macula, or retinal detachment. Antiviral agents are used for the treatment and secondary prophylaxis of CMV retinitis. Ideally, all lesions should be photographed and monitored by slit-lamp examination on a regular basis.

**Blindness** is uncommonly caused by *Toxoplasma* choroidoretinitis, a condition that also implies a high likelihood of cerebral toxoplasmosis. Retinal necrosis can be caused by HSV or herpes zoster virus. Ocular and periocular KS and lymphoma can also occur.

*Toxoplasma* **retinochoroiditis** should be considered if a lesion is initially thought to be CMV but appears atypical or does not respond to conventional CMV therapy. **Multifocal choroiditis**

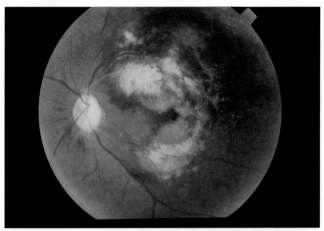

Figure 5.69 Cytomegalovirus retinitis. Greyish-white granular lesions with exudates and retinal opacification are visible. Retinal haemorrhage usually occurs, giving the classic 'pizza' appearance. (Courtesy of Dr Pavesio.)

may be a manifestation of disseminated infection, such as TB, MAC, *P. jirovecii* pneumonia, cryptococcosis, histoplasmosis, candidiasis (particularly in intravenous drug users) or syphilis.

With **herpes virus infections**, the most common presentation is herpes zoster ophthalmicus, but progressive outer retinal necrosis can occur due to varicella-zoster, and acute retinal necrosis can be due to herpes simplex or zoster.

A suspicion of any of these infections should lead to prompt referral to an ophthalmologist.

### Other Lesions

Other ocular conditions include molluscum, KS and lymphoma. **Ocular KS** occurs in 25 per cent of people with AIDS, and 20 per cent of these have periocular involvement, usually on the lid margin or conjunctiva. **Lymphoma** may be intraocular or orbital – the former is rare and notoriously difficult to diagnose. It may present as chronic uveitis, and the diagnosis is dependent on a vitreous biopsy.

## Solid Organ Transplantation

Traditionally, HIV was an exclusion criterion for solid organ transplantation. However, end-stage liver disease due to hepatitis B and/or C co-infection and end-stage renal disease is increasing, while the excellent prognosis of many individuals taking ART means that selected patients are undergoing renal and hepatic transplantation. The risks of immunosuppressive therapy are reduced with various screening measures and with prophylaxis for opportunist infections. So far, survival of the graft and the patient seems to be equivalent to that of non-infected individuals, without any increased risk of progression of the HIV disease.

## The Ageing Patient

Older individuals are increasingly being diagnosed with HIV infection, particularly in areas or groups with a high prevalence of the condition. In addition, as a result of ART, HIV-positive individuals now have a longer life expectancy. Patients can present to surgical specialties with conditions caused by ageing, including those that might compromise operative outcomes. Clinicians are thus being faced with a new spectrum of pathology, and the need for surgical interventions such as coronary revascularization is likely to rise.

### HIV TESTING

HIV may be transmitted by exposure to blood products, bloodstained body fluids, breastfeeding, sexual intercourse or vertical transmission via the placenta. The risk of transmission from other fluids (e.g. faeces, nasal secretions, sputum, saliva, sweat, tears, urine and vomitus) is very low unless they contain blood. The gold standard of routine HIV testing in adults is a fourth-generation test for antibodies and HIV P24 antigen. Exceptions are patients in whom primary HIV infection is suspected and in infants less than 18 months old, when PCR testing for HIV RNA is appropriate.

Considerations surrounding HIV testing have changed in recent years. An increased uptake of testing is seen as being vital for individual and public health. Guidelines such as those in the UK seek to normalize HIV testing (Table 5.3). Routine testing in high-prevalence areas or targeted testing in certain patient

**Table 5.3 Messages on HIV testing from UK national guidelines**

| |
|---|
| HIV is now a treatable medical condition and the majority of those living with the virus remain fit and well on treatment |
| A significant number of people in the UK are unaware of their HIV infection and remain at risk in terms of both their own health and of unwittingly passing their virus on to others |
| A late diagnosis is the most important factor associated with HIV-related morbidity and mortality in the UK |
| Patients should be offered and encouraged to accept HIV testing in a wider range of settings than is currently the case |
| Patients with specific indicator conditions (see Table 5.2) should be routinely recommended to take a HIV test |
| All doctors, nurses and midwives should be able to obtain informed consent for a HIV test in the same way as they currently do for any other medical investigation |

or clinic populations is being adopted. Routine testing has been found to be cost-effective with both patients and their sexual partners where the local prevalence is above 1 per cent.

The surgeon needs to be aware of the local prevalence of HIV and local testing guidelines. In addition, a knowledge of the local pattern of HIV indicator diseases is good practice, as a diagnosis of HIV infection means that patients can be directed into appropriate specialist care. One example of such local variation is disseminated *Penicillium marneffei*, which has substantially increased in incidence in certain Asian countries and is now considered to be an AIDS-defining diagnosis in the presence of HIV infection. Patients with TB, lymphoma, hepatitis B and C or an STI warrant the offer of a HIV test, as do patients with other indicator diseases (see Table 5.2). Once HIV has been detected, antiretroviral treatment, where needed, improves the prognosis for the individual and also reduces HIV transmission.

## Key Considerations for HIV Testing

All doctors, nurses and midwives should be able to obtain informed consent for a HIV test in the same way that they currently do for any other medical investigation. Patients should be offered and encouraged to accept HIV testing in a wider range of settings than is currently the case. Key messages from UK national guidelines include the following:

- HIV is now a treatable medical condition and the majority of those living with the virus remain fit and well on treatment.
- A significant number of people in the UK are unaware of their HIV infection and remain at risk to their own health and of unwittingly passing their virus on to others.
- Late diagnosis is the most important factor associated with HIV-related morbidity and mortality in the UK.
- Informed consent is an ethical and sometimes legal requirement. However, extensive formal counselling is generally not required before tests and for negative results.
- Measuring the CD4 count as a surrogate marker for HIV is unethical without gaining the individual's consent.
- A diagnosis of HIV necessitates urgent referral to specialist HIV services – this link should if possible be made prior to informing the patient of their diagnosis.

- With any individual presenting as a surgical emergency, life-saving treatment should always be instituted immediately without laboratory confirmation of HIV status. There remains no role for urgent HIV testing as the result is unlikely to have any impact on immediate treatment and management. If a patient with a specific indicator condition refuses the recommended test, the surgeon may seek specialist advice from the local HIV service.

## PROTECTION OF HEALTHCARE WORKERS

Surveys from the UK and Africa suggest a high level of concern among surgical trainees about carrying out surgical procedures on HIV-infected patients. There is a potential risk of transmission through percutaneous or mucous membrane exposure to many body fluids and materials, including amniotic fluid, blood, cerebrospinal fluid, exudative or other tissue fluid from burns or skin lesions, human breast milk, pericardial fluid, peritoneal fluid, pleural fluid, saliva in dentistry, semen, synovial fluid, unfixed human tissues and organs, vaginal secretions and any other body fluid if it is visibly bloodstained.

Reports suggest a substantial rate of potential exposures in trainees, many of whom are unaware of appropriate protocols and do not fully utilize protective measures. Double gloves, aprons and goggles or visors are key protective equipment, while non-cutting and non-suturing techniques, as well as a deliberately measured or cautious technique, are also recommended where possible.

## Universal Precautions

Universal precautions are based on the premise that all patients are potentially infectious. Presumptions of a negative HIV, hepatitis B and hepatitis C status based on a patient's age, race or sexual orientation are as potentially dangerous for health workers as they are for the patient.

The application of universal precautions to all patients does not negate the responsibility of hospitals to protect health workers, particularly in operating and emergency rooms. All staff should be familiar with procedures for handling sharp instruments and for protection from the dissemination of body fluids. Theatres and examination areas should be organized to minimize the risk of accidental exposure to hepatitis B, hepatitis C and HIV.

## Occupational Exposure

The risk of blood-borne occupational HIV infection depends on the prevalence in the population under treatment and on the risk of inoculation injuries during the procedures undertaken. According to ten prospective studies, the risk of seroconversion following a single parenteral occupational exposure with a hollow-bore needle is 0.37 per cent. However, the risk is greater with higher HIV prevalence, higher rates of exposure, the nature of the exposure and poorer health of the patient and the exposed individual. In sub-Saharan Africa, the risk of occupational transmission over a surgeon's working life has been estimated as 1–10 per cent, at least 15-fold higher than in first-world countries. Approximately 80 per cent of seroconversions in health workers have been shown to follow percutaneous exposure.

Protocols that clearly define procedures to be followed in the event of needle-stick or other exposure must be readily available. These usually include first aid, reporting, baseline testing, post-exposure prophylaxis with antiretroviral drugs and follow-up. Testing of the patient for any blood-borne viral infections and consent to inform the exposed individual must be achieved, with the consent being obtained by a health worker other than the person who sustained the injury. Routine testing prior to surgery due to concerns over occupational transmission is unethical.

## Post-exposure Prophylaxis

Many exposures result from a failure to follow recommended procedures so prevention of exposure is of prime importance. Where available, post-exposure prophylaxis with combination antiretroviral agents, if initiated early after injury (within hours if possible) and continued for 4 weeks, is strongly recommended. Toxicity and side-effects are common so the use of local guidance is imperative to judge when the benefits of post-exposure prophylaxis outweigh the risks.

## PATIENT PROTECTION

### Ethical Issues

HIV-positive individuals have the same right to equal health care and treatment as non-HIV-positive individuals. Much stigma has been attached to HIV and AIDS, usually because of the association with taboo behaviours or due to fear of infection. Consequences have included discrimination and a reluctance to be tested or to disclose the HIV status. Surgeons need to be aware that HIV cannot be acquired by casual contact and that unnecessary infection control measures are stigmatising and could breach patient confidentiality with regard to other staff, other patients and the individual's family.

### Confidentiality

Confidentiality is the right of every individual under medical care. Permission should be sought from the patient before information is passed to any person who does not *need* to know, including relatives and health workers, or to other services.

### The HIV-positive surgeon

A surgeon may acquire HIV through occupational or other exposure. Confidential advice offered by leading HIV services should be sought in the first instance to protect the surgeon, both medically and professionally. However, it is unethical to knowingly put patients at risk. The risk can be minimized by modifying professional practice. In all instances, the surgeon involved should act on advice from the appropriate governing or professional body, for example the Royal College of Surgeons in England.

The US Centers for Disease Control and Prevention (CDC) have estimated that the risk of HIV transmission from a health worker to a patient during a surgical procedure is between 1 in 2.4 million and 1 in 24 million. CDC guidance from 1991 states that surgical healthcare workers who are infected with HIV may be required to divulge their status to their employer or patients and may be restricted in the types of procedure they can perform, depending on whether such individuals perform exposure-prone invasive procedures. Exposure-prone invasive procedures are defined as the digital palpation of a needle tip in a body cavity, or

the simultaneous presence of the healthcare worker's fingers and a needle or other sharp instrument or object in a poorly visualized or confined anatomical site.

Nine cases of HIV transmission from an infected health worker have been documented, six of these from a dentist in Florida, USA, in 1990. Comprehensive retrospective investigations, particularly among doctors engaged in invasive procedures, have not identified additional cases. As of July 1999, the CDC had analysed HIV test results for more than 22 000 patients of 63 HIV-infected healthcare workers, and no documented case of transmission had occurred. Similarly, in 1997, 1180 surgical patients of an HIV-infected obstetrician/gynaecologist were tested in the UK; none were found to be HIV-positive.

In 1997, the Israeli Ministry of Health conducted an extensive look-back following the report of a HIV-positive cardiothoracic surgeon. The absence of transmission to patients and the availability of effective treatment for the surgeon called into question whether his surgical practice should be restricted. HIV testing was performed on 545 of his former surgical patients who had been operated on in the previous decade. The sample represented roughly one-third of his total number of surgical cases from the previous 10 years; none of the patients was found to be HIV-positive. In addition, none of the 1669 patients operated on in the past decade were listed in Israel's National HIV Registry, indicating that none of them had tested positive for HIV in Israel. After test results on the surgeon's patients became available, an expert panel was convened to review the matter and make recommendations regarding the surgeon's ability to practice.

The surgeon was allowed to resume his surgical practice with no restrictions on the types of surgery he could perform. Furthermore, in contrast to the US position, he was not required to notify patients of his HIV status. As recommended by the Israeli Ministry of Health, the surgeon could resume his surgical practice by agreeing to do the following:

- adhere to standard infection control precautions and hand hygiene requirements;
- double-glove during all surgeries;
- immediately report any cuts in gloves or finger sticks;
- undergo quarterly HIV medical monitoring visits;
- adhere to his antiretroviral drug regimen;
- maintain an HIV RNA level below 50 copies/mL and CD4 cell count above 200/$\mu$L.

In the UK, the Department of Health concluded in 2013 that current restrictions on HIV-positive healthcare workers should be lifted, provided that those healthcare workers are taking effective combination antiretroviral drug therapy, have a very low or undetectable viral load and are regularly monitored by both their treating physicians and occupational health physicians. It remains to be seen how such guidance will be altered in other countries.

## PERIOPERATIVE CONSIDERATIONS

Overall, HIV infection is not an independent risk factor for postoperative complications, the most important risk factor being the general health status. However, HIV is reported to be a significant prognostic indicator for a worse outcome in acute injury to the lung and in adult respiratory distress syndrome patients in intensive care.

The postoperative complication rate of surgical procedures is proportional to the patient's degree of immunodeficiency. There is no value in measuring the CD4 count when a patient is ill since CD4 cells migrate from the bloodstream into the tissue source of inflammation, so their measurement in the peripheral blood gives a falsely low reading. The percentage of CD4 cells may be a better indicator of immune status when compared with previous levels and throughout surgical recovery. Higher complication rates occur with CD4 counts less than 200 cells/$\mu$L and with postoperative viral loads over 10,000 copies/mL. However, other general risk factors, such as nutritional status, might have more influence on the risk of complications of, for example, sepsis and delayed wound healing. In all instances, it is preferable to discuss patients with colleagues who are knowledgeable in the management of HIV disease.

Preoperative assessment is key to identifying the likelihood of postoperative complications, and includes the following.

## History

This should take into account:

- previous and current infections (especially with opportunist pathogens) and malignancies;
- antiretroviral treatment;
- antibiotic medications.

Risk factors include:

- cardiovascular status;
- renal disease and nephrotic syndrome;
- viral hepatitis;
- TB;
- drug and alcohol abuse;
- undernutrition;
- disease status (the latest CD4 count and viral load);
- metabolic syndrome and diabetes.

It is important to note in the work-up prior to surgery some particular considerations, described below, that are important even when the CD4 count is high or normal.

## Fluid and Electrolyte Imbalances

**Hyponatraemia** can occur in patients with advanced diseases and is important as it carries an adverse prognosis postoperatively. Causative factors include gastrointestinal causes of volume depletion, renal disease, inappropriate antidiuretic hormone secretion, medication, low albumin levels and primary and secondary adrenal insufficiency.

**Hypokalaemia** can be secondary to vomiting, diarrhoea and renal tubular acidosis.

**Hypocalcaemia** can result from medication, malignancy and CMV disease.

## Haematology

**Thrombocytopenia** (Figure 5.70) may be one of the first signs of immunological dysfunction in HIV and reportedly occurs in 10–20 per cent of patients, although many factors can be involved. Splenectomy might be warranted to control refractory thrombocytopenia. All patients should have their platelet levels and clotting ability tested. Note that an abnormal adjusted partial thromboplastin time is common and is related to the presence of antiphospholipid antibodies.

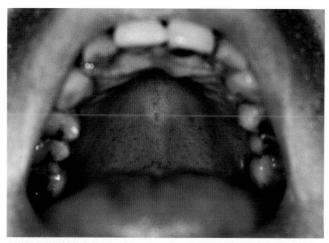

Figure 5.70 Palatal thrombocytopenic purpura in an HIV-positive individual who had no other stigmata of HIV disease. The patient had been admitted for routine surgical naevus removal when this abnormality was noted (platelet count, 6 × 10⁹/L).

**Neutropenia** must be excluded prior to surgery or invasive clinical procedures such as rectal examination or central line insertion. A scrupulous aseptic technique is required at all times.

## Nutrition

Many patients with advanced HIV disease are malnourished, with a low muscle mass. If surgical intervention or the presenting complaint puts the patient in a state of further increased catabolism, early interventional feeding should be considered, for example after polytrauma. The risks of parenteral feeding should always be weighed against the risks of further malnutrition.

## Impact of surgery

Data exist to suggest that even major surgery might not adversely affect disease progression in patients on effective ART, but such treatment regimes must be continued perioperatively, utilizing parenteral routes if required. Prophylaxis for opportunist infections should be optimized.

Important postoperative complications include the following:

- fever; its cause probably being related to the nature of the surgery and the degree of immunosuppression. This includes:
  - bacterial respiratory infections, which are common;
  - intravascular catheter infections;
  - urinary tract infections;
  - hepatitis;
  - thrombophlebitis;
- wound sepsis and poor/delayed wound healing.
- nosocomial infections.
- uncommonly, the unmasking of hypoadrenalism, which causes hyponatraemia, hyperkalaemia and hypotension.
- a reduction in the percentage of CD4 cells post-surgery, which can trigger opportunist infections in untreated patients.

A coexistent diagnosis also needs to be considered, for example active TB at the time of presentation with a lymphoma. It is worth re-emphasizing the importance of multiple pathological sampling, including to check for mycobacteria and fungi.

## Key Points

- Untreated HIV infection results in progressive immunodeficiency, AIDS and death. ART has dramatically improved both morbidity and mortality.
- HIV-positive individuals can present to surgeons with no knowledge of their status. An awareness of common indicator diseases and an index of clinical suspicion assist the surgeon with diagnosis and management.
- HIV-related conditions present to all surgical specialties and can include severe or unusual (opportunist) infections and malignancies. More than one pathogen or disease process often occurs concurrently, and these vary by geographical location. HIV-positive individuals also present with conditions seen in the general population.
- HIV testing can be offered routinely or targeted to an individual or group depending on the local situation. A positive test necessitates immediate referral to specialist HIV services.
- Consultation with HIV clinicians is valuable in all cases where HIV is suspected or proven; there is no place for urgent HIV testing.
- The prevention of occupational exposure requires an awareness of and adherence to local protocols, safer surgery and the use of protective equipment. Post-exposure prophylaxis with antiretroviral medication is recommended under certain conditions.
- Transmission from an HIV-positive surgeon to a patient is extremely rare, but guidance from appropriate bodies needs to be sought by such individuals.
- HIV-related postoperative complications relate to the degree of immunodeficiency present. The general health status of the individual is paramount to their perioperative care.

## QUESTIONS

**1.** A 28-year-old patient attends an accident and emergency department in London, UK, with nausea, sweating and acute abdominal pain against a background of 1 week of general malaise and loose stools. You review the history. Which one of the following would be an indicator for a rapid HIV test (done by fingerprick)?:

**a** A white man with a history of unprotected receptive anal intercourse with another man

**b** A declaration by the patient that they are hepatitis C-positive

**c** The patient requires urgent surgery and could be a high risk to staff

**d** A black woman from Zimbabwe

**e** A 2 year history of intermittent diarrhoea and weight loss

**f** Previous pulmonary tuberculosis

**g** A recent onset of extensive psoriasis

**h** Three admissions in the past year with bacterial pneumonia

**i** None of the above

### Answer

*i* **None of the above.** *Answers a, b, d, e, f, g and h add to an index of suspicion of HIV infection and would warrant asking the patient for verbal consent to do a serum HIV test. Indeed, local protocol might indicate that a serum HIV test is performed as part of a routine work-up. However, rapid HIV testing, carried out via capillary blood testing, currently has a lower sensitivity and specificity than standard serum HIV testing. In addition, rapid (fingerprick) or urgent standard (venous blood) HIV testing has no part to play in the acute management of this patient, whether or not they require surgery. In terms of answer c, universal precautions apply for surgical procedures. It is unethical to test a patient to determine their risk to surgical staff.*

**2.** You examine the patient and do a routine work-up. The following signs might add to your suspicion that the patient could have undiagnosed HIV infection with immunodeficiency. For each of the following signs, select the most likely category from the list below. Each category may be used once, more than once or not at all:

 **1** AIDS-defining diagnosis
 **2** HIV indicator
 **3** Risk factor for HIV infection
 **4** None of the above

**a** Lipoatrophy restricted to the face, with loss of the cheek fat pads

**b** Abscess and scarring in the left antecubital fossa

**c** White striations on the lateral border of the tongue, which cannot be scraped off

**d** Small, shotty lymph nodes in both inguinal regions

**e** Isolated purple/brown papules on the feet with associated lymphodoema

**f** A few scattered lesions of molluscum contagiosum in the pubic region

**g** A raised serum amylase concentration

**h** Splenomegaly

**i** Thrombocytopenia

### Answers

*a* **4 None of the above.** *This is a common side-effect of antiretroviral treatment.*

*b* **3 Risk factor for HIV infection.** *This is an indicator of injection drug use, a risk factor for HIV infection.*

*c* **2 HIV indicator.** *This is hairy oral leukoplakia, which is an indicator of immunodeficiency, although not pathognomonic of HIV infection.*

*d* **4 None of the above.** *This is a non-specific finding and alone is insufficient to diagnose isolated or peripheral generalized lymphadenopathy.*

*e* **1 AIDS-defining diagnosis.** *This could be Kaposi's sarcoma, an AIDS-defining diagnosis, especially as the lesions are raised. If the appearance is not classic, consider vasculitis, chronic thrombophlebitis/venous insufficiency due to intravenous drug use or other causes.*

*f* **3 Risk factor for HIV infection.** *Molluscum contagiosum is a sexually transmitted infection and is an indicator to offer routine HIV testing. However, molluscum contagiosum in the context of HIV-related immunodeficiency is usually extensive.*

*g* **4 None of the above.** *A serum amylase concentration more than three times the normal range is an indicator of pancreatitis, which can occur in both HIV-positive and HIV-negative individuals. Less marked increases can occur with conditions other than pancreatitis.*

*h* **2 HIV indicator.** *Splenomegaly is present in at least a third of individuals with AIDS at autopsy. If the splenomegaly is large, it is indicative of disseminated opportunistic infection or neoplasm. Persistent hepatosplenomegaly in the absence of a known cause is an HIV indicator disease.*

PART 1 | PRINCIPLES

*i* **2 HIV indicator.** *Thrombocytopenia can be due to many factors, but isolated thrombocytopenia is an HIV indicator as well as an important preoperative consideration.*

**3. You construct a differential diagnosis. Which finding or group of findings best matches which diagnosis?:**
1 Acute hepatitis B infection
2 Acute HIV infection
3 Chronic protozoal infection
4 Acute pancreatitis
5 Cytomegalovirus infection
6 Lymphoma
7 Acute appendicitis
8 Acalculous cholecystitis
a Pain isolated to the right inguinal fossa only
b A tender, distended colon and bloody stool
c Markedly raised amylase and lipase levels plus a history of alcohol abuse
d Right upper quadrant tenderness, with a distended gallbladder but no stones on ultrasound scan
e Fever, jaundice, right upper quadrant tenderness and hepatomegaly
f A history of chronic diarrhoea, weight loss, signs of dehydration and vague abdominal tenderness
g Cachexia, splenomegaly, signs of intestinal obstruction and anaemia
h Fever, sore throat, rash, diffuse arthralgia and myalgia

**Answers**

*a* **7 Acute appendicitis.** *Common surgical conditions also present in HIV-positive individuals. Cytomegalovirus and other infections could cause such a presentation but other symptoms and signs would be likely to occur.*

*b* **5 Cytomegalovirus infection.** *Toxic megacolon and perforation are life-threatening complications that are usually the result of cytomegalovirus colitis. As this occurs in very severe immunodeficiency, other AIDS-defining diagnoses should be sought.*

*c* **4 Acute pancreatitis.** *Pancreatitis in HIV-positive individuals can be due to the usual risk factors, opportunist infections, medications or obstruction.*

*d* **8 Acalculous cholecystitis.** *This is a common presentation indistinguishable from gallstone disease on clinical findings. Gallbladder perforation is an important complication.*

*e* **1 Acute hepatitis B infection.** *The most common cause of acute liver disease in HIV-positive patients is viral hepatitis.*

*f* **3 Chronic protozoal infection.** *Chronic protozoal infection, for example cryptosporidiosis, presents as chronic or recurrent gastroenteritis and is a sign of very severe immunodeficiency. Weight loss and dehydration indicate a prolonged history.*

*g* **6 Lymphoma.** *This often affects multiple organs, including the spleen and bone marrow, and is a cause of intestinal obstruction. It may occur earlier or later in the natural history of HIV infection. Disseminated mycobacterial infection is a differential diagnosis.*

*h* **2 Acute HIV infection.** *An index of suspicion is paramount for diagnosing an acute seroconversion illness. Abdominal pain could be due to mesenteric lymphadenopathy.*
*Note: In all these presentations, other opportunists and neoplasms might be present concurrently with the diagnosis if immunodeficiency is present.*

**4. The patient develops focal neurological signs during the admission. An HIV test is positive, with a CD4 count of 86 cells/μL and a viral load of 47 000 copies/mL. A CT scan of the head with contrast demonstrates three ring-enhancing lesions. Which one of the following is the most likely diagnosis?**
a Candidal brain abscess
b Histoplasmosis
c Primary central nervous system lymphoma
d Infarcts due to bacterial endocarditis
e Cerebral toxoplasmosis

**Answer**

*e* *With very severe immunodeficiency (CD4 <100 cells/μL), the most common cause of focal neurological signs and brain lesions is cerebral toxoplasmosis. The CT findings are classic. Although ring-enhancing lesions might be seen in a, b, f and h, candidal brain abscesses are rare, as is histoplasmosis, which also does not occur in the UK. Primary lymphoma of the central nervous system is the second most likely differential diagnosis on the list, although it is much less likely given that the lesions are multiple. The infarcts of bacterial endocarditis and raised*

**f** Cryptococcal meningitis
**g** Raised intracranial pressure
**h** Tuberculoma

*intracranial pressure would usually be differentiated radiologically, as would cryptococcal meningitis, while this and raised intracranial pressure also usually present with diffuse non-focal signs. A tuberculoma might be suspected in a patient from a region where tuberculosis is endemic but is usually seen in patients with less severe immunodeficiency.*

---

**5.** **For the patient in question 4, which one of the following is your next step?**
   **a** Refer the patient to neurosurgery for a brain biopsy
   **b** Initiate infection control procedures
   **c** Order an MRI scan
   **d** Start treatment for toxoplasmosis
   **e** Start treatment for tuberculosis
   **f** Refer to specialist HIV team
   **g** Refer to oncology

**Answer**

*f As soon as an HIV-positive test result is available, the local HIV team should be involved. HIV specialists can advise on medical management, on the samples and specimens required to make the diagnosis/diagnoses, and on the appropriate perioperative care.*

# PART
# 2

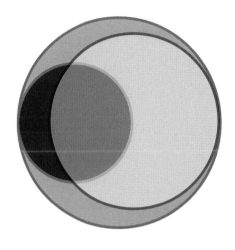

# Trauma and (elective) orthopaedics

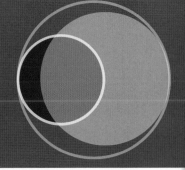

# Management of the Multiply Injured Patient

Ali Hallal and Ahmad Moukalled

## LEARNING OBJECTIVES

- To understand the concept of the 'golden hour' in the trauma patient's journey and its relation to mortality and morbidity
- To appreciate the peculiarities of the history and physical examination as applied to the multiply injured patient

- To understand that the history and physical examination are initially directed at identifying life-threatening conditions
- To be able to comprehend and apply the principles of the primary and secondary surveys

## INTRODUCTION

Injury is an increasingly significant health problem worldwide. The World Health Organization estimates that every day 16 000 people die from injury, and that for every person who dies several thousand are injured with permanent morbidity. Trauma is the leading cause of death in men younger than 45 years of age worldwide. In England and Wales, injury is a major cause of death across all age groups, with over 16 000 deaths per year.

Time is of the essence in the management of multiply injured patients. Mortality from trauma follows a trimodal distribution, with the mortality rate peaking within 1 hour of the injury, when an estimated 50–60 per cent of the fatalities will occur (**Figure 6.1**). This period has been termed the 'golden hour'. The outcome for trauma patients is directly related to the time from injury to definitive care. The rapid assessment of injuries and the institution of life-preserving measures have led to a decrease in the high mortality rate that is seen in the early post-injury period.

The initial assessment of the injured patient focuses on the fact that the history and physical examination should initially be directed at identifying life-threatening injuries. This initial assessment is known as the primary survey and should be followed by a more detailed examination, which is known as the secondary survey. The aim of the secondary survey is to detect and evaluate injuries that are still potentially life-threatening as well as occult injuries. This systematic approach to the initial assessment of the injured patient is the foundation for the Advanced Trauma Life Support course.

## SAFETY FOR HEALTHCARE PERSONNEL

The principle of universal precautions is of paramount importance when attending to an injured patient. The resuscitation area is an environment where blood and other body secretions are abundant, and where the dynamic nature of the resuscitation may lead to an increased chance of contact with these. The doctor caring for the trauma patient should be wearing the following items as standard precautions:

- Cap;
- Gown;
- Gloves;
- Mask and goggles or face shield;
- Shoe covers.

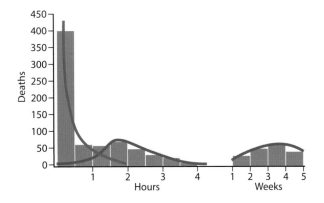

Figure 6.1 Trimodal distribution of deaths in trauma (Adapted from Trunkey DD, Trauma. Accidental and intentional injuries account for more years of life lost in the U.S. than cancer and heart disease. Among the prescribed remedies are improved preventive efforts, speedier surgery and further research. Sci Am 1983;249(2):28–35).

## THE PRIMARY SURVEY

The primary survey is a succession of steps essential for the identification of life-threatening injuries. The sequence of steps follows the mnemonic **ABCDE**, which corresponds to Airway–Breathing–Circulation–Disability–Exposure/Environment. The skills needed in taking an accurate history and conducting a meaningful physical examination differ in a trauma setting compared with a clinic setting. The difference lies in the fact that the history and physical examination should proceed simultaneously with the management of life-threatening injuries during the resuscitation phase. The life-threatening injuries that need to be identified during the primary survey are shown in **Table 6.1**.

## A: Airway and Cervical Spine Protection

All trauma patients should be assumed to have a cervical spine injury and should be initially assessed with a cervical collar on. Securing and maintaining the airway is the first priority in managing the trauma patient as airway obstruction is the most common cause of hypoventilation, which initially lies at the root of the patient's hypoxia. It is of the utmost importance that hypoventilation and hypoxia are promptly identified and corrected in all patients. This is particularly so in multiply injured patients with evidence of head trauma, as these patients are at risk of secondary brain injury from hypoventilation and the ensuing hypoxia and hypercarbia.

The primary survey starts with a quick assessment that consists of asking the patient their name and enquiring briefly about the event that led to the injury. These simple questions allow the doctor to assess both the airway and the patient's mental status. A normal response indicates a patent airway and a relatively intact neurological status. It is important to appreciate the fact that the traumatic insult can be a dynamic process rather than a static one, so a patient who has a patent airway on arrival in the accident and emergency department bay might have a compromised airway 5–10 minutes later for a variety of reasons; a periodical re-evaluation is therefore wise.

Two groups of patients should be identified at this stage to determine whether there is a need for a definitive airway. A definitive airway is defined as a tube in the trachea with the

### Table 6.1 Life-threatening injuries that need to be identified in the primary survey

| | Injuries |
|---|---|
| Airway | Airway obstruction<br>Airway injury<br>Cervical spine injury |
| Breathing | Tension pneumothorax<br>Open pneumothorax<br>Flail chest and lung contusion |
| Circulation | Haemorrhagic shock<br>  Massive haemothorax<br>  Intra-abdominal bleeding<br>  Pelvic bleeding<br>  Bleeding from long bone fractures<br>  Bleeding from vascular injuries to the extremities<br>Cardiac tamponade and cardiogenic shock<br>Neurogenic shock |
| Disability | Intracranial haemorrhage |

cuff of the tube inflated. The first group of patients who require this includes those who are in need of **airway protection**, for example those with:

- severe maxillofacial and midface fractures;
- neck trauma with resulting laryngeal or trachea injury, neck haematoma or stridor;
- foreign bodies in the oropharynx;
- an inhalational injury;
- a risk of aspiration from either blood or vomiting;
- a Glasgow Coma Scale (GCS) score of less than 8 if the patient is unconscious.

The second group include patients who need **ventilation or oxygenation**, which includes those:

- with inadequate respiratory efforts who show any of the following signs:
  - tachypnoea,
  - hypoxia,
  - hypercarbia,
  - central or peripheral cyanosis;
- in shock from massive blood loss;
- with signs of hypoventilation secondary to either medications (e.g. opiates, neuromuscular blockade) or a decrease in level of consciousness;
- with evidence of traumatic asphyxia, suggested by the history and evident from signs of plethora and petechial haemorrhage above the nipple line.

Other helpful symptoms and signs include breathlessness, a weak or absent voice, dyspnoea, the use of short, gasping sentences, dysphonia or hoarseness, stridor, cyanosis, the use of the accessory muscles of breathing, laboured noisy breathing, tachypnoea and hypoxia detected by pulse oximetry.

Several steps should be followed to relieve a suspected airway obstruction. The first is to look inside the oral cavity and inspect for any foreign bodies. This step should be followed by a chin-lift or jaw-thrust manoeuvre with the insertion of an oral or nasal airway. This is a temporizing step until a definitive airway can be secured. It must be remembered that is imperative at all times to protect the cervical spine while securing the airway.

## B: Breathing and Ventilation

Once the airway has been secured, attention should be turned towards assuring appropriate breathing and ventilation. The pathological conditions that jeopardize ventilation and need to be identified at this stage include:

- tension pneumothorax;
- open pneumothorax;
- massive haemothorax;
- flail chest.

Pulse oximetry is a valuable and quick means to assess oxygenation and the effectiveness of ventilation. Ventilation is assessed by inspecting, palpating, percussing and listening to the chest for breath sounds, movement, symmetry and dullness.

The chest wall is inspected for symmetry, the paradoxical movement of a flail segment, contusions, the use of accessory muscles of breathing and the presence of wounds. Any traumatic wound in the chest needs to be classified as a simple or open sucking chest wound. The neck is inspected for distension of the veins or tracheal deviation, which is suggestive of tension pneumothorax. Palpation of the chest identifies surgical emphysema, which is felt as crepitus in the subcutaneous tissue. Surgical emphysema frequently dissects up into the neck and over the torso. Its presence is suggestive of a breach in the pleura of the lung. The chest wall is percussed to identify dullness or hyperresonance.

A **tension pneumothorax** should be suspected if the patient is complaining of difficulty in breathing in the presence of distension of the neck veins, tracheal deviation secondary to a shift in the mediastinum to the contralateral side, and decreased air entry on the ipsilateral side that is resonant to percussion. A tension pneumothorax can cause a decrease in venous return due to the rise in intrathoracic pressure, and this can lead to a life-threatening drop in cardiac output with resulting severe shock and hypotension. Tension pneumothorax has to be corrected promptly without the need for a radiological diagnosis. The situation can be relieved with decompression by a needle inserted into the second intercostal space anteriorly, followed by the rapid insertion of a chest drain. It is occasionally very difficult to differentiate between cardiac tamponade and tension pneumothorax except for the presence of bilateral equal breath sounds in the case of tamponade.

A large **haemothorax** will cause respiratory and circulatory problems at the same time. Examination reveals reduced breath sounds but, contrary to a tension pneumothorax, percussion reveals dullness and the neck veins are flat. The dullness to percussion is associated with a reduced vocal fremitus and vocal resonance. A weak, thready pulse and hypotension, secondary to the massive blood loss into the thorax, will be noted. Treatment consists of aggressive resuscitation with blood and blood products, in addition to the insertion of a chest drain. Thoracotomy and surgical control of the bleeding is indicated if the volume of blood drained by the chest tube exceeds 1500 mL.

A **flail chest** can also cause severe hypoxia. A flail chest occurs when three or more consecutive ribs are broken in at least two places each, or more than one rib fracture along the costochondral edge separates the affected ribs from the sternum. Clinically, a flail chest can occasionally be identified by noting a paradoxical movement of the involved flail segment on inspiration. The extent of the hypoxia caused by a flail segment can be severe, and this needs to be promptly identified and corrected. The hypoxia occurs secondary to the fact that a flail segment is often associated with a lung contusion, a haemopneumothorax or a combination of these pathologies. Treatment consists of oxygen supplementation and occasional positive pressure ventilation.

An **open pneumothorax**, also known as a **sucking chest wound**, can cause severe respiratory difficulties and air hunger. It is defined as a chest wall defect that is greater than two-thirds the diameter of the trachea. In this situation, air passes on inspiration preferentially through the chest wound instead of the anatomical airway, creating the feeling of air hunger. Treatment consist of:

1. immediate coverage of the wound with a gauze fixed to the skin on three sides, leaving the fourth side free;
2. the insertion of a chest tube to prevent a pneumothorax;
3. prompt surgery to cover the soft tissue defect.

## C: Circulation

Haemorrhage is the leading cause of preventable death after injury. The source of the haemorrhage should be identified quickly, and the bleeding should be controlled as soon as possible. There are five sources of bleeding in adult trauma patients: the thorax, the abdomen, the pelvis, the long bones and obvious external bleeding. Some of these sources can be easily identified on physical examination (external bleeding, bleeding into the thigh from a long bone fracture), whereas other sources (thoracic, intra-abdominal, pelvic) may be *more occult and need radiological investigation* with, for example, CT scanning (**Figures 6.2** and **6.3**) or a focused sonography test for trauma (FAST) for their identification.

External bleeding can be arterial, venous or a combination of both. Arterial bleeding is differentiated from venous bleeding by the fact that it is a pulsatile stream of bright red blood that can usually be controlled by either direct pressure or proximal arterial compression. Venous bleeding, on the other hand, presents as a dark, continuous blood flow that responds in most cases to simple pressure.

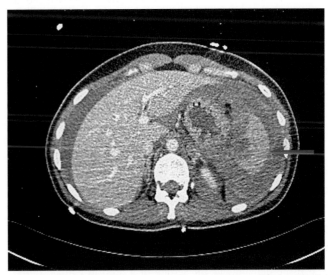

Figure 6.2 CT scan of a young lady involved in a motor vehicle accident who had minimal abdominal tenderness on examination. The CT scan showed a large volume of blood and a splenic injury (arrowed).

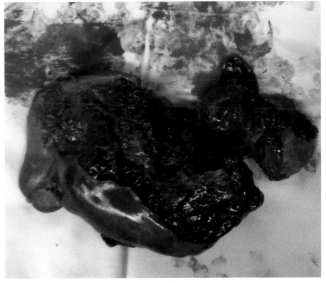

Figure 6.3 Operative findings of the patient in Figure 6.2, which shows a ruptured spleen.

Patients who bleed are at risk of developing hypovolaemic shock as a result of inadequate oxygen delivery to the tissues, with the degree of hypovolaemic shock being directly related to the volume of blood lost. The diagnosis of the haemorrhage is based on detecting the signs and symptoms of hypovolaemic shock. Patients with hypovolaemic shock may demonstrate any of the following: pale cold extremities, a rapid thready pulse, hypotension, tachypnoea and a change in mental status that may present as agitation or obtundation.

Tachycardia results from a compensatory response to a depletion of the intravascular volume in an attempt to maintain the cardiac output. It is caused by stimulation of the sympathetic nervous system that also results in vasoconstriction and a redistribution of the remaining blood volume to vital organs such as the heart and brain, shunting it from other organs such as the skin, the intestine and even the kidneys. The peripheral vasoconstriction causes the skin of the extremities to become pale and clammy. This reflex tachycardia can be concealed in young athletic patients and, if present, might represent an occult sign of significant haemorrhage. The response can, however, be blunted in elderly patients who are taking beta-blockers or calcium-channel blockers.

Hypotension, if present, is an accurate indicator of shock: a systolic blood pressure of less than 90 mmHg is considered to indicate shock, until proven otherwise. A normal blood pressure, however, cannot rule out shock, especially during the initial evaluation. This is because a drop in blood pressure might only appear when a significant amount of blood has been lost. The pulse pressure – the difference between the systolic and the diastolic blood pressure – is a better reflection of the volume of blood loss. Unlike a fall in systolic blood pressure, which can only be detected after 30 per cent of the blood volume has been lost, a narrow pulse pressure might be evident after the loss of only 15 per cent of the blood volume.

The tachypnoea that is often observed in hypovolaemic shock is a compensatory mechanism on the part of the lungs to match the tissue demands in the setting of a drop in cardiac output caused by hypovolaemia. In the absence of obvious lung injury, the presence of tachypnoea is an important sign and might reflect an advanced state of hypovolaemia.

Agitation is especially significant in young patients who do not have a traumatic brain injury, but in all cases, it is another sign that should never be overlooked. In the setting of hypovolaemia, agitation is a reflection of poor cardiac output and brain perfusion despite normally functioning cerebral autoregulation. Haemorrhagic shock is also occasionally associated with paradoxical bradycardia. In this context, it is vital to recognize that bradycardia can occur secondary to a major haemorrhage that demands rapid correction.

The treatment of haemorrhagic shock is **control of the haemorrhage** and resuscitation with fluid, blood and blood components. Type O-negative blood should initially be given until type-specific blood becomes available. The response to resuscitation should be closely monitored. Patients' responses are classified into three categories. In rapid responders, the vital signs are normalized and maintained. In transient responders, the blood pressure and heart rate are normalized for a short period of time, followed by a recurrence of the hypotension and tachycardia. Minimal or non-responders are patients in whom vital signs are not corrected despite adequate initial fluid or blood resuscitation. These three categories correspond to minimal (10–20 per cent), moderate and possibly ongoing (20–40 per cent) and severe and ongoing (more than 40 per cent) blood loss.

The other type of shock that needs to be ruled out in this part of the primary survey is cardiogenic shock resulting from either cardiac tamponade or blunt myocardial injury. Cardiac tamponade should be suspected whenever there is a penetrating injury to the region of the chest bounded by the clavicles superiorly, the nipples inferiorly and the midclavicular lines laterally. Cardiac tamponade is one of the life-threatening injuries that needs to be ruled out and treated promptly. Patients who are conscious and are developing cardiac tamponade are noted to be restless, complaining of air hunger and unable to explain their symptoms but expressing a feeling of doom. Any patient who has a penetrating injury to the chest and is showing these symptoms should be considered to have a pre-cardiac arrest tamponade. The signs to look for are distended jugular veins, muffled heart sounds and hypotension; these signs are classically known as **Beck's triad**. The definitive treatment of cardiac tamponade is either an emergency department thoracotomy or emergency sternotomy.

Blunt cardiac injury can be caused by any blunt trauma to the anterior chest. It might present with anything from minor arrhythmias to life-threatening heart failure. The diagnosis can rarely be confirmed clinically and demands blood tests for cardiac enzymes, electrocardiography and echocardiography. Treatment is supportive with appropriate fluid and pharmacological management of the hypotension and heart failure.

## D: Disability

A brief neurological examination should be performed once the life-threatening injuries have been controlled. The neurological examination at this stage of the initial assessment should include the GCS (**Table 6.2**) and an examination of both pupils for their size, reactivity, symmetry and reaction to light. The rest of the neurological examination should be performed more extensively in the secondary survey. The GCS should be frequently repeated to detect

Table 6.2 The Glasgow Coma Scale

|  | 1 | 2 | 3 | 4 | 5 | 6 |
|---|---|---|---|---|---|---|
| Eye | Does not open eyes | Opens eyes in response to painful stimuli | Opens eyes in response to voice | Opens eyes spontaneously |  |  |
| Verbal | Makes no sounds | Incomprehensible sounds | Utters inappropriate words | Confused, disoriented | Oriented, converses normally |  |
| Motor | Makes no movement | Extension to painful stimuli (decerebrate response) | Abnormal flexion to painful stimuli (decorticate response) | Flexion/withdrawal to painful stimuli | Localizes painful stimuli | Obeys commands |

changes that might signal neurological deterioration and prompt an earlier investigation or intervention. Abnormalities of pupil size, symmetry or reaction to light in the setting of trauma indicate a lateralizing brain lesion, most probably due to an intracerebral bleed.

## E: Exposure and Environmental Control

It is of prime importance that the trauma patient's clothing should be totally removed so that a complete and accurate evaluation can be made. Hypothermia should be prevented by using a blanket, warm air, oxygen and fluids.

## THE SECONDARY SURVEY

Once the primary survey has been completed, all trauma patients who are haemodynamically stable should have a **secondary survey**. This consists of detailed history and a thorough head to toe physical examination, a complete neurological examination, special diagnostic tests and a general re-evaluation. The purpose of the secondary survey is to detect and manage potentially major as well as minor injuries.

It is important to note that even major injuries can be missed, especially in patients who are unconscious or in whom attention has been mainly given to a life-threatening injury. Commonly missed injuries include:

- chest trauma: injury to the aorta and its branches, and oesophageal injury;
- blunt abdominal trauma: injuries to the stomach, small bowel and pancreatoduodenum;
- penetrating abdominal trauma: colorectal and genitourinary injuries;
- trauma to the extremities: fractures, vascular injuries and compartment syndromes.

## History

A detailed history should be obtained from the patient, the pre-hospital personnel and any witnesses to the incident. A quick mnemonic for obtaining a history is **AMPLE**:

- A: Allergies;
- M: Medications (especially anticoagulants, insulin and cardiovascular medications);
- P: Previous medical and surgical history;
- L: Last meal (time);
- E: Events/Environment surrounding the injury, that is, exactly what happened.

A full description of the mechanism, the environment, the circumstances and the sequence of events related to the injury must be sought. This information is extremely important because it directs the clinician towards injuries that are occult. Injuries are classified as blunt (i.e. vehicle or pedestrian impact, falls, assault) or penetrating.

In case of a motor vehicle accident, the clinician should enquire about the speed, seatbelt use, airbag deployment, location of the injured person in the vehicle, deformity, time for extrication and history of injuries or death of the vehicle's other passengers. Seatbelt marks are associated with bowel and mesenteric vessels injuries that may not be obvious on CT scanning (**Figures 6.4** and **6.5**). Pedestrians, cyclists and motorcyclists hit by a car suffer a high incidence of injuries to the extremities and pelvis, as well as brain injuries that need to be investigated.

For falls, the clinician should enquire about the circumstances before the fall, the height of the fall and the type of surface at impact. Penetrating injuries in urban settings are predominantly secondary to gunshot rifle wounds, stabbing and impalement. Various factors affect the extent of body injuries in trauma from firearms, including the distance from the weapon, the type of weapon, the kinetic injuries and the location of the impact. It is

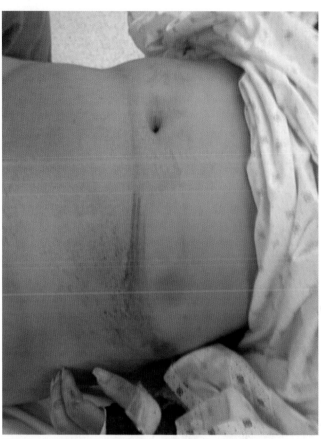

Figure 6.4 A patient involved in a motor vehicle accident with a seatbelt injury to the anterior abdominal wall.

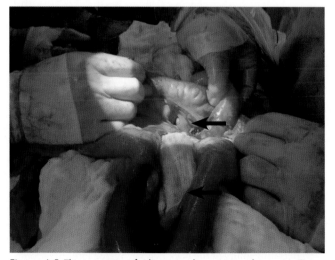

Figure 6.5 The operative findings in the patient shown in Figure 6.4. There are two injuries to the mesentery of the distal small bowel (arrows). This is an injury that is commonly found with seatbelt signs.

PART 2 | TRAUMA AND (ELECTIVE) ORTHOPAEDICS

important to appreciate the fact that firearm injuries are unpredictable in terms of their path and injury pattern. Those from high-velocity projectiles are the most devastating because of the high kinetic energy injuries they dissipate along their path.

The patient's past medical history and current medication may show a connection with the incident, for instance, if there is a history of epilepsy. The patient's medications, allergies, and medical and surgical history should also be noted. The use of anticoagulants and antiplatelet agents increases the risk of bleeding and is a determinant of morbidity and mortality in trauma patients, especially those with head trauma; therefore their use should be clarified and noted. A history of known drug allergies should be sought to avoid any potential allergic reactions. The clinician should also enquire about the most recent meal; this is of particular importance with diabetic patients on insulin therapy and to estimate the risk of aspiration in patients going for emergency surgery.

## Physical Examination

### Head and Face

The whole head and face should be carefully inspected and palpated, looking for tenderness, deformity and bleeding. Palpate the scalp for lacerations as these may be easily missed on inspection. Check for missing teeth as these may have been aspirated. Further examination of the face may reveal depressed facial fractures, mandibular fractures and nasal bone fractures. Both an open bite deformity and numbness of the lower lip suggest a mandibular fracture. A sensory and motor neurological examination should be carried out as the facial nerve and its branches may be injured.

Signs suggestive of a fracture of the base of the skull (e.g. a haemotympanum) should be sought using an otoscope. Retroauricular ecchymosis (Battle's sign) and periorbital ecchymosis (raccoon's eyes) also indicate a base of skull fracture but do not usually appear until at least 24 hours after an injury. Look for nasal septal haematomas and examine the nasal secretions for the presence for rhinorrhoea.

An ocular examination should be performed, evaluating the size, shape and reactivity of the pupils, as well as any movements of the extraocular muscles. Look for signs of globe rupture and intraocular haemorrhage. A fixed dilated pupil occurs with IIIrd cranial nerve compression after a contralateral intracranial bleed or direct injury to the optic nerve. Diplopia on looking upwards is a sign of a fracture of the orbital floor with inward sinking of the eyeball. Loss of upward gaze signifies an intracranial bleed.

Patients with mild traumatic brain injury may not have the above-mentioned external signs of trauma. A CT scan of the brain is indicated when the mechanism of injury and symptoms raise the alarm for intracranial injuries.

### Neck

All patients who have undergone blunt trauma should be assumed to have sustained an injury to the cervical spine. Cervical spine immobilization using a neck collar should be initiated and maintained until an unstable cervical spinal injury has been excluded. The entire neck should be inspected and palpated for signs of injury.

Penetrating injury of the neck may be divided into three zones:

- zone 1: structures at the thoracic outlet;
- zone 2: structures between the clavicle and the mandible;
- zone 3: structures from the angle of mandible to the base of the skull.

The zonal classification is important for both management and prognosis. Mortality in patients with penetrating neck injury appears to be highest with zone 1 injuries. Careful physical examination rules out most arterial wounds but can miss important oesophageal and venous injuries. Therefore, in general, additional evaluation (CT scanning) is necessary for any penetrating neck injury that crosses the platysma. Laryngotracheal injuries can result in respiratory distress, stridor, subcutaneous emphysema, haemoptysis, odynophagia, dysphonia or anterior neck tenderness. Signs of vascular injury include significant bleeding or haematoma, decreased or absent peripheral pulses, global or focal neurological deficits (i.e. stroke) and bruits or thrills. It is important to note that intact pulses do not rule out vascular injury.

### Chest

Inspect and palpate the entire chest wall, especially the sternum and clavicles. Injuries at these sites are often missed, and fractures of these bones suggest the presence of underlying intrathoracic injuries. Clavicular fractures can be associated with injury to the subclavian or axillary vessels. The upper limbs should be examined for signs of decreased blood supply, and the pulses should be palpated. Repeated auscultation can detect a previously missed small haemothorax, pneumothorax or pericardial effusion not yet causing tamponade. All the ribs should be palpated to identify rib fractures and costochondral disruptions. Fractures of ribs 1–3 may be associated with major vascular injury, fractures of ribs 4–9 with intrathoracic injuries, and fractures of ribs 10–12 with injury to the abdominal organs. A haemothorax may be suggested by decreased breath sounds and dullness upon percussion. Further imaging is essential if any changes are noted on physical examination (**Figures 6.6** and **6.7**).

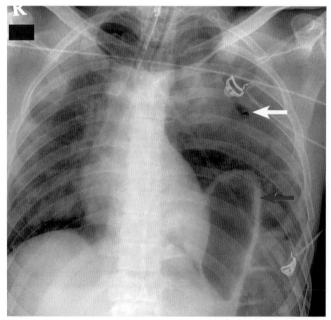

**Figure 6.6** A young man presented after at motor vehicle accident with dyspnoea and decreased air entry on the left side. A chest X-ray showed a pneumothorax (white arrow) and small bowel in the chest (red arrow), suggestive of diaphragmatic rupture.

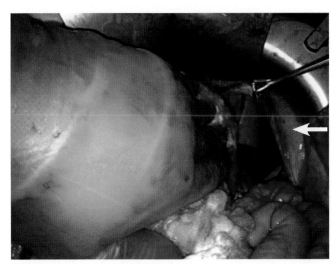

Figure 6.7 The intraoperative findings in the patient shown in Figure 6.6. These confirm the diaphragmatic rupture (arrow) and show the loop of bowel that was reduced back into the abdomen.

## Abdomen

Inspect the abdomen and flanks for lacerations, contusions and bruises. Palpate for tenderness and rigidity. Signs of intra-abdominal injury include a seatbelt sign, rebound tenderness, abdominal distension and guarding. It is important to note that a soft abdomen does **not completely rule out** intra-abdominal injuries (see **Figures 6.2** and **6.3**). The abdomen is a diagnostic black box, and the physical examination is often benign. It is also important to appreciate the fact that an injury can progress and the physical examination can change dramatically over time. Continuous re-evaluation and repeated examination are therefore needed to identify changing alarming signs. Abdominal examination is sometimes unreliable, especially in elderly individuals and patients with an altered mental status. FAST is a non-invasive test that can be carried out and repeated at the bedside to rule out major injury to the intra-abdominal organs.

## Pelvis

Inspect and palpate the pelvis. Look for ecchymosis over the pelvis or tenderness along the pelvic ring that may dictate further imaging. Repeat examinations to assess pelvic stability are unnecessary and are likely to exacerbate any bleeding.

## Rectum and Genitourinary Tract

The perineum should be inspected carefully for signs of injury. Routine rectal examination should not be performed in trauma patients who do not have signs of neurological deficit or pelvic injury as it has a poor sensitivity for injuries of the spinal cord, pelvis and bowel. If it is carried out, check for the presence of blood, a high-riding prostate and abnormalities of sphincter tone. A vaginal examination needs to be carried out on all trauma patients at risk of vaginal injury, especially those with lower abdominal pain, a pelvic fracture or perineal injuries.

## Musculoskeletal System

Inspect and palpate all four extremities looking for areas of tenderness, deformity or decreased range of motion. The neurovascular status of each extremity should also be assessed and documented, and all the joints examined both passively and actively. In the secondary survey, it is important to identify fractures early so that they can be splinted to reduce both pain and ongoing blood loss. The signs of fractures, dislocations and ligamentous injuries on inspection include bruising and deformity, and on palpation include local tenderness, decreased range of movement and crepitus.

An early identification of penetrating injuries, especially those overlying fractures, is essential. Their treatment includes early irrigation and debridement, the application of dressings and antibiotics. Compartment syndromes may develop after trauma and should be identified early. Signs of these include increasing pain, tense compartments and pain on passive stretching of the muscles. This is primarily a clinical diagnosis, commonly associated with long bone fractures. Compartment pressure may be measured, and it should be noted that the presence of a palpable arterial pulse does not exclude a compartment syndrome.

Penetrating or blunt injuries to the extremities may be associated with vascular injuries. Examination should include palpation of all the peripheral pulses and auscultation for bruits or thrills suggestive of an arteriovenous fistula (**Figure 6.8**). A Doppler scan should be carried out, in addition to an assessment of the motor and sensory function of the injured limb. This allows early detection, staging and early management of threatening acute limb ischaemia.

## Neurological System

The patient's neurological status may deteriorate dramatically over time when compared with their initial GCS score, so serial examinations should be performed and compared with previous ones. During the secondary survey, a complete neurological examination is recommended, including the motor, sensory, cranial and peripheral nerves, and the GCS score should be repeated. A decreased level of consciousness is defined as a reduction in GCS score of 2 or more points and should warrant an emergency CT scan.

In cases of a suspected spinal injury, immobilization of the patient is mandatory until the injury has been excluded radiologically.

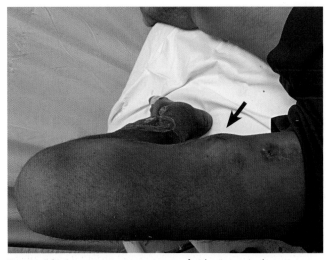

Figure 6.8 A traumatic arteriovenous fistula (arrow) showing as a bulge on the inner aspect of the thigh. This had the typical machinery murmur and easily felt thrill.

## Skin

The skin should be thoroughly inspected for lacerations, abrasions, ecchymoses, haematomas and serosal formation. Lesions, for example of the scalp, axillary folds and perineum, may be missed, especially in obese patients.

## DEFINITIVE CARE

Once the primary and secondary surveys have been completed, thought should be given to the next stage of care of the trauma patient. The decision to transfer the patient or admit them to the same hospital depends on the patient's physiological status, types of injury and comorbidities, as well as the resources that are available locally. If the decision is made to transfer the patient, it is imperative that there should be physician–to–physician communication between the transferring and the receiving hospital. The history, physical findings and treatment received, as well as potentially unresolved problems, need to be clearly communicated. A final check to secure all lines and tubes should be performed prior to the transfer.

### Key points

- Trauma is the leading cause of death in patients between the ages of 1 and 44 and is the third most common cause of all deaths.
- The initial management of the multiply injured patient focuses on the principle of promptly recognizing and treating life-threatening injuries.
- It must be understood that an abbreviated but focused history and physical examination are essential for a successful assessment of these patients.
- The assessment consists of performing the primary survey and clearing life-threatening injuries before proceeding to the secondary survey.
- The clinician should appreciate that these patients may have serious injuries with minimal physical findings and understand the sequence of events leading to the injury as well as the need for adjunct investigations such as blood samples and radiological tests.

# QUESTIONS

## SBAs

1. A 20-year-old man presents to the accident and emergency department with a stab wound to the anterior aspect of his chest medial to the nipple on the left side. He is complaining of shortness of breath and is agitated. His systolic blood pressure is 70 mmHg; he has bilateral neck vein distention and bilateral air entry. What is the best next step in the management of this patient?:
   a   The patient has a tension pneumothorax and you advise needle thoracocentesis followed by insertion of a chest drain
   b   He most likely has cardiac tamponade and needs an urgent cardiothoracic consultation
   c   Taking the low blood pressure into account, this patient probably has a large haemothorax on the left side and needs urgent insertion of a chest drain
   d   An urgent chest X-ray is indicated
   e   None of the above

**Answer**
**b   He most likely has cardiac tamponade and needs an urgent cardiothoracic consultation.** *Answer a is incorrect because a patient with a tension pneumothorax presents with decreased air entry on the ipsilateral side, and resonance to percussion on the affected side. Answer c is incorrect because a patient with a large haemothorax presents with decreased air entry on the affected side in addition to dullness to percussion. Patients with a large haemothorax causing haemodynamic instability do not have neck vein distension as they have hypovolaemia secondary to the haemorrhage. An urgent chest X-ray is not indicated in this instance as the diagnosis is cardiac tamponade, as suggested by the location of the stab wound and the neck vein distension associated with good air entry bilaterally. This patient needs an urgent thoracotomy and decompression of the pericardial haematoma.*

2. A 25-year-old man presents after falling from the first floor and sustaining a direct trauma to his head. When assessed, he opens his eyes to painful stimuli, utters inappropriate words and localizes to pain. What is his Glasgow Coma Scale score?:
   a   12
   b   11
   c   10
   d   9
   e   8

**Answer**
**c   10.** *Opening eye to painful stimuli = 2; utters inappropriate words = 4; localizes to pain = 4 (see Table 6.2).*

3. A patient can develop haemorrhagic shock due to bleeding in many spaces. Bleeding in which of the following spaces will not lead to haemorrhagic shock?:
   a   Abdomen
   b   Mediastinum
   c   Lower extremities
   d   Pelvis
   e   All of the above

**Answer**
**b   Lower extremities.** *The major sites of bleeding that can result in haemorrhagic shock are the chest and pleural cavity, the abdomen and the pelvis, bleeding from a long bone fracture and bleeding to the exterior.*

# Bones and Fractures

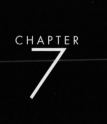

Muhyeddine Al-Taki and Imad S. Nahle

## LEARNING OBJECTIVES

- To successfully perform a physical examination when a bone fracture is present
- To be able to describe a fracture and its overlying soft tissue conditions
- To know the common potential complications following fractures

- To know the differential diagnoses of osteomyelitis
- To be able to describe the generalized diseases affecting bone
- To be familiar with bone tumours

## INTRODUCTION

The bones in the human body are classified into five types: long, short, flat, irregular and sesamoid.

The long bones consist of an epiphysis at each end, a metaphyseal region next to the epiphysis and a diaphysis or shaft connecting the two ends. The outer portion of the bone is made up of dense cortical bone, which is thickest at the diaphysis. The ends of the bone are composed of honeycombed cancellous spongy bone, supported on the outside by a relatively thin cortex. Lining the outer surface of the bones is a dense, irregular connective tissue membrane called the periosteum, which plays an essential role in healing after a bone fracture.

After a thorough history has been taken, a clinical physical examination is carried out. The approach to the musculoskeletal examination can be summarised as 'look, feel and move'. Examination of the extremities becomes more accurate when it is performed systematically and beginning with the contralateral normal extremity.

**Inspection** of a long bone should always include exposure of the proximal and distal joints. Deformities, scars, open wounds, bruises, abrasions, colour changes, swelling and shiny skin should all be noted if they are present.

**Palpation** indicates the skin temperature and helps to detect any tenderness or crepitus on digital pressure and percussion. It is also used to check the pulses and sensation while assessing the neurovascular status of the limb.

At the end of the examination, the **range of motion** at the joints should be checked both actively and passively. In the case of a long bone fracture or joint dislocation, the range of motion will be severely impaired.

After the clinical encounter, imaging and laboratory studies complete the assessment of bones and fractures.

## FRACTURES

A fracture is defined by break in the cartilage or bone accompanied by an insult to the overlying soft tissues. A fracture can result in a discontinuity in the cortical aspect of the bone but may be more subtle if the fracture occurs in cancellous bone. Forces that greatly exceed normal physiological loads cause fractures. In pathological fractures, the bone is so weakened by disease that little or no violence causes the fracture.

The description of a fracture should first include its location. Next, open and closed fractures should be differentiated. Open fractures involve skin breakage and significant soft tissue trauma overlying the bony insult. Then the nature of the fracture (simple, segmented or comminuted – when the bone is fragmented) should be noted.

After that, any displacement and angulation should be described. Displacement of the fracture refers to an abnormal orientation of the distal part in relation to the proximal part. This may occur by translation medially, laterally, anteriorly or posteriorly, or by rotation, shortening, distraction and angulation. Angulation of the fracture occurs when the distal fragment is tilted and is commonly referred to by the direction of tilting of the distal fragment, for example dorsally or medially.

## THE EARLY SIGNS OF A RECENT FRACTURE

### Inspection

The displaced long bone fracture usually shows gross deformity on the clinical examination. Undisplaced fractures, fractures involving joints, and carpal or tarsal fractures can be more difficult to diagnose.

PART 2 | TRAUMA AND (ELECTIVE) ORTHOPAEDICS

The local physical signs on inspection include swelling, bruising, deformity and loss of function. Swelling and bruising are common in both soft tissue injuries and fractures and are not diagnostic of either; both ankle sprains and ankle fractures, for example, present with pain, swelling and bruising.

Deformity of the bone usually implies that there is displacement of the fracture. Several typical patterns are seen in the hip, with shortening and external rotation of the leg or the distal radius with dorsal and radial displacement. The presence of deformity should be confirmed by comparison with the uninvolved side.

Loss of function is often one of the few signs of a fracture in the young child who has been noticed by the parents not to be using a limb after a fall. The patient resists any movement of the limb to avoid further pain from the fracture site.

A fracture is termed 'compound' when there is an adjacent skin wound; this greatly increases the risk of subsequent infection and requires emergency treatment. Wounds are most commonly classified using the Gustilo and Anderson classification, which is best graded after operative exploration of the wound:

- *Type I*: An open fracture with a skin wound that is <1 cm in length and clean;
- *Type II*: An open fracture with a laceration 1–10 cm in length without extensive soft tissue damage or bone loss;
- *Type III*: An open fracture with an open wound >10 cm long, extensive skin and subcutaneous contusion, muscle crush and bone comminution. Type III is subdivided into:

  - IIIa: a comminuted fracture but the bone is still covered by periosteum;
  - IIIb: loss of periosteal cover over the bone;
  - IIIc: fractures with major blood vessel injury.

## Palpation

Palpation comes after inspection. Warmth felt over the fracture is suggestive of an overlying haematoma. Localized tenderness over the bone in a single place is a very valuable sign as it may be the only sign of a crack fracture or greenstick fracture (see below). Palpation over a fracture may elicit crepitus, the grating of bone fragments against each other. Although this is diagnostic, it is usually painful, so local tenderness should deter the clinician from demonstrating the sign. A large effusion palpated with a swollen knee after trauma raises the suspicion of an underlying fracture.

If the bone is subcutaneous, as with the tibia, its entire length should be palpated with the index finger and the patient's expression observed for signs of pain. This may be the only positive finding in a child with an undisplaced fracture. If the bone is deeply placed, the bone is palpated by gently squeezing the affected part between the finger and thumb; deformity of the bone may be palpated in this way.

Finally, the extremity should be assessed for signs of vascular and neurological injury.

## Range of Motion

Fractures are usually accompanied by a loss of function of the affected limb. If the limb has an obvious fracture, no attempt should be made to move the limb to assess crepitus and abnormal movement. If there is no obvious fracture, the limb can be gently moved to assess function and to examine the joints above and below the site of injury. With upper limb fractures, the patient may present with guarding, supporting the arm with the other hand to prevent any painful movement at the fracture site. Angulation and shortening should be documented.

## FRACTURES IN SPECIAL CIRCUMSTANCES

### Impacted Fractures

These are fractures (**Figure 7.1**) where the distal fragment of bone has been driven into the proximal margin of the fracture. They are common in the distal radius, proximal humerus and distal femur. Localized bone tenderness is present, and this should be an appropriate indication for a radiograph. The diagnostic pitfall is that the symptoms and signs are more compatible with a sprain than with a fracture. The fracture is termed comminuted (**Figure 7.2**) when the bone is fragmented.

### Children's Fractures

Buckle fractures (also known as torus fractures) and greenstick fractures are characteristically seen in children. A buckle fracture is a compression seen along the side of the bone. A greenstick fracture (**Figure 7.3**) is incomplete and involves one cortex, or both, but with the periosteum intact on one side of the bone. The cortical bone is more elastic in children than it is in adults and is therefore able to tolerate bending without complete fracture. The bone may be angulated as a result of bending, which is known as plastic deformation.

Fractures may extend into the growth plate, which has not yet closed in children and adolescents. This may have serious consequences for the growth and length of the bone.

### Pathological Fractures

These occur (**Figure 7.4**) when a bone breaks with little or no violence through a weakened area of the bone. This is usually the result of a secondary bone tumour, most commonly from a breast, lung, prostate, thyroid or kidney metastatic cancer. Fractures occurring in osteoporotic or pagetic bone are also considered pathological.

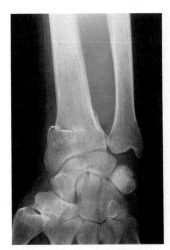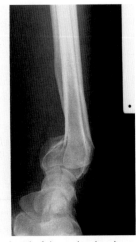

Figure 7.1 An impacted fracture. The distal end of the radius has been driven into the shaft. Note that the radial and ulnar styloid processes are lying at a similar level. In the normal wrist, the radial styloid should lie 1 cm distal to the ulnar styloid (see Figure 12.9), often accompanying the displaced physis. The clinical appearance is identical to that of a bony fracture adjacent to the bone end.

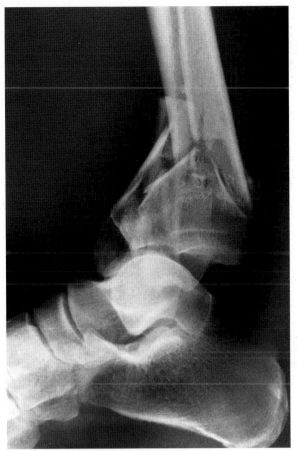

Figure 7.2 A comminuted fracture of the distal end of the tibia and fibula.

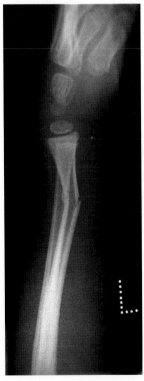

Figure 7.3 A greenstick fracture of the left radius and ulna.

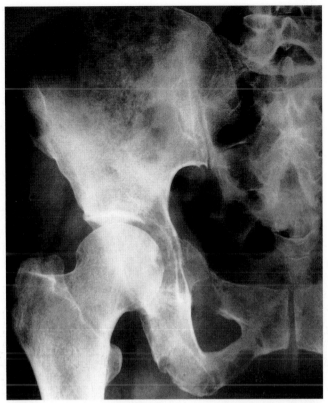

Figure 7.4 A pathological fracture of the superior pubic ramus through a metastatic deposit.

## SIGNS OF COMPLICATIONS OF FRACTURES

### Blisters

Untreated fractures and those associated with severe soft tissue injury may develop serous and blood-filled skin blisters (**Figure 7.5**) that usually appear 3–5 days after the injury. These are most commonly seen around the distal leg.

### Arterial Injury

Pulses distal to a fracture site should always be assessed. If they are not palpable, Doppler examination should be performed. It is not uncommon to have weak or absent distal pulses in open leg fractures or ankle fracture-dislocations following high-velocity motor vehicle accidents. A quick reduction of the dislocated ankle and splintage relieves the tension over the soft tissues, and, in many instances, the pulses are regained. If they are not, arteriography or urgent exploration is warranted.

In the upper limb, supracondylar fractures of the humerus in children put the brachial artery particularly at risk.

### Bleeding

Blood loss can be a concern with fractures (**Figure 7.6**), particularly of the pelvis and the femur. Up to 1.5 L may be lost with a femoral fracture, whereas an unstable pelvic fracture may cause profuse bleeding leading to hypovolaemia and signs of shock, necessitating early resuscitation.

PART 2 | TRAUMA AND (ELECTIVE) ORTHOPAEDICS

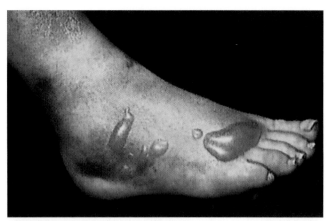

Figure 7.5 Fracture blisters in a patient with a fracture of the right calcaneum.

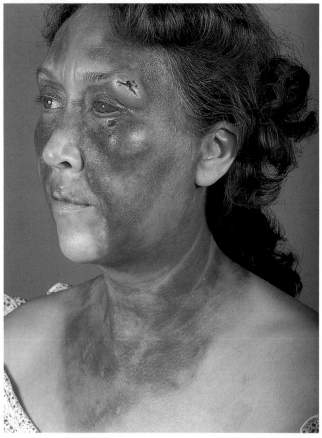

Figure 7.6 A haematoma associated with a facial fracture. The blood loss can be one or more litres in a major fracture, and this may be concealed, as in fractures of the pelvis and thigh.

## Compartment Syndrome

This is a serious, limb-threatening condition. A high index of suspicion is needed as this complication can develop only a few hours after injury (e.g. a fracture) and necessitates prompt intervention.

Compartment syndrome is defined as increased pressure in a muscle compartment compressing the muscle, nerve and vessel inside a closed space. Swelling within the confined fascial envelope around a bone may result in a rise in the compartment pressure to above the capillary tissue perfusion pressure. This leads to muscle ischaemia, with the end result of muscle necrosis, nerve damage, myoglobinuria and toxicity.

The usual cause of a rise in compartment pressure is soft tissue injury followed by swelling and bleeding. It can also result from the swelling of a limb within a tightly constricting dressing or splint.

The cardinal symptom is increasing pain despite reasonable splintage and analgesia. The most important sign is that of pain on a passive range of motion – stretch pain – which is elicited by fully flexing and extending the joints distal to the injury. The diagnosis can be confirmed by measuring the intracompartmental pressures but must be presumed and treated on clinical grounds alone. The pulse is usually preserved unless the pressure within the compartment has reached very high levels.

The long-term result of untreated muscle ischaemia is necrosis leading to repair by fibrosis and subsequent contracture – **Volkmann's ischaemic contracture (Figure 7.7)**. This presents in the forearm with wasting of the muscles and clawing of all the fingers that is relieved by flexing the wrist.

## Nerve Injuries

A complete neurological examination of the affected limb is required. Sensation, motor function and reflexes should be documented. Nerves adjacent to the fracture can be stretched or compressed, leading to neurapraxia or axonotmesis, or, in more serious cases, completely severed.

## Adult Respiratory Distress Syndrome

Adult respiratory distress syndrome is a form of respiratory failure resulting from aspiration, sepsis, shock and particulate emboli.

## Fat Emboli

Fat emboli are partly due the systemic release of bone marrow fat into the circulation. The patient presents with pulmonary distress and neurological symptoms such as agitation, delirium or coma. Anaemia and a low platelet count may be present. A petechial rash, when present, is said to be pathognomonic.

## Delayed Union and Non-union

Union of the fracture is said to be delayed when there is a loss of adequate stability at the fracture site at the time one would normally expect the fracture to have united. Non-union is the absence of union after 12 months. A non-union may be hypertrophic, with abundant palpable callus, or atrophic. Non-union is characterized by persisting movement with pain and tenderness at the fracture site. Although a loss of function is usually present, a stable fibrous non-union can occur that is functionally satisfactory even though the bone has not united.

## Malunion

Malunion (**Figure 7.8**) occurs when a fracture has not united in the anatomical position and gives rise to deformity. This may be the result of delayed diagnosis, delayed treatment or inadequate stabilization of the fracture.

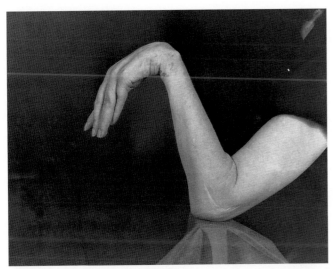

Figure 7.7 Volkmann's ischaemic contracture of the right forearm and hand.

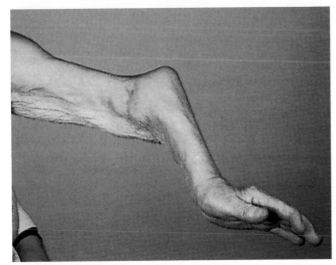

Figure 7.8 Malunion of a fracture of the left elbow.

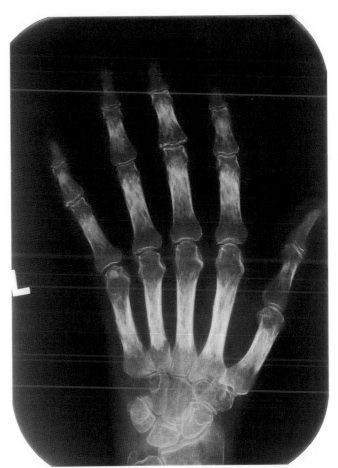

Figure 7.9 Reflex sympathetic dystrophy (Sudeck's osteodystrophy). Rarefaction involves all the joints of the left hand. The changes are particularly marked in the midcarpal region.

## Infection

Infection is a significant risk with any open fracture. The initial infection presents with swelling, redness of the adjacent skin and the presence of a purulent discharge. Chronic osteomyelitis may result.

## Deep Vein Thrombosis and Pulmonary Embolism

Deep vein thrombosis and pulmonary embolism often result from prolonged recumbency or from fractures involving the pelvis, femur or tibia.

## Complex Regional Pain Syndrome

Complex regional pain syndrome (or reflex sympathetic dystrophy) is characterized by severe pain, swelling and skin changes following trauma or surgery. It often presents when mobilization of the joint is attempted at the end of plaster immobilization or internal fixation. Initially, there is pain, out of proportion to the injury, and stiffness in the joint. The pain is exacerbated by movement and this contributes to further stiffness. Subsequently, there are changes in the skin, with the presence of smooth, mottled areas. Radiographs may demonstrate widespread mottling and decalcification of the bone (**Figure 7.9**).

## Myositis Ossificans

Myositis ossificans is the formation of bone within the muscle and is common after elbow and hip fractures and dislocations. There is pain and stiffness in the joint. When the condition is secondary to trauma, it is termed myositis ossificans traumatica. Palpation of the musculature adjacent to the joint demonstrates firm masses that are opaque on radiographs.

## Post-traumatic Osteoarthritis

Intra-articular fractures are often followed by premature osteoarthritis.

### INFECTION

Infection of the bone mostly occurs by direct contamination in the case of an open fracture or by haematogenous spread. Bacterial and tubercular infections account for the majority of cases. Spirochaetal, fungal and parasitic infections can also be present.

## Acute Osteomyelitis in Children

In childhood, acute osteomyelitis it is often secondary to a blood-borne spread of infection. A trivial lesion such as a skin abrasion or cutaneous abscess is usually the source of this. The infection settles in the bone at a region of rich blood supply, usually the metaphysis of a long bone, the most common region being the metaphysis adjacent to the knee. Less commonly in infants, the infection settles in the epiphysis.

Pyrexia and malaise may be present. Local swelling may be seen, but erythema is a late sign. Metaphyseal tenderness is the most reliable sign. Palpable swelling is indicative of subperiosteal pus, and fluctuance suggests a subcutaneous abscess. There is often a loss of function of the neighbouring joint, which may show a sympathetic effusion, but in neglected cases, penetration of infection into the joint can cause a septic arthritis. The initial radiographs are normal but MRI may confirm the diagnosis.

## Acute Osteomyelitis in Adults

This usually results from open fractures. It is occasionally the result of haematogenous spread and affects immunocompromised individuals or intravenous drug abusers. The source of infection may be arterial or venous medical monitoring lines, or multiple venous puncture wounds. The midshaft of the long bones is commonly involved. There are signs of generalized sepsis together with swelling, adjacent cutaneous erythema and a discharge at the site of injury. Localized bone tenderness and warmth are usually also present.

## Differential Diagnosis of Acute Osteomyelitis

The differential diagnosis of acute osteomyelitis includes the following:

- *Acute septic arthritis*: The hallmark of septic arthritis is severe pain on attempting to test the range of motion of the joint in question. This is different from the reactive synovitis seen in osteomyelitis adjacent to a joint. Moreover, localized bony tenderness is usually absent in septic arthritis.
- *Cellulitis*: Cellulitis, which is infection of the dermis and subcutaneous layers of the skin, can be the presenting sign of acute osteomyelitis in a child and should be carefully investigated.
- *Malignant bone neoplasm*: Malignant tumours can present in an identical fashion to an acute osteomyelitis and can only be confirmed by biopsy.
- *Fracture*: The local signs of fractures in infants may be clinically very similar to those of acute osteomyelitis. The absence of systemic features and the radiological findings are usually conclusive.

## Chronic Osteomyelitis

This most frequently presents as a sequel to acute osteomyelitis associated with an open fracture. An area of bone is destroyed by the acute infection and becomes surrounded by reactive dense sclerotic bone – the involucrum. The incarcerated necrotic areas, or sequestra, act as irritants provoking a chronic discharge that escapes through cloacae in the involucrum and hence through a sinus in the soft tissues. The infection may remain dormant or asymptomatic for long periods followed by episodes of acute inflammation.

The patient presents with a history of open fracture or surgery. There is pain, redness and local tenderness. A deformity may be present from the old fracture, and a discharging sinus or healed sinuses may be apparent. Radiographs may show cortical bone erosion (**Figures 7.10** and **7.11**). MRI can confirm the diagnosis.

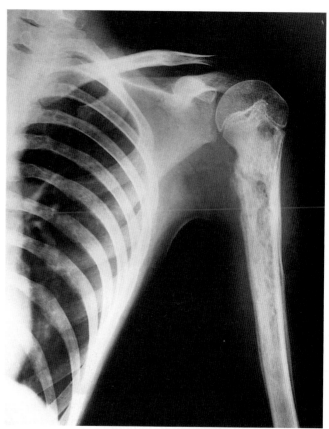

Figure 7.10 Chronic osteomyelitis of the left humerus, showing patchy sclerotic central bone changes and subperiosteal new bone formation.

## Brodie's Abscess

A Brodie's abscess is a subacute osteomyelitis most commonly caused by a staphylococcal infection (**Figure 7.12**). It is a localized, low-grade infection in adults that presents with intermittent episodes of pain, often worse at night, and swelling.

The most common sites are the upper and lower ends of the tibia, the distal femur and the proximal humerus. Plain radiographs demonstrate the architectural changes of the bone where the abscess is present.

## GENERALIZED BONE DISEASES

## Osteoporosis

Osteoporosis or 'porous bone' (see Figure 10.22a) refers to a decrease in bone density of more than 2.5 standard deviations below the mean for an age- and sex-matched healthy population. Osteoporosis is the most common cause of a 'pathological' fracture in adults.

The disease may be classified as primary type 1, primary type 2 or secondary. The form of osteoporosis most common in women after the menopause is referred to as primary type 1 or postmenopausal osteoporosis. Primary type 2 osteoporosis or senile osteoporosis occurs after the age of 75 and is seen in both women and men. Secondary osteoporosis results from chronic predisposing medical problems or disease, or from the prolonged use of medications such as steroids.

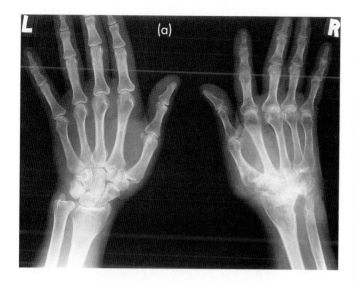

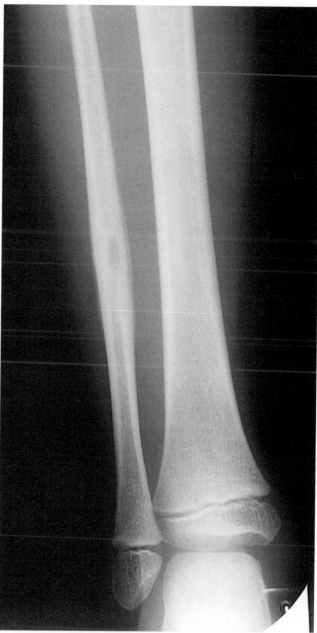

Figure 7.12 Brodie's abscess of the shaft of the fibula.

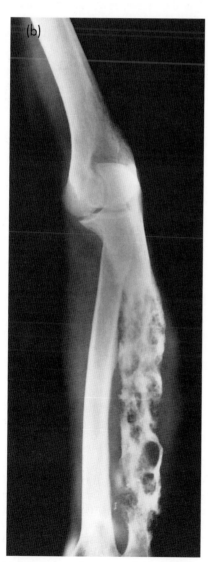

Figure 7.11 (a) Tuberculous destruction of the distal radius, carpal bones and adjacent joints of the right wrist. (b) Syphilitic infection of the ulna.

Individuals suffer a loss of height and a stooped spine as a result of vertebral collapse. Osteoporotic fractures most commonly affect the vertebral bodies, hips and distal radius.

## Paget's Disease of Bone

This is a condition that affects the way bone breaks down and rebuilds, producing bone that is softer and weaker than normal; this can lead to bone pain, deformities and fractures. The condition is a chronic bone dystrophy and 90 per cent of cases are multifocal. There is an association with viral infection but the aetiology has not been demonstrated with certainty. It occurs more often in men than in women and is usually seen after the age of 40. The lumbar vertebrae, sacrum, skull and pelvis are most commonly affected, although the limb bones (**Figure 7.13**) may also be involved.

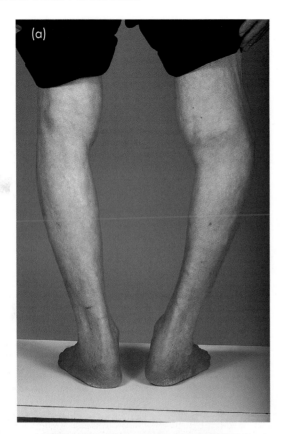

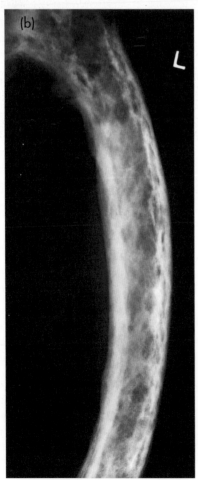

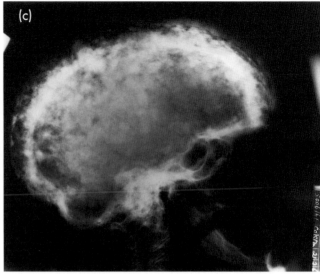

Figure 7.13 (a) Paget's deformity of the right leg, showing lateral bowing that is most marked in the upper third. (b) Paget's disease of the left femur, showing sclerotic changes and bowing. (c) Paget's disease of the skull.

The majority of patients are asymptomatic. They may, however, suffer bone pain and tenderness, bowing of the lower limbs and an increase in skull size, which may become clinically apparent because of blindness or deafness resulting from nerve compression.

Malignant change to osteosarcoma, fibrosarcoma or, occasionally, chondrosarcoma occurs infrequently and the prognosis in these circumstances is very poor. Osteoarthritis results in adjacent joints from abnormal stresses caused by the bone deformity. High-output cardiac failure is described as a result of the highly vascular nature of the bone, although it is very uncommon.

In 10 per cent of cases, the disease is monostotic (involving a single bone), and it is usually the tibia or femur that is involved, with bowing. The diagnosis is confirmed by radiographs demonstrating deformity, cystic changes and stress fractures.

## Fibrous Dysplasia

This is a benign condition comprising 7 per cent of all benign bone tumours. Normal bone is destroyed and replaced by fibrous soft tissue. Fibrous dysplasia normally affects a single bone but can be multifocal. The ribs, jaw, femur and tibia are most commonly affected. In multifocal cases, the femur and tibia are affected together with other bones.

**Albright's syndrome** is congenital multifocal fibrous dysplasia that occurs together with associated precocious puberty and café-au-lait skin patches.

## Osteomalacia

In osteomalacia (**Figure 7.14**), there is softening of the bone due to inadequate bone mineralization, and a large amount of unmineralized osteoid is present. The condition results from an inadequacy of vitamin D as a result of dietary deficiency, gastrointestinal disorders or renal osteodystrophy. In children it is known as rickets (**Figure 7.15**).

The abnormal bone is susceptible to pathological fractures, which may be microscopic stress fracture known as Looser's zones, or a fracture of both cortices. The characteristic

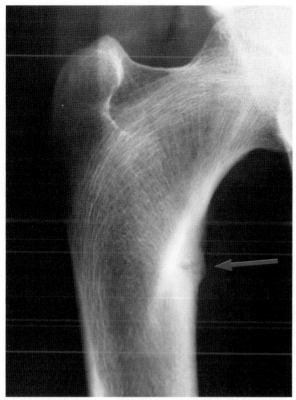

Figure 7.14 Osteomalacia with a transverse stress fracture at the level of the lesser trochanter (arrow).

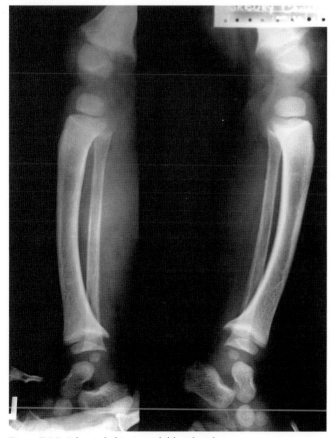

Figure 7.15 A bowed tibia in a child with rickets.

features are enlargement of the costochondral junction, bony deformities – predominantly bowing of the legs – and retarded growth. Radiographs demonstrate biconcave vertebral bodies known as 'codfish vertebrae', as well as abnormal cupped physes. Pathological fracture of the femoral neck occurs in adults with osteomalacia.

## Scurvy

This results from a deficiency of vitamin C (ascorbic acid). There is abnormal collagen growth and repair. Patients present with fatigue, swollen and bleeding gums, bruising, joint effusions and iron deficiency; radiographs may show thin cortices and trabeculae.

## Osteopetrosis (Marble Bone Disease)

This disease (**Figure 7.16**) is characterized by osteoclast dysfunction leading to a failure of bone resorption. The bone hardens and becomes denser and increasingly sclerotic, and the medullary canal is obliterated.

The most severe form of osteopetrosis is the so-called malignant form, which is an autosomal recessive condition leading to dense sclerosis that obliterates the medullary canals on radiographs, hepatosplenomegaly and aplastic anaemia. The 'tarda' form is an autosomal dominant condition and demonstrates generalized osteosclerosis. Radiographs of the spine show the 'rugger jersey' appearance. Pathological fractures occur through the abnormal bone.

## Hyperparathyroidism

Osteitis fibrosa cystica (Von Recklinghausen's disease of bone) is a rare (5 per cent) manifestation of hyperparathyroidism (**Figure 7.17**). The symptoms are those of hypercalcaemia with muscle weakness, gastrointestinal upsets and muscle pains.

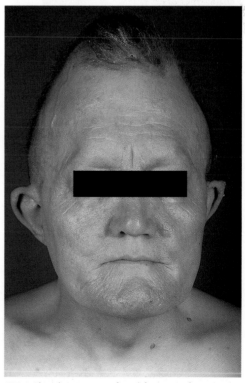

Figure 7.16 The characteristic facial features of a patient with marble bone disease.

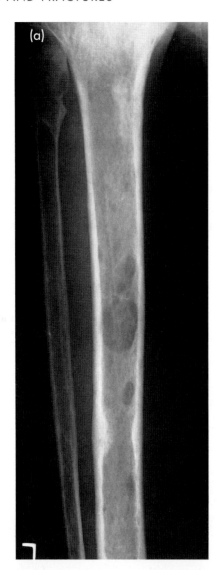

Cystic degeneration of the bone is due to brown tumours of localized osteoclastic resorption and may be evident on radiographs.

## Ochronosis

Ochronosis is a congenital defect of tyrosine and phenylalanine metabolism syndrome caused by an accumulation of homogentisic acid in the connective tissues. The urine turns dark on standing, and pigment is deposited in the auricular cartilages, which look bluish. The sclera and the skin over bony prominences look slate blue. Arthritic changes in the spine are common.

## Osteogenesis Imperfecta

This condition (brittle bone disease, or Lobstein syndrome) (**Figure 7.18**) is a spectrum of conditions in which there is an abnormal cross-linking of collagen leading to a deficiency in type 1 collagen. The condition is usually transmitted as an autosomal dominant trait. The patient may suffer multiple fractures, a short stature, scoliosis, hearing defects and ligamentous laxity. Blue sclera are seen in some forms of the disease. Severe forms are often fatal in infancy.

## Dwarfism

The short stature may be proportionate or disproportionate depending on whether the limbs are of normal length relative to the length of the trunk. Achondroplasia is the most common example of short-limbed, disproportionate dwarfism. The rarer mucopolysaccharidoses give rise to proportionate dwarfism. Skeletal epiphyseal dysplasia can present in different forms with either short trunk or short limb varieties. Involvement of the spine, knees or hips should alert the examiner to the possibility of a dysplasia or dystrophy.

### Achondroplasia

Achondroplasia (**Figure 7.19**) is responsible for 70 per cent of cases of dwarfism. It is inherited as an autosomal dominant condition, but 80 per cent of instances arise from spontaneous mutations. The trunk is of normal length but the limbs are short. Individuals with achondroplasia have prominent foreheads and flat noses. There is often a thoracolumbar kyphosis with lumbar

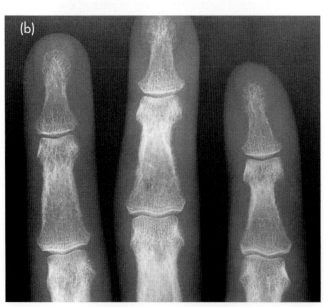

Figure 7.17 Hyperparathyroidism. (a) Cystic lesions within the tibia. (b) Reabsorption of cortical bone in the phalanges.

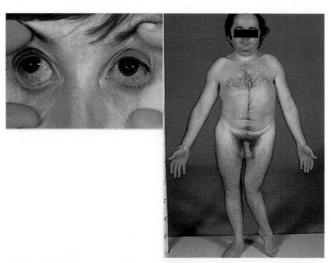

Figure 7.18 Osteogenesis imperfecta. (a) Blue sclera. (b) Limb deformities in a patient with brittle bone disease, showing a short stature with relative sparing of the trunk.

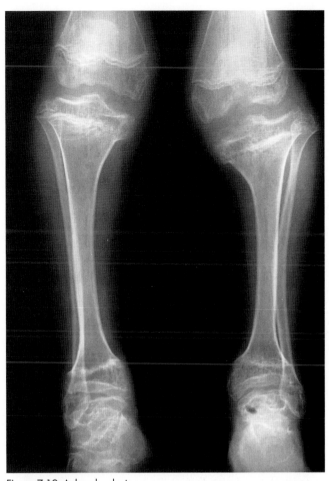

Figure 7.19 Achondroplasia.

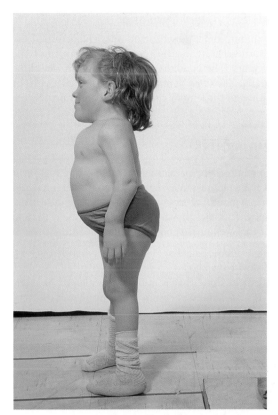

Figure 7.20 Morquio's syndrome (Reproduced with permission of Mr. B. A. Taylor).

hyperlordosis giving rise to prominent buttocks. Intelligence is normal. Adults may develop problems with spinal stenosis.

## Mucopolysaccharidoses

In these conditions, there is an accumulation of mucopolysac-charides resulting from an enzyme deficiency. Type 4 – **Morquio's syndrome (Figure 7.20)** – is the most common. In this, there is short-limbed dwarfism together with a thickened skull, flat pelvis, coxa valga and abnormally shaped metacarpals. In particular, there is instability at the atlantoaxial joint, and the child may present with a progressive deterioration of walking as a result of spinal cord compression.

## Spondyloepiphyseal Dysplasia Congenita

This is an autosomal dominant disorder characterized by a short trunk relative to the length of the limbs. It has an association with cleft palate and increased lumbar lordosis. The vertebrae are flattened (**Figure 7.21**).

## Achondroplasia tarda

This is an X-linked recessive disorder characterized by scoliosis and abnormalities of the major joints, such as the hips, which are liable to early osteoarthritis.

## Pseudoachondroplasic Dysplasia

This is an autosomal dominant disorder characterized by normal facies but with other features similar to those of achondroplasia. There is bowing of the tibia and craniocervical instability.

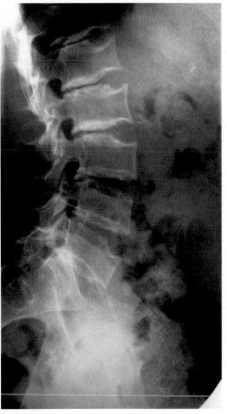

Figure 7.21 Spondyloepiphyseal dysplasia.

## Multiple Epiphyseal Dysplasia

This is an autosomal dominant disorder characterized by short-limbed dwarfism. It may not become apparent until the early teenage years. The condition may present with a waddling gait because the proximal femur is often affected, with bilateral irregularities of the femoral heads and concomitant abnormalities of the acetabula.

## BONE TUMOURS

The age group of the patient and the site of the tumour in relation to the epiphyses may help with the differential diagnosis of a bone tumour. For example, giant cell tumours only arise at the epiphysis. Some physical signs may also help to determine whether the swelling is benign or malignant:

- Benign: Large, painless, a normal temperature over the mass and slow-growing.
- Malignant: Bone that is not greatly enlarged, is often painful, is associated with warm overlying skin and shows rapid recent growth.

## Benign Neoplasms

### Solitary (Simple) Bone Cyst

This is a benign, non-neoplastic, unilocular cystic lesion (**Figure 7.22**) that occurs as a result of abnormal growth at the epiphysis. It is most commonly seen in the region of the metaphysis of the long bones in children aged between 4 and 10 years. The cyst is often seen as an incidental finding on a radiograph. It can present with a pathological fracture occurring through the cyst. Occasionally, it presents as a swelling in the region of the metaphysis.

### Osteochondroma

An osteochondroma (**Figure 7.23a**) is the most commonly encountered benign tumour. It contains both cartilage and bone and commonly occurs at the metaphyses of the long bones. The exostosis (**Figure 7.23b**) may be solitary or multiple, in which case it may be associated with hereditary multiple exostoses – **diaphyseal aclasis**. There is a 10 per cent risk of sarcomatous change in individuals with multiple lesions.

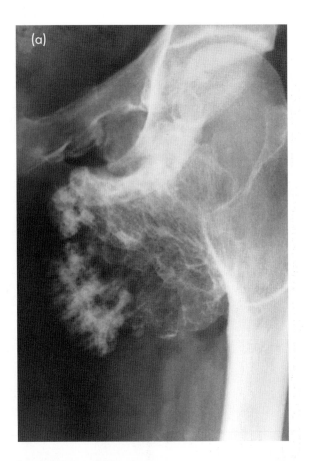
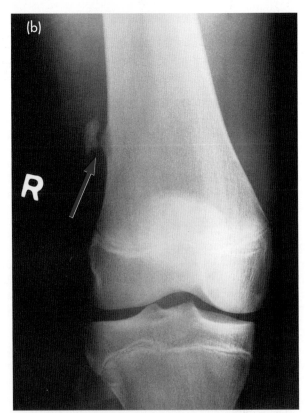

Figure 7.23 Osteochondroma. (a) A large exostosis arising from the neck of the femur. (b) Fractured exostosis of the lower end of the femur (arrow).

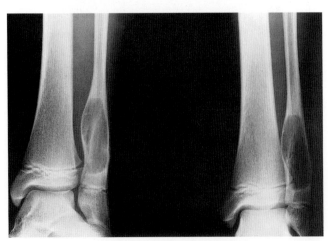

Figure 7.22 A solitary bone cyst at the lower end of the fibula.

## Enchondroma

This is a benign cartilaginous tumour arising from the medullary surface of the bone that usually affects the small bones of the hands and feet (**Figure 7.24**). The tumours may be solitary or multiple (Ollier's disease) or associated with multiple haemangiomas (Maffucci's syndrome). When the phalanges are affected, there is swelling and pain. Malignant transformation is rare in solitary lesions but occurs in a small proportion of cases where multiple lesions are present.

The term 'chondroma' is applied to cartilaginous masses not restricted to the medulla of the bone. Chondromyxoid fibromas and fibromas are rare benign tumours made up of defined tissue and usually presenting as incidental radiological findings. Fibromas differ from fibrous dysplasias in that there is no new bone within them.

## Osteoid Osteoma

Osteoid osteomas are benign tumours with a small sclerotic osteoblastic centre that affect the long bones or spine and present with pain and tenderness in the region of the lesion (**Figure 7.25**). The pain is characteristically present at night and abolished by aspirin.

An **osteoblastoma** (**Figure 7.26**) is a locally aggressive benign lesion made up of mature osteoid cells. Its histological characteristics are similar to those of an osteoma, but the lesion exceeds 1 cm in diameter and may be of a considerable size. Any bone can be affected, but the spine and skull are common sites.

## Aneurysmal Bone Cyst

This is a benign condition affecting children and young adults that causes swelling of the long bones or vertebrae (**Figure 7.27**). The expanding osteolytic lesion contains bloody fluid and may be the site of a pathological fracture.

## Giant Cell Tumour (Osteoclastoma)

These are neoplasms made up of osteoclasts that form osteolytic tumours. They arise more often in the 20–40-year-old age group and occur at the end of the long bones (**Figure 7.28**). The majority of tumours occur around the knee, with local swelling, heat and dilatation of the superficial veins. Pathological fractures are common because of the osteolysis. Some tumours recur after excision, and a small proportion are malignant from the outset.

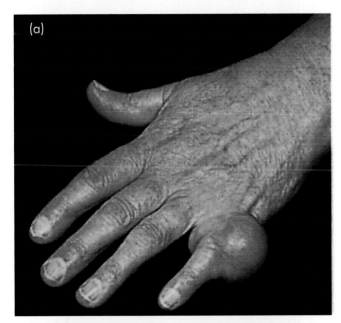
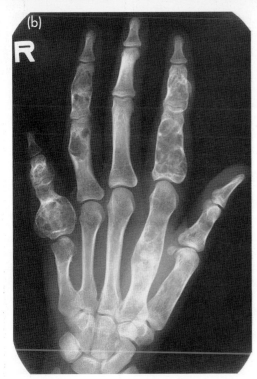

Figure 7.24 Multiple enchondromas (Ollier's disease).

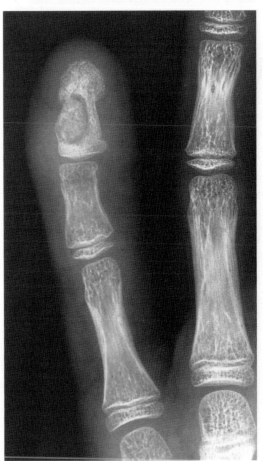

Figure 7.25 Osteoid osteoma of the terminal phalanx of the right index finger, showing dense central bone with a lucent surround.

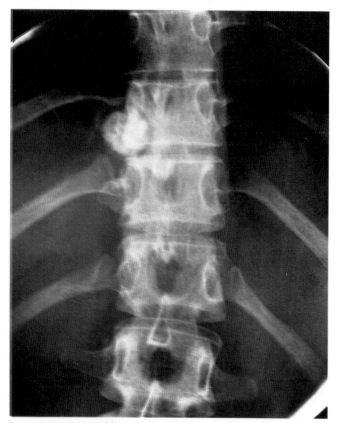

Figure 7.26 An osteoblastoma.

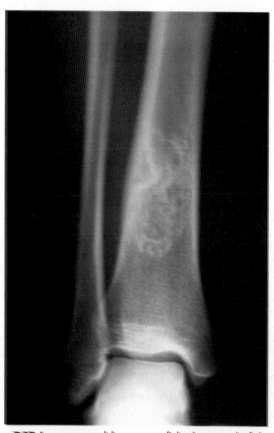

Figure 7.27 An aneurysmal bone cyst of the lower end of the right tibia.

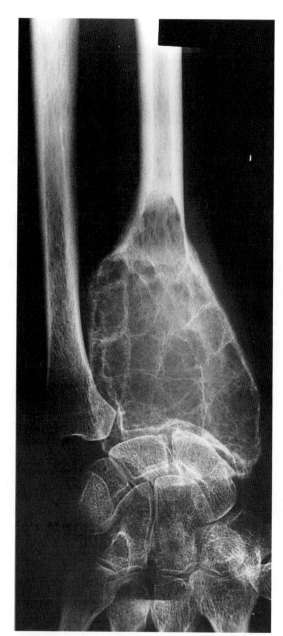

Figure 7.28 An osteoclastoma of the distal radius. Note the characteristic 'soap bubble' appearance.

## Malignant Neoplasms

### Multiple Myeloma

This is the most common primary malignant bone tumour (**Figure 7.29**) and is a neoplastic proliferation of plasma cells or their precursors. It is rare before the age of 40. The common presentation of the bony deposits is with pathological fractures affecting the ribs and vertebrae. The affected areas are osteolytic, and Bence Jones proteins are present. The diagnosis is confirmed on bone marrow biopsy.

### Osteosarcoma

Osteosarcoma (**Figure 7.30**) is a malignant tumour in which osteoid is synthesized by sarcomatous cells. It occurs more commonly in males than females, and 75 per cent of patients are

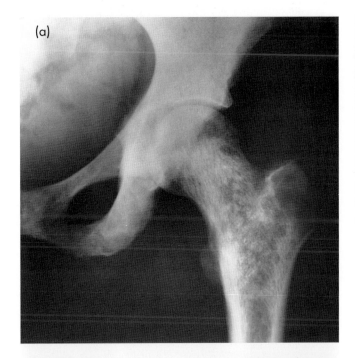

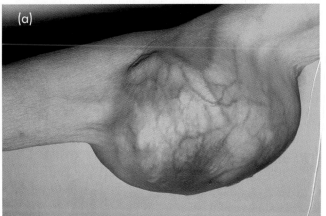

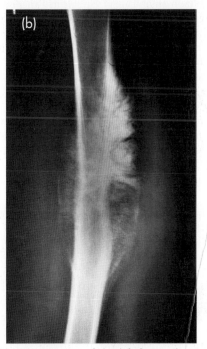

Figure 7.30 (a) Osteosarcoma of the left femur. (b) Osteosarcoma commencing in the left lower humerus. Untreated tumours of this size are relatively rare in the UK.

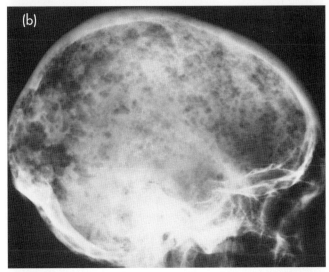

Figure 7.29 Multiple myeloma. (a) Myeloma of the upper left femur. (b) Extensive myeloma of the skull.

between the ages of 10 and 25 years; osteosarcoma in elderly patients often occurs as a complication of Paget's disease. Most sarcomas occur in the metaphyses of the long bones. Many osteoscarcomas occur around the knee and the upper end of the femur and humerus.

Patients present with increasing pain and swelling. Radiographs show characteristic abnormalities of the periosteum with a 'sun-ray' appearance of the bone and a Codman's triangle of reactive bone at the junction with the periosteum. As with most sarcomas, spread of the tumour is usually by the bloodstream to the lungs.

## Parosteal Osteosarcoma

This is an uncommon malignant lesion (**Figure 7.31**) arising from the surface of the bone that often affects the posterior surface of the distal femur and the upper tibia or humerus. There is

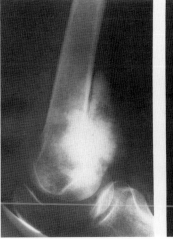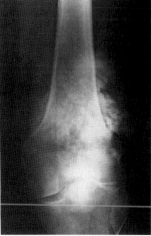

Figure 7.31 A parosteal osteosarcoma of the right lower femur.

a broad-based swelling that grows and can encircle the shaft. Destruction of the cortex and medulla occurs late in the disease.

### Chondrosarcoma

A chondrosarcoma (**Figure 7.32**) is a malignant neoplasm of cartilage. It occurs in an older age group than osteosarcoma, predominantly in the age range 40–70 years. About half of the lesions occur in the pelvic girdle and ribs, together with the proximal femur. The tumour may be situated within the bone or on its periphery. The presentation is usually of an increasing size of a long-standing swelling in the axial skeleton. There is characteristic calcification on radiographs.

### Fibrosarcoma

Fibrosarcomas (**Figure 7.33a**) are usually lytic lesions of the diaphysis or metaphysis and are of variable malignancy. Synovial sarcomas (**Figure 7.33b**) are usually associated with a major joint. They are highly malignant, invading locally and metastasizing to lymph nodes as well as via the bloodstream. Both fibrosarcomas and synovial sarcomas may arise independently of bone, within muscle or subcutaneous tissues.

### Ewing's Tumour

This is a malignant, round-blue-cell tumour (**Figure 7.34**). It usually occurs between the ages of 5 and 20 years. The femur, tibia, humerus and fibula are most commonly involved, but the pelvis and ribs can also be affected. The tumour is usually

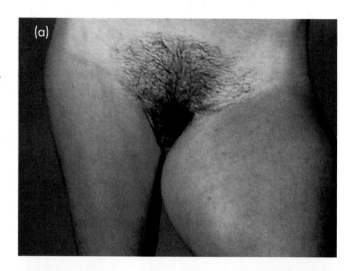

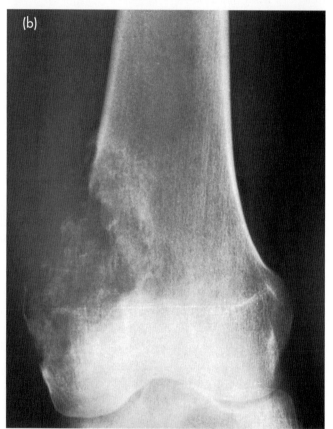

Figure 7.33 (a) A fibrosarcoma of the lower end of the left femur. (b) A synovial sarcoma.

osteolytic, and penetration of the cortex, with raising of the periosteum, may give rise to a mass. The presentation is of pain and swelling of gradual onset. Fever and an elevated white cell count may simulate osteomyelitis.

### Secondary Neoplasia

Metastatic cancers to bone (**Figure 7.35**) are the most common bone tumours. Patients may present with a complication of the metastasis, such as local pain or a pathological fracture. The most common primaries are carcinoma of the breast, bronchus, kidney, thyroid and prostate.

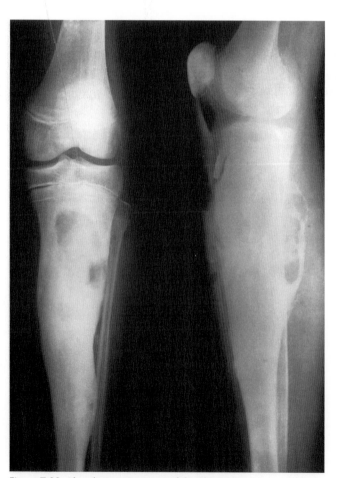

**Figure 7.32** Chondromyxosarcoma of the tibia.

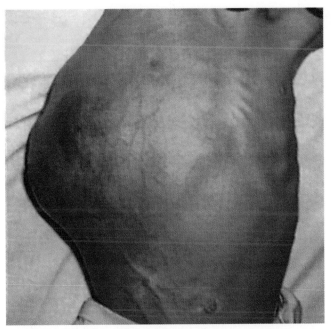

Figure 7.34 Ewing's sarcoma arising in a rib.

**Key Points**

- A fracture is defined as a break in cartilage or bone that is accompanied by an insult to the overlying soft tissues.
- The outer surface of bones is a dense irregular connective tissue membrane called the periosteum. This plays an essential role in healing after a bone fracture.
- The musculoskeletal examination can be summarised as 'look, feel and move'.
- In children, the cortical bone is more elastic than it is in adults and is therefore, as a result of plastic deformation, able to tolerate bending without complete fracture.
- A high index of suspicion is needed to recognize the early development of compartment syndrome, which is a limb-threatening condition that can follow a fracture.
- Osteoporotic fractures most commonly affect the vertebral bodies, hip and distal radius.
- Osteochondroma is the most commonly encountered benign tumour. Multiple myeloma is the most common primary malignant bone tumour. However, metastases are the most common of all malignant bone tumours

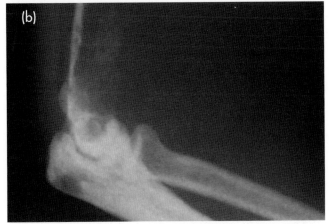

Figure 7.35 (a) Fracture through a metastasis in the right clavicle. (b) Lytic lesion due to secondary deposits from breast neoplasia.

## QUESTIONS

### SBAs

**1. A proximal comminuted fracture of the tibia with a 15 cm open wound, massive tissue devitalization and evidence of popliteal artery transection is classified as which one of the following Gustilo and Anderson types?:**
- a   I
- b   II
- c   IIIA
- d   IIIB
- e   IIIC

**Answer**

**e   Type IIIC.** *An open fracture with a laceration of over 10 cm that associated with a major vessel injury is classified as Gustilo type IIIC.*

**2. The potential complications of a limb compartment syndrome include which one of the following?:**
- a   Muscle necrosis
- b   Nerve damage
- c   Myoglobinuria
- d   Contractures
- e   All of the above

**Answer**

**e   All of the above.** *If left untreated or treated late, compartment syndrome in a limb leads to muscle necrosis, nerve damage, myoglobinuria, contractures, limb loss and systemic toxicity.*

**3. The most common cause of a 'pathological' fracture in adults is which of the following?:**
- a   Multiple myeloma
- b   Osteosarcoma
- c   Simple bone cyst
- d   Osteoporosis
- e   Marble bone disease

**Answer**

**d   Osteoporosis.** *This is the most common cause of a pathological fracture in adults.*

### EMQs

**1. Match each of these conditions with one of the descriptions given below:**
- **1** Osteomyelitis
- **2** Scurvy
- **3** Chronic regional pain syndrome
- **4** Cellulitis
- **5** Septic arthritis
- a   Chronic ankle pain and a discharging sinus following an open fracture
- b   A swollen joint with a painful range of motion
- c   Inflammation of the dermal and subcutaneous layers of the skin
- d   Chronic pain, swelling and skin changes following trauma or surgery
- e   Swollen and bleeding gums, bruising, joint effusions and iron deficiency

**Answers**

**a   1 Osteomyelitis.** *This is infection of the bone that commonly spreads via the bloodstream in children or results from direct contamination in the setting of an open fracture. A discharging sinus may be present in chronic cases.*

**b   5 Septic arthritis.** *This is an emergency condition characterized by a swollen joint, severe pain and limitation of the range of motion.*

**c   4 Cellulitis.** *Cellulitis is suspected when skin erythema, warmth and tenderness are present, sometimes in the absence of systemic toxicity or deeper infections involving the joints, bones or muscles. It is important to inspect the skin for potential ports of entry of microorganisms.*

**d   3 Chronic regional pain syndrome.** *Formerly called reflex sympathetic dystrophy, this refers to chronic pain, swelling and skin changes following trauma or surgery that are usually attributed to an inappropriate response to soft tissue injury.*

**e   2 Scurvy.** *This results from vitamin C deficiency. It initially presents with malaise and lethargy, followed by spots on the skin, spongy gums and bleeding from the mucous membranes.*

**2.** Match each of these conditions with one of the descriptions given below:
   **1** Ewing's sarcoma
   **2** Multiple myeloma
   **3** Osteitis fibrosa cystica
   **4** Enchondroma
   **5** Achondroplasia
   **a** Osteolytic lesions and Bence Jones proteins
   **b** Brown tumours and elevated parathyroid hormone levels
   **c** Disproportinate dwarfism
   **d** A benign cartilaginous lesion arising from the medullary surface of the hand bones
   **e** A malignant round-blue-cell tumour

**Answers**

**a** **2 *Multiple myeloma.*** *This is a cancer of the plasma cells, a subtype of white blood cells that generate antibodies. The common symptoms can be remembered using the mnemonic* **CARB**, *standing for* **c**alcium (elevated), **r**enal failure, **a**naemia, and **b**one lesions.

**b** **3 *Osteitis fibrosa cystica.*** *This is a bone disorder caused by hyperparathyroidism that leads to bone pain and tenderness, deformities and fractures. The commonly associated bone cysts are referred to as brown tumors.*

**c** **5 *Achondroplasia.*** *Achondroplasia is a common cause of dwarfism resulting from a mutation in the fibroblast growth factor receptor 3. This leads to the formation of abnormal cartilage.*

**d** **4 *Enchondroma.*** *An enchondroma is a benign bone tumour arising from cartilage. It is commonly seen in the hands and feet.*

**e** **1 *Ewing's sarcoma.*** *This is a malignant bone tumour that is usually seen in children. It commonly affects the pelvis and the diaphysis of the femur, tibia and humerus. It usually presents with swelling and tenderness. Small-round-blue tumour cells are seen on pathology slides.*

# CHAPTER 8

# Joints and Muscles

Mira Merashli, Rabih Nayfe and Imad Uthman

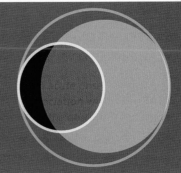

## LEARNING OBJECTIVES

- To identify different joint movements and deformities
- To list the steps involved in a proper musculoskeletal physical examination
- To recognize the different clinical presentations of various arthritides
- To identify different muscular disorders at the level of the muscle, nerve and neuromuscular junction

- To distinguish different types of dyskinesia
- To understand traumatic muscle injuries
- To recognize muscle tumours (rhabdomyosarcoma and leiomyoma)
- To describe the gait cycle

## INTRODUCTION

The diagnosis of nearly all musculoskeletal problems relies upon the demonstration of objective findings, which makes the physical examination enormously important, albeit sometimes poorly understood and inadequately performed by physicians at all levels of training. Without the ability to perform a proper physical examination, the use of additional diagnostic laboratory testing may be excessive, expensive and lacking the precision that comes only from recognizing important musculoskeletal physical findings.

## MOVEMENTS

Body movement falls into the following categories:

- *Flexion*: movement that decreases the angle between two bones. Most flexion movements are forward movements, the major exception being flexion of the knee.
- *Extension*: movement that increases the angle between two bones. Most extension movements are backward movements, the exception being extension of the knee.
- *Lateral flexion*: bending of the spine to the side.
- *Abduction*: moving away from the midline of the body.
- *Adduction*: moving towards the midline of the body.
- *Rotation*: medial (internal) or lateral (external) movement around an axis.
- *Circumduction*: movement in which an extremity describes a 360° circle.
- *Supination*: the lateral rotation of the forearm, bringing the palm of the hand upwards. In this position, the radius and ulna are parallel to each other.

- *Pronation*: medial rotation of the forearm, with the palm in a downward position so that the radius lies diagonally across the ulna.
- *Dorsiflexion*: movement that brings the top of the foot toward the shin.
- *Plantar flexion*: movement that brings the sole of the foot downwards (as in pointing the toes).
- *Depression*: downward movement of the shoulder girdle.
- *Elevation*: upward movement of the shoulder girdle.
- *Scapular adduction*: backward movement of the shoulder girdle with the scapulae pulled toward the midline.
- *Scapular abduction*: forward movement of the shoulder girdle with the scapulae pulled away from the midline.

## Deformities

Hand deformities may be caused by an injury or may result from another disorder (such as rheumatoid arthritis [RA]). They can be of several types:

- *Mallet finger*: The fingertip is curled in and cannot straighten itself. This usually results from injury, which either damages the long extensor tendon or tears the tendon from the bone.
- *Swan-neck deformity*: This deformity comprises a bending in (flexion) of the base of the finger, a straightening out (extension) of the middle joint, and a bending in (flexion) of the most distal joint. It is a feature of RA.
- *Boutonnière deformity* (buttonhole deformity): This is a deformity in which the middle joint of the finger is bent in a fixed position inwards (toward the palm) while the most distal joint of the finger is bent excessively outwards (away

PART 2 | TRAUMA AND (ELECTIVE) ORTHOPAEDICS

from the palm). It is due to a rupture of the central slip of the extensor expansion.

- *Dupuytren's contracture* (palmar fibromatosis): This is a progressive tightening of the bands of fibrous tissue (fascia) inside the palms, causing a curling in of the fingers that can eventually result in a claw-like hand (**Figure 8.1**).
- *Trigger finger/stenosing tenosynovitis*: The finger clicks when it is bent. When the hand is subsequently straightened out, the affected finger remains bent and then straightens with a click. Feel for a tender nodule over the tendon sheath at the distal palmar crease. The condition is caused by inflammatory thickening of the tendon sheath.
- *Z-deformity*: Hyperextension of the interphalangeal joint, fixed flexion and subluxation of the metacarpophalangeal joint gives the thumb a Z appearance.

The two major types of knee or femoral-tibial angular deformity are genu varum (bow legs) and genu valgum (knock-knees).

**Talipes equinovarus**, sometimes called club foot, is characterized by plantar flexion, inward tilting of the heel (relative to the midline of the leg) and adduction of the forefoot (medial deviation away from the leg's vertical axis).

**Kyphosis** (Scheuermann's disease) is an abnormal curving of the spine that causes a humpback.

Scoliosis is an abnormal lateral curvature of the spine. It is often detected during a routine physical examination as an asymmetry in shoulder height, an apparent discrepancy in leg length and asymmetry of the chest wall.

## ROUTINE EXAMINATION OF A JOINT

The examination of a joint should include the following, which can be remembered by the mnemonic 'EIPRS':

- **E**xpose the area or extremity to be examined (and the opposite extremity for comparison).
- **I**nspect for joint asymmetry, deformities, swelling, erythema, scars, rashes and muscle wasting.
- **P**alpate (both the non-involved and the involved extremity) for warmth, tenderness, joint swelling and crepitus.
- **R**ange of motion: test for an active range of motion followed by a passive range of motion, noting any resistance and contractures. In addition, measure and document any deformity of length and angles.
- **S**trength testing should then be carried out.

These tests vary with the patient's complaints and the particular joint(s) involved. Diagnostic manoeuvres and/or stress tests can be used to further assess joint function and stability. Always check for any associated neurological and vascular effects of joint disease, especially after injury.

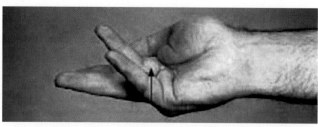

Figure 8.1 Dupuytren's contracture.

## THE ARTHRITIDES

### Osteoarthritis

Osteoarthritis (OA) is not an inflammatory process and is characterized by degeneration of the articular cartilage. This may be primary, resulting from a combination of age and hereditary and environmental factors, or secondary, resulting from trauma, infection or underlying rheumatic inflammatory disorders.

Osteoarthritis usually affects the weight-bearing joints including the hips and knees (from which crepitus can be felt or heard). In OA of the hands, there is bony swelling of the distal interphalangeal joints (**Heberden's nodes**) and/or the proximal interphalangeal joints (**Bouchard's nodes**), as well as the first carpometacarpal joint, usually symmetrically.

On imaging, subchondral sclerosis, osteophytes, bone cysts and joint space narrowing can be seen (**Figure 8.2**).

### Rheumatoid Arthritis

In RA of the hands, there is soft tissue swelling of the metacarpophalangeal and proximal interphalangeal joints. The distal interphalangeal joints are virtually never involved in RA, but inflammatory changes at this site may be seen in psoriatic arthritis

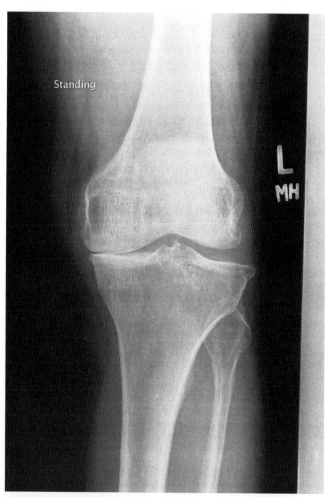

Figure 8.2 Anteroposterior radiograph of the left knee showing a subchondral sclerosis and knee joint space narrowing. (Courtesy of Dr N. Khoury.)

or gout. At the wrist, RA leads to soft tissue swelling around the radiocarpal joint and may result in prominence of the ulnar styloid and a dinner-fork deformity (due to volar subluxation of the carpus in relation to the radius) (**Figures 8.3** and **8.4**). Note also the ulnar deviation of the fingers, Boutonnière, swan-neck and Z-deformities and swelling of the proximal interphalangeal joints, in addition to the wasting of the small muscles of the hand and atrophic skin and purpura (secondary to steroid therapy).

Primary OA never involves the wrist, elbow or shoulder, so swelling of these joints should alert the clinician to the likelihood of RA, gout or chondrocalcinosis. Spinal disease is extremely uncommon in RA, except in the late stages.

## Ankylosing Spondylitis

In ankylosing spondylitis, spinal disease generally occurs early and results in decreased movement in all planes, together with tenderness at the sites where the ligaments insert onto the bones (enthesitis). The peripheral joints may be involved in patients with ankylosing spondylitis, reactive arthritis or psoriatic arthritis. Unilateral uveitis is the most common extra-articular complication of ankylosing spondylitis.

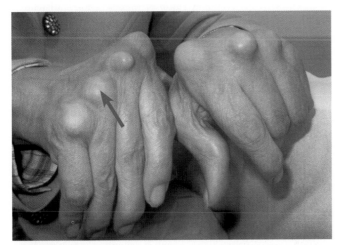

Figure 8.3 Ulnar deviation of the metacarpophalangeal joints and subcutaneous tissue nodules (arrow).

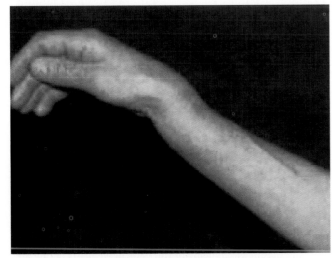

Figure 8.4 Dinner-fork deformity of the hand.

## Psoriatic Arthritis

Psoriatic arthritis occurs in the following patterns:

- *Asymmetrical oligoarticular arthritis*: affects fewer joints on one or both sides of the body. The fingers and toes may be enlarged and tender.
- *Symmetrical polyarthritis*: affects several joints to the same extent on both sides of the body, and can be disabling.
- *Distal interphalangeal arthropathy*: the 'classic' type of psoriatic arthritis. It primarily affects the joints of the fingers and toes closest to the nail, resulting in deformed nails and nail beds.
- *Arthritis mutilans*: affects the small joints of the hands and feet, and is the rarest form of the five types.
- *Spondylitis* with or without sacroiliitis: affects the spinal column between the neck and the lower back.

## Gout

Gout results from the deposition of uric acid crystals in the joints. It commonly occurs in an individual's great toe (podagra; **Figure 8.5**), resulting in sharp pain. Pain caused by gout can also occur in other joints of the body, such as the knees, wrists, ankles and hands, and tends to subside within the first 24 hours of when the attack occurred. Once the sharp pain around the joints has subsided, more subtle pain and general discomfort can be felt around the affected areas. This can last from just a few days to many weeks before all the pain has completely gone. The affected joints are usually red, tender and even swollen. Crystals are also deposited in gouty tophi in the helix of the ear, in the eyelid and around the elbow joint.

**Pseudogout** is similar to gout but tends to affect the knees in individuals aged 50 years or older. Crystal analysis of the joint aspirate reveals monosodium urate crystals in gout and pyrophosphate crystals in pseudogout. Radiographs of pseudogout show chondrocalcinosis.

## Systemic Lupus Erythematosus

This is a chronic autoimmune inflammatory arthropathy that predominantly affects middle-aged women. There is acute tender swelling of the proximal interphalangeal, metacarpophalangeal

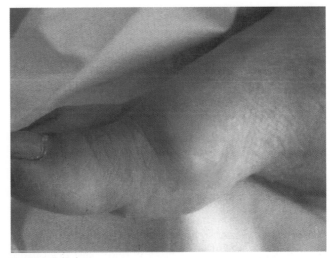

Figure 8.5 Podagra.

and carpal joints of the hand; the knees and other joints may also be involved. Extra-articular manifestations include pyrexia, a butterfly rash on the face, pancytopenia, pericarditis and nephritis.

## Reiter's Syndrome

Reiter's syndrome is an acute non-purulent arthritis complicating an infection elsewhere in the body (other than the joint itself). It is characterized by a triad of symptoms of urethritis, conjunctivitis and arthritis.

## Polymyalgia Rheumatica

Polymyalgia rheumatica is a disorder of the muscles and joints characterized by symmetrical muscle pain and stiffness involving the shoulders, arms, neck and buttock areas. Patients are typically over 50 years of age. Shoulder abduction may be limited by pain. Muscle strength is not usually impaired, but muscle pain may make testing difficult. If the symptoms persist, disuse atrophy of the muscle can occur, leading to muscle weakness. Scalp tenderness and visibly thickened and tender temporal arteries are signs indicative of giant cell arteritis, and may be present in 10–20 per cent of patients with polymyalgia rheumatica.

## Septic Arthritis

The classic picture is a single swollen, warm and tender joint with pain on active or passive movement. The knee is involved in about 50 per cent of cases, but the wrists, ankles and hips are also commonly affected. Septic arthritis may present as polyarticular arthritis in about 10–19 per cent of patients. It is more common in patients with prior joint damage. Fevers and rigors are present in the majority of cases, but their absence does not exclude the diagnosis. Bacteraemia is a common finding and, when present, may cause fatigue, vomiting or hypotension.

Joint aspiration is mandatory when an effusion is present. Empirical treatment with antibiotics should be started once suspected.

## Tuberculous Arthritis

Tuberculous arthritis is caused by the bacterium *Mycobacterium tuberculosis*. The joints most often involved are the ankles, hips, knees, spine and wrists. Most cases involve just one joint. Tuberculosis involving the spine is often referred to as **Pott's disease** and makes up about half of all tuberculosis-related bone infections. Patients usually present with decreased movement in the joints, which are swollen, warm and tender, night sweats, low-grade fever, muscle atrophy and weight loss.

## Haemophilia

The arthropathy of haemophilia is related to destructive changes associated with repeated episodes of intra-articular haemorrhage (haemarthrosis). It is one of the most common causes of joint pain and swelling. The condition typically occurs following an injury to the joint, although it can happen spontaneously in patients with haemophilia. Individuals taking anticoagulants such as warfarin are also prone to developing haemarthrosis.

## Neuropathic Arthropathy (Charcot's Joint)

Any condition that causes sensory or autonomic neuropathy can lead to a Charcot joint. Charcot arthropathy occurs as a complication of diabetes (the most common cause), syphilis, chronic alcoholism, leprosy and renal dialysis. Progressive joint effusion, fracture, fragmentation and subluxation should raise the suspicion of neuroarthropathy. Radiography may be the only imaging required for the diagnosis of neuropathic arthropathy.

## DISORDERS OF MUSCLE

The terms 'muscle disease', 'muscular dystrophy', 'neuromuscular conditions' and 'neuromuscular disorders' describe a large group of conditions that affect the muscles, nerves or neuromuscular junctions. These conditions present with the following symptoms.

## Pain

Muscle pain is most frequently related to tension, overuse or muscle injury from physically demanding work. In these situations, the pain tends to involve specific muscles and starts during or just after the activity; it may also be localized by resisted movement of the relevant group of muscle.

Muscle pain can be a sign of infection (including flu) and disorders that affect the connective tissues (such as lupus erythematosus). One common cause of muscle aches and pain is fibromyalgia, a condition that includes tenderness in the muscles and surrounding soft tissue, sleep difficulties and fatigue.

## Weakness

The term 'weakness' refers to a decrease in strength of the muscles. It may be generalized or localized to one area of the body, limb or muscle. Weakness is more notable when it is localized, which may follow a stroke, a flare-up of multiple sclerosis or injury to a nerve. Measurable weakness may result from a variety of conditions, including primary muscular diseases and metabolic, neurological and toxic disorders.

## Wasting

Muscular atrophy is the wasting or loss of muscle tissue resulting either from neurogenic or disuse atrophy. The extent of the atrophy is determined by clinical observation, noting lack of muscle tone, weakness of the specific muscles and limb circumference measurements. The sensation and reflexes may or may not be abnormal.

## Abnormal Involuntary Movements (Dyskinesias)

Dyskinesias can be classified as follows:

* *Athetosis*: sinuous writhing movement of the fingers and hands.
* *Chorea*: continuous jerky movements in which each movement is sudden and the resulting posture is held for a few seconds. This usually affects the head, face or limbs. The focus may move from one part of the body to another at random.
* *Dystonias*: sustained muscle contractions, frequently causing repetitive twisting movements or abnormal postures. Dystonia may be assessed using a validated rating scale such as the Burke–Fahn–Marsden Dystonia Rating Scale or the Unified Dystonia Rating Scale. They are most useful for measuring the effectiveness of certain treatments, such as deep brain stimulation.
* *Hemiballism*: wild flinging or throwing movements of one arm or leg, usually occurring as a result of a cerebrovascular event.

- *Myoclonus*: rapid muscle jerks that are frequently repetitive.
- *Tics*: repetitive, stereotyped movements.
- *Tremor*: a rhythmic movement of part of the body. There are three types of pathological tremor: resting, postural (which can also remain during movement) and kinetic (which occurs during the voluntary active movement of an upper body part).

## Fasciculation

This is the involuntary contraction and twitching of groups of muscle fibres. Groups of muscle fibres are called fasciculi, hence the name. The contractions are relatively coarse, rather than fine, and are often visible. Fasciculation is usually a feature of disorders of the anterior horn cell, particularly motor neurone disease, but it can occur in thyrotoxicosis and polymyositis.

## Fibrillation

Fibrillation is the rapid, irregular and unsynchronized contraction of muscle fibers.

## Testing of the Muscles
### Passive Movement

Muscle motor power testing depends on a thorough understanding of which muscles are used in performing certain movements. Testing is best performed when the patient is rested, comfortable, attentive and relaxed. Prior to testing muscle strength, the examiner should assess the muscle bulk and the affected muscle to evaluate peripheral nerve and muscle function. Because several muscles may function similarly, it is not always easy for the patient to contract a single muscle on request. Positioning or fixation of parts of the body can emphasize the contraction of a particular muscle while other muscles of similar function are inhibited. The normal or least affected muscles should be tested first to gain the patient's cooperation and confidence. The strength of the muscle tested should always be compared with that of its contralateral counterpart.

The strength of various muscles should also be graded and charted. Scales of various types are used, most commonly grading the strength from 0 (no muscle contraction) to 5 (normal).

### Active Movement

Testing for the active movement of a muscle assesses its range of motion along with any painful limitation. Note the action of the individual muscles and their agonists, checking for trick movements that are being made to overcome the disability.

**Resisted** movement assesses power and discomfort, while **passive** movement demonstrates abnormal mobility due to pain, joint stiffness, contractures, hypermobility and altered tone, for example rigidity and spasticity.

**Coordination** assesses smoothness of movement as well as direction and position sense. Incoordination can interfere with writing and eating, and can produce intention tremors, loss of balance and ataxia. **Reflexes** are reduced in lower motor nerve lesions and muscular dystrophies but may be brisk in myasthenia and polymyositis.

## Motor Neurone Lesions
### Upper Motor Neurone Lesions

Lesions result from damage to the descending motor pathways from the cerebral cortex to the lower end of the spinal cord, which gives rise to upper motor neurone syndrome. The signs associated with this include spastic paralysis, muscle weakness, decreased motor control and increased spinal reflexes, including deep tendon reflexes and the extensor plantar response, known as the **Babinski sign**.

**Extrapyramidal** lesions affect tone, coordination and balance; there may be involuntary movements but usually no loss of power. **Cerebellar disorders** give rise to hypotonia and ataxia.

### Lower Motor Neurone Lesions

These are lesions of the nerve fibers travelling from the anterior horn of the spinal cord to the relevant muscle. The signs include flaccid paralysis, weakness, fibrillation, wasting, hypotonia and areflexia.

## Cerebral Palsy

Cerebral palsy is usually related to a neonatal injury to the developing brain, common causes being anoxia, infection and haemorrhage. The motor damage results in spasticity, which involves the flexor muscles more than the extensor muscles and leads to deformity of the limbs and spine. This may range from a minor equinus deformity of a foot to total body involvement; correspondingly, the symptoms range from minor walking difficulties to a bedridden child. The lesions may be classified into spastic, athetoid, ataxic, atonic, rigid and mixed varieties.

## Multiple Sclerosis

Multiple sclerosis is a chronic, progressive neurological disorder of unknown aetiology, characterized by scattered demyelination of the motor and sensory nerve fibres in the brain and spinal cord (**Figure 8.6**). Autoimmune processes, viral infection and familial tendencies are considered to be risk factors. The lesions may be single or multiple, a common presentation being a monocular optic neuritis, producing diplopia. Other symptoms include numbness, fatigue, motor weakness, tremors and scanning speech. Symptoms can be intermittent, but there is usually a slow progression.

## Motor Neurone Disease

Motor neurone disease is a progressive neurodegenerative disease that attacks the upper and lower motor neurones. The clinical picture is of weakness and wasting, commonly starting in a single upper limb. Painful cramps are common, as is fasciculation of the affected muscles. The disease is progressive, giving rise to

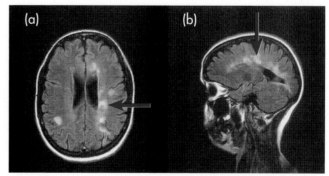

**Figure 8.6** Transverse (a) and sagittal (b) MRI scans of the head showing areas of demyelination (arrows). (Courtesy of Dr N. Khoury.)

difficulties with speech, swallowing and breathing. It is usually fatal in 2–4 years.

## Poliomyelitis

Poliomyelitis is an infectious disease caused by the poliovirus, which attacks the motor nerve cells in the brain and spinal cord. Acute poliomyelitis is usually a mild illness with full recovery in 95 per cent of cases. However, a minority of people experience a serious neurological illness with profound muscle weakness and paralysis – paralytic polio. The disease can be fatal if the muscles of respiration become paralysed. The pattern of paralysis determines the subsequent joint deformity, limb contractures and spinal abnormality.

## Myasthenia Gravis

This is a chronic neuromuscular disorder caused by a defect in the transmission of nerve impulses to the muscles due to an autoimmune blockage of the acetylcholine receptors. It is characterized by muscle weakness that worsens when the muscles are repeatedly used and improves after periods of rest. Although any voluntary muscle can be affected, muscles that control eye and eyelid movement, facial expression and swallowing are most frequently involved. Symptoms may include ptosis (**Figure 8.7**), diplopia, a waddling gait, difficulty in swallowing, shortness of breath, dysarthria and weakness.

## Myositis

Myositis refers to any condition causing inflammation in the muscles, with weakness, swelling and pain being the most common symptoms.

The causes of myositis can be divided into several categories:

- Inflammatory conditions (many of which are autoimmune):
  - Dermatomyositis;
  - Polymyositis;
  - Inclusion body myositis;
- Myositis caused by infection:
  - Viral (the most common cause);
  - Bacterial;
  - Parasitic;
- Myositis due to injury, caused by the vigorous exercise of untrained muscle groups;
- Drug-related myositis, for example with corticosteroids or statins.

Dermatomyositis and polymyositis cause progressive, symmetrical and proximal muscle weakness. Dermatomyositis is associated with characteristic skin manifestations, including Gottron's sign, the shawl sign, the heliotrope rash and generalized erythroderma. On the other hand, inclusion body myositis causes progressive, asymmetrical and distal muscle weakness.

## Trauma
### Muscle Tears

Muscle tears usually occur at the musculotendinous junction, the highest incidence being in the powerful limb muscles that cross two joints, such as the hamstrings, rectus femoris and gastrocnemius. Such muscle tears usually occur in explosive running and in soccer players, but they are also seen in the pectoralis major muscle in weightlifters (**Figure 8.8**).

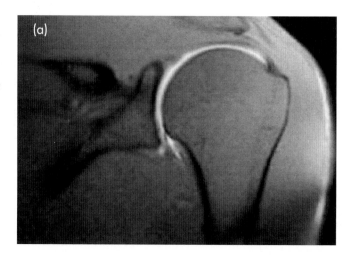

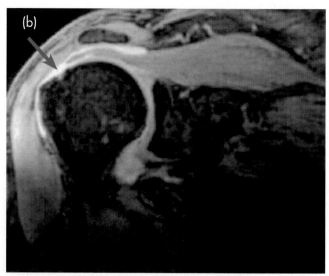

Figure 8.8 MRI of the shoulder. (a) A normal shoulder. (b) A tear in the supraspinatus muscle (arrow). (Courtesy of Dr N. Khoury.)

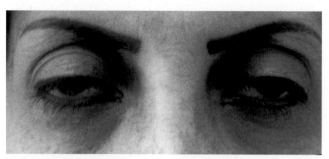

Figure 8.7 Bilateral ptosis.

## Muscular Haematoma

There are two types of muscular haematoma:

- *Intramuscular haematoma*: The bleed is confined within the tissues since the muscle sheath or fascia remains intact. This effectively means that the signs and symptoms will remain localized. An intramuscular haematoma is characterized by tender swelling, and a local cyst may develop. Long-term disabilities include fibrosis and myositis ossificans. Movement is limited, and therefore muscle wasting follows (**Figure 8.9**).
- *Intermuscular haematoma*: In this case, the fascia or sheath is torn. This allows communication of the fluid between the muscles and muscle compartments. The blood is dispersed, leading to dramatic bruising and swelling that tracks along the tissue planes. Pain and long-term complications are usually less severe.

## Repetitive Strain Injury

This disorder has become significant in the workplace due to advances in mechanization in which rapid and repetitive movements, often involving the upper limbs or the hands and wrists alone, are required.

The clinical features include chronic pain in the neck, chest wall, arms and hands, with impairment of full work performance. There may be swelling, as well as poor grip strength and taut proximal muscles.

## Tenosynovitis

Tenosynovitis is inflammation of the synovium surrounding a tendon and is often classified as a repetitive strain injury. The wrists, hands and feet are commonly affected. Suppurative tenosynovitis occasionally develops following an infected cut or wound.

There are variations of tenosynovitis such as **De Quervain's tenosynovitis**, which affects the thumb, and **stenosing tenosynovitis** (sometimes called trigger finger; **Figure 8.10**), which usually affects either the middle finger, fourth finger or thumb. Patients usually feel pain, stiffness, swelling and an inability to straighten the affected area.

## Periarticular Inflammation

Periarticular inflammation at a tendinous attachment to bone is termed **enthesopathy**. The diagnosis of periarticular inflammation is often difficult as other periarticular pathologies may be similar or can coexist.

Pain from an enthesopathy of the common extensor origin from the lateral epicondyle of the humerus – 'tennis elbow' – may be misdiagnosed as pain from a capsulitis or bursitis around the elbow. Similarly, enthesopathic pain from the attachment of the common flexor origin to the medial epicondyle of the humerus – 'golfer's elbow' – may be confused with ulnar nerve compression symptoms.

Inflammation of periarticular structures lined by synovial membrane includes capsulitis of the shoulder joint – frozen shoulder – and bursitis. Fasciitis is characteristically seen in the plantar fascia, and iliotibial band syndrome can be precipitated by running long distances along a road camber.

## Muscle Tumours

These are abnormal tissue growths located in or originating from muscle tissue. Tumours may either arise in muscle tissue or spread to it. The three major types of muscle tumours are leiomyomas, rhabdomyomas, and rhabdomyosarcomas. **Table 8.1** shows a comparison of rhabdomyosarcoma and leiomyoma.

## Sprengel's Deformity

Sprengel's deformity is a complex anomaly that is associated with an elevation and dysplasia of the scapula along with regional muscle atrophy. In this, the scapula is usually tethered to the spine and posterior ribs by tight bands, which restricts abduction of the arm.

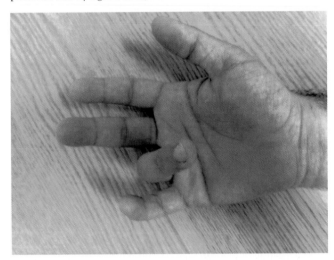

Figure 8.10 Trigger finger.

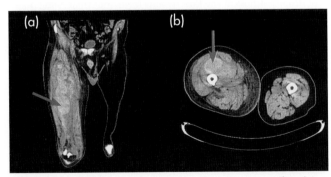

Figure 8.9 Coronal (a) and transverse (b) MRI scans of a lower extremity showing an intramuscular haematoma (arrows). (Courtesy of Dr N. Khoury.)

Table 8.1 Comparison of rhabdomyosarcoma and leiomyoma

| Rhabdomyosarcoma | Leiomyoma |
|---|---|
| Malignant | Benign |
| Striated muscle | Smooth muscle |
| Affects children | Affects adolescents and middle-aged individuals |
| Involves the head and neck, extremities and genitourinary tract | Involves the vascular smooth muscles of limbs, gut mesentery and retroperitoneum |
| Rapidly progressive | Slowly progressive |

## Muscular Dystrophy

The muscular dystrophies are a group of more than 30 genetic diseases characterized by progressive weakness and degeneration of the skeletal muscles that control movement, which initially appear hypertrophied due to fatty infiltration (**Figure 8.11**). Some forms of muscular dystrophy are seen in infancy or childhood, while others may not appear until middle age or later. Sensation is normal, and there is no fasciculation. The disorder is remarkably selective in its pattern of distribution and is classified by the muscles involved, age of onset and rate of progression.

Patients with pelvic girdle disease can only walk slowly, cannot run, have difficulty climbing stairs and climb up their legs with their hands to stand up – **Gowers' sign**.

The most common and severe form of the disease is Duchenne muscular dystrophy, which starts by the age of 2–3 years, children with the condition usually being wheelchair-dependent by the age of 12.

## Metabolic Myopathies

The metabolic myopathies represent a group of heterogeneous muscle disorders characterized by defects in glycogen, lipid, adenine nucleotide and mitochondrial metabolism.

### Endocrine Myopathy

Striated muscle is affected in most disorders caused by hormone dysregulation and is mostly associated with:

- adrenal dysfunction (as in Cushing's disease and Addison's disease);
- thyroid dysfunction (as in myxoedema coma or thyrotoxic myopathy);
- parathyroid dysfunction (as in multiple endocrine neoplasia);
- pituitary dysfunction;
- steroid myopathy (the most common endocrine myopathy).

### Toxic Myopathy

Striated muscle may be damaged by a number of drugs and toxins, including intramuscular bupivacaine, chloroquine, vincristine, corticosteroids, statins, amphetamine, lithium and alcohol.

## GAIT

A person's gait is their manner of walking, and observing a patient's gait upon entering the consulting room can often reveal valuable information. The examination of any lower limb joint

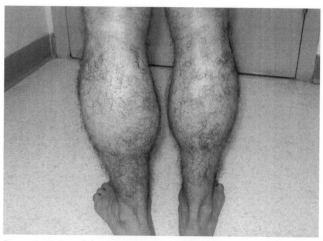

Figure 8.11 Pseudohypertrophy of the calf.

should be preceded by observation of the patient standing and walking. A limp is an abnormal gait.

## The Gait Cycle

### Stance (Support) Phase

The stance phase begins when the heel of the forward limb makes contact with the ground and ends when the toe of the same limb leaves the ground. It has several components:

- *Heel strike*: The heel of the forward foot initially touches the ground before rollover so that the rest of the foot comes into contact with the ground too. A patient with a painful heel avoids weight-bearing on the heel and therefore contacts the ground through the toes and metatarsal heads. A foot drop produces a characteristic slap as the whole foot contacts the ground. The heel strike is violent in tabes dorsalis.
- *Mid-stance*: The foot is flat on the ground and the weight of the body is directly over the supporting limb. If the leg has a painful joint, the patient avoids prolonged weight-bearing during this phase and therefore tends to rush to the next phase.
  - The resulting **antalgic gait** is observed as quick, short, soft footsteps.
  - A **short leg gait** is observed in this phase, showing a pelvic drop, where the vertebral column bends convexly to the short side and the shoulder dips vertically on the long side.
  - If the abductors are insufficiently strong to hold the pelvis upright in the stance phase, the pelvis drops toward the swing leg and there is visible lateral movement of the hip toward the stance leg, known as the **Trendelenburg gait**. If this is bilateral, it produces a characteristic waddle.
- *Toe off*: Only the big toe of the forward limb is in contact with the ground. In this phase, the body weight is transferred forwards and the leg is raised from the ground. If there is a flexion deformity at the hip or knee, the heel rises too soon. If the body is thrown upwards as well as forwards, it suggests that the body is being moved to allow the clearance of a stiff knee.

### Swing (Unsupported) Phase

This phase begins when the foot is no longer in contact with the ground. The limb is free to move. If there is a foot drop, the leg must be lifted up to avoid the toe scuffing the ground. In tabes dorsalis, both legs are elevated rather more than is seen with a foot drop. Stiffness in the knee results in an abnormal swing phase with the leg being thrown out to the side for clearance. The **scissor gait** of spastic diplegia is most noticeable in the swing phase. The **hemiplegic gait** produces a similar picture on one side.

There are two components to this phase:

- *Acceleration*: The swinging limb catches up to and passes the torso.
- *Deceleration*: The forward movement of the limb is slowed down to position the foot for heel strike.

---

### Key Points

- Musculoskeletal problems should be identified based on a proper history and physical examination: inspect, palpate and assess the range of motion.
- Neurological assessment may be a necessary step in completing a rheumatological examination including gait, motor power and sensation.

## QUESTIONS

### SBAs

**1.** A 21-year-old woman has presented to you with a 38 hour history of a red and very swollen right knee, which she cannot bear weight on. No other symptoms are present. She has previously been healthy and has no relevant family history. She denies any history of trauma. The clinic nurse has recorded her temperature as 39.5°C and blood tests have shown a white blood cell counts of $18\,400 \times 10^9$/L with a left shift (82 per cent neutrophils). What is your most likely differential diagnosis?:

**a** Osteoarthritis
**b** Gout
**c** Septic arthritis
**d** Pseudogout
**e** Haemarthrosis

**Answer**

**c Septic arthritis.** The clinical picture of an acute onset of monoarthritis in a young woman in association with a high-grade fever and leukocytosis but in the absence of any other focus of infection suggests septic arthritis. Osteoarthritis is very unlikely given the age of the patient and its acute onset. Gout is more likely to affect men, more commonly involves the first metatarsophalangeal joint and is not usually accompanied by a high-grade fever. Pseudogout does not usually occur before the age of 50 years. Haemoarthrosis is less likely in this patient because of the absence of trauma or any previous coagulopathy disorder.

**2.** A 42-year-old woman is complaining of pain and swelling in both wrists and knees that has been present for the previous 8 weeks. She reports fatigue and lethargy prior to the arthralgia. On examination, her metacarpophalangeal joints are warm and tender but there are no other joint abnormalities. No alopecia, photosensitivity, kidney disease or rash are present. Which one of the following is true?:

**a** The symptoms suggest rheumatoid arthritis so rheumatoid factor should be tested for
**b** The lack of systemic symptoms suggests osteoarthritis
**c** The lethargy suggests chronic fatigue syndrome
**d** Radiographs of the hand are likely to show joint space narrowing and erosions

**Answer**

**a The symptoms suggest rheumatoid arthritis so rheumatoid factor should be tested for.** The presentation of symmetrical polyarthritis lasting more than 6 weeks in a female patient in the absence of other systemic signs suggests rheumatoid arthritis. The next step should be to request testing for rheumatoid factor, which is present in more than two-thirds of affected patients. The metacarpophalangeal joints are not usually affected by osteoarthritis. Fatigue and lethargy are usually part of the rheumatoid arthritis prodrome and do not suggest chronic fatigue syndrome, especially as joint symptoms are present. The radiographic changes described here can be present in rheumatoid arthritis but usually appear at a more advanced stage.

**3.** A 75-year-old woman presents complaining of headaches, fatigue and stiffness of the upper arms and shoulders. The symptoms have gradually increased over the previous 4 weeks. She has previously been healthy and is taking no medication apart from paracetamol for her mild osteoarthritis. What is your most likely differential diagnosis?:

**a** Systemic lupus erythematosus
**b** Rheumatoid arthritis
**c** Sjögren's syndrome
**d** Giant cell arteritis with polymyalgia rheumatica
**e** Fibromyalgia

**Answer**

**d Giant cell arteritis with polymyalgia rheumatica.** The age of the patient, the gradual onset of bilateral shoulder pain and stiffness, and the headache make giant cell arteritis with polymyalgia rheumatica very likely. The affected temporal artery is usually prominent and palpating it will reveal a faint pulse. Systemic lupus erythematosus usually affects middle-aged rather than elderly women and no other criteria are present to support its diagnosis. The absence of dryness of the mouth or eyes makes Sjögren's syndrome unlikely. Fibromyalgia is characterized by diffuse body aches and generalized myalgia, which is not the case with this patient.

## EMQ

1. For each of the following descriptions, select the most likely cause from the list below:
   1 Parkinson's disease
   2 Wilson's disease
   3 Dystonia
   4 Essential tremor
   5 Tic
   6 Huntington's chorea
   a A 76-year-old man with bradykinesia, micrographia and a resting tremor
   b Rapid writing movements in a 40-year-old patient that are associated with dementia

**Answers**

a **1 Parkinson's disease.** The diagnosis of Parkinson's disease is based on the triad of resting tremor, cogwheel rigidity and bradykinesia. The tremor is slow in frequency, occurs at rest and is 'pill-rolling' in nature. Bradykinesia is the most striking feature. Micrographia (small handwriting) is also characteristic. Parkinson's disease is usually accompanied by a shuffling gait.

b **6 Huntington's chorea.** Dementia and non-rhythmic movements should raise the suspicion of Huntington's chorea. This is an autosomal dominant disease that usually affects people in the third and fourth decades of life. The slow and writhing movements of athetosis are usually present in Huntington's disease.

# CHAPTER 9

# Peripheral Nerve Injuries

Badih Adada

## LEARNING OBJECTIVES

- To obtain a solid understanding of the clinically relevant anatomy of the peripheral nerves
- To master the classifications of peripheral nerve injuries
- To become familiar with the physical examination and clinical presentation of specific peripheral nerve injuries
- To understand how each peripheral nerve is prone to different mechanisms of injury

## INTRODUCTION

The human nervous system has two main components: the central nervous system (CNS) and the peripheral nervous system (PNS). The main function of the PNS is to connect the CNS to the limbs and organs. Peripheral nerves are not protected by bone and do not have any equivalent of the blood–brain barrier, which makes them prone to injury secondary to direct trauma or other insults such as toxins.

The sensory, motor and autonomic deficits resulting from peripheral nerve injuries vary, depending on the nerve affected and the location at which it is injured. It is therefore very important for every physician to have a minimum knowledge of the anatomy of the peripheral nerves and a mastery of their physical examination. The motor activity of the nerves is typically evaluated by assessing the associated muscle strength (**Table 9.1**). Pinprick and light touch are used to test the sensory function of a peripheral nerve. The skin is inspected and palpated for vasomotor changes to assess the nerve's autonomic function. The progress of regrowth of a damaged nerve can be monitored by Tinel's sign – paraesthesia on tapping the growing end of the nerve.

## ANATOMY OF THE PERIPHERAL NERVOUS SYSTEM

Peripheral nerves have three functional components: motor, sensory and autonomic. Each peripheral nerve is formed of axons that may or may not be myelinated. A delicate layer of connective tissue known as endoneurium covers the individual axon. Several axons are grouped together and covered by another layer of connective tissue, the perineurium, to form a fascicle.

These fascicles come together to form a nerve root, which is covered by a final layer of connective tissue, the epineurium.

The peripheral nerves include all the spinal nerves (8 cervical, 12 thoracic, 5 lumbar, 5 sacral and 1 coccygeal) and the cranial nerves (except the optic nerve, which is part of the CNS). The brachial and lumbosacral plexuses, which innervate the upper and lower extremities, respectively, are formed by the confluence of branches arising from the spinal nerve roots. The brachial plexus is formed from the ventral rami of cervical nerves C5–C8 in association with the greater part of the first thoracic spinal nerve (T1). The lumbosacral plexus is formed from the anterior rami of lumbar nerves roots L1–L3 and the greater part of nerve roots L4–S4.

Table 9.1 Grading scale for muscle strength

| Grade | Strength |
|---|---|
| 0 | No movement |
| 1 | Flicker or minimal contraction (visible or palpable) |
| 2 | Movement but not against gravity |
| 3 | Movement against gravity |
| 4 | Movement against resistance |
| 5 | Normal strength |
| NT | Not testable |

## CLASSIFICATION OF PERIPHERAL NERVE INJURIES

Two main classification systems of peripheral nerve injuries have been proposed: the Seddon (**Table 9.2**) and Sunderland (**Table 9.3**) classifications. These classification systems are based on the degree of injury to the myelin, axons and connective tissues.

## BRACHIAL PLEXUS INJURY

As described above, the brachial plexus is formed of a network of spinal nerve roots originating from the anterior rami of C5–C8 and the greater part of T1. The plexus sends its branches to the upper limbs and the trunk. The nerve roots forming the brachial plexus join to form the superior, middle and inferior trunks, which in turn each split into a ventral and a dorsal division. Those divisions coalesce to form the lateral, posterior and medial cords.

The first branch of the brachial plexus, the long thoracic nerve innervating the serratus anterior muscle, arises from branches of C5–C7. The upper trunk gives rise to the dorsal scapular nerve, innervating the rhomboids, and the suprascapular nerve, which innervates the supraspinatus and infraspinatus muscles. The thoracodorsal nerve, which innervates the latissimus dorsi, originates from the posterior cord. Finally, the terminal branches of the brachial plexus include the musculocutaneous, axillary, radial, median and ulnar nerves.

The main causes of brachial plexus injuries include penetrating trauma, stretch injuries (which are more likely to affect the posterior and lateral cords), fractures of the first rib and compression by a haematoma.

On initial assessment of the patient with a brachial plexus injury, it is essential to differentiate preganglionic injuries from injuries distal to the dorsal root ganglia as their treatment and prognosis are different. Patients with preganglionic injuries typically present with winging of the scapula (**Figure 9.1**) secondary to injury of the long thoracic nerve causing paralysis of serratus anterior. Winging of the scapula can be tested while the arm is lifted forwards or when the patient pushes the outstretched arm against a wall. Preganglionic injuries also present with early neuropathic pain secondary to nerve root avulsion. Horner's syndrome (**Figure 9.2**) is present in preganglionic injuries involving the T1 level.

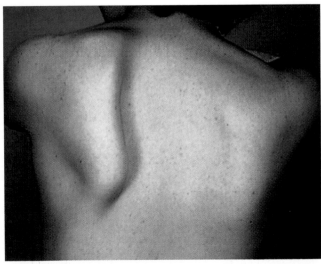

Figure 9.1 Winging of the left scapula.

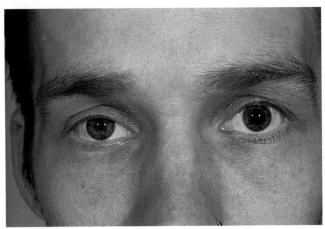

Figure 9.2 Right Horner's syndrome following the removal of a neoplasm from the right side of the neck.

Once the location of the injury in relation to the dorsal root ganglion has been determined, an effort should be made to determine whether the injury involves the upper or lower brachial plexus.

Table 9.2 Seddon classification

| Classification | Neurapraxia | Axonotmesis | Neurotmesis |
|---|---|---|---|
| Common aetiology | Nerve compression | Nerve crush | Nerve transection |
| Description | Local myelin injury, nerve intact | Axonal interruption with intact Schwann cells | Axonal interruption with disrupted surrounding connective tissues |

Table 9.3 Sunderland classification

| | |
|---|---|
| Grade 1 | Neurapraxia |
| Grade 2 | Axonotmesis |
| Grade 3 | Connective tissue injury limited to the endoneurium |
| Grade 4 | Connective tissue injury involving the endoneurium and perineurium |
| Grade 5 | Connective tissue injury involving the endoneurium, perineurium and epineurium (neurotmesis) |

**Upper brachial plexus injuries (Erb's palsy)** include injuries to C5, C6 and C7 secondary to forced lateral flexion of the neck and depression of the shoulder, either in the fetus during delivery or as an adult usually secondary to a motorcycle accident. This results in paralysis of the deltoid, biceps, rhomboid, brachioradialis, supinator, supraspinatus and infraspinatus muscles. Patients typically present with the arm hanging by their side and medially rotated, with the forearm extended and pronated. This posture is known as the bellhop's or waiter's tip position (**Figure 9.3**). The hand movements are normal.

**Lower brachial plexus injuries (Klumpke's palsy)** result from damage to C8 and T1 secondary to traction on an abducted arm (such as grabbing at a structure when falling from a height) or due to involvement by a tumor at the lung apex (Pancoast's syndrome). This presents with a characteristic claw hand due to a loss of function of the ulnar nerve and subsequent weakness of small muscles of the hand, as well as weakness of the flexors of the wrist and fingers. The motor functions of the shoulder and elbow are relatively preserved.

## UPPER LIMB NERVE INJURIES

### Median Nerve

The median nerve has contributions from the C5–T1 nerve roots. It descends in the upper arm adjacent to the lateral side of the brachial artery. It then crosses to the medial aspect of the artery at the level of coracobrachialis. In the cubital fossa, it passes behind the biceps aponeurosis.

The median nerve has no branches in the arm. It supplies all the forearm flexor muscles except for flexor carpi ulnaris and part of flexor digitorum profundus. In the forearm, just distal to pronator teres, it gives rise to the anterior interosseous nerve, a purely motor branch supplying flexor digitorum profundus I and II, flexor pollicis longus and pronator quadratus. At the wrist, the median nerve passes under the transverse carpal ligament, giving rise to its motor branch, which supplies the first and second lumbricals, opponens pollicis, abductor pollicis brevis and flexor pollicis brevis (known as the LOAF muscles). The cutaneous supply of the median nerve covers the thumb and radial two and a half fingers anteriorly and posteriorly as far proximally as the middle phalanx.

The median nerve is prone to entrapment or injury at specific sites along its path. First, above the elbow, it may be compressed by Struthers' ligament (a fibrous bridge between the supracondylar process and the medial epicondyle). Next, at the forearm level, the nerve can be entrapped by one of two structures: the bicipital aponeurosis or the pronator teres muscle. When the nerve is entrapped at either of these sites, patients present with clinical signs of injury to the main trunk of the median nerve. They typically present with a 'benediction hand' (**Figure 9.4**): when trying to make a fist, the index finger stays extended and the middle finger partially flexed as the distal phalanx of the fourth and fifth digits is flexed. This occurs because of weakness of the flexor digitorum sublimis and flexor digitorum profundus I and II, and preservation of flexor digitorum profundus IV and V, which are supplied by the ulnar nerve.

A third site of injury lies deep in the forearm, where the anterior interosseous nerve, a motor branch of the median nerve, can be damaged. This results in a loss of flexion of the distal forefinger and thumb. As a result, the patient is unable to form an O with those two fingers – this is known as the pinch sign. Patients with this injury have no sensory loss.

Finally, compression of the median nerve can occur at the carpal tunnel. This can result from many factors, including trauma and systemic conditions. It presents with painful dysaesthesias in the distribution of the palmar aspect of the first three digits, often wakening the patient at night. There may be

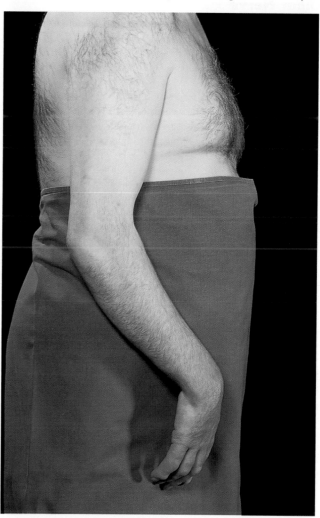

Figure 9.3 A right-sided Erb's palsy.

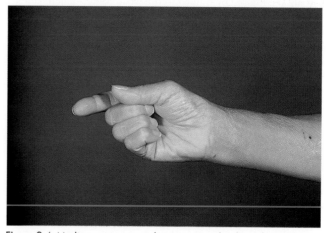

Figure 9.4 Median nerve injury demonstrating the 'benediction sign'.

a weakness of the grip, and in advanced cases atrophy of the thenar muscles is seen (**Figure 9.5**). Patients with carpal tunnel syndrome have a positive Phalen's test (40 seconds of complete wrist flexion reproduce the patient's symptoms) and/or Tinel's sign (paraesthesias and pain along the distribution of the median nerve that are caused by percussion over the carpal tunnel).

## Ulnar Nerve

The ulnar nerve is a direct continuation of the medial cord of the brachial plexus; it has contributions from the C7, C8 and T1 nerve roots. It descends in the arm on the posteromedial aspect of the humerus and does not give out any branches at this level. It then enters the forearm, passing through the two heads of the flexor carpi ulnaris, and runs along the ulna. In the forearm, it gives motor branches to flexor carpi ulnaris and flexor digitorum profundus III and IV. It also gives rise to a palmar and a dorsal sensory branch that innervate the little finger and the ulnar side of the ring finger.

At the wrist, the ulnar nerve passes above the carpal tunnel and through the ulnar canal (Guyon's canal) before dividing into the superficial (sensory) and deep (motor) branches. In the hand, it supplies the hypothenar muscles (flexor, abductor and opponens digiti mimimi), adductor pollicis brevis and all the dorsal and palmar interossei. Injury or entrapment of the ulnar nerve at the elbow usually occurs secondary to trauma or a fracture of the lateral epicondyle of the humerus. Entrapment of the ulnar nerve at the elbow can be idiopathic or arise secondary to arthritis; this condition is known as cubital tunnel syndrome.

Patients with an ulnar nerve injury at this level typically present with pain and discomfort in the ulnar nerve distribution (the inner border of the hand and the fourth and fifth digits), with intrinsic hand muscle weakness. Patients have a positive Froment's sign (**Figure 9.6**): grasping a piece of paper between the index finger and the thumb results in extension of the proximal phalanx of the thumb and flexion of the distal phalanx as the long flexors compensate for the weak abductor pollicis. The muscles of the hypothenar eminence are typically atrophied (**Figure 9.7**).

With severe nerve injuries, a claw hand deformity (main en griffe) develops (**Figure 9.8**). This deformity is apparent when trying to extend the fingers (unlike the deformity secondary to a median nerve injury, which occurs while trying to make a fist).

At the level of the wrist, the ulnar nerve can be entrapped in Guyon's canal or compressed by a ganglion cyst. The nerve can also be injured by trauma to the wrist. Motor deficits due to ulnar nerve injuries at the level of the wrist are similar to those encountered in injuries to the nerve at the level of the elbow. Sensory deficits in patients with ulnar nerve injuries at the level of the wrist typically spare the dorsal aspect of the hand, since the dorsal cutaneous branch of the ulnar nerve originates in the forearm and is usually preserved.

## Radial Nerve

The radial nerve arises from the posterior division of the brachial plexus and carries fibres from C5–C8 and T1. It enters the arm through the triangular space and supplies the triceps muscle. It then turns around the humerus in the spiral groove. In the arm, the radial nerve innervates brachioradialis and extensor carpi radialis longus and brevis.

In the forearm, the nerve divides into a superficial branch that is mainly sensory and a deep branch that pierces the supinator

muscle through a ligamentous structure, known as the arcade of Frohse and becomes the posterior interosseous nerve. The posterior interosseous nerve gives off branches to the supinator, extensor carpi ulnaris, extensor digitorum communis, extensor digiti minimi, abductor pollicis longus, extensor pollicis longus and brevis, and extensor indicis muscles.

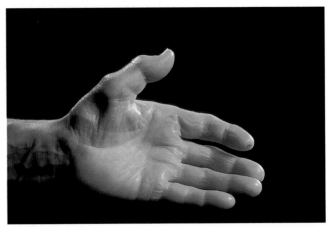

Figure 9.5 Median nerve injury demonstrating wasting of the thenar muscles in a patient with a carpal tunnel syndrome.

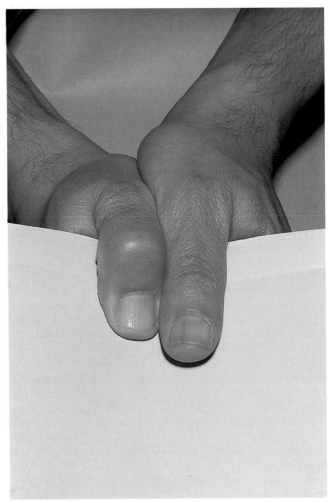

Figure 9.6 Ulnar nerve palsy of the right hand demonstrating Froment's sign.

The cutaneous innervations of the radial nerve include the posterior cutaneous nerve of the arm (which originates in the axilla), the inferior lateral cutaneous nerve of the arm (which originates in the arm), the posterior cutaneous nerve of the forearm (which originates in the forearm) and the superficial branch of the radial nerve, which supplies approximately two-thirds of the dorsum of the hand.

Mid-arm radial nerve injuries can occur secondary to improper positioning of the arm during sleep ('Saturday night palsy') or can occur after a fracture of the humerus. Patients with radial nerve injury at this level present with a wrist drop (**Figure 9.9**) with preservation of the triceps muscle.

Injuries to the nerve in the forearm cause a posterior interosseous neuropathy. This may result from direct compression by a lesion, entrapment at the arcade of Frohse or strenuous muscle exercise. Patients with posterior interosseous neuropathy do not have any sensory loss and usually present with finger drop without wrist drop. This is due to preservation of the wrist extensors (extensor carpi radialis longus and brevis).

Unlike a posterior cord injury in the brachial plexus, a radial nerve injury shows intact axillary nerve and thoracodorsal nerve innervations.

## Musculocutaneous Nerve

The musculocutaneous nerve arises from the lateral cord of the brachial plexus. It passes through the coracobrachialis muscle and then enters the arm between the brachialis and biceps brachii. It provides sensory innervation to the forearm through the lateral cutaneous branch of the forearm.

The musculocutaneous nerve can be injured through stretching, for example after shoulder dislocation, or it can be entrapped between the heads of the biceps. Since the nerve innervates the coracobrachialis, brachialis and biceps brachii muscles, injury causes weakness in elbow flexion and supination of the forearm, with a depressed biceps reflex. The sensory deficit is usually situated along the radial side of the forearm.

## Axillary Nerve

The axillary nerve is a branch of the posterior cord of the brachial plexus and carries nerve fibres from the C5 and C6 nerve roots. It supplies the deltoid and teres minor muscles. It provides sensory innervation to the lateral aspect of the arm through the lateral cutaneous branch of the arm.

The axillary nerve can be injured if the shoulder is dislocated anteroinferiorly. Compression of the axilla by crutches or by a fracture of the surgical neck of the humerus can also damage the axillary nerve. Injury results in a flat shoulder deformity due to paralysis of the deltoid and teres minor muscles. The patient is unable to abduct the arm between 15° and 90°. The initial 15° of arm abduction is preserved since the initiation of abduction is a function of the supraspinatus muscle. Patients with an axillary nerve injury also present with a sensory disturbance over the lateral aspect of the upper arm.

## LUMBOSACRAL PLEXUS

The lumbar plexus supplies the hip flexors, thigh adductors and knee extensors, and the skin over the medial, anterior and lateral thigh, via the obturator, femoral and lateral cutaneous nerves of the thigh, respectively. The sensory continuation of the femoral nerve is the saphenous nerve, which runs across the medial aspect of the knee to supply a long promontory of skin down the medial side of the leg, including the skin over the medial malleolus and, occasionally, part of the medial aspect of the foot.

The sacral plexus supplies the rest of the leg. This plexus forms over the sacroiliac joint and almost immediately leaves the pelvis via the greater sciatic foramen. Its main branches – the gluteal nerve, the sciatic nerve and the posterior femoral cutaneous nerve of the thigh – then lie directly behind the hip joint.

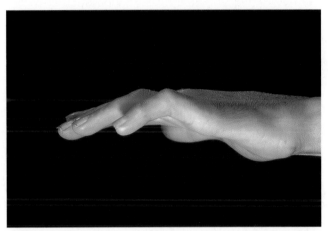

Figure 9.7 Ulnar nerve palsy showing wasting of the hypothenar muscles of the left hand.

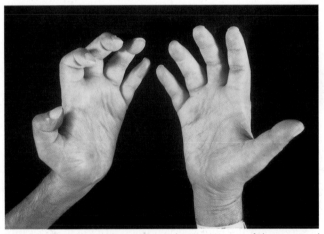

Figure 9.8 Claw-hand demonstrating hyperextension of the wrist and metacarpophalangeal joints, together with muscle wasting.

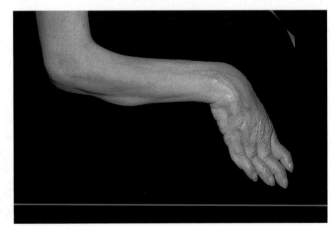

Figure 9.9 Wrist drop from a radial nerve palsy.

Fractures of the upper femur represent a considerable threat to these nerves.

## LOWER LIMB NERVE INJURIES

### Lateral Cutaneous Nerve of the Thigh

This nerve is formed by the L2 and L3 branches. It reaches the thigh by skirting around the pelvic brim, entering the thigh under the lateral part of the inguinal ligament.

The only symptoms of disease in this nerve, which are known as meralgia paraesthetica, are painful paraesthesias – uncomfortable burning, tingling sensations in the anterolateral aspect of the thigh. The symptoms are caused by entrapment or stretching of the nerve under the lateral aspect of the inguinal ligament. The disease is common in people who are gaining or losing weight, or during or after pregnancy. The symptoms are often related to only a single posture, such as sitting or standing.

Examination reveals hyperaesthesia, or rarely hypoaesthesia, in the anterior lateral thigh. The thigh is strong, and the knee reflex is normal.

### Obturator Nerve

The obturator nerve is formed by branches of L2, L3 and L4. It lies on the medial side of the iliopsoas and comes into close relationship with the uterus in the pelvis before passing through the obturator foramen into the medial compartment of the thigh. This muscle supplies the obturator externus and all the adductor muscles of the thigh. The integrity of the nerve can be tested simply by asking the patient to hold their legs together against resistance.

Lesions of this nerve produce a weakness of adduction of the thigh, and pain on the medial aspect from the thigh to the knee. The nerve may be injured during delivery or gynaecological procedures and may be involved by pelvic neoplasms.

### Femoral Nerve

The femoral nerve innervates the iliopsoas and quadriceps muscles. Thus, injury produces a weakness of leg extension and an additional weakness of thigh flexion. The knee reflex is absent, and the sensory loss extends from the anteromedial thigh to the medial malleolus.

Diabetes is the most common cause of femoral neuropathy, although pelvic tumours, a femoral hernia and a femoral artery aneurysm are also possible causes. A retroperitoneal haematoma may compress the nerve, and drainage of the haematoma is an emergency if the nerve is to be saved.

### Sciatic Nerve

The sciatic nerve consists of two discrete components invested by the same fascia: the peroneal nerve and the tibial nerve. There is an important anatomical peculiarity here in that even when the whole nerve trunk is traumatized, the peroneal component is more likely to be damaged than the tibial component. The reason for this is not entirely clear.

Relative to its size, the sciatic nerve supplies a surprisingly small cutaneous area. The area of sensory loss in sciatic nerve injury involves the surface of the limb below the knee except for the area innervated by the saphenous branch of the femoral nerve.

Injury to the sciatic nerve will cause a loss of knee flexion (because of its effects on the hamstrings) and palsy of all the muscles below the knee (**Figure 9.10**). This can be caused by pelvic fractures, posterior dislocation of the hip, penetrating injuries, including misplaced injections, and pelvic tumors.

### Peroneal Nerve

The peroneal nerve, a branch of the sciatic nerve, has to gain access to the anterior and lateral compartments of the leg and in doing so becomes extremely vulnerable as it winds around the neck of the fibula. Injury to the peroneal nerve is the most common peripheral nerve lesion in the lower limb.

The common peroneal nerve divides within the proximal part of the peroneus longus muscle into superficial and deep components. Common peroneal nerve injury presents with foot drop and an area of sensory loss, usually triangular in shape, over the dorsum of the foot and extending upwards just across the ankle joint to the lower leg. Diabetes, sitting with the legs crossed for long periods, trauma and sporting injuries, as well as tightly applied plaster casts, account for most of the identifiable causes.

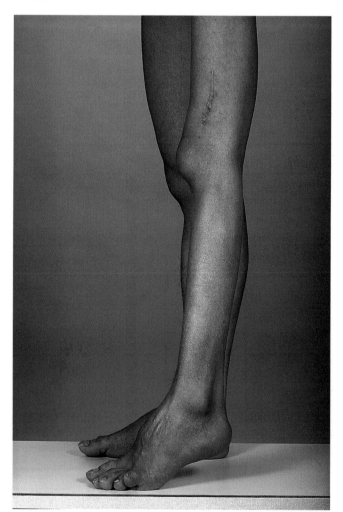

Figure 9.10 Left sciatic nerve palsy showing wasting of the posterior thigh and all lower leg muscle groups. There is also disuse atrophy of the quadriceps and an equinus deformity of the foot.

Injury to the superficial peroneal (musculocutaneous) nerve paralyses the peroneal muscles, with the result that the foot becomes inverted. There is sensory loss over the medial part of the dorsum of the foot. Injury to the deep peroneal nerve paralyses the tibialis anterior and other anterior compartment muscles, and the foot drops due to the unopposed action of the tibialis posterior. There is a sensory loss between the first and second toes.

## Tibial Nerve

The tibial nerve lies deep in the calf and is almost never subject to damage in the leg. Injury to it produces paralysis of the deep and superficial calf muscles and the intrinsic muscles of the sole of the foot. There is a loss of plantar flexion of the ankle and toes, and the patient cannot stand on tiptoe. The foot is held in a calcaneovalgus position by the unopposed action of the extensors and everters. The disability is great and the patient has a pronounced limp due to the difficulty of 'taking off' from the affected foot.

The area of sensory loss is over the sole of the foot and the lateral side of the leg and foot. The ankle jerk is absent.

### Key Points

- Preganglionic brachial plexus injuries need to be differentiated from postganglionic injuries as the prognosis and treatment are different.
- The median nerve is prone to entrapment and injury in four locations. These include Struthers' ligament in the arm, at the pronator teres in the forearm, and deep in the forearm, where the motor branch – the anterior interosseous nerve – can be injured. The most common area of entrapment of the median nerve is, however, at the carpal tunnel in the wrist.
- Injuries of the ulnar nerve at the level of the elbow present with a sensory deficit involving the dorsal aspect of the hand. This area is typically spared when the ulnar nerve injury occurs at the level of the wrist.
- Radial nerve injuries at the level of the arm present with a wrist drop associated with a sensory deficit in the radial nerve distribution, while injuries of the nerve in the forearm present with a finger drop with no sensory deficit.
- Nerve entrapments are not as common in the lower extremities as they are in the upper extremities.
- Injuries to the sciatic nerve will typically present with a predominant deficit in the peroneal distribution.
- Peroneal nerve injuries present with the foot drop associated with the sensory deficit over the dorsum of the foot.

## QUESTIONS

### SBAs

**1. A patient with a positive pinch sign has:**
  a   A posterior interosseous nerve injury
  b   An anterior interosseous nerve injury
  c   An ulnar nerve injury
  d   A radial nerve injury

**Answer**

*b* *An anterior interosseous nerve injury.* The anterior interosseous nerve, a purely motor branch of the median nerve, innervates the flexor digitorum profundus I and II, the flexor pollicis longus and the pronator quadratus. When it is injured, the patient is unable to form an O shape using his thumb and index fingers, which is known as a positive pinch sign.
A posterior interosseous nerve injury causes finger drop.
An ulnar nerve injury presents with a claw hand deformity.
A radial nerve injury presents with a hand drop.

**2. A finger drop occurs secondary to an injury to:**
  a   The trunk of the radial nerve
  b   The posterior interosseous nerve
  c   The median nerve at the carpal tunnel
  d   The anterior interosseous nerve

**Answer**

*b* *The posterior interosseous nerve.* The posterior interosseous nerve gives branches to the supinator, extensor carpi ulnaris, extensor digitorum communis, extensor digiti minimi, abductor pollicis longus, extensor pollicis longus and brevis, and extensor indicis muscles. Patients with posterior interosseous neuropathy do not have any sensory loss and usually present with finger drop without wrist drop. This is due to preservation of the sensory branches of the nerve and the wrist extensors.
An injury to the trunk of the radial nerve presents with a wrist drop.
An injury of the median nerve at the carpal tunnel presents with atrophy of the thenar eminence muscles and hypoaesthesia of the first two digits.
An injury to the anterior interosseous nerve presents with a positive pinch sign.

**3. A patient with entrapment of the ulnar nerve in the cubital tunnel will have all of the following except:**
  a   A positive Froment's sign
  b   Numbness and decreased sensation of the fourth and fifth digits of the hand
  c   A benediction sign
  d   Weakness of the intrinsic muscles of the hand

**Answer**

*c* *A benediction sign.* A benediction sign is seen with injuries to the trunk of the median nerve: when trying to make a fist, the index finger stays extended and the middle finger partially flexed as the distal phalanx of the fourth and fifth digits is flexed due to weakness of the flexor digitorum sublimis and flexor digitorum profundus I and II, and preservation of the flexor digitorum profundus IV and V, which are supplied by the ulnar nerve.

## EMQs

**4.** **For each of the following patients with a brachial plexus injury, select the most likely site of the lesion from the list below. Each option may be used once, more than once or not at all:**

    **1** Upper trunk, preganglionic injury

    **2** Upper trunk, postganglionic injury

    **3** Lower trunk, preganglionic injury

    **4** Lower trunk, postganglionic injury

  **a** A 32-year-old patient has fallen from a second-floor balcony. While falling, he tried to stop his fall by holding onto the balcony's rail with his right arm. He has presented to the accident and emergency department with the right arm in a fixed supinated position and paralysis of the intrinsic muscles of his right hand. He has a ptosis of his right eyelid and his right pupil is smaller than his left.

  **b** After a difficult delivery, a newborn child has been found to have no movement in his left shoulder and weakness in his biceps and triceps muscles on the same side. The strength of the intrinsic muscles of his left hand has been preserved.

  **c** A 24-year-old patient involved in a motor cycle accident presents with his left arm hanging by his side, his forearm extended and pronated, and his hand in a typical 'waiter's tip' position. On physical examination, he also has winging of his left scapula.

### Answers

  **a** **3 Lower trunk, preganglionic injury.** *Severe stretching of the arm while extended can cause significant damage to the lower trunk of the brachial plexus. In extreme cases, the T1 root is avulsed and causes a Horner's syndrome in association with Klumpke's palsy.*

  **b** **2 Upper trunk, postganglionic injury.** *A common cause of upper brachial plexus injury is shoulder dystocia during birth. This causes stretching of the upper brachial plexus. The injury is typically postganglionic.*

  **c** **1 Upper trunk, preganglionic injury.** *In severe trauma, such as a motorcycle accident, the upper brachial plexus can be avulsed from the spinal cord. In such cases, the long thoracic nerve is injured, causing winging of the scapula.*

**5.** **For each of the following patients with a lower extremity weakness, select the most likely nerve injury from the list below. Each option may be used once, more than once or not at all:**

    **1** Tibial nerve

    **2** Common peroneal nerve

    **3** Superficial peroneal nerve

    **4** Femoral nerve

  **a** A 72-year-old patient taking warfarin for atrial fibrillation presents with severe pain in his lower abdomen, right groin and right thigh area. On examination, he has weakness of the right quadriceps muscle, loss of the knee jerk reflex and numbness on the medial aspect of the right thigh and calf. Right hip extension exacerbates the pain.

  **b** A 33-year-old patient being evaluated in the emergency room for a right peroneal fracture has been found to have weakness of eversion of the right foot. The sensation over the dorsum of the foot is decreased, but the sensation at the webbed space between the hallux and second digit is spared.

  **c** A 64-year-old diabetic patient presents to the clinic with a right foot drop. On examination, he is unable to evert or dorsiflex his right foot. He has hypoaesthesia over the dorsum of his right foot.

### Answers

  **a** **4 Femoral nerve.** *Spontaneous haematomas of the psoas muscle can occur in patients taking anticoagulants. They typically present with a femoral neuropathy.*

  **b** **3 Superficial peroneal nerve.** *The superficial peroneal nerve innervates the foot everters and provides sensory branches to the dorsum of the foot. However, the sensory innervation webbed space between the hallux and second digit is provided by the deep peroneal nerve and is thus spared in superficial peroneal nerve injuries.*

  **c** **2 Common peroneal nerve.** *Common peroneal nerve mononeuropathies are frequent in diabetic patients, especially if the nerve is subjected to recurrent microtrauma. The trauma can be as innocuous as habitual leg crossing.*

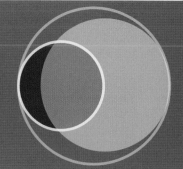

# CHAPTER 10

# The Spine

Rachid Haidar

## LEARNING OBJECTIVES

- To recognize and understand the history, general signs and symptoms observed in spinal disorders
- To be able to identify the different conditions that can affect the spine

## HISTORY

A thorough history is an essential prerequisite to the examination and investigation of spinal disorders. It will include information about the age and maturity of the patient, their family and social/occupational history, as well as their history of previous medical problems. Symptoms such as pain, deformity, its duration and the effects on the patient, their general health and their quality of life should be noted.

The onset, location, nature and radiation of the pain are important, as are any aggravating and relieving factors. The distinction between leg pain and back pain is particularly significant. Exacerbation by coughing or sneezing should be noted, as should its effects on everyday activities and sleep. Neurological symptoms, including bladder and bowel dysfunction, should be identified. Back pain in skeletally immature individuals should always be considered organic and fully investigated, especially if it has lasted for more than a week.

If the patient presents with spinal deformity, determine the time of onset, any precipitating factors, its progression and its effects on the physical and psychological health of the patient. In particular, secondary cardiorespiratory and neurological symptoms should be sought. Previous treatment and the level of compliance with this should be recorded. In children and adolescents, spinal deformities are not usually accompanied by pain, and if it is present, more sinister causes must always be considered and excluded.

Note should be made of any pending industrial or legal complaints related to the patient's presentation as these invariably affect the ultimate prognosis.

In all cases, an accurate recording of the history and examination, including the patient's mental state, will later prove invaluable.

## PHYSICAL EXAMINATION

### Observation

The appearance of the patient in the waiting area, their gait, their communication methods and the ease with which they undress all provide useful information. Adequate exposure is essential.

The patient must be examined in a warm, relaxed and friendly environment and should undress to their underwear for the assessment of their back.

The overall body habitus and facies of the patient can be used as a guide to congenital, endocrine or metabolic diseases. Sitting and standing heights, weight and arm span can be recorded.

An **antalgic gait** is seen when the patient spends less time weight-bearing on one limb due to pain; this is suggestive of hip or knee pathology. A **shuffling gait** may suggest a neurological lesion, and a **flexed gait** spinal stenosis.

Inspection from the side while the patient is standing allows an assessment of their posture. An increase or decrease in the lumbar lordosis or thoracic kyphosis soon becomes evident.

**Kyphosis (Figure 10.1a)** is the general term used to describe an excessive convex posterior curvature of the back such as a round back or humpback deformity. In postural kyphosis, the

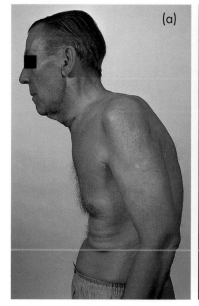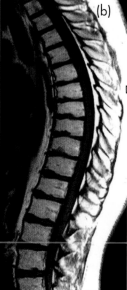

Figure 10.1 (a) Senile kyphosis. (b) Scheuermann's kyphosis.

curve is mobile and regular, and the flow of spinal movement is smooth. This can also be secondary to hip deformity or muscle weakness, both of which also lead to an increased lumbar lordosis. If the kyphosis is fixed, however, other causes such as senile kyphosis due to vertebral collapse, Scheuermann's disease (**Figure 10.1b; see the section on 'Scheuermann's kyphosis', below**) and ankylosing spondylitis should be considered.

A sharp angular kyphosis with a **gibbus** – the exaggerated prominence of a spinous process – points to a vertebral fracture (traumatic, pathological, malignant or osteoporotic); other causes include tuberculosis of the spine and congenital vertebral anomalies (**Figure 10.2**).

**Lordosis** refers to a convex anterior curvature of the spine. Flattening of the normal lumbar lordosis is commonly seen with prolapsed intervertebral discs, vertebral osteomyelitis, ankylosing spondylitis or a degenerative lumbar spine (**Figure 10.3**). The patient who presents with the spine, hips and knees flexed, the 'simian stance' (see the section on 'Spinal Stenosis', below), should be assessed for spinal stenosis. An increase in the lumbar curvature can be a normal racial variant that is more frequently seen in women, notably in pregnancy. It may also be secondary to spondylolisthesis or to a fixed deformity of the thoracic spine or hips, both of which should be examined.

**Scoliosis (Figure 10.4)** is, by definition, a lateral curvature of the spine of more than 10° with a rotational element. Examination is performed by inspecting the patient's back while standing, or

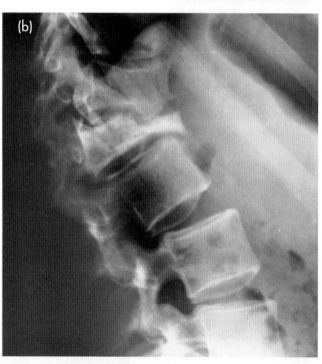

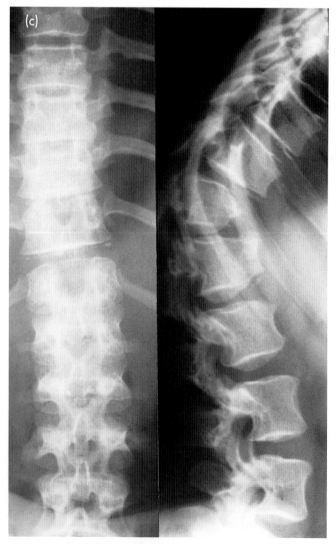

Figure 10.2 Gibbus secondary to: (a) tuberculosis, (b) a compression fracture of the first lumbar vertebra, and (c) achondroplasia.

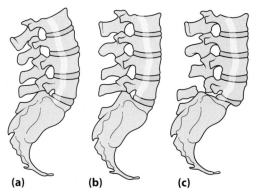

Figure 10.3 Illustration of the lateral contour of the lumbar spine. (a) Normal. (b) Spasm. (c) Spondylolisthesis.

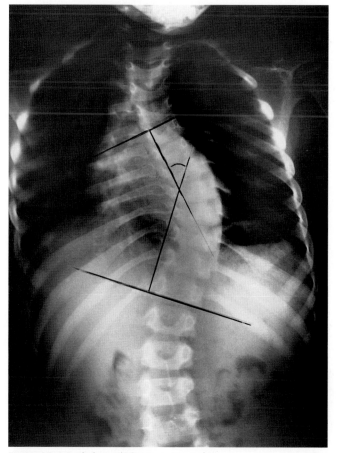

Figure 10.4 Radiological demonstration of the posterior aspect of a long muscular curve in scoliosis.

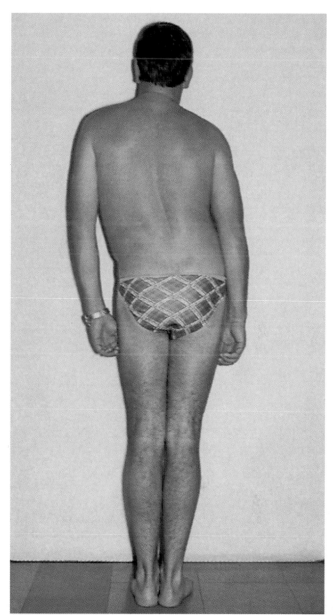

Figure 10.5 A sciatic list secondary to a prolapsed intervertebral disc. (Reproduced with permission from Physical Examination in Orthopaedics, by A. Graham Apley and Louis Solomon, Butterworth-Heinemann, 1997.)

while sitting if the patient has deformities of the lower extremities. A forward-bending test can help to elicit minor scoliosis. Further assessment of such a deformity is necessary to establish whether it is postural, compensatory, structural or related to pain and muscular spasm. In balanced deformities, the occiput lies above the midline; this can be confirmed using a plumb line. The shoulders, breasts and skin creases may also be asymmetrical, and the extent of any difference should be recorded. A scoliometer can be used to record the degree of asymmetry. The pelvic tilt must also be assessed.

A **postural curve** is usually a simple single curve that corrects in flexion; this is managed by observation.

A **compensatory scoliosis** can be secondary to previous thoracic surgery, hip pathology or leg length discrepancy. In the latter, the curve corrects when the patient sits down.

A **sciatic scoliosis** or **list** is due to muscle spasm. Its convexity is usually directed to the side of the intervertebral disc prolapse. It is associated with flattening of the lumbar lordosis and frequently with hip and knee flexion both at rest and on standing **(Figure 10.5)**.

A **structural scoliosis** is fixed in comparison to the flexible curves described above. It is always associated with rotation of the vertebral bodies towards the convexity of the curve. Secondary compensatory curves develop and can in time also become fixed curves. With thoracic curves in particular, vertebral rotation leads to a prominent rib hump deformity that can be measured with a scoliometer.

PART 2 | TRAUMA AND (ELECTIVE) ORTHOPAEDICS

Structural curves can be idiopathic, neuromuscular or congenital. Most scoliosis are idiopathic. These are commonly seen in adolescent girls, with most thoracic curves being right sided, and lumbar curves left sided.

Other causes include neuromuscular curves, such as those seen in cerebral palsy or in the muscular dystrophies. These are typically long, paralytic, C-shaped curves that are convex towards the weaker side (**Figure 10.6**). In neuromuscular curves, there is often significant cardiorespiratory compromise; costopelvic impingement can lead to pain, and sitting becomes progressively more difficult as the curves deteriorate. Congenital curves usually present at a very early stage and are associated with a host of congenital anomalies, including cardiac and renal malformations (**Figure 10.7**).

Inspection of the patient also reveals the scars of previous surgery, sinuses from previous bony sepsis, pigmentation or café-au-lait spots in relation to neurofibromatosis, or hairy patches or fat pads, which are suggestive of spinal dysraphism. The latter represents a failure of fusion of the cartilaginous bars forming the vertebral arch, resulting in a posterior vertebral defect that can have neurological consequences.

During this phase of the examination, the patient is asked to point to the site of greatest pain and the area of its radiation. A suspicion of emotional overlay should be aroused if the patient will not touch their back.

The patient can be asked to stand on tiptoe as a preliminary assessment of gastrocnemius power and hence a motor assessment of the S1 root.

With the patient lying prone, a comparison of the glutei muscles will reveal wasting or atrophy with L5, S1 or S2 lesions. This can also be noted by the observant examiner as a sag in the buttock crease of the standing patient.

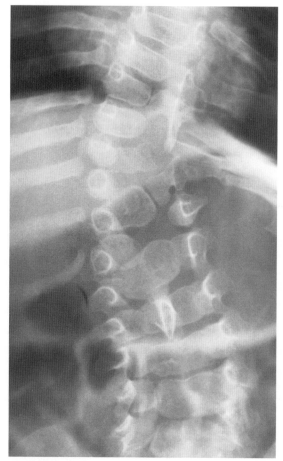

Figure 10.7 Vertebral defects.

## Palpation

The whole spine should be palpated from top to bottom in a systematic way to exclude any sharp irregularities, such as a gibbus, or any steps in the spine, as may be seen at the lumbosacral junction in spondylolisthesis.

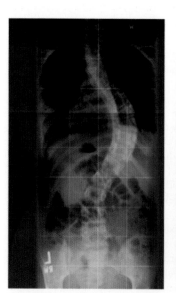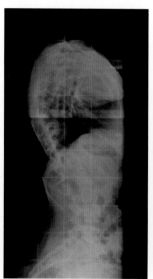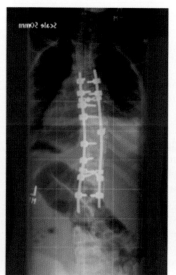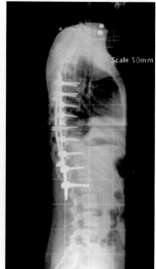

Figure 10.6 Correction of idiopathic scoliosis. Preoperative views: (a) anteroposterior and (b) lateral. Postoperative views showing the correction: (c) anteroposterior and (d) lateral.

Percussion with the examiner's fist is then used in an attempt to elicit tenderness at every spinal/interspinous level and in the paravertebral areas (**Figure 10.8**).

The sacroiliac joints should also be palpated and any tenderness elicited.

## Movement

The range of motion of the spine should be assessed through flexion and extension, lateral bending and rotation.

The patient is asked to touch their toes while keeping their knees extended (**Figure 10.9a–d**). This is a compound movement including thoracic, lumbar and hip flexion. The distance of the fingertips from the floor or from anatomical landmarks, such as the tibial tuberosity or malleoli, can then be recorded. Alternatively, the spine can be marked at predetermined points such as T1–L1 or L1–S1 and the increase in this distance noted with flexion (**Figure 10.10**). Both parameters should increase by approximately 8 cm. Chest expansion can be

similarly measured if rigidity suggests ankylosing spondylitis – an expansion of less than 2.5 cm is almost pathognomonic.

If the patient constantly deviates to one side when bending forwards, this is indicative of an irritative lesion such as a herniated disc, osteoid osteoma or spinal tumour, and should be investigated further. A reversal of the normal spinal rhythm on attempting to regain the erect posture is characteristic of disc degeneration with posterior facet pain.

A similar manoeuvre can be used to measure spinal extension, with the reduction in the measured distance being recorded.

Lateral flexion is assessed by asking the patient to slide their hand down the side of each leg in turn (**Figure 10.9c**). The distance from the floor or from fixed anatomical landmarks can then be recorded.

Rotation is measured by folding the patient's arms across their chest in the seated position and asking them to twist to either side. The rotation usually measures less than 40° and is almost entirely thoracic (**Figure 10.9d**).

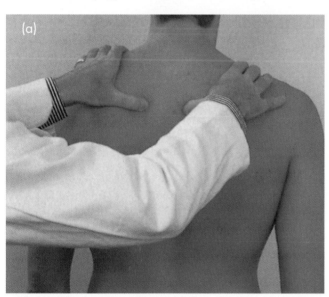
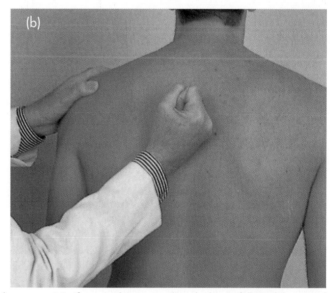

Figure 10.8 Examination for spinal tenderness commences with digital pressure (a). If no tenderness is elicited, this is followed by spinal percussion (b).

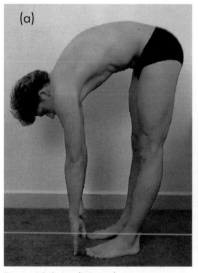
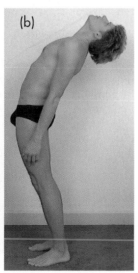
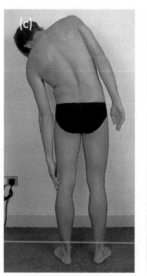
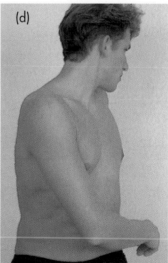

Figure 10.9 (a–d) Spinal movements.

PART 2 | TRAUMA AND (ELECTIVE) ORTHOPAEDICS

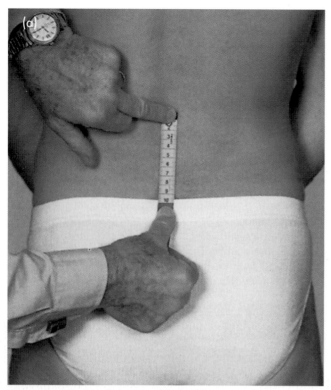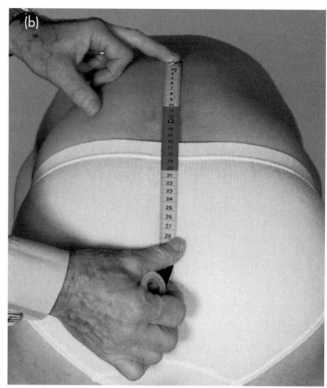

Figure 10.10 (a, b) Schober's test of spinal flexion. (Reproduced with permission from *Physical Examination in Orthopaedics*, by A. Graham Apley and Louis Solomon, Butterworth-Heinemann, 1997.)

Leg lengths with the patient supine, and the range of movement of the hips, are measured to exclude their contribution to the patient's presentation. While the patient is lying flat, compression and distraction of the pelvis can be attempted by grasping the anterior superior iliac spines; reproduction of the patient's pain is suggestive of sacroiliac pathology. The sacroiliac joints can also be stressed by flexing the hip and knee and adducting the thigh – the pump handle test. This is a non-specific test but can suggest sacroiliac pathology including inflammatory and infectious arthropathies.

Examination of the back is incomplete without a full abdominal, rectal and vascular examination.

### Straight Leg Raising (Lasègue's Test)

This is a passive test, with each leg being tested separately, that aims to reproduce pain in the lower extremity by stretching the sciatic nerve. With the patient supine, the hip in neutral and medially rotated and the knee extended, the examiner gently and gradually flexes the hip until the patient complains of pain or tightness (**Figure 10.11a**). The leg is then returned to a level that causes no symptoms and the ankle is dorsiflexed before the leg is again raised (**Figure 10.11b**). If such a manoeuvre recreates pain radiating down the back of the leg, the test is considered positive and indicates stretching of the dura mater or a compressed nerve, primarily at the L5, S1 and S2 levels. Pain that does not increase with ankle dorsiflexion is suggestive of tight hamstrings or a mechanical lumbosacral cause. The test is then repeated on the other side for comparison.

It cannot be overemphasized that it is leg/radicular pain and not merely back pain that signifies a positive test. This distinction between nerve root pain and mechanical back pain is significant in terms of both treatment and prognosis. The level at which the test is positive is recorded for future comparison.

Contralateral pain felt during a straight leg raise – the crossover sign – is highly indicative of a space-occupying lesion in the spinal canal such as a prolapsed intervertebral disc.

Bilateral simultaneous straight leg raising causes the pelvis to rotate and hyperextends the lumbar spine. In the presence of disc degeneration, this leads to pain and is an indicator of painful segmental disorder.

### Bowstring Test

This is carried out in a similar manner to the straight leg raising test. Once the patient is experiencing symptoms during leg raising, the knee is flexed by approximately 20°. This leads to pain relief in a patient with nerve root irritation. Thumb or finger pressure is then applied to the popliteal area. If this pressure recreates the patient's radicular symptoms, it is indicative of nerve root tension due to nerve compression (**Figure 10.12**).

### Femoral Stretch Test

With the patient either prone or in the lateral decubitus position and the back not hyperextended, the knee is flexed while maintaining the hip in neutral rotation (**Figure 10.13**). The hip is then gradually extended. Limited knee flexion/hip extension with pain radiating down the anterior aspect of the thigh is due to stretching of the femoral nerve and is indicative of a lesion at L2, L3 or L4. As with the straight leg raising test, contralateral pain is of considerable significance.

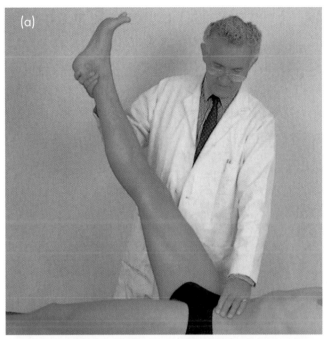

Figure 10.11 (a, b) Straight leg raising to elicit nerve root tension.

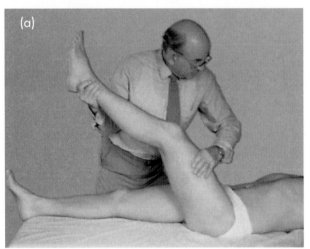

Figure 10.12 (a, b) The bowstring test for nerve root tension. (Reproduced with permission from *Physical Examination in Orthopaedics*, by A. Graham Apley and Louis Solomon, Butterworth-Heinemann, 1997.)

## Stoop Test

This is done to confirm neurogenic spinal claudication. After exertion, the patient's buttock and leg pain is relieved by bending forwards. Conversely, the symptoms are exacerbated by extending the spine.

## Neurological Assessment

A focused neurological examination is vital. Muscle bulk or girth, tone, power, reflexes and sensation are sequentially assessed (Table 10.1).

The girth of the thigh or quadriceps should be compared with that on the contralateral side; it may be decreased secondary to an L4 lesion or to disuse. With lesions of the fourth lumbar root, the quadriceps may be weak and tender to palpation. This is tested by asking the patient to extend the flexed knee against

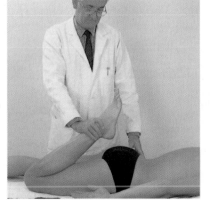

Figure 10.13 The femoral stretch test. This can be performed with the patient prone or lying on their side.

Table 10.1 Potential findings in nerve root dysfunction

| Level | Wasting | Motor weakness | Reflex depression | Sensory disturbance |
|---|---|---|---|---|
| L4 | Thigh/quadriceps | Knee extension | Knee jerk | Medial aspect of calf and ankle |
| L5 | Calf | Extensor hallucis longus (ankle dorsiflexors) | | Lateral aspect of calf and medial dorsum of foot |
| S1 | Calf | Flexor hallucis longus (ankle plantar flexors) | Ankle jerk | Posterior aspect of calf, lateral border of foot and sole |

the examiner's resistance. The knee/patellar tendon jerk may be reduced or absent.

Lesions of the fifth lumbar root may cause weakness of the extensor hallucis longus prior to any demonstrable ankle dorsiflexor weakness. Alternatively, wasting of extensor digitorum brevis is another sensitive sign of an L5 lesion. Ankle dorsiflexion should be tested with the knees flexed, as resisting plantar flexion with the hip and knee extended may exacerbate sciatic pain.

With an S1 lesion, toe and subsequently ankle flexion become weak. In early lesions, the fatiguability of the gastrocnemius should be compared with that of the other side by asking the patient to repeatedly rise on tiptoe. Ultimately, the patient may be unable to stand on tiptoe at all, although this may also be difficult in the presence of quadriceps weakness. With first sacral root irritation, the calf muscles may be tender and the ankle jerk may also become deficient.

Sensory testing, including light touch, pinprick and vibration sense, should be performed in those under 50 years of age. It should be remembered that the distribution of the L4 dermatome comprises the anteromedial thigh and lower leg, the L5 dermatome the dorsum of the foot and anterior lower leg, and the S1 dermatome the sole of the foot and the outer border of the foot and lower leg (**Figure 10.14**). These territories are useful both in interpreting the radiation of the patient's pain and in assessing any root sensory deficit.

Difficulty with micturition, urinary retention, loss of anal sphincter tone or faecal incontinence, progressive motor loss and saddle anaesthesia are all suggestive of central cord compression and require urgent imaging and decompression.

Absence of the superficial abdominal reflex may be the only abnormality noted in the initial presentation of syringomyelia.

At the end of the neurological assessment, the history, general examination findings and motor and sensory findings should be collated to identify the anatomical level of any spinal pathology. This can then be confirmed by radiological investigation before any intervention is planned.

## NEONATAL/CONGENITAL DISORDERS

**Spinal dysraphism** represents a failure of fusion of the cartilaginous bars forming the vertebral arch and results in a posterior vertebral defect. Its incidence is decreasing due to improved prenatal diagnosis and prevention. There are still a variety of forms that can affect any level of the spinal column, although they are most frequently seen in the lumbosacral region:

- *Myelocele*: Both the neural and the vertebral arches fail to close. Clinical examination reveals an oval, raw, uncovered

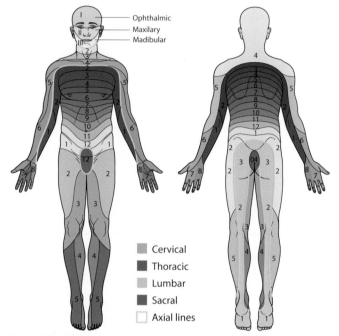

Figure 10.14 Dermatomal maps.

defect communicating with the central canal of the spinal cord. The infant is usually stillborn or dies soon after birth.
- *Syringomyelocele*: The bulging defect includes a dilated cyst of the spinal cord and is associated with dense neurological lesions.
- *Meningocele*: The protruding meningeal sac contains only cerebrospinal fluid and is covered with healthy skin.
- *Meningomyelocele*: A normally developed spinal cord or cauda equina lies within the protruding sac, which is covered by unepithelialized meninges rather than skin (**Figure 10.15**).

A transmitted impulse can be detected from the swelling to the anterior fontanelle. An assessment of the degree of paralysis and anal tone reveals the level of the neurological injury. A general examination of these infants may reveal **hydrocephalus** in relation to the **Arnold–Chiari malformation** in which cerebellar herniation obstructs the cerebrospinal fluid outflow.

**Spina bifida occulta** – a failure of spinal arch fusion, which is often associated with a local patch of hair, skin dimples, sinuses or lipomas, is found in nearly 15 per cent of the population and is asymptomatic. It is frequently an incidental finding when radiographic investigation of the back is undertaken. It may be associated with an abnormal filum terminale or spinal cord tethering, which becomes significant if later operative intervention is planned.

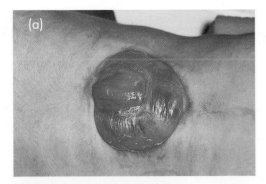

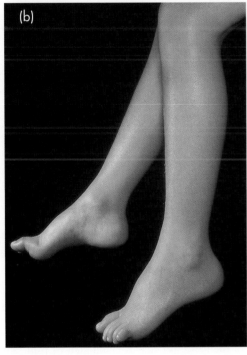

Figure 10.15 (a) Meningomyelocele. (b) Right pes cavus due to neurological damage.

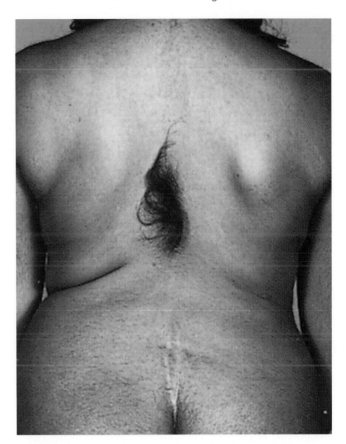

Figure 10.16 Spinal bifida with a faun tail and a scar from previous surgery.

Congenital **osteogenic scoliosis** present a more difficult management problem. Causes include failures of fusion and/or vertebral segmentation. Skin angiomas, dimples, hairy tufts, naevi and fat pads often give a clue to the associated **spina bifida** (**Figure 10.16**) and spinal cord tethering must be excluded or documented by MRI prior to any surgical intervention.

## DIFFERENTIAL DIAGNOSIS OF BACK PAIN

### Back Pain in Children and Adults

Persistent back pain is uncommon in childhood; if it is present, neoplastic and infectious diseases should be ruled out. Although it is often vague and poorly localized, it must be thoroughly investigated as psychosomatic back pain is a diagnosis of exclusion in children. Back pain in children should never be dismissed as non-organic and should always be promptly investigated, especially if it has lasted for more than a week.

The most likely causes of back pain in childhood are infections such as discitis or osteomyelitis, and spinal/paraspinal tumours. As in adults, the most common cause of back pain in children is disc disease in the form of disc degeneration or disc herniation, facet arthroses and other mechanical conditions as spondylolysis and spondylolisthesis. In adolescence, inflammatory disorders such as ankylosing spondylitis or juvenile chronic arthritis must be considered. Mechanical causes such as osteochondritis, Scheuermann's disease, herniated intervertebral discs, spondylolysis and spondylolisthesis must also be excluded. Painful scoliosis should be carefully assessed as many cases have a sinister cause.

In addition, any medical condition that could present itself as back pain should be excluded. This requires a general examination of the patient and an assessment of the abdomen, the pelvis, the lower limbs and the peripheral vascular system to exclude conditions such as peptic ulcer disease, renal or perirenal infections, renal stone disease, gallstones, pancreatitis, intrapelvic tumours, gynaecological infections (pelvic inflammatory disease), arthritis of the hip, an abdominal aortic aneurysm or vascular claudication.

### Discitis

This is usually a childhood affliction, although it can occur as a complication after disc space surgery in adults. The aetiology is not infectious in all cases. The average age of presentation is 2–6 years, with boys and girls being equally affected. The child classically complains of back pain increasing in intensity over 2–4 weeks.

On examination, the child shows some spinal rigidity and maintains a fixed hyperlordosis. A low-grade pyrexia may be

PART 2 | TRAUMA AND (ELECTIVE) ORTHOPAEDICS

noted. Intra-abdominal infection and hip sepsis must be excluded by examination. Plain radiographs can be normal in the early stages of the condition, and MRI scans and bone scintigraphy will allow an early diagnosis.

## Scheuermann's Kyphosis

Scheuermann's disease was described in 1921 as a thoracic kyphotic deformity affecting young males, usually prior to puberty, that is characterized by vertebral wedging and a subsequent growth disturbance of the vertebral end plate (see Figure 10.1b). The aetiology of this condition is not known. Patients usually present with either pain or cosmetic deformity without neurological symptoms or signs. The pain tends to decline following skeletal maturity. The curve is usually rigid, particularly at its apex.

There are two main forms of the disease, thoracic and thoracolumbar. The thoracolumbar type is more common and has its apex between T10 and T11. Scheuermann's disease is radiographically characterized by irregular vertebral end plates, Schmorl's nodes and a reduction in disc height with anterior vertebral wedging.

## Spondylosis and Spondylolisthesis

This is a defect in the pars interarticularis (**Figure 10.17**) in the posterior column of the lumbar spine. It is the most common cause of persistent/recurrent back pain in childhood and adolescence. Bilateral defects in the pars interarticularis may result in spondylolisthesis (**Figure 10.18**), which is a forward slippage of one vertebra on another and is classified into five major types: congenital, isthmic, traumatic, degenerative and pathological.

Acquired defects are known to follow repeated stress on the pars region. This is particularly common in gymnasts, footballers and cricketers. The most common manifestation is back pain aggravated by exercise. Examination reveals localized lumbar back pain, minimal tenderness and some paraspinal muscle spasm. There may be decreased forward flexion of the spine.

Radiological evaluation is usually with plain films, including oblique radiographs. The latter confirm the pars defect as a fracture in the neck of the 'Scotty dog' as the neck of the Scotty dog represents the pars on X-ray (**Figure 10.18c**). As for spondylolisthesis, the severity is graded according to the percentage slip of one vertebra on the other, or the angle of rotation of the slip.

## Disc Herniation

Disc herniation refers to herniation of the central disc material, the annulus pulposus, into the spinal canal. This can be a simple protrusion with an intact annulus fibrosus, extrusion if there is a tear in the annulus fibrosus but the material is still contained by the longitudinal ligament, or sequestration, in which there is a free disc fragment in the canal.

Disc herniation can cause a compression of neural elements, which, depending on the location, can be compression of the spinal cord, dural sac or nerve roots:

- Compression of the *spinal cord* (cervical or dorsal spine) gives rise to the signs and symptoms of upper motor disease, including hyperreflexia, a Babinski reflex and/or clonus; at a later stage, the anal and bladder sphincters might be affected.
- Compression of the *dural sac* by a large central disc herniation in the lumbar area can cause cauda equina syndrome (saddle anaesthesia, bowel and/or bladder dysfunction, and

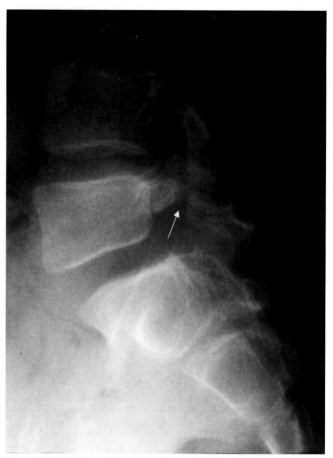

Figure 10.17 Defect of the pars interarticularis.

lower limb sensory and motor deficits), which is a surgical emergency.
- Posterolateral or foraminal disc herniation causes compression of the *nerve root* that is manifested by pain, numbness, weakness and a possible loss of reflexes across the nerve root, with a distribution in the upper or lower extremity depending on the level of the lesion.

## Spinal Stenosis

This condition refers to a narrowing of the spinal canal (**Figure 10.19**) that can compromise the spinal cord and nerve roots. The patient presents with an insidious onset of back and leg pain. The symptoms are usually bilateral with leg pain that is worse on standing and walking; sitting or flexing the spine forwards usually relieves the pain because this increases the area of the spinal canal. The patient often experiences pain on walking a certain distance but can walk further if they lean forwards (the 'simian stance'); with progression of the spinal stenosis, the distance that the patient can walk in one go is decreased. Symptoms are also often severe at night because the supine posture decreases the area in the spinal canal.

Spinal stenosis can be classified into congenital and acquired. The latter can be degenerative, secondary to a spondylolisthesis, iatrogenic, traumatic or related to miscellaneous disorders, such as acromegaly, Paget's disease or ankylosing spondylitis. Moreover, combined causes can be noted in some cases, such as degenerative changes on a background of a congenitally narrow canal. The

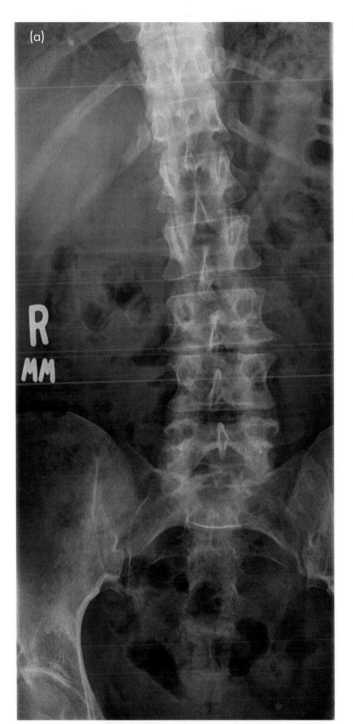

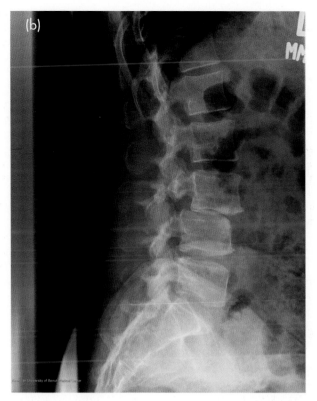

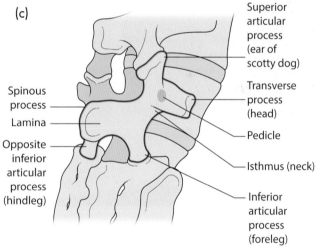

Figure 10.18 Spondylolisthesis at L3–L4 observed from (a) anteroposterior and (b) lateral. (c) An oblique view of the vertebrae will show the 'Scotty dog'.

differential diagnosis of spinal stenosis includes vascular claudication with back pain, and lumbar spondylosis without stenosis.

## Ankylosing Spondylitis

Ankylosing spondylitis (**Figure 10.20**) is a seronegative arthropathy that progresses slowly to bony ankylosis of the joints of the spinal column and occasionally of the major limb joints. It affects two or three per 1000 individuals and has a male preponderance. Although it is related to HLA-B27, the precise cause is not known.

The initial changes are seen in the sacroiliac joints and extend upwards to the lumbar and often the thoracic spine. The hips and shoulders can also be affected. The articular cartilage, synovium and ligaments all show chronic inflammatory changes and eventually become ossified. This condition should always be suspected

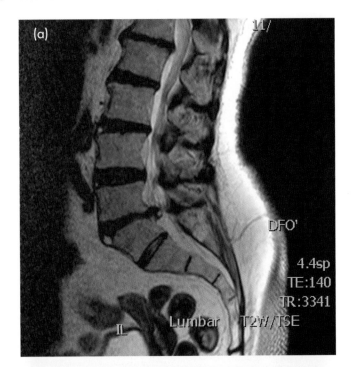

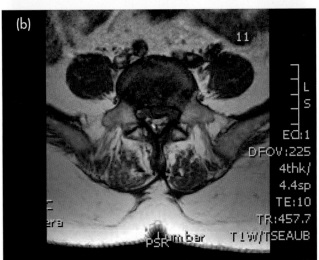

Figure 10.19 (a) Sagittal and (b) axial cuts in MRI of the lumbar spine showing spinal stenosis due to disc herniation, facet arthrosis and hypertrophy of the flavum ligament.

when low back pain, which is worse in the morning and improves as the day progresses, is seen in young male patients.

The diagnosis is usually made on the basis of reduced spinal movement and chest expansion with possible sacroiliac or costochondral tenderness. Typical radiographic features include fuzziness of the sacroiliac joints and squaring or bridging of the lumbar vertebrae. In the early stages, a raised erythrocyte sedimentation rate and increased uptake at the sacroiliac joints on bone scan may be the only positive features.

## Rheumatoid Arthritis

Clinical manifestations from the thoracic and lumbar spine are relatively uncommon. This is unlike the cervical spine, where rheumatoid disease can be extremely severe, can lead to myelopathy and must always be excluded prior to general anaesthesia.

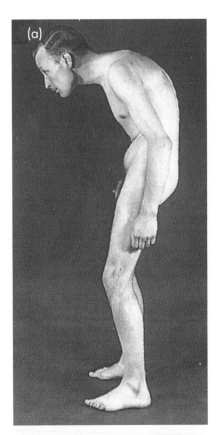

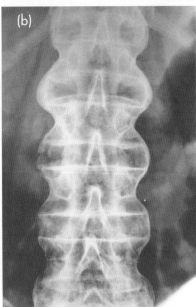

Figure 10.20 Ankylosing spondylitis. (a) A patient with a fixed thoracic kyphosis. (b) A bamboo spine.

## Coccydynia

This refers to any painful condition in the region of the coccyx. In practice, it often refers to patients whose pain persists for weeks or months despite the absence of any demonstrable pathology. There is often a predisposing injury and the coccyx is very tender locally. Enquiry must be made as to whether the patient can pass their faeces normally, and a rectal examination should be performed.

## SPINAL INJURIES

The vertebral column and spinal cord can be injured individually or together (**Figure 10.21**). The spine must be immobilized during the resuscitation phase until a full clinical and neurological assessment has been made and adequate radiographs have been obtained. The patient is therefore examined in a neutral position with the neck held in 'in-line' immobilization or stabilized with a collar and sandbags.

Clinical examination should identify any pain, tenderness, bruising, oedema or deformity. A full autonomic and neurological assessment must also be undertaken. A conscious patient will be able to locate the areas of greatest discomfort and to report any neurological disturbance. The abdomen, pelvis and extremities must be carefully examined as spinal cord injury may render serious pathology asymptomatic. In the unconscious patient, flaccid areflexia, diaphragmatic breathing, hypotension with

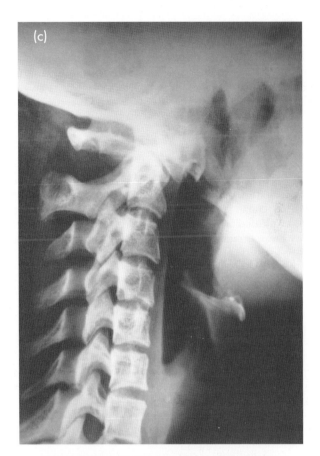

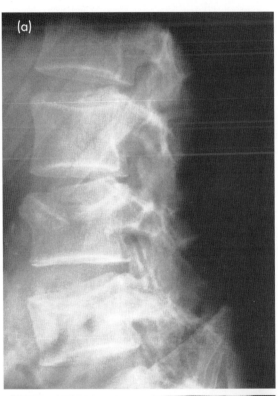

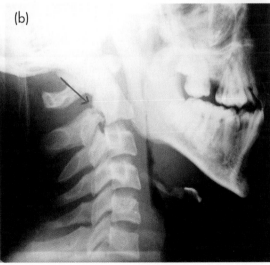

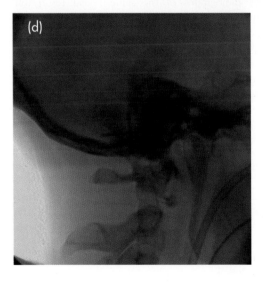

**Figure 10.21** Spinal injuries. (a) Crush fracture of a lumbar vertebra. (b) Fractured neck. (c) Dissociation of the atlantoaxial joint. (d) Sagittal CT view of C1–C2 dissociation.

bradycardia – **neurogenic shock** – and priapism are all suggestive of a spinal cord injury.

**Spinal shock** refers to the flaccidity and areflexia that is seen immediately after spinal cord damage. It lasts up to 48 hours or until the return of the bulbocavernosus reflex. It is replaced in due course by spasticity, increased reflexes and upgoing plantar reflexes. Once this has occurred, the likely residual neurological deficit and prognosis can be determined. A motor and sensory level for the spinal cord injury can then be defined and the appropriate investigation, management and rehabilitation instituted.

Spinal fractures (**Figure 10.21**) can be divided into compression fractures, burst fractures, flexion-distraction injuries and fracture dislocations. The spine can be divided into anterior, middle and posterior columns; if more than one column is involved, the injury is likely to be unstable. The assessment of these injuries requires plain radiographs supplemented by CT and MRI scans.

## OSTEOPOROSIS

This represents a diminution of bone mass (**Figure 10.22**). The composition of the bone is normal, but the amount of bone per unit volume is decreased. With the advent of bone mineral density measurement using dual-energy X-ray absorptiometry, osteoporosis is now defined as a reduction in bone mineral density of more than 2.5 standard deviations from the mean for young adults.

Osteoporosis may be a primary disorder – as is most commonly seen in postmenopausal women – or may occur secondary to nutritional disorders, a variety of hormonal diseases such as thyrotoxicosis, hyperparathyroidism, diabetes mellitus or Cushing's disease, or drug use, most notably with the use of corticosteroids.

**Vertebral compression fractures** (Figure 10.22c) represent one of the most common sequelae of osteoporosis. The clinical presentation may only be of a progressive kyphosis, and the fractures often occur without trauma or with only the mildest stress on the spine. Successive fractures ultimately lead to backache, kyphosis and loss of height.

Plain radiographs of the spine reveal resorption of the horizontal trabeculae with biconcavity of the vertebral bodies. Compression fractures with anterior wedging most commonly occur around the thoracolumbar junction. Involvement of the pedicles suggests malignant pathology.

## SPINAL INFECTIONS

Vertebral osteomyelitis is a not uncommon condition, and it requires a high index of clinical suspicion to identify it. The most common cause is haematogenous spread, although infection can be from a contiguous focus or from direct inoculation during a surgical procedure or therapeutic injection. Most cases affect the lumbar spine. *Staphylococcus aureus* is the most commonly implicated organism, followed by streptococci and Enterobacteriae. Patients with sickle cell anaemia have a known predisposition towards *Salmonella* osteomyelitis, and intravenous drug abusers have a high rate of infection with *Pseudomonas* sp.

The most common presentation is a deep persistent back pain that is not relieved by rest and is unaffected by changes in position. Neurological deficits occur in 30 per cent of patients. As well as a careful examination, a complete blood count, C-reactive protein level and erythrocyte sedimentation rate should be measured and blood cultures taken.

The diagnosis is often delayed as plain radiographic changes may not appear for 2–4 weeks. These include a loss of disc height and paravertebral soft tissue shadows, followed ultimately by end-plate destruction. The differential diagnosis includes renal osteodystrophy, non-pyogenic infection, ankylosing spondylitis and rheumatoid arthritis. In contrast, neoplastic vertebral destruction is more likely to be centered in the vertebral body and spare the disc space. An earlier diagnosis can be reached using MRI scanning or bone scintigraphy; CT scans are also more sensitive than plain radiography.

## Tuberculosis

This remains a common source of vertebral infection on a worldwide scale and is again particularly important with the advent of new strains of resistant mycobacteria; over 50 per cent of cases are reported in the first decade of life. Infection can be acquired either directly from the lungs or by haematogenous spread. The infection begins at the anterior margin of the vertebral body near the intervertebral disc, and the disc can be involved at an early stage. The extent of destruction varies – there is often complete destruction of one intervertebral disc with partial destruction of two adjacent vertebrae. The changes may extend over several spinal segments, and anterior collapse of the infected vertebrae can lead to severe angular kyphosis, called a gibbus (see Figure 10.2a).

Abscess formation is common and can take the form of a solely paraspinal abscess (**Figure 10.23a**) or track down beneath the fascial sheath of the psoas muscle and burst into the compartment behind the iliacus fascia so that part of the abscess forms in the iliac fossa – a **psoas abscess (Figure 10.23b)**. This abscess can also point posteriorly or into the groin. Neurological compromise may occur because of abscess formation within the spinal canal or secondary to a long-standing severe kyphosis.

Tubercular infection differs from pyogenic infection by its multisegment involvement, its spread along soft tissue planes and its propensity to lead to kyphosis and paravertebral abscess formation.

## SPINAL TUMOURS

Tumours in relation to the spinal column can be considered as those of the spinal column itself, those of the meninges and, rarely, those of the spinal cord. There are also neoplasms of the fibrous component of the peripheral nerves and of the adjacent soft tissues. The effects of these tumours can be divided into local destruction of the skeleton, compression of the spinal cord and interference with the peripheral nerves. The degree of each of these components determines the resulting symptomatology. A thorough clinical examination and imaging are necessary before any treatment can be considered.

**Benign tumours** usually affect patients in the second or third decade, although sacral tumours occur in older age groups. The most common types are giant cell tumours, osteoid osteomas, osteoblastomas, haemangiomas, osteochondromas and aneurysmal bone cysts. The most common complaint is pain that may

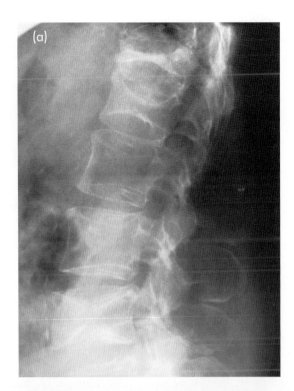

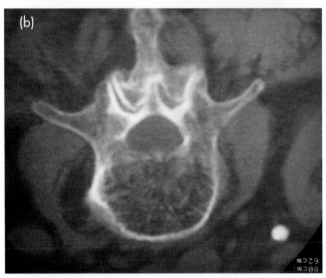

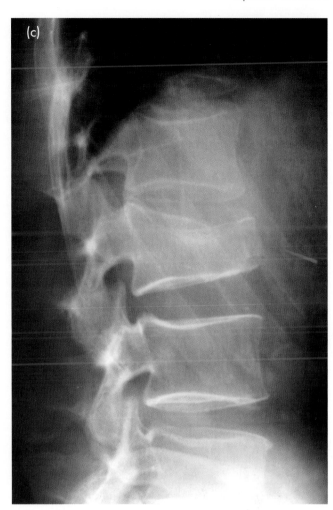

Figure 10.22 Osteoporotic spine. (a) Lateral radiograph. (b) Magnetic resonance image. (c) Crush fracture of the lumbar vertebra.

be local or radicular, and which, particularly in children, must be thoroughly investigated. Night pain is a well-recognized association of osteoid osteoma and osteoblastoma. Scoliosis may also be a presenting feature and is often seen without a compensatory curve.

Most tumours have a characteristic radiographic appearance: osteoid osteomas and osteoblastomas, for example, frequently present as sclerotic lesions in the pedicle. Aneurysmal bone cysts and giant cell tumours are often expansile and lytic, while eosinophilic granulomas can cause vertebral plana or a flat vertebra. Bone scans, CT scanning and MRI are all useful in delineating and defining the lesion.

**Malignant lesions** within the vertebral column are predominantly metastatic (**Figure 10.24**) as opposed to primary tumours such as Ewing's sarcoma and osteosarcoma. Common primary sites are the breast, lung, prostate, kidney, thyroid and gastrointestinal tract, as well as from a lymphoma. The pain associated with these lesions is classically relentlessly progressive and unresponsive to rest and normal conservative measures. The patient often wakes up at night.

There is scant radiographic evidence of the lesions as a 50 per cent destruction of the vertebral body is necessary before an abnormality can be detected on plain radiographs. Biopsy is frequently necessary to reach a diagnosis.

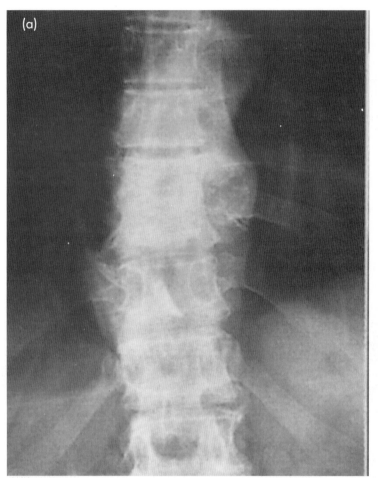

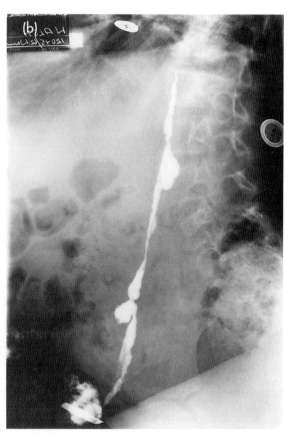

Figure 10.23 Tuberculosis. (a) Collapse of the thoracic vertebrae and abscess formation. (b) Sinogram of a psoas abscess demonstrating the track from the thoracic vertebrae along the psoas sheath to the groin.

## NON-ORGANIC BACK PAIN

Non-organic back or spinal pain represents such a significant clinical and medicolegal problem that it deserves particular attention.

Non-anatomical neurological symptoms and signs, particularly if they are inconsistent, should arouse suspicion that the patient's problems are not entirely organic in nature. Examples include cases in which the pain is multifocal with some features that cannot be ascribed to spinal pathology, when an entire extremity is weak, numb or gives way, or when the patient claims to be 'allergic' to all recommended treatments. These patients must be assessed particularly carefully, both to exclude unusual neurological disorders and to avoid unnecessary investigations that may reinforce the patient's illness behaviour. To this end, a number of manoeuvres and distraction tests – which can easily be incorporated into the standard back examination – have been developed. The following may be seen:

- Pain when the clinician gently touches or pinches the patient's back; alternatively, the patient may refuse to touch their own back because it is too painful. Superficial stimulation does not usually reproduce spinal pain.
- The patient localizes the position of greatest pain to different points at the beginning and end of the consultation.
- Pressure on the hamstrings during the bowstring test, which does not compromise the nerves, should therefore not recreate any nerve root symptoms that these patients may describe.
- The patient is unable to toe their touch by flexing the spine in the standing position but can do so with legs straight when sitting on the examination couch (**Figure 10.25**).
- The 'flip sign' can be elicited: the patient has a very positive straight leg raise but can sit up from a supine position without flexing the knees; this would be very difficult and painful in the presence of nerve root irritation as the tests are identical but merely have different starting points.
- In the Hoover test, the examiner places one hand behind the patient's heel while the patient attempts a straight leg raise on the contralateral side. The absence of downward pressure on the examiner's hand suggests that the patient is not making a significant effort to lift their leg.

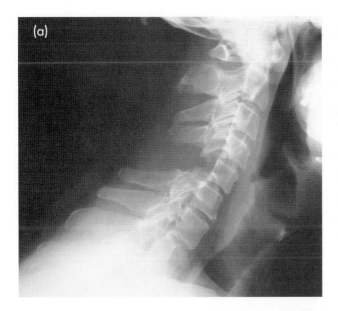

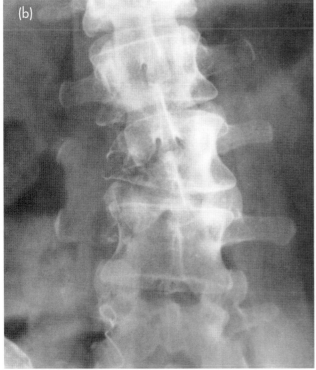

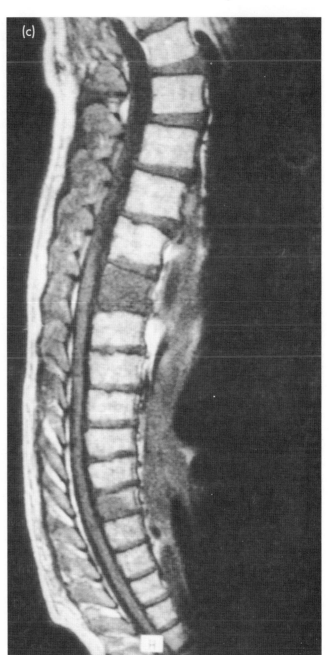

**Figure 10.24** Secondary deposits in the spine. (a) C5. (b) L3. (c) Multiple thoracic sites.

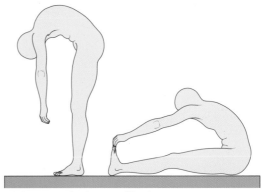

**Figure 10.25** Testing for functional back pain.

**Key Points**

- Clinical examination of the spine should incorporate the patient's chief complaint in light of their age and social status, as well as a history of any trauma, fever, deformity or pain; an observation of the overall habitus, appearance and gait of the patient; palpation to note pain or masses; an assessment of the patient's movement and range of motion through a set of special tests such as straight leg raising (Lasègue's test), the bowstring test, the femoral stretch test and the stoop test; and a neurological assessment.
- The differential diagnosis of back pain in paediatric and adult populations includes: neonatal and congenital disorders; back pain in children from Scheuermann's kyphosis, discitis, disc herniation and spondylosis; and back pain in adults from spondylolysis and spondylolisthesis, disc herniation, spinal stenosis, coccydynia, inflammatory conditions, spinal infections, osteoporosis, spinal injuries, neoplasms and non-organic aetiologies.
- Neoplasms of the spine can be benign or malignant. Benign tumours, commonly giant cell tumours, osteoid osteomas, osteoblastomas, haemangiomas, osteochondromas and aneurysmal bone cysts, usually occur in early adulthood, commonly demonstrate night pain and are diagnosed by imaging. Malignant tumours are mostly metastatic, may be primary, for example Ewing's sarcoma and osteosarcoma, and are diagnosed by biopsy.

## QUESTIONS

### SBAs

**1. The absence of an ankle jerk is a sign of compression of which one of the following nerve roots?:**
  **a** L4
  **b** L5
  **c** S1
  **d** L3

**Answer**
**c S1.** *S1 supplies the triceps surae muscles, so if it is compressed by a disc herniation, the ankle jerk may be absent.*

**2. Which one of the following best describes the symptoms of spinal stenosis?:**
  **a** Leg pain relieved by sitting
  **b** Leg pain aggravated by walking
  **c** Leg pain relieved by bending forwards
  **d** All of the above

**Answer**
**d All of the above.** *Spinal stenosis can cause neurogenic claudication, which is pain in the lower extremity while walking. Sitting for a few minutes will relieve the pain, and bending forwards will relieve the pain by providing more space for the compressed nerve.*

**3. A 5-year-old boy with a history of a febrile illness 1 month previously has presented with back pain of 3 weeks' duration. Which one of the following is the most likely diagnosis?:**
  **a** Disc herniation
  **b** Discitis
  **c** Spinal tumour
  **d** Spondylolisthesis

**Answer**
**b Discitis.** *In febrile illness followed by back pain in children, the most common diagnosis will be discitis, in which bacteraemia has caused infection of the disc space.*

### EMQs

**1. Match the following diseases to the appropriate symptoms in the list below. Each option may be used once, more than once or not at all:**
  **1** Rheumatic problem
  **2** Spinal stenosis
  **3** Tumour
  **4** Spondylolysis and spondylolisthesis
  **a** Night pain
  **b** Morning pain
  **c** Exercise pain
  **d** Walking pain

**Answers**
**a** *3. Night pain is typical of a tumour.*
**b** *1. Morning pain is rather typical of rheumatic problems.*
**c** *4. Spondylolysis and spondylolisthesis are mechanical back problems that will cause pain with activity.*
**d** *2. Neurogenic claudication, which is walking pain, is typical of spinal stenosis.*

**2. A 40-year-old man has presented with disc herniation. Match the location of the disc herniation with the most probable location of signs from the list below. Each option may be used once, more than once or not at all:**
  **1** C4–C5 disc herniation
  **2** C6–C7 disc herniation
  **3** C5–C6 disc herniation
  **a** Triceps
  **b** Wrist extension
  **c** Biceps

**Answers**
**a** *2. C6–C7 disc herniation compresses the C7 nerve root that supplies triceps.*
**b** *2. C6–C7 disc herniation compresses the C7 nerve root that also supplies the wrist extensors.*
**c** *1. C4–C5 disc herniation compresses the C5 nerve root that supplies biceps.*

# The Shoulder Joint and Pectoral Girdle

Muhyeddine Al-Taki and Imad S. Nahle

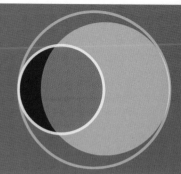

---

## LEARNING OBJECTIVES

- To understand the range of motion of the shoulder and the scapulohumeral rhythm
- To be competent in performing a comprehensive physical examination of the shoulder area, including basic diagnostic tests

- To be able to diagnose impingement syndrome and common rotator cuff tears
- To know about common traumatic fractures and dislocations of the shoulder girdle
- To understand shoulder instability

---

## INTRODUCTION

The shoulder area includes the humerus, glenoid, scapula, acromion, clavicle and surrounding soft tissue structures. Any precise diagnosis of shoulder disorders requires a methodical approach covering all these structures.

## INSPECTION

A complete inspection of both shoulders should be undertaken only after the patient has properly disrobed. The shoulders should be observed from both in front and behind.

Asymmetry, swelling, erythema, scars, bruises and venous distension should be noted if present. Abnormal contours of the trapezius or deltoid muscles can result from denervation of the accessory or axillary nerves. A right angle contour of the deltoid may suggest an anterior shoulder dislocation. Wasting in the supraspinous fossa commonly suggests a tear of the supraspinatus tendon and occasionally a palsy of the suprascapular nerve.

Prominence of the sternoclavicular or acromioclavicular joints occurs as a result of subluxation or dislocation after degeneration or trauma. Swelling that starts in the interval between the tip of the acromion and the humeral head is associated with calcific tendonitis or subacromial bursitis. Winging of the scapula is present if there is a palsy of the nerve to serratus anterior or the accessory nerve, and there may be deformity due to congenital anomalies (see Figure 33.1).

## PALPATION

Palpation should be systematic. Start medially with the sternoclavicular joint, and then pass laterally along the subcutaneous border of the clavicle and along the acromiclavicular joint.

The coracoid process is palpable inferior to the clavicle in the deltopectoral groove (**Figure 11.1**). Any tenderness or crepitus should be noted as this may be associated with a fracture, dislocation, osteoarthritis or non-union of a bone.

Tenderness in the area immediately lateral to the acromion may reveal supraspinatus tendonitis. Crepitus due to a supraspinatus tear can be palpated here, although crepitus from osteoarthritis of the glenohumeral joint will also be palpable. The joint is palpable anteriorly and posteriorly, through the deltoid, and the greater tuberosity is palpable laterally. The axillary artery and medial border of the neck and head of the humerus are palpable in the axilla. In addition, tenderness in the area of the bicipital groove may point towards biceps tendonitis.

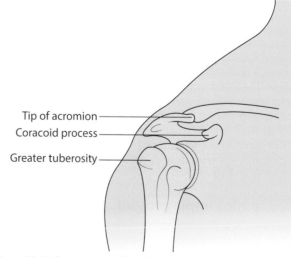

Tip of acromion

Coracoid process

Greater tuberosity

**Figure 11.1** The anatomy of the shoulder region.

## TESTING MOVEMENT

The range of motion of the shoulder can be most accurately assessed by examining the patient from behind as it is then possible to distinguish scapulothoracic from glenohumeral motion.

The active range of motion should be assessed first. If any limitation of active movement is noted, it is essential to evaluate the passive range of motion. The usual range of motion at the shoulder is as follows:

- *Adduction* (50°): This normally allows the elbow to be brought to the midline.
- *External rotation* (70°): This is best compared by testing both sides simultaneously. The range increases when the arm is abducted to 90°.
- *Internal rotation* (70°): This is traditionally described in terms of the vertebral level reached by the thumb behind the patient's back, but this test also requires the presence of a certain amount of extension.
- *Forward flexion* (160°): Forward and lateral elevation are functional terms and refer to forward flexion and abduction, respectively, with the hand outstretched.
- *Abduction* (180°): The scapula contributes 90° of rotation at the shoulder. In order to discern pure glenohumeral movement, the examiner must fix the scapula by placing a hand firmly on the superior border or holding the inferior angle (**Figure 11.2**).

## THE SCAPULOHUMERAL RHYTHM

The majority of movement from 0° to 90° occurs at the glenohumeral joint, and subsequent abduction occurs mainly as a result of scapular rotation. Reverse glenohumeral rhythm, that is, scapular rotation occurring early in abduction, is suggestive of a rotator cuff tear. Pain occurring in the midpart of the range of abduction, the painful arc, is suggestive of supraspinatus tendonitis.

## THE ROTATOR CUFF

The rotator cuff comprises the supraspinatus, infraspinatus, subscapularis and teres minor muscles.

Pathology of the rotator cuff accounts for the majority of shoulder pain. The aetiology of the lesions involved may be different, but a common cycle of pathological processes occurs.

Most problems arise at the supraspinatus. The muscle arises in the supraspinous fossa, passes laterally below the acromion and forms a tendon that inserts into the greater tuberosity of the humerus. The region of the tendon proximal to the insertion is a vascular watershed and is relatively hypovascular, causing it to be at risk of inflammation and tears.

Subacromial impingement or supraspinatus tendonitis can result in a tear of the tendon, and conversely a tear can result in impingement or tendonitis. A systematic examination usually establishes the diagnosis.

## Subacromial Impingement

Impingement is pain resulting from pressure on the supraspinatus tendon as it passes through the outlet between the acromion and the humerus. The pain is aggravated by forward elevation when the tendon is pushed up against the acromion.

The resulting inflammation of the tendon is known as supraspinatus tendonitis.

Primary or outlet impingement is due to a narrow subacromial outlet. This is the result of an abnormal shape or slope of the acromial process, prominence of the underside of the acromioclavicular joint or an anterior acromial spur.

Secondary or non-outlet impingement is due to traumatic or degenerative rupture of an abnormal supraspinatus tendon.

The clinical features of impingement and tendonitis include pain and a painful arc of movement. A number of manoeuvres produce pain and are useful in the diagnosis:

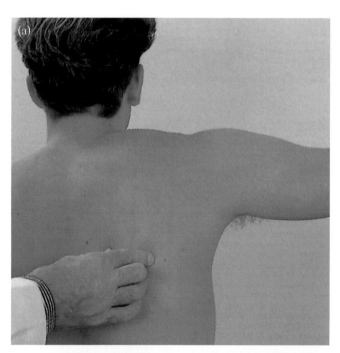

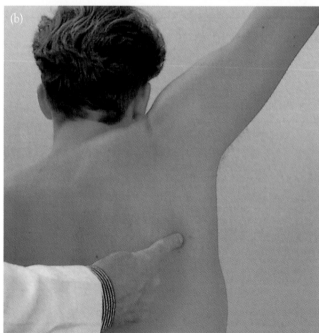

Figure 11.2 Scapular involvement in shoulder abduction. (a) Abduction to 90° with the scapula restrained. (b) Scapular rotation in full abduction.

- *Neer's impingement test*: The scapula is stabilized and the arm is fully pronated (**Figure 11.3**). On forced flexion of the humerus, an increase in pain gives a positive test result.
- *Distraction test*: A decrease in the painful arc is seen with traction of the limb away from the axilla.
- *Injection test*: There is a temporary relief of the pain when local anaesthetic is injected into the subacromial space.
- *Hawkin's test*: This also detects rotator cuff impingement. First, the scapula is stabilized. Next, the shoulder is passively abducted to 90° degrees and flexed to 30° before flexing the elbow to 90°. Pain on internal rotation of the shoulder is a positive result.

## Supraspinatus Tear

A tear of the supraspinatus tendon results from fatty degeneration with age, with attrition from prolonged primary impingement or from trauma. There are two types of tears:

- An **incomplete tear** occurs on the deep or superficial surface, or is intratendinous, but there is no communication between the joint and the subacromial bursa. The tear causes inflammation and gives rise to the signs of secondary impingement.
- A **complete tear** is, in effect, a hole in the tendon, allowing a communication between the joint and the subacromial space. It prevents the muscle from acting.

A positive result on the *drop arm test* suggests a complete tear. With the elbow flexed, the arm is passively abducted to 90° and externally rotated. The patient is asked to keep the arm in this position. The arm drops a little if a tear is present.

## Acute Calcific Tendonitis

Deposits of hydroxyapatite (a crystalline calcium phosphate) in the tendons of the rotator cuff cause pain and inflammation that potentially leads to a frozen shoulder. The diagnosis is confirmed by plain radiographs, which show flecks of calcium (**Figure 11.4**).

### FROZEN SHOULDER (ADHESIVE CAPSULITIS)

The symptoms of frozen shoulder are pain and stiffness in the shoulder joint. The signs and symptoms typically begin gradually, worsen over time and then resolve spontaneously, although this may take up to 2 years. The condition is usually seen in middle-aged and elderly individuals, and is preceded by minor trauma. Frozen shoulder is a diagnosis of exclusion.

### FRACTURES OF THE SHOULDER GIRDLE

Fractures of the clavicle (**Figure 11.5**) are common. The mechanism of injury is usually a fall on an outstretched hand, and the fracture usually occurs in the midshaft. A total 95 per cent of birth fractures involve the clavicle and are associated with breech deliveries.

With midshaft fractures, the medial cord and ulnar nerve, for instance, might be at a slightly increased risk than with other fractures. Distal clavicular fractures may have a higher incidence of non-union or delayed union, but most of these fractures are asymptomatic and only a small number will be severe enough to

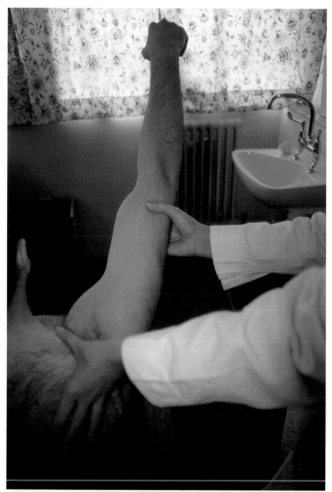

Figure 11.3 Neer's impingement sign. The examiner's left hand is holding the scapula, while the right is flexing and adducting the humerus.

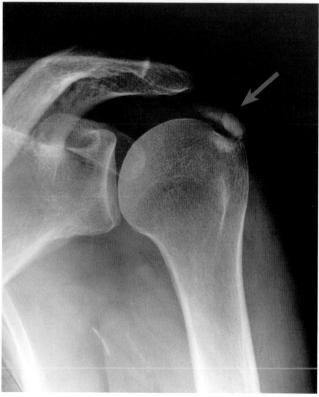

Figure 11.4 Calcification of the supraspinatus tendon.

PART 2 | TRAUMA AND (ELECTIVE) ORTHOPAEDICS

require surgery. Fractures of either end may be accompanied by a dislocation of the joint, with impaction of the fracture.

The rare posterior dislocation of the head of the clavicle can impinge on the great vessels and the trachea in the root of the neck. The patient may be in considerable distress from dyspnoea and cyanosis, and urgent reduction is necessary.

Dislocation of the acromioclavicular joint (**Figure 11.6**) is accompanied by a tear of the coracoclavicular ligaments.

Fractures of the scapular body are usually caused by high-energy trauma and are often associated with injuries to the chest.

A fracture of the neck of the scapula may follow a blow or a fall on the shoulder.

Fractures of the proximal humerus are more common in the older population after a fall (**Figure 11.7**). Sometimes there is no significant displacement of the bone fragments. In other cases, the fracture fragments may be more severely displaced or angulated. Non-displaced fractures can be immobilized. Recovery may require physical therapy to improve motion and strength. Surgery may be the best treatment option for fractures with a significant bone displacement or incongruity of the articular surface.

Fractures of the shaft of the humerus (**Figure 11.8**) may be further complicated by injury to the radial nerve as it lies in contact with the bone in the spiral groove; this may produce a wrist drop.

## SHOULDER INSTABILITY

Patients with shoulder instability complain of the uncomfortable sensation that their shoulder is loose and about to shift out of place. This is known as apprehension. If the joint partially slides out, this is called subluxation. When the joint is completely out of place, this is termed dislocation.

### Acute Anterior Instability

The shoulder is the most commonly dislocated large joint seen in emergency rooms. Acute anterior dislocation (**Figure 11.9**) constitutes over 90 per cent of shoulder dislocations and usually results from forceful injury. Shoulder dislocations can be complicated by a supraspinatus tear or a fracture of the surgical neck or greater tuberosity of the humerus.

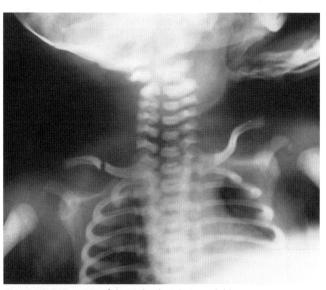

Figure 11.5 Fracture of the right clavicle in a child.

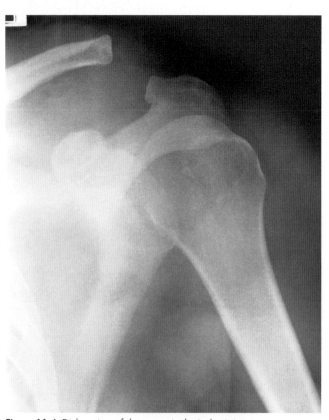

Figure 11.6 Dislocation of the acromioclavicular joint.

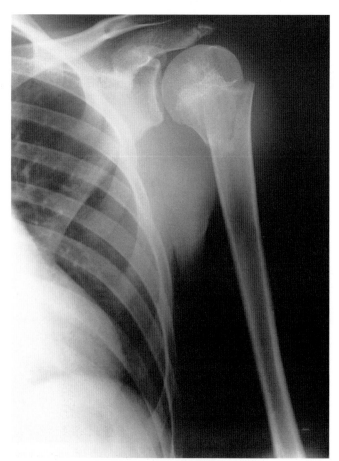

Figure 11.7 Fracture of the neck of the humerus.

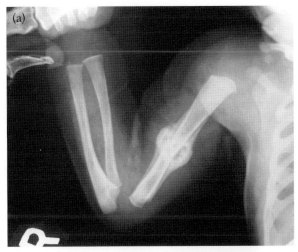

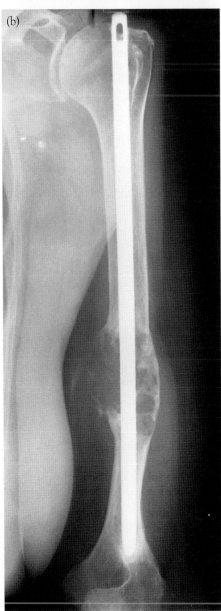

Figure 11.8 Fractures of the shaft of the humerus. (a) A healing birth fracture. (b) A nailed pathological fracture.

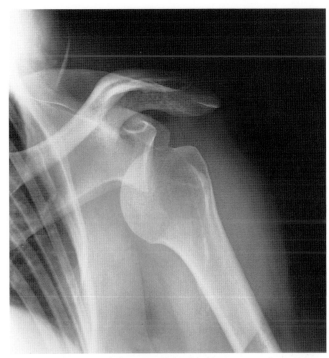

Figure 11.9 Anterior dislocation of the shoulder joint.

There is virtually no movement in acute dislocations, although a surprising range of movement develops over time if the diagnosis is missed. The patient holds the affected arm across the abdomen, supporting it with the good arm. The deltoid contour is lost, and there is almost a right angle at the tip of the acromion; local muscle spasm is present. The head of the humerus is palpable under the lateral aspect of the pectoralis major muscle.

A full neurovascular examination of the upper extremity is warranted. The axillary nerve may be at risk and can be evaluated by testing for sensation in the lateral upper arm.

## Chronic Anterior Instability

After a first dislocation, the shoulder is vulnerable to repeat episodes, leading to shoulder instability. A **Bankart lesion** is an anterior inferior glenoid labral tear associated with chronic anterior instability. In atraumatic instability, the problem is laxity of the capsule.

Patients with recurrent dislocation (**Figure 11.10**) are usually asymptomatic until an incident provokes a painful dislocation. The degree of provocation required declines as the number of episodes increases because the stabilizing mechanisms of the shoulder become more incompetent.

Patients with recurrent subluxation (**Figure 11.11**) have never suffered a dislocation but present either with pain on carrying out heavy or rapid overhead activities or with 'dead arm syndrome'. This is characterized by pain, often of a sudden sharp paralysing nature, clicking, grinding and a heavy feeling. The patient may describe a feeling that the shoulder slips out of place.

Patients with recurrent dislocation and subluxation suffer symptoms of both occasional dislocation and subluxation.

In recurrent atraumatic anterior involuntary instability, the history differs from traumatic instability in that normal physical activities provoke the symptoms of instability. The physical signs are identical.

PART 2 | TRAUMA AND (ELECTIVE) ORTHOPAEDICS

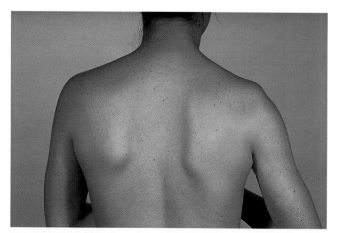

Figure 11.10 Subluxation of the right shoulder with muscle wasting. Note the loss of contour of the deltoid muscle, due to displacement of the underlying head of the humerus, compared with the opposite side.

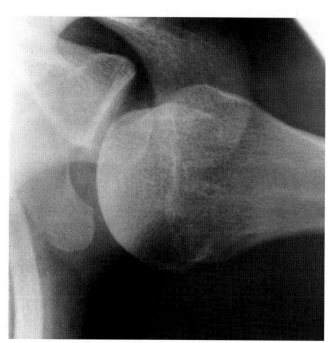

Figure 11.11 Subluxation of the humeral head.

## Posterior Instability

Acute posterior dislocations are uncommon and often related to specific injuries such as lightning strikes, electrical injuries and seizures. This type of dislocation occasionally occurs with minimal injury in the elderly, and often the diagnosis is missed the first time the patient presents for evaluation of the shoulder pain. Characteristically, there is significant loss of passive external rotation of the shoulder. A radiograph shows that the humeral head is forced into internal rotation, giving appearance of a 'light-bulb'.

A missed posterior dislocation is subject to chronic dislocation. Recurrent instability tends to result from subluxation rather than dislocation; there is pain on forward flexion, adduction and internal rotation.

## Multidirectional Instability

Multidirectional instability is present in a minority of patients and is often bilateral. The pathology in these patients is essentially a lax inferior axillary capsular pouch. While the cause may have been traumatic and repetitive overuse, recurrences usually occur without trauma.

Patients with generalized laxity, such as those with Ehlers–Danlos syndrome, provide a good example of multidirectional instability. These patients also have the ability to bend their thumb back to touch their forearm and the ability to hyperextend their knees, elbows and fingers.

## Assessment of Instability

### Apprehension and Jobe's Relocation Test

With the patient supine, the shoulder is abducted to 90° and the arm externally rotated to place stress on the glenohumeral joint. If the patient feels apprehensive that the arm may dislocate anteriorly, this is a positive apprehension test. Jobe's relocation test (Figure 11.12) is then performed, using the examiner's hand to place a posteriorly directed force on the glenohumeral joint. An absence of apprehension that there might be a dislocation, or an increase in external rotation, is a positive test result and suggests anterior glenohumeral instability.

### Anterior Drawer Test

In this test, the scapula is stabilized with one hand while the other hand grasps the humeral head from in front and behind (Figure 11.13). The humeral head is pushed anteriorly, and the extent of translation can then be seen and felt, and compared with that the other side. Increased laxity is suggestive of anterior instability.

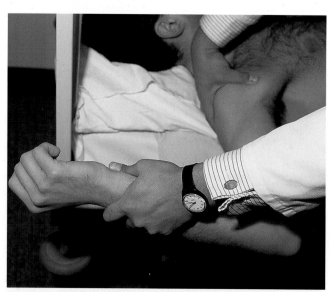

Figure 11.12 Jobe's relocation test. The examiner's right hand is displacing the head of the humerus posteriorly.

## The Sulcus Sign

With the patient's arm in a neutral position, the examiner applies downward traction to the arm while observing the shoulder area for a sulcus or depression lateral or inferior to the acromion (**Figure 11.14**). The presence of a depression indicates inferior translation of the humerus and suggests inferior or multidirectional glenohumeral instability. It is associated with multidirectional instability.

## Load and Shift Test

This tests for anterior and posterior glenohumeral stability. An axial load is placed on the humerus, compressing the glenohumeral joint. The examiner then shifts the humeral head anteriorly and posteriorly. Anterior or posterior displacement is positive for instability. Grade 1 instability involves movement of the humeral head to the rim of the glenoid. Grade 2 instability involves movement of the head over the rim of the glenoid. If it is associated with a sulcus sign, a positive result on the load and shift test may suggest multidirectional instability.

## OSTEOARTHRITIS

Osteoarthritis is a progressive, mechanical and biochemical degeneration of the bone, articular cartilage, capsule and other joint tissues. Risk factors include age, sex, obesity, joint infection, genetic predisposition and previous trauma.

## RHEUMATOID ARTHRITIS

This is a painful erosive arthropathy with deformity and loss of movement. The sternoclavicular joint, that is, the scapulothoracic union, is unaffected, and some patients maintain useful shoulder function even when the glenohumeral joint has been destroyed.

## CONGENITAL ANOMALIES

Interruption in the normal caudad migration of the scapula between the 9th and 12th week of gestation leads to cosmetic and functional impairment. As a result, development of the bone, cartilage and muscle is abnormal. Congenital anomalies of the shoulder girdle include the absence of muscle, Sprengel's deformity and partial or complete absence of the clavicles (**Figure 11.15**). In the latter, there may also be defective ossification of the skull, other bones and teeth – **craniocleidodysostosis**. The abnormal mobility of the pectoral girdle may enable the clavicles to meet in the midline.

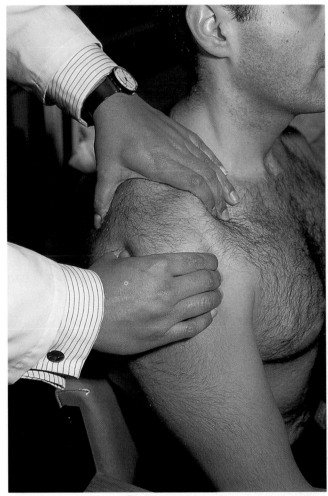

Figure 11.13 Anterior drawer test. The examiner's left hand is fixing the scapula, and the right hand is displacing the head of the humerus anteriorly.

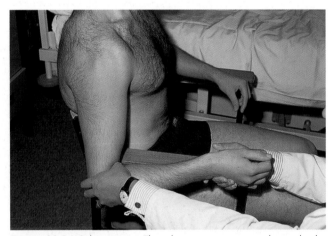

Figure 11.14 Sulcus sign. The depression appears beneath the acromion.

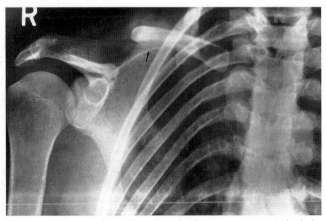

Figure 11.15 Incomplete clavicular development in craniocleidodysostosis.

## Key Points

- The shoulder examination in summarised by 'look, feel and move'.
- The majority of movement from 0° to 90° occurs at the glenohumeral joint, subsequent abduction occurring mainly as a result of scapular rotation.
- Impingement syndrome is pain resulting from pressure on the supraspinatus tendon as it passes through the outlet between the acromion and the humeral head.
- In rotator cuff tears, the supraspinatus is the tendon most commonly implicated, and massive rotator cuff tears can present with a positive drop arm test.
- Calcium deposits in the rotator cuff muscle that are seen on X-ray reflect an inflammatory process that may result in a frozen shoulder.
- Clavicular fractures are common, and the vast majority can be treated conservatively by immobilization in a sling. Humeral fractures can potentially be complicated by axillary nerve injury at the humeral neck or radial nerve injury on the shaft of the humerus.
- Anterior shoulder dislocations are by far the most common dislocations. Posterior shoulder dislocations require a high index of suspicion and tend to be missed on first presentation.
- After a first dislocation, the shoulder is vulnerable to repeat episodes, leading to shoulder instability.

## SBAs

**1.** Which one of the following statements about the clavicle is **incorrect**:

  **a** Most birth fractures involve the clavicle

  **b** Most clavicular fractures occur in the proximal third of the bone

  **c** Birth fractures of the clavicle heal rapidly

  **d** Brachial plexus injuries, vascular injuries and pneumothorax are potential complications

  **e** Clavicular fractures are often caused by a direct blow to the shoulder

**Answer**

**b** *Most clavicular fractures occur in the proximal third of the bone.* The most common clavicular fractures are those of the middle third. The least common are those of the proximal third (sternal side).

**2.** Posterior shoulder dislocation is associated with:

  **a** High-energy trauma

  **b** Lightening strikes

  **c** Seizures

  **d** A 'light-bulb sign' on X-ray

  **e** All of the above

**Answer**

**e** *All of the above.* Posterior shoulder dislocation is associated with high-energy trauma, lightening strikes, seizures and a characteristic 'light-bulb sign' on X-ray.

**3.** Which statement about the supraspinatus muscle is **incorrect**:

  **a** Its origin is the supraspinous fossa

  **b** Its insertion is the superior facet of the greater tuberosity

  **c** It is innervated by the axillary nerve

  **d** It is the most commonly involved tendon in rotator cuff tears.

  **e** Its function is to initiate abduction of the shoulder

**Answer**

**c** *It is innervated by the axillary nerve.* The supraspinatus muscle is supplied by the suprascapular nerve (C5 and C6), which arises from the superior trunk of the brachial plexus.

## EMQs

**1.** For each of the following conditions, select the most likely finding from the list below. Each option may be used once, more than once, or not at all:

  **1** A sulcus sign and positive load shift test

  **2** A positive Hawkin's test

  **3** Electrocution

  **4** Wrist drop

  **5** Multiple joint laxity

  **a** Posterior shoulder dislocation

  **b** Ehlers–Danlos syndrome

  **c** Impingement syndrome

  **d** Multidirectional shoulder instability

  **e** Fracture of the humeral shaft

**Answers**

**a 3** *Electrocution.* Posterior shoulder dislocation is uncommon and often related to specific injuries such as lightning strikes, electrical injuries and seizures. This type of dislocation can occasionally occur with minimal injury in the elderly, and the diagnosis may be missed the first time the patient presents for evaluation of the shoulder pain.

**b 5** *Multiple joint laxity.* Ehlers–Danlos syndrome is a heterogenous group of inherited connective tissue disorders marked by multiple joint laxity, skin extensibility and tissue fragility.

**c 2** *A positive Hawkin's test.* Impingement syndrome of the shoulder is mechanical irritation of the rotator cuff tendon underneath the anteroinferior portion of the acromion, especially when the shoulder is placed in the abducted, forward flexed and internally rotated position. This can be well demonstrated with the Neer's or Hawkin's test.

**d  1  A sulcus sign and positive load shift test.** *Multidirectional shoulder instability is excessive range of motion of the glenohumeral joint in all directions – anterior, posterior and inferior. An anteroinferior or posteroinferior predominance is typically present. Commonly, this is an atraumatic condition affecting both shoulders. The sulcus sign demonstrates the inferior instability, while the load shift test reveals anterior and/or posterior instability.*

**e  4  Wrist drop.** *Humeral shaft fractures are associated with radial nerve palsy in up to 18 per cent of cases. The nerve is especially at risk at the junction of middle and distal thirds of the humeral shaft where is emerges from the spiral groove. Injury to the nerve results in weakness of the wrist extensor muscles, resulting in wrist drop.*

2. **For each of the following conditions, select the most likely association from the list below. Each option may be used once, more than once, or not at all:**
   1  Radial nerve palsy
   2  Axillary nerve palsy
   3  Suprascapular nerve palsy
   4  Long thoracic nerve palsy
   5  Ulnar nerve palsy
   a  Humeral surgical neck fracture
   b  Mid-clavicular fracture
   c  Humerus shaft fracture
   d  Atrophy in the supraspinatus fossa
   e  Medial winging of the scapula

**Answers**

**a  2  Axillary nerve palsy.** *Humeral surgical neck fractures risk injury to the axillary nerve. The nerve winds around the surgical neck of the humerus approximately 7 cm distal to the tip of the acromion. Loss of sensation over the shoulder area and/or or loss of arm abduction is a potential complication resulting from denervation of the deltoid muscle.*

**b  5  Ulnar nerve palsy.** *Mid-clavicular fractures are common and usually heal with no functional deficit. On rare occasions, medial cord injury and ulnar nerve palsy, for instance, can occur.*

**c  1  Radial nerve palsy.** *Fractures of the humeral shaft, especially at the junction of the middle and distal thirds of the humerus, endanger the radial nerve as it emerges from its spiral groove.*

**d  3  Suprascapular nerve palsy.** *Atrophy in the supraspinatus fossa can be appreciated by seeing and palpating a depression over the fossa of the scapula when examining the upper back. It can result from overtension of the nerve secondary to a torn and retracted rotator cuff tendon. It can also result from direct compression of the nerve by a cyst or a soft tissue or bone tumour at specific locations along the nerve's course, such as at the suprascapular and spinoglenoid notches.*

**e  4  Long thoracic nerve palsy.** *Medial winging of the scapula presents with shoulder and scapular pain, weakness when lifting objects and discomfort when sitting on a chair. It is more commonly seen in young athletes due to long thoracic nerve injury from repetitive stretch or chest compression injuries during sports. Iatrogenic injury to the nerve during breast surgery is also possible. The serratus anterior muscle is then denervated and the scapula elevates off the chest wall and migrates medially.*

# The Arm

Muhyeddine Al-Taki and Firas Kawtharani

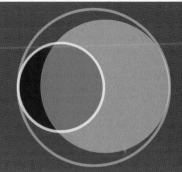

## LEARNING OBJECTIVES

- To be familiar with the anatomy of the elbow and wrist joint
- To think systematically when facing a patient with an upper extremity problem
- To be able to identify the different musculotendinous pathologies affecting the elbow and wrist, for example tennis elbow and de Quervain's tenosynovitis
- To recognize the various fractures of the elbow and wrist, such as Monteggia's and Colles' fractures

- To identify pathologies of a degenerative nature as well as various compression neuropathies of the upper extremity
- To master the different physical examination tests and manoeuvres for the upper extremity that will help lead to the correct diagnosis

## THE ELBOW JOINT

The important landmarks of this joint are easily palpable. The tip of the olecranon and the medial and lateral epicondyles form an equilateral triangle when the elbow is flexed. When the joint is extended, they are positioned in line. This relationship is preserved in supracondylar fractures but lost in dislocations. Effusions are seen as a bulge emphasizing the concavity between the olecranon and the lateral epicondyle. The triangular sulcus is a landmark for access to the elbow joint as it lies between these two structures and the radial head.

The 'carrying angle' is the physiological angulation of the forearm away from the midline when the arm is straight; this is 10° in males and 20° in females. An increased angulation is known as cubitus valgus, and decreased angulation as cubitus varus, a common deformity in the malunion of supracondylar fractures. Flexion and extension occur at the elbow joint, the range of motion being 0–150° degrees. Supination and pronation take place as the radial head rotates, the range of motion being 80°. The radial head, and its rotatory movement, is palpable 1 cm distal to the lateral epicondyle.

### Tennis Elbow (Lateral Epicondylitis)

This is a common overuse condition, often provoked by heavy repetitive physical activity involving rotation at the elbow. The site of the pain is the common extensor origin at the lateral epicondyle.

There is pain along the lateral border of the elbow, which radiates proximally and distally. The origin of the extensor carpi radialis brevis just distal to the lateral epicondyle is tender (**Figure 12.1**).

In **Cozens' test**, ask the patient to clench their fist, keep it clenched and then extend the wrist. Grasp the lower forearm in the left hand and, while the patient continues to try to keep the

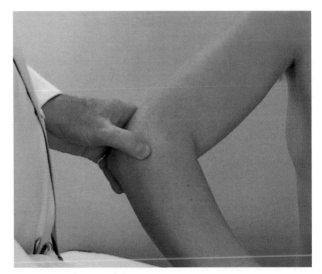

Figure 12.1 Palpation of the common extensor origin.

wrist extended, flex the wrist firmly and steadily. This reproduces the characteristic pain.

In **Mills' manoeuvre**, with the elbow quite straight and the wrist flexed, pronation of the forearm brings on the pain.

### Radial Tunnel Syndrome

This condition causes lateral elbow and radial forearm pain. The problem is produced by radial nerve compression as it passes through the radial tunnel. The maximal point of tenderness is 2–3 cm anterior and distal to the lateral epicondyle. The pain can be provoked by extension of the middle finger against resistance and by supination of the forearm against resistance. There is no motor or sensory loss.

### Golfer's Elbow (Medial Epicondylitis)

This is much less common than tennis elbow. There is pain, aggravated by throwing, and tenderness located at the medial epicondyle at the common flexor origin. Resisted forearm pronation and wrist flexion reproduces the pain.

### Cubital Tunnel Syndrome (Ulnar Nerve Compression)

The ulnar nerve passes in the groove posterior to the medial epicondyle (**Figure 12.2**), with an overlying retinaculum forming the cubital tunnel. The retinaculum, also known as Osborne's ligament, can entrap the nerve. In the vicinity of this landmark are other potential compression sites including the medial intermuscular septum proximally and the flexor carpi ulnaris aponeurosis distally. Cubitus valgus or varus deformities, burns and occupational or athletic overuse also predispose to developing this condition.

Paraesthesias may pass distally along the ulnar one and a half digits. There may be wasting of the muscles of the hypothenar eminence, as well as of the intrinsic muscles of the hand.

Palpation of the nerve in its groove causes pain, and there is a positive Tinel's sign (see p. 232). There is decreased sensation in the ulnar nerve distribution. Clawing of the ulnar digits is a late finding.

### Arthritis of the Elbow Joint

#### Osteoarthritis

Osteoarthritis is manifest by pain, swelling and a loss of range of motion. Occasionally, there are severe degenerative changes including osteophytes, subchondral cysts and intra-articular loose bodies that lead to the symptoms of intermittent locking. Bony changes may be considerable in individuals who move the elbow in repetitive throwing movements, when the sensation to the joint is reduced (Charcot's joint) and in syphilis (Clutton's joint).

#### Rheumatoid Arthritis/Tuberculosis

Rheumatoid arthritis is not uncommon in the elbow, with pain due to intra-articular manifestation, ranging from synovial hypertrophy to soft tissue involvement such as adjacent rheumatoid nodules and periarticular tendon ruptures. The muscle wasting associated with **tuberculous infection** and joint swelling produces a fusiform configuration across the elbow joint.

### Rupture of the Biceps

The biceps is subject to rupture of its muscle belly at both the proximal and distal attachment. Rupture of the belly is usually

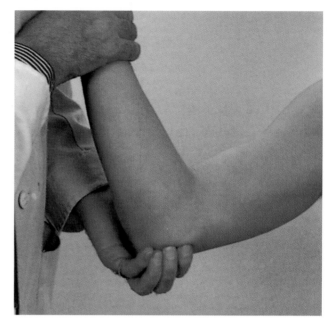

Figure 12.2 Palpation of the ulnar nerve behind the medial epicondyle of the humerus.

painful and dramatic, and caused by heavy lifting, producing two midarm bulges separated by a gap.

Rupture of the long head of biceps occurs in the elderly and is due to attrition of the tendon as it passes through the bicipital groove. The rupture may be spontaneous or caused by minor trauma, and the symptoms mild. The signs are more obvious, a bulge being present in the lower third of the arm, on flexion of the elbow against resistance (**Figure 12.3**). There is a moderate loss of supination power. Rupture of the radial attachment of the biceps follows forced flexion. There is marked pain and bruising of the cubital fossa.

### Biceps and Triceps Tendinitis

Bicipital tendinitis causes pain, either proximally along the bicipital groove in the upper arm or distally at the insertion of the tendon over the antecubital fossa. **Yergason's sign** is positive when the elbow is flexed to 90° and the patient tries to supinate the forearm against resistance.

Tricipital tendinitis causes posterior elbow pain and tenderness at the triceps insertion. Extension of the elbow against resistance exacerbates the pain.

### Valgus Extension Overload (Pitcher's Elbow)

This condition is caused by overuse of the elbow in recurrent throwing or repetitive overhead activities, such as pitching in baseball or javelin throwing. The syndrome has a number of components:

- *Ulnar collateral ligament injuries*: Valgus stresses can cause a partial or complete rupture There is medial elbow pain and tenderness, just distal to the medial epicondyle. If a valgus stress is applied with the elbow in 30° of flexion, there is increased laxity and provocation of the pain. Valgus instability is a dynamic process; the moving valgus stress test of **O'Driscoll** is highly sensitive and specific in detecting the injury.

- *Medial epicondylar apophysitis*: In young people with open epiphyses, there can be pain during sporting activities with tenderness over the medial epicondyle.
- The lax ulnar collateral ligament allows the transmission of excessive compressive forces into the radiohumeral joint, and results in damage to the articular surfaces of the radius and capitellum. This repetitive microtrauma leads to osteochondritis dissecans and even the appearance of osteochondral loose bodies, resulting in locking and crepitus.
- *Posterior olecranon impingement*: Repetitive forceful extension with valgus stress results in impingement of the posteromedial aspect of the olecranon against the medial aspect of the olecranon fossa. This extension overload may lead to the development of osteophytes, chondromalacia and loose bodies. There is posterior pain, tenderness over the olecranon, loss of extension, and pain when the examiner passively extends the elbow with a valgus force.
- *Olecranon bursitis* (**Figure 12.4**): Inflammation of the olecranon bursa as a result of repeated trauma results in a painless swelling. Infection results in a painful olecranon bursitis; this is also referred to as student's or miner's elbow.

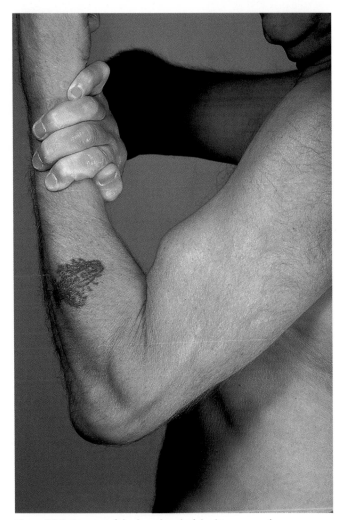

Figure 12.3 Rupture of the long head of the biceps muscle.

## Acute Injuries
### Supracondylar Fractures

Supracondylar fractures (**Figure 12.5**) are a common injury in children and adolescents, resulting from falling on an outstretched hand. The distal fragment of the humerus is usually displaced posteriorly and tilted dorsally (an extension-type injury). The relationship of the bony landmarks of the elbow is maintained.

The presence of the radial pulse must be ascertained because the brachial artery is easily compromised at this site, with the risk of a Volkmann's contracture if it is not corrected. Pain on passive stretch of the fingers is an important red flag for compartment syndrome. Less commonly, the median, radial or ulnar nerve is affected, and these usually undergo a gradual recovery. Malunion is common and may present with an elbow in a valgus, varus, extension or flexion deformity.

### Intercondylar T-shaped Fractures

These fractures constitute adult elbow fractures that are sustained through a fall on the elbow. Such fractures involve the articular surface, and, as in children, the neurovascular structures are also at risk. The relationship of the bony landmarks of the elbow is preserved.

### Fractures of the Epicondyles

Fractures of the lateral epicondyle in adults and the epiphysis in children are produced by lateral angulatory forces applied to the fully extended elbow. The same forces can avulse the medial epicondylar epiphysis in children. The lateral epicondyle is subject to delayed or non-union, and healing of the medial epicondylar epiphysis is usually by a fibrous union. Cubitus valgus or varus, degenerative joint disease and ulnar nerve injury are potential complications of these injuries.

### Fractures of the Olecranon

Fractures of the olecranon can range from simple avulsion to a comminuted fracture-dislocation. There is swelling and tenderness of the olecranon. In a significant fracture, the ability to extend the elbow against gravity, as a result of the action of triceps, is lost. A considerable joint effusion develops. The gap across the fracture line is usually palpable and even visible.

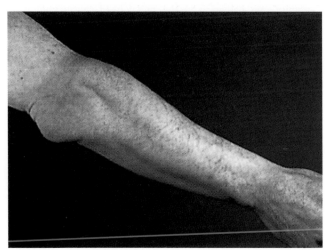

Figure 12.4 Olecranon bursitis.

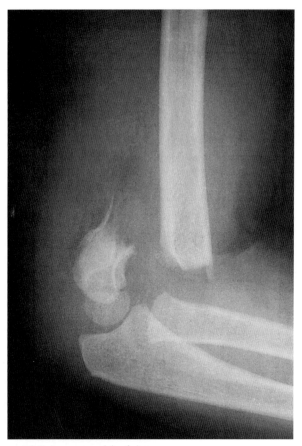

Figure 12.5 A supracondylar fracture.

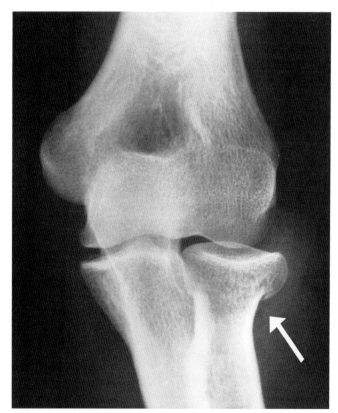

Figure 12.6 A fracture (arrow) of the head of the radius.

### Fractures of the Radial Head

Fractures of the radial head (**Figure 12.6**) follow a fall on an outstretched hand, particularly in children. An effusion is present, and the elbow is painful in flexion, extension, and mostly supination and pronation. The radial head is tender to palpation. There may be an associated impaction of the capitellum and its overlying cartilage.

A **pulled elbow** is a subluxation of the radial head through its annular ligament in a toddler, resulting from an ascending force on a stretched arm. There is an inability to range the upper extremity, and palpation of the radial head causes pain. The injury is less common in adults as the radial head conforms to the conical shape of the ligament.

### FOREARM FRACTURES

These fractures interfere with pronation and supination. They are usually accompanied by deformity and are often palpable, the posterior border of the ulna lying subcutaneously. Combined fractures of both the radius and the ulna are common in direct trauma. When the fractures are complete, there is usually an angular and translation deformity, but this is less so in the case of greenstick forearm fractures of children. It is important to remember that angular deformity in the fracture of a single bone cannot occur without an associated dislocation at one end or the other. A displaced ulnar fracture is accompanied by dislocation of the head of the radius – a Monteggia fracture-dislocation.

Isolated fractures of the **shaft of the radius** are less common than those of the ulna. Displacement is accompanied by dislocation of the distal radioulnar joint – a Galeazzi fracture-dislocation.

### Dislocation

Dislocation (**Figure 12.7**) involves mostly posterolateral displacement of the olecranon. The relationship between the bony landmarks of the elbow is lost. The injury may be complicated by fractures of the medial epicondyle, coronoid process or radial head. Other complications include median and ulnar nerve injury, brachial artery injury, flexion contracture and myositis ossificans.

### Myositis Ossificans

This condition is also known as heterotopic ossification. This is an uncommon complication of fractures (see p. 151) but is characteristically associated with elbow injuries.

### THE WRIST

### Anatomy of the Wrist

In the anatomical position, the radial and ulnar styloid processes are palpable on the sides of the wrist joint, the tip of the radial styloid being 1 cm distal to that of the ulna in most people (**Figure 12.8a**). This relationship may change with fractures of the lower end of the radius. On pronation, the lower end of the radius rotates around the anterior surface of the head of the ulna, which becomes palpable (**Figure 12.8b**).

On flexion of the wrist against resistance, the flexor carpi radialis and ulnaris tendons stand out on either side of the anterior surface of the wrist. They are attached to the second metacarpal head and pisiform bones, respectively. Upon opposition of

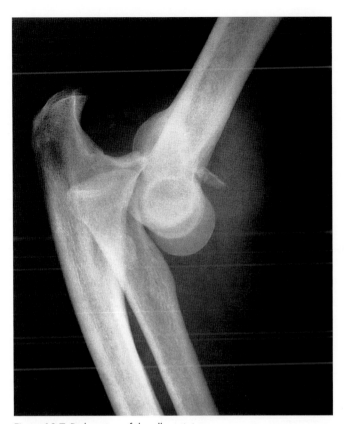

Figure 12.7 Dislocation of the elbow joint.

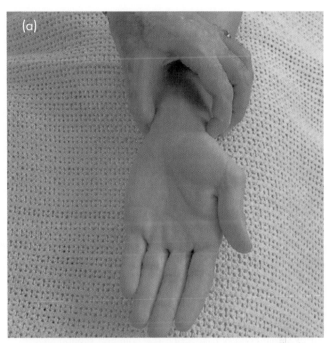

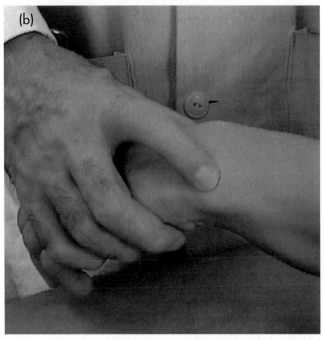

Figure 12.8 (a) The relative positions of the radial and ulnar styloid processes. (b) The head of the ulna.

thumb and little finger in flexion, the palmaris longus tendon may stand out between the carpal flexors as it passes into the flexor retinaculum. If it is absent, the median nerve becomes palpable.

Extension of the thumb demonstrates the tendons bordering the anatomical snuffbox. The abductor pollicis longus and extensor pollicis brevis lie radially, and the extensor pollicis longus ulnarly. Within the snuffbox, the radial styloid and scaphoid bone are palpable on either side of the wrist joint. The radial artery passes across the floor and the cephalic vein across the roof of the snuffbox.

In young adults, the normal range of movement between full extension and full flexion is 150°, but as age increases, this range becomes slightly less. Although it is customary to attribute these movements to the wrist joint, they cannot be dissociated from movements at the midcarpal and intercarpal joints. These joints are also involved in radial and ulnar deviation, the sum of these movements being 60°.

## Soft Tissue Lesions of the Wrist

**Carpal tunnel syndrome (Figure 12.9)** denotes a compression neuropathy of the median nerve as it passes beneath the flexor retinaculum. This can be acute, associated with a fracture, chronic due to a systemic disease, such as diabetes or renal failure, or merely occupational from overuse. It is prevalent in elderly women. It may be bilateral but mostly affects the dominant hand.

The complaint is of progressive weakness and clumsiness due to an impairment of finer movements of the hand – for example, picking up a pin, sewing or knitting, which are associated with attacks of pain, tingling and numbness of the lateral three digits. Characteristically, the attacks are nocturnal. The aching or pain occasionally radiates proximally even as far as the shoulder, but sensory and motor changes are limited to the hand, the latter being the late onset of wasting of the thenar eminence and interossei muscles.

A positive result in the **wrist flexion test** – Phalen's sign – for carpal tunnel syndrome is the exacerbation of paraesthesia when the patient is asked to maintain full wrist flexion for 60 seconds. The **tourniquet test**, when the cuff is pumped to systolic pressure for 60 seconds, has a similar effect. The diagnosis is supported by abnormal median nerve conduction studies.

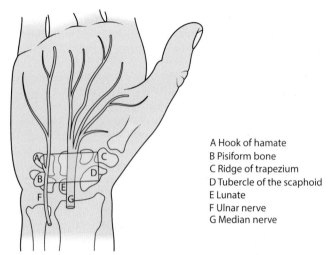

A Hook of hamate
B Pisiform bone
C Ridge of trapezium
D Tubercle of the scaphoid
E Lunate
F Ulnar nerve
G Median nerve

Figure 12.9 The carpal tunnel, demonstrating the attachments of the flexor retinaculum and its relationship to the median and ulnar nerves.

**De Quervain's disease – stenosing tenosynovitis –** is a painful disabling condition affecting the common tendon sheath of the first dorsal wrist compartment (abductor pollicis longus and extensor pollicis brevis). It is caused by inflammatory changes that may proceed to fibrosis and limitation of movement of the thumb. The condition only occurs in adults, usually women. There is always marked tenderness over the radial border of the anatomical snuffbox, and there may be associated swelling and fine crepitus. Pain is produced by ulnar deviation of the wrist and thumb (Finkelstein's test).

A **ganglion** (**Figure 12.10**) is a myxomatous degeneration of connective tissue adjacent to a joint capsule. A cyst forms, which is filled with crystal clear gelatinous fluid. The most common situation is on the dorsal aspect of the wrist over the scaphoid–lunate articulation. The swelling is rounded and sessile, becomes tense and prominent when the wrist is flexed, and may partially or wholly disappear on extension. The tensely filled cyst feels solid, but fluctuation is occasionally elicited, and if the swelling is large enough to be tested, it is translucent. Other common sites of ganglia are on the anterior aspect of the wrist, between the tendons of flexor carpi radialis and brachioradialis, along the finger and on the dorsum of the ankle and foot.

**Arthritic** changes around the wrist produce swelling, tenderness and limitation of movement. Osteoarthritis, following injury, and rheumatoid arthritis are common findings, and the joint is often affected in tuberculosis in regions where the disease is prevalent. In the latter condition, there is spindle-shaped enlargement across the joint, together with palmar flexion; abscess and sinus formation occur early because of the superficial nature of the joint surfaces.

## Ulnar Tunnel Syndrome

This is caused by compression of the ulnar nerve in Guyon's canal (a fascial compartment anterior to the flexor retinaculum), often by a ganglion cyst. The condition can result in sensorimotor involvement, such as paraesthesias in the ulnar digits or wasting of the hypothenar eminence.

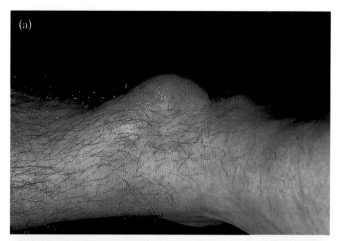

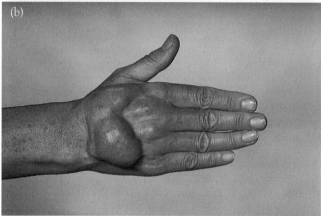

Figure 12.10 Ganglia (a) of the wrist, (b) of the dorsum of the hand.

## Kienböck's Disease

Kienböck's disease (**Figure 12.11**) is an avascular necrosis of the lunate bone that is usually diagnosed radiologically. It is often associated with a relatively shorter ulna, which is also called negative ulnar variance. The condition is attributed to repetitive microtrauma and venous congestion. There is pain and a limited range of motion in the wrist, and tenderness on the dorsum of the lunate. The grip strength may be affected in late stages.

## Fractures of the Distal Radius

A **Colles' fracture** (**Figure 12.12**), which occurs in the radial metaphysis, is produced by a fall on an outstretched hand and is a very common extra-articular fracture. There is a dorsal displacement of the distal fragment together with shortening. There might be distortion of the anatomical landmarks, such as the volar tilt, and the radial height and inclination. Clinically, there is a 'dinner-fork' deformity with local bony tenderness.

Immediate complications include median nerve compression from direct pressure on the nerve and Volkmann's ischaemic contracture. Late malunion, with dorsal tilting and shortening of the radius, may be asymptomatic or lead to pain from the radiocarpal or distal radioulnar joint, or even from instability and degeneration within the carpal bones.

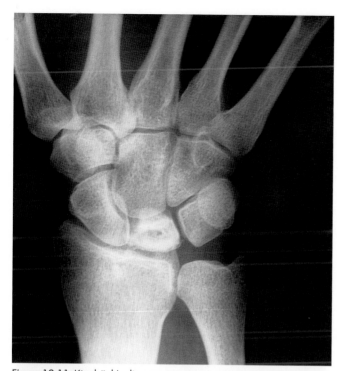

Figure 12.11 Kienböck's disease.

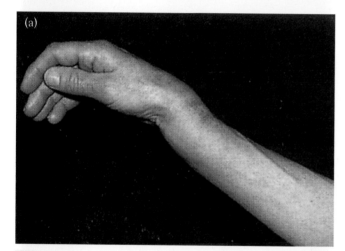

(a)

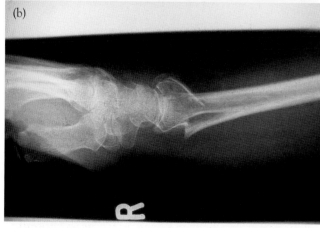

(b)

Figure 12.12 A Colles' fracture. (a) The typical 'dinner-fork' deformity. (b) Lateral view.

Late attrition rupture of the extensor pollicis longus tendon may occur as it passes over the fracture site; active extension at the thumb interphalangeal joint is lost.

**Smith's fracture (Figure 12.13)** is caused by a fall onto a flexed wrist. The distal radius is tilted and displaced in a volar direction, and the fracture line often extends into the joint. Other wrist fractures include a comminuted fracture of the distal radius (**Figure 12.14**) and displacement of the distal radial epiphysis in children (**Figure 12.15**). In the latter, the deformity is similar to that of a Colles' fracture.

**Barton's fracture** is an intra-articular fracture involving a dorsal or volar rim of the distal articular surface of the radius.

**Radial styloid fracture** – a **chauffeur's fracture** – is frequently caused by high-energy trauma to wrist in young adults. There is tenderness over the scaphoid fossa along the anatomical snuffbox.

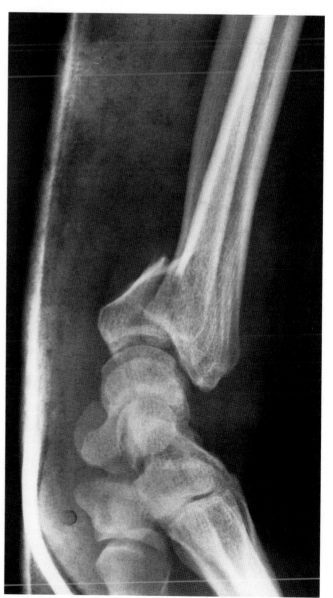

Figure 12.13 A Smith's fracture.

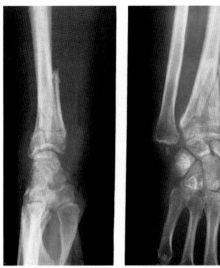

Figure 12.14 A distal comminuted fracture of the end of the radius, involving the wrist joint.

## Scaphoid Fracture

This common fracture is easily missed, resulting in serious consequences for the patient and the physician. It results from a fall onto an outstretched hand. The presentation may be immediate or delayed, with pain in the wrist and on gripping objects. Passive wrist movements may also be painful. Palpation in the anatomical snuffbox (**Figure 12.16**) is more painful than on the unaffected side. Pain may be provoked by a tractive or compressive force applied to the thumb in its long axis and on direct pressure on the tubercle of the scaphoid.

The diagnosis can be confirmed radiologically with wrist and scaphoid views. The fracture may involve the neck, waist, body or proximal pole of the scaphoid. In cases that present soon after injury, the diagnosis should be made on clinical grounds even if radiographs do not demonstrate a fracture, and the scaphoid should be immobilized with a thumb spica cast.

A chronic painful wrist may result as there is a relatively high rate of non-union and avascular necrosis of the proximal pole (**Figure 12.17**) due to the retrograde blood supply to the scaphoid.

## Carpal Dislocation

This also occurs through a fall onto an outstretched hand. There are two main categories:

- In *peridislocations*, the entire carpus and hand are dorsally dislocated, with the exception of one or more of the proximal carpal row of bones. Most commonly, it is the lunate that remains in the normal position – perilunate dislocation (**Figure 12.18**). On examination, there is gross deformity of the wrist and minimal movement present. Radiographs are confirmatory.
- In *proximal row dislocation*, the carpus and hand remain in alignment with the radius, but one or more of the proximal carpal row of bones are dislocated, most commonly the lunate – lunate dislocation. The lunate is usually displaced anteriorly and there can be direct compression of the median nerve, leading to pain and diminished sensation in its distribution. Radiographs are essential to establish the diagnosis.

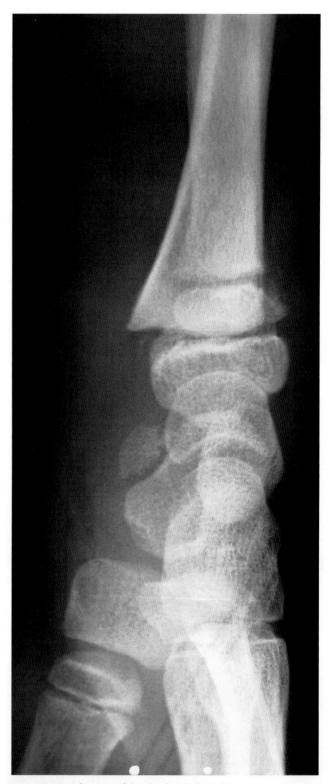

Figure 12.15 A fracture of the distal radial epiphysis.

## Carpal Instability

This is a group of conditions resulting from injury in which a loss of normal alignment of the carpal bones develops, either early or late, causing chronic pain and weakness.

The **pseudostability test** (**Figure 12.19**) is a non-specific indicator of carpal instability. The examiner firmly grasps the carpus with one hand and the distal forearm with the other, and applies an anteroposterior translation force. Reduced translation compared with the normal side is suggestive of instability. Point tenderness located over a carpal interosseous ligament is suggestive of its injury.

**Dorsal intercalated segment instability** results from a fall onto the thenar eminence of an outstretched hand, with

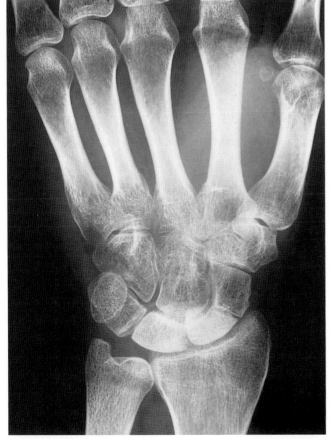

A Distal phalanx  G Abductor pollicis longus
B Proximal phalanx  H Extensor pollicis brevis
C First metacarpal  I Extensor carpi radialis longus
D Trapezium  J Extensor carpi radialis brevis
E Scaphoid  K Extensor pollicis longus
F Radius

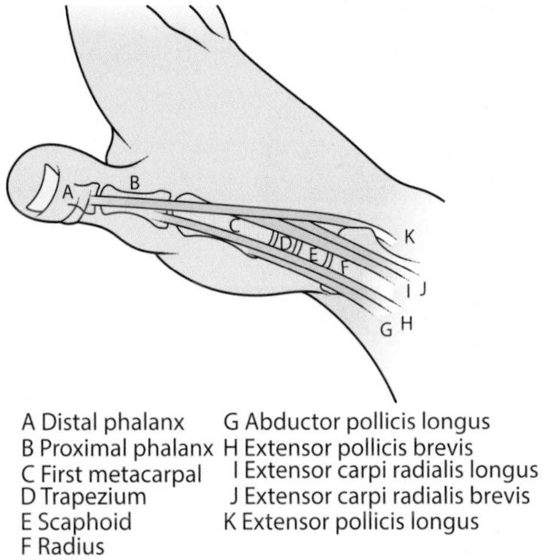

Figure 12.16 Markings of the anatomical snuffbox.

Figure 12.17 A scaphoid fracture with proximal sclerosis from avascular necrosis.

disruption of the scapholunate ligaments possibly associated with a scaphoid fracture. In the **Watson test**, the examiner presses firmly on the tubercle of the scaphoid when the wrist is in ulnar deviation (**Figure 12.20a**). The wrist is then rotated into radial deviation (**Figure 12.20b**). In scapholunate dissociation, a painful 'clunk' occurs. A posteroanterior radiograph of the clenched fist confirms the presence of a wide scapholunate interval or 'Terry-Thomas sign'. The lateral film shows an increased scapholunate angle.

**Volar intercalated segment instability** often follows a fall onto the hypothenar eminence, causing rupture of the lunotriquetral and radiocarpal ligaments of the ulnar side of the wrist. Intermittent traction across the wrist joint produces tapping of the mobile bones – lunotriquetral ballotement. The lateral radiograph shows a decreased scapholunate angle.

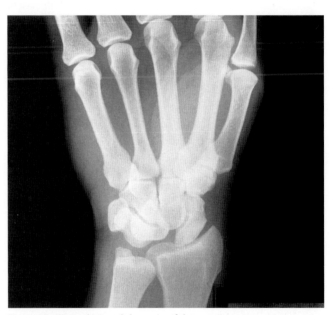

Figure 12.18 Perilunate dislocation of the wrist.

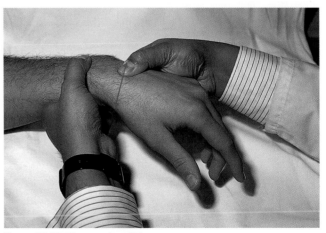

Figure 12.19 The pseudostability test.

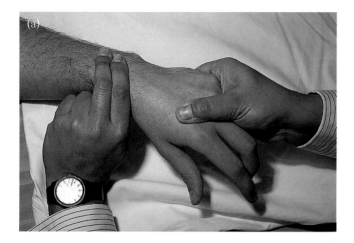

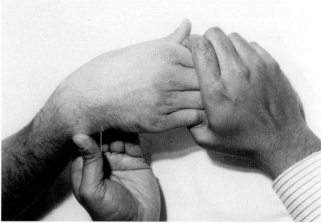

Figure 12.21 The piano key sign.

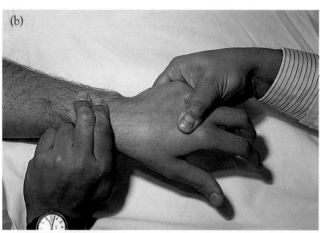

Figure 12.20 The Watson test. (a) The examiner's left thumb is applying pressure to the scaphoid. (b) Radial deviation of the wrist.

Instability of the distal radioulnar joint is characterized by pain over the ulnar aspect of the wrist and weakness in some movements. The piano key sign (subluxation of the head of the ulna due to ligament degeneration, which is prominent in hand pronation) demonstrates pain or increased movement at the distal radioulnar joint (**Figure 12.21**).

Tears of the triangular fibrocartilage complex cause ulnar-sided wrist pain that is made worse with ulnar deviation of the wrist. There is tenderness in the sulcus distal to the ulnar styloid – the ulnar snuffbox.

## Key Points

- Periarticular elbow pathologies can be the result of overuse, as in tennis or golfer's elbow, or due to compression neuropathies, as in radial tunnel and cubital tunnel syndromes.
- The elbow joint can be involved in degenerative conditions such as inflammatory processes invading the synovium, for example in rheumatoid arthritis. In addition, wear and tear due to osteoarthritis can ensue, leading to mechanical failure of the joint, ligaments (ulnar collateral) and tendons (biceps brachii).
- Traumatic pathologies of the elbow and forearm may lead to fractures and dislocations. These injuries follow a predictable pattern according to their mechanism; be sure to check for vascular and nerve injuries. Their treatment is systematic, involving closed and open procedures according to the patient's age and the displacement of the bones.
- The wrist is a complex joint prone to a myriad of injuries. Mastering the surface anatomy over the dorsal and volar aspects of the joint should aid in diagnosing these injuries.
- Soft tissue and degenerative conditions of the wrist are also encountered. Due to its relatively narrow hour-glass configuration, structures in the wrist might be subjected to compression neuropathy as in carpal tunnel syndrome, overuse as in de Quervain's disease and traumatic ganglion cysts.
- Traumatic injuries to the wrist and carpus may be obvious on radiography, as in a Colles' or Smith's fracture, or subtle, as in scaphoid fracture and carpal instability. One should keep a high index of suspicion when addressing wrist injuries.

# QUESTIONS

## SBAs

**1. Which one of the following is true regarding Colles' fractures?:**

a They are extra-articular in nature

b They result in a dorsal displacement of the distal forearm

c They are produced after a fall onto an outstretched hand

d In some patients, they can lead to an attrition rupture of the extensor pollicis longus tendon

e All of the above

**Answer**

e ***All of the above.*** *A Colles' fracture is an extra-articular fracture of the distal radius resulting from a fall on an outstretched hand that more often occurs in the elderly. The displacement is dorsal, described as a 'dinner-fork' deformity on radiographs. Some patients develop an attrition rupture of the extensor pollicis longus tendon that is associated with the insult to the wrist from the fracture.*

---

**2. In tennis elbow, which one of the following is true?:**

a The culprit is the origin of the extensor carpi radialis longus tendon over the medial epicondyle

b There is rarely tenderness over the common extensor tendon just distal to the lateral epicondyle

c Overuse and heavy physical activity over the elbow joint trigger the symptoms

d Cozen's test describes the reproduction of symptoms after pronating the forearm while flexing the wrist

e None of the above

**Answer**

c ***Overuse and heavy physical activity over the elbow joint trigger the symptoms.*** *Tennis elbow is an overuse syndrome consisting of pain and tenderness over the common extensor tendon just distal to the lateral epicondyle. The culprit is the origin of the extensor carpi radialis brevis tendon. The Mills manoeuvre reproduces the pain upon pronation the forearm while flexing the wrist.*

---

**3. Which one of the following is true about carpal tunnel syndrome?:**

a It is the least frequent compression neuropathy of the upper extremity

b Attacks can lead to numbness and tingling of the ulnar three fingers

c It is sometimes associated with systemic diseases such as diabetes and chronic kidney disease

d It is usually more common in men than women

e It results from compression of the median nerve under the extensor retinaculum

**Answers**

c ***It is sometimes associated with systemic diseases such as diabetes and chronic kidney disease.*** *Carpal tunnel syndrome is the most common compression neuropathy of the upper extremity. It is more common in women rather than men. It can be associated with systemic diseases such as diabetes mellitus, thyroid disease and chronic kidney disease. Symptoms result from the compression of the median nerve under the flexor retinaculum over the wrist area. The patient complains of numbness and tingling over the radial three fingers, mostly at night. Over the long term, motor function can be impaired, as witnessed by atrophy of the thenar eminence, weakness and loss of fine movements.*

PART 2 | TRAUMA AND (ELECTIVE) ORTHOPAEDICS

## EMQs

**1. Match each of the following patient presentations to the correct diagnosis in the list below. Each option may be used once, more than once or not at all:**

    **1** De Quervain's tenosynovitis
    **2** Attrition rupture of the long head of biceps
    **3** Dorsal intercalated segment instability
    **4** Cubital tunnel syndrome
    **5** Kienböck's disease
  **a** Atrophy of the intrinsic muscles of the hand
  **b** Widening of the scapholunate distance
  **c** Avascular necrosis of the lunate
  **d** Pain along the first dorsal wrist compartment
  **e** Presence of a bulge in the lower third of the arm

**Answers**

**a 4 Cubital tunnel syndrome.** *Compression of the ulnar nerve in the cubital tunnel at the level of the medial elbow may lead to sensory and motor disturbance along the distribution of the ulnar nerve in the upper extremity, mainly in the hand, and lead to atrophy of the intrinsic muscles.*

**b 3 Dorsal intercalated segment instability.** *Dorsal intercalated segment instability is due to a traumatic disruption of the scapholunate ligament. A wide scapholunate interval, or Terry-Thomas sign, is a diagnostic radiological sign on an anteroposterior view.*

**c 5 Kienböck's disease.** *Kienböck's disease is also known as avascular necrosis of the lunate. It is usually attributed to either repetitive microtrauma or a vascular insult to the lunate and produces progressive pain, stiffness and mid-wrist tenderness*

**d 1 De Quervain's tenosynovitis.** *This is a painful disabling condition affecting the common tendon sheath of the first dorsal wrist compartment. It usually starts with inflammation but may progress to fibrosis and stiffness of the thumb.*

**e 2 Attrition rupture of the long head of biceps.** *Bulging of the flexor side of the distal arm is also known as the Popeye sign. It reflects a failure at the myotendinous junction of the proximal biceps in the elderly, which results in an attrition rupture and the appearance of the pathognomonic bulge.*

**2. Match each of the physical tests with the correct diagnosis from the list below. Each option may be used once, more than once or not at all:**

    **1** Dorsal intercalated segment instability
    **2** De Quervain's tenosynovitis
    **3** Biceps tendonitis
    **4** Carpal tunnel syndrome
    **5** Pitcher's elbow
  **a** Yergason's test
  **b** Phalen's test
  **c** Finkelstein's test
  **d** Watson's test
  **e** O'Driscoll's test

**Answers**

**a 3 Biceps tendonitis.** *Yergason's test involves the supination against resistance of a elbow flexed to 90°. Pain indicates the presence of proximal biceps tendinitis.*

**b 4 Carpal tunnel syndrome.** *Phalen's test in carpal tunnel syndrome is the exacerbation of paraesthesia when the patient is asked to maintain full wrist flexion for 60 seconds.*

**c 2 De Quervain's tenosynovitis.** *The Finkelstein test involves ulnar deviation of the wrist when the fist is clenched over the thumb. If the test positive (causing severe pain), it reflects the presence of inflammation over the first dorsal compartment – de Quervain's tenosynovitis.*

**d 1 Dorsal intercalated segment instability.** *Watson's test is positive when there is apprehension upon exerting pressure on the scaphoid tubercle in a radially deviated wrist. A clunk may be heard. This is a sign of a dorsal intercalated segment instability resulting from a disrupted scapholunate ligament.*

**e 5 Pitcher's elbow.** *The moving valgus stress test of O'Driscoll entails applying a constant moderate valgus torque to the fully flexed elbow and then quickly extending it. Apprehension at the medial elbow reflects the presence of a valgus extension overload, a condition known as pitcher's elbow.*

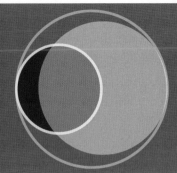

CHAPTER

13

# The Hand

Hamed Janom, Elie Ramly and
Ghassan S. Abu-Sittah

## LEARNING OBJECTIVES

- To understand the unique anatomical and functional features of the hand
- To know the general approach to the history-taking and physical examination of the hand
- To be aware of the distinctive signs and symptoms of specific acquired hand conditions

- To know the significance of diagnostic tests that are relevant to specific hand conditions
- To know how to manage specific conditions of the hand

## INTRODUCTION

> We ought to define a hand as belonging exclusively to man ... corresponding in sensibility and motion with that ingenuity which converts the being who is the weakest in natural defences to the ruler over all animated nature.
> (Sir Charles Bell)

The essential value of the hand for human beings is illustrated by the very beginning of a person's life, infants relying almost entirely on this organ to interact with and learn about their surroundings. Throughout a person's productive years, the hand continues to be of vital importance as an exceptionally useful tool in almost every experience. The essential components of effective hand function are strength, pain-free mobility and sensation. Thumb opposition is the key feature of the human hand that allows for various configurations of grip and pinch movements.

This chapter demonstrates an organized and thorough approach to the examination of the hand. Careful enquiry and a detailed assessment of signs and symptoms are essential for the examiner to reach the correct diagnosis. The pillars of this approach are history-taking and physical examination.

## HISTORY-TAKING

History-taking should cover the important elements of the patient's social history, including their age, sex, occupation and hand dominance. A hand injury may have devastating consequences for a young worker whose productivity directly depends on manual dexterity. Occupational considerations are important when discussing treatment options and prognosis. For example, a right-handed writer with right hand weakness or numbness may not tolerate conservative treatment as they would if the debilitating condition involved their left hand.

In the assessment and management of hand conditions, priority should be directed to mobility, pain and numbness rather than cosmesis. Smoking and alcohol consumption are important social habits that need to be addressed during history-taking for being significant modifiable factors that may alter the prognosis.

The medical history should be carefully gathered as systemic medical conditions could be directly related to the complaint. Diabetes mellitus, pulmonary and cardiac diseases, renal insufficiency, vascular diseases, autoimmune diseases and many other conditions may have hand-related signs or symptoms that are typically recognizable during a simple assessment.

The examiner should collect all the relevant details that are related to the complaint. In a traumatic hand injury, it is important to identify the time, place, mechanism of injury and any interventions undertaken prior to the patient's presentation. It is useful to address the symptoms by asking about their characteristics. Patients may present with pain, muscle weakness, numbness, a mechanical derangement of motion or a change in colour or temperature of the hand. A good description of these symptoms helps in reaching an accurate diagnosis. The examiner should enquire about details of the symptom's location, duration, frequency, intensity and radiation, as well as any associated symptoms.

## PHYSICAL EXAMINATION

The hand is a complicated anatomical unit that is designed to perform a spectrum of functions ranging from the finest and most delicate movements, such as those involved in performing surgery and playing music, to the simple coarse motion that is involved in handling common objects. Its examination requires a thorough knowledge of its anatomy and excellent examination skills that have been gained through practice.

PART 2 | TRAUMA AND (ELECTIVE) ORTHOPAEDICS

## Inspection

The examination starts with a simple inspection of the hand. It is always beneficial to compare the affected hand with the contralateral hand. Through inspection, the examiner should identify old or new scars that indicate trauma or previous surgery. Colour changes in the hand usually reflect traumatic injury, vascular insult or skin disease (**Figure 13.1**).

Gross deformities or asymmetry of the hands, such as an abnormal alignment of the digits in flexion and extension, should raise the possibility of a bone fracture, tendon laceration, tumour or arthritis, as in autoimmune diseases (**Figures 13.2** and **13.3**). Swelling of the hand can result from trauma, infections, compression and less often lymphatic or venous obstruction, for example after breast surgery. Chronic nerve compression, which occurs in carpal tunnel syndrome and ulnar tunnel syndrome, can result in muscle atrophy of the thenar and interosseous muscles, respectively, which should be recognized by simple inspection.

## Palpation

Palpation plays a large role in assessment of the hand following traumatic injury. It is important to spot tenderness over fractured bones, and to identify inflamed joints or tendons, as in the case of tenosynovitis. In addition, superficial or deep space hand infections can manifest as an increase in hand temperature, which will be detected by palpation, while compromise of the vascular supply to the hand will manifest as coldness.

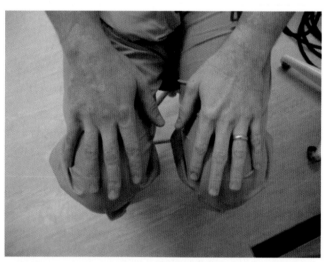

Figure 13.1 Vascular insult: proximal arterial injury may present with drastic whitening of the skin of the affected hand.

(a)             (b)

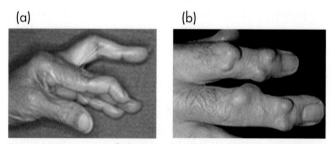

Figure 13.2 Features of rheumatoid arthritis. (a) Characteristic joint appearances including the swan-neck (index finger) and boutonnière (middle finger) deformities. (b) Rheumatoid nodules, which are firm lumps in the skin of patients with rheumatoid arthritis that usually occur over the pressure points, most commonly the elbows but also the joints of the hand.

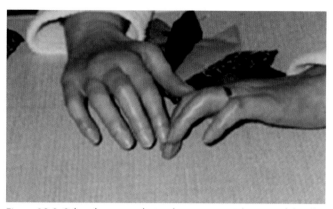

Figure 13.3 Scleroderma results in characteristic tightening of the skin that ultimately significantly hampers motion at the joints.

The examination of hand function includes an assessment of the range of motion of all the joints, the stability of the joints and the motor function of the tendons (**Figures 13.4** and **13.5**). The range of motion during active movement allows the examiner to assess the function of the tendons, muscles and nerves. Passive movement of the joints provides information about their intrinsic condition, for example fibrosis, inflammation, bone deformity and instability.

The ligaments around the joint provide its stability. Consequently, any change in the tone of these ligaments, whether loosening or tightening, causes joint laxity and stiffness, respectively. This is usually examined by manipulation of the joint between two fixed points in both the flexed and extended positions.

The mechanics of the hand are governed by the action of intrinsic and extrinsic muscles, conveyed through their tendons. To perform a complete assessment of the hand, especially in the setting of trauma or complex laceration, each of these muscles should be examined.

## DISTINCTIVE FEATURES OF SELECTED HAND CONDITIONS

### Dupuytren's Disease

This is a hereditary connective tissue disorder that occurs most commonly in older men. It is characterized by fibrosis of the normal palmar and digital fascia, resulting in fascial thickening and gradual contracture of the digital joints. It can present with either unilateral or bilateral involvement of the hands, soles of the feet or the penis depending on the severity of the disease.

#### History and Presentation

Common in men aged 40–60, this condition is associated with diabetes mellitus, smoking, alcohol intake and antiepileptic medications. Patients usually present with a long-standing history of palmar thickening and a gradual decrease in hand function, as shown by problems using a key or undoing buttons due to flexion contractures of the joints, mainly the metacarpophalangeal and proximal interphalangeal joints of the middle and ring fingers.

#### Physical Examination

The examination should start by inspecting both hands to rule out bilateral disease. On the volar aspect of the hand,

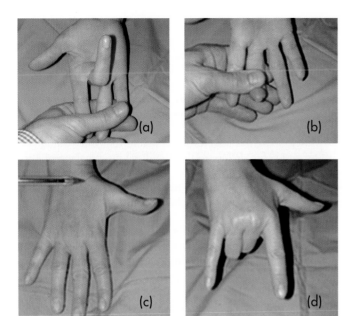

Figure 13.4 (a) Flexor digitorum superficialis is tested by asking the patient to flex the proximal interphalangeal joint while the remaining three fingers are held fully extended. (b) Flexor digitorum profundus is tested by asking the patient to flex the distal interphalangeal joint against resistance while the proximal interphalangeal joint and remaining three fingers are held fully extended. (c) Extensor pollicis longus testing. The palm is placed flat on the examining table while the patient is asked to lift their thumb towards the ceiling (retropulsion). (d) Extensor digiti minimi and extensor indicis proprius are tested by asking the patient to point with their little finger or index finger while making a fist with the rest of their fingers.

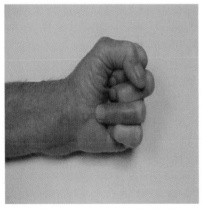

Figure 13.5 Isolated flexor digitorum profundus injury results in an apparent deficiency of flexion of the distal interphalangeal joint.

palmar nodules, longitudinal cords over the fingers and transverse cords over the web space become obvious in advanced disease. Pretendinous and natatory cords (from the pretendinous bands and the natatory ligaments in the palm), as well as central and lateral cords (from the volar superficial fascia and the lateral digital sheets of the digits, respectively), can be detected by palpation. On the dorsal aspect of the hands, ectopic deposits appear as Garrod's pads over the metacarpophalangeal and proximal interphalangeal joints.

The range of motion and stiffness of the joints should be assessed to rule out involvement of the collateral ligaments,

flexor sheath and volar plate. Possible involvement of the feet (in Ledderhose's disease) or penis (in Peyronie's disease) should be kept in mind and looked for in every patient as, along with Garrod's knuckle pads, they usually indicate a strong Dupuytren's diathesis.

## Compartment Syndrome of the Hand

Compartment syndrome occurs when the compartmental pressure rises above the perfusion pressure, causing compromise of the blood supply to the tissues within the compartment, which may lead to tissue necrosis. There are multiple causes for compartment syndrome, including trauma, open and closed fractures, reperfusion injury after arterial laceration and repair, external compression by a cast and snake bites.

The diagnosis of compartment syndrome is clinical and treatment should be prompt. Several methods can be used to measure the pressure inside the compartment, and this is usually done in the absence of strong clinical evidence of the condition. An intracompartmental pressure within 30 mmHg of the mean arterial pressure is considered to provide the diagnosis of compartment syndrome.

### History and Presentation

- Patients present with pain out of proportion to the clinical picture.
- The hand is oedematous and tense in the safe position.
- A loss of sensation occurs first, followed by a loss of motor power.

### Physical examination

- Inspect the hand for oedema, colour changes and apparent injuries. Pallor is usually a late presentation.
- Assess the pulses using palpation or Doppler scanning, keeping in mind that the presence of pulses does not rule out compartment syndrome, while their absence indicates a very late presentation and a very high compartmental pressure.
- Assess for severe pain, elicited by flexion of the interphalangeal joints.
- Examine sensation and motor power.

### Management

- The treatment is emergency fasciotomy.
- All the hand compartments should be decompressed and repeatedly followed up to undertake debridement.
- Closure of the wounds is carried out at a later stage, either via a split-thickness skin graft or by primary closure if possible.

## NERVE INJURIES

## Median Nerve Compression: Carpal Tunnel Syndrome

This is the most common nerve entrapment syndrome and is much more common in women. Carpal tunnel syndrome is usually associated with conditions such as rheumatoid arthritis, hypothyroidism, diabetes mellitus, pregnancy and carpal and distal radius fractures. Median nerve compression occurs in the compartment beneath the (transverse ligament) flexor retinaculum.

### History and Presentation

Patients usually present with a history of numbness and pain in the thumb, index finger, middle finger and radial aspect of the ring finger. Symptoms often occur bilaterally during the night and in the early morning. Activities that involve wrist extension may aggravate these symptoms, while placing the hand in the dependent position as if shaking hands will alleviate them. Patients who have been suffering from these symptoms for a long time might also have hand grip weakness and clumsiness, which may significantly affect their function.

### Physical Examination

Bilateral hand inspection should be carefully undertaken to detect any scars, swelling of the hands and wrists or wasting of the thenar muscles. Joint swelling and deformity as well as skin nodules are sometimes found in patients with severe rheumatoid arthritis.

Sensory assessment reveals decreased sensation over the area innervated by the median nerve. The two-point discrimination test is usually abnormal in moderate to severe cases. The symptoms can be provoked by several tests:

- In *Phalen's test* – the most sensitive of the tests – the patient is asked to fully flex the wrist for 60 seconds. The test is considered positive if the patient reports numbness or aggravation of the symptoms.
- *Tinel's sign* is positive if the patient reports pain and paraesthesia upon percussion over the median nerve at the wrist.
- In *Durkan's compression test*, pressure is applied over the median nerve at the carpal tunnel, which will provoke the symptoms in patients with carpal tunnel syndrome.
- In terms of motor power, functional tests will demonstrate weakness in opposition and thumb flexion, which usually occurs in severe cases. Patients show or report difficulty in undoing their buttons or signing their name.

## Ulnar Nerve Compression: Cubital Tunnel Syndrome

This is the second most common entrapment syndrome of the upper extremity. The ulnar nerve passing between the medial epicondyle and the olecranon beneath Osborne's ligament at the elbow becomes compressed at that point. It is also subjected to traction forces during elbow flexion; this is especially true when there is a loosening of Osborne's ligament.

### History and Presentation

Patients usually present with numbness and a tingling sensation over the little finger and the ulnar aspect of the ring finger. Patients may report a history of trauma to the elbow with or without a fracture. Moreover, sleeping with the elbow flexed beneath the head or neck and diseases such as rheumatoid arthritis are also considered risk factors.

### Physical Examination

During the physical examination, the elbow and hand should be inspected for scars, lumps or masses and hypothenar wasting.

Clawing of the ring and small finger may be evident in severe disease.

The sensation on the palmar aspect of the ulnar digits will be altered; however, the dorsal aspect should also be examined to make sure the compression is not at the level of the wrist. The symptoms are provoked by hyperflexion of the elbow for 30 seconds and by percussion over the ulnar nerve at the level of the elbow (Tinel's sign).

Muscle weakness manifests as a failure to abduct the fingers against resistance, failure to flex the distal interphalangeal joint of the little finger and a positive Froment's sign. Froment's sign is demonstrated by asking the patient to hold a piece of paper between the thumb and index finger and resist its being pulled out. The patient will experience difficulty maintaining a hold and will compensate by using the flexor pollicis longus of the thumb to maintain the pressure of the grip. This compensation manifests as flexion, rather than adduction, of the interphalangeal joint of the thumb.

## Radial Nerve Compression: Radial Tunnel Syndrome

This is caused by compression of the posterior interosseous nerve, a division of the radial nerve, at the lateral intermuscular septum of the arm; it occurs in repetitive strain injuries.

### History and Presentation

- Pain occurs on the dorsal (extensor) surface of the forearm and elbow.
- The pain increases with elbow extension, wrist flexion and forearm pronation.
- Weakness, if reported, is due to pain.
- Numbness over the dorsal forearm is a rare presentation.

### Physical examination

- Scars, lumps or oedema should be noted.
- Muscle wasting at the level of the extensors, triceps or brachioradialis muscle may indicate upper radial nerve injury.
- Wrist drop is a sign of upper radial nerve injury and not radial tunnel syndrome.
- Tenderness may be present over the extensor area and radial neck.

### Special Tests

- *Middle finger test*: Increasing pain can be elicited when the elbow is extended while the examiner applies resistance to middle finger extension.
- *Supination test*: Pain is elicited upon resisting hand supination with the elbow extended.

## HAND INFECTIONS

## Felon (Pulp Infection)

A felon is an infection of the finger or thumb pulp. It accounts for 15 per cent of hand infections. The infective organism is introduced through a puncture wound and subsequently gets trapped between the vertical septa in the pulp. *Staphylococcus aureus* is the most common cause, but gram-negative organisms can be involved if an abscess has formed.

## History and Presentation

- The patient reports a puncture injury from a thorn or sharp metal object.
- Local cellulitis occurs initially and is followed by swelling.
- The pain is throbbing in nature and is caused by an increase in local pressure in the pulp.
- A purulent discharge is sometimes reported.

## Physical Examination

- Inspect the finger for a foreign body, purulent discharge, nail and nail bed changes to rule out any concurrent injury.
- Palpate the pulp and joint for tenderness to check for any coexisting fracture in the setting of fingertip trauma.
- Examine the motion of the joint and look for associated pain in cases of fracture or tendon sheath involvement (flexor tenosynovitis).

## Management

- The felon should be incised and drained with adequate debridement.
- The contents should be cultured.
- The wound should be packed for a few days and left to heal by secondary intention.
- Antistaphylococcal antibiotics should be initiated until cultures are available.

## Paronychia

Paronychia is the most common infection of the hand. It is a superficial infection that involves the soft tissue around the nail. If it extends from the lateral nail fold distally to the eponychial fold proximally, it is then termed eponychia. It is caused by repetitive trauma, the most commonly involved pathogen being *S. aureus*. However, *Candida albicans* and mycobacteria might be involved in chronic cases. In children, paronychia is caused when repetitive biting and thumb sucking leading to anaerobic infection.

### History and Presentation

- Patients report a history of trauma to the digit, improper nail care or thumb biting.
- Presentation is with pain and increasing tenderness over the surrounding soft tissues.
- Erythema and swelling are common, and a purulent discharge is reported in severe cases.

### Physical Examination

- Inspect the nail and surrounding tissues to determine the extent of the infection.
- Assess for fluctuation and severe tenderness on palpation, which suggests abscess formation.
- Examine the proximal joint's mobility for a possible spread of infection to the bones or tendons.

## Management

- An X-ray should be arranged if the physical examination does not rule out involvement of the bone.
- Early infection that is still restricted to the skin is treated with warm water irrigation, dressings and oral antibiotic coverage.
- If there is abscess formation, incision and drainage are required, with proper antibiotic coverage.
- Nail care should be undertaken properly. However, in cases of repeated infection, a partial nail plate excision should be undertaken to prevent lateral nail growth.

## Acute Flexor Tenosynovitis

Acute flexor tenosynovitis is an infection that involves the flexor tendon sheath and the surrounding synovial space (**Figure 13.6**). It usually results from penetrating trauma but can be caused by haematogenous seeding of bacteria. It accounts for 10 per cent of hand infections and most commonly occurs in the index, middle and ring fingers. The most common pathogen is *S. aureus*.

### History and Presentation

- The patient presents with generalized finger oedema and erythema associated with pain that is exacerbated by motion.
- Trauma to the digit is reported in most cases, but some patients report a history of infection elsewhere with systemic manifestations, for example a gonococcal urinary tract infection.
- A history of vascular and autoimmune diseases must be ruled out.

### Physical Examination

- Inspect the hand for penetrating trauma and any apparent foreign body.
- Inspect the infected digit for oedema along the flexor sheath, and erythema when the finger is in the flexed position.

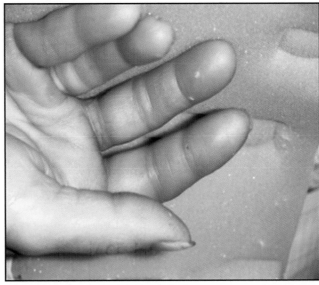

Figure 13.6 Flexor sheath infection is often accompanied by a vague history of injury. It presents with fusiform swelling and tenderness along the whole tendon sheath. Patients hold their finger flexed to avoid the pain that is experienced upon extension.

- Palpate the finger to elicit tenderness. Pain is severe with passive extension of the finger.
- Examine the palm to rule out spreading of the infection through the flexor sheath. The palmar, radial and ulnar bursae are at risk for contiguous spread if the infection involves the thumb and the little finger because of their continuity with the flexor sheaths of these two digits.

## Management

- Early infection should be treated with intravenous antibiotics depending on the cause.
- Splinting and elevation of the hand are important to decrease oedema and pain.
- If no improvement is noticed after 24 hours, incision and drainage should be considered.

## Deep Space Infections

The three deep, potential spaces of the hand are the thenar, midpalmar and hypothenar spaces, which are separated by facial septa. Infectious agents can reach these spaces via penetrating trauma, haematogenous spread or contiguous spread from the flexor tendon sheaths of the digits. If the infection is left untreated, an abscess eventually forms. These infections account for 2 per cent of hand infections and are mostly due to *S. aureus* and streptococci.

### History and Presentation

- Patients present with a painful and oedematous hand, with most of the symptoms being in the palm.
- Normal motion is restricted due to pain.
- Patients may report a history of tenosynovitis or penetrating trauma.

### Physical Examination

- Inspect the hand for any penetrating trauma and foreign body.
- Look for swelling. The oedema is usually palmar, with a loss of palmar concavity; however, it can also be dorsal, which may mislead the examiner.

- Examine the digits and web spaces. This is important to rule out spread of the infection, which can result in the formation of a collar stud abscess.
- Palpate the hand for tenderness. The pain usually increases with passive flexion and extension of the fingers.

## Management

- Broad spectrum intravenous antibiotics should be initiated immediately.
- Incision and drainage of abscesses with adequate debridement should be undertaken.

### Key Points

- A thorough history, systematic bilateral comparative inspection and palpation are the cornerstones of hand examination.
- A colour change should alert the examiner to skin or vascular conditions that may be traumatic in origin.
- An adequate examination of every joint and digit includes an assessment of the range of motion, strength, sensation including pain and numbness, alignment and symmetry.
- Dupuytren's disease classically involves the hand but can also affect the feet or penis. A full physical examination should always be performed.
- Compartment syndrome is an emergency that should be treated with fasciotomy.
- Median, ulnar or radial nerve compression can present with pain, paraesthesia, weakness or muscular atrophy in advanced cases. Remember Phalen's test, Froment's sign and the supination test, respectively, for these conditions. Electromyography may be useful as an adjunct.
- Antibiotics do not replace incision and drainage for abscesses.

# QUESTIONS

## SBAs

1. A patient presents with local cellulitis and swelling of his right index finger. He reports throbbing pain that increases when pressing the pulp. Which one of the following is true?:
   a This is most likely to be caused by a puncture injury from a thorn or a sharp metal object
   b The most common cause is *Staphylococcus aureus*
   c Treatment is conservative and antibiotics should be administered
   d Answers a and b are both correct

**Answer**

d ***Answers a and b are both correct.*** *A felon is an infection of the finger or thumb pulp. It accounts for 15 per cent of hand infections. The infective organism is introduced through a puncture wound and subsequently gets trapped between the vertical septa in the pulp.* Staphylococcus aureus *is the most common cause, but gram-negative organisms can be involved if an abscess has formed. The felon should be incised and drained with adequate debridement. Antistaphylococcal antibiotics should be initiated until cultures results have been received.*

2. A 3-year-old boy has been brought to the accident and emergency department with swelling of the tip of his left thumb, especially around the nail. This is very tender and fluctuant when pressed. Which one of the following is true?:
   a The cause might be an anaerobic infection
   b Incision and drainage should be carried out
   c An X-ray can be considered to rule out bone involvement
   d All of the above

**Answer**

d ***All of the above.*** *Paronychia, a superficial infection that involves the soft tissue around the nail, is the most common infection of the hand. In children, paronychia is caused by repetitive biting and thumb sucking, leading to anaerobic infection. An X-ray should be taken if the physical examination cannot rule out involvement of the bone. In cases of abscess formation, incision and drainage are required, with proper antibiotic coverage.*

3. The treatment of choice for acute compartment syndrome of the hand is which one of the following?:
   a Elevation of the hand above heart level
   b Fasciotomy if pulses are not detectable
   c Splinting
   d None of the above

**Answer**

d ***None of the above.*** *Compartment syndrome occurs when the compartmental pressure rises above the perfusion pressure, causing compromise of the blood supply to the tissues within the compartment, which may lead to tissue necrosis. Emergency fasciotomy is the treatment once the condition is suspected. All the hand compartments should be decompressed, and the patient should be repeatedly followed up for debridement of the area.*

## EMQs

**1.** **For each of the following descriptions, select the most likely sign or cause from the list below. Each option may be used once, more than once or not at all:**

    **1** Positive Phalen's test

    **2** Positive Tinel's sign

    **3** Ulnar nerve compression

    **4** Median nerve compression

    **5** Radial nerve compression

    **6** Tenosynovitis

    **7** Palmar nodules

    **8** Thenar atrophy

**a** A 55-year-old man who is a heavy smoker presents to the clinic with a gradual decrease in hand function and an inability to extend his ring finger. Physical examination of the hand shows normal sensation, and the patient reports no numbness.

**b** A 47-year-old woman presents with a long-standing history of numbness and pain in the thumb, index and middle finger of her right hand. Symptoms often occur during the night and in the early morning. Paraesthesia is elicited upon percussion over the volar aspect of the wrist.

### Answers

***a* 7 Palmar nodules.** *Dupuytren's disease is a hereditary connective tissue disorder that occurs most commonly in older men. It is characterized by fibrosis of the normal palmar and digital fascia, resulting in fascial thickening and a gradual contracture of the digital joints. Common in men aged 40–60 years, this condition is associated with diabetes mellitus, smoking, excessive alcohol intake and antiepileptic medications. Palmar nodules, longitudinal cords over the fingers and transverse cords over the web space become obvious on the volar aspect of the hand in advanced disease.*

***b* 4 Median nerve compression.** *Median nerve compression (carpal tunnel syndrome) is the most common nerve entrapment syndrome and is much more common in women. It is usually associated with conditions such as rheumatoid arthritis, hypothyroidism, diabetes mellitus, pregnancy and carpal and distal radial fractures. Median nerve compression occurs in the compartment beneath the transverse ligament. Patients usually present with a history of numbness and pain in the thumb, index finger, middle finger and radial aspect of the ring finger. Symptoms often occur bilaterally and are particularly frequent during the night and in the early morning.*

# CHAPTER 14

# The Pelvis, Hip Joint and Thigh

Firas Kawtharani and Bernard H. Sagherian

## LEARNING OBJECTIVES

- To identify basic traumatic injuries of the pelvis, acetabulum and hip
- To conduct a basic hip examination
- To recognize the main congenital, inflammatory and infectious pathologies affecting the paediatric hip
- To identify common adult intra-articular and extra-articular conditions of the hip
- To acknowledge the main reconstructive options for the hip and their implications

## PELVIC FRACTURES

### Anatomy

The pelvic girdle is composed of two innominate bones and the sacrum. Each innominate bone is formed from three bones: the ilium, the ischium and the pubis. The innominate bones are held together anteriorly by the ligaments of the symphysis pubis, inferiorly by the pelvic floor ligaments and posteriorly by the strong posterior sacroiliac ligamentous complex. The latter consists of the strong interosseous ligaments, the anterior and posterior sacroiliac ligaments. The pelvic floor ligaments are the sacrotuberous and sacrospinous ligaments. The iliolumbar ligaments attach the pelvis to the lumbar spine.

Contained within the pelvis are the rectum and urogenital organs as well as neurovascular structures. Injury to these structures is the main source of morbidity and mortality emanating from pelvic ring fractures.

### Injuries to the Pelvis

Injuries to the pelvis are usually caused by falls or road traffic accidents. The mechanism of the injury determines the energy imparted to the pelvis, and this is usually associated with the degree of injury. Minor falls, particularly in the elderly, may produce isolated fractures of the pubic rami. Falls from a horse may cause severe ligamentous disruption or a fracture in the pelvis that is associated with visceral injuries. In road traffic accidents, the force transmitted along the femur or from the tightening of a lap seatbelt can cause significant injury to the bony pelvis. Sporting activity in adolescence can cause avulsion fractures of the pelvis.

Fractures of the pelvis may lie outside the pelvic ring and therefore do not compromise its stability. Fracture or ligamentous disruption within the pelvic ring itself usually occurs at two simultaneous sites, producing two fragments. The smaller fragment of the ring is unstable and may lead to displacement and later disability. The anterior ring fails along the symphysis pubis or through the pubic rami. The posterior ring fails at the sacroiliac joint or can produce vertical fractures of the sacrum.

Fractures of the pelvis are thus classified into three types:

- *Type A* fractures or injuries lie outside the pelvic ring. These lesions do not lead to instability of the pelvic ring or any long-term problems with weight-bearing. They are not usually associated with other morbid injuries. Examples include fractures of the iliac wing, avulsion fractures and transverse fractures of the sacrum or coccyx.
- *Type B* injuries give rise to partial instability of the pelvic ring, that is, they are rotationally unstable but vertically stable. Typically, the injury renders one hemipelvis unstable on either external or internal rotation. Examples include separation of the symphysis pubis associated with a posterior lesion, such as a partial injury to the strong posterior sacroiliac ligament complex. The remaining ligamentous connections prevent a vertical migration of the involved hemipelvis. An 'open book' injury is described when there is a wide diastasis or opening at the level of the symphysis pubis; this rotational displacement may be associated with a shearing injury to the pelvic vessels and thus haemodynamic instability.
- *Type C* injuries also involve the pelvic ring in two places. In contrast to type B injuries, the posterior injury is complete, there being little or no ligamentous connection between the sacrum and the innominate bone. The fracture is rotationally and vertically unstable. These injuries are often associated with visceral and vessel injury.

### Presentation of Pelvic Fractures

The history of the mechanism of the accident often indicates whether the trauma is of low or high energy. In high-energy injuries, the patient may have multiple injuries and be

PART 2 | TRAUMA AND (ELECTIVE) ORTHOPAEDICS

haemodynamically unstable. The assessment of such a patient includes resuscitation in accordance with the guidelines relating to advanced trauma life support (ATLS). The primary survey must address life-threatening issues such as airway, breathing and blood pressure support. An anteroposterior radiograph of the pelvis is one of the cornerstones of the trauma series of ATLS.

Examination during the secondary ATLS survey should involve examination of the skin for haematoma, bruising and degloving injuries. Rectal and genital examinations may suggest the perforation of a viscus or a urethral injury. A neurological assessment of the lower extremities should be undertaken, and major long bone deformities and limb length discrepancies noted.

The stability of the pelvis should be assessed in both the rotational and vertical displacement planes. The anteroposterior compression test over the iliac crests may detect rotational instability (**Figure 14.1**). The assessment of vertical stability requires two people – one needs to hold the two iliac crests to

detect movement, while the other applies longitudinal traction and compression through the leg to cause vertical displacement of the hemipelvis. This procedure needs to be undertaken with each leg in turn.

The clinician should be alert for neurological abnormalities in type C injuries as they are seen in nearly 50 per cent of cases. The early diagnosis of such an injury is important and should be documented.

Further radiographic evaluation is often carried out by pelvic inlet and outlet radiographs, and by CT scanning.

## ACETABULAR FRACTURES

### Anatomy

The acetabulum consists of the anterior and posterior columns, extending in an inverted Y shape in the sagittal plane from the ilium down to the pubis anteriorly and the ischium posteriorly. Superiorly, there is a weight-bearing domed area, and medially a quadrilateral plate of bone separating the acetabulum from the inside of the pelvis. Injuries to the acetabulum most commonly occur with severe trauma, such as is sustained in heavy falls or road traffic accidents. Low-energy trauma affects mostly the elderly.

The direction of the force vector and the position of the femoral head at the time of injury may predict the fracture pattern. Letournel devised a classification that groups fractures into simple wall fractures, column fractures and complex fractures involving both columns. A fall onto the greater trochanter applies a force along the femoral neck, fracturing the medial quadrilateral plate, often in association with anterior and posterior column fractures, and forcing the head into protrusion (**Figure 14.2**).

A longitudinally applied force along the femoral shaft, often produced by a dashboard injury to the knee, results in a posteriorly directed force, leading to fracture of the posterior column. This injury is often associated with posterior dislocation of the hip and injury to the adjacent sciatic nerve.

### Assessment of Acetabular Fractures

The history of the mechanism of injury often alerts the examining doctor to the diagnosis. The patient may be haemodynamically unstable because of an associated injury or severe pelvic

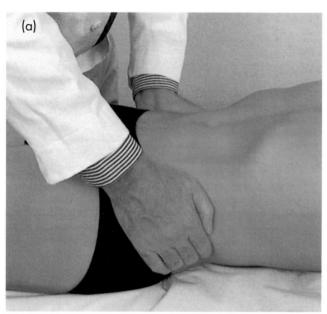

(a)

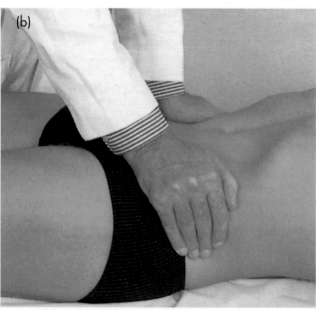

(b)

Figure 14.1 Assessing the rotational stability of the pelvis. (a) Side-to-side compression. (b) Backward pressure at the iliac crests.

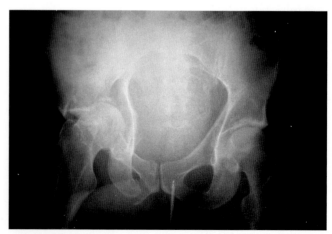

Figure 14.2 A fracture of the pubic ramus with disruption of the sacroiliac joint.

haemorrhage. As with pelvic fractures, the ATLS protocol should be implemented.

Contusion or bruising over the hip joint and pelvis should be sought. Gross deformity of the lower extremities, shortening and abnormal rotation may indicate accompanying fractures and hip dislocation. Palpation in the groin often reveals tenderness, and any attempt at movement of the affected hip causes severe pain.

An assessment of the stability of the pelvic ring, a thorough assessment of the distal pulses and a neurological examination must be carried out and the findings documented. Sciatic nerve injury is not uncommon following posterior column fractures. Further assessment involves a review of the six cardinal lines (iliopectineal, ilioischial, anterior rim, posterior rim, teardrop and dome) on an anteroposterior radiograph. Additional information is obtained from 45° Judet views of the pelvis and hip, roof arc measurements and CT scanning (**Figure 14.3**).

## GAIT

The examination of a hip joint must, unless there is a suspected fracture, begin with an observation of the patient's gait. A **coxalgic gait**, which results from pain in the joint, involves a shortening of the stance phase of the affected limb with an associated lurch of the shoulders to the affected side and a more rapid swing phase of the contralateral limb. Despite these changes, the pelvis remains level.

A **Trendelenburg gait** occurs as a result of weakness of the abductors of the affected hip joint, which causes the pelvis to drop to the contralateral side. There is also a lurch of the upper body to the affected side in order to maintain the centre of gravity while the affected leg is in the stance phase. If this is bilateral, the waddle of bilateral congenital dislocation of the hips should be suspected.

A **short leg gait** occurs as a result of an inequality in leg length and is characterized by an excessive rise and fall of the ipsilateral shoulder with each full gait cycle.

## EXAMINATION OF THE STANDING PATIENT

### Inspection

Examine the standing patient from the front and look for a pelvic tilt, which points to the presence of a limb length discrepancy, hip contracture or spinal deformity. Limb shortening may be compensated by plantar flexion of the foot on the affected side, flexion of the knee on the contralateral side or pelvic tilting as mentioned above.

Inspection along the sagittal plane may show an increase in the lumbar lordosis that may be related to a hip contracture. Look for wasting of the gluteus muscles, which is apparent where there has been chronic arthritis. Scars and sinuses indicate previous surgery or sepsis.

To demonstrate the **Trendelenburg sign (Figure 14.4)**, observe the patient from behind and ask them to lift their affected leg by bending their knee to the back, keeping the hip extended. The iliac crest on the affected side is elevated as a result of the normal functioning of the abductor mechanism of the opposite hip. The patient is then asked to lift up the good leg while

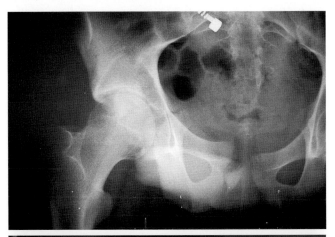

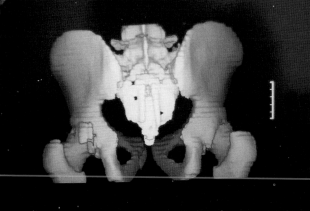

Figure 14.3 (a) Acetabular fracture of the left hip. (b) CT reconstruction of the fracture shown in (a). The orientation is reversed from left to right.

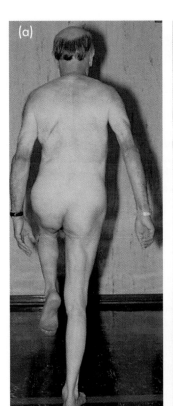
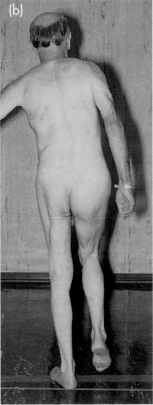

Figure 14.4 (a, b) The Trendelenburg test. (Reproduced with permission from *Physical Examination in Orthopaedics*, by A. Graham Apley and Louis Solomon, Butterworth-Heinemann, 1997.)

PART 2 | TRAUMA AND (ELECTIVE) ORTHOPAEDICS

standing on the affected leg. If the iliac crest on the unaffected side is seen to drop towards the floor due to weak abductor muscles, the patient may be forced to throw their shoulders towards the affected side in order to maintain their centre of gravity.

A positive Trendelenburg sign may be due to weak abductor muscles, a shortened femoral neck reducing the lever arm for the muscles, the lack of a fulcrum in congenital dislocation of the hip or pain on movement of the abductors caused by arthritis, inflammation or injury.

## EXAMINATION OF THE SUPINE PATIENT

### Position

The patient should lie flat, preferably with only one pillow supporting their head. The anterior superior iliac spines should be palpated to ensure that the pelvis is square to the examining table. The patient's legs are then positioned by the examiner so that they lie with the medial malleoli adjacent to the centre line of the examination table.

### Inspection

A further inspection for scars and sinuses is performed, and any deformity is noted. The state of the skin over the rest of the leg is assessed for signs of peripheral vascular disease or infection.

### Palpation

The normal bony landmarks of the hip are identified. The bony prominences at the insertion of the major muscles are palpated for tenderness; this will mainly involve the greater trochanter (abductors), the lesser trochanter (iliopsoas), the pubic tubercle (adductors) and the ischial tuberosity (hamstrings). The hip joint itself is palpated just below the inguinal ligament and lateral to the pulsation of the femoral artery. An absence of the femoral head may be obvious in congenital dislocation of the hip.

The anterior superior iliac spines are palpated with the examiner's thumbs, which are hooked under the spines with the index fingers placed over the greater trochanters (**Figure 14.5**). A decrease in distance between the anterior superior iliac spine and trochanter compared with the normal side signifies shortening of the femoral neck or dislocation of the hip.

### Measurement

#### Leg Length

Shortening may be true or apparent due to hip contracture, for example if there is a compensatory pelvic tilt. This can be detected by comparing the levels of the two anterior superior iliac spines. The tape measure technique can be used to evaluate for true shortening. The measurement is made from the anterior superior iliac spine to the medial malleolus. It is important to position the legs in the same attitude as any discrepancy constitutes a real shortening of the limb (**Figure 14.6**).

If shortening is present, it is important to know if it is above or below the trochanters. With the patient lying supine, measure the distance between the greater trochanter and the anterior superior iliac spine by placing a thumb and index finger on each and comparing the two sides. If the distances are equal, the shortening lies below the trochanters.

To measure distally, both the hips and the knees are flexed (with the knees at 90°) (**Figure 14.7**). The knees are then observed from the side of the couch. Shortening of the tibia is demonstrated by a decrease in the level of the anterior surface of the distal femur on the affected side. Shortening of the femur is demonstrated by a relative depression of the proximal anterior surface of the tibia on the affected side.

### Girth

Similar points are measured on the two legs by marking a specific distance – for the thigh from the anterior superior iliac spine, and for the shin from the tibial tuberosity. The circumference at these points monitors the wasting of muscles in the thigh or calf.

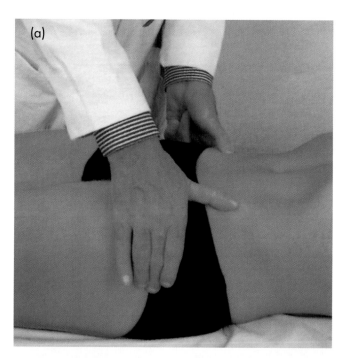

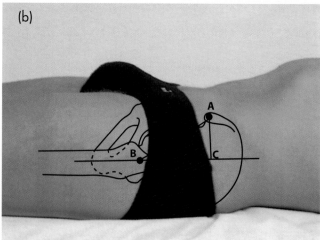

Figure 14.5 (a) Palpation of the anterior superior iliac spines and greater trochanters. (b) A, anterior superior iliac spine; B, cranial limit of the greater trochanter; C, Bryant's triangle. The distance BC is shortened in fractures of the head of the femur, which can be demonstrated by comparing the distance AB on the two sides.

## Thomas's Test

This test **(Figure 14.8)** is designed to demonstrate a fixed flexion deformity or a loss of the ability to fully extend the hip. The examiner passes one hand, palm upwards, under the patient's lumbar spine. The examiner then flexes the normal contralateral hip to its full extent and confirms that the lumbar lordosis has flattened. If there is a fixed flexion deformity, the free affected limb becomes flexed at the hip and the knee rises from the couch. The degree of flexion of the hip when the lumbar lordosis is flattened constitutes the amount of the fixed flexion deformity.

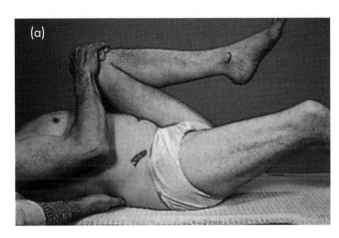

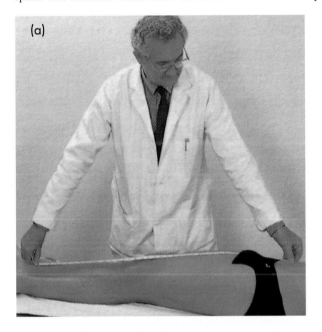

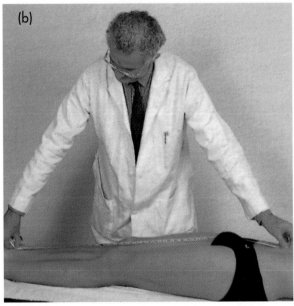

Figure 14.6 Measurement of leg length. (a) Looking for real shortening. (b) Looking for apparent shortening.

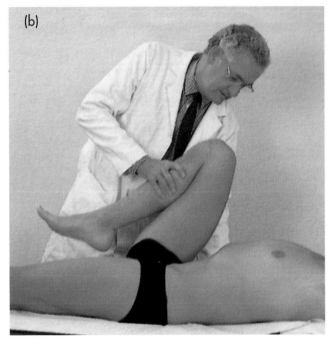

Figure 14.8 Thomas's test. (a) The patient flexing their own right knee and demonstrating how pelvic rotation takes place. The abnormality of the left hip does not allow the leg to remain in extension on the couch. (b) The left hand is placed behind the lumbar spine and demonstrates the moment at which the lumbar curve is flattened.

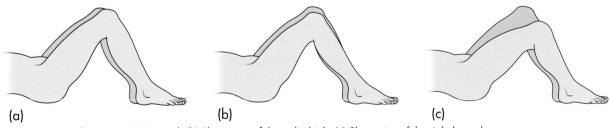

Figure 14.7 Leg shortening. (a) Normal. (b) Shortening of the right thigh. (c) Shortening of the right lower leg.

## FABER Test

The FABER test is done through **f**lexion, **ab**duction and **e**xternal **r**otation of the lower extremity. If pain is elicited in the contralateral lower extremity this suggests the presence of inflammation around the sacroiliac joint, which must be differentiated from true intra-articular pathology of the hip.

## Movements

Having confirmed that the pelvis is square to the examination table, the following movements can be tested (**Figure 14.9**).

### Rotation

The examiner stands at the end of the table and, holding both the patient's feet, rotates the hips internally and externally with the knees flexed to 90°. The normal angle of internal and external rotation is approximately 45°. The patella can be used as a reference point to compare the rotation of the lower extremities. A limitation of internal rotation is indicative of intra-articular pathology of the hip. If there is debilitating pain, as in a suspected fracture, rotation can be measured in extension.

### Adduction and Abduction

The examiner grasps the contralateral anterior superior iliac spine firmly with one hand in order to fix the pelvis against the examination table. Grasping the lower tibia or ankle with the other hand, the examiner then moves the leg away from the midline to test for abduction, and towards the midline to test for adduction.

### Flexion and Extension

The hip is flexed as much as possible in supination, keeping the pelvis fixed against the table, and the angle achieved is recorded. Testing of extension is done with the patient prone. A loss of extension alone may be an early sign of a hip effusion. Extension may be very limited in the presence of a fixed flexion contracture with a positive Thomas's sign.

## PAEDIATRIC HIP CONDITIONS

# Developmental Dysplasia of the Hip

This is a common condition in children, with an incidence of 1 in 1000 live births (**Figure 14.10**). Girls are affected four times more often than boys, and it is associated with 'packaging problems' – disorders that stem from an adverse intrauterine environment – such as torticollis and metatarsus adductus. There is often an associated family history of developmental dysplasia of the hip, and an increased incidence is seen in breech presentations and with oligohydramnios. It covers a spectrum of diseases ranging from dysplasia to subluxation and instability to complete dislocation.

Widespread screening was originally mainly clinical, consisting of Ortolani's test at birth (see below), but this is now supplemented with ultrasound imaging. Despite all of these efforts, however, there is a significant incidence of missed or late diagnosis of this condition. It is advisable that two experts examine every child on two occasions to increase the yield from screening. The clinical presentation depends on the child's age.

### Neonate (0–6 Months)

Most cases are diagnosed by routine screening in this age group. The correct diagnosis and treatment results in a 95 per cent cure rate.

The key physical signs are as follows:

- There is *limited abduction in flexion*.
- *Ortolani's test*: This demonstrates a dislocated hip. The infant lies supine on a flat surface, and the examiner flexes the knees and hips to 90°. The examiner then pushes the greater trochanters anteriorly with their fingers, while abducting the hips. The examiner's thumbs will be positioned over the femoral heads, and a palpable jerk will be felt as the femoral head reduces.
- *Barlow's test*: With the baby's hips and knees flexed to 90°, the examiner adducts the legs and applies a posteriorly directed force longitudinally through the femur. This causes a palpable jerk if the femoral head dislocates.

The examiner should be aware that neither Barlow's nor Ortolani's test will be positive if the dislocation is irreducible. These clinical tests should not be repeated unnecessarily because of the risk of a vascular necrosis of the head of the femur. If there is doubt, the definitive diagnosis is made by early ultrasound or plain radiographs taken at 3 months of age, when the upper femoral epiphysis is calcified and visible on radiographs. If the hip is found to be dislocated, prompt splinting is recommended.

### Infant (6–18 Months)

At this age, the infant is crawling or walking. The key signs are:

- *limited abduction* as stiffness sets in;
- a positive *Galeazzi's sign* marked by shortening and external rotation of the affected lower extremity;
- *asymmetrical gluteal skin folds*.

The hip is usually no longer reducible, and the acetabulum undergoes further dysplasia because the femoral head cannot be optimally contained. The condition may be associated with excessive anteversion of the femoral head with increased internal rotation of the hip on the affected side. Imaging will confirm the diagnosis. Beware, however, that bilateral dislocation with symmetrical physical signs may make diagnosis difficult. Bilateral involvement may be suggested by widening of the perineum and an increased lumbar lordosis.

### Toddler (18 Months to 3 Years)

These children present with a delay in walking, a limp, leg length discrepancy, increased shoulder sway and hyperlordosis of the spine.

### Adult Life

Symptoms usually start in the early 30s with pain, weakness and a limp. The leg is often short and a Trendelenburg gait or sign is present. Compensatory scoliosis and hyperlordosis in the lumbar spine may predispose to degenerative changes and even instability. In the hip, limited abduction and internal rotation is characteristic due to intra-articular degeneration and underlying increased femoral anteversion.

# Septic Arthritis of the Hip

This condition develops usually as a result of trauma, adjacent osteomyelitis or direct haematogenous spread. It is a surgical emergency because the infective process results in destruction of the articular cartilage. The common organisms are

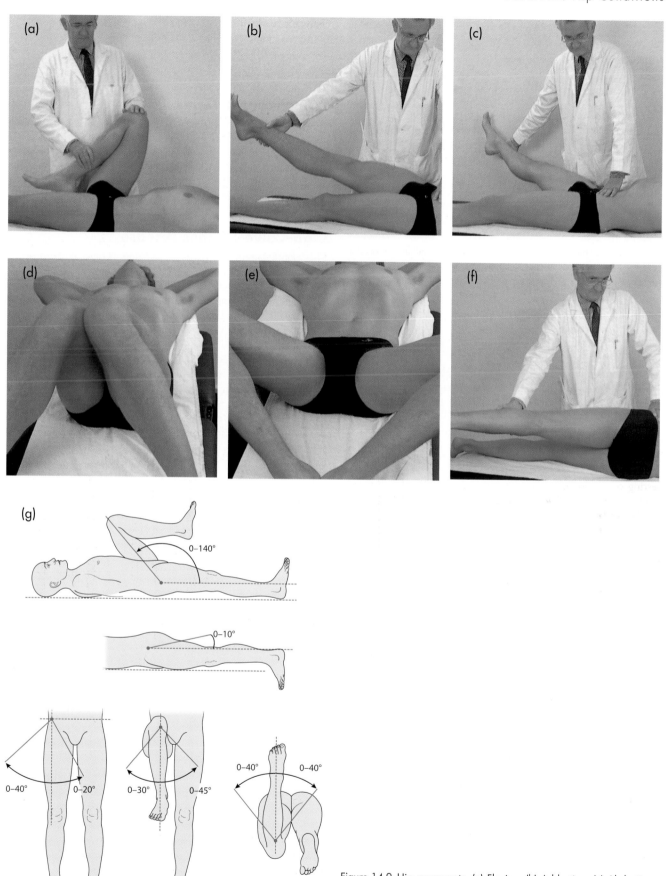

Figure 14.9 Hip movements. (a) Flexion. (b) Adduction. (c) Abduction. (d) Internal rotation. (e) External rotation. (f) Extension. (g) Normal ranges of movement at the hip.

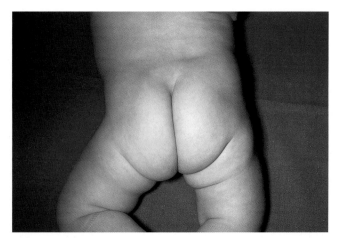

Figure 14.10 Congenital dislocation of the right hip. Note the difference in the skin creases. The legs do not abduct and externally rotate equally, which can affect nappy changing.

staphylococci, group B streptococci, *Haemophilus influenzae* and *Neisseria gonorrhoeae*.

The symptoms are pain in the hip and a decreased active and passive range of movement in all directions, with accompanying protective muscle spasm. Radiographs may show a widened joint space or even dislocation. The generalized signs of sepsis may be present, and infants may present with high-grade fevers with an unclear focus.

A thorough observation of the child often reveals that the leg is immobile – pseudoparalysis – due to pain. The hip may be held in the characteristic posture in infants – the 'frog position' – with the hip flexed, abducted and externally rotated. This position maximizes the intracapsular space and reduces the pain that results from excessive fluid pressure within the joint capsule.

The hip is tender on palpation in the groin. Any movement of the hip is resisted and causes the child to scream in pain. The presence of hip pain, an inability to ambulate, an increased white cell count and inflammatory markers is diagnostic of this condition.

## Transient Synovitis of the Hip

This is a common condition of the hip in childhood and should be a diagnosis of exclusion. There may be a history of trauma (<5 per cent), an antecedent viral illness (30 per cent) or even an allergic reaction. The child has a limp (85 per cent).

Pain is felt in the hip (80 per cent) and may radiate to the knee (25 per cent). All hip movements but specifically extension and internal rotation cause pain, and the range of movement is limited, although not as severely as in septic arthritis. **Gauvain's test** – in which sudden passive internal rotation of the leg is associated with a reflex contraction of the abdominal muscles – is often positive.

The pathological process is a traumatic or immunologically mediated aseptic inflammation of the synovium, leading to an effusion within the hip joint. Infection should be excluded by looking for the symptoms and signs of sepsis and by haematological investigations. Raised interferon levels have been found, but the erythrocyte sedimentation rate is usually below 20 mm per hour. Radiographs and ultrasound scans of the hip can demonstrate the presence of synovitis and effusion. If real doubt exists, the hip should be aspirated for microscopy and culture.

If a septic arthritis has been excluded, the child should be observed and rested; the application of skin traction can be of benefit in preventing the child from mobilizing. Transient synovitis normally improves within a few days of its onset, resolution being indicated by a negative Gauvain's sign.

## Tuberculous Arthritis

Tuberculosis of the hip joint is now rarely seen in developed countries. It presents with a limp and pain that is felt in the thigh or knee. Night pain is characteristic. Hip rotation becomes limited, and muscle wasting and a fixed flexion deformity – Thomas's sign – are important features. Radiographs of the hip show a widened joint space early on before joint destruction ensues. Neglected cases may develop an abscess or sinus.

## Legg–Calvé–Perthes Disease

This condition is known as *coxa plana*. There is necrosis of the head of the femur due to an unknown vascular insult. This process is followed by revascularization and resorption of the bone with fragmentation (**Figure 14.11**). Flattening of the femoral head and lateral subluxation are ominous signs. The severity of the condition is dependent on the extent of femoral head involvement.

The condition occurs most often in the age group between 4 and 8 years. Boys are affected more commonly than girls, with a ratio of 4:1, and in 10 per cent the problems are bilateral. An increased incidence is seen in association with a positive family history, a low birth weight and an abnormal birth presentation.

The pain is often felt in the knee rather than the hip or thigh. The child has a limp, and a Trendelenburg gait is common. There is a decreased range of movement at the hip joint, particularly abduction and internal rotation.

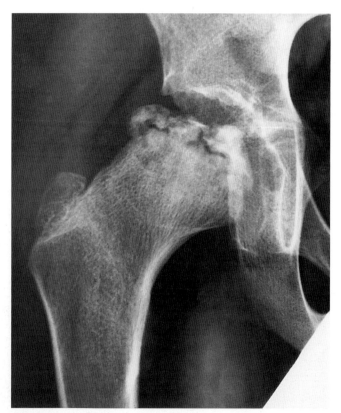

Figure 14.11 Legg–Calvé–Perthes disease.

The diagnosis can be confirmed at the time of presentation by plain radiographs. The differential diagnosis can include juvenile rheumatoid arthritis, proximal femoral osteomyelitis, irritable hip and hypothyroidism. Bilateral disease may mimic hypothyroidism and multiple epiphyseal dysplasia. Radiographic findings vary with the stage but include cessation of growth of the ossific nucleus, medial joint space widening and the crescent sign, which represents a subchondral fracture.

Revascularization and remodelling of the head of the femur occur over a period of some years. A good outcome results from restoration of the sphericity of the head during healing.

## Slipped Upper Femoral Epiphysis

This is a common condition in adolescents and affects boys more frequently than girls, with a ratio of 3:2 (**Figure 14.12**). The classical description is of a child who is obese from hypogonadism, although many children are in fact tall and thin. The patient presents with a limp and often complains only of pain in the knee. There may be a history of acute injury, but the majority will have had symptoms for weeks or months. On examination, there is an antalgic or Trendelenburg gait. There may also be an external rotation deformity. There is a painful limitation of internal rotation and of abduction of the hip.

The diagnosis is based on radiographs. The usual direction of slippage of the epiphysis is posteriorly and medial to the femoral neck. The most sensitive investigation is the lateral 'frog-leg' radiograph; this demonstrates the posterior slippage before the medial slippage of the head becomes apparent on an anteroposterior film. The other hip is involved in 40 per cent of cases, but only 50 per cent of these will produce symptoms.

## ADULT HIP CONDITIONS

## Osteoarthrosis of the Hip

This is a common condition whose incidence increases with age (**Figure 14.13**). The condition is more prevalent with increased weight and high joint stress activities. The patient complains of pain that is often felt in the groin, buttock or greater trochanter and may radiate to the knee. Stiffness, particularly after a long period of rest, results in difficulty in putting on shoes, socks and stockings. As the condition deteriorates, the walking distance is reduced and walking is associated with a limp. The patient goes on to suffer pain at night or at rest.

Examination of the hip demonstrates an antalgic or Trendelenburg gait. A small amount of shortening of the leg is often present. This may be due to **real shortening**, as the

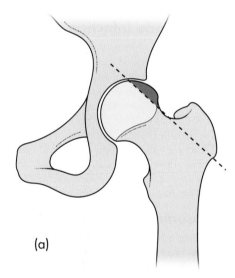

(a)

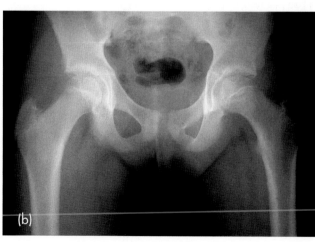

(b)

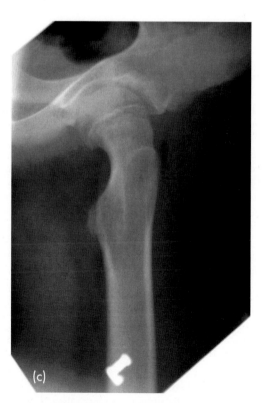

(c)

Figure 14.12 A slipped upper femoral epiphysis. (a) A line drawn along the superior margin of the neck of the femur on an anteroposterior radiograph intersects a small area of the supralateral part of the upper femoral epiphysis (shaded) in normal individuals. With a slipped upper femoral epiphysis, a smaller area or no part of the epiphysis projects superior to this Trethowan's line. However, the lateral radiograph is a more sensitive guide to an early slip. (b) Anteroposterior view of a slipped epiphysis of the left hip. (c) Lateral views of a slipped epiphysis.

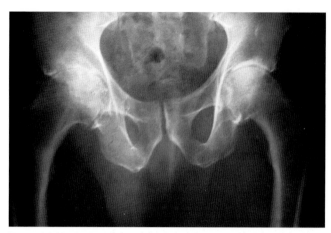

Figure 14.13 Osteoarthritis of the right hip.

joint space is eroded, or may be an **apparent shortening** of the leg resulting from an adduction or flexion deformity of the hip (see p. 240). If the legs are placed in the same orientation and the length is measured from the anterior superior iliac spine to the medial malleolus, the only shortening that is detected is real shortening due to a loss of joint space. Any apparent shortening is eliminated by placing both legs in the same orientation with respect to the pelvis. There is a limitation of all hip movements.

The majority of cases of osteoarthrosis of the hip constitute a primary condition. Premature osteoarthrosis of the hip can result as a secondary process in younger individuals from developmental dysplasia of the hip, Legg–Calvé–Perthes disease, a slipped upper femoral epiphysis or osteonecrosis of the head of the femur.

## Osteonecrosis of the Femoral Head

This condition results from an interruption of the blood supply to the head of the femur. There is death of the trabecular bone and bone marrow, followed by collapse of the bony architecture. Revascularization does not occur in adults.

Causes include a subcapital fracture of the neck of the femur (see p. 248), which leads to a traumatic interruption of the blood supply. Atraumatic causes of osteonecrosis are corticosteroid use, alcohol consumption, sickle cell anaemia, Gaucher's disease, myeloproliferative disorders, chronic pancreatitis, Caisson disease – inadequate decompression after deep sea diving – and irradiation.

The usual feature is severe pain at night. In the early stages, there may be only a slight restriction of movement. Later on, after the femoral head bone has collapsed, the signs are similar to those of an arthritic hip. The diagnosis is confirmed in later cases by plain radiographs as these show the collapse of the femoral head and narrowing of the joint space. Early cases are best detected by MRI.

## Meralgia Paraesthetica

This is a compressive neuropathy of the lateral femoral cutaneous nerve of the thigh when it becomes entrapped under the inguinal ligament or occasionally through the fascia lata. The symptoms are rarely due to direct trauma, a stretch injury or ischaemia.

This nerve is purely sensory, resulting in an area of hyperaesthesia and tingling over the lateral aspect of the thigh. This is worse on standing and walking but is relieved by sitting as flexion of the hip shortens the course of the nerve. Percussion over the inguinal ligament may result in an exacerbation of the symptoms – Tinel's sign.

## Psoas Bursa

This condition is rare but should be considered in those patients who present with pain and swelling in the groin that sometimes radiates to the anterior hip and knee. It occurs most commonly in athletes as a result of overuse.

The swelling is located in the femoral triangle but is too lateral to be a femoral hernia. There is pain with flexion and abduction of the hip as the psoas tendon rubs against the inflamed bursa. Tenderness over the anterior hip is a feature, and stretching exercises are the recommended treatment. See also p. 200 for psoas abscess.

## The Snapping Hip

Occasionally patients present with a spectacular condition in which they can, with volition, bring about a distinct 'snap' with certain hip movements. This is sometimes associated with pain. The condition usually results from the iliotibial tract passing over the greater trochanter. It is common in women who have a wide pelvis and/or trochanters. The snapping hip can be reproduced with passive flexion from an adducted position. This condition should be differentiated from intra-articular snapping, which stems from the iliopsoas tendon impinging on the hip capsule.

## COMPLICATIONS OF TOTAL HIP REPLACEMENT

Four complications are shown in **Figure 14.14**.

## Chronic Low-grade Infection

The patient complains of a continuous ache in the groin or thigh, usually starting some weeks or months after hip replacement. There is an accompanying limp, leading to abductor weakness and a Trendelenburg gait if the condition is not treated promptly.

A physical examination of the skin sometimes reveals an inflamed hip wound and possibly a sinus with chronic discharge, and there is a noticeable limitation of range of motion in all directions. The erythrocyte sedimentation rate and C-reactive protein level are elevated. Plain radiographs may show some signs of loosening, and a bone scan shows an increased uptake in keeping with infection. The diagnosis is confirmed by hip aspiration.

## Aseptic Loosening of the Hip

Some patients have a satisfactory outcome of their hip replacement for several years before progressively increasing pain develops in the groin or thigh. There is an associated stiffness, an inability to bear weight and a progressive limitation of the range of motion. The pain may be exacerbated by getting up from rest in a chair.

Examination involves flexing the hip and the knee to 90° and applying axial compression or traction to the femur. This often produces pain as the femoral component of the prosthesis pistons or subsides within the femur. Rotation of the hip causes pain and may be associated with a 'clunking' sensation as the loose femoral component moves inside the femoral shaft. A plain radiograph will show a defined sclerotic line around the loose stem and, in advanced cases, migration of the prosthetic components. The same situation can occur with the acetabular component.

## Acute Dislocation of the Hip

The majority of successful total hip replacements use a prosthetic femoral head that has a much smaller diameter than the

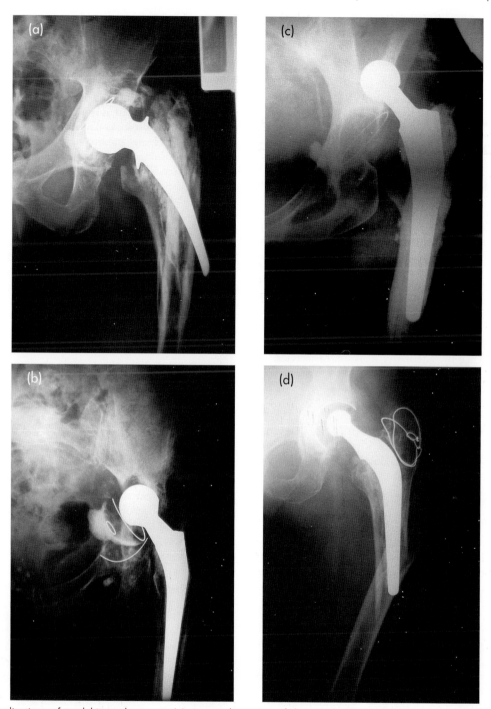

Figure 14.14 Complications of total hip replacement. (a) Aseptic loosening of the prosthesis. (b) A loose cup. (c) A dislocated prosthesis. (d) A periprosthetic fracture.

natural head. This affords particular advantages in allowing a good range of movement and reducing the frictional torque within the hip. However, it also produces an increased risk of dislocation.

The direction of the dislocation is governed by the alignment of the acetabular and femoral components, as well as the surgical approach used. With the commonly used lateral surgical approach, the risk of dislocation is greatest when the hip is flexed and adducted. The patient complains of sudden severe pain in the hip and feels the hip popping out of the socket. In a posterior dislocation the leg is short and internally rotated, while in an anterior dislocation it is short and externally rotated.

## Trochanteric Bursitis

This is inflammation of the trochanteric bursa that occurs mainly after increased physical activity. Palpation over the greater trochanter causes pain, as may getting the patient to abduct their leg against resistance. Laboratory tests are not usually indicated in this condition. It can also occur in patients who have not had hip surgery.

PART 2 | TRAUMA AND (ELECTIVE) ORTHOPAEDICS

## Heterotopic Bone Formation

This occurs when abnormal bone is formed in the soft tissues. It can be seen on plain radiographs 3–8 weeks after hip surgery. In extensive cases, there is a progressive limitation of movement as bony islands can coalesce between the femur and pelvis.

### TRAUMATIC INJURIES OF THE HIP

## Fracture of the Neck of the Femur

Two types of fracture occur here, but the clinical picture is similar. The capsule of the hip joint extends down the neck of the femur as far as the top of the trochanters, and fractures may occur inside or outside this capsule.

**Intracapsular fractures** – also known as subcapital or cervical fractures (**Figure 14.15a, b**) – occur through the femoral neck. At this point, the blood supply to the head of the femur is often interrupted, resulting in a loss of blood supply to the head. Reduction and internal fixation of the fracture may not always result in satisfactory union of the bone, and a prosthetic replacement is often the treatment of choice in the elderly.

**Extracapsular fractures** (**Figure 14.15c**) occur outside the hip capsule, usually at the base of the femoral neck or between the trochanters, hence the alternative name of 'basicervical' or 'intertrochanteric' fractures. The blood supply to the femoral head is not transgressed so reduction and internal fixation of the fracture usually leads to a satisfactory union.

The majority of fractures occur through osteoporotic bone and are seen in the elderly. Patients present having suffered a fall, often with a benign cause. There is pain in the hip, and there may be bruising in the region of the greater trochanter. The leg is held in external rotation and there is usually shortening. If the leg is severely externally rotated (90°) and short, the fracture is probably extracapsular. Lesser degrees of external rotation and shortening are seen in intracapsular fractures due to the constraints of the hip capsule. Some intracapsular fractures are undisplaced, or the bone ends are impacted, giving rise to little or no deformity; the patient may even be able to raise their leg from the bed. The diagnosis of a fracture is confirmed by anteroposterior and lateral radiographs.

## Isolated Trochanteric Fractures

A direct fall onto a hip can cause an isolated fracture of the greater trochanter. There is usually bruising and swelling around the trochanter, with local tenderness. The hip movements are usually reasonably well preserved, although painful, and the diagnosis is confirmed radiologically. Avulsion of the lesser trochanter in isolation tends to occur in schoolchildren who hurdle and is due to violent contraction of the psoas. If this fracture is seen in an elderly individual, the clinician should think of a pathological fracture. The patient is unable to actively flex the hip but other movements are intact – **Ludloff's sign**.

## Fractures of the Shaft of the Femur

These result from a severe mechanism of injury, such as a high-velocity motor vehicle accident, and range from simple transverse or spiral undisplaced fractures to severe, shattered, comminuted lesions, which may be open and also accompanied by vascular compromise.

The fractures occur in all ages but are most common in young adults. In infants and toddlers, child abuse must be ruled out. In the elderly, pathological fractures (**Figure 14.16**) occur in the upper third of the shaft, usually through secondary deposits but also with osteomalacia, in osteoporotic bone or in Paget's disease, where the brittle bone produces a characteristic transverse fracture. Observation of the patient in bed shows that the lower leg is laterally rotated and cannot be moved, and there is true shortening of the limb.

Displacement is related to the direction and severity of the injury. In the upper third of the femur (**Figure 14.17**), unopposed action of the iliopsoas and gluteal muscles flexes, externally rotates and abducts the proximal fragment, while the quadriceps and hamstring muscles draw the distal fragment proximally. In fractures of the mid and distal (**Figure 14.18**) thirds, the distal

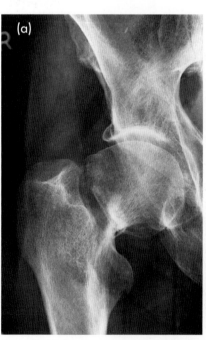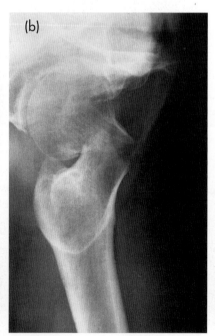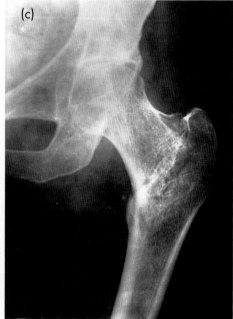

Figure 14.15 Fractures of the neck of the femur: (a, b) intracapsular, and (c) extracapsular.

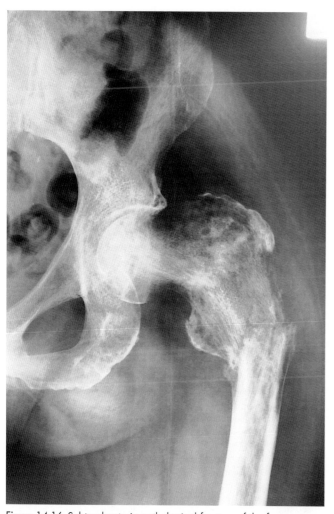

Figure 14.16 Subtrochanteric pathological fracture of the femur.

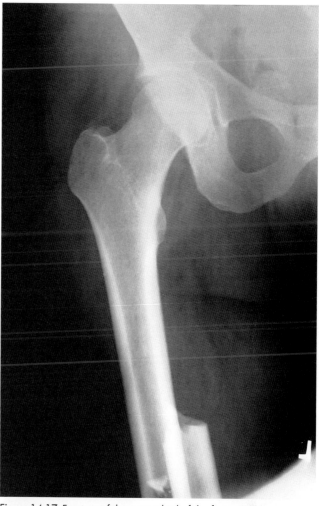

Figure 14.17 Fracture of the upper third of the femur.

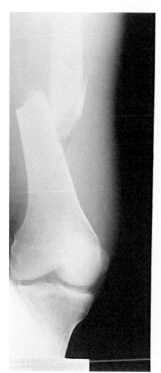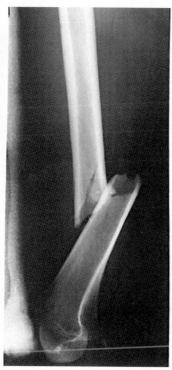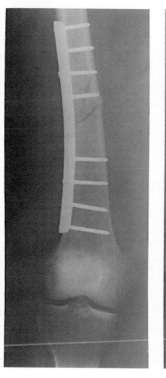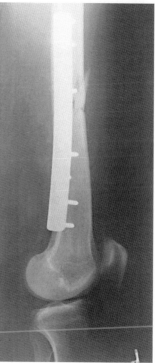

Figure 14.18 Fracture of the lower third of the femur.

fragment angulates posteriorly due to the unopposed pull of the quadriceps.

There can be a considerable blood loss in these types of injury, and prompt resuscitation may be required.

## Traumatic Dislocations of the Hip

These are relatively rare and usually require a severe mechanism of injury. The most common form is the posterior dislocation, which usually results from a road traffic accident, when the victim's knee hits the dashboard and a longitudinal force is directed up the femur. The head of the femur is dislocated, and the posterior rim of the acetabulum is often fractured (**Figure 14.19**). There is severe pain in the groin.

The leg lies internally rotated, is shortened and is often slightly flexed at the hip. The greater trochanter appears unduly prominent. The sciatic nerve is injured in up to 10 per cent of cases.

In a central dislocation of the hip, the head of the femur is driven through the floor of the acetabulum, which is fractured, creating a protrusio acetabuli type of injury. There may be signs of a direct blow to the side of the hip and the leg tends to be abducted. Movements are painful.

Anterior dislocation is very rare and usually occurs after a fall from a height onto the feet. The leg is abducted, externally rotated and slightly flexed. The femoral head is palpable in the groin. There is usually no shortening because upward migration of the hip is prevented by the iliofemoral ligament.

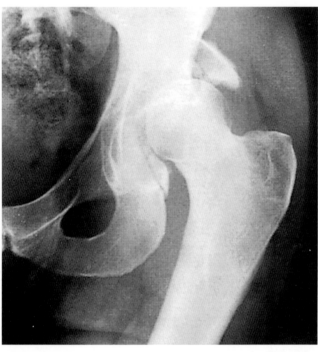

Figure 14.19 Dislocation of the hip with an associated acetabular fracture.

### Key Points

- The pelvis and acetabulum form a solid unit that usually fails in significant traumatic stress. A systematic approach to these injuries should be adopted.
- As with all other joints, examination of the hip starts with inspection, palpation and assessment of the range of motion. Special diagnostic tests and manoeuvres such as the Trendelenburg sign and Thomas's test should be conducted.
- Paediatric hip pathologies vary according to the age of presentation and frequency of the condition. They may be divided into hereditary or developmental pathologies, such as developmental dysplasia of the hip, Legg–Calvé–Perthes disease and inflammatory or infectious conditions, such as toxic synovitis and septic arthritis.
- Adult hip pathologies range from intra-articular conditions, such as osteoarthritis and avascular necrosis, to compressive neuropathy, such as meralgia paraesthetica, and mechanical problems, for example psoas bursitis and hip snapping.
- The devastating complications of hip arthroplasty consist of dislocation, aseptic loosening and infections. The more tolerable ones include trochanteric bursitis and heterotopic ossifications.
- Traumatic hip injuries include fractures of different anatomical areas of the hip such as the femoral neck, trochanters and femoral shaft. Another major culprit is traumatic dislocation.

PART 2 | TRAUMA AND (ELECTIVE) ORTHOPAEDICS

## QUESTIONS

### SBAs

**1.** Which one of the following statements about developmental dysplasia of the hip is incorrect?:

a  It is more common in girls than boys
b  Abduction of the thighs is limited
c  The gluteal folds are symmetrical
d  Ortolani's test may be positive
e  Radiography of the hip is not indicated at birth

**Answer**

c  *The gluteal folds are symmetrical. Developmental dysplasia of the hip is a 'packaging problem' that affects a wide range of patients. It is vital to detect the condition as early as possible to salvage the function of the lower extremity. It is more common in females. The hip relocation test or Ortolani test is usually positive in infancy. Abduction of the hip is limited, the gluteal folds are asymmetrical and a leg length discrepancy can be noted. Radiography of the hip is postponed until the physis begins to ossify at 3–6 months of age.*

**2.** Which one of the following correctly describes osteoarthrosis of the hip?:

a  Pain is mostly felt in the groin and is most exacerbated by internal rotation
b  Pain is mostly mechanical and leads to a gradual decrease in the tolerated walking distance
c  It may cause a true limb length discrepancy due to loss of the joint space
d  It can be a primary process or arise secondary to another entity such as trauma or hip dysplasia
e  All of the above are true

**Answer**

e  *All of the above are true. Osteoarthrosis of the hip is a degenerative process that develops with age as a primary condition or can be secondary to a previous insult to the hip joint such as in osteonecrosis of the femoral head or hip dysplasia. The joint space gradually narrows and may be obliterated, causing stiffness and shortening of the involved lower extremity. The pain is mostly mechanical and is exacerbated by walking; however, in severe cases it may be continuous at rest and at night. Pain and apprehension upon internal rotation of the hip may be indicative of hip osteoarthrosis as it largely suggests an intra-articular pathology.*

**3.** In a traumatic hip dislocation, which one of the following is true?:

a  The force is posterior, causing an anterior dislocation
b  The involved lower extremity is shortened and externally rotated
c  It may be associated with a posterior acetabular wall fracture
d  The risk of nerve injury is close to zero
e  The mechanism of injury is usually mild, such as a fall on the hip

**Answer**

c  *It may be associated with a posterior acetabular wall fracture. Traumatic hip dislocation usually results from a severe mechanism of injury such as a high-speed road traffic accident. The knee hits the dashboard, resulting in a posterior hip dislocation with a possible posterior acetabular wall fracture and a sciatic nerve injury in 10 per cent of cases. On examination, the involved extremity is shortened and internally rotated.*

### EMQs

**1.** For each of the following conditions, select the sign or test that will produce the proper diagnosis. Each option may be used once, more than once or not at all:

1  Barlow's manoeuvre
2  Thomas's test
3  Trendelenburg sign
4  Gauvain's test
5  FABER test

a  Flexion contracture of the hip
b  Abductor weakness

**Answers**

a  *2 Thomas's test. This is a physical examination to detect hip flexion contracture. With the patient supine on the examination table, the hip is flexed towards the abdomen. Any flexion in the contralateral hip is a sign of flexion deformity at the hip.*
b  *3 Trendelenburg sign. This test detects weakness in the abductors of the hip joint. It is performed by asking the patient to stand on the affected side. The Trendelenburg*

c Transient synovitis
d Sacroiliitis
e Developmental hip dysplasia

test is positive if the pelvis drops on the unaffected contralateral side.

c **4 Gauvain's test.** This is used to detect synovitis of the hip joint. The test is positive if there is involuntary contraction of the abdominal muscles upon internal rotation of the extended hip.

d **5 FABER test.** FABER stands for **f**lexion, **ab**duction, and **e**xternal **r**otation of the hip. The test is used to evaluate pain or pathology in the sacroiliac joint. Pain elicited on the opposite side is a sign of sacroiliitis.

e **1 Barlow's manoeuvre.** This is a screening examination for developmental dysplasia of the hip in newborns. It is performed by adducting the hip and applying posterior pressure on the knee, thus attempting to dislocate the hip. The test is considered positive if the hip is dislocatable.

2. **For each of the following pathological entities, select the correct location of the hip pain:**
    1 Lateral
    2 Inguinal
    3 Anterior
    4 Posterior
    5 Mons pubis
 a Degenerative arthritis of the hip
 b Impingement syndrome
 c Ischial bursitis
 d Fracture of the superior pubic ramus
 e Trochanteric bursitis

Answers

a **2 Inguinal.** Inguinal or groin pain is most often a sign of arthritis in the hip joint.

b **3 Anterior.** Anterior hip pain typically occurs due to hip impingement. The pain becomes worse after prolonged periods of sitting.

c **4 Posterior.** Patients with ischial bursitis commonly present with pain in the posterior hip or lower buttock region.

d **5 Mons pubis.** Pain in the mons pubis area can be a sign of a fracture of the superior pubic ramus.

e **1 Lateral.** Lateral hip pain is a common presenting symptom of trochanteric bursitis, which can further be confirmed by tenderness over the greater trochanter of the hip.

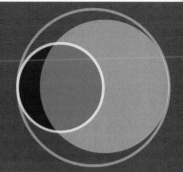

# The Knee Joint

Muhyeddine Al Taki and Firas Kawtharani

## LEARNING OBJECTIVES

- To identify abnormalities of the knee by an observation of gait, malalignment and the presence of deformities
- To carry out a systematic examination of the knee, including the viscoelastic and bony structures
- To recognize various ligamentous pathologies affecting the stability of the knee

- To identify the different degenerative and inflammatory conditions that affect the knee joint
- To be efficient in evaluating the aetiology of anterior knee pain
- To recognize traumatic knee injuries

## GENERAL EXAMINATION OF THE KNEE

### Gait

An antalgic or apprehensive gait can stem from a myriad of painful knee conditions, resulting in muscle wasting around the joint. The straight leg gait, in which the patient circumducts the affected leg during its swing phase, results from knee fusion or from a flexion deficit in cases of effusion or advanced arthritis.

There is a resulting shortening of step length as well as an increase in metabolic demands. In long-standing weakness of the quadriceps muscle, control of the knee is diminished and hyperextension of the knee may be present during the stance phase.

### Observation with the Patient Standing

Childhood deformity may result from congenital bone dysplasias, paralytic disorders or developmental growth plate abnormalities. In adults, it may result from previous traumatic injuries or compartmental knee arthritis.

Deformities in the coronal plane, i.e. varus/valgus angulation, are better elicited with the patient standing and weight-bearing. The normal physiological angulation between the shafts of the tibia and femur is 5–7° of valgus. An angulation in excess of this is genu valgum, or knock knees (**Figure 15.1**), whereas an angulation of less than this constitutes genu varum – bow legs (**Figure 15.2**). Deformities in the sagittal plane are also better elicited in the standing position. Examples are a flexion deformity due to arthritis or a mechanical block to full extension resulting from a complex meniscal tear. Another example is a recurvatum or hyperextension deformity, which is evident in cases of hypermobility, ligamentous injury or long-standing quadriceps weakness.

The presence of scars or sinuses should also be noted.

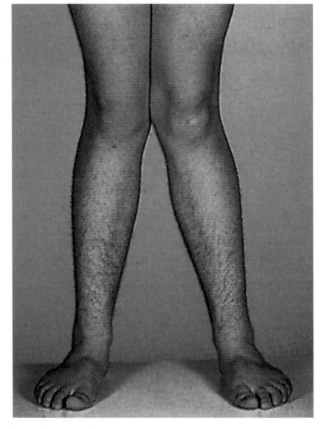

Figure 15.1 Knock knees.

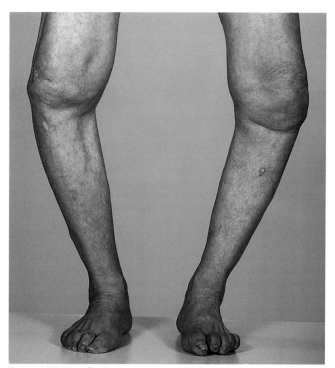

Figure 15.2 Bow legs.

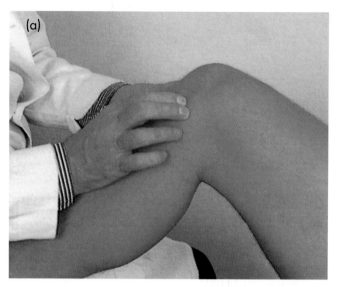

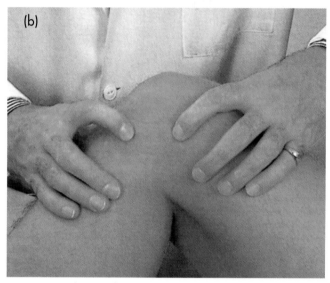

Figure 15.3 Palpation of the knee joint. Palpation of proximal and distal ends of the medial ligament.

## Examination with the Patient Supine

The back of the examination couch can be placed at 45° so that the patient is comfortable and the posterior structures of the lower limb are relaxed when the knee is extended. The thigh and calf should be observed for wasting of the quadriceps muscle and gastrocsoleus complex, respectively. Circumferential measurements can be made with a measuring tape for a comparative evaluation (see Figure 29.4).

Observations should be made for generalized and local swelling around the knee. Generalized swelling suggests that a joint effusion is present, whereas localized swelling with bruising at a specific region of the knee may point to a limited bony or ligamentous injury. Swelling at the level of the joint line may indicate osteophyte formation or a meniscal cyst depending on the presentation. A swelling confined to the popliteal area is usually due to a fluid-filled popliteal bursa or Baker's cyst. Redness of the skin, effusion and an increased temperature indicate an inflammatory or infectious process in the knee.

## Palpation

Palpation is preferably done in a systematic way whether in extension or in flexion (**Figures 15.3** and **15.4**).

The examiner can palpate the anatomical landmarks along the longitudinal axis, starting proximally with the suprapatellar pouch, patella, patellar tendon and tibial tuberosity. Along the mediolateral axis at the joint line, the structures to be palpated are the medial collateral ligament, medial meniscus, patellar tendon, lateral meniscus and lateral collateral ligaments. Pain may also be elicited from bony prominences, such as the tibial and femoral condyles, as well as entheses such as the pes anserinus (see p. 263) and Gerdy's tubercle (the tibial attachment of the iliotibial tract).

Finally, the popliteal fossa should be palpated to detect any fullness.

## Testing for an Effusion

Excess fluid within the knee joint cavity translates into an effusion. The first signs are bulging at the medial and lateral parapatellar gutters. Further swelling creates fullness in the suprapatellar pouch. In the **patellar tap test or ballottement test** (**Figure 15.5**), the suprapatellar pouch is emptied by pressing above the patella with one hand, which will induce 'floating' of the patella. In the presence of a significant effusion, axial compression on the patella with the other hand produces a click as it strikes the trochlear groove.

The **stroke or fluid displacement test (Figure 15.6)** is used to detect small effusions. The suprapatellar pouch is emptied as in the ballotement test. The examiner then uses their other hand to stroke the medial parapatellar gutter to displace the fluid to the lateral side. The lateral parapatellar gutter is then sequentially

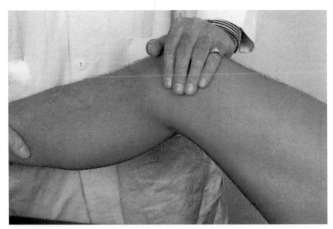

Figure 15.4 Eliciting crepitus. The examiner's left hand is palpating the joint while the right is used to passively flex and extend the knee.

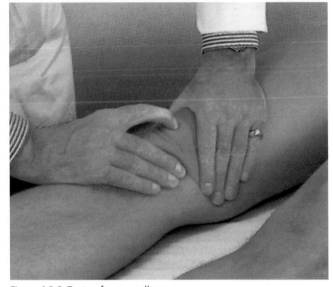

Figure 15.5 Testing for a patellar tap.

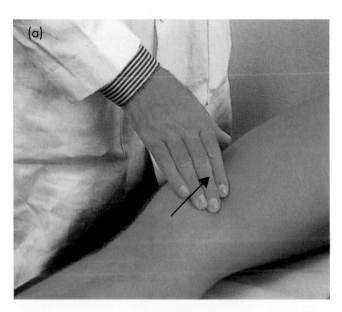

(a)

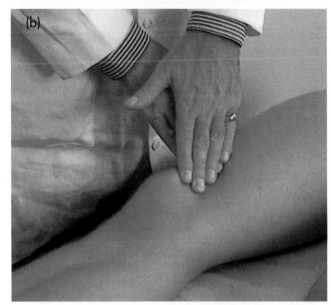

(b)

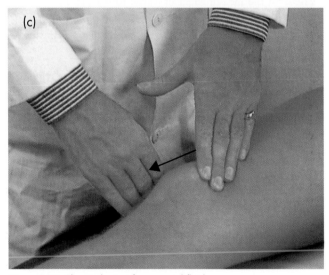

(c)

Figure 15.6 The stroke test for synovial fluid.

stroked and the medial side observed for movement as fluid passes from the lateral gutter into the medial gutter.

## Range of Motion

The patient should first be asked to demonstrate the limits of active flexion and extension. Then, with the patient lying in the supine position, the examiner grips the dorsiflexed ankle with one hand while pushing downwards on the patella with other hand (**Figure 15.7**). An inability to fully extend the knee is a flexion deformity. A non-rigid flexion deformity may be due to a mechanical block to extension, suggestive of a bucket-handle meniscal tear or loose body. A rigid or fixed flexion deformity is the result of capsular contracture, as in degenerative conditions.

If the knee extends 5–10° beyond a straight tibiofemoral line while pushing downwards on the patella as described above, a recurvatum or hyperextension deformity exists. This condition is seen mostly in joint laxity and patellofemoral pathologies, as well as in ligamentous injuries.

An inability of the patient to fully extend the knee despite the success of the examiner in doing so points to the presence of an extensor lag related to a deficient quadriceps.

PART 2 | TRAUMA AND (ELECTIVE) ORTHOPAEDICS

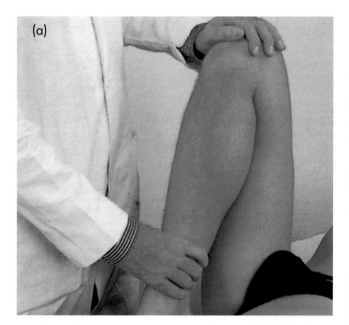

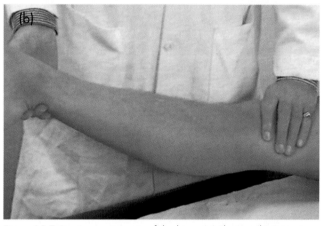

Figure 15.7 Passive movements of the knee. (a) Flexion. (b) Extension.

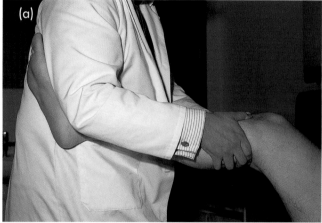

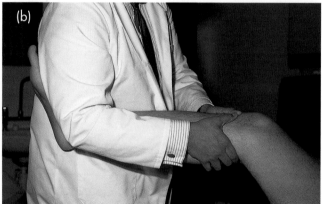

Figure 15.8 (a) Varus and (b) valgus stress test (method 1).

Flexion is regarded as normal if the examiner obtains 130–135°of flexion from a fully extended knee. A periodic increase in the measurement of a heel to buttock distance can evaluate the progress of a flexion deficit. Loss of flexion is mostly associated with an effusion or an arthritic process.

## Tests for Ligamentous Laxity
### Collateral Ligaments

**Varus and valgus stress tests** are used to determine if there is injury to the lateral or medial collateral ligaments, respectively. Two methods can be used:

- A varus or valgus force can be applied by stressing the medial or lateral side of the knee, respectively. The patient's ankle can be stabilized between the examiner's elbow and trunk (**Figure 15.8**), allowing the examiner's hands to be placed either side of the knee. Movement in excess of that seen in the normal knee is noted.
- The second more sensitive method involves placing one examining hand behind the knee with the fingers and the thumb on either side of the knee (**Figure 15.9**). The other

hand grasps the ankle and applies a varus or valgus force while the femur is restrained by the hand behind the knee, which applies an opposing force.

Any opening at the joint line is felt using the thumb.

The test should be carried out in both full extension and slight flexion. Full extension of the knee causes tightening of the posterior capsule and the posterior cruciate ligament, adding stability to the knee. Abnormal movement in full extension indicates a major ligamentous/capsular rupture in addition to damage to the collateral ligament. Carrying the test out using 30° of flexion is more specific for an injury limited to the collateral ligaments.

An arthritic knee may demonstrate a fixed deformity of the knee into varus or valgus due to loss of the articular cartilage on either the medial or lateral side of the knee, respectively.

These tests are complemented by inspection for bruising and tenderness at the most common area of detachment of the involved collateral ligament – the medial femoral condyle in the case of a medial collateral ligament injury, and the fibular head in a lateral collateral ligament injury.

### Anterior Cruciate Ligament

In the **Lachman test** (**Figure 15.10**), the knee is relaxed and flexed to 20° and the examiner grasps the thigh and upper calf, one in each hand. A forward translational force is applied to the tibia while the femur is stabilized. The knees are compared, an

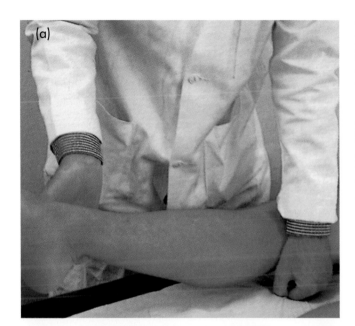

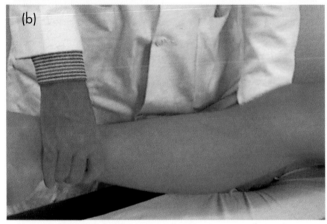

Figure 15.9 (a) Varus and (b) valgus stress test (method 2).

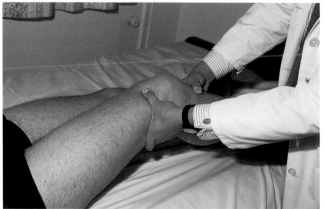

Figure 15.10 Lachman test.

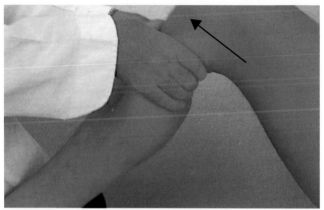

Figure 15.11 Anterior drawer test.

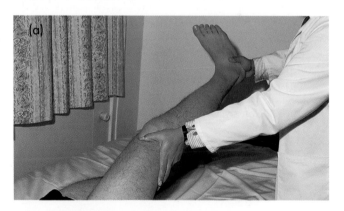

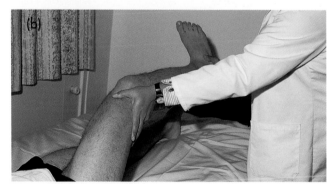

Figure 15.12 Pivot shift test.

increase in movement suggests a complete or partial rupture of the anterior cruciate ligament.

To perform the **anterior drawer test (Figure 15.11)**, the knees are flexed to 90°. The examiner steadies the patient's feet by sitting lightly on their toes and grasps the leg with both hands at the level of the tibial tubercle with the fingers palpating the hamstring tendons to confirm that they are relaxed. An anterior force is applied; a displacement of more than 1 cm suggests a high possibility of a tear involving the anterior cruciate ligament. Note that a false positive anterior drawer test may be elicited if the posterior cruciate ligament is already ruptured.

The **pivot shift test (Figure 15.12)** is used to confirm instability of the knee resulting from rupture of the anterior cruciate ligament. The patient lies supine with the hip in neutral rotation and slightly flexed. The knee is held in full extension. The examiner holds the foot internally rotated in one hand and applies a valgus stress to the knee with the other. If there is a rupture of the anterior cruciate ligament, this manoeuvre will lead to a forward subluxation of the lateral tibial condyle on the femur. The knee is then flexed smoothly from full extension. A positive test result occurs if there is a palpable clunk at about 20–30° as the tibia reduces into its normal position.

### Posterior Cruciate Ligament

In the **posterior drawer test (Figure 15.13)**, both knees are flexed to 90° with the feet placed together. The knees are observed from the lateral side: a posterior sag of the tibia on the femur of the involved extremity indicates that there has been a rupture of the posterior cruciate ligament. A posteriorly directed force on the tibia is confirmatory, and an anterior force on the tibia should reduce the tibia to its normal position.

### The Arcuate Ligament Complex

The **arcuate ligament** is a thickening of the posterior capsule. It arises from the fibular head and diverges such that one limb is attached to the femoral condyle and popliteus tendon, while the other limb curves over the popliteus and is attached to the back of the lateral meniscus.

**Posterolateral rotatory instability** of the knee results from disruption of the arcuate ligament complex, which is made up of the arcuate ligament, the lateral collateral ligament, the tendoaponeurotic portion of the popliteus muscle and the lateral head of the gastrocnemius. The posterior cruciate ligament is also injured in the majority of cases. This usually occurs after a sporting injury or a traffic accident.

The **external rotation recurvatum test** is positive in posterolateral rotatory instability. With the patient supine, the legs are elevated from the examining table by grasping the great toes and lifting them. The test is positive if the involved knee falls into external rotation, varus and recurvatum.

In the **posterolateral drawer test**, the knee is flexed to 90° and the examiner sits gently on the patient's toes. The tibia is pushed posteriorly, a positive test result occurring when the lateral side of the tibial plateau is subluxed posteriorly in relation to the femoral condyle. The medial side of the tibial plateau remains stationary.

## Signs of a Meniscal Injury

There may be wasting of the quadriceps muscle if the tear has been present for some weeks. A block to full extension may also be present. Tenderness can be elicited at the level of the joint line over the torn meniscus. Oedema over the involved joint line may be present in recent meniscal injuries.

In the **McMurray test (Figure 15.14)**, the hip is flexed to 90° and the knee to over 90°. The examiner uses one hand to grasp the knee with their fingers over both joint lines, and the other hand to grasp the foot. The knee is taken from a position of abduction and external rotation to adduction and internal rotation by applying force to the foot. The test is repeated in varying degrees of flexion. The test is positive if there is a palpable click in the appropriate compartment of the knee as the torn meniscus becomes entrapped within the knee. A comparative test should be carried out on the normal knee to rule out the presence of a non-pathological click.

In **Apley's test (Figure 15.15)**, the menisci are challenged by applying rotational and compressive forces over the knee. The patient lies prone with the knee flexed to 90°. The thigh is fixed by the examiner's knee, and the foot is externally rotated and then internally rotated in extension. The torn meniscus elicits sharp pain on various degrees of rotation. The examiner then exerts an axial downward force over the flexed knee while externally and internally rotating the foot. A sharp pain is indicative of a tear in the medial meniscus on external rotation and the lateral meniscus in internal rotation.

The **Thessaly test** has recently been designed to detect the presence of a meniscal tear with a high sensitivity and specificity. The examiner holds the patient by his outstretched hands while

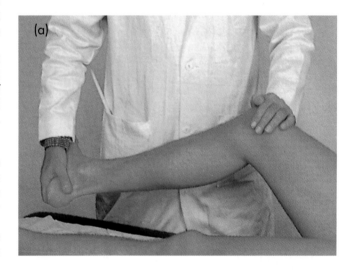

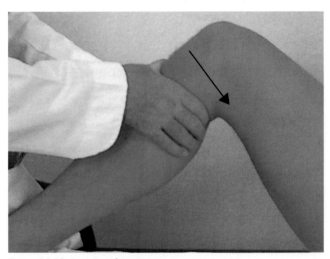

Figure 15.13 Posterior drawer test.

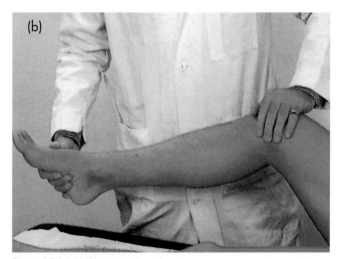

Figure 15.14 McMurray test.

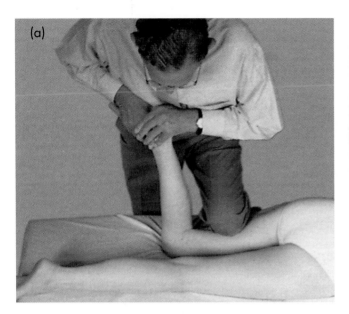

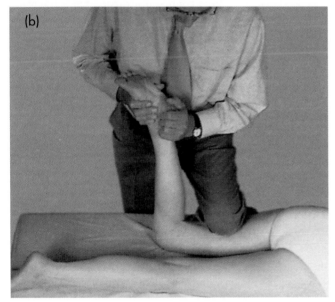

Figure 15.15 Apley's grinding test. (Reproduced with permission from *Physical Examination in Orthopaedics*, by A. Graham Apley and Louis Solomon, Butterworth-Heinemann, 1997.)

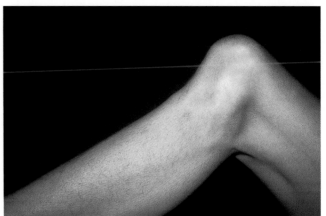

Figure 15.16 Long-standing cruciate ligament damage. Note the joint laxity.

An injury to the intra-articular elements leads to swelling. It is important to know the time period between the injury and the onset of swelling. Immediate swelling of the knee usually results from bleeding into the joint cavity – haemarthrosis – due to tearing of the vascularized structures inside the knee. This leads to great discomfort. There could be a tear of a cruciate ligament or peripheral detachment of the meniscus, but an intra-articular fracture may have occurred and radiographs should therefore be taken.

Symptomatic haemarthrosis is usually aspirated using an aseptic technique. The fluid can be investigated to detect the presence of globules of fat as this strongly suggests a fracture. An effusion that occurs some hours after the injury is suggestive of a traumatic synovitis, which usually does not involve any major structure in the knee, although this scenario may mask the presence of a meniscal tear in the avascular zone. Muscle spasm and swelling make interpretation of the limitation of movement difficult, while pain and apprehension limit testing for a ligamentous laxity (**Figure 15.16**). In these circumstances, it is important to re-examine the knee some days later when a more accurate assessment can be made.

## The Locked Knee and Meniscal Injury

The menisci transmit a significant proportion of the body weight through the knee, and meniscal tears are the most common injuries to the knee that necessitate surgery. These injuries occur most commonly in athletes where there is sudden twisting motion of the flexed weight-bearing knee, leading to a tear in the substance of the meniscus.

When the displaced fragment crosses or gets settled in the intercondylar notch, true locking of the knee usually occurs. This is strongly suggestive of a displaced bucket-handle tear of the meniscus. The locked knee is one of the few conditions in which a reasonable presumptive diagnosis can be made after an acute knee injury. The patient is unable to fully extend the knee. Passive knee extension by the examiner comes up against a firm elastic resistance, preventing full extension. The other causes of a locked knee are a loose body, a torn remnant of the anterior cruciate ligament and a symptomatic discoid meniscus.

The usual initial presentation of a torn meniscus is of an acute knee injury. In middle age, however, the menisci undergo degenerate change with loss of elasticity whereby the slightest trauma can cause a tear.

the patient stands on his symptomatic foot. The patient then rotates his knee, internally and externally, at 5° and then 20° of flexion. Pain, catching or locking is indicative of a torn meniscus.

## ACUTE INJURIES OF THE KNEE

These are a common occurrence and involve either a direct blow to the knee or a twisting injury with or without a 'pop' being felt. The patient presents with pain, swelling and a limited range of motion of the knee. It is often difficult to make an accurate diagnosis at the initial assessment. Certain features should, however, be sought.

In the case of injury during a sporting event, it is useful to know whether the patient was able to finish the event; if so, it is less likely that there is a serious injury.

These tears may cause pain and discomfort but are usually self-limiting. In certain cases, however, there is interference with movement between the joint surfaces due to a loose meniscal fragment, especially when the knee is flexed and twisted during normal activities. The patient thus complains of intermittent true 'locking' of the knee.

The patient's complaint of 'locking' should be carefully compared with the precise medical meaning of locking, which means an inability to fully extend the knee because of a mechanical obstruction to movement:

- *True locking* of the knee occurs as a result of a mechanical obstruction from a loose body obstructing the joint surfaces. The patient may be able to overcome the locking by shaking the limb or twisting the knee, resulting in a sudden freeing of knee movement.
- '*Pseudolocking*' often arises from patellofemoral joint disorders when the patient finds it painful to move the knee to change from a flexed position; there is no true mechanical obstruction to joint movement.

Only 40 per cent of all meniscal tears are displaced into the joint, causing locking of the knee. Other symptoms include pain at the joint line, especially on twisting or kneeling, repeated swelling and giving way of the knee. The other signs of a meniscal tear are quadriceps wasting, intermittent mild effusion, tenderness at the joint line and a positive McMurray, Apley's or Thessaly test.

## Rupture of the Ligaments

Ligamentous rupture requires a considerable degree of violence following direct trauma such as a traffic accident or a sports-related injury. The mechanism is usually a non-contact pivoting injury with an audible 'pop'. There is usually haemarthrosis if the ligament is intra-articular, or bruising if the ligament is extra-articular. An immediate diagnosis often cannot be made with certainty due to the patient's generalized apprehension, and therefore a little time must be allowed for these acute symptoms to settle.

Rupture of the **medial collateral ligament** results from vigorous ball games and skiing, in which a severe valgus force is applied to the knee. If the knee is examined a few days after the injury, there may be visible swelling and bruising on the medial side of the knee. There is tenderness over the ligamentous attachments, the medial aspect of the knee and the joint line. When a valgus stress is applied to the knee at 30°, there is excessive laxity and pain. Incomplete injuries are often more painful than complete ruptures on valgus stress, due to stretching of the remaining injured but intact ligament fibers, but marked instability is noted with complete injuries.

Rupture of the **lateral collateral ligament** of the knee occurs when severe varus forces are applied to a knee in 30° of flexion. The discrete cord-like ligament runs from the femoral condyle to the head of the fibula. When it is torn, there may be swelling and bruising laterally, tenderness over the ligamentous attachments and lateral joint line, and excessive movement when a varus stress is applied to the knee. The injury can be associated with a palsy of the common peroneal nerve.

Rupture of the **anterior cruciate ligament** occurs in hyperextension injuries, when the ligament is tented over the intercondylar notch in the femur. It is also ruptured in severe valgus injuries of the knee when there is associated rupture of the medial collateral ligament of the knee and tearing of the medial meniscus – O'Donoghue's triad. The physical signs of anterior cruciate ligament injury are of an effusion (often a haemarthrosis), a positive anterior drawer test, a positive Lachman's test (the most sensitive test) and a positive pivot shift test.

Rupture of the **posterior cruciate ligament** results from a violent injury such as striking the dashboard of a car in an accident, hyperflexion or hyperextension. In an acute injury, there may be swelling and bruising in the popliteal fossa. The knee exhibits more hyperextension than the uninjured side when the legs are lifted off the couch by holding the heels. The posterior drawer test reveals a posterior sag of the tibia, which can be increased by a posteriorly directed force and reduced to normal by an anterior force.

Injury to the **arcuate ligament complex** and the posterior cruciate ligament gives rise to **posterolateral rotatory instability** of the knee. This usually occurs after a sporting injury or motor accident. The external rotation, recurvatum and posterolateral drawer tests are positive.

## Loose Bodies

Loose bodies may appear after long-term osteoarthritis, osteochondral defects, synovial chondromatosis and rarely traumatic events. The patient often describes something moving in the joint and can sometimes even feel the loose body. There is often a history of the knee giving way or of painful clicking. The physical findings are often non-specific unless the joint is locked at the time of consultation. Radiographs are required to demonstrate the loose body.

## Osteochondritis Dissecans

This is a common cause of loose bodies in young people, predominantly men. The inciting event is mostly an occult trauma. The site of the lesion is usually the medial femoral condyle, adjacent to the intercondylar notch. There is an area of osteonecrosis and partial detachment of articular cartilage resulting from intra-articular impingement upon movement.

The patient has symptoms of pain and recurrent effusion; catching and locking can occasionally occur if a loose body detaches in the joint. A false-positive patellar grind test is usually present due to rubbing of the patella against the lesion upon flexion and extension of the knee. This condition is rarely seen in the patella, in which it gives rise to anterior knee pain.

### ANTERIOR KNEE PAIN

Pain in the anterior aspect of the knee occurs mostly in middle-aged and elderly patients. It is worsened by prolonged sitting, walking and going up and down stairs. Changes in the articular cartilage of the patella and trochlea are the primary problems. The spectrum ranges from minor cartilage fibrillation via chondromalacia to frank patellofemoral arthritis. Anterior knee pain can also present as well in the younger population due to different underlying aetiologies, described below.

## Patellar Malalignment

Patients may show an altered quadriceps angle (Q angle), that is, the angle between the line joining the anterior superior iliac spine to the centre of the patella and the line joining the centre of the patella to the tibial tuberosity. Other causes are weakness of the vastus medialis muscle and tightness of the hamstring muscles. These conditions can alter the mechanics of the patellofemoral joint, leading to excessive forces across it and producing anterior knee pain.

## Chondromalacia Patellae

This is a usually self-limiting condition that is seen in young adults and adolescents. There is softening and fibrillation involving the articular cartilage of the patella. On examination, there may be wasting of the quadriceps muscle and an effusion. A patellar grind test is usually positive in flexion and extension. The condition is likely to be a late sequel a of a traumatic event.

## Synovial Shelf Syndrome

The medial synovial shelf or fold is an embryological remnant. Impingement of this synovial shelf on the femoral condyle can cause abrasions affecting the condylar cartilage and thus antero-medial knee pain. It should be suspected when tenderness can be elicited along the medial patellar retinaculum during flexion and extension of the knee.

## Lateral Facet Compression Syndrome

This condition is due to a tight lateral patellar retinaculum and excessive lateral tilt. Patellofemoral tenderness is exacerbated when the lateral facet of the patella is pushed laterally against the femur, and is reduced when the examiner pushes it medially. The mobility of the patella is usually compromised.

## Patellar Tendonitis (Jumper's Knee)

This condition involves the patellar tendon near its origin at the inferior pole of the patella, and is seen in jumping athletes such as basketball or volleyball players. It is associated with pain and tenderness at the torn tendon fibers.

## Osgood–Schlatter's Disease

This is a traction apophysitis of the tibial tubercle (**Figure 15.17**). It occurs in adolescents during their growth spurt and is most common in athletic youngsters. The tibial tuberosity is tender and unusually prominent. The diagnosis is confirmed with radiographs.

## Sinding-Larsen–Johansson Disease

This occurs predominantly in children under 10 years of age and is characterized by tenderness of the lower pole of the patella and the adjacent patellar tendon. The aetiology is similar to Osgood–Schlatter's disease.

## Patellar Instability

In normal circumstances, the patella engages the trochlear groove at 30–40° of flexion, and when the quadriceps muscle contracts with the knee in the extended position, the patella should be pulled superiorly in a straight direction. At terminal extension with an unstable patella, however, the patella may be seen to sublux laterally out of the trochlear groove. As the knee goes into flexion again, the patella may be noted to jump back into the groove. This is called the patellar **J sign** and indicates abnormal tracking of the patella.

**Sage's sign** is indicative of a tight lateral retinaculum. The patient lies supine and relaxed with the knee flexed to 20°. The examiner then attempts to displace the patella medially – excursion of the patella of less than one-quarter of its maximum width is considered a positive result, while 10 mm of displacement medially is considered normal, and 5 mm or less abnormal.

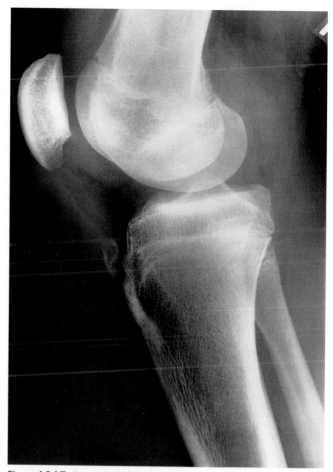

Figure 15.17 Osgood–Schlatter's disease.

The **patellar apprehension test** is indicative of dynamic instability and recurrent dislocations. The patient lies supine with the knee flexed to 20°. The examiner displaces the patella laterally. Patients with instability fire their quadriceps in response to the painful gliding motion of the patella.

The **quadriceps (Q) angle** indicates the relative angle of insertion of the quadriceps mechanism. It is measured, as described above, by drawing two imaginary lines connecting the centre of the patella to the anterior superior iliac spine proximally and the tibial tuberosity distally. The angle of intersection of these lines is the Q angle. The average Q angle in males is 14°, and in females 17°. A Q angle greater than 20° is considered abnormal and is associated with patellar instability.

## Patellar Dislocation

Many factors can contribute to patellar instability and ultimately recurrent lateral dislocations. These can include, for example, abnormal patellar tracking and an increased Q angle due to excessive femoral anteversion, genu valgum and a wide pelvis. Other factors are related to poor patellofemoral contact due to hypoplasia affecting the condylar groove or the patella itself. The patella may be high-riding and thus fail to engage in the femoral sulcus. Tight lateral structures or lax medial structures may contribute to lateral patellar dislocation.

Acute dislocations also occur laterally and are usually the result of a traumatic event in an athlete. When examined a few days after reduction of the patella, there is usually bruising and swelling medial to the patella due to tearing of the medial capsule and medial patellofemoral ligament (**Figure 15.18**).

Radiographs should be carefully examined for evidence of a fracture of the patella or lateral femoral condyle. Not infrequently, an osteochondral fragment is sheared off during the dislocation and should be removed or fixed back into place. Examine the lateral radiograph for evidence of a lipohaemarthrosis, that is, fat floating on top of the effusion, seen in the suprapatellar bursa. If in doubt, aspirate the knee and look for fat globules floating on the haemarthrosis. A lipohaemarthrosis indicates that a fracture is present.

In cases of recurrent dislocation, the signs suggestive of patellar instability are Sage's sign, a positive patellar apprehension test and a patellar J sign. The diagnosis can be confirmed by examination under anesthesia.

## Anterior Fat Pad (Hoffa's) Syndrome

There is a substantial fat pad lying deep to the patellar tendon. This may be injured by direct trauma to the knee, with resulting fibrosis and oedema. In the chronic condition, there is pain when the knee is fully extended as the fat pad is compressed between the articular surface of the femur and tibia. There is also tenderness to palpation on examination. Premenstrual fluid retention in women may lead to swelling of the fat pad and an exacerbation of the symptoms.

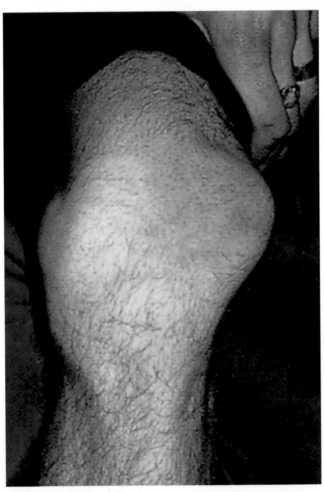

Figure 15.18 Patellar dislocation.

## Prepatellar Bursitis (Housemaid's Knee)

This is the most common bursitis affecting the knee. It is brought on by trauma and overuse in activities such as prolonged kneeling. Swelling in the prepatellar bursa ensues. Redness, swelling and tenderness anterior to the patella are the usual signs (**Figure 15.19**).

If a penetrating injury has occurred, this bursa may be infected with pyogenic organisms, leading to a surrounding cellulitis. The range of movement in the knee should, however, be well preserved, differentiating this condition from septic arthritis.

## Infrapatellar Bursitis (Clergyman's Knee)

There is a cystic subcutaneous swelling overlying the patellar tendon and tibial tuberosity that is caused by activities similar to those causing prepatellar bursitis. The signs are similar but the swelling is more distal.

## CYSTS AROUND THE KNEE

### The Semimembranosus Bursa

This cyst lies between the medial head of the gastrocnemius and semimembranosus tendon and is found on the medial side of the popliteal fossa. It is tense when the knee is extended and flaccid when the joint is flexed. It does not communicate with the joint and cannot be emptied by compression.

### Popliteal (Baker's) Cyst

The swelling is more central and is lower in the popliteal fossa than the semimembranosus bursa. The patient is likely to be of middle age or above. The cyst is formed from synovium that herniates through a hiatus in the capsule of the joint, and is associated with rheumatoid arthritis or osteoarthritis. Although the cyst is in communication with the cavity of the knee joint, the channel may be very small and it may not be possible to express fluid from the cyst into the knee itself.

The popliteal cyst is prone to rupture spontaneously or after minor trauma (**Figure 15.20**) or strenuous exercise – which results in pain, swelling and tenderness in the calf – and has a clinical picture that is similar to deep vein thrombosis. Swelling and bruising in the dorsum of the foot may, however, differentiate a Baker's cyst from a deep venous thrombosis.

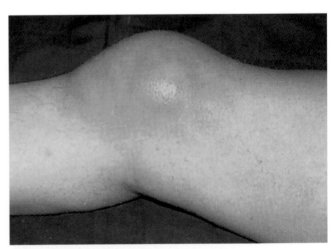

Figure 15.19 Prepatellar bursitis.

## The Bursa Anserina

This is located about 6 cm distal to the joint line medially between the tendons of the sartorius, gracilis and semitendinosus muscles superficially, and the medial collateral ligament of the knee deep to the bursa. When distended and swollen, it is apparent over the anteromedial tibia. It is also referred to as breast-stroker's knee.

## Meniscal Cysts

This is a swelling on the medial or lateral aspect of the knee at the level of the joint line (**Figure 15.21**). The aetiology of the lesion is a degenerate tear within the meniscus that creates a

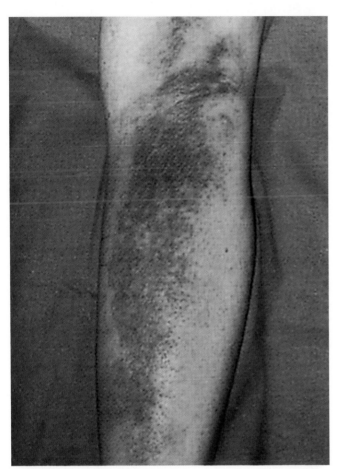

Figure 15.20 A ruptured Baker's cyst.

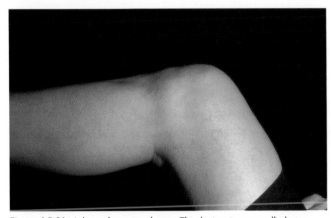

Figure 15.21 A lateral meniscal cyst. This lesion is unusually large.

one-way valve mechanism. The synovium herniates through the tear, creating a cystic outgrowth filled with joint fluid. Depending on the nature of the opening between cyst and joint, there may be intermittent or progressive enlargement. In the '**disappearing sign**', the cyst is apparent when the knee is extended and less apparent or absent when the knee is flexed.

## ARTHRITIS OF THE KNEE

### Septic Arthritis of the Knee

The knee is swollen and held in 20–30° of flexion. The overlying skin is often red and hot. A tense effusion is present, effacing the anatomical landmarks of the knee and preventing the patient from engaging in any sort of movement at the joint. There may be systemic symptoms such as fever, chills and lethargy. Any patient presenting in this manner must be presumed to have a septic arthritis until proven otherwise.

The differential diagnosis includes osteomyelitis of the adjacent femur or tibia and inflammatory conditions such as rheumatoid or crystal arthropathies. Blood studies including a complete blood count, erythrocyte sedimentation rate, C-reactive protein level and blood cultures should be carried out. Joint aspiration using a sterile technique is mandatory. The sample is sent for microscopy, cell count, Gram staining and culture to tailor a treatment plan.

### Osteoarthritis of the Knee

This is a common condition in advancing age. It may result from senile degeneration and overuse or may be secondary to malalignment, ligamentous or meniscal injuries, osteochondritis dissecans, previous infections or trauma. The disease is expressed in the subchondral bone by osteophytes, bony eburnations and cystic degeneration, and subsequently affects the cartilage, leading to severe pain, immobility and joint deformities (**Figure 15.22**). Involvement of the medial compartment is more common than that of the lateral and patellofemoral compartments.

The patient walks with an antalgic gait. Examination of the patient standing may reveal a varus or valgus thrust depending on the compartment involved. Examination in the sagittal plane may show the knee to be held in fixed flexion due to capsular contraction. An effusion is often present, mainly during a flare-up of the disease. Osteophytes are palpable and there is joint line tenderness, crepitus and restriction of movement. The varus or valgus deformity can usually be corrected passively to neutral by doing a valgus or varus stress test.

### Rheumatoid Arthritis

In rheumatoid arthritis, the disease starts in the synovium and subsequently moves to the cartilage, causing severe inflammation and widespread destruction in all three compartments of the knee (**Figure 15.23**). Other joints are also involved – look for ulnar deviation in the patient's hands – and there may be extra-articular manifestations of rheumatoid arthritis such as subcutaneous nodules (see p. 230). The knee may be warm to the touch, and tenderness may be easily elicited. Note the muscle wasting surrounding the knee as well as the more common valgus deformity that is usually associated with a fixed flexion deformity. Thickening of the synovium may be palpable in the suprapatellar bursa.

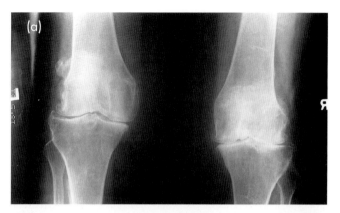

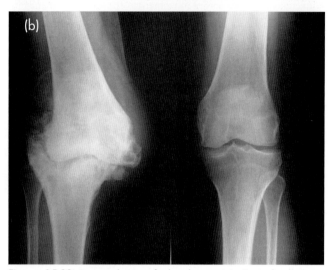

Figure 15.22 Osteoarthritis of the knee. (a) Typical changes. (b) Destruction from wear and tear when the protective sensation of the joint is lost. (Charcot's joint.)

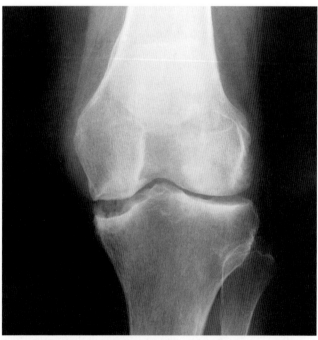

Figure 15.23 Rheumatoid changes of the knee joint.

## Tuberculosis

This condition is now rare in the Western world but is still common in less developed countries. The patient, who is usually aged 10–30 years, presents with a painful, swollen knee of several months' duration. A fixed flexion deformity and synovial thickening may be present. There is usually a good range of movement. Diagnosis is usually achieved by performing a synovial biopsy as well as a knee aspiration. Additional tests are a purified protein derivative skin test and a chest radiograph.

## THE POPLITEAL FOSSA

### Popliteal Aneurysm

The popliteal pulse is usually difficult to palpate. When it can be very easily palpated, particularly in a middle-aged or elderly male, an aneurysm should be suspected.

### Tumour of the Common Peroneal Nerve

The common peroneal nerve leaves the popliteal fossa and winds around the neck of the fibula. The rare tumour of the nerve is palpable in this area. It has the particular characteristic that it is mobile from side to side but not proximally and distally. Percussion over the nerve may elicit a Tinel's sign with pain radiating to the dorsum of the foot and paraesthesias.

## INJURIES TO THE EXTENSOR MECHANISM

### Rupture of the Quadriceps Tendon

This condition occurs most commonly in elderly individuals after indirect trauma. There is pain around the patella and a characteristic hollow in the quadriceps tendon where the fibers have been avulsed. A patella *baja*, or low-riding patella, may be noticed. If the patient has deficient extension, operative repair should be considered.

### Patellar Fractures

Fractures (**Figure 15.24**) may be transverse or stellate. Transverse fractures are due to powerful contraction of the quadriceps and are avulsion fractures. A lipohaemarthrosis will be present. Separation of the fragments occurs if the medial and lateral retinacular expansions of the quadriceps tendon are also torn. In these cases, a gap is palpable in the patella and the patient is unable to raise their straight leg.

Stellate fractures are usually caused by a direct blow to the anterior aspect of the knee, giving rise to local bruising. The retinacular expansions are rarely torn, and marked separation of the fragments is less common than in transverse fractures; the straight leg raise is usually intact.

### Ligamentum Patellae Ruptures

These occur in young adults as a result of sporting injuries or violent trauma. The injury can occur in the substance of the ligament or through an avulsion fracture of the tibial tuberosity in children or the lower pole of the patella in adults. A puffy swelling develops over the ligament, and the patella is *alta* or high-riding. The straight leg raise is absent.

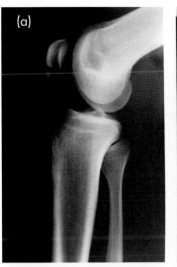
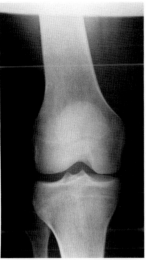

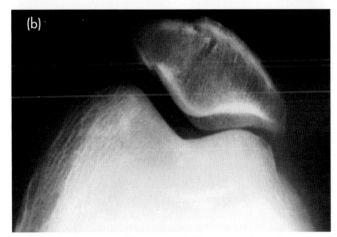

Figure 15.24 Fractures of the patella. (a)Transverse. (b) Stellate.

## FRACTURES AROUND THE KNEE

Patellar fractures have been mentioned above. Other fractures of the knee usually involve significant violence in children and young adults. In the elderly, osteoporosis significantly weakens the bone and fractures can occur with minimal trauma. As with all fractures, good quality radiographs are essential for an accurate diagnosis.

## Supracondylar Fracture of the Femur

This fracture is usually clinically obvious as it is accompanied by pain, swelling, tenderness and an inability to move the leg. The gastrocnemial attachments to the distal fragment may produce posterior angulation at the fracture site. The foot pulses should always be assessed in view of the close relation of the fracture to the popliteal vessels. A distal neurological assessment should also be carried out. The comparable injury in children is a fracture separation of the lower femoral epiphysis.

## Fracture of a Femoral Condyle

Fracture of a femoral condyle (**Figure 15.25**) results in a lipohaemarthrosis. One or both condyles can be involved in a T or Y form and may be displaced, such as after a direct blow when the patella is driven backwards, splitting the two femoral condyles.

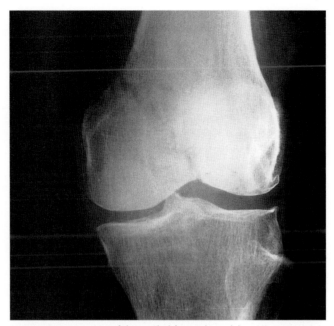

Figure 15.25 Fracture of the medial femoral condyle.

## Fractures of the Tibial Plateau (Condyles)

Tibial plateau fractures are relatively common and may be articular or non-articular. The lateral condyle is most frequently involved during falls or from a side impact, typically from a car bumper – a valgus force. A tear of the opposite collateral ligament is often present. A depression may affect the condyle leading to bone loss and incongruity. Involvement of the medial condyle is a more serious injury and calls for a prompt vascular evaluation of the lower extremity.

### Key Points

- The knee is examined systematically through observation, palpation and testing of the range of motion.
- Different examination tests are adopted for the extra-articular and intra-articular structures of the knee. These include the varus and valgus stress tests for the collateral ligaments, the Lachman test for the anterior cruciate ligament and the McMurray test for the menisci.
- Acute injuries of the knee may affect the viscoelastic structures, such as the ligaments and menisci, as well as the osteochondral structures, as in articular cartilage injuries or fractures. The presentation varies from a nearly normal knee to one with an acute effusion and immobility.
- Anterior knee pain results from an abnormal patellofemoral articulation in addition to proximal and distal patellar tendonitis and various types of peripatellar bursitis.
- Cysts around the knee can develop from either bursae such as the semimembranosus bursa, or from cysts that communicate with the joint and the menisci, for examples Baker's cysts and meniscal cysts.
- Intra-articular knee conditions can be infectious, osteoarthritic or inflammatory, as in rheumatoid arthritis.
- Traumatic injuries to the knee may affect the extensor mechanism, resulting in a patella *alta* or *baja* deformity. Injuries to the bony structures, for example fractures of the patella, femoral condyles or tibial plateau, are well documented in the knee and necessitate immediate attention.

## SBAs

**1.** Which one of the following is true of malalignment of the knee in the coronal plane?:

a In adults, it is never related to previous traumatic events

b In paediatric patients, it is solely associated with growth plate defects

c It is accentuated in varus when the medial collateral ligament is injured

d It is accentuated in valgus when the lateral collateral ligament is injured

e It is not present when the angle between the femur and tibia in the adult is 5–7° of valgus

**Answer**

**e** *It is not present when the angle between the femur and tibia in the adult is 5–7° of valgus. In adults, malalignment in the coronal plane or varus–valgus malalignment is usually related to post-traumatic deformities or degenerative arthritis of one or more compartments of the knee. In children, the aetiology of coronal deformities can be congenital bone dysplasias, paralytic disorders or growth plate abnormalities. The valgus stress test may unravel a medial collateral ligament injury, and a varus stress test may unmask an injury to the lateral collateral ligament. The normal angle between the femur and tibia in the adult is 5–7° of valgus.*

**2.** Which one of the following is correct in relation to a meniscal injury of the knee?:

a It is never associated with a knee effusion

b It will cause locking of the knee in extension

c It may illicit tenderness over the joint line

d The Apley test to detect a meniscal injury is conducted with the patient in the supine position

e It is usually of traumatic origin in the elderly

**Answer**

**c** *It may illicit tenderness over the joint line. Injury to the meniscus, especially if the vascularized periphery is involved, may cause an acute swelling of the knee due to a spontaneous haemarthrosis. When a bucket-handle tear of the meniscus is trapped in the intercondylar notch, the knee locks in flexion and a mechanical block to extension may be felt. The knee sometimes also becomes locked in extension. Joint line tenderness is a very common finding in meniscal pathology. The Apley maneuver consists of rotation and downward compression of the flexed knee when the patient is in the prone position. Meniscal tears in the young are usually of traumatic origin, while in the elderly they usually have a degenerative aetiology.*

**3.** Patellar instability is caused by which one of the following?:

a An increased Q angle

b Hypoplasia of the condylar groove

c Laxity in the medial structures with tightness in the lateral structures

d Failure of the patella to engage the trochlear groove at 30–40° of flexion

e All of the above

**Answer**

**e** *All of the above. The normal value of the angle between a line extending along the axis of the quadriceps tendon and another extending along the patellar tendon, or Q angle, is 14° in males and 17° in females. All values higher than this, such as may be seen with genu valgum or a wide pelvis, predispose the patella to subluxation in a lateral direction. Other causes of patellar subluxation are anatomical factors such a shallow trochlear groove or traumatic events affecting the medial muscular and retinacular structures. The patella in a healthy person should engage in the trochlea at 30–40° of flexion.*

## EMQs

**1.** For each of the following clinical diagnoses, select the correct diagnostic test from the list below:

  1 McMurray's test
  2 Pivot shift test
  3 Sage's sign
  4 Patellar ballotement
  5 Disappearing sign
  a Tight lateral retinaculum
  b Knee effusion
  c Meniscal cyst
  d Anterior cruciate ligament tear
  e Meniscus injury

**Answers**

**a 3 Stage's sign.** *In Sage's sign, the patella displays decreased excursion at 20° of knee flexion. It is indicative of a tight patellar lateral retinaculum.*

**b 4 Patellar ballotement.** *This can be demonstrated by pressing on the suprapatellar pouch to float the patella, and then producing a clicking sound upon axial compression against the trochlear groove. Patellar ballottement is a sign of a knee effusion.*

**c 5 Disappearing sign.** *With the disappearing sign, a meniscal cyst is present when the knee is extended but disappears when the knee is flexed.*

**d 2 Pivot shift test.** *In this, the tibia is reduced over the femur upon flexion, valgus and internal rotation. The test is a marker of instability in the presence of a defective anterior cruciate ligament.*

**e 1 McMurray's test.** *The McMurray test demonstrates the trapping of a torn meniscus when rotating the foot in 90° of flexion.*

**2.** For each of the following causes of anterior knee pain, select the most likely area of tenderness from the list below:

  1 Insertion of the patellar tendon
  2 Over the mid-patella
  3 Origin of the patellar tendon
  4 Lateral facet of the patella
  5 Lower pole of the patella
  a Housemaid's knee (prepatellar bursitis)
  b Osgood–Schlatter's disease
  c Lateral facet compression syndrome
  d Jumper's knee (patellar tendonitis)
  e Sinding-Larsen–Johansson disease

**Answers**

**a 2 Over the mid-patella.** *Housemaid's knee is inflammation of the prepatellar bursa from overuse.*

**b 1 Insertion of the patellar tendon.** *Osgood–Schlatter's disease is traction apophysitis of the tibial tubercle in adolescents at the insertion site of the patellar tendon.*

**c 4 Lateral facet of the patella.** *Lateral patellar facet compression syndrome is one of the culprits of a poor patellofemoral articulation. It is due to lateral patellar tilt from a tight lateral patellar retinaculum.*

**d 3 Origin of the patellar tendon.** *Jumper's knee is an overuse syndrome that affects jumping athletes. The condition involves the patellar tendon near its origin at the inferior pole of the patella.*

**e 5 Lower pole of the patella.** *Sinding-Larsen–Johansson disease is characterized by tenderness of the lower pole of the patella and the adjacent patellar tendon. It typically occurs in children under 10 years of age.*

# The Leg and Ankle Joint

Karim Masrouha and Bernard H. Sagherian

## LEARNING OBJECTIVES

- To be able to carry out an inspection of the leg and ankle with an understanding of the unique anatomy of the ankle joint and its range of motion
- To recognize that both lower extremities should always be examined so that a comparison can be made
- To be able to assess soft tissue injuries including sprains, strains, tendon ruptures and compartment syndrome

- To know how to evaluate the leg and ankle for specific fractures and fracture patterns
- To understand the different degenerative conditions that occur in the ankle joint
- To recognize the different inflammatory conditions that affect the ankle joint, as well as the tendons and bursae
- To understand how benign and malignant tumors of the bone and soft tissue present

## BASIC EXAMINATION OF THE ANKLE JOINT

The leg and ankle joint are subject to a number of traumatic, inflammatory as well as oncological conditions of the soft tissue and bones.

The leg and ankle are particularly vulnerable to trauma. The tibia and fibula are often injured during sports or motorcycle accidents and are among the most commonly fractured bones in the body. The injuries range from tendon injuries, such as ruptures of the Achilles tendon, ligamentous injuries around the ankle, muscle tears of the gastrocsoleus complex and fractures of the tibia, fibula and malleoli, to compartment syndrome secondary to trauma to the muscles in the compartments of the leg. Some injuries, such as tibial plafond fractures, can result in long-term functional deficits due to post-traumatic osteoarthritis.

As with the evaluation of complaints in any part of the body, an excellent knowledge of the relevant anatomy and an adequate history and physical examination are essential for formulating an appropriate differential diagnosis. Importantly, even if the complaint is unilateral, both lower extremities should be exposed when examining the leg and ankle for comparison.

The ankle joint is a particularly complex joint, and its examination requires a strong knowledge of its anatomy. On inspection, the two malleoli are the most prominent surface markings at the ankle (**Figure 16.1**). The lateral malleolus is a little less prominent and descends 1 cm lower than, and posterior to, the medial malleolus. The joint line of the ankle is 1 cm above the tip of the medial malleolus. The neutral position of the ankle joint occurs when the foot is at a right angle to the leg.

The ankle joint should be examined with the knee in slight flexion to decrease the tension on the Achilles tendon. To examine flexion movements of the left foot, hold the heel with the left hand, and the forefoot with the right hand. For dorsiflexion, pull down with the left hand and push up with the right. For plantar flexion, this movement is reversed. These movements occur principally at the ankle joint.

Inversion (turning the sole inwards) and eversion (turning the sole outwards) occur principally at the subtalar joint and should also be tested (**Figure 16.2**). Varus and valgus rotation occur at the midtarsal joint when the ankle joint is in plantar flexion. Supination is the combination of internal rotation and inversion, while pronation is external rotation plus eversion.

## TRAUMATIC CONDITIONS

### Soft Tissue Injuries

#### Ankle Sprains

Sprains are a particularly common complaint in the accident and emergency department, as well as in orthopaedic and primary care clinics. These injuries are typically secondary to inversion and plantar flexion of the foot, or are rarely eversion injuries.

Patients usually present with pain over the dorsum of the midfoot extending to the lateral malleolus, due to an injury to one or more of the ligaments around the ankle joint, such as the anterior tibiofibular ligament. A haematoma develops at the site of the ligamentous injury, followed by progressive oedema. Ankle sprains can be classified into three grades, according to

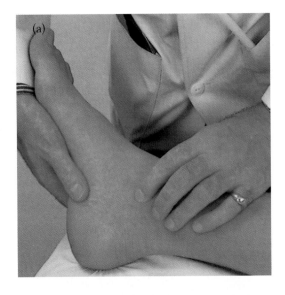

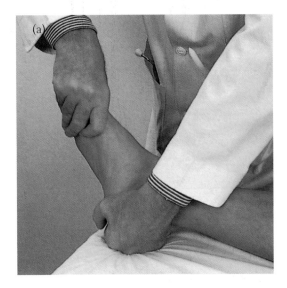

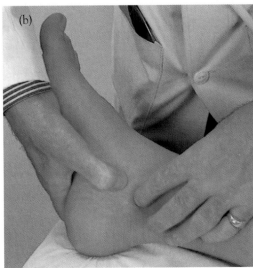

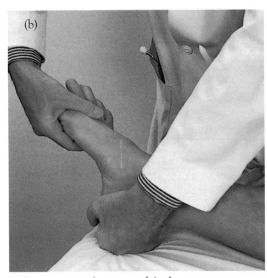

Figure 16.1 Surface markings (a) of the medial malleolus, (b) of the medial ligament.

Figure 16.2 Inversion and eversion of the foot.

swelling, tenderness and functional impairment (**Table 16.1**). Ankle sprains can be differentiated from ankle fractures using the Ottawa Ankle Rules (**Figure 16.3**).

### Achilles Tendon Rupture

Rupture of the Achilles tendon is a common sports injury in young and middle-aged men, but may occur after minimal strain in elderly patients, particularly those taking fluoroquinolone antibiotics or corticosteroids and those with renal compromise. Patients typically present with the complaint of a sudden severe pain in the posterior aspect of the ankle and leg with an inability to bear weight, even when limping.

On examination, the foot is somewhat more dorsiflexed than the contralateral foot, and a gap may be felt along the superficial Achilles tendon approximately 5 cm proximal to its insertion on the calcaneus. The **Thompson test** (also called Simmonds' test) is a highly sensitive and specific test for complete rupture of the Achilles tendon (**Figure 16.4**). It is performed with the patient lying prone and their feet hanging off the edge of the examination table. The calf muscles are then squeezed in the mediolateral

plane. In patients with an intact Achilles tendon, the foot will plantar-flex; however, the foot will not move if there is a complete rupture.

### Calf Muscle Strains

These usually occur secondary to sports injuries or in individuals who are not accustomed to exercise. The gastrocnemius is most commonly involved, with varying reports of the incidence of soleus muscle tears. The mechanism is usually rapid extension of the knee with the foot in dorsiflexion, making this injury common in soccer players.

The muscle that is involved can be isolated by physical examination. Gastrocnemius tenderness usually occurs along the medial border of the muscle bulk, while soleus muscle tenderness is usually lateral to it. In addition, due to the insertion of the gastrocnemius above the knee and the soleus below it, the site of injury may be identified by the following: if the knee is placed in maximal flexion, the soleus will be the primary muscle that is involved in plantar flexion, while with the knee in full extension, it is the gastrocnemius. Conversely, passive dorsiflexion of

Table 16.1 Grading of ankle sprains

| Grade | Swelling | Tenderness | Functional deficit | Injury extent |
|---|---|---|---|---|
| 1 | Mild | Minimal | Minimal | Tiny ligamentous tears |
| 2 | Moderate | Moderate | Moderate | Partial full-thickness tears |
| 3 | Severe | Significant | Severe | Complete ligamentous rupture |

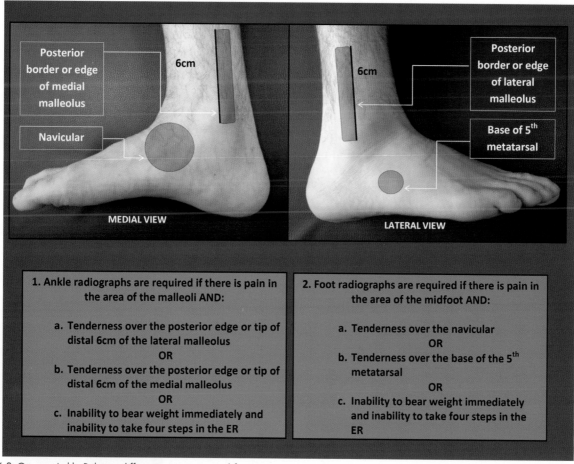

Figure 16.3 Ottawa Ankle Rules to differentiate sprains and fractures.

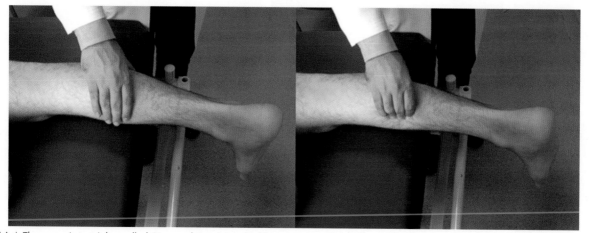

Figure 16.4 Thompson's test (also called Simmonds' test) is a highly sensitive and specific test for complete ruptures of the Achilles tendon.

PART 2 | TRAUMA AND (ELECTIVE) ORTHOPAEDICS

the foot in flexion and extension of the knee can stretch each in isolation and elicit a painful stimulus in only the injured muscle. In severe cases, a palpable defect may be present.

### Shin Splints

Shin splints cause pain over the anterior part of the leg secondary to small extensor muscle tears after strenuous activity in individuals who are not accustomed to exercising. There are usually no abnormal findings on physical examination, but local tenderness may occur over the tibia. It is important to differentiate this condition from more serious ailments such as compartment syndrome or stress fractures of the tibia.

### Compartment Syndrome

Compartment syndrome of the leg is a condition in which increased pressure builds up within its muscle compartments, decreasing the blood flow to the muscles themselves. This condition can be acute or chronic.

Acute compartment syndrome occurs after major trauma that results in swelling of the muscle compartments. Patients typically present with pain beyond what is expected for the injury, tightness of the muscle and paraesthesias. This is a surgical emergency that is treated by opening the compartments in a procedure called a fasciotomy, as muscle death can quickly ensue.

Chronic or exertional compartment syndrome is less dangerous and typically occurs in athletes who perform rigorous repetitive exercises. They present with pain that occurs during exercise and is relieved by rest, as well as swelling and difficulty with dorsiflexion and plantar flexion of the foot. Other conditions such as stress fractures or soft tissue injuries, as described above, need to be ruled out. In both acute and chronic compartment syndrome, the diagnosis is confirmed by measuring the intracompartmental pressures.

## Bony Injuries

### Stress Fracture of the Tibia

This occurs due to overuse in professional athletes, dancers and soldiers in training. It is an incomplete fracture involving a single bone cortex on orthogonal radiographs. There is usually localized tenderness over the medial aspect of the tibia. The diagnosis is confirmed by plain radiographs, or a bone scan if no fracture is seen on a radiograph but there is a high clinical suspicion of one.

### Fractures of the Tibia and Fibula

Fractures of these bones, either together or in isolation, occur due to a direct blow or, when they occur around the ankle, possibly an inversion/eversion injury (**Figure 16.5**). In severe injuries,

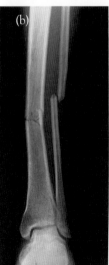
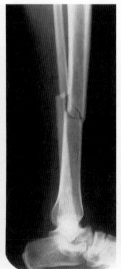
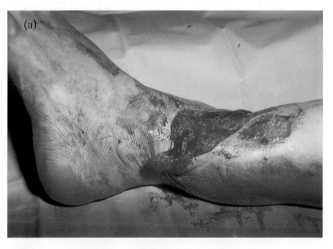
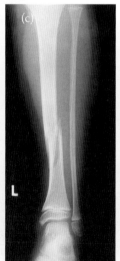
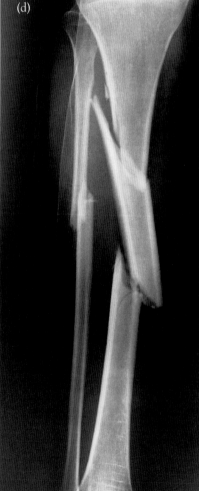
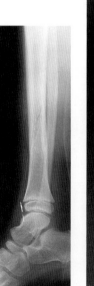
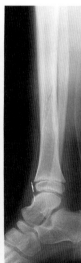

Figure 16.5 Fractures of the tibia and fibula. (a) Compound. (b) Transverse. (c) Spiral. (d) Segmented.

there may be a deformity of the foot, ankle and leg. The straight line through the medial aspect of the first toe, medial malleolus and medial patella is usually lost. Typically, there is localized swelling and tenderness, with or without deformity, and the patient cannot ambulate on the extremity. When both bones are fractured, the fibula is fractured at a higher level than the tibia. In high-speed motor vehicle accidents, these fractures may be open and are classified using the Gustillo–Anderson classification (**Table 16.2**).

It is imperative that an adequate neurological and vascular examination is performed, confirming the distal pulses so as not to miss possible distal ischaemia, and sensation to rule out nerve injury. If the injury occurs around the ankle, the Ottawa Ankle Rules (see Figure 16.3) are a useful method to assess the need for radiographic evaluation (**Figure 16.6**).

## Fractures of the Talus

Fractures of the talus (**Figures 16.7** and **16.8**) are uncommon but can occur due to a fall from a height or secondary to a motor vehicle accident. The fractures usually occur at the neck of the talus and can be confirmed by plain radiographs. The talus is particularly susceptible to avascular necrosis following a fracture, which results in non-union and arthritic changes.

## Maisonneuve Fractures

These are fractures of the fibula above the syndesmosis, potentially as high as the neck, along with diastasis of the ankle joint.

Such fractures are important as they can easily be missed and left untreated. There is typically swelling and tenderness of the ankle joint anteriorly, as well as tenderness over the fibular fracture. The diagnosis is made primarily by plain radiographs involving the whole leg and ankle joint.

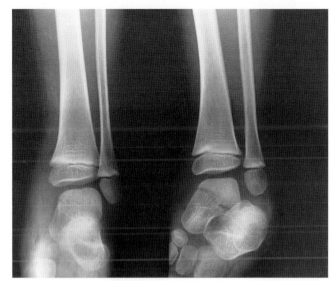

Figure 16.7 Fracture of the talus.

Table 16.2 Gustillo–Anderson classification

| Type | Wound size (cm) | Fracture pattern | Soft tissue loss | Periosteal stripping | Wound status | Neurovascular status | Skin and soft tissue coverage |
|---|---|---|---|---|---|---|---|
| I | <1 | Simple | Minimal | None | Clean | | Simple |
| II | >1 | Moderate comminution | Moderate | None | Contaminated | Normal | Local coverage |
| IIIA | | | | | | | Local coverage |
| IIIB | >10 | Severe comminution | Extensive | Yes | Extensive contamination | | Free or rotational flap |
| IIIC | | | | | | Arterial injury | |

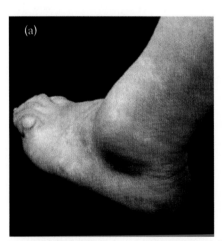
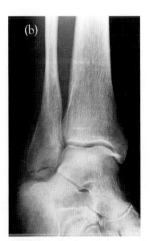
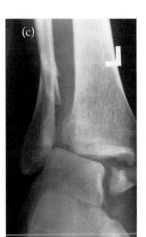
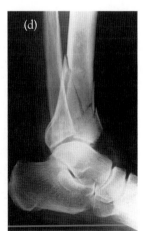

Figure 16.6 Ankle fractures. (a) Fracture of the lateral malleolus demonstrating marked local swelling. (b) Fracture of the lateral malleolus. (c) Fracture of the medial malleolus with a spiral fracture of the lower end of the fibula. (d) Comminuted fracture of the lower end of the tibia.

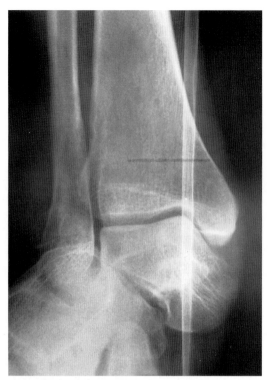

Figure 16.8 Subtalar dislocation.

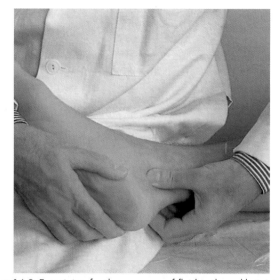

Figure 16.9 Examining for the presence of fluid in the ankle joint.

## DEGENERATIVE AND INFLAMMATORY CONDITIONS

### Osteoarthritis of the Ankle Joint

This may occur prematurely, secondary to repeated trauma or a previous fracture involving the ankle joint. Patients usually present with swelling (**Figure 16.9**), and there is decreased dorsiflexion and/or plantar flexion due to the osteophytes that form over the anterior and posterior lip of the anterior aspect of the talus, respectively.

### Rheumatoid arthritis

Rheumatoid arthritis can occur in the ankle joint, leading to a loss of cartilage and joint destruction, followed by bony collapse and deformity (**Figure 16.10**).

### Achilles Tendonitis

Inflammation of the paratenon of the Achilles tendon can occur due to pressure from the heel of the shoes (**Figure 16.11**). The patient presents with pain and tenderness of the tendon above the line of pressure from the shoe, and occasionally with a red, tender nodule at its insertion on the calcaneus.

### Retrocalcaneal Bursitis

This is an inflammation of the bursa between the calcaneus and the Achilles tendon; therefore the tenderness lies deep to the tendon, and the swelling is on either side of it (**Figure 16.12**). It is commonly associated with other inflammatory conditions, such as rheumatoid arthritis and gout, or with trauma. It may also be secondary to **Haglund's deformity**, which is a bony enlargement between the calcaneus and the Achilles tendon. In this case, there is usually pain, swelling, erythema and a visible

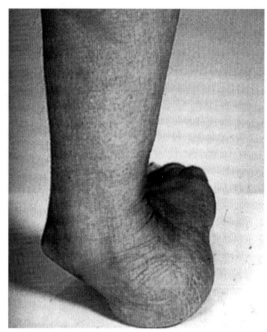

Figure 16.10 Rheumatoid arthritis.

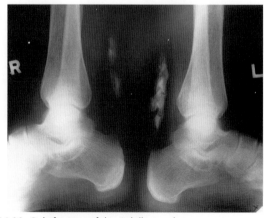

Figure 16.11 Calcification of the Achilles tendon.

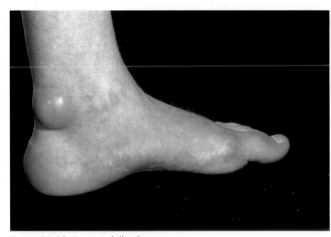

Figure 16.12 Retro Achilles bursa.

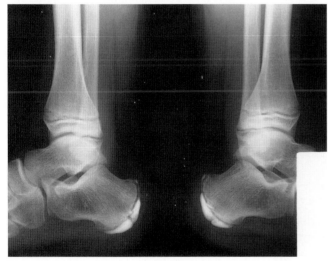

Figure 16.13 Calcaneal apophysitis (Sever's disease).

bump at the heel. It is common in women who wear high-heeled shoes.

## Calcaneal Apophysitis (Sever's Disease)

Calcaneal apophysitis occurs in children aged 8–12 years as a result of increased physical activity. Patients usually present with a limp and pain over the posterior aspect of the calcaneus. There may be some swelling over the insertion of the Achilles tendon, and there is tenderness on squeezing the back of the heel transversely from medial to lateral. Radiographs are usually normal, so it is primarily a clinical diagnosis (**Figure 16.13**).

## ONCOLOGICAL CONDITIONS

There are a number of soft tissue and bony benign and malignant tumours that occur in the leg. Soft tissue tumuors usually do not present with symptoms at an early stage; however, they may present with painless swelling over the leg, and at later stages may result in pain due to compression of the nearby nerves or muscles. Bony tumours may present with bone pain or pathological fractures, which occur due to a weakened bone structure at the site of the tumour.

### Key points

- The leg and ankle can be affected by traumatic, inflammatory and oncological conditions of the soft tissue and bone.
- Evaluation of the leg and ankle begins with adequate knowledge of the anatomy and a careful history, followed by a physical examination that starts with inspection. Note the poor blood supply of the skin over the shin.
- Ankle sprains are typically secondary to inversion and plantar flexion of the foot, and are divided into three grades. The Ottawa Ankle Rules should be used to determine the need for radiographs to rule out a fracture.
- Muscle strains occur after physical activity in patients unaccustomed to sports. Stretching the muscle can elicit pain.
- Tendon ruptures can be traumatic in young patients or occur after minimal strain in elderly individuals. The Thompson test is used to assess for rupture of an Achilles tendon.
- Shin splints need to be differentiated from compartment syndrome and stress fractures of the tibia (which occur in high-stress physical activity).
- Acute compartment syndrome is a surgical emergency, usually following severe injury, in which patients present with severe pain, paraesthesia and tight muscles. Chronic or exertional compartment syndrome occurs in athletes after repetitive motion and the symptoms are typically relieved with rest.
- In high-energy trauma, fractures of the tibia and fibula may be open. The Gustillo–Anderson classification divides these according to soft tissue, bone loss and vascular compromise. Adequate neurovascular examination is essential.
- The fractured talus is particularly susceptible to avascular necrosis.
- Pain, swelling and decreased dorsiflexion/plantar flexion are the key findings in osteoarthritis of the ankle.
- Bursitis and tendonitis are inflammatory conditions of the bursa and paratenon, respectively, and are diagnosed clinically.
- Calcaneal apophysitis occurs in patients aged 8–12 years after increased physical activity.
- Bone and soft tissue tumors typically present with a painless mass, but may become painful if nearby muscles or nerves are compressed or there is a pathological fracture.

## QUESTIONS

### SBAs

**1. Which one of the following is among the Ottawa Ankle Rules?:**
  a Bony tenderness along the posterior edge of the distal 6 cm of the tibia
  b Bony tenderness along the posterior edge of the distal 6 cm of the fibula
  c An inability to bear weight immediately or to take four steps in the emergency department
  d All of the above

**Answer**
**d All of the above.** *Bony tenderness in these tibial and fibular areas and an inability to bear weight or take four steps are all included in the Ottawa Ankle Rules.*

**2. Which one of the following is not a risk factor for the rupture of an Achilles tendon?:**
  a Corticosteroid use
  b Fluoroquinolone antibiotics
  c Diabetes mellitus
  d Renal compromise

**Answer**
**c Diabetes mellitus.** *Corticosteroids, fluoroquinolones and renal compromise are all known risk factors for Achilles tendon ruptures. Diabetes mellitus is known to cause structural changes and thickening of the Achilles tendon but does not result in an increased rate of rupture.*

**3. Retrocalcaneal bursitis is associated with all of the following except:**
  a Rheumatoid arthritis
  b Gout
  c Trauma
  d Infection

**Answer**
**d Infection.** *Rheumatoid arthritis, gout and trauma may all may play a role in the development of retrocalcaneal bursitis, but infection does not.*

### EMQs

**4. For each of the following conditions, select the appropriate diagnostic criterion from the list below. Each option may be used once, more than once or not at all:**
  1 Pain on passive muscle stretch
  2 Thompson test
  3 Overuse injury
  4 Gustillo–Anderson type IIIC classification
  a Stress fracture
  b Open fracture with vascular injury
  c Calf muscle strain
  d Achilles tendon rupture

**Answers**
a **3 Overuse injury.** *A stress fracture is a bone bruise or microfracture caused by overuse or repetitive trauma. It is common in runners, army recruits and ballet dancers.*
b **4 Gustillo–Anderson type IIIC classification.** *A Gustillo–Anderson type IIIC fracture is by definition an open fracture with associated vessel and/or nerve injury.*
c **1 Pain on passive muscle stretch.** *Calf pain elicited by passive gastrocnemius stretching is a sign of muscle strain.*
d **2 Thompson test.** *A positive Thompson test is diagnostic of an Achilles tendon rupture. It is performed with the patient lying face down with the foot hanging off the examination table. The test is deemed positive if there is no movement of the foot when the corresponding calf muscle is squeezed.*

# The Foot

Karim Masrouha and Bernard H. Sagherian

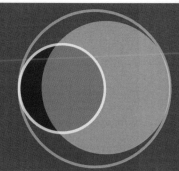

## LEARNING OBJECTIVES

- To be able to undertake a comparative inspection of the two feet, with an understanding of the unique anatomy and range of motion of the foot
- To evaluate the patient's gait and look at the arches, alignment and skin condition of the feet
- To understand conditions that involve the whole foot, such as club foot, metatarsus varus, equinus deformity, pes cavus and pes planus
- To recognize conditions that involve the hindfoot, such as subtalar/talonavicular arthritis, sinus tarsi syndrome and calcaneal fractures
- To distinguish conditions that involve the midfoot, such as rocker bottom foot, Lisfranc injury,

- tarsal stress fracture, tarsal tunnel syndrome and Köhler's disease
- To understand conditions that involve the forefoot, such as hallux valgus, hallux rigidus, bunionette, Morton's neuroma, metatarsalgia and march fracture
- To know about conditions that involve the toes, such as hammer toes, subungal haematoma, subungal exostosis, subungal glomus tumour, onychogryphosis and congenital abnormalities
- To understand specific conditions of the heel and sole, such as plantar fasciitis, callosities, hard and soft corns, and neuropathic ulcers

## BASIC EXAMINATION OF THE FOOT

The foot is subject to a number of infectious, inflammatory and traumatic conditions, as well as acquired and congenital deformities. These are discussed by region, dividing the chapter into conditions involving the whole foot, hindfoot, midfoot, forefoot, toes and superficial tissues of the foot.

The foot is a particularly complex region of the body and, as with other parts of the body, a detailed knowledge of the anatomy and a good history are essential prior to performing a physical examination. When examining the foot, make sure the lower extremity is exposed to the mid-thigh and, even if the complaint is unilateral, expose both sides so that an adequate comparison can be made.

Start by examining the patient's gait, if their condition permits. Observe for a limp and try to ascertain if it is due to pain, deformity or weakness. Observe the patient in the standing position and examine the arches of the feet to ascertain whether a flat foot or a high arch is present. Look at the feet from behind to determine the alignment of the calcaneus relative to the tibia.

With the patient supine, look for obvious skin lesions, masses and deformities. Palpate for local tenderness, and then assess the active and passive movement of the foot in dorsiflexion, plantar flexion, inversion and eversion; the movement of the toes should also be ascertained.

## CONDITIONS INVOLVING THE WHOLE FOOT

### Talipes Equinovarus and Equinovalgus

**Talipes equinovarus** (club foot) (**Figure 17.1**) is a congenital deformity with four distinct abnormalities: equinus (**Figure 17.2**), varus, cavus and metatarsus adductus. It can be diagnosed by fetal ultrasonography or at birth. The gastrocsoleus complex is generally underdeveloped, with proximal migration and fanning of the musculotendinous junction. It is associated with other conditions such as developmental dysplasia of the hip or spina bifida, and may be part of a syndrome such as Edwards' syndrome (trisomy 18).

**Talipes calcaneovalgus** (**Figure 17.3**) occurs with a congenitally long Achilles tendon – a vertical talus is present and it can be classified as a form of this abnormality.

### Metatarsus Varus

Metatarsus varus, or pigeon toes, is a congenital condition in which the forefoot is medially deviated and the foot is plantigrade. It generally corrects spontaneously by the age of 4 years.

### Isolated Equinus Deformity

This is usually acquired secondary to a nerve injury that results in extensor muscle paralysis. If physical therapy is not initiated

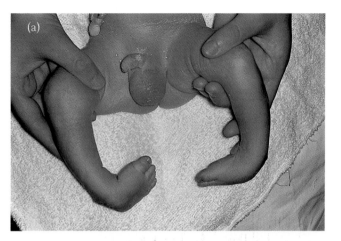

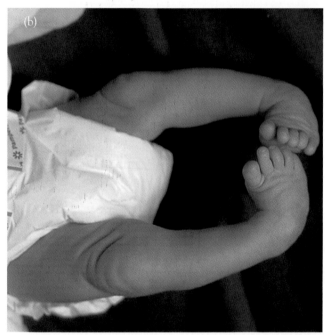

Figure 17.1 (a, b) Talipes equinovarus.

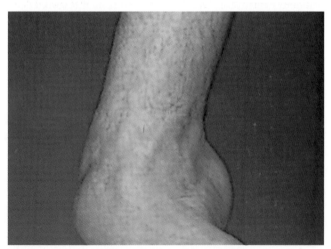

Figure 17.2 Equinus deformity.

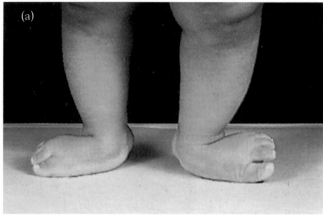

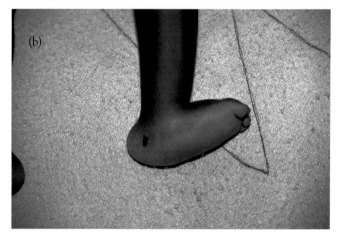

Figure 17.3 (a, b) Talipes valgus.

early, contractures can develop in the Achilles tendon, leading to a fixed deformity.

Examine the plantar aspect of the foot to look for calluses over the metatarsal heads, which are often associated with this deformity.

## Pes Cavus

Pes cavus is a deformity consisting of an abnormally high medial longitudinal arch associated with claw toes and calluses over the metatarsal heads (**Figure 17.4**). It is usually idiopathic, but can be associated with neuromuscular disorders such as Friedreich's ataxia, muscular dystrophies, Charcot–Marie–Tooth disease and peroneal nerve palsy.

## Pes Planus

Pes planus (flat foot) (**Figure 17.5**) involves a fallen longitudinal arch, but may also involve the transverse arch with splaying of the metatarsals. It is usually bilateral and asymptomatic, and can be corrected by standing on the tips of the toes. A rigid flat foot implies that there is an underlying associated pathology, such as a post-traumatic tarsal abnormality or rupture of the tibialis posterior tendon.

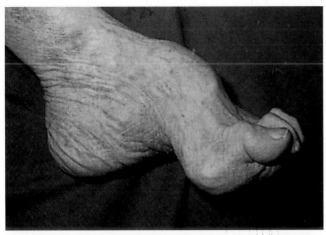

Figure 17.4 Pes cavus following poliomyelitis.

## THE HINDFOOT

### Subtalar/Talonavicular Arthritis

This commonly occurs in patients with rheumatoid arthritis but can be post-traumatic. Patients usually present with hindfoot swelling and pain, with a planovalgus deformity and collapse of the medial longitudinal arch.

### Sinus Tarsi Syndrome

This occurs when there is an injury to the interosseous talocalcaneal ligament, which is located in the depression on the lateral side of the tarsus, distal to the lateral malleolus. There is typically pain and tenderness over the lateral side of the hindfoot and a feeling of instability when walking over uneven ground.

### Calcaneal Fractures

These fractures occur when patients fall from a height onto their feet, meaning that it is frequently bilateral (**Figure 17.6**). Patients typically present with an inability to ambulate, heel swelling, bruising and pain. Tenderness is elicited by palpation over the medial or lateral side of the bone. The fracture is usually intra-articular, involving the subtalar joint, so there is significant pain and limitation of motion in inversion and eversion. These fractures frequently result in post-traumatic osteoarthritis.

## THE MIDFOOT

### Rocker Bottom Foot

This condition involves the collapse of the longitudinal arches of the foot, which occurs in diabetic patients with neuropathic arthropathy and sensory neuropathy. The autonomic neuropathy results in dry and inelastic skin. There may be ulcerations over the metatarsal heads.

### Tarsometatarsal Dislocation (Lisfranc Injury)

Tarsometatarsal dislocation (**Figure 17.7**) occurs from a rotational injury in the fixed foot or is due to axial loading onto a plantar-flexed or vertical foot. Patients present with significant pain and swelling of the midfoot. On inspection, there is oedema and ecchymosis. A careful vascular examination is warranted as there is occasional distal ischaemia. This is a commonly missed injury, but there are particular signs on plain radiographs such

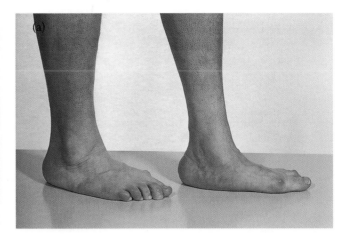

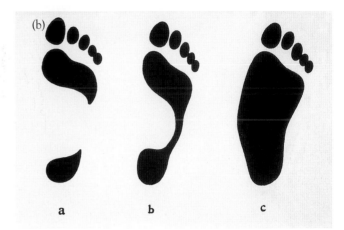

Figure 17.5 (a) Flat feet. (b) a. High arch; b. Normal foot; c. Flat foot.

as the 'fleck' sign, which is the avulsion of the Lisfranc ligament from the base of the second metatarsal, and an increased distance of the second metatarsal base from the medial cuneiform.

### Tarsal Stress Fractures

These fractures typically occur in professional athletes and soldiers in training. They usually occur at the navicular or cuboid, and the patient presents with generalized pain over the midfoot. There is typically tenderness over the fractured bone. These fractures may be missed on plain radiographs, and if the index of suspicion is high, a bone scan is the study of choice to confirm the diagnosis.

### Tarsal Tunnel Syndrome

Tarsal tunnel syndrome is due to compression of the tibial nerve as it passes into the foot posterior to the medial malleolus with the posterior tibial artery, deep to the flexor retinaculum in the fibro-osseous tunnel. As with carpal tunnel syndrome, the presenting symptoms involve the nerve supply, which include pain, paraesthesia and a burning sensation over the sole of the foot extending to the toes, particularly the first three toes. The cause can be anything that results in compression of the nerve within the tarsal tunnel, including trauma, inflammation or benign tumours. The symptoms can be reproduced by inflating a sphygmomanometer cuff over the ankle for a minute in order to occlude the blood supply to the foot. The diagnosis is then confirmed by electromyography.

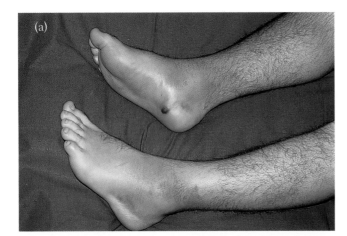

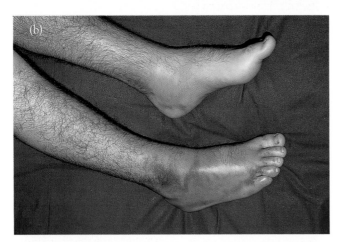

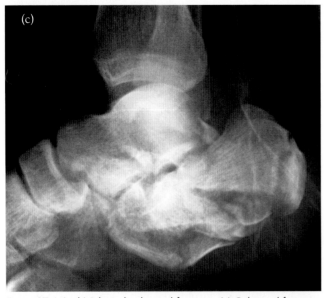

Figure 17.6 (a, b) Bilateral calcaneal fractures. (c) Calcaneal fracture.

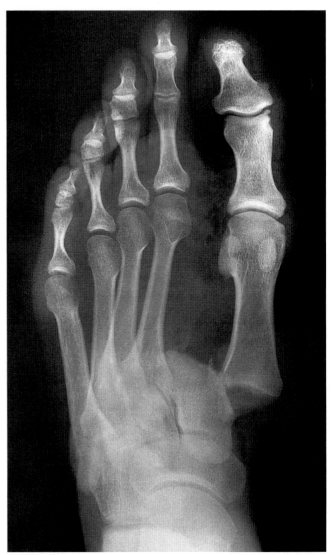

Figure 17.7 Tarsometatarsal dislocation.

present with a limp, associated with pain, swelling and tenderness over the midfoot. Upon ambulation, the weight is shifted to the lateral aspect of the foot to avoid placing pressure on the navicular bone. Plantar flexion and inversion of the foot can reproduce the pain. The diagnosis is confirmed by plain radiographs of both feet, which may show sclerosis and possible flattening of the navicular bone (**Figure 17.8**).

## THE FOREFOOT

### Hallux Valgus

Hallux valgus is an acquired, frequently bilateral, lateral deviation of the big toe that is commonly seen in women (**Figure 17.9**). A **bunion**, which is a swollen bursa, is usually present and can be erythematous and painful. On inspection, the laterally deviated phalanx may result in a dorsally displaced and over-riding second toe, which may result in pressure symptoms. There may be associated widening of the foot due to loss of the transverse arch.

## Köhler's Disease

Köhler's disease is a temporary, self-limiting avascular necrosis of the navicular that occurs in children, mostly boys, between the ages of 4 and 6 years. It is typically unilateral. Patients usually

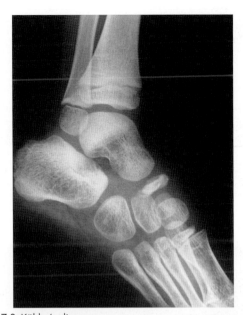

Figure 17.8 Köhler's disease.

## Hallux Rigidus

This occurs due to degenerative osteoarthritis of the metatarsophalangeal joint. The condition can be idiopathic, secondary to trauma, or may be a consequence of a long history of hallux valgus deformity. On examination, the metatarsophalangeal joint is stiff and pain is elicited on attempted plantar flexion or dorsiflexion. When asked to curl the toe, patients will only have motion of the interphalangeal joint of the big toe.

## Bunionette

A bunionette is a bursal inflammation of the lateral aspect of the head of the fifth metatarsal. This occurs in patients with broad feet due to pressure from tight-fitting shoes.

## Morton's Neuroma

Morton's neuroma is a benign swelling of the intermetatarsal branches of the medial plantar nerve (usually those of the second and third web spaces). Transversely squeezing the metatarsal heads together or palpating between the two metatarsal heads can elicit pain and paraesthesia.

## Metatarsalgia

Metatarsalgia is pain over one or more metatarsal heads, most commonly affecting the first and/or second metatarsals. It is

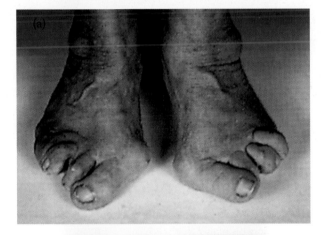

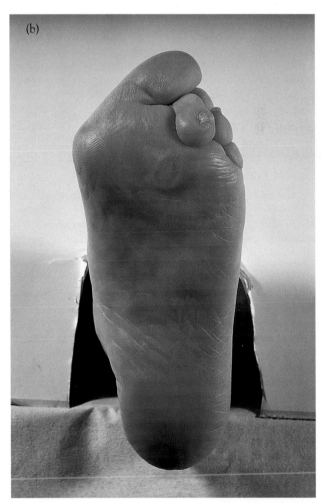

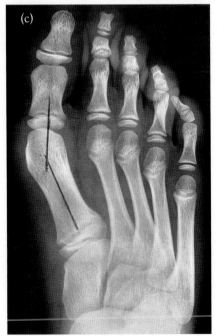

Figure 17.9 (a) Hallux valgus. (b) Hallux valgus in a patient with rheumatoid arthritis. (c) Markings added to a radiograph to demonstrate the angle of deformity.

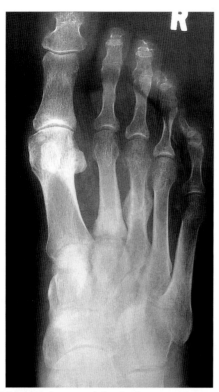

Figure 17.10 March fracture of the third metatarsal. Repair has often commenced by the time of diagnosis: callus is seen on this radiograph.

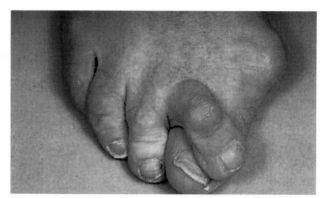

Figure 17.11 Hammer toe. Displacement secondary to hallux valgus.

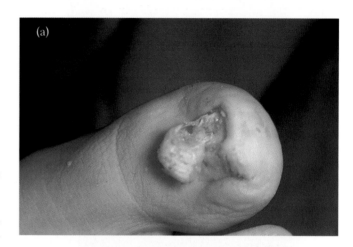

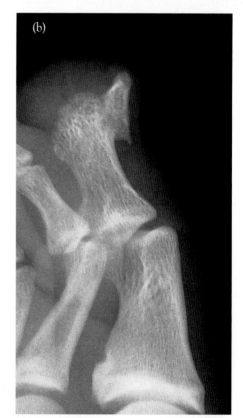

Figure 17.12 Subungual exostosis.

usually due to uneven loading of the metatarsal heads secondary to poorly fitting shoes, stress fracture, cavus foot deformity or flattening of the transverse arch, as well as rheumatoid arthritis, hallux rigidus, Morton's neuroma and diabetic neuropathy. Patients usually present with pain just proximal to the toes that increases during walking or standing (especially if barefoot) and is relieved by rest. The patient may also complain of paraesthesias and shooting pain in the corresponding toes.

## March Fracture

This is a stress fracture of the metatarsal secondary to increased and repeated physical stress (**Figure 17.10**). On examination, there is swelling and tenderness over the painful metatarsal. Plain radiographs may initially be negative, but if the clinical suspicion is high, a bone scan will reveal the fracture.

### THE TOES

**Hammer toe** is a deformity in which the toe is dorsally displaced, with a hyperextended metatarsophalangeal joint and a flexed proximal interphalangeal joint (**Figure 17.11**). Patients present with pain over the dorsum of their toe, as well as corns over the flexed proximal interphalangeal joint.

A **subungal haematoma** is a collection of blood between the toenail and the nail bed secondary to trauma. The diagnosis is generally straightforward. Patients present with pain and swelling of the toe with dark discoloration underneath the nail.

A **subungal exostosis** is recognized as a bony extension of the distal phalanx that usually appears as a painless discoloration and elevation of the distal half of the nail (**Figure 17.12**). It may become painful if it undergoes trauma and/or becomes infected.

A **subungal glomus tumour** is a benign tumour that occurs under the nails, usually of the smaller toes. Patients can present with bouts of severe pain.

The nail deformity of **onychogryphosis** occurs secondary to nail bed trauma (**Figure 17.13**). It occurs mostly in the big toe and results in a nail that is detached from the tissues deep to it and has a keratinized and curled horn. Patients present with pain when wearing closed shoes, or as a result of secondary infection or trauma.

**Gout** (**Figure 17.14**) is a systemic disorder resulting from elevated uric acid levels and most commonly affects the first metatarsophalangeal joint. There is exquisite tenderness in the joint, which is dusky red and swollen from the deposition of urate crystals; the patient resists any movement. The diagnosis is aided by the absence of a bunion, the male predominance and the presence of gouty tophi, usually on the helix of the ear, but also in olecranon bursae and the tendon sheaths of the hands and feet. Blood tests will reveal the abnormally high uric acid levels.

**Congenital abnormalities** can include adactyly (absent toes), polydactyly (extra toes), syndactyly (joined toes), ectrodactyly (an abnormal number and/or arrangement of toes) and overriding or curly toes (**Figures 17.15** and **17.16**). These deformities may be part of a syndrome and may be associated with talipes deformities.

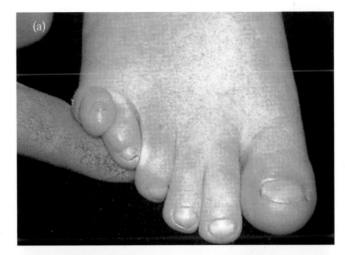

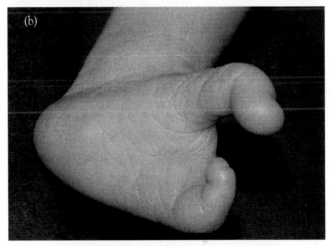

Figure 17.15 (a) Polydactyly. (b) Absent toes.

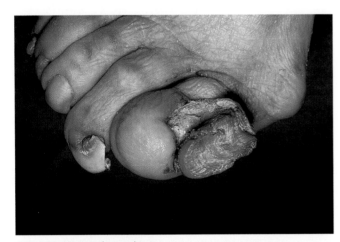

Figure 17.13 Onychogryphosis.

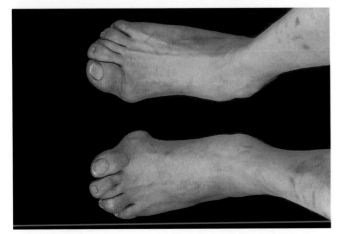

Figure 17.14 Gouty deformity of the metatarsophalangeal joints.

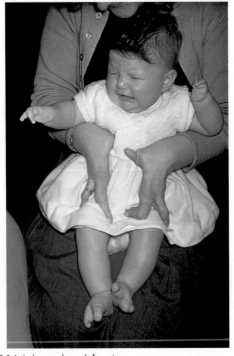

Figure 17.16 Lobster claw deformity.

## SOFT TISSUES OF THE FOOT

### Plantar Fasciitis

This is an inflammation of the plantar fascia over the medial calcaneal tuberosity. It occurs secondary to overuse, particularly in overweight individuals. Patients present with pain proximally at the insertion and along the plantar fascia. The pain is increased on plantar flexion of the toes. An incidental heel spur is commonly found on plain radiographs.

### Callosities

Callosities occur on the plantar aspect of the foot, usually over the metatarsal heads (particularly with a cavus foot), the heel, or on the medial aspect of the big toe. The skin becomes hard and thickened due to the increased pressure over a large surface area.

### Hard Corns

Unlike callosities, hard corns occur over the dorsum of the foot, are painful and are caused by pressure over bony prominences with small surface areas. They are seen in patients with hammer toes and can occur over the fifth toe.

### Soft Corns

Soft corns are also painful but they occur between the digits, usually between the fourth and fifth toes, and are caused by the friction between the toes (**Figure 17.17**).

### Neuropathic Ulcers

Neuropathic ulcers occur in patients with diabetic neuropathy, spinal cord injuries or diseases, or sciatic nerve palsies (**Figure 17.18**). They usually occur over the first and fifth metatarsal heads with surrounding callosities, and are associated with sensory deficits.

### Other Conditions

The capillary networks of the extremities constrict in the cold, preserving heat. In very low temperatures, the blood flow may stop altogether, and if this is prolonged it can lead to digital ischaemia (**frostbite; Figure 17.19a**). The networks are also sensitive to the effects of vasoconstrictor drugs, as seen with the inadvertent intra-arterial injections of recreational or other medications. Although this is usually an upper limb problem, overdoses of powerful vasoconstrictors such as **ergot** may also affect the extremities of the lower limb (**Figure 17.19b**).

Prolonged exposure of the feet to an unhygienic wet environment (such as in trench warfare) produces swelling of the skin and subcutaneous tissues. When these damaged tissues become secondarily infected, often with superadded capillary cold responses, gangrene may set in – a condition termed **trench foot** (**Figure 17.19c**).

### Cutaneous Tumours

The superficial tissues of the foot are subject to the same skin and subcutaneous lesions that occur elsewhere in the body, but of particular note are ganglia over the dorsum and cutaneous malignancies of the sole (**Figure 17.20**). **Ganglia** arise on the dorsum of the foot, particularly around the tarsus. They have the same clinical features as ganglia of the hand and wrist (see Chapter 13) but are less common.

**Malignant melanoma** of the foot is uncommon but mostly appears on the instep. The lesions usually have pigmentation as a distinguishing feature but may go unnoticed until ulceration occurs. When a melanoma is suspected, the groin nodes and

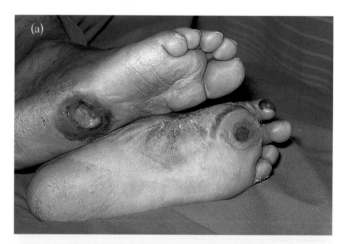

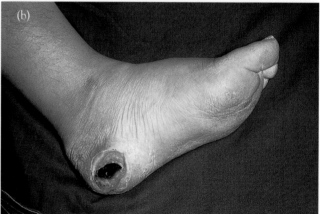

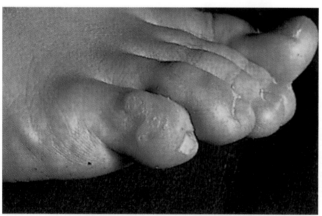

Figure 17.17 A soft corn.

Figure 17.18 (a) Diabetic ulcers. (b) Bed sores.

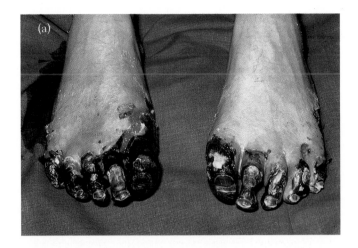

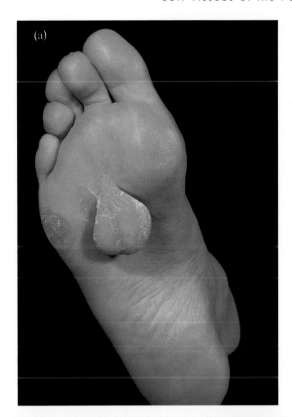

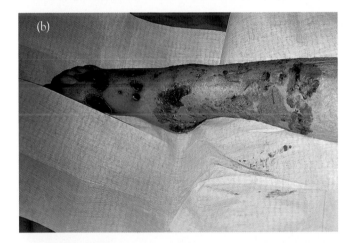

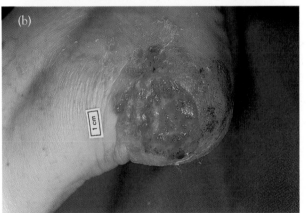

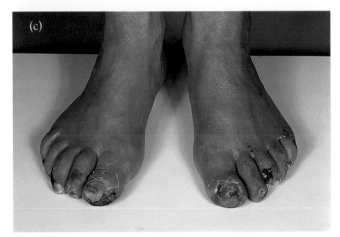

Figure 17.19 (a) Frostbite of the toes. (b) Ergot poisoning. (c) Bilateral trench foot.

liver must be examined. **Squamous cell carcinoma** of the foot (**Figure 17.20b**) occurs over the weight-bearing areas of the foot and rapidly infiltrates the deep tissues. Other rare malignancies are occasionally encountered.

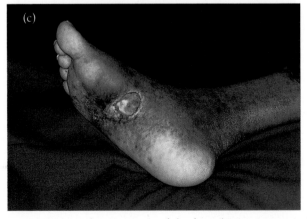

Figure 17.20 (a) A benign tumour of the foot. (b) A squamous cell carcinoma of the heel (c) Radionecrotic ulcer following treatment of a Kaposi's sarcoma of the sole.

**Key Points**

- The foot is subject to a number of infectious, inflammatory and traumatic conditions, as well as acquired and congenital deformities.
- Evaluation of the foot begins with adequate knowledge of the unique anatomy of the foot and a careful history, followed by a physical examination that starts with inspection.
- A number of congenital and acquired conditions involve the whole foot. These include club foot, pes cavus, pes planus, metatarsus varus and isolated equinus deformity.
- The hindfoot is subject to arthritis as well as soft tissue and bony traumatic injuries.
- The midfoot is subject to a variety of conditions including those that result from neuropathies such as rocker bottom foot, a decreased blood supply such as in Köhler's disease, trauma such as with Lisfranc injuries and tarsal stress fractures, or conditions affecting the peripheral nerves such as tarsal tunnel syndrome.
- The forefoot is subject to a variety of common conditions such as hallux valgus, hallux rigidus, bunionette, Morton's neuroma and march fracture.
- The toes are subject to acquired deformities such as hammer toes or subungal exostosis, trauma such as subungal haematomas and onychogryposis (which results from trauma to the nail bed), tumourous growths such as subungal glomus tumours, and congenital abnormalities.
- The soft tissues of the heel and sole can become inflamed with activity, such as with plantar fasciitis, can develop hard and soft corns as well as callosities from pressure on bony prominences or friction, and can develop ulcers secondary to diabetes, central or peripheral nerve injuries.

# QUESTIONS

## SBAs

**1.** Which one of the following deformity is **not** seen in patients with club foot?:

- a Equinus
- b Valgus
- c Cavus
- d Metatarsus adductus
- e Varus

**Answer**

**b Valgus.** The four deformities seen in club foot are equinus, cavus, varus and metatarsus adductus.

**2.** Which one of the following is associated with a Lisfranc injury?:

- a Plantar ecchymosis
- b An increased distance of the second metatarsal base from the medial cuneiform
- c Axial loading onto a plantar-flexed or vertical foot
- d A fleck sign on a plain radiograph
- e All of the above
- f Answers a, b and d

**Answer**

**e All of the above.** Lisfranc injuries typically occur as a result of axial loading onto a plantar-flexed or vertical foot. Patients present with plantar ecchymosis and swelling on inspection. An increased distance of the second metatarsal base from the medial cuneiform and a 'fleck' sign (avulsion of the Lisfranc ligament from the base of the second metatarsal) are seen on plain radiographs.

**3.** Which one of the following occurs secondary to pressure on bony prominences in the foot?:

- a Hard corn
- b Soft corn
- c Callosities
- d Neuropathic ulcers
- e All of the above
- f Answers a, c and d

**Answer**

**f Answers a, c and d.** Pressure on bony prominences results in hard calluses, callosities and neuropathic ulcers (in patients with diabetes or central/peripheral nerve injuries). Soft calluses result from friction between two toes.

## EMQs

**1.** For each of the following conditions, select the most likely structure to be injured from the list below. Each option may be used once, more than once or not at all:

- 1 Navicular bone
- 2 Tibial nerve
- 3 Interosseous talocalcaneal ligament
- 4 High medial longitudinal arch
- a Pes cavus
- b Sinus tarsi syndrome
- c Tarsal tunnel syndrome
- d Köhler's disease

**Answers**

- a **4 High medial longitudinal arch.** Pes cavus is characterized by fixed plantar flexion of the forefoot that does not correct with weight-bearing.
- b **3 Interosseous talocalcaneal ligament.** Sinus tarsi syndrome is characterized by pain and tenderness on the lateral side of the foot. It is caused by injury to the interosseous talocalcaneal ligament, most commonly due to an ankle sprain.
- c **2 Tibial nerve.** Tarsal tunnel syndrome is caused by compression of the tibial nerve by the flexor retinaculum at the level of the medial ankle. Patients may present with pain, numbness or a burning sensation in the medial or plantar aspect of the foot.
- d **1 Navicular bone.** Köhler's disease is avascular necrosis of the navicular bone in the foot. It occurs in the paediatric age group between the ages of 4 and 9 years, and is more common in boys. Patients present with pain and swelling in the dorsal-medial midfoot area with difficulty walking.

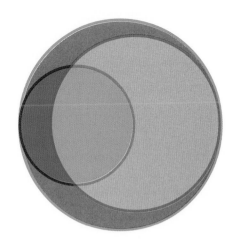

# PART
# 3

# Skin

# The Skin

Abdel Kader El Tal

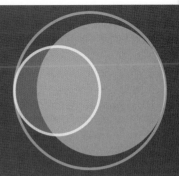

## LEARNING OBJECTIVES

- To be able to describe and differentiate the different morphological skin lesions including the macule, papule, plaque and nodule
- To become familiar with common cutaneous lesions of epithelial, mesenchymal and adnexal origin and know the differentiating features of acrochordons, seborrhoeic keratoses, warts, molluscum contagiosum and the different benign cysts
- To know the difference between the malignant and premalignant lesions of the skin and

- the characteristics and prognosis of basal cell carcinoma, squamous cell carcinoma, keratoacanthoma and Paget's disease.
- To learn the different benign melanocytic lesions and the possible associated syndromes, in addition to mastering the ABCDEs of malignant transformation, the different types of melanoma and their associated stages and prognostic survival
- To become familiar with the different vascular and neural lesions

## INTRODUCTION

The skin functions as a barrier against potentially harmful physical, chemical and microbiological agents. It is important in heat regulation and neurosensory perception. It also plays a minor role in excretion, absorption and metabolism.

This chapter reviews and solidifies the principles of the history and examination of skin conditions that are of surgical relevance, in particular benign premalignant and malignant lesions. Cutaneous manifestations of malignant and systemic disease (Tables 18.1 and 18.2), skin pigmentation (Tables 18.3 and 18.4), purpura and pruritus (Table 18.5) and abnormalities of the hair (Table 18.6) are tabulated for the reader's ease and reference.

Table 18.1 Skin manifestations of non-malignant systemic disease

| Manifestation | Disease |
| --- | --- |
| Erythema | Collagen disease |
| | Carcinoid |
| | Mitral valve (malar flush) |
| | Polycythaemia or hyperviscosity syndrome |
| | Superior vena cava obstruction |
| | Liver disease |
| Erythema multiforme | Fever |
| | Inflammatory bowel disease |
| | Rheumatoid arthritis |

contd...

| Manifestation | Disease |
| --- | --- |
| | Thyrotoxicosis |
| | Virus and mycoplasma infections |
| Urticaria | Collagen disorders |
| | Xanthomatoses |
| | Hereditary angioneurotic oedema |
| | Urticaria pigmentosa |
| | Henoch–Schönlein purpura |
| | Cold agglutinins |
| Scaling | Vitamin deficiencies |
| | Hypothyroidism |
| | Acromegaly |
| | Malabsorption |
| | Refsum's and Reiter's diseases |
| Papules and nodules | Behcet's disease |
| | Erythema nodosum |
| | Erythema induratum |
| | Gardner's syndrome |
| | Necrobiosis lipoidica |
| | Neurofibromatosis |
| | Polyarteritis nodosa |
| | Pseudoxanthoma elasticum |
| | Sarcoid |
| | Tuberous sclerosis |
| | Xanthoma |

contd...

Table 18.1 **Skin manifestations of non-malignant systemic disease** (*contd...*)

| Manifestation | Disease |
|---|---|
| Blisters | Dermatitis herpetiformis |
| | Drugs |
| | Glucagonoma |
| | Pemphigus |
| | Porphyria |
| | Vascular disease |
| Angiomas | Multiple vascular malformations |
| Pruritus | See p. 620 |
| Purpura | See p. 30 |

Table 18.2 **Cutaneous manifestations of malignancy**

| Cutaneous manifestation | Malignancy and/or site |
|---|---|
| Primary skin malignancy | |
| Secondary malignant deposits **or** infiltration – leukaemia, lung | |
| Paget's disease of the breast | |
| Weight loss and cachexia | Loss of subcutaneous tissue in the skin |
| Pruritus, particularly associated with lymphoreticular disease | |
| Clubbing and hypertrophic pulmonary osteoarthropathy | Lung |
| Superficial or deep venous thrombosis | Sometimes an occult primary, e.g. lung, gastric, pancreas |
| Dermatomyositis | 50% associated with malignancy |
| Acanthosis nigricans | Gut and bronchus |
| Ichthyosis | Commonly gut |
| Alopecia | Gastric |
| Purpura | Thrombocytopenia |
| Exfoliative erythroderma | Lymphoma |
| Erythema gyratum repens | Breast, lung |
| Erythema nodosum, erythema multiforme | |
| Eczematous dermatitis | |
| Herpes zoster | Lymphoreticular disease |
| Flushing of carcinoid syndrome | |
| Skin lesions | Genodermatoses (Table 18.7), Gardner's syndrome |
| Pyoderma gangrenosum | Leukaemia and multiple myeloma |
| Palmar keratosis | Bladder and lung |
| Disseminating intravascular coagulation | Leukaemia, lymphoma, cancer of the pancreas; also as a generalized terminal malignant event |
| Hypertrichosis languinosa | Gut |

Table 18.3 **Local skin discoloration**

| Colour change | Cause |
|---|---|
| Haemorrhage/bruising | Trauma, blood dyscrasias, increased capillary fragility, old age, lower limb venous hypertension |
| Brown pigmentation | Freckles, moles, melanoma, basal cell carcinoma |
| | Café-au-lait spots – neurofibromatosis |
| | Oral spots – Peutz–Jeghers syndrome with small gut polyps |
| | Erythema ab igne – fires and hot water bottles |
| | Pregnancy – areolar and midline abdominal |
| | UV light |
| | Radiotherapy |
| | Warts, senile keratosis, keratoacanthoma, callosities |
| Black pigmentation | Eschar, burns and other scabs |
| | Gangrene |
| | Anthrax |
| | Pyoderma gangrenosum |
| Yellow pigmentation | Xanthelasma, pus |
| Purple pigmentation | Campbell de Morgan spots |
| | Capillary naevus – port wine, strawberry |
| | Spider naevi |
| | Telangiectasia |
| | Pyogenic granuloma |
| | Stria – pregnancy, Cushing's, sudden weight loss |

Table 18.4 **Diffuse skin discoloration**

| Colour change | Cause |
|---|---|
| Brown pigmentation | UV light |
| | Acanthosis nigricans (suspected malignancy) |
| | Addison's disease |
| | Nelson's syndrome |
| | Cushing's disease |
| | ACTH secretion |
| | Haemochromatosis (bronze diabetes) |
| | Arsenic and silver poisoning |
| | Gardner's syndrome |
| | Pellagra – nicotinic acid deficiency |
| | Rheumatoid arthritis |
| | Gaucher's syndrome |
| | Lichen planus |
| | Fixed drug reaction |
| Pallor | Anaemia, hypoalbuminaemia |
| Cyanosis | Deoxygenated haemoglobin |
| Blue pigmentation | Methaemoglobin |
| Jaundice | Liver disease |

*contd...*

Table 18.4 Diffuse skin discoloration (*contd...*)

| Colour change | Cause |
|---|---|
| Purplish pigmentation | Polycythaemia |
| Pale brown/yellow pigmentation | Chronic renal failure |
| Orange pigmentation | Carotenaemia |
| Yellow pigmentation | Mepacrine |
| Purpura | Bleeding disorders<br>Vasculitic disorders – collagen diseases, diabetes<br>Septicaemia – especially meningococcal<br>Systemic malignancy<br>Cushing's disease<br>Ehlers–Danlos syndrome |
| Depigmentation | Albinism – absence of melanocytes<br>Vitiligo – destruction of melanocytes<br>Idiopathic<br>Pernicious anaemia<br>Gastric cancer<br>Hypo- and hyperthyroidism<br>Addison's disease<br>Late-onset diabetes<br>Autoimmune disease (Hashimoto's)<br>Scleroderma<br>Syphilis<br>Leprosy |

Table 18.5 Pruritus

| Association | Cause |
|---|---|
| Secondary to local skin conditions | Parasites – fleas, scabies, bites, pediculoses<br>Eczema – local irritants, clothing, washing powder<br>Urticaria<br>Rectal and vaginal discharge<br>Lichen planus<br>Dermatitis herpetiformis<br>Miliaria rubra (prickly heat) |
| Secondary to systemic disease | Neoplasia – Hodgkin's disease, leukaemia<br>Chronic cholestasis – typically biliary cirrhosis and obstructive jaundice<br>Chronic renal failure, particularly late stage and dialysis patients<br>Drug reactions and food sensitivity<br>Polycythaemia, anaemia<br>Psychological<br>Endocrine – hyper- and hypoparathyroidism<br>Heroin addicts |

Inflammatory conditions, although frequently seen, are discussed only briefly since these are mostly addressed by the primary care physician or the dermatologist. Some local diseases have serious or life-threatening consequences and the specific features of these conditions are also covered in this chapter. Diseases and conditions that create lumps and ulcers (see Chapter 3) are particularly relevant to the skin.

Table 18.6 Hair changes

| Decrease/increase | Cause/reason |
|---|---|
| Decrease (alopecia) | Age<br>Genetic – myotonia<br>Damage from chemical treatment<br>Severe illness, malnutrition<br>Immunosuppressive drugs<br>Radiotherapy<br>Lichen planus<br>Psoriasis<br>Systemic lupus erythematosus<br>Fungal |
| Increase | Racial<br>Endocrine – virilizing from ovarian tumours, precocious puberty, adrenogenital syndrome, Cushing's disease, acromegaly, drugs<br>Steroids, anabolic steroids<br>Anti-epileptic drugs<br>Minoxidil, diazoxide<br>Anorexia nervosa |

## THE HISTORY IN SKIN DISORDERS

### Onset

The time of onset of the skin disorder is of critical importance. Congenital and atopic conditions are those present from birth, although they may not necessarily present in their florid state until later. A family history of similar problems may also be elicited.

Note the relation of the onset to any exposure to physical and chemical agents, and remember that the exposure may antedate the skin disorder by a number of months. Similarly, a history of drug or supplement exposure is of essence when a drug eruption is suspected. These diffuse pruritic rashes are usually preceded by the introduction of the drug or supplement around 2–4 weeks prior to the eruption, but the duration can vary from 1 week to 1 year in certain particular drug eruptions. Seek a source for infective lesions, including human and animal contacts at home and abroad. Ask whether the onset of the disorder coincided with times of stress. The rate of onset and progression to other sites can indicate the degree of reaction to the precipitating cause and continued exposure.

### Morphology of Skin Lesions

Rashes may be discrete or continuous – that is, confluent – and the lesions may be primary or secondary.

**Primary lesions** have specific features:

* Macules are flat, circumscribed areas of abnormal skin colour; they may also have a characteristic texture or markings.
* Papules are circumscribed areas of abnormal skin raised in a dome-shaped fashion and are usually less than 1 cm in diameter.
* Larger papules are termed nodules or tumours when they are greater than 1 cm in diameter.
* Raised areas that appear flat or as a plateau may be referred to as plaques. They may result from increased cellular content or oedema.
* Vesicles are raised papules containing clear fluid. Larger collections are termed blisters or bullae.

PART 3 | SKIN

- Pustules are raised papules containing pus.
- Wheals are raised papules with pale centres.
- Purpura indicates haemorrhage within the skin.
- Annular lesions may indicate spreading and infiltration or may have a healing centre.

**Secondary lesions** develop from the expansion or decline of primary lesions or may be related to their mechanical effect. Examples are desquamation or crusting, infiltration, ulceration and scarring. Ichthyosis is thickening of the skin; lichenification is accentuation of the skin lines or dermoglyphics with depigmentation. Scratching produces specific longitudinal, reddened areas and there may be some associated skin thickening. The finding of primary lesions is essential in order to diagnose skin conditions, as most descriptions of skin rashes or eruptions refer to the description of the primary lesion(s) and not the secondary ones.

## Distribution

The distribution is characteristic for many disorders, a specific example being Paget's disease of the nipple (see p. 421) in which the lesion is central on the nipple and overlies a deeper malignancy. In contact disorders, the infective skin may be limited to a ring finger or an ear lobe. Wider areas of potential contact include the hands, feet and axillae.

The mode of spread provides further clues to the diagnosis. Annular spread suggests erythema annulare (Figure 18.1), erythema multiforme (Figure 18.2), pityriasis rosea (Figure 18.3) and fungal infections (Figure 18.4), whereas other diseases, such as malignancy and pyoderma gangrenosum, spread in a much more irregular fashion (Figure 18.5).

**Other common symptoms** include itching, which is usually a sign of eosinophil and mast cell involvement and is seen with, for example, drug eruptions, atopic states and scabies (Table 18.5). Pain is a feature of inflammation and can be seen particularly with infective lesions and some benign tumours, and following a herpes zoster eruption. Erosion indicates superficial skin (epidermal) loss, as seen in acute dermatitis, while ulcers indicate a deeper loss of skin structure (epidermal and dermal). Locally associated symptoms include regional lymph node tenderness and swelling. General symptoms include fever and malaise and possibly those of the underlying associated disease (see Tables 18.1 and 18.2).

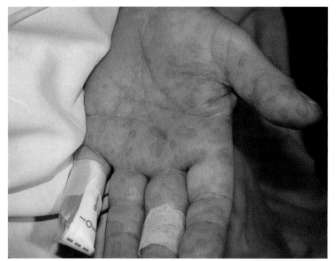
Figure 18.2 Erythema multiforme.

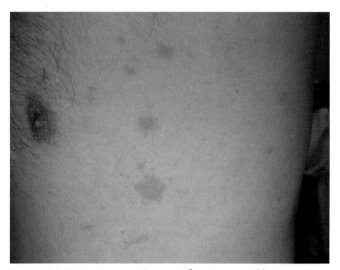
Figure 18.3 Pityriasis rosea (Courtesy of Dr Ossama Abbas).

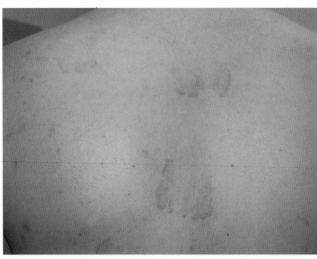
Figure 18.1 Erythema annulare.

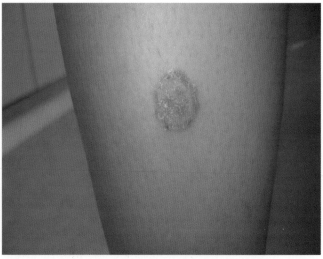
Figure 18.4 Tinea corporis (Courtesy of Dr Ossama Abbas).

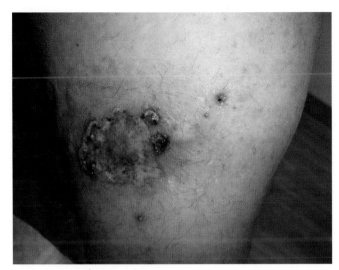

Figure 18.5 **Pyoderma gangrenosum.**

## HISTOLOGY OF THE SKIN

The skin is composed of an outer layer of stratified squamous epithelium – the epidermis – and a deeper layer of dense connective tissue – the dermis. The epidermis is composed of four main layers. The first is the basal layer, or stratum basale, which is found at the lower border of the epidermis. It is composed of actively dividing cells with stem cells, Langerhans cells and melanocytes intercalated between keratinocytes.

This layer attaches to the basement membrane. The derivatives of the basal cells start maturing as they move upwards in the epidermis and become progressively flattened and spinous, hence the name of this second main layer – the stratum spinosum (the prickle cell layer).

The third important layer is the stratum granulosum, which is found overlying the stratum spinosum and is characterized by purple dense granules called keratohyaline granules. The final layer is the stratum corneum, which consists of closely packed, flattened, dead keratin cells that desquamate.

The dermis gives considerable strength to the skin, due to an extensive interweaving collagen mesh, and some resilience due to its elastic component. A rich network of vessels and nerves lies superficially within the dermis and more deeply are the skin appendages, hair follicles and sebaceous and sweat glands. The dermis is divided into the outer, thinner papillary dermis and the deeper reticular dermis. The parallel collagen bundles in the latter are sited along the lines of skin cleavage. There is great regional variation in the amount of keratin, hair, pigment, vessels, nerves and glands among the different body sites. At most sites, the skin is freely mobile over the underlying subcutaneous fatty tissue.

The skin is subject to a large number and variety of focal and generalized diseases, many of which are cutaneous manifestations of systemic disorders. They can usually be diagnosed on the history and physical findings alone, although a great diversity of signs can make this diagnosis very difficult.

The diversity of structures making up the skin and subcutaneous tissue gives rise to a variety of lumps, which are difficult to classify. Most of these have characteristic features and it is important to make a diagnosis in order to confirm or exclude premalignant and early malignant conditions. Carefully apply the system used for examining lumps (see Table 3.1; p. 54) and particularly

note whether the lump is in the skin or attached to it, or whether the skin is mobile over it. Abnormalities of the skin surface and colour changes are particularly helpful, and remember to examine for enlarged regional lymph nodes.

The following sections consider benign and malignant lesions arising from the skin, its appendages and the subcutaneous tissues. Pigmented lesions are considered separately in view of the importance of diagnosing a malignant melanoma; ulcers are considered on Table 3.1; p. 54 and Table 4.1; p. 77.

The description of cutaneous and subcutaneous lesions follows the order given in Table 1.1, including all applicable features. The table is based on the description of lumps and ulcers and is considered in Chapter 3.

## CLASSIFICATION OF SKIN DISORDERS

It is useful to classify skin diseases into the broad categories of inflammatory, infectious and proliferative processes. Although this classification follows a simplistic approach, most skin conditions and eruptions will fall under one of these categories.

The inflammatory conditions, as the name implies, involve primarily the immune response in the skin eruption. Inflammatory skin reactions to external agents (physical or chemical), otherwise known as physical dermatoses, are usually unilateral in nature, in contrast to inflammatory conditions related to systemic conditions such as atopic dermatitis (Figure 18.6) or psoriasis (Figure 18.7). An example of a physical agent is exposure to cold, producing cold urticaria and chilblains (Figure 18.8). Heat and sweating produce some dermatoses, aggravate infective lesions and increase itching. Ultraviolet light from the sun and tanning beds can produce severe burns and other reactions in sunbathers. Irritant and allergic chemical agents may be encountered in the home or industrial environment (Figure 18.9). Examples may be found in exposure to new clothing (Figure 18.10), jewellery, soaps, cosmetics, hair dyes and products for use in the garden and drugs.

Infectious conditions are mostly bacterial but may also be due to fungal or parasitic infections. The vast majority of bacterial skin infections are staphylococcal infections, which are responsible for most folliculitis (Figure 18.11), carbuncles (Figure 18.12) and furuncles (Figure 18.13), as well as

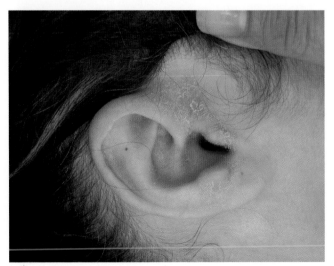

Figure 18.6 **Atopic dermatitis.**

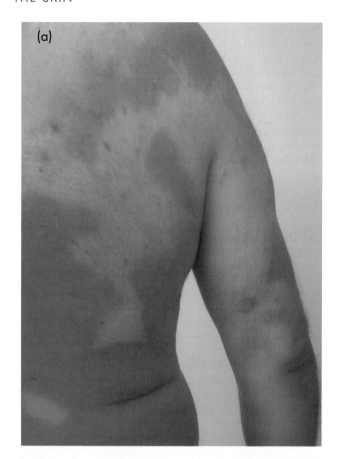

Figure 18.7 Psoriasis with (a) well-demarcated erythematous plaques and (b) thickened grey whitish scale.

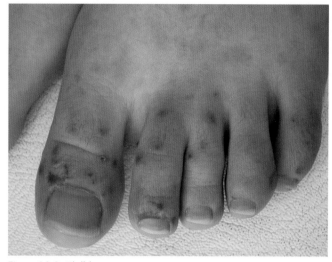

Figure 18.8 Chilblain or perniosis.

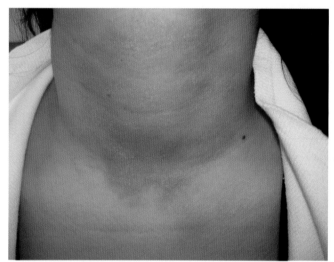

Figure 18.9 Contact dermatitis (Courtesy of Dr Ossama Abbas).

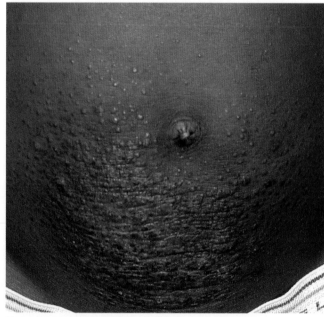

Figure 18.10 Contact dermatitis to nickel in a belt.

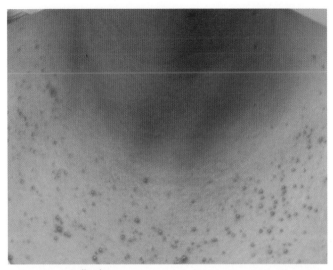

Figure 18.11 **Folliculitis.**

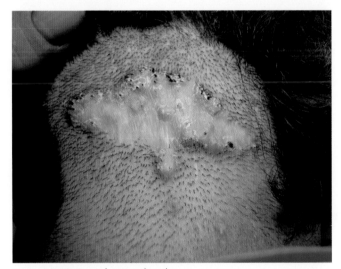

Figure 18.12 **A resolving carbuncle.**

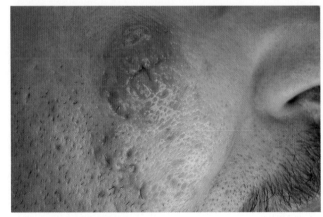

Figure 18.13 **A furuncle.**

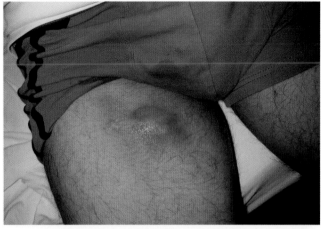

Figure 18.14 **A skin abscess.** (Courtesy of Dr Shukrallah Zaynoun.)

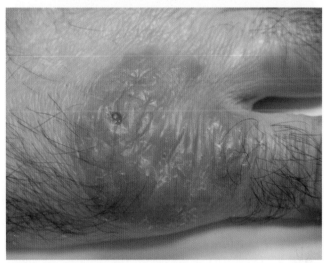

Figure 18.15 **Primary cutaneous tuberculosis.** (Courtesy of Dr Shukrallah Zaynoun.)

unilateral erythematous, scaly patch referred to as tinea. These are located most commonly over the feet, groins and buttocks. They mostly originate from human reservoirs but animal and plant reservoirs are less common culprits. Communal sports activities facilitate the transfer of fungal infections. Parasitic infections include most commonly scabies infestations, which are cause by the mite *Sarcoptes scabiei*. This form of infection is most commonly sexually transmitted but can occur following a close skin-to-skin contact.

Proliferative conditions are discussed below. These are mostly subclassified into benign or malignant. Cutaneous proliferative lesions may originate from keratinocytes, melanocytes or fibroblasts. They may also be vascular or neural in origin, or may be a combination of these.

## CUTANEOUS LESIONS OF EPITHELIAL, MESENCHYMAL AND ADNEXAL ORIGIN

### Benign Lesions of the Skin and its Appendages

#### *Benign Papilloma – Skin Tags or Acrochordons*

Papillomas (Figure 18.16) are hamartomas consisting of an overgrowth of all the skin layers and its appendages; they have a

skin abscesses (Figure 18.14) and cellulitis. Less commonly, streptococcal infection can produce a more demarcated, cellulitis-like lesion such as erysipelas. Infections by atypical mycobacteria such as *Mycobacterium tuberculosis* can cause primary cutaneous tuberculosis (Figure 18.15), which may look like a verruca or an ulcerated plaque. Fungal infections cause a

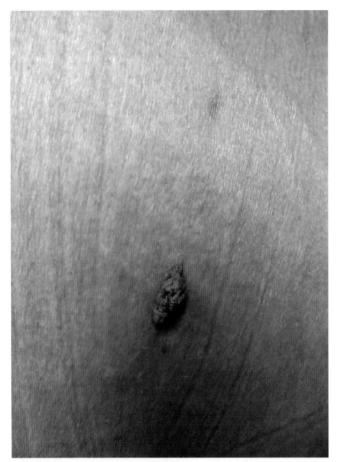

Figure 18.16 A papilloma or skin tag

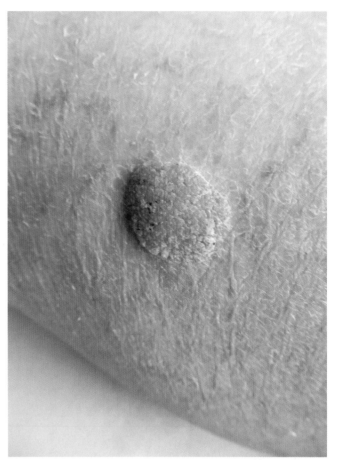

Figure 18.17 Seborrhoeic keratosis.

central core and normal sensation. The lesions can occur at any age but are usually seen in the elderly. The symptoms are mostly cosmetic but the papillomas may catch in clothing and if repeatedly traumatized may bleed and become inflamed, swollen and painful, and sometimes ulcerate.

Papillomas can be seen anywhere on the body but are predominantly present over flexural areas such as the neck and groin. They are well-defined, hyperpigmented to skin-coloured papules, usually pedunculated and ranging from a few millimeters to a few centimetres in size. The surface may be flat or deeply fissured.

Acrochordons are solid, usually firm, but may be soft if there is a large, central, fatty component. They are non-invasive and not indurated unless there is associated inflammation and ulceration, in which case they may be mistaken for malignant lesions. They tend to occur mostly in obese individuals as well as patients with diabetes mellitus and those with a familial history of acrochordons.

Intradermal naevi and pedunculated seborrhoeic keratosis may simulate skin tags and are sometimes difficult to differentiate on a clinical basis. Nodular melanomas may present as pedunculated papules or nodules but are usually dark brown to black in coloration.

### Seborrhoeic Keratosis – Seborrhoeic Warts, Senile Warts and Verruca Senilis

Seborrhoeic keratoses (Figure 18.17) are overgrowths of the upper part of the hair follicle (infundibulum) so they are not seen over non-hairy or glabrous skin such as the palms and soles.

They are very common and usually multiple in the elderly of both sexes, but are occasionally seen in the young. The lesions slowly increase in size over many years and may fall or be rubbed off. They give rise to cosmetic problems and can catch on clothing. Although they rarely bleed, bleeding into the lesion can produce the appearance of a pyogenic granuloma or a squamous cell carcinoma (SCC). The lesion may become infected.

Seborrhoeic keratoses predominantly occur over the trunk, particularly the back, but also over the arms and neck. They have the appearance of 'stuck-on', well-defined, firm, slightly raised, verrucous (i.e. wart-like) plaque lesions. The surface is usually rough and hyperkeratotic but can occasionally be smooth and flat. They are usually light brown to skin coloured but may become deeply pigmented and be mistaken for a malignant melanoma. The lesions can be peeled or scraped off, leaving a pale pink patch of underlying skin, sometimes with a few fine bleeding points.

The sudden eruption of multiple seborrhoeic keratoses in an individual might be a herald sign of an internal malignancy, most commonly colon cancer. This sign is referred to as the sign of Leser–Trélat.

### Warts

Warts are epidermal growths resulting from infection with the human papillomavirus of the papovavirus group. A number of different viruses are involved. Common and plantar warts (Figure 18.18) – called verruca vulgaris and verruca plantaris, respectively – are most commonly produced by the same viral subtypes and differ from the flat wart (verruca plana), genital wart (Figure 18.19) and oropharyngeal wart subtypes. Warts are contagious, the virus probably entering through minor abrasions. The wart virus needs the keratinocyte machinery in order to grow and multiply and hence does not survive in areas below the epidermis.

Warts occur at all ages but are most common in children between 12 and 16 years old. They develop to their full size within a few weeks but there is probably an incubation period of several months. Approximately one-third disappear spontaneously within 6 months and two-thirds within 2 years. Warts cause cosmetic problems and when on the fingers interfere with fine movements of the hand; they can cause pain and irritation. Associated inflammation is usually due to attempts to pick them off.

Warts commonly occur over the knuckles and nail folds of the fingers, on the backs of hands, over the knees and on the face. They are usually multiple and may coalesce. They are hard, 3–8 mm in diameter and raised by 1–2 mm. Facial warts are often of the smoother – plain/juvenile – variety. Plantar warts occur on the sole of the foot, where they are commonly inverted into the skin and painful during walking.

When warts grow over the palms and soles, there is characteristically a loss of the skin lines (dermoglyphics), and black dots are seen within the papules, corresponding to thrombosed blood vessels.

## Molluscum Contagiosum

Molluscum contagiosum lesions (Figure 18.20) are produced by the poxvirus. The molluscum papule is smooth, shiny and pearly white to skin coloured. It is a few millimeters in diameter and characteristically becomes umbilicated as it matures. The lesions occur on the abdomen, genitalia, face and arms, and undergo spontaneous regression after several months. In adults, the infection is most commonly sexually transmitted. In children, transmission is by skin-to-skin contact with peers or parents. Sexual abuse should be kept in mind in a minor with genital molluscum.

## Hypertrophic Scars and Keloids

Hypertrophic scars and keloids (Figures 18.21 and 18.22) are caused by the overproduction of normal collagen or the

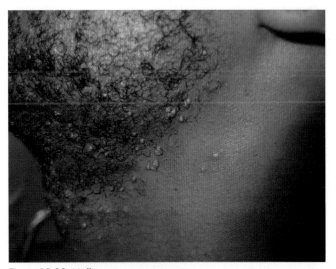
Figure 18.20 Molluscum contagiosum.

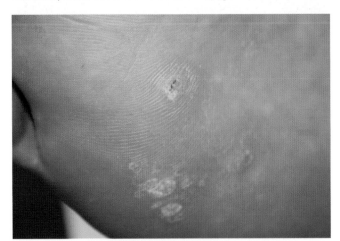
Figure 18.18 Plantar warts (Courtesy of Dr Osama Abbas).

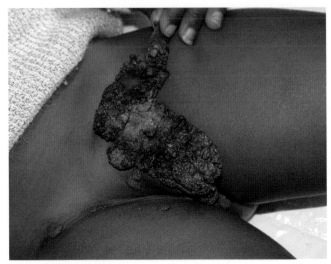
Figure 18.19 Genital warts.

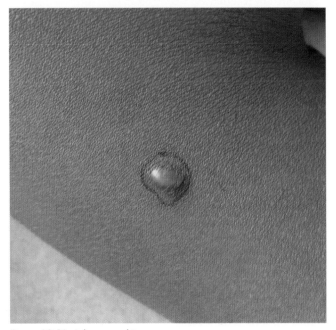
Figure 18.21 A hypertrophic scar.

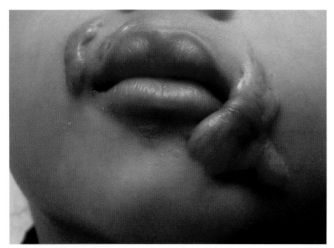

Figure 18.22 A keloid scar.

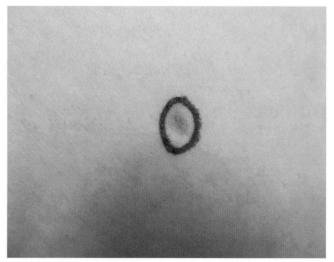

Figure 18.23 Dermatofibroma.

production of abnormal collagen tissue in a wound. With hypertrophic scars, the cause is often abnormal local conditions such as infection, a foreign body, undue tension across the wound and incisions across the skin creases. The scar continues to increase in width and thickness for up to 2–3 months but, unlike keloids, does not tend to grow over the margin of the initial incision. Within a year, however, there is often shrinkage and the initial browny-red discoloration fades. The abnormality does not necessarily include the whole length of the scar, and excision is not usually followed by recurrence.

Keloid is often familial and commonly seen in darker skinned individuals. The hypertrophy includes the wound and also the tissues on either side. Proliferation continues for 6–12 months and can produce a tumour-like overgrowth. The scar is often itchy, tender and painful. Keloid is rare in infancy and in old age, and reduces in severity from about 30 years of age onwards. In extreme examples, the overgrowth can be pedunculated, especially over the ear lobes; the epithelial covering is usually thin and gives it a shiny appearance. Excision of the lesion is likely to be followed by recurrence.

### Histiocytoma – Dermatofibroma

Dermatofibromas (Figure 18.23) are benign, dermal tumours predominantly of fibrous origin that are covered with normal epithelium. They are asymptomatic and take a number of years to grow to their full size, which can be 5–20 mm in diameter. They are sited predominantly on the limbs and are well circumscribed, red to brown, firm, smooth-surfaced lesions. Lateral compression characteristically leaves a dimple-like depression in the overlying skin, hence the name 'dimple sign'.

Their main importance is that, as the lesions increase in size, their pigmentation can be mistaken for that of a malignant melanoma. In addition, the presence of multiple dermatofibromas (more than 15 lesions) has been associated with immune status disturbances such as lupus erythematosus and human immunodeficiency virus (HIV) infection. A sclerosing angioma is a variant containing prominent vascular elements.

### Callosities and Corns

Callosities (Figure 18.24) are due to excessive skin keratinization and occur as a protective measure over an area of intermittent pressure. This is commonly on the feet – especially the

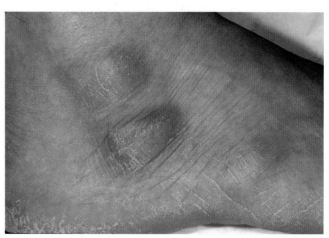

Figure 18.24 Callus over the heel and corns over the lateral ankle. (Courtesy of Dr Shukrallah Zaynoun.)

inframedial aspect of the great toe and the heel – but may also occur over the dorsal aspect of deformed toes and pressure sites with other limb deformities.

Corns (Figure 18.25) are callosities over focal pressure points, usually over a bony prominence. A central core of keratin is compressed into the skin in the same way as a plantar wart, producing pain.

On examination, the keratin of callosities marks out the pressure area, and the lesion is continuous around its margins with normal skin. The callosities surrounding neuropathic ulcers can be particularly prominent. The central core of a corn is palpable as a nodule of whitish degenerate cells.

Callosities, unlike warts, tend to maintain the dermoglyphics of the skin.

### Dermoid Cysts

Dermoid cysts (Figure 18.26) are due to the sequestration of epithelial elements deep to the skin surface. Congenital dermoid cysts occur along the lines of embryological skin fusion. Common sites are at the medial and lateral ends of the eyebrow (internal and external angular dermoids), sublingually (deep or superficial to the mylohyoid muscle) and in post-auricular and pre- and post-sacral sites. The latter may expand within the spinal canal,

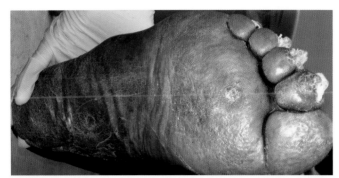

Figure 18.25 A corn over the anterior heel (Courtesy of Dr Marijana Atanasovski).

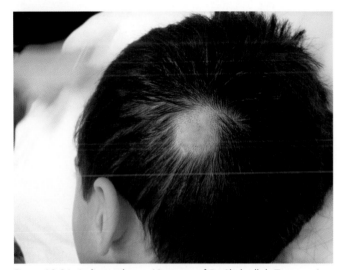

Figure 18.26 A dermoid cyst. (Courtesy of Dr Shukrallah Zaynoun.)

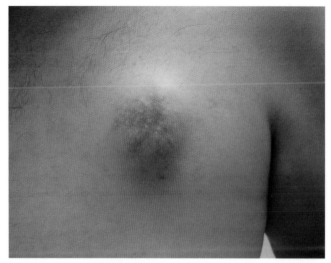

Figure 18.27 An epidermal cyst.

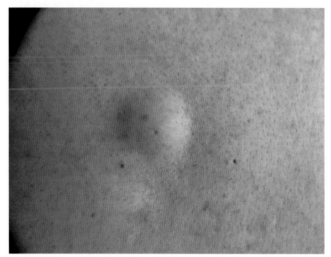

Figure 18.28 An epidermal inclusion cyst (Courtesy of Dr Marijana Atanasovski).

causing compression of the cauda equina. The lesions may be present at birth but are usually noted in the first 2 years of life; they are occasionally first seen in adulthood. Their prime symptom is their unsightly appearance, but they rarely give rise to pain, infection or discharge.

The lesions are usually single and slow-growing. They are smooth, spherical and mobile, enlarging to 1–2 cm in diameter; sublingual cysts can reach 3–5 cm. The cysts are lined with keratinized stratified squamous epithelium and may contain other epithelial elements, such as hair and sebaceous material. These influence their physical signs since they do not usually transilluminate and may indent rather than be fluctuant.

With post-traumatic inclusion dermoids, the injury is usually remembered and the overlying scar is visible. These typically occur on the fingers, are 4–6 mm in diameter and are firm in consistency. They contain keratinized, squamous epithelium but not usually sebaceous material. They may be confused with a sebaceous cyst, but although there is often skin tethering, no punctum is present.

## Sebaceous Cysts – Epidermoid Cyst, Wen

Sebaceous cysts (Figures 18.27 and 18.28) are derived from hair follicles and are usually filled with altered keratin so they are more appropriately called epidermal cysts. They represent one of the most common skin lesions, occurring at any age after childhood. They are often multiple and occur at any hair-bearing site

on the body, commonly the trunk, face and neck, and particularly the scalp and scrotum; they do not occur on the palms and soles. If seen over toes or fingers, they are associated with osteomas and intestinal polyps in the setting of Gardner's syndrome. They are unsightly and may become painful if there is secondary inflammation or abscess formation. The inflammatory response is usually a foreign body, granulomatous reaction. When ruptured, they may discharge toothpaste-like, whitish, granular material with an unpleasant smell.

The lesions are well defined and tethered to the overlying skin but freely mobile over the deep tissues, growing slowly up to 12 cm in diameter. They lie in the dermis and can extend to the subcutaneous tissue. An opening to the outer skin is sometimes seen through a black punctum, but a punctum is often not seen.

Sebaceous cysts may occasionally ulcerate and in these circumstances can look very much like a malignant skin lesion. They are then termed a Cock's peculiar tumour. The concretions of a sebaceous cyst can be gradually excreted and build up into a hard, conical sebaceous horn.

PART 3 | SKIN

### Other Tumours of Skin Appendages

These are rare. They include steatocystomas (which are true sebaceous cysts containing oily material; Figure 18.29), leiomyomas from the smooth erector pili muscle of the hairs (Figure 18.30) (which are usually painful and contract upon being touched), hidradenomas (benign tumours of the eccrine glands that might simulate a pyogenic granuloma), sebaceous adenomas, cylindromas and trichoepitheliomas.

Cylindromas (Figure 18.31) are tumours of the sweat glands, frequently multiple and commonly found on the scalp. They can range from a few millimeters to several centimetres across, the latter producing disfigurement. They are soft, boggy swellings but do not fluctuate or indent. They are rarely malignant. Cylindromas are one of the causes of turban tumours of the scalp, the deformity being better known for its title than for its incidence.

Trichoepitheliomas are benign growth of the hair follicle epithelium. Clinically, they consist of skin-coloured papules that can be confused with a basal cell carcinoma (BCC).

## Premalignant and Malignant Lesions of the Skin

Exposure to sunlight can produce a number of skin disorders and aggravate many existing conditions. Scantily clad sun-worshippers are at risk; blonde and red-headed individuals are particularly susceptible. There is a high incidence of skin disorders in Australia, South Africa and the southern states of the USA. Also at risk are outdoor workers such as fishermen, farmers and labourers.

Sunburn can occur within an hour of exposure in sensitive-skinned individuals, producing erythema, blistering and later peeling. Continued exposure may give rise to severe, permanent skin damage even at an early age, leading to premature skin ageing, although the changes are usually degenerative and age-related. The signs of ageing are fragile skin with loss of elasticity, increased keratosis, vascular changes such as spider navi and angioma, telangiectases, venous lakes and pronounced sebaceous glands. Of particular concern is the predisposition to premalignant and malignant skin lesions, including solar keratosis, Bowen's disease, BCC, SCC and malignant melanoma. The risk of developing malignant melanoma increases mostly with sunburn-related incidents before age 18, while the risk of developing basal and squamous cell carcinomas is related to chronic sun exposure that accumulates during a person's lifetime.

### Actinic Keratosis (Solar Keratosis)

Actinic keratoses (Figure 18.32) are painless, hyperkeratotic, skin-coloured to erythematous, 'rough', non-indurated macules, related to prolonged exposure to sunlight. Because of their rough surface, these lesions are more commonly felt than seen. The risk of these lesions undergoing malignant transformation is 1–5 per cent. The lesions usually occur in elderly persons and outdoor workers, and are seen over the tops of the ears, on the face and on the backs of the hands and fingers. The lesions are usually painless.

Actinic keratosis, SCC *in situ* and SCC fall within a spectrum of the disease. Microscopically, actinic keratosis reveals a dysplasia at the lower level of the epidermis (the basal and spinous layer). Once full-thickness involvement of the epidermis has occurred, this becomes SCC *in situ* or Bowen's disease. Invasion of the dermis by such tumours denotes a SCC.

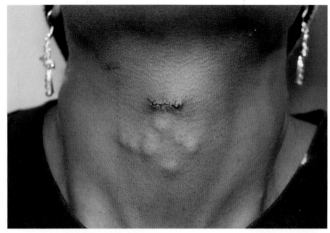

Figure 18.29 Multiple steatocystomas.

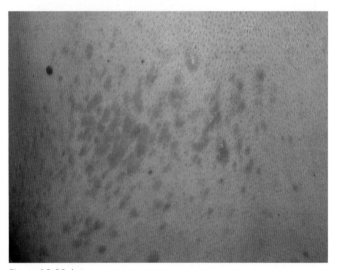

Figure 18.30 Leiomyomas.

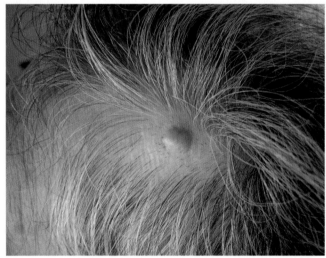

Figure 18.31 A cylindroma.

### Bowen's Disease and Erythroplasia of Queyrat

The lesions of Bowen's disease or SCC *in situ* (Figure 18.33) are irregularly shaped, well-defined plaques that may be mistaken for a patch of eczema or psoriasis. They therefore present late and

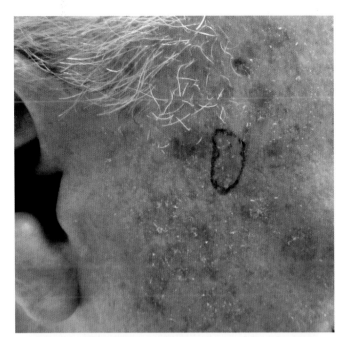

Figure 18.32 **Multiple actinic keratoses.**

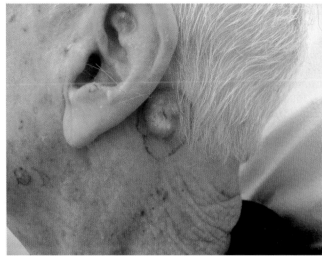

Figure 18.34 **Squamous cell carcinoma behind the ear.**

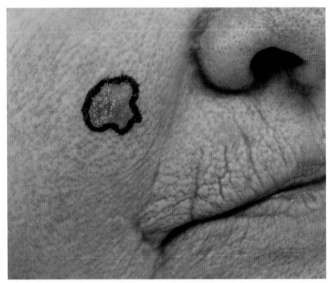

Figure 18.33 **Squamous cell carcinoma** *in situ.*

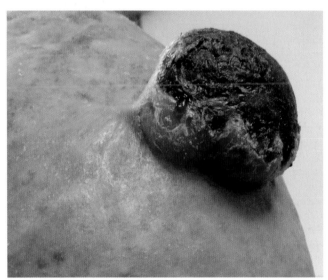

Figure 18.35 **A fungating squamous cell carcinoma.**

any such lesion that does not respond to topical steroids should be biopsied.

The lesions vary in size from 5 mm to a few centimetres in diameter. They are beefy red, erythematous areas that are slightly raised and have a scaly crust on their surface. The skin beneath the crust is moist and papilliform. Malignant changes produce papules and nodules.

Erythroplasia of Queyrat (see p. 651) has features identical to those of Bowen's disease but is situated on the penis.

### Leukoplakia

Leukoplakia can occur along the margins of the lips (see p. 17) and on the vulva, although it is most common in the oral cavity. It is a white coating of the mucous membrane that does not rub off, unlike *Candida* and some other infections. The lesions are the result of multiple traumas such as from sharp teeth and dentures,

spicy foods, sepsis, syphilis, pipe smoking and betel nut (areca nut) chewing.

The majority of lesions are benign, but some may show dysplastic changes, and there is an incidence of 13 per cent change to SCC. This incidence rises to two-thirds in the floor of the mouth, where all lesions must be biopsied and carefully monitored. **Erythroplakia** is a pink to red discoloration underlying the white coating, the cellular abnormality in this instance showing *in situ* or invasive SCC in all cases.

### Squamous Cell Carcinoma

Cutaneous SCC (**Figures 18.34** and **18.35**) is the second most common skin malignancy following BCC. The sun is considered to be the most important culprit in inducing these tumours, but there are a number of other predisposing factors including exposure to chemical hydrocarbons, tar and mineral oils. There is a high incidence of cutaneous SCC in patients living in tropical countries due to the high ultraviolet index in these areas. When seen in sun-exposed skin, SCCs are mostly due to sun damage, whereas on the genitalia they are mostly due to chronic

PART 3 | SKIN

human papillomavirus infection, and in the oral cavity they are mostly due to chronic alcohol ingestion and cigarette smoking. Cutaneous SCCs occasionally arises from areas of chronic radiation damage or a chronic ulcer or scar and are then referred to as Marjolin's ulcers. Chronic immunosuppression (e.g. in organ transplantation) is associated with an increased risk of SCC.

If any nodularities or changes in the skin edges are seen in a chronic non-healing ulcer, they must be biopsied to rule out SCC. The behaviour of SCCs of the genitalia and oral mucosa is more aggressive and the risk of metastasis is higher compared with SCCs arising in sun-exposed skin.

Clinically, SCCs can initially present as a firm, round erythematous nodule that progressively enlarges and ulcerates. The enlargement usually takes place over a few months. The ulcer has a crusty or horny covering but as it becomes deeper it penetrates the dermis, exposing underlying tissues such as tendons, bones, cartilage and joints; the base of the ulcer bleeds easily and is very necrotic. The ulcer's edge is everted and local invasion of the surrounding tissues produces induration that is visible beyond the ulcer margin.

The rate of onset, progressive deepening and increased eversion are typical of malignant change. There may be associated thrombosis and the ulcer may penetrate the adjacent vessels, producing severe and possibly fatal haemorrhage. Metastasis is usually via the lymphatics, and the local nodes are commonly involved. However, one-third of these prove to be due to infection rather than secondary malignancy. Metastases can occur via the bloodstream but this is uncommon.

Histologically, there is full-thickness atypia of the epidermal cells together with invasion into the dermis. According to the degree of atypia and differentiation, SCCs are divided into well, moderately or poorly differentiated tumours. The degree of differentiation carries a prognostic indicator for their behaviour. With well-differentiated SCCs, keratin deposition, often arranged in onion-like, concentric layers termed keratin pearls, may be seen within the masses extending into the dermis and are not to be confused with the keratin pearls that can be seen within the epidermis in a seborrheic keratosis.

The differential diagnosis of SCC includes solar keratosis, pyogenic granuloma, seborrhoeic keratosis, BCC and malignant melanoma.

### Keratoacanthoma

Keratoacanthoma (Figure 18.36) is an overgrowth of an unknown aetiology. It has a characteristic rapid development to its full size in 3–5 weeks, and spontaneous regression occurs in 2–12 months. Besides these two hallmarks of keratoacanthoma, differentiation from well-differentiated SCCs is extremely difficult both clinically and histologically. The lesions are usually single and can occur anywhere on the body, although particularly on exposed areas such as the arms and around the nose.

The lesion is a discrete, dome-shaped nodule 1–2 cm in diameter and 2–3 mm high. The firm, smooth outer rim is skin coloured, but the central core is of hard, irregular, keratinized white or black material.

Multiple keratoacanthomas are also encountered with familial inheritance (Ferguson-Smith syndrome) or as part of other syndromes such as Muir–Torre syndrome, in which colonic polyps, sebaceous tumours and keratoacanthomas are seen. The major problems with keratoacanthomas are the possible disfigurement and the difficulty of differentiating them from SCCs, both

clinically and histologically. For these reasons, keratoacanthomas are better excised in order not to miss an SCC counterpart.

### Basal Cell Carcinoma

Basal cell carcinomas (Figures 18.37 and 18.38) are the most common type of skin cancer. The ratio of BCC to SCC is 2:1 but this is reversed in chronic immunosuppression. BCC reflects a

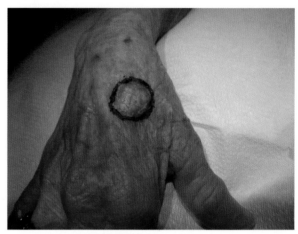

Figure 18.36 **Keratoacanthoma.**

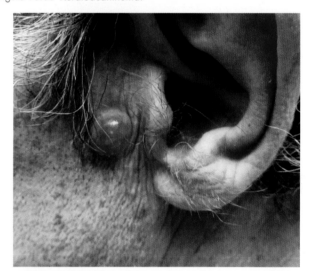

Figure 18.37 **Basal cell carcinoma.**

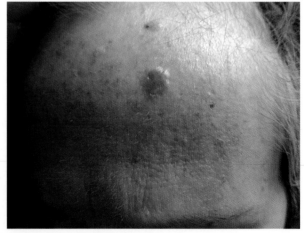

Figure 18.38 **Basal cell carcinoma.**

malignant change in the basal layer of the epidermis. The lesions undergo slow, steady enlargement, invading the adjacent skin, and are very destructive if left untreated. They metastasize in less than 1 per cent of the cases, and metastases to the lymph nodes, lung and brain are most common. Lesions are most common in the elderly, being twice as common in men than women. There is also a high incidence in sun-worshippers.

Although the lesions are most commonly seen on sun-exposed areas, BCCs can occur over sun-spared areas such as the genitals and buttocks, reflecting that although the majority are secondary to sun-induced mutations, a few are due to genetic mutations.

Clinically, BCC starts as a nodule with a slightly transparent, superficial epidermal layer giving a cystic appearance. Lesions are occasionally pigmented. The next stage is central erosion with intermittent bleeding. The edge is characteristic and diagnostic, being raised and rolled, with a pearly appearance. It may also be slightly pinkish due to telangiectases running over the surface. If the lesion is untreated, local invasion progresses into both the underlying tissues and the peripheral edges of the tumour, making them irregular. The presence of ulceration and irregular borders gave rise to the original nomenclature of 'rodent ulcer'. The lesions can be differentiated from SCCs by the pearly translucent papules and the rolled pearly border, which are not present in cutaneous SCCs.

Histologically, BCC starts as a nidus of basal cells extending into the dermis. The nidus grows into larger masses consisting of basaloid cells that display little atypia with only few mitoses, form characteristic palisades at the periphery and surround themselves with a concentric thin stroma from which the tumour frequently detaches or clefts.

The differential diagnosis of BCC is similar to that mentioned above for cutaneous SCC.

## Paget's Disease

Paget's disease (see p. 421) consists of eczema-like skin patches over the nipple area that arise secondary to intraductal carcinoma. A similar eruption – extramammary Paget's disease – may occur over the anogenital area secondary to an adenocarcinoma of the gastrointestinal or genitourinary system.

The lesions are red, weeping, crusty and scaly plaques involving the nipple and surrounding areola. Because of its eczema-like appearance, the lesion may be disregarded by the patient until there is retraction, ulceration and destruction of the nipple or until an underlying mass or regional lymph node becomes palpable.

## Cutaneous Lymphoma

Lymphomas may affect any organ in the body but some forms predominantly affect the skin. Unlike those in the body, cutaneous lymphomas are most commonly of the T-cell type and less commonly of the B-cell type. The name 'mycosis fungoides', which used to be used to describe these cases, is a misnomer and has now been replaced by the name 'cutaneous T-cell lymphoma' (CTCL). The name 'Sézary syndrome' is still used to describe the leukaemic form of the disease.

CTCL is most commonly found in middle-aged men. Early lesions begin as non-specific, asymptomatic, flat, red, scaly eruptions suggestive of chronic eczema or psoriasis. However, they have a typical distribution, often over non-exposed areas. Lesions progress to become plaques (Figure 18.39),

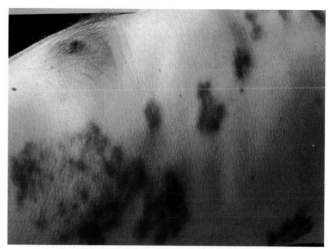

Figure 18.39 Plaque-stage cutaneous T-cell lymphoma.

nodules and tumours. Involvement of the bone marrow produces Sézary syndrome, which consists of diffuse redness over the skin, otherwise known as erythroderma. There may be up to 20 years of progression before tumour formation, lymphadenopathy and visceral involvement occurs.

## CUTANEOUS LESIONS OF MELANOCYTIC ORIGINS

The pigment melanin is produced by melanocytes. These are derived from neural crest cells that migrate during development and are scattered throughout the basal layer of the skin epidermis. Although the number of melanocytes is similar in all races, the amount of melanin produced varies between black- and white-skinned individuals, and also increases in response to ultraviolet light.

Benign overgrowths of melanocytes are termed moles or pigmented naevi. Pigmented lesions may also be produced by an overproduction of melanin from a normal number and distribution of melanocytes – for example, a freckle – or by an increased number of melanocytes within the basal layer of epidermis, as seen in lentigo and the pigmentation of Peutz–Jeghers syndrome.

In order to diagnose and treat malignant melanoma as early as possible, it is important to recognize typical benign lesions and to examine all doubtful lesions histologically.

## Benign Melanocytic Lesions
### Pigmented Naevi – Moles

Moles or naevi (Figures 18.40 and 18.41) are very common and most white individuals have at least one at birth, the number increasing throughout life. Moles may regress or disappear during childhood; pigmentation may also increase but malignant change is very rare before puberty. Moles are less obvious in black-skinned individuals but are seen on the palms and soles.

The lesions may occur anywhere on the body and are usually discrete and 2–4 mm in diameter. The colour varies from very pale to black, as does the amount of hair in the mole. The symptoms are usually cosmetic but rough and protruding lesions may catch on clothing. Although pain can occur because of trauma to the lesion or due to the inflammation of sebaceous glands within it, this is an unusual symptom, as are bleeding and itching.

PART 3 | SKIN

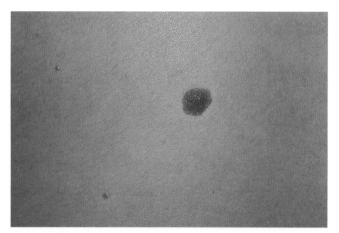

Figure 18.40 **A junctional naevus.**

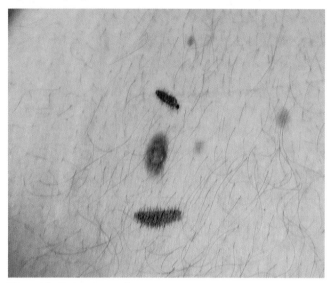

Figure 18.41 **A compound naevus.**

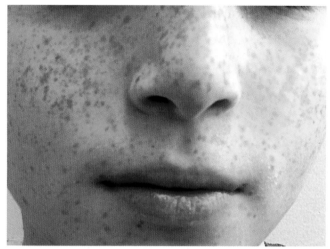

Figure 18.42 **Freckles.**

The clinician must always be on the lookout for any changes in a lesion suggesting malignant change. The clinical signs of malignant transformation can be remembered using ABCDE:

- A – Asymmetry (note whether one side is larger than the other).
- B – Border (jagged borders are suggestive of transformation).
- C – Colour (multiple colours within a naevus should raise suspicion).
- D – Diameter (any naevus that has grown to more than the size of the pencil eraser or 6 mm in diameter should be examined).
- E – Evolution (a lesion that is changing with time should be checked).

Another easy method is the 'ugly duckling' sign, where patients' naevi are examined and moles that show changes that are not present in most others are considered for biopsy.

## Freckles

A freckle (Figure 18.42) is an overproduction of melanin from a normal population of melanocytes. Freckles are common and occur particularly on exposed areas such as the face and the dorsum of the hands. They are pale brown lesions, 2–4 mm in diameter, and are usually multiple. They have no malignant potential. They frequently arise with sun exposure and may disappear with disciplined protection against the sun. Individuals with freckles are more likely to develop skin cancers at later stages in their lives.

## Lentigo

A Hutchinson's lentigo or solar lentigo (Figure 18.43) results from an increased number of melanocytes within the basal layer of the epidermis. It is usually found in elderly people (reflected in the name 'senile lentigo'), grows slowly usually over sun-exposed areas (hence the alternative name 'solar lentigo') and is darkly pigmented. The irregular area may be a number of centimetres in diameter and is usually flat, but it may be a slightly raised plaque or have flat nodules within it. Lentigines are usually found on the neck and the back of the hand.

## Café-au-lait Spots

These pale brown, flat, multiple patches (Figure 18.44) are usually a few millimeters in diameter but may be larger in size; they are present at birth. The lesions can be associated with neurofibromatosis – particularly if there are more than five of them – and occasionally phaeochromocytomas. Histologically, the lesions can be due to increased melanin production or sometimes an increased number of basal melanocytes. However, they have no malignant potential.

## Pigmented Lesions in Peutz–Jeghers Syndrome

These lesions (Figure 35.53; p. 571), associated with multiple intestinal polyposis, are usually found over the mucous membrane of the lips and circumoral area. They are 1–2 mm in diameter and asymptomatic. Although they are to the result of an increased number of basal melanocytes, they have no malignant potential.

## Malignant Melanocytic Lesions: Malignant Melanoma

Malignant melanomas are highly malignant tumours of melanocytic origin. Approximately half develop in pre-existing benign naevi, while the rest occur spontaneously in previously normal skin.

Melanoma occurs most commonly in white individuals, particularly those exposed to the sunlight of subtropical zones.

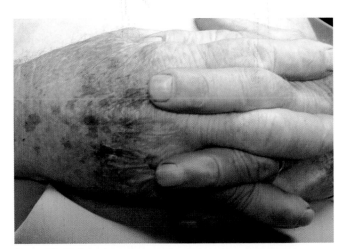

Figure 18.43 Solar lentigines.

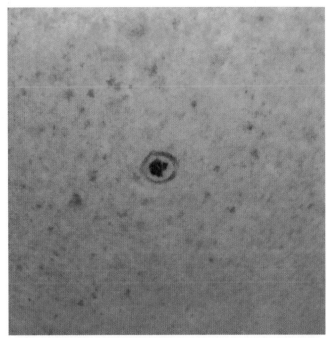

Figure 18.45 A superficial spreading melanoma.

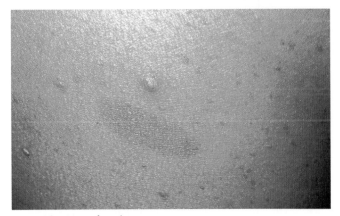

Figure 18.44 A café-au-lait spot.

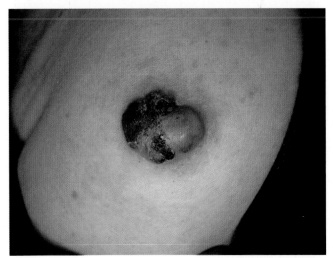

Figure 18.46 Nodular melanoma. (Courtesy of Dr Shukrallah Zaynoun.)

The highest incidence is seen in northern Australia but the incidence is increasing in northern Europe. Melanomas are unusual in black-skinned individuals, although Africans are susceptible to malignant melanomas of the palms and soles.

Short, sharp, repeated exposures to ultraviolet light are more harmful than an accumulated effect. This suggests a possible immunological carcinogenic response. In keeping with this is the fact that the lesions can occur anywhere on the body. They may occur at any age but are very rare before puberty and are unusual under 20 years of age; they are most common between 40 and 60 years old. The lentiginous group occurs in elderly individuals. There is often a family history of atypical or multiple pigmented naevi or malignant melanoma, and it is essential that individuals with this history avoid the sun or use appropriate screening agents.

Although the lesions can occur anywhere, they are common over the trunk in men and lower legs in women. Be suspicious of pigmented lesions on the palms and soles and under the nails. Choroidal melanoma occurs in the eye, and lesions may also be seen in the oral or anal mucosa. Men have a slightly higher incidence than women, but women have a better prognosis. Multiple lesions are rare.

Clinically, four main varieties of lesions occur. The first is the superficial spreading melanoma (Figure 18.45), which is the least aggressive and the most common variant, while nodular melanoma (Figure 18.46) is the second most common.

The lesions of nodular melanoma are more invasive, produce early nodal involvement and have the worst prognosis. The third type is lentigo maligna melanoma (Figure 18.47), a variant form that occurs in the elderly over the head and neck region. Finally, acral lentiginous melanoma (Figure 18.48) is a rare form that occurs beneath a nail and is the form seen in Afro-Asian races, often on the palms and soles.

Pathologically speaking, the lesions are generally poorly differentiated with abundant mitotic figures and can increase rapidly in size over a few weeks. They are highly malignant and usually relentlessly progressive, yet they can also be unpredictable: the spontaneous regression even of nodal metastases has been recorded. Secondary spread may become evident after removal of the primary lesion.

A number of clinical features should alert the clinician to a suspicion of primary malignant melanoma or malignant change

PART 3 | SKIN

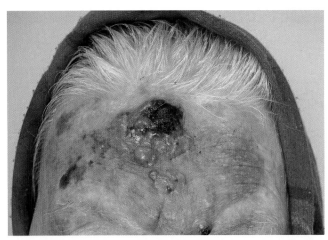

Figure 18.47 Lentigo maligna melanoma. (Courtesy of Dr Shukrallah Zaynoun.)

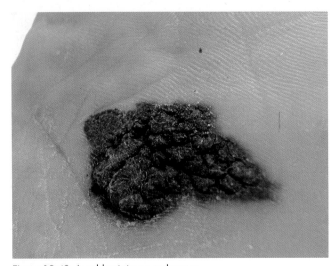

Figure 18.48 Acral lentiginous melanoma.

in a pre-existing naevus. The ABCDE rule and the ugly duckling sign described above are helpful. An amelanotic variety of melanoma is occasionally encountered and these lesions, although not pigmented, can still produce melanin and are dopamine-positive. A pink halo is suggestive of an inflammatory response to a developing malignant lesion.

Pain is a late sign but itching, together with bleeding, is not uncommon once ulceration has occurred. Nodal involvement is highly suggestive of malignant change, as are systemic symptoms such as weight loss, the dyspnoea of pulmonary involvement and pleural effusions, and jaundice, suggesting liver metastases. A number of attempts have been made to classify malignant melanomas on clinical grounds. More useful classifications take into account the thickness of the lesion, either measured directly (Breslow thickness) or related to the depth of cutaneous involvement (Clark level). Clark describes five levels:

1. Lesion confined to the epidermis.
2. Lesion extending into the superficial papillary dermis.
3. Lesion reaching the junction of the reticular dermis.
4. Lesion reaching the base of the reticular dermis.
5. Subcutaneous spread.

The Breslow thickness is considered to be the most reliable factor for assessing the prognosis of the tumour.

The American Joint Committee on Cancer staging for melanoma, with the 5 year corresponding survival rates, is as follows:

- **Stage 0**: Melanoma *in situ* (Clark Level I), 99.9 per cent survival;
- **Stage I/II**: Invasive melanoma, 89–95 per cent survival;
  - T1a: Less than 1.0 mm primary tumour thickness, without ulceration, and with mitosis $<1/mm^2$;
  - T1b: Less than 1.0 mm primary tumour thickness, with ulceration or mitoses $\geq 1/mm^2$;
  - T2a: 1.01–2.0 mm primary tumour thickness, without ulceration;
- **Stage II**: High-risk melanoma, 45–79 per cent survival;
  - T2b: 1.01–2.0 mm primary tumour thickness, with ulceration;
  - T3a: 2.01–4.0 mm primary tumour thickness, without ulceration;
  - T3b: 2.01–4.0 mm primary tumour thickness, with ulceration;
  - T4a: Greater than 4.0 mm primary tumour thickness, without ulceration;
  - T4b: Greater than 4.0 mm primary tumour thickness, with ulceration;
- **Stage III**: Regional metastasis, 24–70 per cent survival;
  - N1: Single positive lymph node;
  - N2: Two to three positive lymph nodes *or* regional skin/in-transit metastasis;
  - N3: Four positive lymph nodes *or* one lymph node and regional skin/in-transit metastasis;
- **Stage IV**: Distant metastasis, 7–19 per cent survival;
  - M1a: Distant skin metastasis, normal lactate dehydrogenase (LDH);
  - M1b: Lung metastasis, normal LDH;
  - M1c: Other distant metastasis *or* any distant metastasis with elevated LDH.

## CUTANEOUS LESIONS OF VASCULAR ORIGIN

Cutaneous vascular lesions involve any one of or combinations of arteries, capillaries, veins and lymphatics. Combinations are often termed haemangiomas or lymphangiomas, although they are actually overgrowths of embryonic tissue rather than neoplasms. Vascular lesions can usually be emptied of their blood content and are therefore compressible. On emptying, they blanch, although there may be some fixed haemorrhagic brown staining. Telangiectases can be blanched and observed by compression with a glass slide.

### Benign Vascular Lesions
*Telangiectasia*

Telangiectases (Figure 18.49) are dilated, single arterioles, capillaries or venules. One or two are found in most individuals. They can be congenital and familial, an example being Rendu–Osler–Weber syndrome (hereditary haemorrhagic telangiectasia). This syndrome is transmitted as an inherited dominant trait, and the telangiectases are seen periorally and along the length of the gut. The latter lesions occasionally give rise to haemorrhagic problems.

Telangiectases are common in collagen disorders (systemic lupus erythematosus, scleroderma, dermatomyositis,

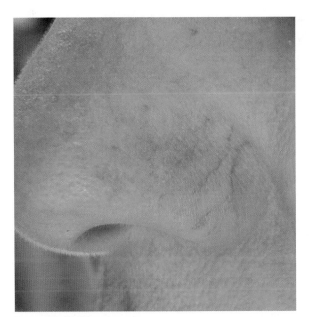

Figure 18.49 **Telangiectasia.**

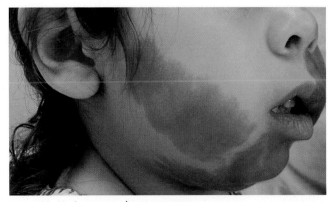

Figure 18.50 **A segmental port wine stain.**

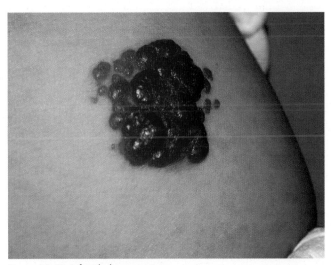

Figure 18.51 **Infantile haemangioma.**

post-radiotherapy) but worse with blushing (rosacea, carcinoid, oestrogen imbalance, pregnancy, liver disease) and with loss of the supporting tissues (steroid atrophy, Cushing's disease, exposure to the sun and wind, solar elastosis, ageing).

The abnormality is of the supporting tissue rather than the endothelial lining of the vessel. The lesions are flat and red or red–purple in colour. They vary in size from a pinpoint to a pinhead and may be punctate, linear or spider-like in form. Spider naevi are particularly common in liver disease. Telangiectases are occasionally larger, raised and scaling. They do not thrombose and rarely ulcerate or bleed. They persist into old age.

## Port Wine Stain

This vascular malformation is a deep purple, irregular area of disfiguring discoloration that occurs in early childhood and persists throughout life (Figure 18.50). The lesion may become darker but does not enlarge relative to the rest of the body unless there is an associated arterial shunt. The latter may accompany other vascular malformations (see p. 351). The lesions are usually flat and compression produces blanching. There may be some surrounding prominent veins.

## Infantile Haemangiomas

Infantile haemangiomas (previously known as strawberry naevi; Figure 18.51) are intradermal collections of blood vessels that usually present within a few days up to the first year after birth. They then grow rapidly and often alarmingly for 4–6 weeks and eventually stabilize at 6–12 months. The majority of lesions regress spontaneously but this may take up to 9 years or more. As a general rule, 30 per cent regress at 3 years, 50 per cent at 5 years, 70 per cent at 7 years and over 90 per cent at 9 years. They are usually 1–2 cm in diameter but may be much larger. As they are often visible in the head, neck and limbs, they cause much parental concern.

The lesions are covered with smooth epidermis, and their pink, red and pitted surface provides the typical strawberry appearance; they may be multiple. Strawberry naevi are well demarcated, mobile over the subcutaneous tissue and compressible.

The lesions can bleed with minor trauma – for example if under a nappy (diaper) – but this can be controlled by gentle pressure. The bleeding tendency can be accentuated by platelet sequestration in some larger lesions. On resolution, there may be some wrinkling of the skin but only a few residual telangiectases.

## Cherry Angiomas

Campbell de Morgan spots, also known as cherry angiomas (Figure 18.52), are bright red, well-circumscribed capillary abnormalities, 2–3 mm in diameter. They occur in most individuals after middle age and are usually found on the trunk, occasionally on the limbs but rarely on the face. Although they arrive individually, they are usually multiple. The aetiology of the spots is unknown and they have no clinical significance.

## Angiokeratomas

An angiokeratoma (Figure 18.53) is a single red–blue to black papule that is covered by a hyperkeratotic or wart-like surface. It can occur in any area but most commonly on the legs. Variants such as the angiokeratoma of Fordyce are commonly seen as multiple purple to black papules over the scrotum of elderly men. These may occasionally bleed but are otherwise asymptomatic. The eruption of multiple angiokeratomas over the legs, lower abdomen and buttocks in addition to shooting pain in the

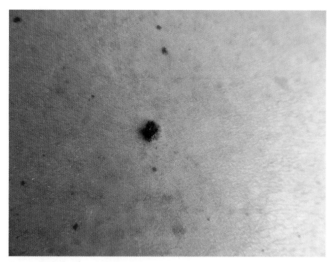

Figure 18.52 **Cherry angiomas.**

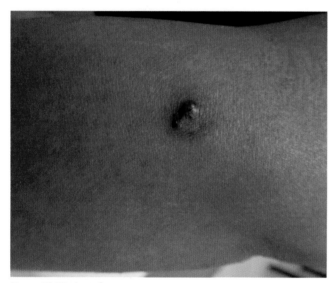

Figure 18.53 **Angiokeratoma.**

Table 18.7 Genodermatoses – inherited skin disorders

| Type of disorder | Condition |
| --- | --- |
| Chromosomal | Down syndrome – alopecia, ichthyosis |
| | Klinefelter's syndrome – leg ulcers, altered hair distribution |
| | Turner's syndrome – lymphoedema |
| | XYY – acne |
| Autosomal dominant | Ehlers–Danlos syndrome |
| | Erythropoietic protoporphyria |
| | Gardner's syndrome |
| | Gorlin's syndrome |
| | Hereditary haemorrhagic telangiectasia |
| | Ichthyosis vulgaris |
| | Neurofibromatosis |
| | Peutz–Jeghers syndrome |
| | Tuberous sclerosis |
| | Tylosis |
| | Urticaria pigmentosa |
| Autosomal recessive | Acrodermatitis enteropathica |
| | Albinism |
| | Ataxia telangiectasia |
| | Lipoid proteinosis |
| | Pseudoxanthoma elasticum |
| | Xeroderma pigmentosum |

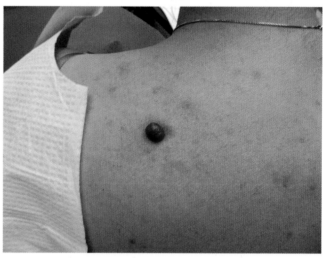

Figure 18.54 **Pyogenic granuloma.**

extremities is suggestive of a metabolic abnormality, referred to as Fabry's disease. In Fabry's disease, there is a mutation of the alpha-galactosidase enzyme. In addition to the pain and skin lesions, whorled opacities of the cornea are a common sign in this disease.

## Pyogenic Granuloma

'Pyogenic granuloma' (Figure 18.54) is a misnomer – this growth was originally thought to be infectious in origin, hence the name 'pyogenic'. It is an exuberant overgrowth of granulation tissue producing a sessile or polypoid papule, typically 7–10 mm in diameter. The abnormal inflammatory response usually occurs in response to a foreign body, such as a splinter or insect bite, and develops within a few days. The trauma may be minor and not remembered by the patient. Resolution is very slow and excision is sometimes necessary.

Pyogenic granulomas are usually single and sited on exposed areas such as the hands, arms and face. They can also occur in the oral mucosa (Figure 18.55), particularly during pregnancy, and are then called granulomata gravidarum. They are initially soft, friable and beefy red in colour and bleed easily. Most will have a colarette of thick skin surrounding them. As they mature, they tend to become firmer and less friable once surface epithelialization is complete, and they ultimately turn skin coloured. Ulceration can make the differential diagnosis from malignant lesions, particularly malignant melanoma, more difficult.

## Glomus Tumours

A glomus is a specialized arteriovenous anastomosis found particularly around the nail beds and concerned with heat regulation. It is surrounded by large, pale cells and is heavily innervated.

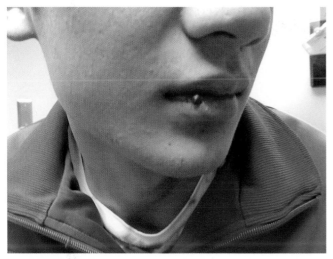

Figure 18.55 Pyogenic granuloma – oral.

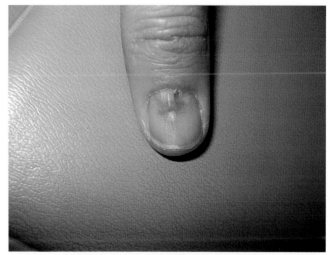

Figure 18.56 A glomus tumour with the nail plate removed secondary to biopsy.

Glomus tumours (Figure 18.56) are discrete, small, firm, benign nodules rarely greater than 1 cm in diameter and made up of the same components. They would go unnoticed if it were not for the extreme sensitivity of some lesions in which even gentle trauma or a temperature change can precipitate severe, sharp or throbbing pain.

The tumours are often found in a subungual position. The symptoms are dramatically abolished by tumour excision.

## Malignant Vascular Lesions

### Lymphangiosarcoma and Angiosarcoma

These are rare, highly malignant tumours (Figure 18.57). Their relevance to the skin is that they may develop in long-standing, massive lymphoedema, whether primary or secondary, including that of the upper limb, post-radical mastectomy. The course of the tumours is massive, relentless enlargement. They are very vascular, may bleed and produce early pulmonary metastases. Although they are radiosensitive, radical amputation is the only curative option when this is possible. Angiosarcomas may also produce massive tumours in the liver, spleen or bone. Both tumours are usually seen in young adults.

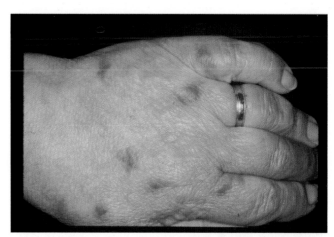

Figure 18.57 Angiosarcoma. (Courtesy of Dr Shukrallah Zaynoun.)

### Kaposi's Sarcoma

Kaposi's sarcoma (Figure 18.58) is a form of angiosarcoma characterized by endothelial and fibroblastic proliferation together with haemorrhage. Human herpes virus-8 is known to be the cause in the vast majority of cases. The typical skin lesions arise as purple–brown patches that progress to become discrete nodules or plaques that may ulcerate and bleed. The condition may also progress to nodal and visceral involvement, with the gastrointestinal tract being the most common involved organ.

Before the HIV era, Kaposi's sarcoma was generally seen in the Mediterranean area, where it commonly involved the skin of the lower limb in men over the age of 60. It ran a relatively benign course. An African form of the disease occurred in young children (Figure 18.59), with widespread involvement of the lymphatic system and usually running a slow, fatal course. With the advent of acquired immune deficiency syndrome (AIDS), it is now the most common opportunistic neoplastic lesion. HIV-positive

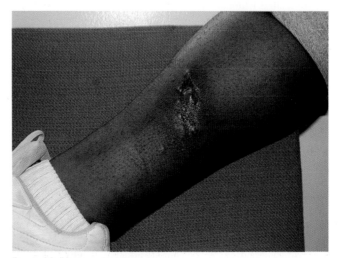

Figure 18.58 Kaposi's scarcoma.

individuals, unlike those with the classical Mediterranean Kaposi, tend to develop their lesions mostly over the head and neck area as well as the oral mucosa.

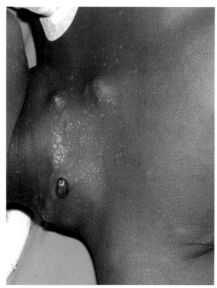

Figure 18.59 Kaposi's sarcoma – African type.

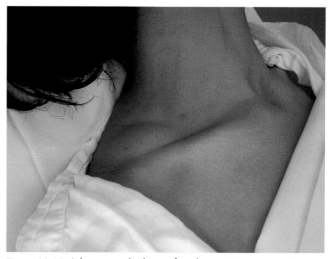

Figure 18.60 A lipoma at the base of neck.

## CUTANEOUS LESIONS OF OTHER ORIGINS

### Lipomas

Lipomas (Figure 18.60) are very common, benign, subcutaneous tumours. They occur at any age but are less common in children. They are usually asymptomatic but large lesions can present with cosmetic problems. The lesions grow slowly, and as they have features similar to the surrounding fat, they have usually reached 2–3 cm in diameter before a patient presents.

Lipomas have characteristic signs. They are smooth, soft and slightly lobulated due to thin fibrous septa. The edge slips away from the examining finger – the 'slip sign'. They transilluminate and fluctuate, and are mobile with no attachments to the skin or deep fascia. They are non-tender and non-reducible, and there is no associated lymphadenopathy. The overlying skin is generally normal, but there may be stretch marks, thinning or prominent veins with large lesions.

### Xanthomas

Xanthomas (Figure 18.61) are yellow cutaneous polypoid lesions of lipid-filled macrophages sited within the dermis. They commonly occur in the upper eyelid and are particularly prominent in patients with hyperlipidaemia.

### Neurofibromas

Neurofibromas are common, benign tumours containing both fibrous and neural tissue elements. Other fibroid lesions are occasionally encountered. More than one neurofibroma may be present but multiple lesions usually indicate the existence of von Recklinghausen's disease (see below).

Isolated neurofibromas usually occur in adults and can be found anywhere over the body but are attached to a nerve sheath. They are usually asymptomatic but pressure applied to the lesion may produce distal tingling and, if they are in a confined space such as an intervertebral foramen, they may produce nerve compression and symptoms from the damaged nerve. Single lesions are often fusiform and 4–6 mm in diameter.

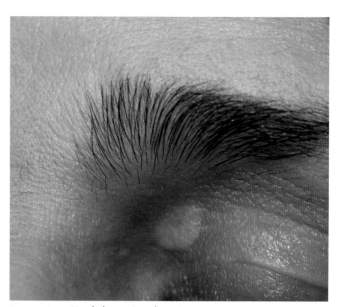

Figure 18.61 Xanthelasma (xanthoma).

### Neurofibromatosis

Von Recklinghausen's disease – type 1 neurofibromatosis – is a congenital and familial disease that is inherited as an autosomal dominant trait. Any patient is likely to have one parent and siblings with the disease. However, different members of the family may display a wide range of abnormalities ranging from a few nodules or pigmented areas to gross deformity. The degree of parental involvement is not a good predictor of the degree of expression in the next generation.

The neurofibromas are present at birth and increase in number. Lesions vary from a few millimeters to a few centimetres in diameter. They may be pedunculated (Figure 18.62). They are usually softer than single lesions. They are not usually painful, and there is no nodal involvement.

There are a number of associated abnormalities. Café-au-lait spots (Figure 18.63) are characteristic and diagnostic of von Recklinghausen's disease if there are more than six of them or there is a patch more than 1.5 cm in diameter.

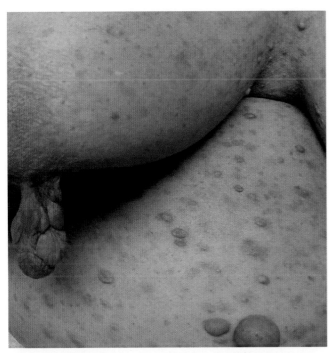

Figure 18.62 Neurofibromatosis with pedunculated fibromas.

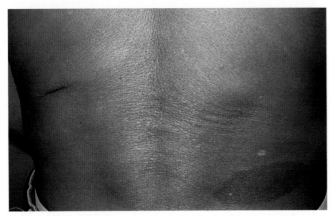

Figure 18.63 A café-au-lait spot.

About 5 per cent of patients develop neurofibrosarcoma. Other associated tumours are ganglioneuromas, phaeochromocytomas, gliomas and meningiomas. Phaeochromocytomas present in 1 per cent of cases of von Recklinghausen's disease, making up 5 per cent of the total; any patients with unexplained hypertension should be examined for café-au-lait spots. There is diffuse cerebral dysgenesis in 10 per cent of patients, accompanied by varying degrees of mental retardation.

Central neurofibromatosis – type 2 neurofibromatosis – is characterized by bilateral acoustic and spinal neuromas. Hearing should be checked and the possibility of nerve root compression considered since spinal tumours may be dumb-bell-shaped and partly inside and partly outside the vertebral canal. This condition also shows autosomal dominant inheritance.

## Plexiform Neurofibromatosis

Plexiform neurofibromatosis is a primary abnormality in which an area of the body is involved in a diffuse and often very extensive subcutaneous enlargement (Figure 18.64). The overlying skin is thickened and pigmented, and the deformity may resemble lymphoedema, although in severe cases the overgrowth gives a picture of the classic 'Elephant Man'.

## Schwannomas

Schwannomas are benign, painless, firm nodules 1–2 cm in diameter that develop from the Schwann cells of peripheral nerve sheaths. They are usually tethered to a nerve and therefore mobile only from side to side. They are asymptomatic and not tender, and are not associated with any nodal involvement or malignant potential. The diagnosis is usually made histologically after excision of an asymptomatic lump.

## Ganglia, Bursae and Synovial Protrusions

These benign lesions are lined with synovial membrane and present in characteristic sites.

A ganglion (Figure 18.65) is produced by cystic myxomatous degeneration of the fibrous tissue. It lies adjacent to a joint or tendon sheath but debate exists as to whether it has any communication with these structures or whether it has arisen as an embryonal remnant.

Ganglia occur at any age but are unusual in children. The lesions grow slowly over a number of years, usually reaching

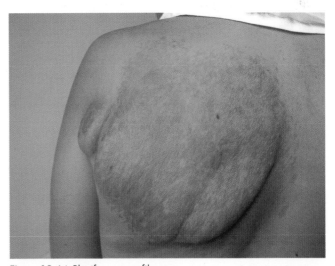

Figure 18.64 Plexiform neurofibroma.

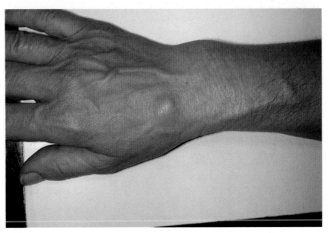

Figure 18.65 A ganglion.

1–2 cm in diameter. They are painless unless knocked and asymptomatic unless they get in the way of some activity. They may disappear spontaneously or after a sharp blow but return in 50 per cent of cases.

Ganglia are usually sited over the dorsum of the hands or feet and are tethered to the site of origin. During certain movements, they may disappear underneath adjacent tendons. The lesions are smooth and spherical and may be loculated. They contain a clear, colourless, gelatinous fluid that does not empty on pressure, shows some fluctuation if the lesion is not too tense, and transilluminates.

Bursae occur in relation to joints but may also develop over pressure points that are subject to repeated trauma; the latter are termed adventitious bursae. The bursae and synovial protrusions around joints are sited beneath adjacent structures, such as muscles and tendons, and act to prevent friction during joint movement. They often communicate with the joint and are not usually mobile. They become symptomatic if the synovial fluid is increased due to joint disease such as rheumatoid arthritis or osteoarthritis, in which case the lesions are often symmetrical and other joint abnormalities are present. They usually occur in middle age.

Examples of adventitious bursae are prepatellar ('housemaid's knee'), infrapatellar ('clergyman's knee') and olecranon ('student's elbow') (Figure 18.66), the bunions lateral to the deformed head of the first metatarsal in hallux valgus and an ischial bursa over the ischial tuberosity. The repeated trauma that produces symptomatic adventitious bursae also produces changes in the overlying skin. This may be dry, wrinkled and keratinized, and there may be superadded inflammation, eczema and cracking. The bursa is well circumscribed, hemispherical and tethered to the skin and deep tissues. The diameter and fluid content are variable depending on the duration, the extent of the stimulus producing it and any associated infection. Fluctuation and transillumination may be demonstrable. If infection is present, there may be signs of inflammation and abscess formation.

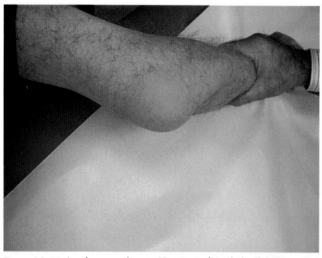

Figure 18.66 An olecranon bursa. (Courtesy of Dr Shukrallah Zaynoun.)

## Key Points

- The differentiation of skin lesions by morphology is crucial and essential.
- Skin tags tend to occur mostly in obese individuals as well as patients with diabetes mellitus and those with a family history of acrochordons.
- The Leser–Trélat sign – the sudden eruption of multiple seborrheic keratoses – may be a herald sign of an internal malignancy, most commonly colon cancer.
- Warts are caused by the human papillomavirus and are subtyped according to the area that is infected. Warts are at risk of malignant transformation when present in the genital area. Newer vaccines are being developed against the subtypes of genital warts.
- Molluscum contagiosum is caused by the pox virus and is common in children. In adults, it is most commonly sexually transmitted.
- Sebaceous cysts are commonly derived from the hair follicle. They are filled with keratin. Steatocystomas are benign cysts filled with oily material.
- Actinic keratoses are 'rough' macules that are more often felt than seen. They can progress into SCC *in situ* and SCC.
- Bowen's disease is SCC *in situ*.
- Cutaneous SCC carries the highest risk of metastasis over the lip and ears.
- Basal cell carcinoma is the most common type of skin cancer and is a slow growing tumour. Its characteristic feature is its 'pearly bordered' appearance. It can occur in younger individuals in the setting of basal cell naevus syndrome.
- Paget's disease consists of eczema-like skin patches over the nipple area that arise secondary to intraductal carcinoma. A similar eruption, called extramammary Paget's disease, may occur over the anogenital area secondary to an adenocarcinoma of the gastrointestinal or genitourinary system.
- The clinical signs of malignant transformation of a melanocytic lesion can be remembered using ABCDE: asymmetry, border, colour, diameter and evolution.
- Café-au-lait spots are pale brown, flat patches that are present at birth. If multiple in number, the lesions may be associated with neurofibromatosis.
- Infantile haemangiomas commonly involute at 1 year of age. Most are left to involute naturally, except for ulcerating lesions and lesions obstructing organ structures or vision. Beta-blockers are the first-line treatment.
- Kaposi's sarcoma is a form of angiosarcoma that has a benign course in Mediterranean individuals, but a more progressive one in African or HIV-associated disease.

## QUESTIONS

### SBAs

**1. A 40-year-old man who has been suffering from severe weight loss and cachexia for the past 3 months has presented to the clinic with multiple stuck-on verrucous brownish plaques over his trunk. The most likely cause of his symptoms is:**

a Anorexia nervosa
b Colon carcinoma
c Factitial disease
d Neurofibromatosis
e Basal cell carcinoma

**Answer**

*b **Colon carcinoma.** The presence of stuck-on verrucous plaques is the description of seborrhoeic keratoses. The setting of eruptive seborrhoeic keratoses with cachexia suggests the presence of a carcinoma, most likely a colon carcinoma. This sudden eruption of seborrhoeic keratoses is called the Leser–Trélat sign.*

**2. A 67-year-old woman presents to the clinic with weight loss and an asymptomatic eczema-like eruption of the right nipple that has been growing for the past year. She does not have a past history of eczema. The most likely diagnosis is:**

a Eczema
b Lipoma
c Melanoma
d Haemangioma
e Paget's disease

**Answer**

*e **Paget's disease.** Paget's disease is an asymptomatic eczema-like eruption of the nipple that is associated with intraductal breast carcinoma. Eczema is usually an itchy rash on dry skin. A lipoma is a skin-colored soft nodule and not an eczema-like rash. A melanoma appears as a brownish atypically pigmented plaque, and a haemangioma is an erythematous cherry red plaque.*

**3. The most common area of metastasis for a melanoma is:**

a Lymph nodes
b Lung
c Brain
d Liver
e Bone

**Answer**

*a **Lymph nodes.** Although malignant melanoma can metastasize to all the areas mentioned here, the most common area of metastasis is the lymph nodes – hence the sentinel lymph node assessment that is commonly undertaken during melanoma surgery.*

### MCQs

**1. Which of the following are signs of malignant melanocytic transformation?:**

a Asymmetry
b Border
c Colour
d Diameter
e Evolution
f Flat surface

**Answer**

*a, b, c, d and e. Asymmetry, border, colour, diameter and evolution. 'Flat surface' is not an answer as flat-surfaced lesions can be benign or malignant.*

**2. Which of the following lesions are sexually transmitted in the adult setting?:**

a Skin tags
b Warts
c Seborrhoeic keratoses
d Molluscum contagiosum
e Neurofibroma

**Answer**

*b and d. Warts and molluscum contagiosum. Skin tags, seborrhoeic keratoses and neurofibromas are benign lesions that can occur spontaneously in normal individuals.*

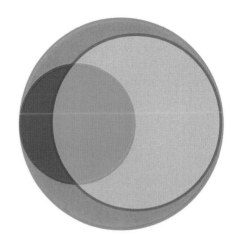

# PART
# 4

# Head and neck

# The Head

Murad Lala and Basant K. Misra

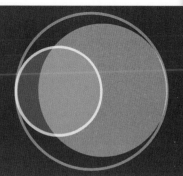

- To be able to identify the presence of a neurological problem
- To identify whether the problem is confined to the nervous system or is part of a systemic problem
- To identify the anatomical location (single or multiple sites) of the lesion or injury that is causing symptoms
- To elucidate and understand the pathophysiology of the lesion involved
- To construct a list of differential diagnosis based on the patient's signs and symptoms
- To guide the relevant investigations leading to a proper diagnosis and timely intervention

## THE SCALP

Lesions of the scalp are often not apparent due to the presence of hair, so parting the hair will enable a closer inspection. Look for any congenital malformations, characteristic facies, prominences, lumps, nodules, scars, rashes, areas of seborrhoeic dermatitis, naevi, hair loss or other lesions. Look for facial asymmetry, involuntary movements and the presence, absence and symmetry of oedema and wrinkling. Palpate the scalp to identify any tenderness or deformity.

Scalp lesions superficial to the galea aponeurotica can be moved, and move with the skin when the patient voluntarily contracts the frontalis or occipitalis muscle. Any lesion deep to the galea aponeurotica or invading it and the adjacent pericranium will remain fixed with no movement.

Capillary malformations appear as a red-purple skin discoloration. Venous malformations appear as swellings that can be emptied, as can other fluid-containing communicating swellings such as meningoceles. A sinus pericranii (a haemorrhagic cyst of the intracranial dural venous sinus) also shows this sign. It appears as a soft swelling in the midline, usually on the occiput, contains blood instead of cerebrospinal fluid (CSF) and communicates with a venous sinus through a defect in the skull.

A **sebaceous cyst (Figure 19.1a)** is the most common swelling of the scalp. It is a retention cyst of a hair follicle, is often multiple **(Figure 19.1b)**, is round and is attached to the overlying skin. The contents are cheesy in nature, non-fluctuant and firm on palpation. A punctum is usually visible in the centre of the cyst.

It may discharge pus when infected, and the swelling also becomes painful and swollen. These lesions are known to recur frequently.

**Lipomas** and **dermoids** may also occur in the scalp.

**Plexiform neurofibromas** may occur on the head. They may also hang in festoons and are hair-bearing.

**Basal cell carcinomas** and **squamous cell carcinomas (Figure 19.2)** can arise in the scalp but are more common on

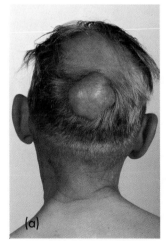
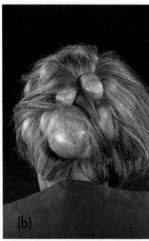

Figure 19.1 (a) A large sebaceous cyst of the scalp. (b) Turban tumours, which are rare multiple cystic tumours of the scalp.

the face. Examination of the draining lymph nodes is important, particularly in the case of squamous carcinoma.

**Cirsoid aneurysms** are pulsatile swellings over the scalp; there may be a bruit on auscultation. These so-called aneurysms are in fact traumatic arteriovenous fistulas, which commonly arise from a birth injury or a blow to the head. Pressure atrophy can result in erosion of the underlying bone. Similarly, a caroticocavernous fistula can arise from fractures or injuries to the base of the skull; these cause engorgement of the orbital veins resulting in oedema of the orbit and conjunctiva, a pulsatile exophthalmos and a bruit.

**Lacerations** and **haematomas** may result from trauma to the scalp. Wounds usually only gape if the underlying galea aponeurotica has been divided, and in such cases the exposed skull should be palpated for fractures.

Birth injuries in neonates can result in various scalp injuries. **Caput succedaneum** is oedema of the scalp secondary to pressure on the head during the delivery process. The oedema can extend across the midline and cross the suture lines. A **cephalhaematoma** is the most frequent cranial injury in the neonate and is seen following instrumental delivery or vacuum extraction. It presents as a soft scalp swelling confined by the cranial sutures due to haemorrhage beneath the periosteum; it is rarely associated with fractures. A **subgaleal haemorrhage** secondary

to rupture of the veins running between the scalp and the dural sinuses may extend from the orbital ridges to the nape of the neck and ears depending upon the severity.

## THE SKULL OR CRANIUM

### Congenital and Developmental Abnormalities

The size of the skull is measured from the supraorbital ridges anteriorly to the most prominent point on the occipital protuberance posteriorly. The size of the vault is determined by the volume of the brain. Malformations of the central nervous system (CNS) are therefore associated with abnormalities of the size and shape of the skull.

The vault grows rapidly in the first year of life and reaches almost adult size by the seventh; however, the sutures do not close until 30–40 years of age. The fibrous membrane that initially formed the skull remains unossified in the angles between the bones – the fontanelles. The anterior fontanelle is the most prominent and at birth is palpable as a soft area at the junction of the sagittal, frontal and coronal sutures. The posterior fontanelle lies between the sagittal, parietal and occipital bones. These fontanelles later become ossified. The posterior fontanelle closes at about 6 months and the anterior fontanelle by about 18 months of age.

Tension in the fontanelles is increased during crying or any condition that increases intracranial tension, and is reduced in dehydration. In the hydrocephalic infant, the fontanelles are wide and bulging. Metabolic diseases such as rickets delay the closure of the fontanelles.

**Macrocephaly or macrocrania** is said to occur when the head circumference is more than 98th percentile. It can be familial (with no neurological signs or symptoms) or pathological (associated with developmental delay, mental retardation, focal neurological deficits, a bulging fontanelle, split sutures and/or the features of raised intracranial tension).

**Microcephaly** is a condition in which the skull is very small in relationship to the size of the body (**Figure 19.3**). Microcephaly is defined as a head circumference of more than 3 standard deviations below the mean for the corresponding age and sex. It may be due to cerebral agenesis, syndromic malformations or intrauterine infections and is generally associated with mental

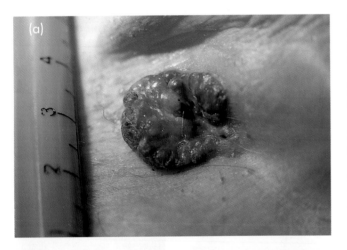

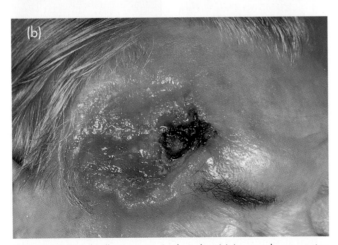

Figure 19.2 Basal cell carcinoma (rodent ulcers) (a) unusual presentation (b) extensive lesion.

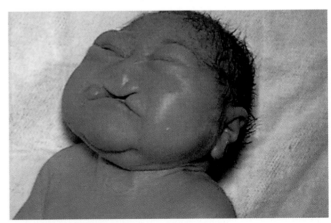

Figure 19.3 Microcephaly.

retardation. There is a secondary premature closure of the sutures and fontanelles.

Craniofacial deformities may result from developmental defects, premature fusion of the sutures, craniosynostosis or craniofacial dysplasia.

In **anenecephaly**, the infant is stillborn with a large defect in the skull and meninges, and absence of the hemispheres and cerebellum (**Figure 19.4**).

**Craniosynostosis** occurs when there is premature fusion of one or more of the cranial vault sutures, resulting in abnormal calvarial growth and an abnormal shape of the skull. The skull enlarges rapidly in the first 2 years of life, so premature fusion results in skull deformities and sometimes a raised intracranial pressure if more than one suture is involved.

The sutures involved can generally be discerned by the characteristic deformity: scaphocephaly (sagittal), plagiocephaly (coronal or lambdoid), trigonocephaly (metopic), brachycephaly (bicoronal), cloverleaf skull (Kleeblattschädel syndrome), acrocephaly or oxycephaly (multiple sutures). Premature fusion of all the sutures – pansynostosis – results in a severely raised intracranial pressure causing developmental delay or visual loss. The fused suture is prominent and feels like a ridge on palpation, in contrast to a fused suture in microcephaly, which is flat.

**Craniofacial dysplasia** occurs when the vault stenosis extends into the base of the skull. As the name implies, the deformity involves not only the cranium, but also the face. These deformities occur as part of a variety of syndromes such as Crouzon's and Apert's syndromes (**Figure 19.5**).

Exophthalmos, hypertelorism (an abnormally wide separation of the orbits), a beaked nose and low-set ears characterize Crouzon's syndrome. Atresia of the external auditory meatus and middle ear abnormalities result in conductive deafness. There is raised intracranial pressure with mental retardation, progressive worsening of the exophthalmos and visual loss.

In Apert's syndrome, the middle third of the face is underdeveloped with a small nose, hypertelorism, shallow orbits, proptosis and strabismus. There is syndactyly with complete fusion of all the digits of the hands and feet, skeletal defects, congenital heart disease and anal atresia. It may be associated with clefting defects and meningoencephalocoeles (**Figure 19.6**).

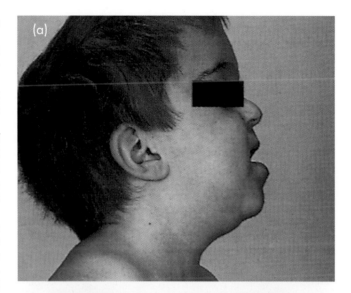

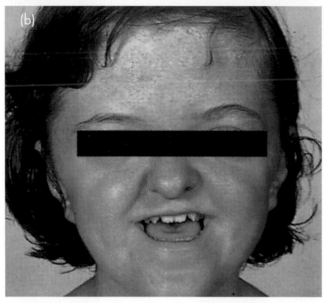

Figure 19.5 (a) Crouzon's syndrome. (b) Apert's syndrome.

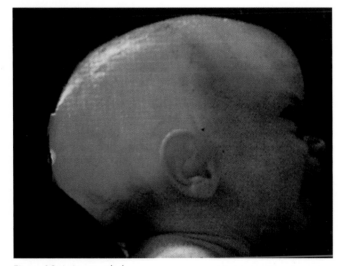

Figure 19.4 Anencephaly.

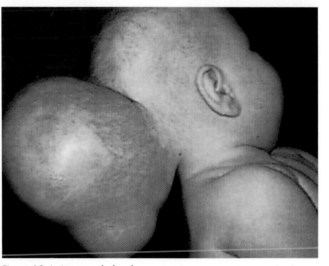

Figure 19.6 An encephalocele.

In **hydrocephalus**, there is an enlargement of the ventricles and an increase in CSF volume (Figures 19.7 and 19.8). The CSF is formed in the ventricular system by the choroid plexus and exits through foramina in the fourth ventricle into cisterns at the base of the brain. It then flows over the brain and is reabsorbed by the arachnoid villi. The balance between the production and absorption of CSF is very important. Because CSF production is a continuous process, any condition that blocks the normal flow or absorption of CSF results in an excessive accumulation, causing excessive pressure over the brain tissue.

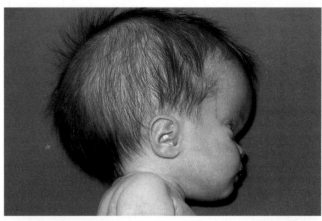

Figure 19.7 Hydrocephalus.

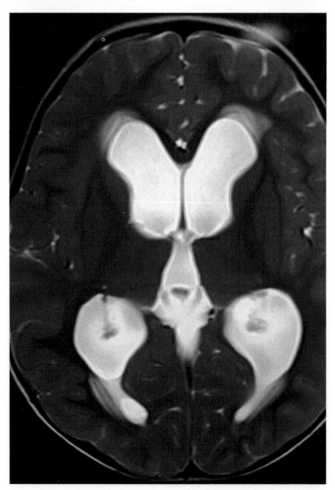

Figure 19.8 **MRI of the brain showing gross hydrocephalus with periventricular ooze.**

Hydrocephalus can be congenital or acquired. It can result from obstruction within the ventricular system – obstructive or non-communicating hydrocephalus – from an impaired reabsorption of CSF due to a malfunction of the arachnoid villi or rarely from overproduction of CSF from the choroid plexus – non-obstructive or communicating hydrocephalus.

Clinically, the symptoms vary with age, disease progression and the underlying aetiology. Hydrocephalus in the infant is manifest as an enlargement of the head, a wide, bulging anterior fontanelle and dilatation of the scalp veins. The forehead is broad and the eyes may deviate downwards, resulting in the sclera being visible above the iris: the 'setting sun' sign. In the older child, a deteriorating mental ability may be noted, but hydrocephalus in the adult is less apparent clinically – here it is the ventricles that enlarge rather than the cranium. Patients present with symptoms relating to the underlying cause or to the raised intracranial pressure.

**Craniotabes** (abnormal softening of the skull) may be due to, for example, rickets, osteogenesis imperfecta, hydrocephalus, congenital syphilis or hyperparathyroidism.

**Neural tube defects** may affect the cranium and result from failure of the neural tube to close in the third or fourth week of intrauterine development. They take the form of a protrusion of tissue through a midline bony defect – a cranium bifidum. **Meningocoeles and meningoencephalocoeles** are congenital midline swellings that usually occur in the occipital region and less commonly in the frontal region. A careful neurological examination is mandatory, as is a thorough evaluation to determine the extent of neural tissue involvement and any associated anomalies. A meningocoele is a meningeal protrusion containing only CSF. It is fluctuant and translucent, and transmits a cough impulse on crying; the scalp or only a thin epithelial layer may cover it.

Meningomyelocoeles and encephalocoeles also contain neural tissue. These defects most commonly occur in the occipital region, but frontal and nasofrontal encephaloceles are also seen. Asymptomatic children with normal neurological findings and full-thickness skin covering the lesion can have their surgery delayed. Those with leaking CSF or a thin skin covering the lesion should undergo immediate surgical treatment to prevent contamination and spread of infection.

Other disease processes can also result in craniofacial deformities. Fibrous dysplasia of the frontal bone may result in inferior displacement of the globe and optic nerve compression. Haemolymphangiomas may occur in the orbit and communicate intracranially. Localized craniofacial plexiform neurofibromas may occur in neurofibromatosis.

## Infections

**Osteomyelitis** of the skull is rare; most cases are secondary to trauma or the spread of infection from adjacent sites, such as the air sinuses or mastoid air cells. **Pott's puffy tumour** is a localized area of oedema that forms over an area of osteomyelitis. It usually occurs in the frontal region due to incompletely treated frontal sinusitis. Epidural empyemas are usually associated with osteomyelitis of the skull. Subperiosteal abscess is the most common complication of skull osteomyelitis.

## Neoplasms

The majority of skull tumours are malignant in nature (Table 19.1). Metastatic deposits are the most common type of skull tumour. They may either appear as hard lumps or be soft to palpation; very vascular deposits may even be pulsatile.

Table 19.1 Tumours of the skull

| Origin | Examples |
| --- | --- |
| Bony | Osteoma, osteoid osteoma, ossifying fibroma, osteoblastoma, osteosarcoma |
| Cartilaginous | Chondroma, chondromyxofibroma, chondroblastoma, chordoma, chondrosarcoma |
| Connective tissue | Desmoplastic fibroma, fibrosarcoma |
| Histiocytic | Eosinophilic granuloma, giant cell granuloma, Ewing's sarcoma, giant cell tumour, xanthoma |
| Vascular | Haemangioma, lymphangioma, angiosarcoma |
| Other | Squamous cell carcinoma, dermoid, epidermoid, Paget's disease, multiple myeloma |

Osteomas are benign tumours (**Figure 19.9**) that appear as radio-opaque protuberances. Chordomas are midline malignant destructive tumours that affect the base of the skull and appear radiologically as lytic lesions (**Figure 19.10**). In contrast, a chondrosarcoma is a lateralized lesion (**Figure 19.11**). Multiple myeloma causes multiple 'punched-out' lytic lesions in the skull – the 'pepperpot skull'. Fibrous dysplasia and eosinophilic granulomas are tumour-like lesions that also appear as lytic areas radiologically (**Figure 19.12**).

Paget's disease of the bone – osteitis deformans – most frequently affects the long bones of the lower extremity and the skull, and occurs in middle or later life. The skull becomes thickened and its circumference enlarges. Deafness, vertigo and failing vision may result from compression of the brain and of the cranial nerves at their foramina. Sarcoma complicates 1 per cent of cases.

## Trauma

In order to appropriately diagnose and manage trauma and injuries to the skull, the clinician must understand the mechanisms involved, be able to identify the clinical manifestations of extradural, subdural and diffuse brain injuries, cautiously monitor the progress of the patients and provide immediate definitive management.

Many skull fractures are associated with maxillofacial injuries and intracranial injuries with underlying subdural or epidural haematomas. A blow to the skull causes a fracture if the elastic tolerance of the bone is exceeded; most fractures are linear and extend from the point of impact to the base of skull.

### Comminuted Fractures

Comminuted fractures occur when multiple linear fractures radiate from a point of impact and may produce free bone fragments. In compound fractures, there is a risk of meningitis or a brain abscess.

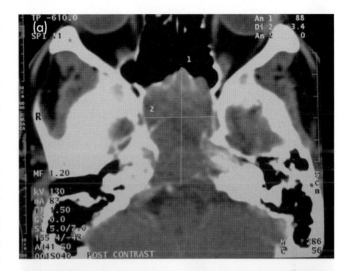

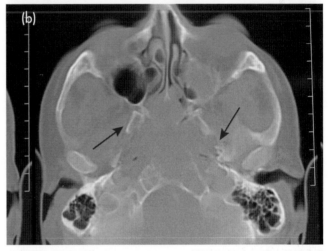

Figure 19.10 (a, b) CT scan contrast and bone window showing skull base demonstrating lytic lesions (arrows) and destruction of the clivus.

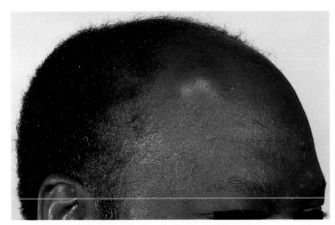

Figure 19.9 An osteoma of the right side of the skull.

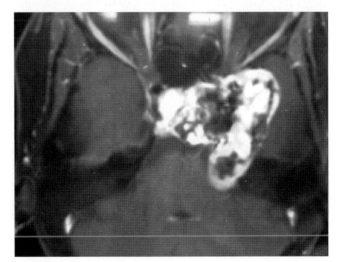

Figure 19.11 MRI brain showing a skull base chondrosarcoma.

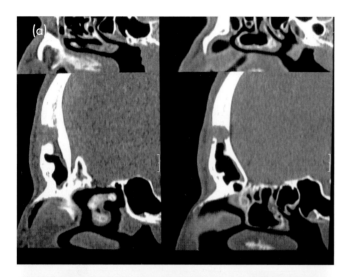

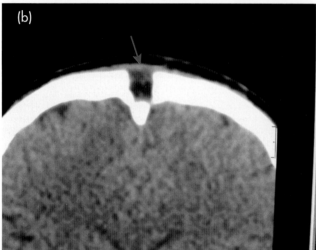

Figure 19.12 A fracture of the frontal bone (a), with associated haematoma causing marked cerebral compression. (b) CT scan of the brain (sagittal and coronal) showing a punched-out lesion of the skull in a case of eosinophylic granuloma (arrow).

### Linear Vault Fractures

These may not be apparent externally except for a history of significant injury or the presence of a contusion or laceration of the scalp. Radiologically, they may be visible in only one plane. Fractures crossing the temporal bone may result in injury to the middle meningeal artery or vein that can give rise to an extradural haematoma. Fractures through air sinuses may lead to pneumocephalus with a risk of a CSF leak and meningitis.

### Depressed Fractures

Depressed fractures result from a relatively focused source of trauma, for example a blow from a hammer. Clinically, they may appear as a depressed area surrounded by a boggy haematoma. In a compound depressed fracture, there is an overlying laceration or an area of tissue loss, and the fracture may be directly palpable. It is therefore good practice to palpate the skull through the scalp laceration while the patient is locally anaesthetized prior to wound 1 closure. The severity of the depressed area can be assessed radiologically, preferably with CT scanning. Patients with a depressed fracture have a greater incidence of underlying brain injury and a greater risk of subsequent epilepsy.

### Pond Fractures

Pond fractures are depressed areas of the skull in the neonate resulting from moulding in the birth canal or from forceps deliveries.

### Basal Skull Fractures

These fractures are difficult to diagnose both clinically and radiologically. They should be suspected in severe head injuries, but a number of specific signs help to identify less obvious cases. Anterior fossa fractures may pass through the paranasal sinuses and therefore be internally compound; CSF rhinorrhoea may occur and there is a risk of meningitis. Bloodstained CSF may be distinguished from blood by placing a drop on filter paper: blood produces only a single ring, whereas bloodstained CSF separates into two rings. Sneezing or blowing the nose can result in air being forced into the cranium, producing a pneumocephalus.

The presence of a 'black eye' without direct injury also raises the suspicion of such a fracture. The discoloration is caused by blood tracking through the tissues and is limited by the attachments of the orbicularis oculi, whereas in a true 'black eye' there is no such limitation. In addition, in a traumatic 'black eye', there may be intraconjunctival haemorrhage, which moves with the conjunctiva when the eyelid is moved with the examiner's finger. In a fracture, blood can track into the subconjunctival space, forming a fan of blood extending from the iris with no outer limit: a subconjunctival haemorrhage (Figure 19.13a). Bilateral 'black eyes' with no history direct trauma to the region is a fairly certain sign of an anterior fossa fracture: the 'panda' or 'raccoon' sign (Figure 19.13b).

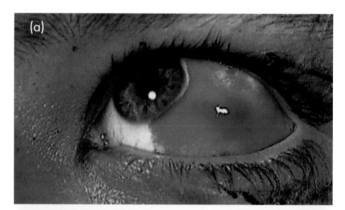

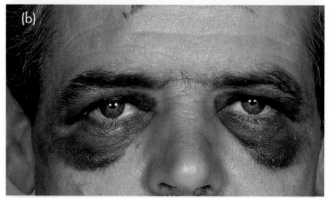

Figure 19.13 An anterior fossa fracture showing (a) subconjunctival haemorrhage and (b) bilateral 'black eyes' (the 'panda sign').

## Middle Cranial Fossa Fractures

Fractures may result in blood and CSF escaping from the external auditory meatus. Rupture of the tympanic membrane may also result in such bleeding, but here the blood tends to clot in the meatus as it is not mixed with CSF. Facial paralysis, nystagmus or deafness may result from cranial nerve entrapment. A late sign is the appearance of bruising over the mastoid process 2 days after the injury: **Battle's sign**. Posterior fossa fractures are often associated with injury to the venous sinuses and brainstem. In injuries to the brainstem, the patient is usually deeply unconscious and the outcome is frequently fatal.

## INTRACRANIAL CONDITIONS

## Trauma

### Birth Injuries

Intraventricular haemorrhage may occur in the premature infant due to capillary fragility and is associated with hypoxia. Ultrasound examination reveals that this is a common problem, occurring subclinically in about 50 per cent of premature babies. Severe cases result in developmental delay and hydrocephalus.

### Head Injury

Injuries to the head can be classified as closed or penetrating based on the mechanism causing the injury, as mild, moderate or severe depending on the severity, or as skull fractures and intracranial lesions based on the morphology. The principal objectives are to identify the severity of the primary brain injury, to record a baseline of neurological disability, to cautiously monitor the patient's subsequent progress and to rectify treatable causes immediately.

Initial information from witnesses and from the ambulance crew, such as the nature and velocity of the trauma and the patient's initial state of consciousness, indicate the potential severity of the head injury. The patient is likely to suffer from other life-threatening injuries that are of more immediate relevance. The advanced trauma life support system protocol should therefore be followed, with airway, breathing and circulation ('ABC') being stabilized. The cervical spine should be immobilized as there is a high incidence of associated injury.

An initial neurological assessment of consciousness level and pupils should be assessed, as drugs, hypoxia and endotracheal intubation may soon influence these. Later, a detailed neurological examination should be performed for focal neurological signs. The Glasgow Coma Scale (GCS; Table 19.2) is a reproducible method of assessing the level of consciousness. Eye opening, motor response and verbal response are quantified. The head injury is considered mild if the GCS score is 14–15, moderate if it is 9–13 and severe if it is 8 or less.

Factors other than cerebral injury may also influence the score. Eye opening may be limited by facial trauma and periorbital oedema. The motor response is the most reliable indicator of neurological injury, and the best motor response should be recorded. If there is no response to commands, painful stimuli are applied in the form of supraorbital or sternal pressure. A hand moving purposefully to the stimulus is regarded as localizing. Arm flexion and extension at the elbow are the lower levels of response.

Verbal performance is graded as orientated conversation, confused conversation, inappropriate words, sounds (e.g. grunts) or nothing at all, but language difficulties, endotracheal intubation and facial trauma may greatly influence these findings.

Table 19.2 Glasgow Coma Scale

| Response | Criterion | Score |
| --- | --- | --- |
| Eye opening | Spontaneous | 4 |
| | Speech | 3 |
| | Pain | 2 |
| | None | 1 |
| Verbal response | Oriented | 5 |
| | Confused | 4 |
| | Inappropriate words | 3 |
| | Incomprehensible sounds | 2 |
| | None | 1 |
| Best motor response | Obeys commands | 6 |
| | Localizes pain | 5 |
| | Withdrawal from pain | 4 |
| | Flexion to pain | 3 |
| | Extension to pain | 2 |
| | None | 1 |

Focal neurological signs may be observed in the eyes or the limbs, or as the effects of medullary dysfunction on the patient's vital signs. The pupils are examined for size, inequality and reactivity to light. An acute compressive intracranial haematoma presses the ipsilateral third nerve against the free edge of the tentorium as it expands. After an initial slight contraction, the ipsilateral pupil begins to dilate and the reaction to light becomes sluggish: Hutchinson's pupil, a sign of coning (see 'Raised Intracranial Pressure', below). Eventually, as the mass increases, the contralateral pupil also becomes dilated and unreactive. In a Hutchinson's pupil, the consensual light reflex is also lost. Thus, pupillary dilatation from optic nerve injury or intraocular haematoma may be distinguished, as in these cases the consensual reflex is present.

The development of a hemiplegia is also indicative of an acute compressive intracranial haematoma. The hemiplegia is most likely to be contralateral to the lesion.

### Raised Intracranial Pressure

Symptoms of rising intracranial pressure are headache, vomiting and double vision. The headache is typically worse in the morning, or on bending or stooping. Papilloedema may be observed on fundoscopy. Coning eventually occurs when the pressure forces the brain through the tentorium or foramen magnum. This distorts the brainstem and the oculomotor nerve, resulting in coma and an ipsilateral, dilated unreactive pupil. Bradycardia, rising blood pressure and slow, irregular respiration are features of medullary compression (Cushing's triad).

Causes of raised intracranial pressure include the following:

- localized mass lesions such as traumatic haematomas (extradural, subdural or intracerebral);
- neoplasms: gliomas, meningiomas and metastases;
- abscesses;
- focal oedema secondary to trauma, infarction or tumour;
- disturbances of CSF circulation, for example obstructive hydrocephalus and communicating hydrocephalus;
- obstructions to the major venous sinuses after depressed fractures overlying major venous sinuses or cerebral venous thrombosis;
- diffuse brain oedema or swelling, for example with encephalitis, meningitis, diffuse head injury, subarachnoid haemorrhage,

Reye's syndrome, lead encephalopathy, water intoxication or near-drowning;

• idiopathic: idiopathic intracranial hypertension.

## Hypoxia and Oedema

A deterioration in the patient's condition may not only be the result of an intracranial haematoma because in severe brain injury, a vicious circle of oedema and hypoxia develops. Medullary compression then results in respiratory depression. The fall in cerebral $P_{O_2}$ causes tissue oedema, and the rise in $P_{CO_2}$ causes vasodilation with an increase in cerebral blood volume. These changes further increase the intracranial pressure and thus the cycle continues. Intracranial pressure can be monitored by various methods, with a pressure greater than 20 mmHg being abnormal.

## Intracranial Lesions Following Head Injury

These lesions can be focal or diffuse, although both coexist in most cases of head injury. Focal lesions include epidural haematomas, subdural haematomas and contusions.

## Diffuse Axonal Injury

This refers to the microscopic axonal damage caused by the distortion of brain tissue during the impact of an injury. The term covers the wide range of states that are seen after a head injury. It may manifest clinically as nothing more than a mild concussion or, at the other end of the spectrum, the patient may be in a profound coma. Contrary to previous thinking, such brain injury is diffuse.

## Contusions and Lacerations

Macroscopic damage occurs as contusions and lacerations, these being most common on the undersurfaces of the frontal and temporal lobes where the brain moves over the bony ridges on impact.

## Acute Extra (Epi) Dural Haematomas

These haematomas usually result from bleeding from the middle meningeal vessels into the extradural space. They may occur in severe head injury (**Figure 19.14**) but, more importantly, it must be recognized that the condition may arise from a more moderate injury. The classical scenario is that the patient suffers only a light blow to the side of the head, but this is still sufficient to fracture the relatively thin squamous temporal bone over which the artery runs.

The patient may initially only be dazed or may have lost consciousness for a short while. Consciousness is then regained, and after a 'lucid interval' the patient gradually deteriorates over several hours as the haematoma slowly collects in the extradural space, with symptoms of rising intracranial pressure – worsening headache, vomiting, visual disturbances and drowsiness. The level of consciousness deteriorates and localizing signs develop.

The pattern of presentation of an extradural haematoma is the underlying reason for admission for observation after relatively mild to moderate head injuries, especially when they are associated with a skull fracture. The prognosis is excellent if they are treated early.

## Acute Subdural Haematomas

Acute subdural haematomas commonly occur from tearing of the bridging veins between the cortex and the draining sinuses, and are usually associated with significant brain injury (**Figure 19.15**). Lacerations of the surface of the brain result in bleeding into the subdural space. The patient may be deeply unconscious on initial assessment. There is usually no associated lucid interval. Localizing signs may be present. Patients presenting in this state require transfer to a neurosurgical unit for a CT scan and subsequent management.

The prognosis is guarded, with significant risks of morbidity and mortality. The deeply unconscious, flaccid patient with only

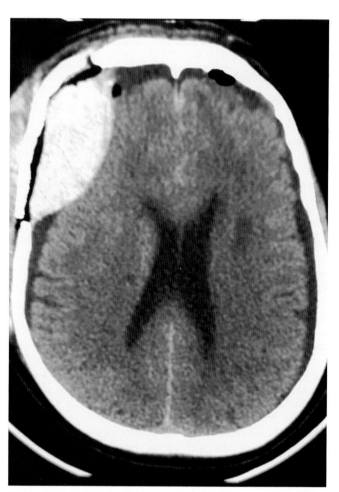

Figure 19.14 A CT scan of the brain showing a biconvex, high-density extra-axial lesion in the right frontal area with a fracture that is classical of an extradural haematoma.

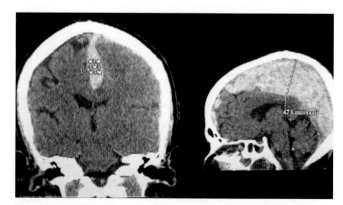

Figure 19.15 Plain CT scan of brain coronal and sagittal images demonstrating an interhemispheric corcavo-convex high extra-axial lesion characteristic of acute subdural hematoma.

primitive reflexes and bilateral fixed dilated pupils is likely to have suffered brainstem shearing, and the situation is probably irretrievable.

## Chronic Subdural Haematomas

These usually occur after a minor injury in the elderly, those who abuse alcohol and individuals with clotting disorders, and are not associated with significant head injury (**Figure 19.16**). A small collection of blood gradually enlarges by osmosis, and the symptoms develop over days, weeks or even months. Headache, vomiting, mood change, irritability, incontinence and drowsiness may occur, and senility may be wrongly suspected. The signs vary, but pupillary inequality, long tract signs, upgoing plantar reflexes, dysphasia and fits may result. The prognosis following evacuation is usually excellent.

## Post-concussion Syndromes

These are persisting symptoms of headache, dizziness, seizures, memory impairment and lack of concentration following a head injury.

# Cerebrovascular Diseases

## Vascular Malformations

Vascular malformations affecting the CNS include arteriovenous malformations, capillary telangiectasias, cavernous malformations, venous malformations, haemangiomas and dural arteriovenous fistulas. They usually develop early in life due to maldevelopment of the vascular channels (**Figure 19.17**). The symptoms may vary with the location. Seizures and haemorrhage are the common presenting features of arteriovenous and cavernous malformations. Headache and progressive neurological deficit because of 'steal syndrome' are the other uncommon presentations. Blood sucked into a high-flow **arteriovenous malformation** deprives the surrounding brain of an adequate blood supply, resulting in ischaemia – the so-called 'steal syndrome'. Telangiectasias and venous malformations are usually detected incidentally.

## Stroke

A stroke is the abrupt and dramatic onset of a neurological deficit resulting from a vascular mechanism and is defined by the World Health Organization as 'rapidly developing clinical signs of focal disturbance of cerebral function, lasting for more than 24 hours or leading to death'. Atherosclerosis, hypertension, diabetes,

smoking, hyperlipidaemias and familial tendencies constitute major risk factors.

The majority of strokes are ischaemic in origin and occur when the normal blood flow to the brain is blocked, typically because of an embolism or thrombosis. The symptoms reflect the vascular territory involved and give a clue to the localization of the vessel involved and the pathology. An ischaemic deficit that rapidly resolves (within 24 hours) is termed a transient ischaemic attack.

Haemorrhagic stroke comprises two main types:

- intraparenchymal haemorrhage, in which there is bleeding within the brain parenchyma;
- subarachnoid haemorrhage, which is characterized by vessel rupture in the CSF-filled subarachnoid space surrounding the brain.

**Subarachnoid haemorrhage** results from the rupture of a cerebral aneurysm in the subarachnoid space, with trauma being the most common cause (**Figure 19.18**). Berry aneurysms occur at the junctions of the cerebral vessels in the circle of

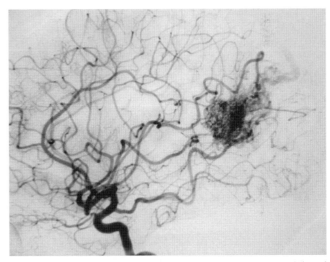

Figure 19.17 A lateral projection of internal carotid injection in digital subtraction angiography, demonstrating an abnormal cluster of vessels (the nidus of an arteriovenous malformation supplied by the middle cerebral artery).

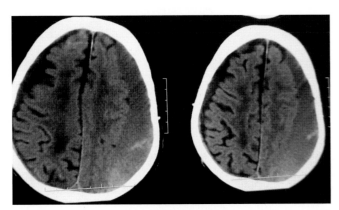

Figure 19.16 A plain CT scan of the brain showing a left extra-axial, concavo-convex hypodense lesion, suggestive of a chronic subdural haematoma.

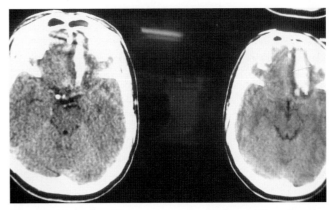

Figure 19.18 A plain CT scan of the brain showing a bifrontal patchy, hyperdense, intra-axial lesion in a case of traumatic brain injury, suggesting contusion.

Willis (**Figure 19.19**). These may rupture, which most commonly occurs in the 35–60-year-old age group. Patients present with a sudden, severe, headache 'like never before' and signs of meningism caused by blood in the CSF: neck stiffness, photophobia, nausea and vomiting. There may be signs of cerebral compression and raised intracranial pressure with papilloedema.

**Intracerebral haemorrhage** may be primary (spontaneous) caused by essential hypertension (**Figure 19.20**), or secondary due to arteriovenous malformations, aneurysms (**Figure 19.21**), blood dyscrasias, tumours or drugs (anticoagulants or thrombolytic agents). Vomiting and headache are common features, along with focal neurological deficits that depend on the location of the intracranial haemorrhage. The signs and symptoms are generally not confined to a single vascular territory.

## Infections

Infections of the CNS can be bacterial, mycobacterial, viral or fungal in origin (**Table 19.3**). Regardless of the aetiology, symptoms usually include headache, lethargy, fever, vomiting, anorexia, restlessness, irritability, photophobia, meningism and focal neurological deficits. The anatomical distribution of the infection may be diffuse (encephalitis or meningitis) or focal. The patient's age, mode of onset, presence of associated typical comorbid conditions (malnutrition, HIV, rash and malignancies), clinical examination and laboratory evaluation may act as pointers to the underlying aetiology. Infections frequently present as medical emergencies requiring prompt recognition and management.

### Tuberculosis

*Mycobacterium tuberculosis* can cause neurotuberculosis, which begins with the development of small tuberculous foci (**Rich foci**) in the brain, spinal cord or meninges. The location of these foci and the capacity to control them ultimately determine which form of CNS tuberculosis occurs. It usually manifests as tuberculous meningitis and less commonly as tubercular encephalitis, intracranial tuberculoma or a tuberculous brain abscess. Immunocompromised subjects have a higher risk of developing not only infection of greater severity, but also atypical mycobacterial infections (*Mycobacterium avium* or *Mycobacterium intracellulare*).

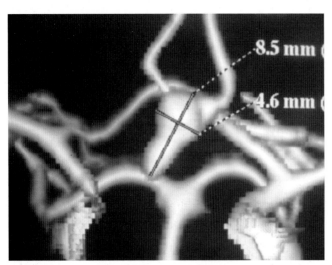

Figure 19.19 A CT angiogram of the brain vessels demonstrating an aneurysm arising from the anterior communicating artery.

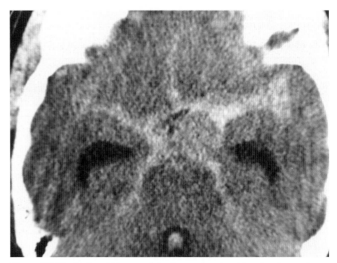

Figure 19.21 A plain CT scan of the brain showing blood as hyperdense areas in the basal subarachnoid space; this was caused by a subarachnoid haemorrhage.

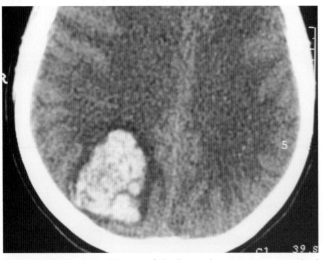

Figure 19.20 A plain CT scan of the brain showing an intracerebral hyperdense lesion that is suggestive of an intracerebral haematoma.

Table 19.3 Pathogens in central nervous system infection

|  | Examples |
|---|---|
| Bacterial | *Streptococcus pneumoniae, Neisseria meningitidis, Haemophilus influenzae, Listeria monocytogenes,* gram-negative bacilli, *Escherichia coli, Staphylococcus, Pseudomonas aeruginosa, Shigella* |
| Viral | Polio, coxsackie, ECHO, influenza, parainfluenza, Japanese B, varicella, Epstein–Barr, cytomegalovirus, rabies, HIV, mumps, measles, rubella, slow viruses |
| Fungal | *Cryptococcus, Aspergillus, Histoplasma, Blastomyces, Coccidioides, Candida,* zygomycosis |
| Other | Mycobacteria, plasmodia, *Treponema, Amoeba, Toxoplasma, Trypanosoma, Taenia echinococcus, Schistosoma, Toxocara, Strongyloides* |

**Tubercular meningitis** often presents with the classic symptoms of fever, headache and meningismus (a stiff neck) along with focal neurological deficits, behavioural changes and alterations in consciousness. Depending on the stage of presentation, neurological symptoms range from lethargy and agitation to coma.

The clinical manifestations of **tuberculoma** and **tuberculous brain abscess** depend largely on their location, size, number, stage of evolution and extent of surrounding reaction; patients often present with headache, seizures, papilloedema or other signs of increased intracranial pressure. The symptoms develop over weeks or months.

## Pyogenic Abscesses

Pyogenic abscesses are intracranial collections of pus that present as space-occupying lesions. They may be extradural, intradural or intracerebral. Brain abscesses can result from:

- direct extension of cranial infections: osteomyelitis, mastoiditis, sinusitis and subdural empyema;
- penetrating head injuries: severe head injury, gun shots, stab wounds and neurosurgical procedures;
- haematogenous spread: bacterial endocarditis, congenital heart disease with a right-to-left shunt or intravenous drug abuse;
- unknown causes.

In the case of extradural lesions, there may be evidence of overlying osteomyelitis: a Pott's puffy tumour. Intracerebral abscesses and multiple abscesses may result from the systemic spread of serious infection. Intracerebral abscesses may be secondary to lung abscesses, bronchiectasis or other pyaemic states. The symptoms result from increased intracranial pressure and a mass effect associated with fever. The diagnosis is established by contrast-enhanced MRI or CT and culture. Treatment is with appropriate antibiotics and surgical drainage.

## Subdural Empyema

A surgical empyema is a collection of pus between the dural and arachnoid membranes secondary to aerobic, anaerobic or tubercular infections. Coexisting signs and symptoms of meningitis, paranasal sinusitis, mastoiditis, otitis, cranial osteomyelitis and trauma may give a clue to the source of infection. Subdural empyema can be life-threatening. The signs and symptoms include those of antecedent infection, meningeal irritation, a focal CNS lesion and increased intracranial pressure.

## Neoplasms

Primary brain tumours can arise from the brain tissue, meninges, nerves, pituitary gland and various embryonic tissues and developmental abnormalities (**Table 19.4**). Gliomas (**Figure 19.22**) are the most common, astrocytomas being the most common of the gliomas. Meningiomas (**Figure 19.23**) are slow-growing and benign; schwannomas most commonly arise from the VIIIth cranial nerve (as acoustic neuromas) (**Figure 19.24**); and pituitary tumours are usually benign adenomas (**Figure 19.25**). AIDS is associated with the appearance of rare intracranial granulomas and primary lymphoma of the brain.

In adults 80 per cent of tumours are supratentorial, whereas in children infratentorial lesions are the most common. Brain tumours may be primary or metastatic lesions. The most common metastatic tumours originate in the breast and lungs, although melanoma has the greatest propensity for metastasizing to the

Table 19.4 Neoplasms in the brain

|  | Examples |
|---|---|
| Congenital | Craniopharyngioma, germinoma, teratoma, dermoid cyst, angioma |
| Children | Primary: cerebellar astrocytoma, medulloblastoma, ependymoma, germinoma<br>Metastatic: neuroblastoma, leukaemia |
| Adults | Primary: glioma, meningioma, schwannoma, lymphoma<br>Metastatic: from bronchogenic carcinoma, carcinoma of the breast, malignant melanoma |

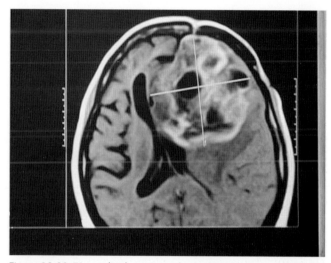

Figure 19.22 T1-weighted contrast-enhanced MRI image of the brain demonstrating a left posterofrontal intra-axial lesion with irregular margins and heterogenous contrast enhancement suggestive of a malignant glioma.

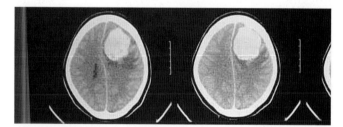

Figure 19.23 A contrast-enhanced CT scan of the brain showing a dural-based, extra-axial, uniformly enhancing lesion with a regular margin in the left front convexity, suggestive of a meningioma.

brain. Symptoms of raised intracranial tension, headache, an altered sensorium, focal neurological deficits, endocrine disturbances and seizures may occur.

Malignant tumours grow fairly rapidly and therefore result in rising intracranial pressure. Midline tumours may obstruct the CSF pathways, causing hydrocephalus.

## Headache

Headache is one of the most commonly encountered symptoms and has a long list of differential diagnoses. Primary headaches are benign headaches in which no examination or investigation

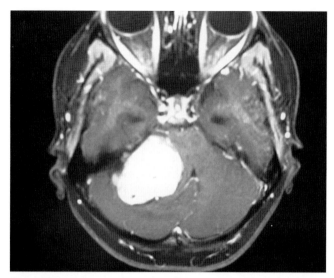

Figure 19.24 Contrast-enhanced axial MRI images of the brain demonstrating an enhancing, extra-axial lesion in the right cerebellopontine angle, which was suggestive of a vestibular schwannoma.

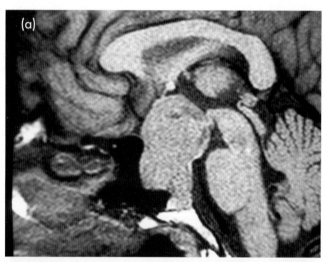

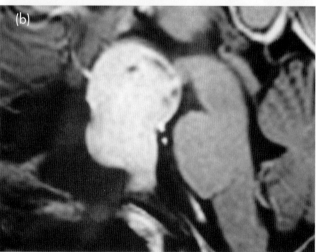

Figure 19.25 (a) Plain and (b) contrast-enhanced MRI of the brain. A sagittal sequence demonstrating a sellar and suprasellar mass that showed contrast enhancement and was suggestive of a pituitary adenoma.

is needed, nor will this yield a clue to the possible aetiology; migraine, tension headache and cluster headache are common examples.

In secondary headaches, an underlying structural, vascular, metabolic or infective cause can be detected. The associated symptoms and signs often provide a clue to the cause, for example vomiting (migraine or increased intracranial pressure), fever (infections), visual symptoms (blurring of vision, photophobia), infection, acute closed-angle glaucoma, migraine, cluster headaches, space-occupying lesions, idiopathic intracranial hypertension, preceding aura (migraine), focal neurological deficits (intracerebral haemorrhage, subdural haematoma, a mass lesion or infection) or seizures (epilepsy, infection or mass lesions).

## Epilepsy

Epilepsy is a common disorder of the CNS and is characterized by a recurrence of unprovoked seizures. Epilepsy can be idiopathic/cryptogenic with no known aetiology, or symptomatic with a known structural abnormality. The identifiable risk factors include congenital malformations, head injury, cerebrovascular causes, metabolic disorders, infections, tumours, Alzheimer's disease and drugs. Syncope, breath-holding spells, pseudoseizures, panic attacks and paroxysmal rapid eye movement sleep can all mimic epilepsy.

Tumours in the posterior strip of the frontal lobe – the motor strip – may cause focal motor seizures: Jacksonian epilepsy. Here the fit begins in a localized region of the contralateral half of the body but then spreads to affect the whole half and may become generalized.

## Brain Death and the Vegetative State

Brain death and a vegetative state may result following delayed resuscitation after a cardiorespiratory arrest, severe head injury or primary intracerebral catastrophe such as an intracranial haemorrhage.

The cerebral cortex is the organ most vulnerable to hypoxic injury, followed by the brainstem. The myocardium is much more resistant, so in any of the above crises the heart and other body organs survive preferentially. Where such hypoxic injury occurs, the usual result is cortical death. The brainstem survives so spontaneous respiration occurs and the heart continues to beat independently; this is termed a vegetative state.

If hypoxia is further prolonged, the brainstem also dies. The heart can still beat spontaneously, but spontaneous respiration does not occur and artificial ventilation is required. This state is referred to as brain death.

As defined by the UK Royal Colleges, as well as many US states, if the brainstem is dead, the cortex is also considered to be dead. Death can therefore be declared when brainstem death is diagnosed rather than when the heart stops. This has important implications for the withdrawal of ventilatory support and for organ donation.

Brain death results from head injury in approximately 50 per cent of cases and from subarachnoid haemorrhage in about 30 per cent more. It should be noted that alcohol, neuromuscular relaxants and hypothermia may cause a temporary absence of brainstem function so must be withdrawn or corrected before the diagnosis can be made. In brain death, the patient is apnoeic and in a deep coma. The examination findings confirming brainstem death are:

- the lack of a pupillary response to light;
- absence of the corneal reflex;

- no motor response to pain;
- a lack of laryngeal response to movement of the endotracheal tube;
- no caloric or vestibulo-ocular response – syringing the external auditory meatus with ice cold water normally results in vestibular nystagmus.

Once these criteria have been met, the final test is that there should be no respiratory movement after disconnection of the ventilator for a duration that allows the arterial $P\text{CO}_2$ to exceed 60 mmHg when 6 L/min of oxygen is being delivered via the endotracheal tube.

**Key Points**

A complete neurological examination evaluates the higher mental functions, cranial nerves and motor, sensory and reflex functions, and is essential:

- to understand the pathophysiology of any lesions involved;
- to outline a differential diagnosis depending on the patient's signs and symptoms;
- to allow relevant investigations that will lead to an accurate diagnosis and timely management.

## SBAs

**1. Which one of the following is true of a sebaceous cyst?:**
a　It is an uncommon scalp swelling
b　It is a retention cyst of a hair follicle
c　It lies deep to the galea aponeurotica
d　It is never attached to the skin

**Answer**
b　*It is a retention cyst of a hair follicle.* A sebaceous cyst is a closed sac under the skin, filled with a cheese-like, oily material, that most often arises from a swollen hair follicle.

**2. Which of the following is not related to craniostenosis?:**
a　Plagiocephaly
b　Scaplocephaly
c　Brachycephaly
d　Macrocephaly

**Answer**
d　*Macrocephaly.* Macrocephaly literally means large head. All the other options are examples of craniostenosis, where the head size is usually small in some dimension, depending on the suture involved.

**3. Cerebrospinal fluid is formed by which one of the following?:**
a　Choroid plexus
b　Archnoid villi
c　Venous sinus
d　Internal cerebral vein

**Answer**
a　*Choroid plexus.* The epithelial cells of the choroid plexus secrete cerebrospinal fluid (CSF) from the blood in to the ventricles of the brain.

**4. With regard to a meningoencephalocoele, which one of the following is not correct?:**
a　It is a midline swelling
b　It contains only cerebrospinal fluid
c　It transmits a cough impulse on crying
d　It contains neural tissue

**Answer**
b　*It contains only cerebrospinal fluid.* A meningo-encephalocoele is a hernial protrusion of brain substance, meninges and CSF through a congenital or traumatic opening of the skull; compare this with a meningocoele, which only contains CSF.

**5. Features of raised intracranial pressure include all of the following except:**
a　Early morning headache
b　Vomiting
c　Papilloedema
d　Scalp swelling

**Answer**
d　*Scalp swelling.* The triad of raised intracranial pressure comprises early morning headache, vomiting and papilloedema.

**6. Cushing's triad arises from which one of the following?:**
a　Medullary compression
b　Frontal lobe damage
c　Parietal lobe damage
d　Thalamic compression

**Answer**
a　*Medullary compression.* 'Cushing's triad' is the presence of hypertension, bradycardia and irregular respiration. The irregular respiration is due to reduced perfusion of the brainstem from swelling or possible brainstem herniation.

**7. Acute extra-axial haematoma is commonly due to which one of the following?:**
a　Brain contusion
b　Carotid artery injury
c　Middle cerebral artery injury
d　Middle meningeal artery injury

**Answer**
d　*Middle meningeal artery injury.* Brain contusion or middle cerebral artery injury may produce an intracerebral haematoma. Carotid artery injury may produce cerebral infarction. Middle meningeal arteries are vessels in the dura mater; injury to these may produce an extradural haematoma.

**8.** Seizures and intracerebral haemorrhage are common modes of presentation of which one of the following:
   a Dermoid
   b Arteriovenous malformations
   c Venous malformation
   d Telangiectasia

Answer

b **Arteriovenous malformations.** *Arteriovenous malformations are an abnormal cluster of vessels in the brain, and are usually congenital. They may rupture spontaneously, resulting in intracerebral haemorrhage or seizures.*

**9.** The most common malignant primary brain tumour is:
   a Pituitary tumour
   b Chordoma
   c Acoustic neuroma
   d Glioma

Answer

d **Glioma.** *The most common primary brain tumour – those that begin in the brain and tend to stay in the brain – is a meningioma. The most common malignant primary brain tumour is a glioma.*

**10.** The final test to confirm brain death is which one of the following?:
   a No motor response
   b No vocal response
   c No eye opening
   d No respiratory movement after increasing the $P\text{co}_2$ to above 60 mmHg

Answer

d **No respiratory movement after increasing the $P\text{co}_2$ to above 60 mmHg.** *There are a series of bedside clinical tests to assess brainstem function. In the absence of any brainstem function, the patient is declared brain dead, which is legally considered to be dead. The final confirmatory test for declaring brain death is the apnoeic test, a test to observe for respiratory movement after increasing the $P\text{co}_2$ to above 60 mmHg.*

PART 4 | HEAD AND NECK

# 20 The Face and Jaws

Gouri H. Pantvaidya, Abhishek Vaidya
and Sagar Vaishampayan

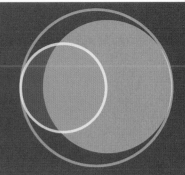

## LEARNING OBJECTIVES

- To recognize the signs and symptoms of various pathologies of the face and jaws
- To understand the pathognomonic facial features of certain clinical conditions
- To have an overview of the inflammatory and neoplastic lesions of the face and jaws

- To be able to provide a differential diagnosis for common signs and symptoms relating to the face and jaws

## CONGENITAL ABNORMALITIES

Facial deformities occur due to abnormal development of the maxillofacial skeleton and the mesenchymal components. Any part of the face may be affected. Abnormalities of eyes include anophthalmos (absent eye), microphthalmos (small eye) and buphthalmos (congenital glaucoma). Defects of the pinna can range in severity from microtia (a small rudimentary pinna) to anotia (complete absence of the pinna).

Midfacial, jaw and palatal abnormalities include micrognathia (mandibular hypoplasia) or macrognathia/megagnathia (large mandible), retrognathia (retracted hypoplastic mandible), cleft lip and cleft palate. The differential diagnosis of a congenital midline nasal swelling includes the following lesions:

- *Dermoids* are solid, non-compressible and non-transilluminant. They often present with infection, discharge and a visible sinus tract.
- *Nasal gliomas* are also firm, non-compressible and non-transilluminant. They may be associated with overlying telangiectasia.
- *Encephaloceles* may be bluish or red, soft and compressible, and enlarge with crying. They are associated with a positive Furstenberg test (enlargement on compression of the jugular veins).

Some deformities may be a part of well-defined syndromes such as Pierre Robin syndrome, in which the mandibular ramus is congenitally shortened. Facial abnormalities occur with cranial deformities in Crouzon's and Apert's syndromes. Down syndrome is characterized by a round face, microgenia (small chin), macroglossia (large tongue) and upslanting palpebral fissures.

## THE FACIES IN SYSTEMIC DISORDER

Certain systemic disorders are associated with characteristic facies that may point towards the diagnosis:

- *Acromegaly*: This occurs due to an increased secretion of growth hormone. The facial features include a generalized expansion of the skull at the fontanelles, prominent brow protrusion, pronounced lower jaw protrusion and macroglossia.
- *Cushing's syndrome*: This produces a 'moon face' resulting from the redistribution of fat due to excessive levels of adrenocorticotropic hormone.
- *Hypothyroidism*: A dull face, puffiness of the face and eyes and a loss of the lateral third of eyebrows (madarosis) are seen. In infancy and childhood, there may be widely spaced eyes with puffy eyelids, a broad depressed nasal bridge, thick lips and macroglossia.
- *Multiple endocrine neoplasia type IIB*: This is characterized by patulous lips, thickened eyelids and mucosal neuromas (**Figure 20.1**).
- *Neurofibromatosis type 1 (von Recklinghausen's disease)*: Characteristics include the presence of dermal neurofibromas, which are sessile or pedunculated masses on the skin (cutaneous) or smooth bumps just below the skin (subcutaneous), which may vary in size, number and distribution. They usually begin at puberty and may continue to increase in number and size throughout adulthood. The presence of

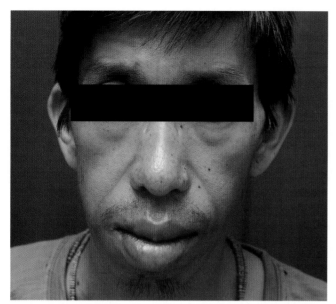

Figure 20.1 The characteristic facies of multiple endocrine neoplasia (MEN) type II syndrome.

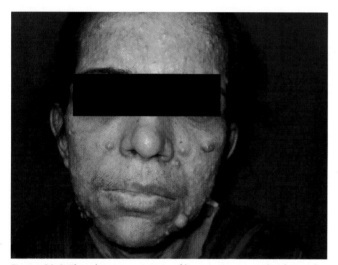

Figure 20.2 The characteristic neurofibromas seen on the face of a patient with neurofibromatosis type 1.

neurofibromas forms one of the diagnostic features for this disorder (Figure 20.2).

## INFLAMMATORY CONDITIONS

### Sinusitis

**Acute sinusitis** is an infection of the mucosal lining of the paranasal sinuses of less than 4 weeks' duration. It is usually precipitated by a preceding upper respiratory tract infection, generally of viral origin. Among infections of bacterial origin, the most common causative agents are *Streptococcus pneumoniae*, *Haemophilus influenzae* and *Moraxella catarrhalis*.

Sinusitis most commonly affects the maxillary sinus and is characterized by pain in the cheek or upper teeth that may be referred to other areas of the face. The pain typically worsens on bending or lying down. It may occasionally follow dental extraction or an abscess of the upper molars.

Sinusitis of the frontal and ethmoidal sinuses usually occurs secondary to maxillary sinusitis. Frontal sinusitis may cause pain or fullness in the forehead or above the eyes, while ethmoid sinusitis can cause pain or pressure pain between or behind the eyes, as well as headaches. Isolated sphenoid sinusitis is rare. Rarely, an infective pathology in the sphenoid sinus may cause lateral rectus palsy due to an associated osteitis affecting the abducens nerve.

**Chronic sinusitis** is an inflammation of the nasal airway and sinuses that lasts for more than 12 weeks. It may be a sequela of acute sinusitis or secondary to other conditions that predispose to chronic inflammation of the sinuses such as allergic rhinitis, cystic fibrosis, ciliary dyskinesia or an immunocompromised state. Anatomical variations that hinder the normal drainage of a sinus may lead to chronic sinusitis. Diagnosis is clinical and is confirmed by the following symptoms:

* Mucopurulent drainage;
* Nasal obstruction;
* Pain, pressure or fullness in the face;
* A decreased sense of smell.

The complications of sinusitis are varied and may occur due to osteitis or a spread of infection along the veins or lymphatics. The proximity of the sinuses to the orbit may give rise to orbital complications, which have been described as passing through five stages: preseptal cellulitis, orbital cellulitis, subperiosteal abscess, orbital abscess and cavernous sinus thrombosis. The signs and symptoms worsen progressively through lid oedema, chemosis (conjunctival oedema), a restriction of movement of the extraocular muscles and, finally, ophthalmoplegia.

**Pott's puffy tumour** is a rare complication of frontal sinusitis that is characterized by osteomyelitis and a subperiosteal abscess of the frontal bone. It presents as a firm, non-compressible, mildly tender swelling on the forehead (**Figure 20.3**).

## Chronic Infections

Chronic infections are often seen in the paranasal sinuses, face and jaws, and are more common in the tropics. **Tuberculosis** of the sinuses usually occurs secondary to infection at a primary location elsewhere. Tuberculosis may also involve the skin of the face and is known as lupus vulgaris. This is characterized by painful cutaneous lesions with a nodular appearance that are most often seen on the face around the nose, eyelids, lips, cheeks and ears. If left untreated, they may cause disfiguring scars.

**Actinomycosis** is a chronic infection most commonly affecting the face and the jaws (lumpy jaw). It is characterized by multiple sinuses and abscesses around the mouth and jaws that often discharge sulphur granules (**Figure 20.4**).

## Deep Infections

Deep infections of the face and neck are in almost all cases secondary to dental infection or tonsillitis.

A **buccal space abscess** (**Figure 20.5**) is usually seen secondary to infection of the upper second and third molars. It is characterized by a pus collection between the buccinator muscle and the subcutaneous tissue. There is brawny oedema on the cheek, tenseness of the skin, pain and often trismus. The pus occasionally points onto the skin.

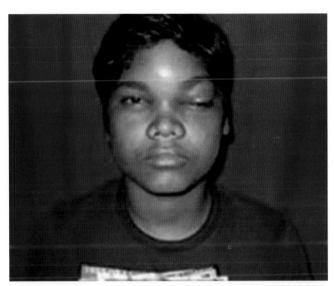

Figure 20.3 A subperiosteal abscess of the frontal sinus – 'Pott's puffy tumour'.

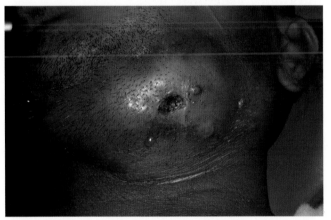

Figure 20.4 Actinomycosis of the lower jaw with discharging sinuses and abscess formation.

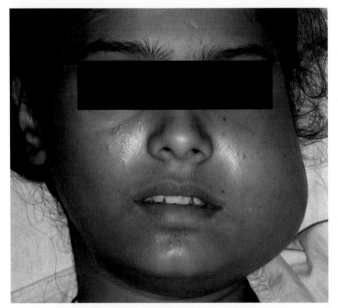

Figure 20.5 A left buccal space abscess with tense skin, erythema and brawny induration.

**Ludwig's angina** is a severe, potentially life-threatening cellulitis of the floor of mouth secondary to infection of the mandibular molars. Patients have an elevated floor of the mouth, fever, trismus, odynophagia and, in severe cases, breathing distress or even stridor.

## TUMOURS

### Cysts

**Cystic lesions of the jaws** are quite common. They may be associated with defects of fusion of the embryonic elements forming the facial skeleton and maxilla, or they may occur secondary to an unerupted tooth or dental conditions. They are more common in the mandible. They present as slow-growing, painless swellings of the jaws. These dental cysts are submucosal, bony hard and, usually, non-tender.

**Dermoid cysts** are developmental cysts that usually arise at the lines of embryological fusion. The most common location is in the midline of the root of the nose, and the cysts may even extend intranasally. Dermoids may also occur at the orbital margins.

### Benign Tumours

A large variety of benign jaw tumours may be encountered in the bones of the jaws. These may be broadly classified into odontogenic (arising in relation to the dental structures) and non-odontogenic tumours.

**Ameloblastoma** is the most prevalent of all the odontogenic tumours. It is a locally aggressive, slow-growing, epithelial odontogenic neoplasm. The mandible is the most common site of occurrence. It is usually painless and remains asymptomatic until it enlarges, producing a gradual jaw expansion that causes facial asymmetry. Most ameloblastomas appear as a submucosal mass surrounding the mandible without obvious overlying ulceration of the mucosa (**Figure 20.6**).

Non-odontogenic jaw tumours include osteomas, exostoses and tori. **Osteomas** arising in these regions take two forms. Localized compact osteomas occur in the frontal sinuses of young adults.

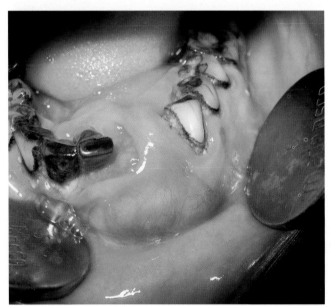

Figure 20.6 Ameloblastoma of the mandible. Note the submucous nature of the tumour.

They may cause displacement of the eye owr give rise to a mucocele of the sinus as a result of frontonasal duct obstruction. Localized cancellous osteomas occur in the maxillary and ethmoidal sinuses.

Exostoses may occur in the midline of the hard palate as a torus palatinus.

## Malignant Tumours

**Squamous carcinomas** are the most common malignant tumours of the upper aero-digestive tract. They may occur in any part of the upper airway lined by stratified squamous epithelium. Although the commonest sites are the oral cavity and oropharynx, they may also appear in the jaws and face. Here they may occur in the paranasal sinuses and nasal passages, or in the upper or lower jaw.

The symptoms of malignancy vary and may mimic sinusitis. Unilateral nasal obstruction, unilateral epistaxis and nasal discharge are suspicious of malignancy. There may be swelling of the cheek, alveolar margin or nasal bridge. Loosening of the teeth, ulceration of the palate and facial skin involvement may occur in advanced cases (**Figure 20.7**). Unilateral proptosis (**Figure 20.8**) that is not accompanied by the signs of sinusitis should arouse the suspicion of an underlying tumour. Invasion of the maxillary division of the trigeminal nerve may result in facial pain or facial paraesthesias.

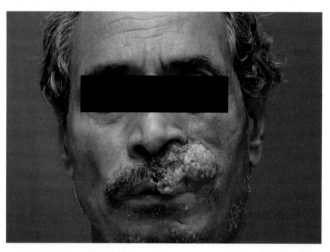

Figure 20.7 Characteristic ulceration in a patient with squamous cancer of the facial skin.

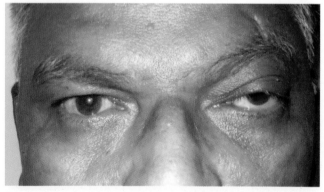

Figure 20.8 Left unilateral non-axial proptosis in a patient with a lacrimal gland tumour.

**Malignant melanomas** arise as polypoidal masses on the septum or lateral walls of the nose. These are characteristically dark or black in colour, although they can occasionally be pale (amelanotic melanoma). Metastases from other tumours may rarely occur in these regions.

Ohngren's line is an imaginary line joining the medial canthus of the eye to the angle of the mandible. This divides the maxilla into a superior and an inferior portion. Tumours arising above Ohngren's line (suprastructure tumours) have a poorer prognosis than those arising below this line.

**Basal cell carcinomas** (rodent ulcers) are usually seen on the face above a line joining the angle of the mouth to the ear lobe. They occur on skin exposed to sunlight but may also involve the scalp. Morphologically, there are three forms: superficial, infiltrative and nodular. The lesion usually starts as a raised papule, which may ulcerate with pearly white beaded edges as it progresses.

## TRAUMA

## Maxillary Fractures

Fractures of the maxilla are described according to the Le Fort classification, which relates to the plane of injury. This classification is based on the course of the fracture line that defines the level above which the midfacial skeleton is intact:

- *Line I* runs transversely, just above the floor of the nose and through the lower third of the nasal septum.
- *Line II* runs through the bridge of the nose and medial orbital walls via the lachrymal bones, and then crosses the inferior orbital rim at the junction of its medial one-third and lateral two-thirds. It passes through the infraorbital foramen and runs beneath the zygomaticomaxillary suture to extend backwards through the lateral pterygoid plates. The zygomatic arches remain intact (**Figure 20.9**).

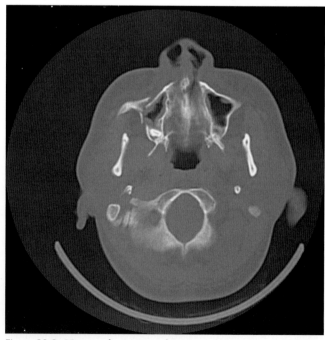

Figure 20.9 CT scan of a Le Fort II fracture

- *Line III* runs parallel to the base of the skull. The fracture line runs through the nasal bone and continues posteriorly through the ethmoid bone, crosses the lesser wing of the sphenoid and then runs laterally upwards to the frontozygomatic suture. It usually passes below the optic foramen, but rarely may run through it. There is total craniofacial disconnection in this type of fracture.

All these fractures are open to the nose, the paranasal sinuses or the mouth. Le Fort III fractures involve the cribriform plate and should therefore be regarded as communicating with the subarachnoid space. Le Fort II and III fractures affect the attachments of the orbital contents.

The general features of all three fracture types are periorbital bruising (the 'panda sign'), bilateral gross facial oedema and lengthening of the middle third of the face. There may be malocclusion in the molar region, and the nose is filled with blood.

Sensory loss can result if the fracture lines run through nerve canals. Infraorbital nerve injury gives rise to anaesthesia in the area between the inferior orbital margin and the upper lip, the side of the nose being spared. Inferior alveolar nerve injury results in anaesthesia of the mental region, while supraorbital nerve injury results in anaesthesia above the eye.

Examination for instability of the maxilla may be possible in the unconscious or anaesthetized patient. When steadying the frontonasal junction with one hand, it may be possible to illustrate mobility in a Le Fort II or III fracture by lifting the premaxillary region upwards with the other hand. In the mouth, the mandibular, maxillary and lingual sulci should be palpated for abnormalities of the bony contour, but maxillary fractures are not often compound to the mouth. Percussion of the maxillary teeth may illustrate a change in the normal resonance to a 'cracked cup' sound. There is a loss of occlusion in one or both molar regions.

## Zygomatic Fractures

Fractures of the zygoma may be part of Le Fort fractures or occur as isolated injuries. The injury may involve the temporomandibular joint, the infraorbital canal and the frontozygomatic suture with resultant painful mastication, numbness of the cheek and diplopia.

## Mandibular Fractures

Mandibular fractures are usually multiple. The most common sites are the condylar region and the angle of the mandible. For isolated fractures, however, the angle is the principal site. Fractures of the body and opposite condyle or angle are the most likely combination, but bilateral subcondylar fractures can also occur. Bilateral involvement of the angles or bodies, or three or more fracture sites, is uncommon.

Condylar fractures are usually indirect, while direct impact produce fractures of the body. This is because the condylar region is well protected by the zygomatic arch. The displacement in condylar fractures is relatively slight, and the mandible tends to deviate to the side of the injury on opening the mouth, the lateral pterygoid no longer being able to influence the main fragment of the mandible. Movement at the temporomandibular joint is painful and limited because of the protective muscle spasm. Bilateral condylar fractures classically result when patients lose consciousness and fall onto their chins. In combination with

a parasymphyseal fracture and a characteristic laceration beneath the chin, this injury is called a parade ground fracture.

Temporomandibular joint dislocation can be distinguished from a condylar fracture in that it produces a prominence anterior to the articular eminence and a hollow in the glenoid fossa. In unilateral cases, the mandible deviates to the opposite side. There is an inability to close the mouth. In a combined fracture-dislocation of the condyle, the balance between the elevator muscles and the lateral pterygoid is disturbed, and the jaw deviates towards the injured side.

Fractures of the angle of the mandible tend to occur anterior to the attachment of the masseter. The elevator muscles therefore tend to pull the posterior fragment upwards, forwards and inwards, leaving them unable to have any effect on the remainder of the mandible.

Fractures of the body of the mandible tend to occur in the region between the canine and first molar teeth (**Figure 20.10**). If the fracture site is more anterior, the upward pull of the jaw retractor muscles is countered by the downward pull of the mylohyoid muscle, thereby reducing the degree of displacement.

In examining the mandible, the lower border should be palpated from behind, and the temporomandibular joint regions inspected from the front. Movement of the condylar heads can be assessed by placing the little fingers in the external auditory meatuses with the pulps pointing forwards while the patient attempts to move the mandible in all directions. A compression test will elicit pain from an undisplaced fracture by applying gentle compression in two planes.

Mandibular fractures are often open to the buccal cavity, bloodstained saliva being a common finding. However, when this finding accompanies maxillary fractures, it is more likely to be due to nasopharyngeal bleeding. There may be ecchymoses of the buccal sulci near the zygomatic prominences or in the region of the greater palatine foramen – Guérin's sign. A sublingual haematoma is indicative of a fracture involving the lingual plate.

## Bell's Palsy

Bell's palsy (**Figure 20.11**) is a unilateral lower motor neuron facial palsy of unknown cause. It may start as a pain below the ear or in the mastoid region, followed by a rapid onset of facial

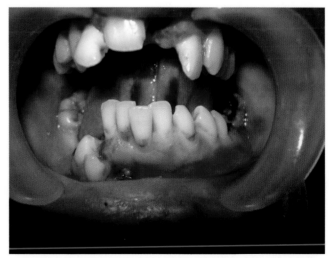

Figure 20.10 Fracture of the body of the mandible with displacement.

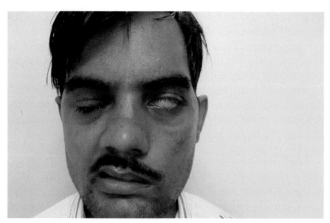

Figure 20.11 Left lower motor neurone palsy (Bell's palsy).

**Key Points**

■ A large variety of lesions may be seen in the face and the jaws. These can be classified as congenital, developmental, systemic, inflammatory, neoplastic and traumatic.
■ Congenital anomalies may be syndromic or non-syndromic, and a brief understanding of these is necessary.
■ Certain systemic disorders may be associated with characteristic facial features, which point to the underlying condition.
■ The paranasal sinuses and dentition may be the seat of several infections involving the face and the jaws.
■ Facial and jaw trauma is common. Owing to the complex anatomy of the bones and soft tissues in this region, a detailed understanding of the characteristic features, clinical signs, mechanism of trauma and underlying disorders is required.

paralysis. In severe cases, there may be a loss of taste in the anterior two-thirds of the tongue, and paralysis of the stapedius resulting in an intolerance to high-pitched or loud sounds.

In Ramsay Hunt syndrome, facial nerve paralysis is associated with herpes zoster infection. This may affect both the otic and the geniculate ganglion, and classically includes the triad of sensori-neural deafness, vertigo and facial paralysis.

# QUESTIONS

## SBAs

1. A 40-year-old woman presents with lethargy and weight gain. Her face appears dull and expressionless, and is puffy. There is thinning of her eyebrows in the lateral one-third. The most likely diagnosis is:
   a  Acromegaly
   b  Cushing's syndrome
   c  Hypothyroidism
   d  Hyperthyroidism

**Answer**

c  *Hypothyroidism. This presents with facial features of puffiness, madarosis, dry skin and a dull face. Other findings include weight gain, depression, lethargy, cold intolerance, bradycardia and menstrual irregularities. Hyperthyroidism presents with palpitations, resting tachycardia, eye changes (including proptosis), increased sweating, heat intolerance and often fine tremors. The facial features of acromegaly are generalized expansion of the skull at the fontanelles, prominent brow protrusion, pronounced lower jaw protrusion and macroglossia. A 'moon face' is the characteristic facial feature in Cushing's syndrome.*

2. A 50-year-old sawmill worker presents with left nasal obstruction and discharge that has lasted for 2 months. He complains of a recent-onset spontaneous falling of his upper left molar, and painful restricted mouth opening (trismus). He gives a past history of facial trauma. The most likely cause is of his symptoms is:
   a  Chronic maxillary sinus infection
   b  Maxillary sinus malignancy
   c  Tuberculosis of the sinuses
   d  Long-term effects of the facial injury

**Answer**

b  *Maxillary sinus malignancy. The initial features of maxillary sinus malignancy may mimic sinusitis and include nasal obstruction, discharge and dull pain. Spontaneous falling of the teeth indicates extension to the maxillary alveolus, while trismus indicates involvement of the pterygoid musculature. These features strongly point towards an underlying malignancy. Tuberculosis of the sinuses or face may produce indolent features of pain, discharge, obstruction and swelling, and may also cause a disfiguring scar; trismus is, however, rare. A history of trauma may sometimes be elicited, and the patient will often wrongly attribute his symptoms to this.*

3. Which one of the following most correctly describes the fracture line of a Le Fort III fracture?:
   a  A fracture line in the facial skeleton running parallel to the base of the skull
   b  A fracture line running horizontally just above the floor of the nose
   c  A fracture line running across the mandibular condyles
   d  A fracture line running across the nasal bridge

**Answer**

a  *A fracture line in the facial skeleton running parallel to the base of the skull. The Le Fort classification system of fractures describes fractures of the maxilla. The Le Fort III fracture line runs parallel to the base of the skull. It runs through the nasal bone and continues posteriorly through the ethmoid, crosses the lesser wing of the sphenoid and then runs laterally upwards to the frontozygomatic suture.*

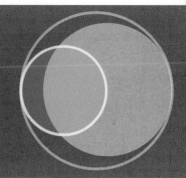

Deepa Nair, Arpit Sharma and
Shraddha Deshmukh

## LEARNING OBJECTIVE

- To identify the symptoms and signs of common ear diseases

- To understand the wide variety of pathology that can affect different parts of the ear

## MALFORMATIONS OF THE EAR

The external, middle and inner ear differ in terms of their embryonic development (Table 21.1), accounting for the wide variations in the type of malformations that can be encountered.

Malformations of the external and middle ear are often combined and include microtia (Figure 21.1), anotia (Figure 21.2), macrotia, bat ear, stenosis or atresia of the external auditory canal, malformed or fixed ossicles, and missing pneumatization of the middle ear or mastoid. Accessory auricles (Figure 21.3) may arise from abnormally sited tubercles. Preauricular sinuses (Figure 21.4) result from incomplete fusion of the tubercles and are usually situated at the root of helix; they are asymptomatic unless they become infected.

Table 21.1 Embryological development of the ear

|  | Tissue of origin | Adult structure |
|---|---|---|
| External ear | Fusion of the six tubercles of His around the first branchial cleft | Pinna |
|  | First branchial cleft | External auditory meatus |
| Middle ear | First branchial arch (mesoderm) | Malleus Incus |
|  | Second branchial arch (mesoderm) | Stapes |
| Inner ear | Otic placode (ectoderm) | Membranous labyrinth |
|  | Mesoderm surrounding otic vesicle | Bony labyrinth |

Malformations of the inner ear usually occur independently of those of the outer ear, but may be associated with other craniofacial abnormalities and hereditary syndromes. They include Michel's dysplasia, cochlear aplasia, common cavity and Mondini's dysplasia. Common craniofacial syndromes with involvement of ear are the Waardenburg, Pierre Robin, Treacher Collins–Franceschetti and Goldenhar syndromes.

## DISEASES OF THE OUTER EAR

### Trauma

Blunt trauma (from contact sports or an assault) or sharp trauma to the pinna results in an accumulation of serous fluid or blood between the perichondrium and the auricular cartilage, causing **seroma or haematoma auris**. The resultant necrosis of the cartilage due to the disrupted blood supply leads to scarring and deformity – known as a **cauliflower ear** (Figure 21.5). Other causes of trauma include lacerations, bite wounds, frostbite and burn wounds.

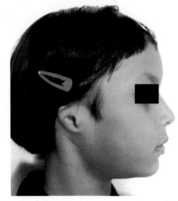

Figure 21.1 Microtia of the right pinna. (Courtesy of Dr Hetal Patel.)

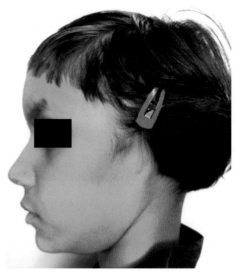

Figure 21.2 Congenital absence of the left pinna (anotia) with absence of the external auditory canal. (Courtesy of Dr Hetal Patel.)

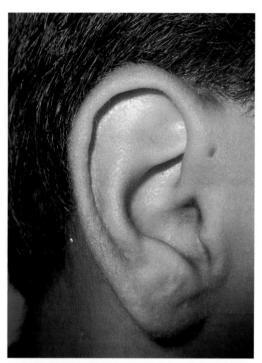

Figure 21.4 A right preauricular sinus.

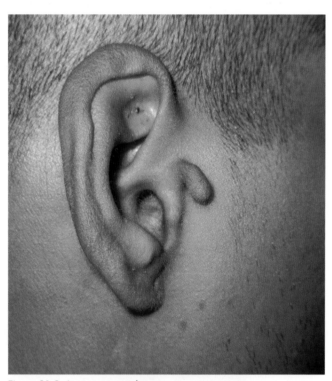

Figure 21.3 Accessory auricles.

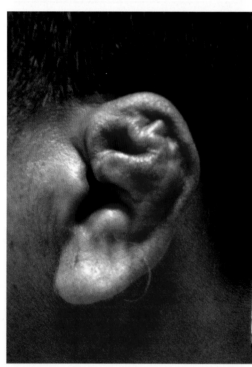

Figure 21.5 A resolved haematoma with deformity of the left ear causing a cauliflower ear.

## Infections and Inflammations of the Auricle

- In *erysipelas*, a streptococcal infection causes the whole auricle, including the ear lobe, to become inflamed and swollen.
- *Perichondritis* is a bacterial infection of the auricular cartilage, the ear lobe being spared.
- *Relapsing polychondritis* is an autoimmune, recurrent inflammation of cartilaginous structures. In most cases, it starts with inflammation of the auricular cartilage, but other cartilages (the nasal septum, larynx, trachea and bronchi) may be involved.

## Otitis Externa

**Furunculosis** is a staphylococcal infection of the hair follicle of the cartilaginous external auditory canal. Individuals with diabetes are particularly susceptible to recurrent furunculosis.

**Acute diffuse otitis externa (swimmer's ear)** is a spreading dermatitis involving the external auditory canal and auricle that is characterized by desquamation and crusting. It is associated with swimming in infected public pools, and is also seen in moist humid conditions.

**Fungal otitis externa/otomycosis** is characterized by intense pruritus, a smelly ear discharge and hearing loss due to impacted debris. Examination reveals abundant fungal debris embedded in thick, cheesy material (resembling wet newspaper) that may contain fungal hyphae and spores (**Figure 21.6**).

**Ramsay Hunt syndrome** is herpes zoster oticus accompanied by facial palsy that occurs because of reactivation of the varicella zoster virus. There is a painful vesicular eruption on the pinna, concha, external auditory canal, tongue and palate. The VIIIth cranial nerve may be involved, resulting in hearing loss, tinnitus and/or vertigo.

**Malignant necrotizing otitis externa** is an aggressive and potentially life-threatening infection of the external ear that spreads rapidly to involve the periosteum and bone of the skull base. *Pseudomonas aeruginosa* is the most common pathogen, mainly affecting elderly patients with diabetes or individuals who are immunocompromised. The condition is characterized by severe otalgia, granulations in the external auditory canal and involvement of the facial and lower cranial nerves. Fatal complications include meningitis, epidural abscess and thrombophlebitis.

**Contact dermatitis** is an inflammatory response triggered by contact with an irritant such as hairspray or shampoo, the use of neomycin-containing ototopical agents (**Figure 21.7**) or earrings (especially nickel), which may result in inflammation of the pinna and external auditory canal.

## Obstructions of the External Auditory Canal

- *Impacted wax* causes earache and deafness.
- A variety of *foreign bodies*, such as inanimate matter or even live insects, may be present in the external auditory canal.
- *Exostoses* are broad-based, localized bone growths in the osseous external auditory canal. They are usually multiple and bilateral, and are common among water sport enthusiasts.
- An *osteoma* is a solitary, benign, narrow-based bony tumour of the external auditory canal.

- *Keratosis obturans* is the accumulation of a large plug of desquamated keratin in the external auditory canal due to abnormal epithelial migration of the skin of the ear canal. It presents with otalgia and conductive hearing loss.
- A *primary cholesteatoma of the external auditory canal* is seen when there is an invasion of squamous tissue from the ear into a localized area of bony erosion. It presents with otorrhoea, itching and minimal hearing loss.

## Tumours of the Auricle

**Squamous cell carcinoma** usually occurs in fair-skinned people with a history of a long exposure to sunlight. It presents as a rapidly growing ulcer that is usually fixed to the underlying structures (**Figure 21.8**). The regional nodes may be involved. **Basal cell carcinoma** presents as a slow-growing, raised, indurated nodule with firm, pearly edges that is usually not associated with regional metastasis.

## Miscellaneous Conditions

**Keloids** present as a firm painless mass at the site of ear piercing (**Figure 21.9**) or secondary to surgical incisions. It can be differentiated from a hypertrophic scar as the latter remains within the confines of the wound, whereas keloid extends beyond the site of the original injury.

**Gouty tophi** are painless sodium urate concretions at the margin of helix in patients with gout.

The causes of **referred pain** are outlined in Table 21.2.

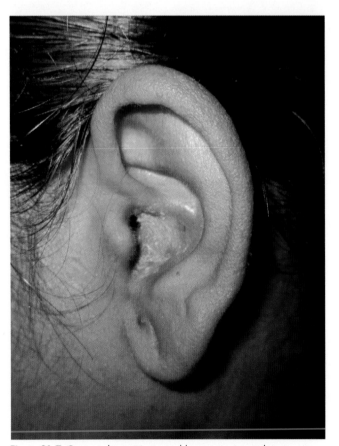

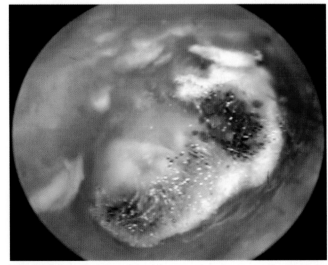

Figure 21.6 Otomycosis of the left external auditory canal with fungal spores.

Figure 21.7 Contact dermatitis caused by neomycin eardrops.

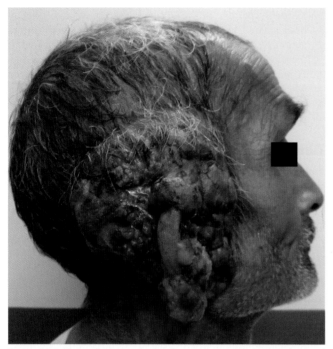

Figure 21.8 Fungating squamous cell carcinoma of the right pinna and mastoid.

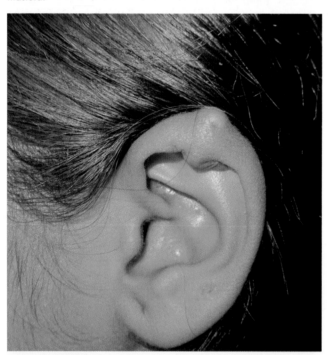

Figure 21.9 A keloid at the site of ear piercing in the left pinna.

## DISEASES OF THE MIDDLE EAR

### Traumatic Rupture of the Tympanic Membrane

Foreign bodies, unskilled instrumentation or syringing, sudden changes in air pressure (from flying, diving or nose-blowing), fractures of the skull base that pass through the petrous temporal bone and electrocution may all result in perforation of the

Table 21.2 Referred ear pain

| Site of referred otalgia | Involved nerve | Possible causes |
| --- | --- | --- |
| Anterior around the tragus and anterior wall of the EAC | Trigeminal nerve (auriculotemporal) | Dental problems Temporomandibular joint problems Trigeminal neuralgia |
| Posterior EAC wall | Vagus nerve (Arnold's nerve) | Acute tonsillitis/ post-tonsillectomy Supraglottic carcinomas |
| Posterosuperior EAC | Facial nerve | Ramsay Hunt syndrome (herpes zoster oticus) |
| Deep-seated otalgia | Glossopharyngeal nerve (Jacobson's plexus) | Oropharyngeal carcinoma Elongated styloid process (Eagle's syndrome) |
| Retroauricular | Cervical C1–C2 | Cervical spondylosis Cervicofacial syndrome |

EAC, external auditory canal.

tympanic membrane, causing pain, deafness, tinnitus, vertigo and blood in the meatus. Many traumatic perforations heal spontaneously within 3 months.

## Infections of the Middle Ear

**Bullous myringitis** is inflammation of the outer epithelial layer of the tympanic membrane caused by the influenza virus or by *Mycoplasma pneumonia*. Otoscopy reveals blood-filled, serous or serosanguinous blisters involving the tympanic membrane.

**Granular myringitis**, which produces granulations on the external surface of the tympanic membrane, can follow manipulations or local trauma (e.g. from cotton buds).

**Acute otitis media** is a viral or bacterial infection of the mucosal lining of the middle ear and the mastoid air cell system. It presents with severe earache, hearing loss, discharge and tinnitus. General symptoms include fever, irritability and nocturnal agitation. Otoscopy reveals a red, lustreless, bulging drum (Figure 21.10).

In infants, acute suppurative otitis media is a common cause of pyrexia and meningeal irritation. The natural history is of spontaneous recovery. If untreated, the drum may perforate. There may be marginal or central perforations that may heal or persist to cause hearing loss. Scarring of the tympanic membrane (tympanosclerosis) and adhesions between the ossicles (adhesive otitis) following infection may also result in conductive deafness.

**Acute mastoiditis** may follow inflammation of the mastoid air cell system, with purulent effusion, demineralization of the bony cellular walls and necrosis of the bone (coalescent mastoiditis). Clinically, there is inflammation over the mastoid region (Figure 21.11) and a more pronounced systemic response to infection.

Rarely, the infection may spread to the apex of the temporal bone (petroapicitis), causing abducens nerve palsy and trigeminal neuralgia of the first and second branches of the nerve. This triad of abducens palsy, retrobulbar pain and suppurative otorrhoea constitutes **Gradenigo's syndrome**, which, together with radiographic evidence of an abscess in the petrous temporal bone,

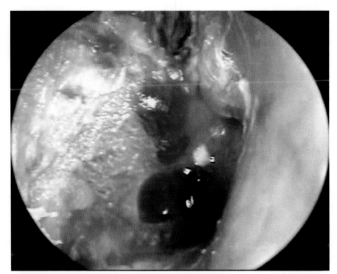

Figure 21.10 Acute suppurative otitis media of the left ear.

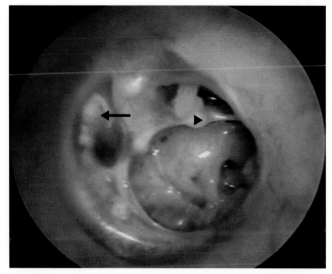

Figure 21.12 Chronic suppurative otitis media with a large central perforation of the left tympanic membrane. The arrowhead points to the head of the stapes, and the arrow points to tympanosclerosis on the remnant drum.

Otitis media is often asymptomatic and detected during screening. Clinically, it presents with a feeling of pressure with occasional earache, hearing loss, tinnitus and developmental or behavioural problems, such as a delayed development of language. Otoscopy reveals a dull, relatively immobile tympanic membrane, and a fluid level is sometimes visible.

The term 'chronic suppurative otitis media' covers two unrelated conditions with markedly different outcomes. The first form is **tubotympanic disease**, in which there is chronic inflammation of the middle ear mucosa characterized by long-standing central perforation of the tympanic membrane (**Figure 21.12**). Repeated reinfection may occur via the perforation or due to an upper respiratory tract source. Sequelae include ossicular resorption, fixation, tympanosclerosis and conductive or mixed hearing loss.

The second form is **atticoantral disease**, characterized by the presence of a cholesteatoma, that is, keratinizing stratified squamous epithelium within the middle ear cleft, which appears as white flakes (**Figure 21.13**). The exact aetiology is unknown but it may arise as a retraction pocket of the tympanic membrane, perhaps drawn inwards by negative pressure due to a blocked Eustachian tube. Retractions are usually located in the pars flaccida or in the posterosuperior region of the pars tensa of the eardrum (**Figure 21.14**).

A cholesteatoma is locally destructive and can cause the destruction of any of the structures within the temporal bone, leading to serious consequences. Patients present with a foul-smelling discharge, bleeding and hearing loss. Earache in chronic otitis media is alarming and may indicate an impending intracranial complication.

## Complications of Otitis Media

These occur in association with cholesteatoma and less frequently with chronic otitis media without cholesteatoma (Table 21.3).

Infection spreading through the temporal bone may manifest itself externally as a **subperiosteal abscesses**. These are usually postauricular (mastoid abscesses) or preauricular (zygomatic abscesses), lie in the substance of the sternocleidomastoid muscle (von Bezold's abscess), lie along the posterior belly of the digastric

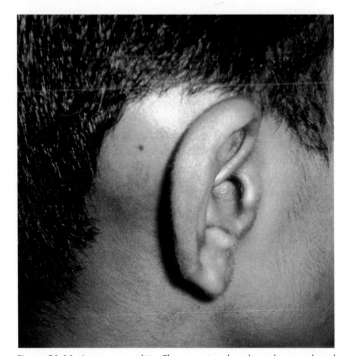

Figure 21.11 Acute mastoiditis. The associated oedema has produced a 'bat ear' appearance.

is diagnostic of petrositis. Other complications include acute labyrinthitis (deafness and vertigo), facial palsy, sigmoid sinus thrombosis, meningitis and subdural/epidural abscess.

**Recurrent otitis media** may indicate a nidus of infection elsewhere, such as sinusitis, or it may occur in immunodeficiency. Some recurrent cases show a persisting effusion in the middle ear between attacks.

**Otitis media with effusion** (serous or secretory otitis media or glue ear) is an accumulation of non-purulent fluid within the middle ear cavity, usually accompanied by Eustachian tube dysfunction. It is commonly seen in children, in whom it usually occurs secondary to recurrent adenoidal infection. Other aetiologies include recurrent upper respiratory tract infection, nasopharyngeal pathologies, allergy, cleft palate, radiation in the area of the ear/nasopharynx, barotrauma and environmental smoking.

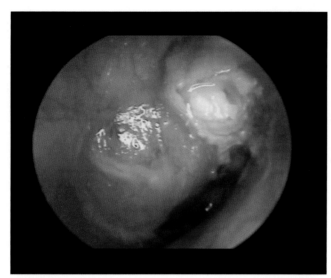

Figure 21.13 Chronic suppurative otitis media with a cholesteatoma in the pars flaccida.

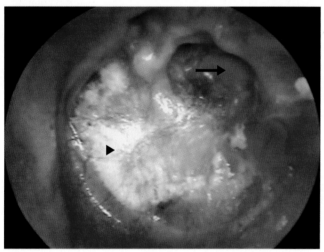

Figure 21.14 Chronic suppurative otitis media with a posterosuperior retraction pocket (arrow) and tympanosclerosis (arrowhead).

muscle (Citelli's abscess) or break through the deep part of bony meatus (Luc's abscess).

**Intracranial infection** may result from a direct spread from temporal bone osteomyelitis, by retrograde thrombophlebitis via small veins from the brain substance that communicate with the Haversian canals, through the various foramina or via old basilar fractures. Outcomes include extradural or epidural abscess, meningitis, subdural abscess, lateral sinus thrombophlebitis, brain abscess and otitic hydrocephalus.

Ear and sinus infections account for half of all **brain abscesses**, most of these being otogenic. Brain abscesses arising from middle ear infection may be in either the ipsilateral temporal lobe or the ipsilateral cerebellar hemisphere. Symptoms may be acute or insidious, with systemic evidence of sepsis, raised intracranial pressure and focal signs specific to the region involved. In the case of the temporal lobe, this may take the form of temporal lobe epilepsy, nominal aphasia and upper quadrantic

Table 21.3 Complications of otitis media

| Mastoid infection | Extracranial complications | Intracranial |
|---|---|---|
| Mastoiditis | Petrositis | Extradural abscess |
| Mastoid abscesses | Facial nerve palsy | Subdural abscess |
| Subperiosteal abscess | Labyrinthitis | Meningitis |
| Bezold's abscess | | Brain abscess |
| Zygomatic abscess | | Sigmoid sinus thrombophlebitis |
| Luc's abscess | | Otitic hydrocephalus |
| Citelli's abscess | | |

hemianopia for the opposite field of vision. Cerebellar abscesses may cause vertigo, nystagmus and balance problems.

## Otosclerosis

This hereditary condition causes conductive deafness in the young adult, with a normal eardrum on otoscopy. It results from new spongy bone formation in the region of the stapes footplate, which limits its mobility. Inheritance is as an autosomal dominant condition with incomplete penetrance, about 50 per cent of affected patients having a family history. Pregnancy may promote its development, more females being affected than males. There is an association with osteogenesis imperfecta as **van der Hoeven's syndrome**.

## Tumours Involving the Middle Ear

**Paragangliomas** are rare, benign tumors arising from nonchromaffin paraganglionic tissue in the head and neck. In the temporal bone, these may be in the middle ear (glomus tympanicum), in the jugular bulb (glomus jugulare) or with the vagus nerve (glomus vagale). They classically cause pulsatile tinnitus and sensorineural deafness. Palsies of the facial, glossopharyngeal and hypoglossal nerves may occur. Otoscopy may reveal a pulsatile mass behind the tympanic membrane – the **rising sun sign** (Figure 21.15) – and there may be an audible bruit over the temporal bone.

**Squamous cell carcinomas** arising primarily from the middle ear are rare and have a presentation similar to that of the external ear, as described above.

## DISEASES OF THE INNER EAR AND VESTIBULOCOCHLEAR NERVE

## Conditions Causing Sensorineural Deafness or Vertigo

A range of conditions may lead to sensorineural deafness or vertigo.

### Presbyacusis

This term describes age-related hearing loss. It is a progressive, sensorineural hearing loss that is bilateral and symmetrical, and

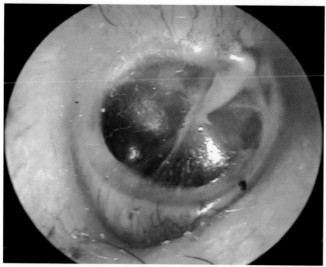

Figure 21.15 Glomus tympanicum of right middle ear seen behind an intact tympanic membrane (the 'rising sun' sign).

affects the higher frequencies. Speech discrimination is reduced, mainly in ambient noise. Tinnitus is common.

## Ototoxic Drugs

Ototoxic drugs, such as aminoglycosides, high-dose salicylates, loop diuretics, quinines and certain chemotherapeutic agents may produce tinnitus, sensorineural deafness and vertigo. Some, such as streptomycin, selectively affect the vestibular system, whereas others, such as gentamicin, affect both the cochlear and vestibular systems.

## Noise-induced Hearing Loss

Hearing loss may result from exposure to a sudden, severe noise or from prolonged exposure, such as industrial exposure. Patients can recover if the damage is not too severe.

## Ménière's Disease

This is a condition of unknown aetiology characterized by recurrent attacks of fluctuating low-frequency sensorineural hearing loss, vertigo, tinnitus and aural fullness. It affects more females than males and is generally unilateral. An accumulation of endolymphatic fluid is thought to result in rupture of the inner ear membrane with subsequent mixing of the endolymph and perilymph. This disturbance of electrolyte balance gives rise to vestibulocochlear failure.

## Labyrinthitis

Labyrinthitis is an acute or chronic, serous or purulent inflammation of the labyrinth that is caused by bacteria, viruses, spirochaetes or fungi. Complications include meningitis, encephalitis, brain abscess and complete deafness.

## Trauma

Sensorineural hearing loss may also occur as a result of **transverse basal skull fractures** causing damage to the inner ear.

**Barotrauma** refers to damage caused by sudden pressure changes as in unpressurized flying or diving. It may cause rupture of the inner ear membranes with the formation of an endolymph fistula. Patients present with sensorineural deafness, vertigo and tinnitus. There may be a **positive fistula test**, in which raising and lowering the external ear pressure by a Seigel's speculum or manual pumping action on the tragus induces nystagmus and vertigo.

## Viral Infections

Viral infections can be related to sudden sensorineural hearing loss. They may also give rise to acute vestibular failure or **vestibular neuronitis** characterized by sudden severe vertigo that resolves spontaneously over a few days. **AIDS** may be associated with auditory nerve neuropathy and a resultant hearing loss.

## Acoustic Neuroma

An acoustic neuroma is a slowly growing, benign tumour arising from the Schwann cells of the vestibular nerve within the internal auditory canal. It presents with hearing loss, tinnitus and vertigo. Neuromas are either sporadic (95 per cent) or part of the familial disorder neurofibromatosis type 2 (5 per cent), in which case they are usually bilateral. The trigeminal nerve may become involved, causing pain or numbness in any nerve division and loss of the corneal reflex. The tumour may compress the fourth ventricle, causing headache due to rising intracranial pressure. Cerebellar symptoms, diplopia and facial palsy may also develop later.

---

### Key Points

- Congenital malformations of the ear are present at birth. Hearing assessment and rehabilitation should be prioritized to avoid the sequelae of auditory deprivation.
- Malignant otitis externa is an important cause of otalgia in immunocompromised individuals, and a high index of suspicion should be borne in mind to allow for early diagnosis and treatment.
- Cholesteatoma is a form of chronic suppurative otitis media with serious consequences. A thorough examination supplemented with imaging gives important information regarding the extent of the disease and the presence of any intracranial complications.
- Unilateral sensorineural hearing loss should be investigated further with MRI to rule out retrocochlear pathology such as an acoustic neuroma.

## QUESTIONS

### SBAs

**1. Gradenigo's triad consists of all of the following except which one?:**
   **a** Abducens palsy
   **b** Retrobulbar pain
   **c** Facial palsy
   **d** Suppurative otorrhoea

**Answer**

**c** *Facial palsy. Gradenigo's triad is diagnostic of petrositis in which the facial nerve is not affected.*

**2. All of the following are causes of sensorineural hearing loss except which one?:**
   **a** Acoustic neuroma
   **b** Ménière's disease
   **c** Early otosclerosis
   **d** Noise-induced hearing loss

**Answer**

**c** *Early otosclerosis. Early otosclerosis will show conductive hearing loss, but advanced otosclerosis will have a mixed hearing loss.*

**3. Pain referred to the posterior wall of external auditory canal can be due to which one of the following?:**
   **a** Supraglottic malignancy
   **b** Elongated styloid process
   **c** Dental caries
   **d** Temporomandibular joint arthritis

**Answer**

**a** *Supraglottic malignancy. The pathway of referred pain in supraglottic malignancy is via the vagus nerve (pharyngeal plexus) and radiates to the posterior canal wall, which it supplies (Arnold's nerve).*

### EMQ

**1. For each of the following cases, select the most likely diagnosis from the list below. Each option may be used once, more than once or not at all:**
   **1** Acute otitis media
   **2** Chronic suppurative otitis media – tubotympanic
   **3** Chronic suppurative otitis media – atticoantral
   **4** Malignant otitis externa
   **5** Temporal bone malignancy
   **6** Paraganglioma
   **7** Ménière's disease
   **a** An elderly diabetic man presents with severe and persistent otalgia. Otoscopic examination demonstrates foul-smelling, purulent otorrhoea and a mass lesion of the external ear canal. Biopsy of the mass demonstrates granulation tissue. What is the most likely cause?
   **b** A 56-year-old woman presents with tinnitus of 1 year's duration with decreased hearing in the right ear. On enquiry, this is found to be pulsatile in nature, and there is no giddiness. On otoscopy, there is a reddish mass behind the intact drum. A pure tone audiogram shows right-sided mild conductive hearing loss. What is the most likely diagnosis?

**Answers**

**a** *4 Malignant otitis externa. This condition tends to occur in elderly or immunocompromised individuals. A typical presentation is of severe otalgia and otorrhoea. Facial nerve and other lower cranial nerve palsies may be present. Biopsy, which is mandatory to rule out malignancy, typically shows just granulation tissue.*

**b** *6 Paraganglioma. Paragangliomas of the jugular foramen – glomus jugulare tumours – typically present with pulsatile tinnitus and mild conductive hearing loss in the early stages. The presence of a mass behind the intact tympanic membrane confirms the diagnosis clinically.*

# The Orbit

Mandar S. Deshpande and Parul M. Deshpande

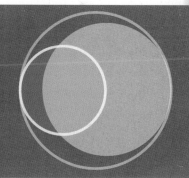

## LEARNING OBJECTIVES

- Although most eye conditions are the province of the ophthalmic surgeon, it is essential that all clinicians recognize that visual loss, ocular pain and red eye require urgent diagnosis and management

## PERIORBITAL DISEASES

### Dermoid Cysts

These are benign teratomas that present as a solid painless mass and represent 3–9 per cent of all orbital tumours. They result from an inclusion of ectodermal elements during closure of the neural tube adjacent to the fetal suture lines.

The cyst wall is lined by cutaneous epithelium that rests on dermal tissues containing skin appendages. It may have pedicular attachments to the periorbita that may cause hollowing of underlying bone.

The cysts are usually found near the lateral canthus at the temporofrontozygomatic suture above the superior orbital margin (**external angular dermoid**). The outer part of the eyebrow overlies the cyst, differentiating it from a swelling of the lacrimal gland, which causes fullness in the upper lid below the eyebrow. The second most common site is the superomedial orbital rim (**internal angular dermoid**). The cyst is initially small and enlarges with age.

**Deep orbital dermoid cysts** usually present in teens or adults with proptosis. Inflammation can occur due to cyst leakage or rupture, resulting in pain and discoloration. Goldenhar's syndrome is a condition with multiple dermoid (eye and ear) and lid defects (Figure 22.1).

### Venous Malformations

#### Superficial Capillary Haemangiomas

The lesions are usually seen as red or bluish purple lesions or swellings of the eyelids at birth or within a few months afterwards. They initially increase in size but are known to undergo spontaneous resolution by the age of 7–8 years. Treatment is indicated only if the lesions are large or involve the upper lid, causing amblyopia, ulceration or severe disfigurement.

Capillary haemangiomas are more frequent in premature or low-birth-weight infants. There is an approximately 10-fold

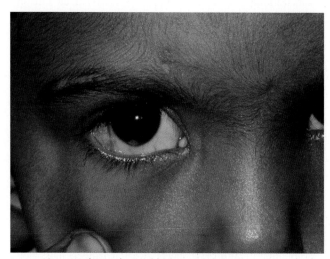

Figure 22.1 Lipodermoid in Goldenhar's syndrome.

increase in infants born to women who have undergone chorionic villus sampling during pregnancy.

#### Sturge–Weber Syndrome

Sturge–Weber syndrome is a hamartomatous malformation affecting the central nervous system (CNS), skin and eye, usually in a unilateral distribution. It is characterized mainly by a unilateral naevus flammeus or a port wine stain around the eye with glaucoma, ipsilateral leptomeningeal angiomatosis and possible brain vascular malformations.

### Preseptal Cellulitis and Orbital Cellulitis

These can result from the spread of infection from the lids, frontal and ethmoidal sinuses or lacrimal glands. The ethmoidal sinus is commonly implicated as it is separated from the orbital contents by the thin lamina papyracea.

Clinically, it presents with a painful inflammatory oedema of the lids and periorbital tissues (preseptal cellulitis) (**Figure 22.2**), protrusion of the globe (orbital cellulitis) and a purulent conjunctival discharge. In neglected cases, there is a high risk of optic nerve damage, meningitis and cavernous sinus thrombosis.

## Dacryocystitis

Dacryocystitis is inflammation of the lacrimal sac and can present as *acute dacryocystitis* with sudden painful swelling of the lacrimal sac (limited to below the inner canthus) and discharge into the conjunctival cul de sac. Untreated cases may result in spread to the preseptal region or orbit, resulting in orbital cellulitis.

*Chronic dacryocystitis* presents with persistent watering and mucoid discharge in the affected eye with a chronic mucocele (a cystic mass along the side of the nose below the inner canthus), which with pressure results in a regurgitation of the mucoid discharge through the punctum into the conjunctival fornix. This needs to be differentiated from a lacrimal sac tumour.

## Lacrimal Sac Tumours

Lacrimal sac tumours are malignant tumours, in which the obstruction lies proximal instead of distal to the sac, as seen on nasolacrimal sac syringing and probing. The sac is usually hard, becomes irregularly enlarged over months to years and may be attached to the surrounding tissues. They are relatively rare and usually occur in midlife.

Mixed tumours are the most common, but adenoid cystic carcinomas, lymphomas and lymphosarcomas also occur. Involvement of the gland in lymphoma is usually associated with widespread reticulosis. Other differential diagnoses are tumours of the frontal or ethmoid sinuses, which can destroy the orbital wall and present with a hard, non-tender swelling that extends above the medial canthus.

## THE EYELIDS

## Inflammations

An **external hordeolum** (stye) is an infection of the glands of Zeis, clinically appearing as a sudden painful swelling at the lid margin that may rupture. Recurrent styes may indicate the presence of underlying blepharitis, uncontrolled diabetes or a refractive error.

**Meibomian gland cysts** appear as a soft painless mass along the lids (along the tarsal plate), resulting from obstruction of the Meibomian gland ducts (**Figure 22.3**). An **internal hordeolum** usually presents as a painful, localized lid swelling due to infection within a Meibomian gland cyst.

**Molluscum contagiosum** appears as multiple umbilicated, translucent, vesicular swellings along the lid margin. Similar swellings may appear on the face or body. They may cause recurrent red eyes (blepharoconjunctivitis).

**Blepharitis** is inflammation of the anterior lid margin. Sebaceous blepharitis presents as greasy scales at the base of eyelashes. Staphylococcal blepharitis appears as matted lashes with a haemorrhagic crust at the base of the lashes and lid margin ulceration.

**Meibomian gland disease** is inflammation of the posterior lid margins (**Figure 22.4**). The lid margins show occluded gland openings with turbid or thick white secretions, or even cysts at the mouth of the ducts.

**Canaliculitis** is inflammation of the vertical or horizontal canalculus that appears as a painful red swelling along the inner canthus with a mucopurulent discharge in the conjunctival cul de sac.

**Ptosis** is unilateral or bilateral drooping of the upper lids. A common cause is congenital ptosis, which is associated with lid lag on vertical eye movements (looking down) due to a dystrophic levator palpebral superioris muscle in children (**Figure 22.5**). Myogenic ptosis is seen in patients with myasthenia gravis or myotonic dystrophies. Traumatic or neurogenic ptosis is seen in cases of IIIrd cranial nerve palsy along with other extraocular

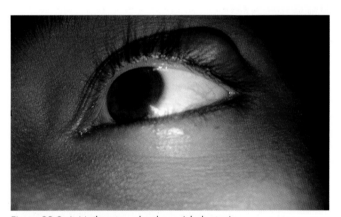

Figure 22.3 A Meibomian gland cyst (chalazion).

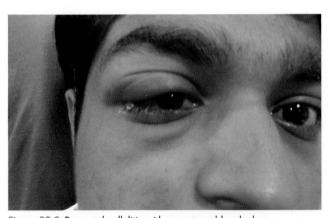

Figure 22.2 Preseptal cellulitis with an external hordeolum.

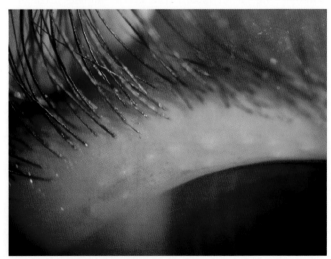

Figure 22.4 Meibomian gland disease of the posterior lid margin.

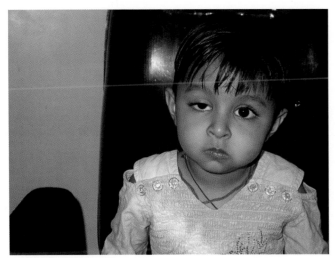

Figure 22.5 Congenital ptosis.

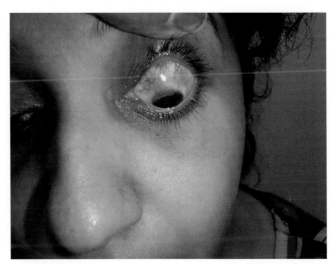

Figure 22.6 Sclerokeratitis.

muscle limitations. Aponeurotic ptosis is usually unilateral or bilateral, and is seen in elderly individuals due to disinsertion of the levator palpebrae superioris complex.

## Miscellaneous Facial Palsies

Palsies can occur following middle ear disease, such as Bell's palsy, or after parotid gland surgery or disease. There is lagophthalmos with incomplete closure of the eye on blinking on the affected side.

## THE EYE

### Red Eyes

Red eyes can occur with or without visual loss.

#### Red Eyes without Visual Loss

**Conjunctivitis** can occur following bacterial, viral or parasitic infections:

- *Bacterial conjunctivitis* presents with acute redness and mucopurulent discharge with conjunctival chemosis.
- *Adenoviral conjunctivitis* results in redness, a mucoid discharge and conjunctival chemosis with a follicular reaction. Pseudomembrane formations with preauricular lymphadenopathy may occur.
- Parasitic-like *microsporidial conjunctivitis* is either sporadic or epidemic and usually presents with unilateral follicular keratoconjunctivitis that may mimic viral conjunctivitis.
- *Neonatal conjunctivitis* can occur secondary to infections with herpes simplex, *Neisseria gonorrhoeae* or *Chlamydia trachomatis*.

**Subconjunctival haemorrhage** results in localized redness of the affected eye. It can occur secondary to trauma or in patients with hypertension or atherosclerosis.

#### Red Eyes with Visual Loss

**Keratitis** is inflammatory necrosis of the cornea that can be bacterial, viral, fungal or parasitic. It appears as dry or wet yellow-white, central or peripheral infiltrates with surrounding corneal oedema and a hypopyon (leukocytic exudate) in the anterior chamber (**Figure 22.6**). It commonly occurs with exposure keratopathy in intensive care units or following trauma.

With viral keratitis, herpes simplex keratitis shows classical dendritic epithelial lesions, while herpes zoster keratitis results in pseudo-dendrites or mucous plugs and stromal keratitis.

Inflammation of the iris is termed **iritis**, and inflammation of both the iris and ciliary body is termed **iridocyclitis**. This presents as a painful red eye with a diminution of vision and intolerance of light (photophobia). There is circumciliary congestion with a flare and cells in the anterior chamber. The pupil is small and miotic, with a sluggish reaction to light. Iridocyclitis is usually idiopathic but may be associated with autoimmune diseases such as collagen vascular disorders (rheumatoid arthritis, ankylosing spondylitis and Wegener's granulomatosis) or chronic infections like tuberculosis or sarcoidosis.

**Episcleritis** and **scleritis** are inflammation of the episclera and sclera, respectively. They present as a painful, nodular or diffuse congestion of the sclera under the bulbar conjunctiva. The causes are similar to those of iridocyclitis.

**Acute congestive glaucoma** is described with glaucoma (see below).

**Endophthalmitis** or **panophthalmitis** is inflammation of the vitreous cavity of the eye (endophthalmitis) or may even involve the outer coats of the eye and periocular tissues (panophthalmitis). It occurs following intraocular surgery or trauma (**Figure 22.7**).

Other causes of a red eye with visual loss are **trauma** and a **foreign body** (**Figure 22.8**).

### Acute Visual Loss Without Red Eyes

The causes of acute visual loss without red eyes are:

- retinal detachment;
- optic neuritis;
- anterior ischaemic optic neuropathy;
- central retinal artery occlusion;
- central retinal vein occlusion;
- branch retinal vein occlusion;
- subluxation or dislocation of the lens.

### Glaucoma

Glaucoma refers to a group of eye diseases characterized by damage to the optic nerve usually due to an excessively high

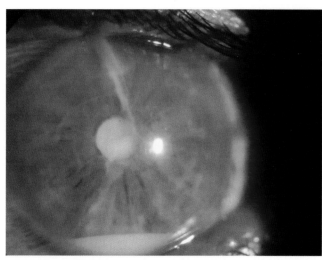

Figure 22.7 Endophthalmitis with a corneal tear.

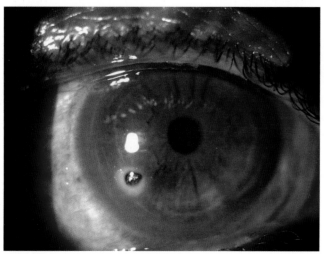

Figure 22.8 A corneal foreign body.

intraocular pressure. It may, however, also be associated with a normal or low pressure.

## Primary Glaucoma

Glaucoma is one of the most common causes of vision loss worldwide.

**Open-angle glaucoma** is usually seen in adults above the age of 40 years. Predisposing factors include a family history of glaucoma, hypertension or diabetes. It is usually asymptomatic in the initial stages and progresses to loss of vision in the later stages. Patients frequently present with headaches or frequent change of prescriptions for spectacles.

The intraocular pressure is high. The optic disc shows progressively increased cupping in its initial stage that can only be picked up on routine ophthalmic examination. It is therefore recommended that individuals with no apparent risk of glaucoma undergo a routine check-up every 5 years, and those who are at risk have a check-up every year. Findings include arcuate (Bjerrum's) or comma-shaped (Seidel's) scotomas on automated visual field testing.

**Angle-closure glaucoma**, commonly known as acute congestive glaucoma, usually presents in elderly hyperopic individuals with a shallow anterior chamber or occludable angles. It manifests as sudden-onset redness, severe headache with nausea and vomiting, pain in the eyes and a reduction in vision. The cornea is oedematous with a semi-dilated fixed pupil resulting from ischaemia or paralysis of the papillary sphincter. It is usually preceded by episodes of coloured haloes or transient diminution of vision, due to temporary closure of the anterior chamber angles.

**Congenital glaucoma** usually manifests at or immediately after birth with enlargement of the eye, especially the cornea (buphthalmos), and a cloudy cornea in persistent untreated cases.

### Secondary Glaucoma

Angle recession (post-traumatic) glaucoma usually occurs after direct trauma to the eye. It can present in the acute stage or even months after the initial trauma.

Drugs such as steroids (local or oral) and oral topiramate can induce open or acute glaucomatous episodes, respectively.

## The Lens

A **cataract** is clouding or opacification of the lens due to ageing, trauma or diseases such as uncontrolled diabetes and hyperparathyroidism.

**Subluxation and dislocations of the lens** is the partial or complete displacement of the natural lens. It occurs following trauma or with Marfan's syndrome or homocystinuria; alternatively, it may be associated with ectopia pupillae. It results in diminution of vision.

## The Retina

Systemic diseases such as diabetes and hypertension cause retinovasculopathy, resulting in the appearance of haemorrhages and exudates on the central part of retina.

**Central retinal artery occlusion** is an acute emergency with a sudden loss of vision in one eye. There is usually only light perception with an absent or sluggish direct pupillary reaction. A retinal examination shows a pale retina with a bright red macula, giving the appearance of a cherry red spot. This is sometimes preceded by transient attacks of vision loss. It is usually seen in atherosclerosis or trauma.

**Retinoblastoma** is described on p. 359.

## Strabismus

The ocular movements are usually well coordinated, keeping the eyes aligned. Any deviation from the primary gaze is termed strabismus. The eye may turn inwards (esotropia) or outwards (exotropia).

A **concomitant or non-paralytic** squint is one in which the angle of deviation does not change irrespective of the fixation taken by a normal or squinting eye, and is the same in any direction of gaze. It may be congenital or acquired at a later age. There are various causes of concomitant squint, including hereditary, ametropic, anisometropic and amblyopic.

In **non-comitant or paralytic squint**, the angle of the squint is variable, depending on which eye takes up fixation (the angle of squint being larger when the paralytic eye is fixating than when the normal eye is fixating) and which direction the patient is looking in (Figure 22.9).

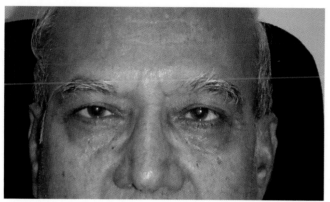

Figure 22.9 A paralytic squint.

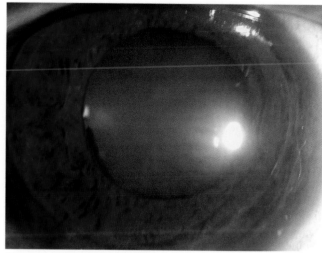

Figure 22.10 Traumatic mydriasis.

It occurs following a IIIrd, IVth and VIth cranial nerve palsy or may be congenital. Duane's syndrome is a restrictive type of non-comitant squint in which there is congenital fibrosis of the lateral rectus muscle. A IIIrd nerve palsy results in a restriction of all movements except those of the lateral rectus and superior oblique muscles. A IVth nerve palsy results in a restriction of the superior oblique muscle. A VIth nerve palsy results in an abduction deficit. Head injury, thyroid gland disease and myasthenia gravis are among the common causes of a paralytic squint.

## The Pupil
### Neurological causes

Abnormal pupillary responses may be a sign of a central nervous system disease but may also result from disease of the optic and oculomotor nerves, and from the effects of disease and drugs on the eye itself.

An **Argyll Robertson pupil** is a small pupil that is non-reactive to light but reacts to convergence. It shows a poor response to mydriatic drugs. It is commonly seen in neurosyphilis, trauma affecting the Edinger–Westphal nucleus or aneurysms compressing the IIIrd cranial nerve.

A **Holmes–Adie pupil** is a large pupil that has a poor or abnormal reaction to light or near reflex but may slowly dilate in a darkened room or with mydriatics. The cause is unknown but it results from myotonia, occurring in association with depressed tendon reflexes and anhidrosis of the limbs.

**Horner's syndrome** results from damage to the cervical sympathetic chain. It is characterized by ipsilateral miosis (pupillary constriction), ptosis (drooping of the eyelid), vasodilatation (flushing of the face, with increased temperature) and anhidrosis of the face, all occurring on the same side as the underlying lesion.

Horner's syndrome can be congenital, may occur secondary to birth trauma or can result from preganglionic lesions (a Pancoast tumour of the lungs or thyroid disease). Eye signs may occur in isolation with interruption of the intracranial sympathetic plexus around the carotid artery. The combination of Horner's syndrome and loss of the first division of the trigeminal nerve – Raeder's syndrome – may result from invasion of a tumour at the skull base.

Acute intracranial haematomas may compress the ipsilateral oculomotor nerve against the edge of the tentorium, resulting in dilatation of the ipsilateral pupil – **Hutchinson's pupil**. The pupil is poorly reactive in both the direct (light in the affected eye) and consensual (light in the other eye) light reflexes. Coning of the brain results in bilateral pupillary dilatation.

A **Marcus Gunn pupil** has a relative afferent pupillary defect, that is, an absent direct pupillary reflex but a good consensual reflex on the affected side. The unaffected eye has a diminished response to stimulation of the affected eye by light. It is usually seen in optic nerve diseases.

**Optic tract disease** usually does not affect the resting pupillary size but results in absent pupillary reflexes on the side opposite to the lesion when either eye is stimulated by light (**Behr's phenomenon**, which occurs when the anterior two-thirds of the optic tract is involved).

**IIIrd cranial nerve paresis** (which can involve or spare the pupil, differentiating ischaemic from non-ischaemic causes) gives rise to a dilated pupil that is unreactive to light stimulation of either eye, along with a divergent paralytic squint.

### Non-neurological causes

Abnormalities of the shape of the pupil may result from colobomas – congenital notching of the iris – or be secondary to globe injury or glaucoma.

**Traumatic mydriasis** may result in a dilated pupil that is unreactive to light shone in either the affected or the unaffected eye following trauma to the globe (**Figure 22.10**).

**Drug-induced pupillary constriction** occurs with miotic eye drops, such as pilocarpine, and opiates. Drug-induced pupillary dilatation occurs with anticholinergic drugs, including mydriatic eye drops, such as atropine, and cocaine.

## Nystagmus

Nystagmus is rhythmic, involuntary oscillations of the eye and may be congenital, voluntary or physiological. As a localizing sign, it is most often described in relation to vestibular and cerebellopontine angle disease.

Eye movements are controlled by the paired vestibular nuclei. Each nucleus drives the eye towards the opposite side, and hence the opposing forces keep the eyes in a stable position. If a pathological process affects one side, the other nucleus drives the eye slowly to the opposite side (the slow phase of nystagmus). This is then rapidly corrected (the fast phase of nystagmus). The direction of the nystagmus is defined by the fast phase.

Horizontal nystagmus results from disease processes affecting the vestibulocochlear system. The fast phase is towards the healthy side. The nystagmus is accentuated by deviating the eyes in the direction of the fast phase (Alexander's law).

In vertical nystagmus, the abnormal movements occur in the vertical plane. In fourth ventricle lesions, the nystagmus is characteristically described as upbeat (with the fast phase upwards), while in cervicomedullary junction lesions resulting in tonsillar herniation, the nystagmus is downbeat (with the fast phase downwards).

Tumours of the cerebellopontine angle initially result in vestibular horizontal nystagmus in which the fast phase is away from the tumour. In the later stages, however, the fast phase is directed towards the lesion and is evoked by turning the gaze in that direction.

Drugs such as lithium, anticonvulsants and sedatives are known to induce nystagmus.

## TRAUMA

### Orbit

Orbital fractures are most commonly blow-out fractures, occurring after a fist blow or an injury involving a ball. Fractures of the inferior and medial wall (through the lamina papyracea) are common. Most orbital floor fractures occur medial to the infraorbital canal, anterior to the inferior orbital fissure where the orbital floor is relatively weak. Other sites of fractures are the roof of the orbit or posterolaterally through the greater wing of the sphenoid. Periorbital fat and the inferior rectus and inferior oblique muscles may become trapped in the maxillary antrum through the fracture site.

The patient may present in the acute phase with lid crepitus after nose-blowing, soft tissue entrapment being suggested by severe pain or headache with vomiting. The presence of enophthalmos (Figure 22.11) or binocular diplopia on a vertical upward gaze indicates soft tissue or muscle entrapment and a need for surgical correction. Coronal CT scans are important in determining the extent and site of the fracture and the degree of soft tissue involvement. Acute optic nerve compression, causing traumatic optic neuropathy, can occur in compound fractures involving the optic nerve foramen.

### Depressed Fractures of the Zygomatic Bone

These fractures result from a direct blow to the zygoma. Fracture separations occur at the infraorbital rim, the zygomaticofrontal suture and the zygomatic arch. The wall of the related maxillary sinus may be shattered. There may be unilateral epistaxis from tearing of the mucous membrane of the maxillary sinus, a black eye with subconjunctival haemorrhage from the orbital floor injury and flattening of the contour of the cheek, which may be masked by oedema.

Additional physical signs can assist in the clinical diagnosis. The fracture may be palpable as a notch or irregularity of the lateral orbital margin at the zygomatic suture line, or tenderness may be noted at this point. If the fracture extends through the orbital floor across the path of the infraorbital foramen, there may be anaesthesia or hyperaesthesia over the lower eyelid resulting from infraorbital nerve injury. These sensory changes may be temporary in the case of a neuropraxia or permanent if there is complete shearing of the nerve.

There may also be diplopia from entrapment or displacement of the attachments of the extraocular muscles and the lateral attachment of the suspensory ligament of the eyeball to the zygoma. Air may enter the overlying tissues from the maxillary sinus, resulting in surgical emphysema.

Zygomatic fractures are not always easily seen on radiography, but if the orbital floor is involved, blood may obliterate the normal radiolucency of the maxillary sinus. This is particularly evident on an occipitomental view (a Waters' projection).

### Lid Injury

Although usually insignificant, lid injury can sometimes be critical. It usually occurs after trauma from a sharp or blunt object, from a fall or following a fight. A full-thickness tear of the lid needs suturing in layers with meticulous approximation of the lid margin.

Injury to the medial third of the eyelid may be associated with a canalicular tear and demand recanalization during repair. Lid ecchymosis is seen commonly following head injury due to gravitation of blood into the soft tissue.

### Globe Injury

Subconjunctival haemorrhage results in localized redness of the affected eye. It occurs secondary to trauma, or in patients with hypertension or atherosclerosis.

Hyphaema occurs with trauma or rarely in neovascular glaucomas (Figure 22.12). Traumatic hyphaema appears as blood within the anterior chamber. It may be associated with

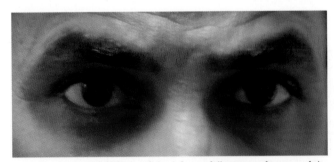

Figure 22.11 Enophthalmos of the left eye following a fracture of the medial orbital wall.

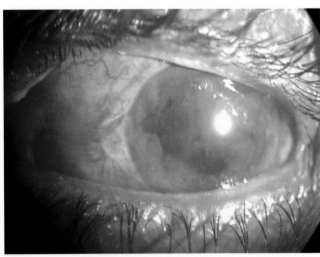

Figure 22.12 Hyphaema (a blood clot in the anterior chamber).

**iridodialysis** (separation of the iris root) (**Figure 22.13**) or **cyclodialysis** (disinsertion of the ciliary body). The intraocular pressure needs to be checked as associated glaucoma can result in permanent staining of the cornea by the blood (**Figure 22.14**) or optic nerve damage resulting in permanent visual loss. It may also be associated with vitreous haemorrhage.

**Retinal detachment** usually presents acutely or subacutely with complaints of a curtain-like shadow in the field of vision. This may be preceded by symptoms such as floaters; flashes of light may indicate a retinal tear secondary to vitreous traction on the retina. Myopia and trauma are common predisposing factors. The treatment is mostly surgical.

**Rupture of the globe** can occur following blunt or penetrating injury. A corneal, corneoscleral or scleral tear can occur leading to collapse of the globe and demanding urgent repair (**Figure 22.15**).

**Traumatic or compressive optic neuropathy** is usually seen with an orbital fracture involving the orbital apex. It presents with an afferent pupillary defect on the side of the injury, with severe visual loss. Immediate treatment can prevent permanent blindness.

## TUMOURS

### Lid Tumours

In Asians populations, basal cell carcinomas (**Figure 22.16**) are the most common tumours (40–60 per cent), followed by sebaceous gland carcinomas (23–30 per cent) and squamous cell carcinomas (10 per cent). In white individuals, the most common tumour is also the basal cell carcinoma (75–90 per cent), and this is followed by the squamous cell carcinoma (8–19 per cent). Sebaceous cell carcinoma (1–3 per cent) is very rare in this group.

**Sebaceous gland carcinoma** is the most common tumour affecting the ocular surface of the eyelid and is more frequent in Asians than white individuals.

**Squamous cell carcinomas** (**Figure 22.17**) most often appear on the lower lids. Risk factors include exposure to ultraviolet light, arsenic, hydrocarbons, radiation and immunosuppressive drugs, albinism, pre-existing chronic skin lesions and genetic skin disorders (e.g. xeroderma pigmentosum and epidermodysplasia verruciformis).

**Sebaceous gland carcinomas** usually affect elderly women and are characterized by a high rate of local recurrence,

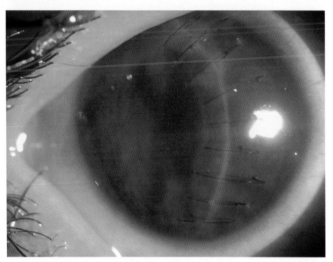

Figure 22.13 Iridodialysis (between the 7 and 10 o'clock positions) and a repaired corneal tear.

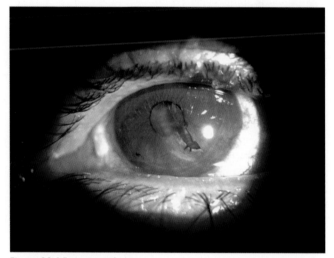

Figure 22.15 A corneal tear.

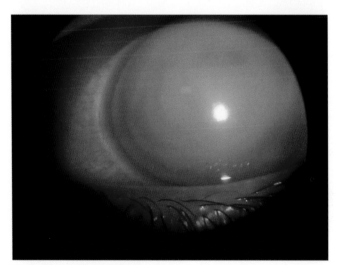

Figure 22.14 Corneal blood staining.

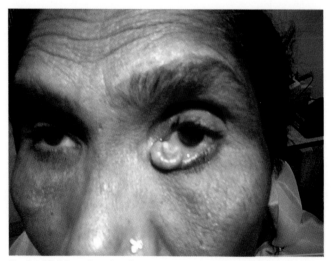

Figure 22.16 A basal cell carcinoma of the medial canthus and lower lid.

PART 4 | HEAD AND NECK

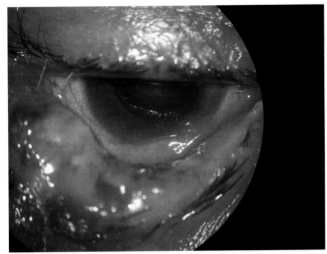

Figure 22.17 A squamous carcinoma of the eyelid and conjunctiva.

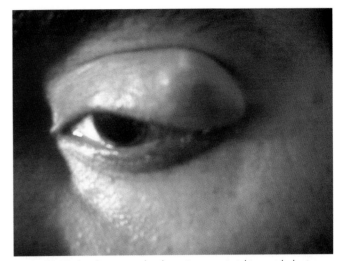

Figure 22.18 A sebaceous gland carcinoma mimicking a chalazion.

with regional and distant metastases. They are two to three times more common in the upper eyelids.

There are two form of sebaceous gland carcinoma:

- In the *nodular* form, the lesion forms a discrete, hard, immobile nodule that is commonly located in the upper tarsal plate. It is yellowish in colour due to its lipid content. Any chalazion of unusual consistency or its recurrence after incision should raise the suspicion of a sebaceous gland carcinoma (**Figure 22.18**).
- *Diffuse* forms may appear slowly as diffuse thickenings of the lid margin and loss of the eyelashes, and are often misdiagnosed as benign blepharoconjunctivitis.

Two important characteristics of both forms of sebaceous gland carcinoma are their multifocal origin (in the Meibomian glands, glands of Zeis or caruncle) and their pagetoid spread. Such spread may involve both palpebral and bulbar conjunctival epithelium. Hence a conjunctival map biopsy is essential in cases of sebaceous gland carcinoma. Muir–Torre syndrome is characterized by squamous differentiation of the tumour, multiple sebaceous adenomas or carcinomas in the skin, and visceral malignancies.

## Conjunctival Tumours

Ocular surface squamous neoplasia (OSSN) may range from conjunctival dysplasia and carcinoma *in situ* to invasive squamous cell carcinoma (**Figures 22.19** and **22.20**). The tumour usually occurs at or near the limbus and may progress to involve the cornea.

Clinically, tumours appear as elevated lesions with a gelatinous, papillary surface. They are locally invasive (of low-grade malignancy) and rarely disseminate to the regional (preauricular) lymph nodes. Impression cytology can be a useful method to diagnose OSSN. Recurrence rates are generally higher for more severe grades of OSSN (invasive squamous cell carcinoma) and are also related to inadequacy of initial excision of the tumour margins. Solar injury is recognized as a major risk factor for conjunctival squamous cell carcinoma, and human papillomavirus infection, especially genotype 16, is also implicated.

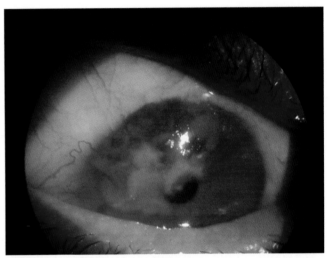

Figure 22.19 A pigmented corneal squamous neoplasia (ocular surface squamous neoplasia).

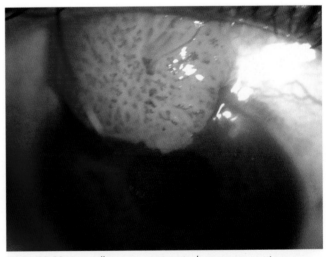

Figure 22.20 A papillomatous conjunctival squamous carcinoma.

## Uveal Tumours

Melanocytic lesions of the conjunctiva and cornea include benign naevi (**Figure 22.21**), primary acquired melanosis (PAM) of the conjunctiva with or without atypia, and malignant melanoma.

**Primary acquired melanosis** is typically characterized by a unilateral, flat, superficial, brown discoloration of the bulbar conjunctiva. It may also involve the fornix or the tarsal conjunctiva. Primary acquired melanosis without atypia is usually benign, but PAM with atypia may show a malignant transformation.

**Malignant melanoma** of the periocular skin or conjunctiva (**Figures 22.22** and **22.23**) may arise *de novo*, from a pre-existing naevus or from PAM with atypia. Its incidence is low, less than 1 per million per year in white populations.

The melanoma typically presents unilaterally and is found at the limbus. Both melanotic (brown, elevated, vascular lesions) and amelanotic variants are known. Prominent blood vessels may be visible. Any change in thickness of a pre-existing PAM or any change in the size, shape, colour or vascularity of a naevus should raise a suspicion of malignant transformation.

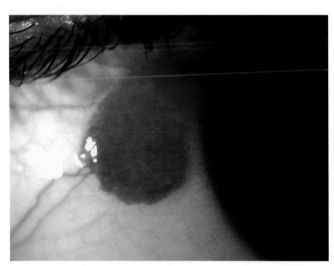

Figure 22.21 A benign conjunctival naevus.

Malignant melanoma carries a 10-year risk of death (with treatment) of up to 30 per cent. Poor prognostic features include a multifocal presentation, recurrent disease, involvement of the caruncle, eyelid margin, tarsal or forniceal conjunctiva, regional and systemic metastases and surgical margins that are positive for invasion by tumour cells. Larger tumours are associated with a higher risk of recurrence and death.

## Retinoblastoma

Retinoblastoma is the most common intraocular tumour affecting the retina that is seen in children. Approximately 95 per cent of cases occur in children younger than 5 years, with a mean age of 18 months.

The tumour may be unilateral or bilateral, and classically presents as a white reflex in the pupil. Fundoscopy shows an elevated white tumour with calcification. More advanced cases present with squint, proptosis and/or a fungating mass. The tumour may spread along the optic nerve to the brain. Distant metastasis is known to occur via haematogenous spread.

Retinoblastomas show four different growth patterns: endophytic (towards the vitreous), exophytic (towards the choroid), mixed exophytic and endophytic (the most common type) and diffuse infiltrating. The condition has a recessive inheritance with a point mutation on chromosome 13. It only occurs in homozygotes. There is also an associated risk of developing second, unrelated malignancies, especially osteogenic sarcoma, in later life.

Treatment is usually chemotherapy combined with laser therapy or enucleation, with a long excision of the optic nerve in advanced stages of disease.

### PROPTOSIS AND EXOPHTHALMOS

Proptosis refers to protrusion of the entire orbital contents (**Figure 22.24**), whereas exophthalmos is a protrusion of the globe alone (seen as lower lid retraction with showing of the inferior sclera). This distinction is, however, rarely made and the terms are often used synonymously. Proptosis is demonstrated

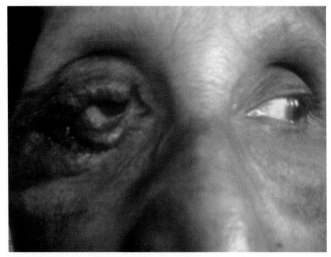

Figure 22.22 A malignant melanoma of the periocular skin.

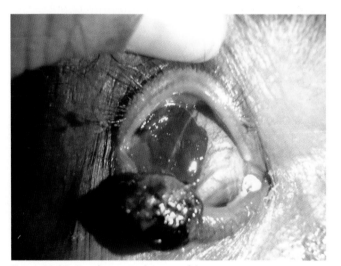

Figure 22.23 A malignant melanoma of the conjunctiva.

by examining the patient from behind while tipping their head backwards. Common causes of proptosis are congenital abnormalities, infection, orbital masses, arteriovenous fistulae and thyrotoxicosis.

**Congenital proptosis** occurs in craniofacial deformities such as Apert's and Crouzon's syndromes.

**Orbital cellulitis** is described in more detail on p. 351.

**Cavernous sinus thrombosis** results from a spread of infection from the face along the angular ophthalmic vein, from the middle ear along the lateral and petrosal venous sinuses, from a peritonsillar abscess via the pterygoid venous plexus, or from orbital cellulitis via the ophthalmic vein. The symptoms progress rapidly from a severe headache and rigors to delirium. Proptosis, conjunctival chemosis (oedema), ophthalmoplegia and a loss of pupillary reactions are found. Blindness and death may ensue.

**Retro-ocular and ocular neoplasms** may displace the globe, causing proptosis, strabismus and diplopia from interference with the extraocular muscles, and decreased visual acuity from optic nerve compression. Primary retro-ocular tumours include haemangiomas, optic nerve gliomas, neurofibromas, meningiomas, lymphomas and osteogenic sarcomas. In addition, dermoid cysts, lacrimal gland tumours (**Figure 22.25**) and swellings of the lacrimal sac may displace the globe. Secondary tumours include direct intraorbital extension of nasopharyngeal malignancies and metastatic deposits from breast and lung carcinomas.

**Orbital cysticercosis** affects the extraocular muscles, leading to painful limitations of ocular movement with isolated redness overlying the affected muscles.

**Malignant melanoma of the choroid** is seen on fundoscopy as a raised brown area near the posterior pole of the fundus. A gradually increasing shadow may be noted in the visual field, but a more rapid deterioration of vision may occur with secondary retinal detachment. Benign choroidal naevi occur as a flat, pigmented areas on the fundus near the posterior pole. There is no field defect, and the lesion is incidentally discovered on fundoscopy.

**Retinoblastomas** also occur and are described on p. 359.

**Carotid cavernous fistulae** (see **Figure 22.26**) arise when an aneurysm of the intracranial carotid artery ruptures into the cavernous sinus. This may occur spontaneously or as a result of trauma. There is a rapid onset of throbbing orbital pain, a buzzing noise in the head and blurred vision. Examination reveals a pulsating proptosis with a loud orbital bruit, the pulsation ceasing when the ipsilateral carotid artery in the neck is occluded. Pulsating proptosis may also be a feature of a highly vascular orbital neoplasm or an aneurysm of the ophthalmic artery.

**Thyroid eye disease**, also known as thyroid ophthalmopathy, Graves' ophthalmopathy or thyroid-related orbitopathy, describes a complex constellation of ophthalmic signs and symptoms that occur with hyperthyroidism. Thyroid disease more commonly affects women than men, with a 4:1 ratio.

Ocular involvement is the most common extrathyroidal manifestation of hyperthyroidism, and is present on clinical examination in 10–45 per cent of patients. Thyroid ophthalmopathy can present with soft tissue involvement, eyelid retraction, proptosis, strabismus (from involvement of the superior rectus, medial rectus and inferior oblique muscles) and optic neuropathy.

Thyroid eye disease can be staged using the 'NOSPECS' classification:

- Stage 0: **N**o eye findings.
- Stage 1: **O**nly lid retraction and stare (with lid lag on following the examiner's finger up and down – von Graefe's sign).
- Stage 2: **S**oft tissue involvement.
- Stage 3: **P**roptosis.
- Stage 4: **E**xtraocular muscle involvement.
- Stage 5: **C**orneal involvement.
- Stage 6: **S**ight loss secondary to optic nerve compression.

The clinical course of thyroid eye disease can be highly variable, and severe disease is thought to occur in 3–5 per cent of patients with the condition.

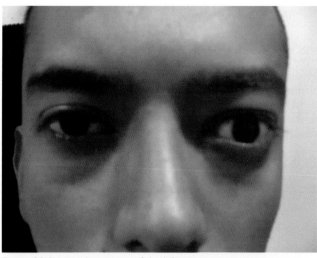

Figure 22.24 Axial proptosis of the left eye.

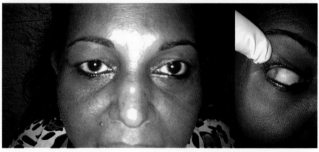

Figure 22.25 A lacrimal gland tumour.

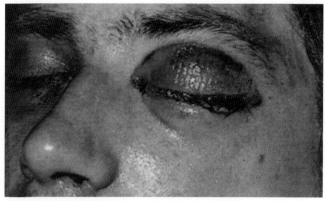

Figure 22.26 Carotid cavernous fistula.

## MISCELLANEOUS CONDITIONS

A range of other conditions should also be remembered for the differential diagnosis of ocular presentations.

### Sudden Changes in Refractive Error

Sudden changes in refractive error can be the result of:

- drugs such as topiramate, and possibly acetazolamide;
- uncontrolled diabetes;
- nuclear sclerosis;
- subluxation of the lens;
- corneal ectasia, for example keratoconus and pellucid marginal degeneration.

### Ophthalmic Emergencies

Emergency situations include:

- central or branch retinal arterial occlusion;
- retinal detachment;
- acute congestive glaucoma;
- endophthalmitis or panophthalmitis;
- corneal ulcers or infections;
- any red eye;
- trauma;
- foreign body in the eye.

### Visual Pathway Defects

With defects of the **optic nerve**, the visual field shows unilateral or bilateral enlarged blind spots, centrocecal scotomas, generalized depression of the fields, arcuate scotoma or altitudinal scotoma. These are usually associated with abnormalities of the pupil such as afferent pupillary defects (a non-reactive direct reflex but a reactive consensual reflex in the affected eye).

**Optic chiasm defects** present with bitemporal hemianopia if a pituitary gland tumour is present. Binasal hemianopia is very rare and occurs secondary to vascular malformation compressing the optic chiasm.

**Optic tract defects** produce homonymous hemianopia. No pupillary abnormality is seen in these patients.

**Temporal and occipital lobe lesions** produce homonymous quadrantanopias.

### Refractive Errors

Table 22.1 describes the main refractive errors that may be encountered.

Table 22.1 **Refractive errors**

| Condition | Description |
| --- | --- |
| Myopia (short sightedness) | Long eyeballs so light is focused in front of the retina<br>Produces headache and decreased vision for distance |
| Hyperopia (long sightedness) | Short eyeballs so light is focused behind the retina<br>Produces headache and decreased vision for near objects |
| Astigmatism | Blurred vision for all distances<br>Produces headache and eye strain |
| Presbyopia | Decreased near vision after the age of 40 years |

### Key Points

- Glaucoma and traumatic disruption of the globe require emergency management, and visual loss needs urgent diagnosis and referral.
- Foreign bodies need to be removed, and a red eye diagnosed and followed up to ensure it is not progressing.

## QUESTIONS

### SBAs

**1. Retro-orbital pain is a characteristic feature of which one of the following?:**
  a  Diabetic eye disease
  b  Conjunctivitis
  c  Glaucoma
  d  Retinal detachment
  e  Cataract

Answer
*c  Glaucoma.*

**2. A bitemporal hemianopia is due to which one of the following?:**
  a  A pituitary tumour
  b  Horner's syndrome
  c  Diabetic retinopathy
  d  Optic atrophy
  e  Hypertensive retinopathy

Answer
*a  A pituitary tumour.*

### EMQ

**1. For each of the case histories, choose the most appropriate diagnosis from the list below. Each option may be used once, more than once or not at all.**
  1  Glaucoma
  2  Cataract
  3  Horner's syndrome
  4  Retinal detachment
  5  Amaurosis fugax
  6  Hypertensive retinopathy
  7  Diabetic retinopathy
  8  Chalazion
  9  Thyroid eye disease
  10  Abducens nerve palsy

  a  A 60-year-old man with known type 2 diabetes and prostatic cancer was watching TV late one night when a curtain seemed to drop over part of his left eye. He decided to sleep it off, but the symptom was unchanged the next morning. When he visited his doctor, his pulse was regular at 84 beats per minute, he was normotensive and his blood sugar level was normal.

  b  A 54-year-old woman presented to her doctor with intermittent headache and blurring of vision in her right eye. She said her mother was diabetic and her sister hypertensive, and that both had visual problems. Her pulse was regular at 78 beats per minute, she was normotensive, and she had a normal blood sugar level. Perimetry showed an arcuate defect in the upper outer part of her right visual field, and there was mild cupping of the right optic disc.

  c  A 57-year-old man, who suffered from intermittent claudication, visited a bar on the way home from work.

Answers
a  4  **Retinal detachment.** *This gentleman had a detached retina.*
b  1  **Glaucoma.** *The lady had open-angle glaucoma, which can be familial and linked to diabetes and hypertension.*
c  5  **Amaurosis fugax.** *This is a typical history of amaurosis fugax. It was probably caused by disease at the carotid artery bifurcation. There may be a bruit and the arteries should be scanned.*
d  2  **Cataract.** *This lady has cataracts.*
e  3  **Horner's syndrome.** *An apical lung cancer can involve the T1 nerve root and the sympathetic chain, giving rise to a Horner's syndrome, with myosis, ptosis and loss of sweating on the ipsilateral side of the face.*

After the second glass of wine, he lost the vision in his right eye, but it returned after another drink. He had no further episodes of this but decided to visit his doctor for a check-up a few days later; no new physical signs were present.

d An 83-year-old woman visited her doctor because of deteriorating vision in her left eye. Her pulse was regular at 74 beats per minute, her blood pressure was 135/90 mmHg and her blood sugar level was normal. There was reduced visual acuity in both eyes, and fundoscopy was not possible.

e A 51-year-old man attended his doctor on account of pins and needles in his right arm and weakness of his right hand. He was found to have an abnormal right pupillary response, but his visual fields were normal.

# The Mouth

Devendra Chaukar and S. Girish Rao

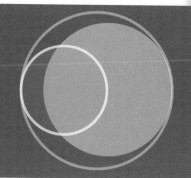

## LEARNING OBJECTIVES

- To describe the characteristic or unique clinical features of the most common and important diseases of the mouth

- To perform a step-by-step clinical differential diagnosis, using the decision tree, for patients with oral lesions

## INTRODUCTION

The mouth is like a mirror that reflects the patient's general health. Examination of the mouth thus forms an important clinical aspect of the diagnosis of local and systemic conditions affecting the body.

## THE TEETH AND GUMS

Human beings have two sets of teeth. There are 20 deciduous and 32 permanent teeth. The chronology of tooth eruption of both the deciduous and permanent teeth is listed in Table 23.1.

## Congenital and Developmental Abnormalities

**Anodontia** refers to congenitally missing teeth. This condition can be partial, where one or more teeth are absent, or all the teeth can be missing (**Figure 23.1**).

**Supernumerary and supplementary teeth** may occur. The additional teeth can be abnormal, conical supernumerary teeth, most often in the midline, which are called mesiodens or supplementary, and have the appearance of normal teeth (**Figure 23.2**).

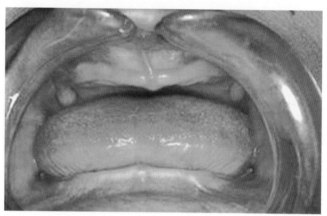

Figure 23.1 Anodontia.

Table 23.1 Chronology of teeth eruption

| Teeth | Deciduous (months) | Permanent (years) |
|---|---|---|
| Lower incisors | 6–9 | 6–8 |
| Upper incisors | 6–9 | 7–9 |
| Lower canines | 16–18 | 9–10 |
| Upper canines | 16–18 | 11–12 |
| Premolars | Absent | 10–12 |
| First molars | 12–14 | 6–7 |
| Second molars | 20–30 | 11–13 |
| Third molars | Absent | 18–25 |

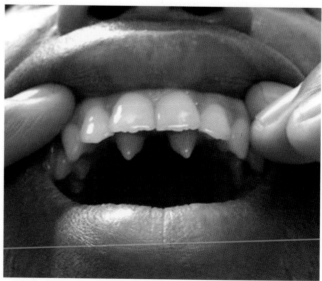

Figure 23.2 Supernumerary teeth.

### Impacted Teeth

The wisdom teeth, or the third molars, are the teeth that most commonly fail to erupt. With evolution, human jaw sizes are receding so the third molars, which erupt during the late teens, have a tendency to become impacted (**Figure 23.3**). Depending on the position, this is classified as horizontal, mesio-angular, distal, vertical, buccal or lingually impacted.

Food and debris collect between the gingival tissue covering the wisdom tooth, which becomes infected, leading to **pericoronitis**. This can be a recurrent problem and may lead to an abscess, facial space infections or Ludwig's angina.

Maxillary and mandibular canine and premolars may also fail to erupt and be a cause of impacted teeth.

### Morphological Changes in the Tooth

Dentinogenesis imperfecta represents a group of hereditary conditions that are characterized by abnormal dentin formation (**Figure 23.4**). This condition may affect only the teeth or may be associated with osteogenesis imperfecta, in which all the bones are hypoplastic and brittle.

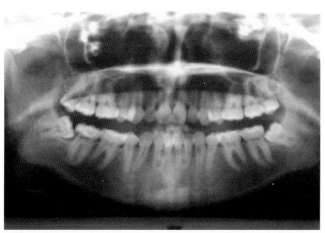

Figure 23.3 An orthopantomogram showing an impacted tooth; note the growth direction of the third molars ('wisdom teeth').

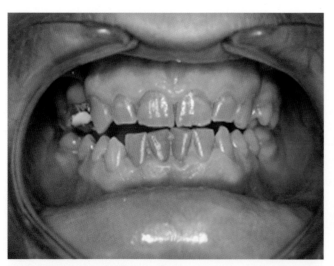

Figure 23.4 Dentinogenesis imperfecta.

The teeth are often discolored blue-grey or yellow-brown and are translucent. They are weaker than normal and prone to rapid wear, breakage and loss.

## Dental Fluorosis

An excessive ingestion of fluoride during early childhood may damage the tooth-forming cells, leading to a defect in the enamel known as dental fluorosis (**Figure 23.5**). These teeth have visible discoloration, ranging from white spots to brown and black stains.

The intake of drugs such as tetracycline in early childhood can also lead to discoloration and hypoplastic teeth.

## Dental Caries, Pulpitis and Periapical Periodontitis and Toothache

Tooth decay is one of the most common of all disorders, second only to the common cold.

Bacteria are normally present in the mouth. The bacteria convert all foods – especially sugar and starch – into acids. Bacteria, acid, food debris and saliva combine in the mouth to form a sticky substance called plaque that adheres to the teeth. Plaque that is not removed by brushing mineralizes into tartar. The acids in plaque dissolve the enamel surface of the tooth and create holes in the tooth (cavities).

### Dental Caries

Caries develops in the presence of three factors: bacterial plaque, bacterial substrate (sugar) and a susceptible tooth surface. *Streptococcus mutans* is the most common cariogenic organism.

Caries is usually painless in the initial stages when it is confined to the enamel. As it progresses further and the dentine becomes involved, there may be symptoms of sensitivity or mild discomfort to hot and cold.

### Pulpitis

The progression of dental caries involves the tooth pulp, leading to inflammation of the pulp, and is termed pulpitis. This causes severe pain in the tooth, jaw and surrounding area. Percussion of the involved tooth with a dental probe localizes the affected tooth.

### Periapical Periodontitis

Infection from the pulp may spread through the apical foramen to the periapical tissues, producing a periapical periodontitis.

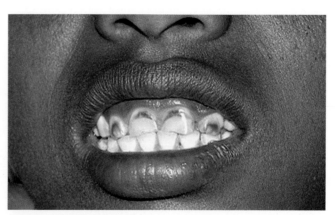

Figure 23.5 Dental fluorosis.

This inflammation and oedema of the periodontal membrane surrounding the apex of the tooth may slightly lift the tooth, and the patient may experience severe pain on biting.

As the process continues, the infection may further spread into the alveolar bone, leading to a **dento-alveolar abscess**. A sinus may develop intraorally in the alveolar mucosa or may drain extraorally through the facial skin over the jaws. Dental caries and its sequelae are the most common cause of the loss of teeth in young adults.

## Gingivitis

Gingivitis is inflammation of the gums caused by plaque. Red, oedematous gingiva, bleeding on brushing or on probing, and halitosis are the clinical signs and symptoms of gingivitis.

**Necrotizing ulcerative gingivitis** is an acute condition associated with poor oral hygiene, malnutrition, smoking, upper respiratory infection and general debilitation. This is also known as Vincent's angina or trench mouth disease. It is caused by *Spirochaeta denticola* in an immunocompromised host. It can be a rapidly progressive condition that begins at the tips of the interdental papillae, spreads along the gingival margins and destroys the periodontia, which sometimes leads to **cancrum oris**.

In acute leukaemia of childhood, gingivitis may be a presenting sign due to the abnormal white cell function. The region requires a defence from infection but the only response the cells can mount is to infiltrate the gums in large numbers. Gingivitis may also occur in uraemia, scurvy and pregnancy.

## Periodontitis

Untreated, gingivitis leads to a more advanced condition called **periodontitis** (Figure 23.6). In this, a pocket forms between the teeth and gums in which plaque and food debris accumulate. There is a progressive loss of alveolar bone, and the tooth gradually becomes mobile and is eventually lost. Chronic periodontitis is the most common cause of loss of teeth in the elderly.

### Juvenile and Rapidly Progressing Periodontitis

Aggressive periodontitis can occur even before puberty or in early adult life. This is characterized by early bone loss around the first molars and incisors. The classical clinical signs, such as inflammation, bleeding and a heavy accumulation of plaque, are not present. If untreated, this condition leads to very early loss of teeth.

## Heriditary and Drug-induced Gingival Hyperplasia

Heriditary gingival hyperplasia is a rare autosomal dominant condition that is commonly associated with epilepsy, hypertrichosis and mental retardation. The gums may become grossly enlarged and completely engulf the teeth.

Drugs such as phenytoin (an antiepileptic), ciclosporin (an immunosuppressant) and nifedipine (an antihypertensive) can cause gingival hypertrophy or hyperplasia (Figure 23.7). There is an overgrowth of the interdental papilla, which becomes bulbous and surrounds the entire tooth.

## Dental Cysts and Gingival Tumours

A cyst is a fluid-filled cavity lined with epithelium, and dental cysts are very common in the oral cavity. They occur either due to an infected tooth or are associated with an impacted or missing tooth. Rarely, cysts can also be developmental in origin, developing from epithelial remnants of the dental follicle. A classification of common dental cysts and tumours is given in Table 23.2.

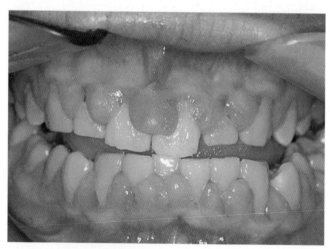

Figure 23.7 Phenytoin-induced gingival hyperplasia.

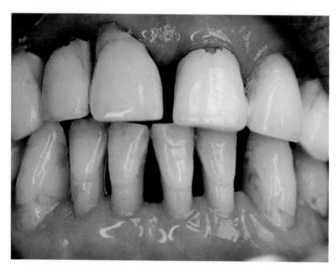

Figure 23.6 Periodontitis.

Table 23.2 Cysts and tumours of the teeth and jaws

| Cysts | Primordial, dentigerous, periodontal, periapical, odontogenic keratocyst, eruption, nasopalatine, globulomaxillary, solitary bone, aneurysmal, haemorrhagic |
| --- | --- |
| Benign tumours | Teeth – enameloma, dentinoma, cementoma, complex and composite odontomas, ameloblastoma<br>Jaw– fibroma, osteoma, chondroma, myxoma, giant cell granuloma |
| Malignant tumours | Osteogenic sarcoma, fibrosarcoma, chondrosarcoma, secondary carcinoma, ameloblastic carcinoma |

PART 4 | HEAD AND NECK

A dental abscess may develop, which may point and discharge externally (Figure 23.8).

## Epulis

Epulis is a non-specific benign lesion situated on the gingiva (Figure 23.9). It is generally a fibrous, granulomatous or firm swelling that is either sessile or pedunculated.

## Odontomas

Odontomas are hamartomas of aborted tooth formation and account for 22 per cent of odontogenic tumours (Figure 23.10). They are the most common benign odontogenic tumours of epithelial and mesenchymal origin. They can be broadly classified into two categories: compound odontomes, which resemble a tooth structure, and complex odontomes, which consist of a haphazard conglomerate of enamel, dentine and pulp.

## Ameloblastomas

Ameloblastomas (previously known as an adamantinomas) are benign but locally aggressive tumours arising from the mandible, or less commonly from the maxilla.

They are slow-growing and tend to present in the second to fifth decades of life, with no gender predilection. If untreated, the tumour can become enormous in size or undergo malignant transformation. The shell of the bone cracks on palpation, a phenomenon referred to as 'eggshell cracking', which is pathognomonic of a long-standing ameloblastoma.

## Malignant Tumours

Malignant tumours arising from dental tissue are rare, but oral squamous cell carcinoma is quite common and arises from the oral mucosa and gingiva. This is dealt with in detail later in this chapter.

# MUCOSAL LESIONS

## Herpes Simplex

Herpes simplex viruses are categorized into two types: type 1 (HSV-1, or oral herpes) and type 2 (HSV-2, or genital herpes). Herpes is transmitted by mucosal contact, usually kissing or the sharing of objects such as toothbrushes and utensils.

Primary infection commences with a sore throat and fever-like symptoms. There may be cervical lymphadenopathy and splenomegaly. Vesicular lesions appear on the lips, palate and gingiva, and sometimes on the surrounding facial skin, and break down to form shallow, painful ulcers (Figure 23.11). These

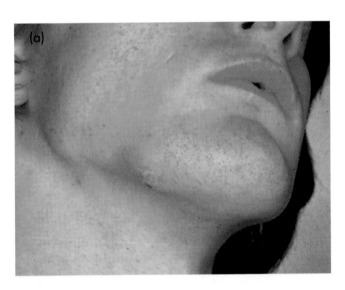
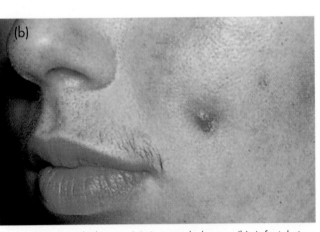

Figure 23.8 Dental abscess. (a) An apical abscess. (b) A facial sinus of dental origin.

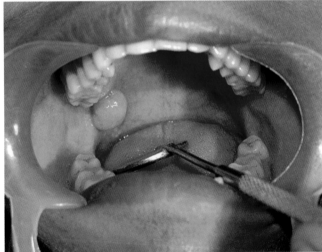

Figure 23.9 Epulis.

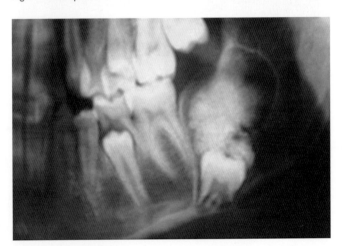

Figure 23.10 Odontoma.

ulcers normally heal in a few weeks. However, the virus may lie dormant in the sensory ganglia of the trigeminal nerve, and recurrence may occur when the individual's immune system is compromised.

## Herpes Zoster

Herpes zoster is caused by varicella-zoster virus. Lesions typically occur in the cutaneous distribution of one or more branches of the trigeminal nerve. There is a prodromal phase of itching and tingling followed after hours or days by the eruption of a cluster of small blisters filled with clear fluids and involving only one side of the face along the distribution of the branch of the trigeminal nerve.

The lesions heal in about 2 weeks, but they may get secondarily infected or, in rare circumstances, lead to a neuralgic type of pain in the distribution of the involved nerve. The virus occasionally also involves the VIIth and VIIIth cranial nerves, adding facial weakness and deafness to the cutaneous blistering and pain of a Vth cranial nerve infection (Ramsay–Hunt syndrome).

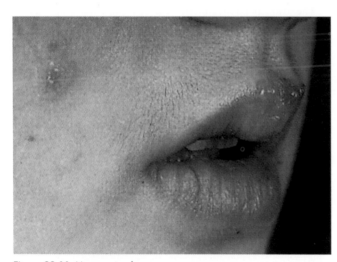

Figure 23.11 Herpes simplex.

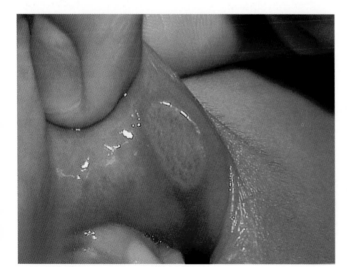

Figure 23.12 An aphthous ulcer.

## Herpangina

Herpangina is an acute, virally induced, self-limiting illness that is often seen in young individuals and is caused typically by Coxsackie virus. Vesicles or ulcers develop at the back of the throat and palate, and last for about 10–14 days.

## Aphthous Ulcers

Aphthous ulcers are one of the most common mouth ulcers (Figure 23.12). The aetiology is unknown. They are characterized by a round or oval ulcer involving any part of the oral mucosa.

There are three types of apthous ulcer:

- *Minor apthous ulcers*, which are smaller than 10 mm, usually last for 7–10 days and heal without scarring.
- *Major apthous ulcers* are 10 mm or larger, very painful, last from 2 weeks to several months and heal leaving a scar.
- *Herpetiform ulcers* are multiple, tiny 1–2 mm ulcers that sometimes join together and form irregularly shaped ulcers. They usually heal in about 2 weeks without scars.

## Oral Candidiasis

Oral candidias, also known as thrush, is frequently caused by *Candida albicans* or less commonly by *Candida glabrata* or *Candida tropicalis*.

The infection usually appears as thick white or cream-coloured deposits on mucosal membranes such as the tongue, inner cheeks, gums, tonsils and palate (Figure 23.13); the membrane can be peeled off, leaving behind a red, inflamed mucosa.

## Syphilis

Syphilis is a sexually transmitted infection caused by the spirochaete *Treponema pallidum*. Oral manifestations may be seen in all the three stages of this disease:

- In the primary stage, a painless sore, open, wet ulcer called a **chancre** affects the lip and tongue.
- In the secondary stage, a mucous patch may appear on the oral mucosa as a '**snail track ulcer**', which lasts for 2–6 weeks.

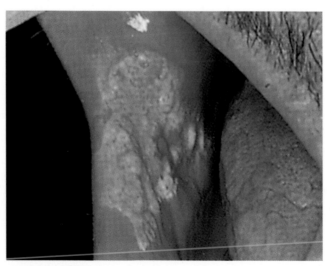

Figure 23.13 Chronic candidal infection of the mouth.

- In the tertiary stage, a **gumma** may appear on the palate or tongue, usually in the midline. Destruction of the tissue may result in a hole in the palate (**Figure 23.14**).

## Behçet's Syndrome

Behçet's syndrome is classically characterized as a triad of symptoms that include recurring crops of mouth ulcers (aphthous ulcers), genital ulcers and inflammation of a specialized area around the pupil of the eye, the uvea, which is known as uveitis.

## Pemphigus and Pemphigoid

Pemphigus is the term given to a group of potentially lethal disorders that are all characterized by autoantibodies directed against intercellular substances or stratified squamous cell epithelium. Large bullae first appear on the skin or mucous membranes, and then rupture to leave an ulcer (**Figure 23.15**).

Pemphigoid is a non-fatal condition that is otherwise similar in character to pemphigus. It is a subepithelial immune disease in which the autoantibodies act against zones of the epithelial basement membrane zones. Although typically arising idiopathically, pemphigoid may be drug-induced, particularly by penicillamine.

## Lichen Planus

Lichen planus is a common idiopathic lesion that affects the skin and oral mucosa. It has many variations. The most common variant is the striated or lace-like appearance involving both sides of the buccal mucosa (**Figure 23.16**). A characteristic clinical feature that aids diagnosis is the presence of fine whitish lines extending from posterior to anterior in the buccal mucosae (Wickham's striae). The erosive or atrophic forms of lichen planus may present as irregular erosions on the tongue or palate; this is potentially malignant in less than 3 per cent of cases.

## Leukoplakia

Leukoplakia is a potential premalignant condition that appears as a white patch involving the oral mucosa. It cannot be scraped off and cannot be attributed to other known conditions. Approximately 3 per cent of leukoplakia lesions undergo malignant transformation over time.

The two common varieties are homogenous, which has a regular appearance and a flat or slightly raised surface, and non-homogenous, which has an irregular, raised, thick or erythematous appearance. Malignant transformation is more likely in the non-homogenous variety. Leukoplakias of the tongue and floor of the mouth are more likely to undergo malignant transformation (**Figure 23.17**).

Sublingual keratosis is a white patch seen on the floor of the mouth and has a higher incidence of malignant transformation.

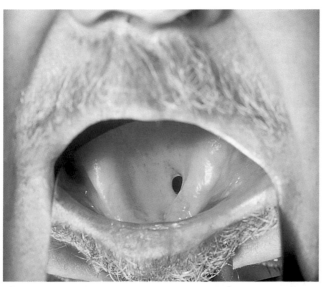

Figure 23.14 A palatal fistula following a syphilitic gumma.

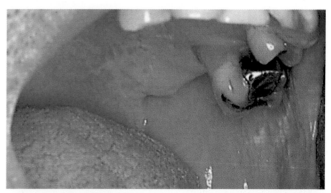

Figure 23.16 Lichen planus.

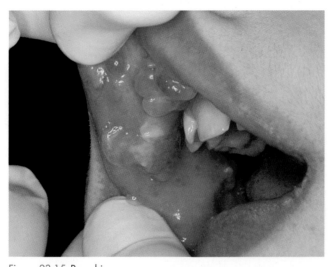

Figure 23.15 **Pemphigus.**

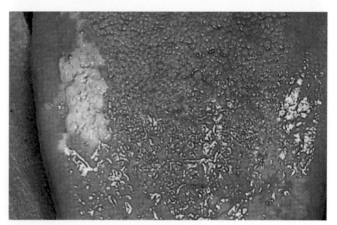

Figure 23.17 Leukoplakia.

## Erythroplakia

Erythroplakia is defined as a fiery red patch that cannot be characterized either clinically or pathologically as any other definable lesion. It is mostly associated with the use of tobacco and has a high potential to undergo malignant transformation.

## Submucous Fibrosis

Submucous fibrosis is a peculiar condition, commonly seen in the Indian subcontinent, that is caused by the chewing of areca nut, betel leaves and slaked lime, also called betel quid.

There is a progressive reduction in mouth opening with stiffness and a band-like formation in the buccal mucosa and glossopalatal folds (Figure 23.18). There is also a severe burning sensation in the oral cavity, with intolerance to spicy food. This is a premalignant condition with a 5 per cent incidence of malignant transformation to oral squamous cell carcinoma over a 15 year period.

## Leukoedema

Leukoedema is a benign abnormality of the buccal mucosa characterized by a filmy, opalescent-to-whitish grey appearance due to folding of the mucosa.

## White Spongy Naevus

White spongy naevus is an autosomal dominant lesion that appears more commonly in childhood or early adult life. There is a typical shaggy white patch in the buccal mucosa that can be peeled away leaving a red raw area (Figure 23.19).

## Peutz–Jeghers Syndrome

Peutz–Jeghers syndrome, also known as hereditary intestinal polyposis syndrome, is an autosomal dominant genetic disease characterized by the development of polyps in the gastrointestinal tract and hyperpigmented macules on the lips and oral mucosa (Figure 23.20).

The risks associated with this syndrome include a strong tendency to develop cancer in multiple sites. While the hamartomatous polyps themselves have only a small malignant potential (less than 3 per cent), patients with the syndrome have an increased risk of developing carcinomas of the pancreas, liver, lungs, breast, ovaries, uterus, testes and other organs.

## Multiple Endocrine Neoplasia Syndrome

Multiple endocrine neoplasia (MEN) syndromes are rare, inherited conditions in which several endocrine glands such as the parathyroids, pancreas, pituitary, adrenal and thyroid develop tumours or excessive growth and activity. Multiple endocrine neoplasia syndromes occur in three patterns – types 1, 2A and 2B – although the types occasionally overlap.

MEN type 2B is associated with multiple nodules (neuromas) of the oral mucosa, phaeochromocytoma and medullary thyroid carcinoma (Figure 23.21).

## Fordyce Spots

Multiple, pinhead-sized, whitish to yellowish papules on the buccal mucosa or lips caused by ectopically located sebaceous glands. They are of no clinical significance.

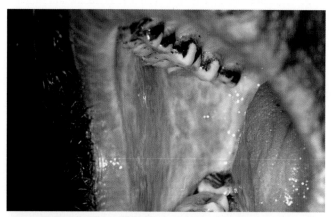

Figure 23.18 Submucous fibrosis.

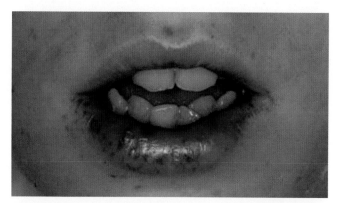

Figure 23.20 Peutz–Jeghers syndrome.

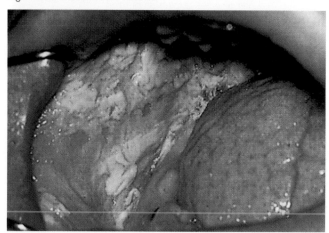

Figure 23.19 A white spongy naevus of the mouth.

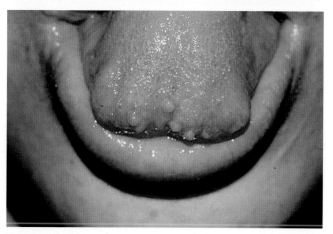

Figure 23.21 Mucosal neuromas associated with multiple endocrine neoplasia syndrome type 2B.

## Oral Squamous Cell Carcinoma

Oral squamous cell carcinoma is one of the most common cancers in the Indian subcontinent and is caused by chewing tobacco and areca nut. Genetic factors, smoking, alcohol intake and chronic irritation from the sharp cusp of a tooth are the other aetiological factors.

A squamous cell carcinoma may arise from any part of the oral mucosa, although the buccal mucosa, tongue and floor of the mouth are more common (**Figure 23.22**). It may present as an indurated non-healing ulcer or a swelling that is painless in the initial phase. In the next stage, the tumour spreads to the cervical lymph nodes. Features of the local invasion of an oral squamous cell carcinoma are outlined in **Table 23.3**.

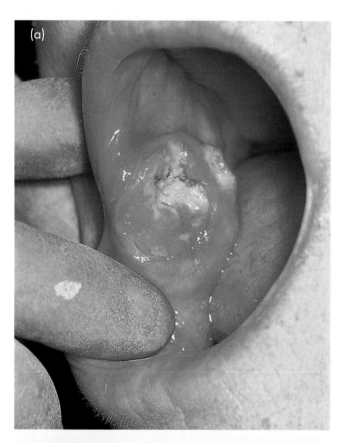

Figure 23.22 Squamous cell carcinoma. (a) The buccal mucosa. (b) The floor of the mouth.

## Basal Cell Carcinoma

A basal cell carcinoma may present as an indolent, non-healing ulcer on the lip (**Figure 23.23**) or any exposed part of the face. It is locally aggressive and generally does not metastasize.

Most basal cell carcinomas are thought to be caused by long-term exposure to ultraviolet radiation from sunlight. Avoiding the sun and using sunscreen may help to protect against the condition.

## THE TONGUE AND FLOOR OF THE MOUTH

### Geographic and Fissured Tongue

**Fissured tongue,** also known as scrotal tongue, is a benign condition characterized by deep grooves and fissures on the dorsum of the tongue. Although these grooves may look unsettling, the condition is painless and individuals experience no physical discomfort (**Figure 23.24**).

**Geographic tongue** (benign migratory glossitis) is an inflammatory condition of the tongue characterized by discolored regions of taste buds or sometimes even cracks on the surface of the tongue (**Figure 23.25**). The condition is chronic and usually exacerbated by eating certain foods or during times of stress, illness or hormonal surges (particularly in women before menstruation).

### Macroglossia

Macroglossia, an unusual enlargement or hypertrophy of the tongue, is commonly seen in amyloidosis, cretinism, acromegaly and Down syndrome. There may be speech abnormalities, and patients keep their mouth open, causing drooling of saliva. At times, benign tumours or malformations, such as haemangiomas, lymphangiomas or neurofibromas, can lead to enlargement of the tongue.

Table 23.3 Features of local invasions by oral carcinoma

| Structure | Feature |
| --- | --- |
| Muscles of mastication | Trismus |
| Inferior alveolar nerve | Mandibular anaesthesia |
| IXth and Xth cranial nerves | Referred otalgia and palsy of the soft palate |
| XIIth cranial nerve | Ipsilateral tongue weakness/wasting |
| Base of tongue | Deviation to the affected side on protrusion or fixed |

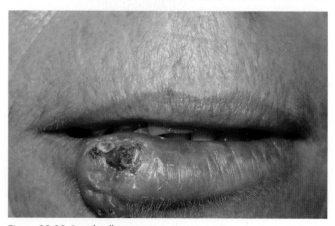

Figure 23.23 Basal cell carcinoma.

## Ankyloglossia

Ankyloglossia, commonly known as tongue tie, is a congenital anomaly that may decrease the mobility of the tongue tip and is caused by an unusually short, thick lingual frenulum (Figure 23.26). It varies in severity from mild cases characterized by mucous membrane bands to complete ankyloglossia in which the tongue is tethered to the floor of the mouth.

## Median Rhomboid Glossitis

Median rhomboid glossitis is the term used to describe a smooth, red, flat or raised nodular area in the midline in relation to the circumvallate papillae. Characteristically, the filliform papillae are absent in this area. It probably results from candidal infection.

## Hairy Tongue

Hairy tongue is a condition caused by elongation of the filliform papaillae on the dorsal surface of the tongue. The black discoloration is due to staining by certain bacteria, and the condition occurs in response to some antibiotics and antiseptics (Figure 23.27).

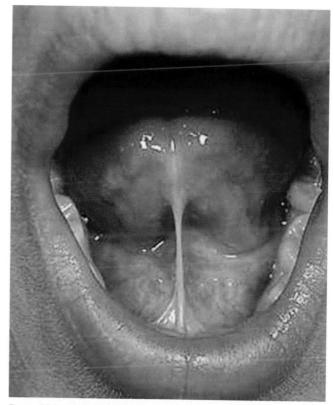

Figure 23.26 Ankyloglossia.

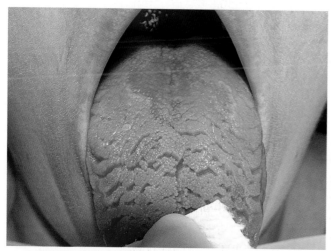

Figure 23.24 A fissured tongue.

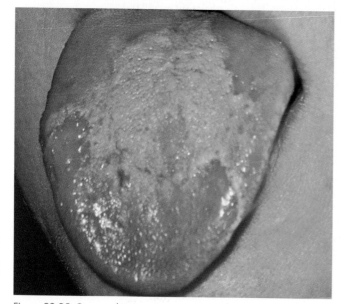

Figure 23.25 Geographic tongue.

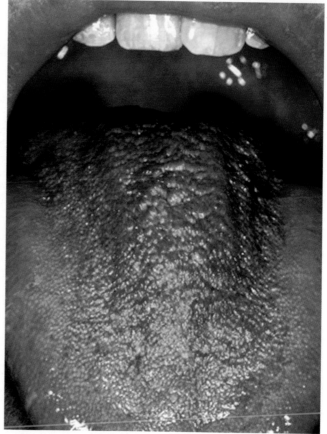

Figure 23.27 Hairy tongue.

PART 4 | HEAD AND NECK

## Hairy Oral Leukoplakia

Hairy oral leukoplakia is seen in severe defects of immunity, particularly in HIV infection. The cause of this condition is an opportunistic infection by the Epstein–Barr virus. It is a white patch on the side of the tongue with a corrugated or hairy appearance.

## Pernicious Anaemia

Pernicious anaemia is characterized by the triad of paraesthesia, sore tongue and weakness. The tongue shows a characteristic baldness and inflammation that is described as Hunter's glossitis. There may also be angular cheilitis and pallor of the mucous membrane.

## Pellagra

Pellagra is a vitamin deficiency disease commonly caused by a chronic lack of niacin (vitamin $B_3$) in the diet. It is classically described by 'the four Ds': diarrhoea, dermatitis, dementia and death. Oral findings include angular cheilitis, glossitis and fissured tongue.

## Agranulocytosis

Agranulocytosis is an acute condition involving severe and dangerous neutropenia. It may present as with a sudden onset of sore throat and ulceration. There is often severe gingivitis, and at times stomatitis. The ulcers are necrotic, with a whitish or greyish surface, often without signs of inflammation.

## Wasting and Deviation of the Tongue

Unilateral wasting of tongue is associated with long-standing hypoglossal nerve palsy, with the tongue deviating to the affected site. Bilateral weakness of the tongue occurs in bulbar and pseudobulbar palsy.

## Lingual Thyroid

A lingual thyroid is a specific type of ectopic thyroid and results from a lack of normal caudal migration of the thyroid gland. It appears as a reddish purple swelling in the midline of the back of the tongue. It may represent the only functioning thyroid tissue, and its removal may render the patient hypothyroid.

## Carcinoma of the Tongue

Carcinoma of the tongue usually occurs on the lateral border of the anterior two-thirds of the tongue but can occasionally involve the posterior one-third. Deviation of the tongue to the side of the lesion and ankyloglossia are signs of deep tumour infiltration. Nodal spread to the cervical lymph nodes is usually unilateral in the initial stage but can be bilateral in advanced tumours (Figure 23.28).

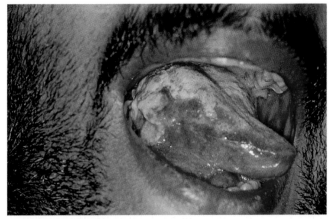

Figure 23.28 Advanced squamous cell carcinoma of the tongue.

## Ranula

A ranula is a fluctuant swelling with a bluish translucent colour that somewhat resembles the underbelly of a frog (Figure 23.29). The classical bluish appearance may not be seen in deep-seated ranulas. It commonly arises from the sublingual salivary gland and occasionally from the submandibular gland.

## Lingual Torus

A mandibular torus is a compact bony lesion that occurs along the lingual side of the mandible, usually on both sides of the midline. It is asymptomatic and is not treated unless it gets in the way of denture fixation.

## Sialolith

A sialolith is a stone in the submandibular duct (Figure 23.30). This can result in an obstruction of the flow of saliva from the gland, leading to recurrent swellings of the submandibular gland.

## Sublingual Dermoid

A sublingual dermoid is a cyst that is painless and slow-growing. It has a soft, doughy consistency, is well encapsulated and has no associated cervical lymphadenopathy.

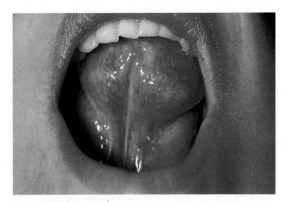

Figure 23.29 A ranula.

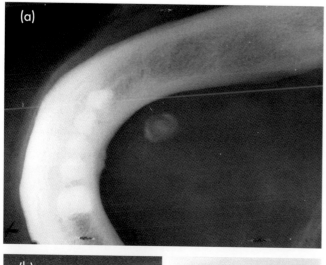

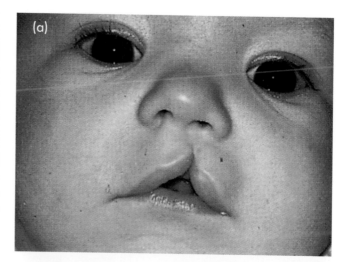

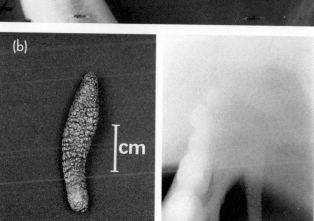

Figure 23.30 A submandibular calculus (sailolith). (a) *In situ*. (b) On removal.

## THE PALATE

### Clieft Lip and Palate

Cleft lip and palate are congenital deformities that occur in approximately 1 in 800 births. They result from a failure of the mesenchyme to penetrate the junctions between the primary processes (the frontonasal and maxillary process) that fuse to form the nose, lips and palate. The condition may be partial or complete, unilateral or bilateral and involve the lip, alveolus and hard and soft palate (**Figure 23.31**).

A cleft lip is primarily a cosmetic problem, but a cleft palate may cause problems with feeding and speech, as well as an increased risk of respiratory and ear infections. A submucosal cleft is a rare form of cleft palate in which the mucosal covering is intact but there may be abnormal muscle positioning or an underlying bony cleft. There is severe nasality of speech, a blue line may be seen in the midline of the palate, and the condition is occasionally associated with a bifid uvula.

A cleft palate may occur in association with micrognathia and glossoptosis in a condition known as **Pierre Robin syndrome**. In these babies, the tongue may fall backwards, leading to respiratory obstruction or sleep apnoea.

### Palatal Torus

The palatal torus or torus palatinus is a localized overgrowth of the bone, usually in the midline of the palate. It appears as a

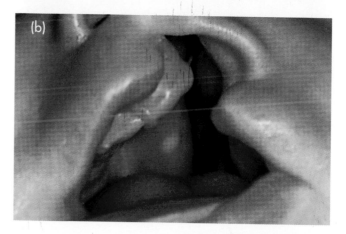

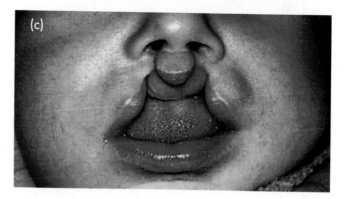

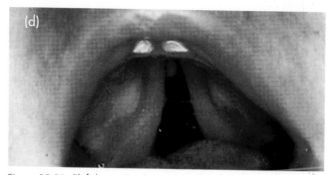

Figure 23.31 Cleft lip and palate. (a) Left-sided cleft lip. (b) Left-sided cleft lip and palate. (c) Bilateral cleft lip and palate. (d) Cleft palate.

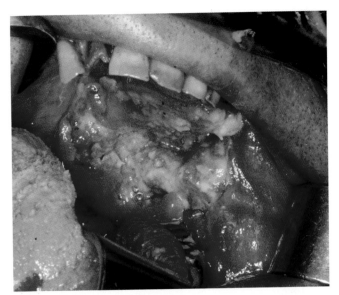

Figure 23.32 Carcinoma of the palate.

slow-growing, hard, asymptomatic, rounded swelling that is usually less than 2 cm in size.

## Paralysis

Paralysis of the soft palate may be unilateral from a lesion of the vagus nerve or bilateral in bulbar poliomyelitis. There is an absence of movement of the soft palate associated with problems of speech and deglutition.

## Carcinoma

Carcinoma in the palatal region is commonly seen to arise from either the minor salivary glands in the palate or the maxillary sinus. It presents in the oral cavity after perforating or expanding the palate (Figure 23.32). Squamous cell carcinoma can also arise in chronic smokers.

### Key Points

- An incredible variety of lesions may involve the oral cavity. These can be classified as congenital, developmental, inflammatory or neoplastic.
- The diagnosis of oral lesions depends on the age of presentation, the characteristic morphological appearance and the clinical features.
- Lesions of the dentition comprise an important part of the lesions of the mouth and a knowledge of these conditions is essential.
- Non-healing ulcers, particularly those which are indurated, warrant a biopsy.
- It is important to recognize premalignant lesions, namely leukoplakia, erythroplakia and submucus fibrosis, as they have a potential for malignant transformation.

## QUESTIONS

### SBAs

**1.** A college student presents with a week-long history of oral lesions. He has also been suffering from malaise and a sore throat. An examination reveals several lesions on the lips and buccal mucosae; some are tiny and vesicular, while some have broken down to form shallow ulcers. He is mildly febrile. The most likely diagnosis is which one of the following?:
   **a** Herpes zoster
   **b** Herpes simplex
   **c** Oral malignancy
   **d** Aphthous ulcers

**Answer**

*a* **Herpes simplex.** *The infection is usually transmitted by mucosal contact such as kissing. Initially, there may be fever and malaise. The lesions are in the form of small vesicles that break down to form shallow ulcers. Herpes zoster lesions are usually unilateral, and lie along the distribution of a particular branch of the trigeminal nerve; they may be quite painful. Aphthous ulcers are not associated with prodromal symptoms or vesicles. Oral malignancy presents with non-healing ulcers or frank growths that bleed to the touch, are often indurated and may be accompanied by enlarged neck nodes.*

**2.** All of the following are premalignant lesions of the oral cavity except which one?:
   **a** Leukoplakia
   **b** Erythroplakia
   **c** Submucous fibrosis
   **d** Pemphigoid lesions

**Answer**

*d* **Pemphigoid lesions.** *Pemphigoid lesions are vesicobullous lesions of autoimmune origin and have no malignant potential. Leukoplakia appears as a whitish plaque-like lesions in the absence of any obvious cause, and carries a small but definite malignant potential. Erythroplakia carries a very high risk of malignant transformation. Submucous fibrosis, or progressive stiffening of the oral mucosa, with trismus may transform into malignancies.*

**3.** All are true about ameloblastoma except which one of the following?:
   **a** They commonly arise from the mandible
   **b** They are malignant lesions
   **c** They were previously referred to as adamantinomas
   **d** The lesions can be treated by surgery

**Answer**

*b* **They are malignant lesions.** *This statement is untrue as ameloblastomas are usually benign tumours that are locally aggressive.*

### EMQ

**1.** For each of the following descriptions, select the most likely diagnosis from the list of lesions and tumours of the oral cavity below:
   **1** Dental cyst
   **2** Leukoplakia
   **3** Oral squamous cell cancer
   **4** Pemphigus
   **5** Ranula
   **6** Submucous fibrosis
   **7** Erythroplakia
   **8** Epulis
   **a** A 5-year-old girl presents with a swelling in her oral cavity. On examination, a fluctuant swelling can be seen on the ventral side of the tongue, extending to the floor of the mouth. There is also some bulging in the submental region. The surface of the oral swelling shows distended veins, and clear fluid can be aspirated from the swelling.

**Answers**

*a* **5 Ranula.** *A ranula is a cystic swelling that arises from the sublingual salivary gland, and its usual position is in the anterior floor of mouth. The swelling may become large enough to produce a bulge in the submental region.*

**b** A 25-year-old man has been complaining of painful mouth opening for a month. He gives a history of smokeless tobacco usage. The patient has trismus, and a complete oral examination is not possible due to his restricted mouth opening. A firm to hard node can be felt in the submandibular region.

**b 3 Oral squamous cell cancer.** *While trismus is also characteristically seen in submucous fibrosis, it is usually of a long-standing duration in comparison with trismus caused by oral malignancy. The finding of a hard neck node in the submandibular region (which is the usual draining region of oral cavity) further substantiates the diagnosis.*

LEARNING OBJECTIVES

- To understand the clinical presentations of various congenital and acquired conditions
- To develop a differential diagnosis for similar clinical presentations
- To describe the characteristic physical signs for these conditions
- To understand the aetiologies of and various methodologies for diagnosing these conditions

## THE NOSE

### Congenital Abnormalities

Defects of embryological midline fusion may rarely give rise to a **bifid nose**. This is commonly associated with hypertelorism (Figure 24.1). **Dermoid cysts** may occur on the bridge of the nose.

**Atresia of the posterior nares**, which may be bony or membranous, may result from persistence of the primitive bucconasal membrane. Unilateral atresia may go unnoticed, but bilateral atresia presents soon after birth with intermittent asphyxia or asphyxia during feeding. The child may show cyanosis at rest but an improvement on crying (paradoxical cyanosis). It may be one of the components of CHARGE syndrome. An absence of condensation after placing a cold spatula beneath the nostrils and an inability to pass a soft plastic tube through the nose are seen in atresia.

### Rhinitis

#### Acute and Chronic Rhinitis

Acute rhinitis presents with rhinorrhoea, nasal obstruction and constitutional disturbances. It is mainly due to the common cold or influenza. Chronic rhinitis may present as relapsing attacks of acute rhinitis (lasting more than 12 weeks) or secondary to sinusitis. The nasal mucosa may hypertrophy, fibrose, atrophy and degenerate. On posterior rhinoscopy, a mulberry-like enlargement of the posterior end of the inferior turbinate is seen.

#### Allergic Rhinitis

Allergic rhinitis usually occurs in response to allergens. Clinically, the condition is identifiable as an 'allergic crease' over the

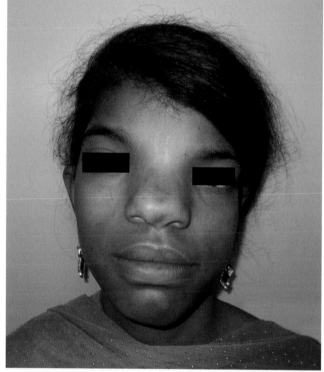

Figure 24.1 A bifid nose with hypertelorism. (Courtesy of Dr Jyoti Dabholkar.)

external nose, a profuse, watery rhinorrhoea with paroxysms of sneezing and a poor sense of smell. Pale or bluish, swollen mulberry turbinates may be seen.

### Atrophic Rhinitis

Primary atrophic rhinitis is common in women. Secondary atrophic rhinitis can follow granulomatous infection, extensive nasal surgery and trauma. There is 'merciful' anosmia (which means patients are spared the foul smell emanating from their own nose), atrophy of the turbinates and a roomy nasal cavity with greenish crusting.

### Vasomotor Rhinitis

Vasomotor rhinitis presents with sneezing, watery rhinorrhoea and nasal obstruction of unknown aetiology. Hereditary factors, psychological factors, atmospheric conditions and dusty environments may trigger paroxysmal symptoms.

### Mucocoeles

Frontoethmoidal mucocoeles are common due to the complexity of the drainage. They appear following infection, polyps or trauma. They present as headache, orbital displacement and visual disturbances in the late stages.

## Granulomatous Conditions

### Sarcoidosis

The external nose shows a 'lupus pernio' (frostbite) appearance and the nasal mucosa shows a 'strawberry skin' appearance. It presents with nodules on the septum, nasal obstruction, crusting, anosmia and a purulent discharge.

### Wegener's Granulomatosis

This is an autoimmune disorder with multiple organ involvement in which vasculitis and granulomas develop. Subtle features include splinter haemorrhages in the nails, a fleeting arthritis, haemoptysis, renal failure, septal perforation and punched-out ('tick-bite') skin lesions.

### T-cell Lymphoma (Stewart's Midline Granuloma)

Rather than having an inflammatory origin, Stewart's midline granuloma is now regarded as a T-cell lymphoma. The initial prodromal stage presents with nasal obstruction and rhinitis. This is followed by a necrotic stage in which there is crusting, discharge and destruction of the nose, before the terminal stage presents with haemorrhage and mutilation of the midface region.

### Tuberculosis

Low-virulence bacilli may affect the nose as **lupus vulgaris** (a cutaneous, nodular type), which has a characteristic glistening, reddish-brown nodule with an 'apple jelly' appearance when a glass slide is pressed against it. More virulent forms of tuberculosis affecting the nose may give rise to a **tuberculoma** (a mucosal, ulcerative type), which erodes the cartilaginous septum and inferior turbinate. **Isolated sinus involvement** can present with soft tissue infiltration and bony destruction.

### Leprosy

Leprosy may present as nasal obstruction, hyposmia or crusting. It may cause atrophic rhinitis, septal perforation or dorsal saddling in the late stages.

### Diphtheria

Diphtheria may cause rhinitis secondary to pharyngeal involvement.

### Scleroma

Scleroma is a chronic inflammatory condition. In the atrophic stage, it presents with rhinitis, crusting and a foul smell. After progressing to the nodular stage, ulcerative bluish-red, mobile nodules develop over the anterior part of septum (**Figure 24.2**). Adhesions and stenosis occur during the cicatrization stage.

### Syphilis

Congenital syphilis causes a purulent rhinitis, vestibule excoriation and other stigmata in infants up to about 3 months of age. In the acquired form, it may cause a chancre as a hard, painless, ulcerated papule with non-tender rubbery nodes at about 3–6 weeks of age. A secondary form may cause persistent rhinorrhoea, with crusting and fissuring of the vestibule at about 6–9 weeks. The gumma occurs in the tertiary stage after 1–5 years and affects the periosteum of the septum, leading to perforation of the bony septum and resulting in the characteristic saddle deformity.

**Yaws** is a tropical condition affecting the nose that is clinically indistinguishable from syphilis.

### Rhinosporidiosis

Rhinosporidiosis gives a bleeding, raspberry-like polyp appearance (**Figure 24.3**) and results from a sporozoal infection.

### Leishmaniasis

Nasopharyngeal leishmaniasis causes ulceration of the mucosa and may recur years after the original infection, destroying the facial tissues.

## Fungal Infections

Fungal infections occur in immunocompromised individuals. A non-invasive fungal ball frequently presents as a unilateral postnasal discharge and allergic fungal rhinosinusitis. **Aspergillosis** gives rise to grey areas on the mucosa with a musty discharge. **Mucormycosis** can present as an invasive or non-invasive form. Orbital involvement can occur following destruction of the lateral wall of the nose, along with proptosis, headache or cranial nerve deficits (**Figure 24.4**).

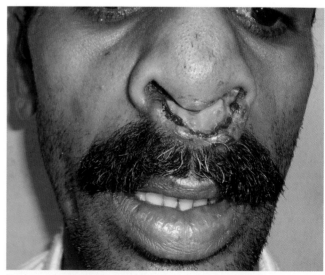

Figure 24.2 Rhinoscleroma. (Courtesy of Dr Arpit Sharma.)

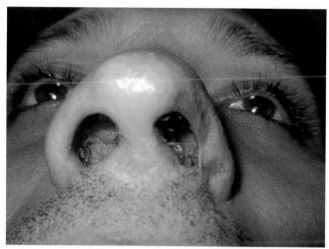

Figure 24.3 Rhinosporidiosis. (Courtesy of Dr Arpit Sharma.)

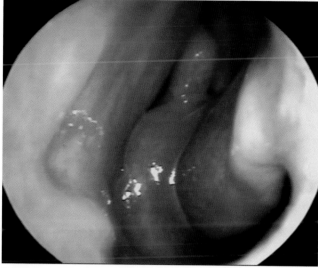

Figure 24.5 Antrochoanal polyp. (Courtesy of Dr Jyoti Dabholkar.)

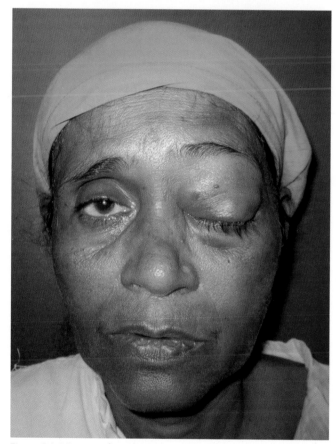

Figure 24.4 Invasive fungal sinusitis with orbital cellulitis. (Courtesy of Dr Jyoti Dabholkar.)

## Nasal Tumours

### Benign Tumours

**Capillary haemangiomas** may occur on the nose as a strawberry naevus, or on the septum, causing epistaxis. **Rhinophyma** is a benign swelling involving the nasal tip ('potato nose'). It results from hyperplasia and fibrosis of the sebaceous glands in the skin, and occurs in relation to acne rosacea. **Nasal polyps (Figure 24.5)** may occur in isolation or associated with vasomotor rhinitis, asthma, an intolerance to non-steroidal anti-inflammatory drugs, cystic fibrosis, allergic fungal infections and ciliary dyskinesia.

### Angiofibroma

This is a locally invasive vascular tumour that arises in the sphenopalatine foramen. More aggressive tumours may extend to the orbit and cavernous sinus. Adolescent boys present with repeated epistaxis, nasal obstruction, anosmia, broadening of the nose and facial swelling. Later there is serous otitis media secondary to blockage of the Eustachian tube, proptosis and diplopia. On examination, a fleshy pinkish nasal and nasopharyngeal mass bulging over the soft palate may be seen, with rhinolalia clausa (abnormal speech attributable to a nasal and nasopharyngeal block) and poorly developed secondary sexual characteristics.

### Malignancy of the Nose and Paranasal Sinuses

These tumours present mainly in the advanced stages, the maxilla being the most common site. Occupational exposure to wood dust, chemical inhalation, smoking and genetic factors are predisposing factors. Histologically, squamous cell carcinoma is more common, followed by adenocarcinoma, adenoid cystic carcinoma and aesthesioneuroblastoma (**Figure 24.6**). The tumour may extend:

- to the nasolacrimal duct (causing epiphora);
- medially to the nasal cavity (leading to a blocked nose, anosmia and bleeding);
- inferiorly to the hard palate (giving rise to loose teeth, the need for a change of dentures and lesions over the palate);
- posteriorly to the infratemporal fossa and pterygopalatine fossa (causing trismus and trigeminal nerve deficits);
- laterally to the cheek (producing fullness);
- superiorly to the orbit (resulting in proptosis and diplopia).

Ethmoidal tumours lead to anosmia, widening of the distance between the eyes, proptosis, nasal blockage and diplopia. Sphenoidal sinus tumours may extend into the cavernous sinus and lead to nerve deficits, most commonly lateral rectus palsy (from damage to the abducent nerve).

PART 4 | HEAD AND NECK

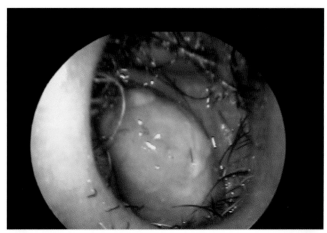

Figure 24.6 Aesthesioneuroblastoma. (Courtesy of Dr Jyoti Dabholkar.)

## Nasal Trauma

### Fractures

Fractures (**Figure 24.7**) may take three forms:

- *Type 1*: The distal thin portion of the nasal bone is displaced, and the nasal septum is fractured vertically. This results from frontal trauma and is also known as a Chevallet fracture. There is minimum nasal deformity. In subluxation of the septum, caudal deviation of the septum is seen on lifting the nose.
- *Type 2*: Lateral trauma produces a C-shaped fracture of the perpendicular plate of the ethmoid and quadrilateral cartilage. This is also known as a Jarjavay fracture. The frontal process of the maxilla and the septum are sometimes also fractured.
- *Type 3*: These fractures are caused by a more significant blow. There is marked depression, the perpendicular plate of the ethmoid rotating backwards and the septum collapsing inwards. The tip of the nose turns upwards (producing a 'pig-like' face). A naso-orbito-ethmoidal fracture may result in telecanthus. Severe forms of fracture may cause cerebrospinal fluid leaks with dural tears and pneumocephalus due to a fracture of the anterior skull base and posterior wall of the frontal sinus.

### Haematoma of the Septum

Following injury, a bilateral haematoma appears because of a collection of blood beneath the mucoperichondrium. On nasal examination, this appears as soft, red, septal swellings (giving an 'hour-glass' appearance) with complete nasal obstruction. Haematomas occasionally give rise to a septal abscess, with fever. Absorption of the cartilage may occur if this is not treated.

### Perforation of the Septum

Perforations of the septum (**Figure 24.8**) commonly follow trauma and septal surgery. Erosion may occur from acid fumes in chromium platers, cocaine abuse and chronic inflammatory conditions, or after a haematoma. The perforation may manifest as crusting, epistaxis, nasal blockage, whistling noises on nasal breathing (with smaller defects) and rhinolalia (with larger defects). Anterior perforations are more symptomatic than posterior perforations.

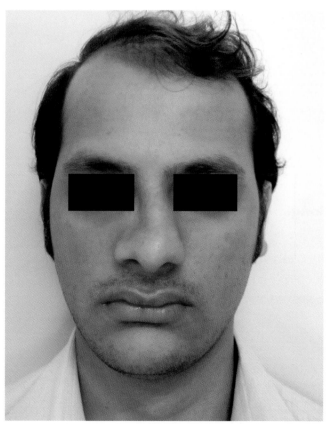

Figure 24.7 A compound nasal fracture. (Courtesy of Dr Arpit Sharma.)

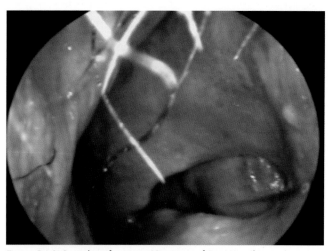

Figure 24.8 Septal perforation. (Courtesy of Dr Arpit Sharma.)

### Foreign Bodies

A foreign body in the nose should be suspected if a child is brought in with a unilateral, purulent nasal discharge. Inspection with a nasal speculum is usually diagnostic.

## Miscellaneous Conditions

### Epistaxis

This commonly arises in Little's area (from Kiesselbach's plexus) in old age. Epistaxis is caused by trauma, surgery, inflammatory and neoplastic conditions, a low atmospheric pressure with dry weather at high altitude, systemic disorders with a deranged coagulation profile, and non-steroidal anti-inflammatory drug and anticoagulant overdose. Osler–Weber–Rendu disease and arteriosclerosis lead to uncontrollable bleeding.

## Snoring and Sleep Apnoea

Snoring, obesity, diabetes and cardiovascular and cerebrovascular diseases may be associated with sleep apnoea, in which there is a cessation of airflow for more than 10 seconds. There may be an identifiable cause of nasal obstruction such as a polyp or septal deviation.

## THE PHARYNX

## Congenital Abnormalities

A bifid uvula is the most common malformation in this area, probably constituting a minor degree of cleft palate. Congenital strictures of the pharynx may cause speech difficulties or dysphagia.

## Pharyngitis

### Acute Pharyngitis

Acute pharyngitis may be due to bacterial, viral or candidal infection or result from non-infectious causes (allergy, gastric reflux, smoking or chemical fumes). Group A beta-haemolytic streptococcal infection presents with tonsillopharyngeal palatal petechiae, tender cervical lymphadenopathy, fever, purulent exudates in the tonsillar crypts and a 'sandpaper rash'. Viral infection presents with sneezing, rhinorrhoea or conjunctivitis. **Vincent's angina** is an acute ulcerative infection of the tonsils spreading to the oropharynx that is associated with a high fever and a grey membranous slough; it occurs in overcrowded conditions in debilitated, malnourished people. A number of organisms have been implicated, including a spirochaete.

**Diphtheria**, due to *Corynebacterium diphtheriae* infection, presents with a sore throat, malaise, pyrexia, cervical lymphadenopathy and a grey-white membrane covering the pharynx. The pharyngeal wall bleeds on separation of the membrane and may obstruct the upper airway. Candida may cause painless, white patches (pseudomembranous lesions) on the pharynx, and removal of the whitish patches leave an erythematous ulcer. It is seen following prolonged systemic antibiotic treatment, after radiotherapy or in immunocompromised individuals.

**Herpes simplex** may cause painful papulovesicular lesions, ulceration, tonsillopharyngeal exudates and lesions on the lips and face. **Infectious mononucleosis**, caused by the Epstein–Barr virus, is also known as glandular fever, or as 'kissing disease' as transmission is via the saliva. It presents with tender cervical lymphadenopathy along with follicular tonsillitis with exudates and the formation of a false membrane.

### Chronic Pharyngitis

Chronic pharyngitis is caused by chronic irritation (smoking, dusty working environments, acid reflux, allergic postnasal drip and post tonsillectomy).

Primary pharyngeal tuberculosis is rare and may be seen in children; it affects the tonsils, adenoids and cervical lymph nodes. Secondary tuberculosis is mainly due to coughing up heavily infected sputum. It presents as multiple, shallow ulcers or widespread miliary tuberculosis of the pharynx.

In the primary stage of syphilis, a chancre develops over the tonsils as a papule and then breaks down into an ulcer with indurated margins. In the secondary stage, syphilitic ulcers are 'serpiginous' or 'snail track' in shape and covered with a whitish-grey membrane, which on scraping has a non-bleeding pink base. In the tertiary stage, syphilitic gumma formation results in a firm, red swelling of the posterior pharyngeal wall or palate. Tissue destruction may result in perforation of the soft palate, regurgitation and changes in the voice.

Leprosy, sarcoidosis and Wegener's granulomatosis are rare causes of painless pharyngeal ulceration. The inflammatory masses produced in scleroma may involve the nasopharynx and palate, producing nasal obstruction.

## Globus Pharyngeus

This mainly affects women in middle age and has a functional cause. It presents as a lump in the throat on swallowing saliva rather than swallowing food or fluid. It may be associated with gastro-oesophageal reflux, increased upper oesophageal sphincter pressure or an inferior constrictor strain swallow because of irritation from the lingual tonsil/epiglottis area and increased muscle tension.

## Tonsillitis and Adenoidal Hypertrophy

### Acute and Chronic Tonsillitis

Acute tonsillitis results from group A haemolytic streptococcal infection. Sore throat, earache and difficulty swallowing are common complaints. Most cases resolve spontaneously, but some give rise to a peritonsillar abscesses, rheumatic fever, otitis media or chronic tonsillitis.

Chronic tonsillitis (**Figure 24.9**) represents a chronic inflammatory hypertrophy causing a persistent sore throat, odynophagia, a chronic cough, cervical lymphadenopathy and problems from blockage of the Eustachian tube.

### Peritonsillar Abscess (Quinsy)

A quinsy is an abscess lying between the capsule of the tonsil and the lateral pharyngeal wall. It causes a high pyrexia, progressive pain in the throat, dysphagia to solids followed by liquids, otalgia, drooling of saliva, a plummy voice and recent-onset trismus. It

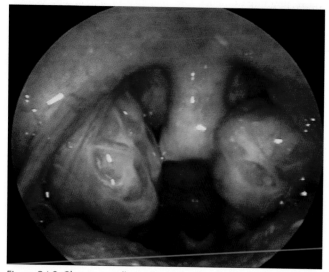

Figure 24.9 Chronic tonsillitis. (Courtesy of Dr Arpit Sharma.)

may be visible in the soft palate, above a hyperaemic, medially displaced tonsil and tender upper jugulodiagastric nodes.

## Adenoids

Adenoids are hypertrophied, nasopharyngeal tonsils. They may cause nasal obstruction resulting in breathing through the mouth, crowding of the front teeth, a toneless voice and nostrils with a pinched appearance. Eustachian tube obstruction causes serous otitis media leading to conductive deafness. An egg-white plug of mucus visible behind the uvula is diagnostic. Spontaneous regression usually occurs during adolescence.

## Parapharyngeal Abscess

A parapharyngeal abscess lies on either side between the pharynx and the parotid gland, and extends from the skull base to the greater cornu of the hyoid bone. The most common causes are tonsillitis, quinsy and dental infection due to gram-negative aerobic infection. Intraoral swellings behind the tonsil, fluctuant abscess in the neck and torticollis are salient features.

## Retropharyngeal Abscess

An abscess lies in the potential space between the buccopharyngeal and prevertebral fascia. Acutely, the condition may be caused by suppuration of the retropharyngeal lymph nodes or be secondary to penetration by a foreign body, the site then becoming infected. This usually occurs in the infant and is manifested as fever, neck stiffness, breathing and suckling difficulties. Spontaneous rupture of the abscess may cause death due to aspiration.

Tuberculosis of the retropharyngeal nodes or spread from tuberculous involvement of the cervical vertebrae may give rise to a chronic retropharyngeal abscess. The collection is effectively a 'cold abscess' and presents with dysphagia, cervical adenitis or mediastinitis. A plain lateral radiograph shows a loss of the normal curvature of the cervical spine with a soft tissue bulge in front of the spine. On imaging, the parapharyngeal space is displaced from posteromedially to anterolaterally.

## Parapharyngeal Tumours

These are rare tumours, the majority of which are benign. Neoplasms of the deep lobe of the parotid gland are the most common prestyloid tumours, whereas neurogenic tumours followed by paragangliomas are the most common poststyloid tumours. Malignant tumours are mainly direct extensions from the nasopharynx, tonsil, parotid and oral cavity. Common metastatic tumours are from the nasopharynx, thyroid and breast. Large parapharyngeal tumours may present with neck swelling, dysphagia, otalgia, trismus due to pterygoid muscle involvement and obstructive sleep apnoea. On examination, there is an oropharyngeal bulge with lower cranial nerve palsies (cranial nerves IX, X and XI at the jugular foramen, in addition to the XIIth cranial nerve) and a middle ear effusion.

## Pharyngeal Tumours

### Benign Tumours

Benign tumours are uncommon. Transsphenoidal meningoencephaloceles, Rathke's pouch remnants and congenital gliomas are benign congenital nasopharyngeal lesions that occur due to defective fusion of the base of the skull. Adenoiditis, nasopharyngeal tuberculosis and a Thornwaldt's cyst may present as acquired lesions.

### Malignant Tumours

Squamous cell carcinoma is most the common tumour arising in the pharynx. Adenocarcinoma, lymphoma (non-Hodgkin's large B cell type-oropharyngeal tumour), salivary malignancy and sarcoma occur less commonly.

### Carcinoma of the Nasopharynx

This is associated with the Epstein–Barr virus, being of Chinese race and certain environmental factors, such as occupational exposure and diets containing salty fish (nitrosamines). It presents with cervical lymphadenopathy, epistaxis, obstruction and a postnasal drip. On posterior rhinoscopy, a nasopharyngeal mass may be visible.

The tumour may cause symptoms from local invasion. A combination of such features comprises **Trotter's triad:** conductive deafness due to Eustachian tube invasion, pain on the side of the head due to invasion of the trigeminal nerve, and unilateral elevation and fixity of the soft palate. Invasion of the orbit and paralysis of the IInd, IVth and VIth cranial nerves may occur. Jugular foramen syndrome, with paralysis of the IXth, Xth and XIth cranial nerves, presents along with nasal obstruction and epistaxis.

### Carcinoma of the Oropharynx

A sore throat, dysphagia, blood in the saliva, enlarged cervical nodes, referred otalgia and altered speech and swallowing may be the presenting symptoms, and are classically seen in elderly men who smoke and show alcohol addiction. If the patient is a young man without a history of addiction, human papillomavirus is the likely aetiology.

### Carcinoma of the Laryngopharynx and Hypopharynx

These may cause a 'foreign body sensation', referred otalgia, dysphagia and stridor. Bilateral cervical lymphadenopathy, a poorly differentiated tumour, thyroid gland invasion and distant metastases are the peculiarities of hypopharyngeal cancer. Indirect laryngoscopy shows pooling of the saliva in hypopharyngeal tumours (Jackson's sign). Laryngeal crepitus is absent (Bocca's sign) in advanced tumours. Widening of the laryngeal framework suggests spread beyond the larynx.

Post-cricoid carcinoma presents with dysphagia, but is distinct from the other squamous malignancies of these regions in that it almost exclusively affects women (Figure 24.10). Plummer–Vinson (Paterson–Kelly) syndrome predisposes to the development of post-cricoid carcinoma. There is a relationship with iron deficiency, angular stomatitis, glossitis and koilonychia. Pyridoxine deficiency, abnormal tryptophan metabolism and gastrectomy are also associated. Dysphagia for solids and later liquids develops as a result of a chronic, atrophic inflammation of the cricopharyngeal region and concentric stenosis along with a web.

## Pharyngeal Pouch

Pharyngeal pouches can be congenital or acquired. Posterior herniation of the pharyngeal mucosa at Killian's dehiscence (the area between the thyropharyngeal and cricopharyngeal parts of

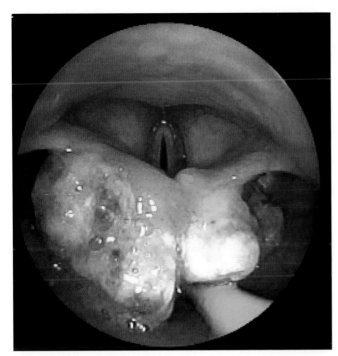

Figure 24.10 Post-cricoid cancer.

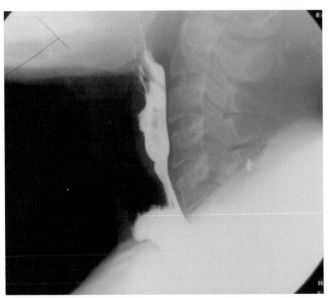

Figure 24.11 A Zenker's diverticulum. (Courtesy of Dr Jyoti Dabholkar.)

the inferior constrictor muscle) is called a Zenker's diverticulum (**Figure 24.11**). This may occur due to an anatomical weakness, spasm of the cricopharyngeus muscle or incoordination of the pharyngeal muscles. It may be associated with gastro-oesophageal reflux or a lower oesophageal carcinoma.

Patients are usually elderly and malnourished, and complain of a long-standing dysphagia and regurgitation of undigested food. The lesion may gurgle and empty on pressure (Bryce's sign). Patients may present with pulmonary complications due to aspiration, including pneumonia, lung abscess, bronchiectasis or lung collapse. Rarely, a carcinoma may develop in a long-standing pouch.

## THE LARYNX

### Congenital Abnormalities

Complete occlusion of the larynx by a laryngeal web results in a stillbirth; lesser obstruction presents with stridor at or soon after birth, depending on the size and location of the web. Laryngeal cysts, subglottic haemangiomas and laryngomalacia cause reduction of the laryngeal inlet. Unilateral vocal cord palsy presents with hoarseness and aspiration, but bilateral paralysis presents mainly with stridor. Laryngeal clefts, tracheo-oesophageal fistulas and vascular anomalies give rise to dysphagia. Congenital subglottic stenosis and post-intubation stenosis also lead to laryngeal obstruction. Infants with cri-du-chat syndrome (trisomy 5) develop a high-pitched cat-like cry due to developmental abnormalities in the larynx.

### Laryngocoele

A laryngocoele is an elongation of the laryngeal vestibule that is typically seen in elderly men and is related to occupations involving forced expiration (e.g. glassblowers and trumpet players). An internal laryngocoele is confined to the framework of the larynx, whereas an external laryngocoele passes through the thyrohyoid membrane, probably via the points of entry of the superior laryngeal nerve and artery; the two types are sometimes combined.

Lesions present with dysphagia, hoarseness and an expanding swelling in the neck on coughing, and are sometimes associated with carcinoma (**Figure 24.12**) of the larynx. The swelling can be compressed, and can be emptied by digital pressure, producing a hissing sound (Bryce's sign). Bacterial infection of a laryngocoele leads to a laryngopyocoele.

### Laryngitis

#### Acute Laryngitis

Acute laryngitis causes hoarseness, a sore throat, cervical lymphadenitis, breathlessness and a dry cough. In adults, viral infection resolves uneventfully. As well as upper respiratory

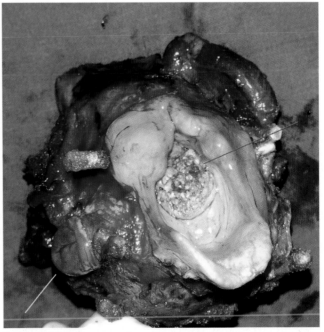

Figure 24.12 A laryngocoele with transglottic cancer.

tract infection, gastro-oesophageal reflux, inhalation of chemical fumes, lung infections, smoking and alcohol are also associated with laryngitis.

In children, upper respiratory tract infections produce a more pronounced obstruction of the subglottic area because of the greater quantity of surrounding lymphoid tissue. These conditions present with acute biphasic stridor and a barking cough, the most common being acute laryngotracheobronchitis (viral 'croup'). This usually occurs in the 1–2 years age group and is the result of infection with parainfluenza virus, respiratory syncytial virus or rhinovirus. Adult croup is rare but can be seen in immunocompromised individuals. A frontal X-ray shows narrowing of the subglottic airway (the church steeple sign).

A serious form of this condition is called acute epiglottitis. This is caused by *Haemophilus influenzae* and tends to affect 2–3-year-old old boys. The children are unwell with a high fever, tachycardia, dysphagia, odynophagia, cervical lymphadenopathy, drooling of saliva, a tender larynx and an acute onset of stridor. They are anxious, sitting and leaning forwards (the tripod sign). There is a danger of life-threatening upper airway obstruction; this may be precipitated by inspecting the throat and may warrant rapid intubation. A lateral radiograph shows the swollen epiglottis (the thumb sign) and absence of the deep vallecula (the vallecula sign).

### Pertussis/Whooping Cough

Pertussis mainly affects infants and is caused by *Bordetella pertussis*. It is a communicable disease. The child presents initially with a runny nose and fever, and later develops a prolonged acute spasmodic cough known as a 'whooping cough'.

### Diphtheria

Diphtheria presents with a sore throat, fever, nasal discharge and cervical lymphadenopathy. On examination, a grey-white inflammatory membrane is seen to involve the vocal cords. Progressive stridor and croup may be seen. This is particularly dangerous in young children because it can lead to respiratory distress.

### Chronic Laryngitis

Chronic laryngitis produces persisting hoarseness and cough after chronic exposure to irritants. It is graded according to the presence of erythema, diffuse oedema, a granular and ulcerated mucosa and granuloma formation. Radiation-induced chronic laryngitis is related to the dose of and response to the radiotherapy.

Tuberculous laryngitis usually results from infected sputum. The posterior portion of the larynx tends to be involved, having a nodular ulcerated appearance (**Figure 24.13**). There is impaired adduction of the cords and they appear 'moth-eaten'. A turban-shaped epiglottis is present due to pseudo-oedema. Untreated infection leads to stenosis and cord fixity.

Syphilis may also affect the larynx – in the secondary stage as erythematous papules, and in the tertiary stage as painless nodular infiltrates. The most common laryngeal finding is a gumma of the epiglottis, but diffuse infiltration may occur. Leprosy may result in cartilaginous destruction, scarring and stenosis with stridor due to vocal weakness. Sarcoidosis and Wegener's granulomatosis lead to inflammation and a granulomatous ulcer over the subglottis.

### Mycotic Infection

Mycotic infection of the larynx can occur in immunocompromised individuals and is mainly caused by *Candida* and

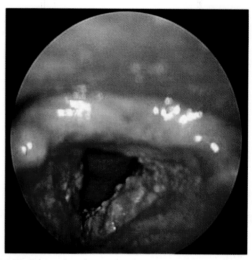

Figure 24.13 Tuberculous laryngitis. (Courtesy of Dr Hetal Marfatia.)

*Aspergillus*. It presents with curdy, white patch on the mucosa with erythema and oedema. It is necessary to rule out coexisting pulmonary mycotic infection.

## Benign Vocal Cord Lesions

A variety of benign lesions may be encountered:

- 'Singer's nodes' may result from excessive use of the voice (**Figure 24.14**). On indirect laryngoscopy, the nodes appear as small nodules (less than 3 mm in diameter) at the junction of the anterior third and posterior two-thirds of the cord, giving an 'hour-glass' appearance.
- At the free edge of the vocal cord, polyps (larger than 3 mm) (**Figure 24.15**) may present due to vocal abuse.
- *Contact ulcers* may take the form of depressions over the vocal processes and are thought to be the result of the hammering of one vocal process of the arytenoid cartilage against the other (**Figure 24.16**).
- Lesions may also occur due to the mechanical trauma of intubation (in women), secondary to hyperfunction (in men), as a result of reflux, after surgery or post radiotherapy.
- *Reinke's oedema* may present as bilateral, chronic, diffuse oedema of the membranous part of the vocal cords. It may result from allergy, reflux, inflammation or hypothyroidism.
- A *laryngeal web* may present as congenital or post-traumatic acquired lesions. A child with a congenital web may present with cyanosis, stridor, feeding problems, breathlessness and hoarseness.
- A *vocal sulcus* presents as a mucosal groove or fold.
- *Relapsing polychondritis* is an autoimmune, chronic inflammatory process that presents with dysphagia and pain in the throat.
- Primary or secondary *amyloidosis* may deposit submucosal amyloid in a diffuse pattern.

## Laryngeal Tumours
### Benign Neoplasms

Recurrent respiratory papillomatosis is the most common neoplasm seen in children and is caused by human papilloma virus types 6 and 11 (**Figure 24.17**). Fibromas, chondromas and angiomas can also occur. The usual symptom is hoarseness.

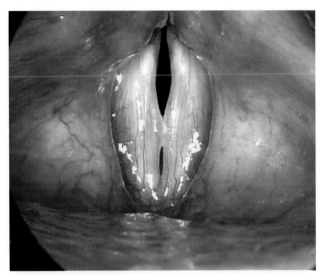

Figure 24.14 Singer's nodes. (Courtesy of Dr Hetal Marfatia.)

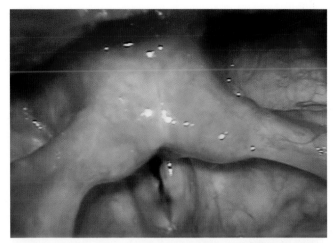

Figure 24.16 A contact ulcer. (Courtesy of Dr Hetal Marfatia.)

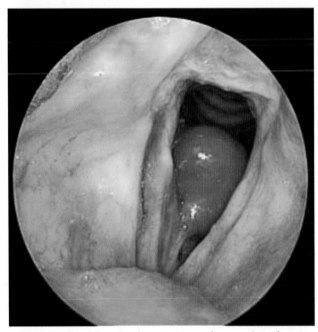

Figure 24.15 A vocal cord polyp. (Courtesy of Dr Hetal Marfatia.)

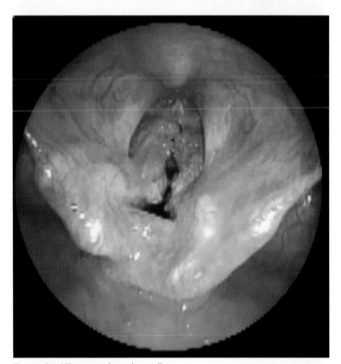

Figure 24.17 A vocal cord papilloma.

## Leukoplakia

Leukoplakia, or hyperkeratosis of the larynx, is a premalignant condition that appears as raised white patches on the vocal cords. It may appear due to reflux or smoking.

## Carcinoma of Larynx

The most common site for glottic carcinoma is the true vocal cords (Figure 24.18). Rarely, the carcinoma is subglottic and involves the undersurface of the cords.

Glottic carcinoma invades locally but does not show early nodal metastases because of the paucity of lymphatics. These lesions tend to present with early hoarseness and stridor. Subglottic lesions are also mainly locally invasive but tend to present late. The tumour may initially be concealed when the cords are viewed on indirect laryngoscopy. Bilateral cervical lymph node metastases are much more likely in supraglottic tumours as a result of the better lymphatic drainage (Figures 24.19).

## Referred Otalgia

Unexplained ear pain must raise the suspicion of laryngeal or oropharyngeal conditions (neoplastic or inflammatory). The laryngeal mucosa is innervated by the internal branch of the superior laryngeal nerve. The pain pathway goes via the jugular ganglion at the jugular foramen, and may be referred to the auricular branch of the vagus (Arnold's nerve), which supplies the posterior wall of the external auditory canal. The oropharynx is innervated by the glossopharyngeal nerve. The afferent nerve goes via the petrosal ganglion at the jugular foramen. Ear pain is deep seated, and the efferent nerve is the tympanic nerve (Jacobson's nerve).

## Paralysis of the Larynx

The cause of this condition is mostly unknown. Lesions of the vagus and superior or recurrent laryngeal nerves, malignancies of the cervical structures, surgical injury to the laryngeal nerve (e.g. in thyroidectomy) and peripheral neuritis from chemical and bacterial toxins may all result in paralysis.

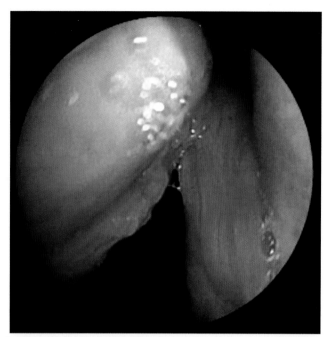

Figure 24.18 Early glottic cancer.

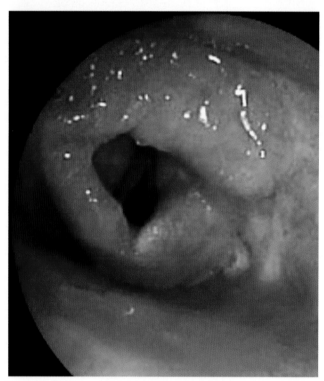

Figure 24.19 Cancer of the supraglottis (epiglottis).

In unilateral recurrent laryngeal nerve palsy, the patient may be asymptomatic if the active cord compensates, or hoarse if it does not. Paralysis may be seen in Ortner's syndrome due to enlargement of the left atrium (Figure 24.20). In bilateral recurrent laryngeal nerve palsy, there may still be some compensation but dyspnoea may result on exertion or with laryngitis. Superior laryngeal nerve palsy results in a low-pitched voice that tires easily. In combined lesions, the voice may be very weak and food aspiration may be a problem. On laryngoscopy, the cords are seen to be lying in the 'cadaveric' (intermediate) position. In an isolated recurrent laryngeal nerve palsy, the affected cord lies near to the midline.

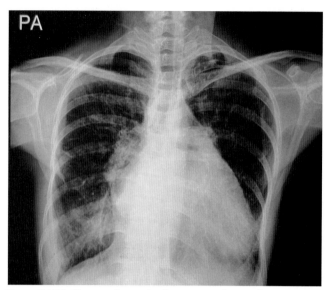

Figure 24.20 Chest radiograph showing cardiomegaly in Ortner's syndrome. (Courtesy of Dr Arpit Sharma.)

## Laryngeal Trauma

- Laryngeal injury can occur due to a blunt or penetrating injury.
- Low-velocity blunt trauma from a blow or strangulation may result in hoarseness, dyspnoea, dysphagia and surgical emphysema in severe case. High-velocity trauma causes calcified laryngeal cartilages to fracture, which may lead to fatal subglottic oedema and airway obstruction. Separation of the trachea and cricoid cartilage can lead to death.
- Isolated laryngeal penetrating injuries are common at the thyrohyoid or cricothyroid membrane. They may present with dyspnoea and haemorrhage.
- Cricothyroid membrane injuries mainly lead to surgical emphysema with mediastinum and respiratory distress.

### Burns

Thermal and chemical burns may result in an oedematous larynx and upper airway obstruction. Burns may heal by fibrosis with stricture formation and lead to progressive dysphagia.

### Key Points

- Different infective and neoplastic pharyngeal conditions should be differentiated from globus pharyngeus, which is a functional disorder.
- Trotter's triad, which is seen in carcinoma of the nasopharynx, comprises conductive deafness, pain on the side of the head and a unilateral palsy of the soft palate.
- Plummer–Vinson syndrome predisposes to the development of post-cricoid carcinoma, which is characterized by iron deficiency, angular stomatitis, glossitis and koilonychia.
- A posterior herniation between the thyropharyngeal and cricopharyngeal parts of the inferior constrictor muscle is known as a Zenker's diverticulum.
- Laryngeal and oropharyngeal cancers can cause referred otalgia.
- Malignancies are usually associated with tobacco and alcohol, but there is a rising association with human papillomavirus infection.

## SBAs

1. A 45-year-old obese woman has been admitted to the cardiothoracic department with palpitations, chest pain, dyspnoea on exertion and orthopnoea. She gives a history of a change in her voice over the past 2 weeks. Indirect laryngoscopy reveals a left vocal cord palsy with no lesions in the larynx and pharynx. There is no obvious swelling in the neck. Which one of the following symptoms is most likely to be responsible for this lady's condition?:
   a  Churg–Strauss syndrome
   b  Mendelson's syndrome
   c  Jervell and Lange-Nielson's syndrome
   d  Ortner's syndrome
   e  Stickler's syndrome

**Answer**

d  **Ortner's syndrome.** In Ortner's syndrome, left atrial enlargement produces a unilateral left recurrent laryngeal nerve palsy. Churg–Strauss syndrome is an autoimmune condition with vasculitis and atopy. Mendelson's syndrome is chemical aspiration pneumonitis during anaesthesia. Jervell and Lange-Nielson's syndrome is an autosomal recessive disorder that is a type of long QT syndrome with severe bilateral sensorineural hearing loss. Stickler's syndrome is a hereditary progressive collagenopathy characterized by facial abnormalities, ocular problems, hearing loss and joint problems.

2. A 30-year-old woman presents with progressive dysphagia to solids that has progressed over the last few months. Examination reveals that she is anaemic and has angular stomatitis and spoon-shaped nails. Which one of the following types of cancer is most likely to be responsible for this?:
   a  Post-cricoid cancer
   b  Vocal cord cancer
   c  Oropharyngeal cancer
   d  Oral cancer
   e  Nasopharyngeal cancer

**Answer**

a  **Post-cricoid cancer.** This presents with dysphagia and almost exclusively affects women. Paterson–Kelly (Plummer–Vinson) syndrome predisposes to it. There is a relationship with iron deficiency anaemia (pallor), angular stomatitis (fissures at the angles of the mouth), glossitis and koilonychia (spoon-shaped nails). Dysphagia for solids and later liquids develops as a result of a chronic, atrophic inflammation of the cricopharyngeal region and concentric stenosis, along with a web.

3. A 10-year-old child has presented to his general practitioner with left-sided chest pain. The history is of a recent onset of joint pain, a small swelling over his right wrist joint and a red rash over his trunk. He also had a sore throat 3 weeks ago. Which one of the following is the most likely diagnosis?:
   a  Acute coronary syndrome
   b  Rheumatic fever
   c  Myocardial infarction
   d  Osteoarthritis
   e  Carpal tunnel syndrome

**Answer**

b  **Rheumatic fever.** This may follow acute infection of throat with group A beta-haemolytic streptococci. It affects children 1–3 weeks after a sore throat. There may be upwardly migrating polyarthritis, subcutaneous, painless, rheumatoid nodules lying over bony prominences and a reddish macular rash called known as erythema marginatum, which has a snake like appearance. Carditis may also develop, manifesting as an apical systolic murmur due to mitral regurgitation, or an early diastolic murmur due to aortic regurgitation following valvulitis. Myocarditis may impair cardiac function, and the accompanying pericarditis may cause chest pain and a pericardial rub.

## EMQs

**1.** For each of the following patients with malignancy of the nose and throat select the most likely diagnosis from the list below. Each option may be used once, more than once or not at all:

    **1** Squamous cell carcinoma
    **2** Mixed cellularity type Hodgkin's lymphoma
    **3** Non-Hodgkin's large B cell type lymphoma
    **4** Epstein–Barr virus infection
    **5** Human papillomavirus
    **6** Melanoma
    **7** Human immunodeficiency virus infection
    **8** Adenoid cystic carcinoma
    **9** Aesthesioneuroblastoma

**a** A 28-year-old man presents with the chief complaint of 2 months of dysphagia. Examination reveals the presence of an oropharyngeal mass 2 cm in diameter, and a 3 cm upper jugulodiagastric lymph node on the right side. He is non-smoker and has an average alcohol intake.

**b** A 40-year-old man from China is complaining of bilateral neck nodes, pain on the right side of his head, blockage of his right ear and nasal regurgitation for the last month. On examination, a nasopharyngeal mass is visualized.

**c** A 38-year-old lady comes to the clinic with a history of tonsillar enlargement and slight pain while swallowing for which she underwent tonsillectomy. The histopathology is suggestive of lymphoma.

### Answers

**a  5  Human papillomavirus.** *In a young man without any history of addiction, this pictures suggests a diagnosis of oropharyngeal cancer caused by human papillomavirus infection.*

**b  4  Epstein–Barr virus infection.** *This occurs particularly in Chinese individuals and the history may shown infection with Epstein–Barr virus. It often presents with cervical lymphadenopathy or epistaxis, obstruction and a postnasal drip. A nasopharyngeal mass may be visible on posterior rhinoscopy. It may cause symptoms from local invasion. Trotter's triad is the combination of conductive deafness, pain in the side of the head, and elevation and unilateral fixity of the soft palate.*

**c  3  Non-Hodgkin's large B cell type lymphoma.** *This is the most common type of lymphoma involving the tonsil.*

**2.** For each of the following descriptions, select the most appropriate physical or radiological sign from the list below. Each option may be used once, more than once or not at all:

    **1** Tripod sign
    **2** Church steeple sign
    **3** Bryce's sign
    **4** Thumb sign
    **5** Jackson's sign
    **6** Bocca's sign

**a** A 2-year-old child is admitted with an upper respiratory tract infection with a cough, a change in his voice and fever. He developed biphasic stridor and barking cough for 1 day. A frontal X-ray shows narrowing of the subglottic airway.

**b** A 60-year-old man has presented with a right-sided neck swelling that becomes prominent on coughing. He also gives a history of loss of weight, halitosis and regurgitation after eating. He can empty the swelling by digital pressure.

**c** A 38-year-old man presents with dysphagia, neck swelling and a change in his voice. Indirect laryngoscopy shows pooling of saliva, mainly on the right side.

### Answers

**a  2  Church steeple sign.** *This sign appears due to narrowing at the subglottic level, which is seen in viral croup.*

**b  3  Bryce's sign.** *This is seen with a laryngocoele. The swelling can be compressed and emptied with a hissing sound by digital pressure.*

**c  5  Jackson's sign.** *Indirect laryngoscopy shows pooling of the saliva with hypopharyngeal tumours.*

# Salivary Glands

Sudhir Nair and Shivakumar Thiagarajan

## LEARNING OBJECTIVES

- To understand and recognize the symptoms of common pathological conditions affecting the salivary glands
- To be able to identify and explain the signs seen in conditions commonly affecting the salivary glands

## NON-NEOPLASTIC CONDITIONS

### Congenital Disorders

**Agenesis** or **aplasia** (Table 25.1) of one or more major salivary glands is uncommon. Depending on the number of glands that are absent, the spectrum of symptoms can range from asymptomatic to severe xerostomia.

An **ectopic salivary gland** occurs when normal salivary gland tissue is found in a location other than in its normal anatomical locations due to a developmental malformation; this is a rare phenomenon. Common locations include the periparotid nodes (intranodal), the soft tissue of face and neck, the middle ear and the tonsil (extranodal).

### Infection
#### Viral Infections

**Mumps** is a contagious disease caused by a viral infection that produces painful swelling of predominantly the parotid glands, and affects children aged between 4 and 12 years. There is general malaise followed by a bilateral or unilateral painful parotid swelling, with fever and arthralgia. The swelling spreads down the neck, giving a double chin appearance (Figure 25.1). Rarely, there may be associated orchitis, meningoencephalitis, pancreatitis, thyroiditis or sensorineural hearing loss. In most cases, however, the condition subsides uneventfully.

**HIV-associated salivary gland disease** occurs in 4–8 per cent of HIV-positive patients and predominantly affects the parotid glands. The major manifestation is unilateral or often bilateral cystic parotid enlargement. These cysts are painless and soft, and can be single or multiple. The cysts gradually increase in size and can cause severe cosmetic deformity.

#### Bacterial Infections

**Acute bacterial sialadenitis** – This is commonly seen in elderly patients and those with poor oral hygiene. Other predisposing

Table 25.1 Disorders of the salivary glands

| Category | Examples |
|---|---|
| Developmental | Agenesis/aplasia<br>Aberrant salivary gland |
| Inflammatory | Sialolithiasis<br>Sialoadenitis<br>– Bacterial (acute bacterial, tuberculosis, actinomycosis, cat-scratch disease)<br>– Viral (mumps) |
| Autoimmune | Sjögren's syndrome<br>Mikulicz's syndrome<br>Sarcoidosis |
| Metabolic disorders | Diabetes (uncontrolled)<br>Alcoholism<br>Malnutrition<br>Obesity |
| Benign neoplasms | Pleomorphic adenoma<br>Monomorphic adenoma<br>Warthin's tumour<br>Oncocytoma<br>Lymphoepithelial lesion<br>Benign cysts |
| Malignant neoplasms | Mucoepidermoid carcinoma<br>Adenoid cystic carcinoma<br>Acinic cell tumour<br>Malignant mixed tumour<br>Squamous cell carcinoma<br>Adenocarcinoma<br>Undifferentiated carcinoma<br>Lymphoma |

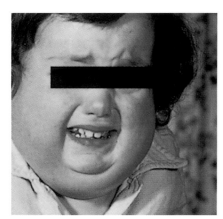

Figure 25.1 Mumps giving rise to bilateral facial oedema over the infected parotid glands.

Table 25.2 Drainage of the salivary glands

| Salivary gland | Name of the duct | Location of the duct opening |
|---|---|---|
| Parotid | Stenson's duct | Opposite the crown of the second maxillary molar |
| Submandibular | Wharton's duct | On either side of the lingual frenulum |
| Sublingual | Via short independent ducts or Wharton's duct | Floor of the mouth |

factors include dehydration, general debilitation and stricturing or stones in Stensen's duct (Table 25.2). Typically, there is a sudden, painful swelling of one of the parotid glands with trismus, dysphagia and fever. An intraoral inspection of Stensen's duct may reveal the discharge of purulent or particulate saliva. Less commonly, the submandibular gland is also affected.

**Parotid abscess** – Acute infection may lead to abscess formation that produces throbbing pain along with erythema and swelling over the parotid region (Figure 25.2). Unlike abscess of the other sites, fluctuation is a very late feature since, to become fluctuant, the abscess has to breach the strong parotid fascia covering the parotid.

**Chronic sialadenitis** – Obstruction or narrowing of Stensen's or Wharton's duct by a calculus or stricture may cause chronic sialadenitis of the corresponding gland. The symptoms are recurrent swelling and aching of the gland, especially before eating.

## Sialolithiasis

Calculus formation commonly occurs in the submandibular duct (see Figure 23.30). The characteristic features are pain and swelling of the gland before and during meals. Pressing the gland may release foul-tasting purulent saliva. The symptoms can be elicited by giving the patient lemon juice. Examination of the duct orifice may reveal an inflamed duct ampulla exuding pus, or occasionally a stone in the duct orifice. There is often a pattern of remission and relapse over days or weeks as the stone moves in the duct; the stone may eventually pass.

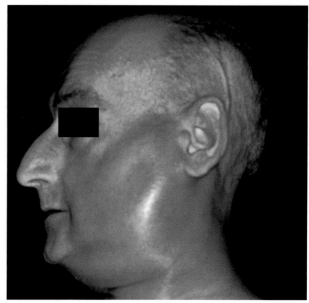

Figure 25.2 Parotid abscess in an ageing patient.

## Systemic and Metabolic Conditions Affecting the Salivary Glands (Table 25.3)

**Sjögren's syndrome** is a rare autoimmune condition affecting the salivary glands. It can occur in combination with other autoimmune connective tissue disorders (Figure 25.3) and may take many forms. Typical features are as follows:

- It is characterized by xerostomia and xerophthalmia.
- It takes two main forms:
  - Primary – with symptoms of only the eyes and mouth.
  - Secondary – associated with connective tissue disorders such as rheumatoid arthritis or systemic lupus erythematosus, as well as with eye and mouth symptoms.
- There is an association with an increased incidence of dental caries and infection (e.g. candidiasis).
- Also associated are dysgeusia or loss of taste and intermittent swelling of the gland.
- There is an increased risk of developing lymphoma (24 per cent).

Table 25.3 Bilateral parotid gland enlargement

| Category | Examples |
|---|---|
| Systemic/metabolic disease | Diabetes mellitus Sarcoidosis Alcoholism Malnutrition Eating disorder (bulimia) Sjögren's syndrome Mikulicz's syndrome Mucosa-associated lymphoid tissue lymphoma Sialosis Hypothyroidism HIV salivary gland disease |
| Benign tumours | Warthin's tumours |
| Malignant tumours | Acinic cell carcinoma |

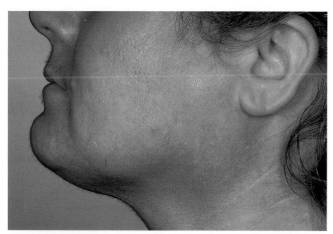

Figure 25.3 Sjögren's syndrome.

**Mikulicz's syndrome** affects both the salivary and the lacrimal glands. According to some authors, it is a variant of Sjögren's syndrome, but it is associated with sarcoidosis, lymphoma and other systemic disorders.

## NEOPLASTIC CONDITIONS

A number of benign and malignant tumours can affect both the major and minor salivary glands (Table 25.4).

### Benign Tumours

**Pleomorphic adenomas** (mixed salivary tumours) are the most common benign tumours of the parotid gland and usually present as firm, lobulated, painless swellings that gradually increase in size (**Figure 25.4**). Facial nerve and skin involvement may suggest malignant transformation, which occurs in 3–5 per cent of cases. Involvement of the deep lobe can push the tonsil medially (**Figure 25.5**). The key differential diagnosis is that of an enlarged preauricular lymph node. A useful feature in their distinction is mobility – the parotid gland, and tumours arising from it, is relatively fixed, whereas preauricular nodes usually occur outside the capsule of the gland and so are very mobile. The clinical features of parotid lesions are outlined in the Table 25.5.

**Adenolymphomas** (Warthin's tumours; **Figure 25.6**) are the second most common benign salivary tumours and are found exclusively in the parotid gland. They usually affects men in their 50s, forming a slow-growing, painless swelling over the angle of the jaw. The tumour surface is smooth and often soft in consistency, with well-defined margins. Bilateral involvement is seen in 10 per cent of cases.

Less common benign tumours include **monomorphic adenomas** and **oncocytomas**.

Table 25.4 Distribution of benign and malignant tumours in various salivary glands

| Salivary gland | Benign (%) | Malignant (%) |
| --- | --- | --- |
| Parotid | 80 | 20 |
| Submandibular | 60 | 40 |
| Sublingual and minor salivary glands (most commonly, soft palate) | 20 | 80 |

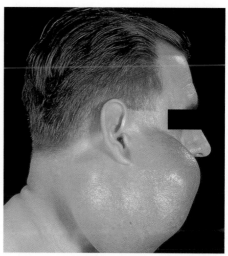

Figure 25.4 A large, mixed parotid tumour.

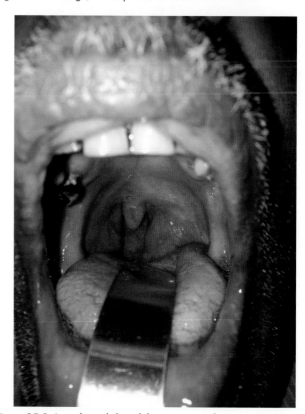

Figure 25.5 An enlarged deep lobe in a parotid tumour. (Courtesy of Pankaj Chaturvedi MS, Professor of Surgical Oncology, Tata Memorial Hospital, Mumbai, India.)

### Malignant Tumours

Malignant tumours of the salivary gland can be categorized as low-risk, high-risk or intermediate-risk tumours (**Tables 25.5** and **25.6**). It is frequently not possible to establish the cell type derivation and whether or not the tumour is malignant until cytology is available. Lymph node metastases are very common with high-grade tumours and require postoperative adjuvant radiotherapy. Typically, malignant tumours produce indistinct, rapidly growing masses and malignant cervical lymphadenopathy. For the submandibular gland, numbness of the anterior two-thirds of the tongue from lingual nerve infiltration is diagnostic,

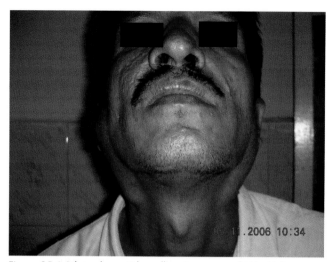

Figure 25.6 Bilateral parotid swelling in a case of Warthin's tumour. (Courtesy of Pankaj Chaturvedi MS, Professor of Surgical Oncology, Tata Memorial Hospital, Mumbai, India.)

Table 25.5 Clinical features suggestive of parotid tumours

| Type of parotid tumour | Clinical features suggestive of this tumour |
|---|---|
| Benign parotid neoplasm | Slow growing painless swelling<br>Raised ear lobule<br>Curtain sign – the swelling cannot be lifted above the zygoma because the superior attachment of the strong parotid fascia is on the zygoma<br>Deviation of the uvula and pharyngeal wall towards the midline, indicating involvement of the deep lobe |
| Malignant parotid tumour | Rapid increase in size<br>Hard consistency<br>Facial nerve palsy<br>Skin ulceration<br>Palpable neck nodes<br>Pain<br>Fixity to underlying structure |

Table 25.6 Common malignant tumours of the salivary glands

| Category | Examples |
|---|---|
| Low risk | Acinic cell carcinoma<br>Low grade mucoepidermoid carcinoma<br>Epithelial-myoepithelial carcinoma<br>Polymorphous low-grade adenocarcinoma<br>Low-grade salivary duct carcinoma<br>Oncocytic carcinoma |
| Intermediate risk | Intermediate-grade mucoepidermoid carcinoma |
| High risk | High-grade mucoepidermoid carcinoma<br>Adenoid cystic carcinoma<br>Sebaceous carcinoma<br>Mucinous adenocarcinoma<br>Carcinoma ex pleomorphic adenoma (high grade)<br>Carcinosarcoma |

whereas sublingual tumours may cause deviation of the tongue from invasion and fixation.

**Adenoid cystic carcinomas** are common malignant tumours affecting both the major and minor salivary glands. Perineural invasion is typically seen so the tumour is more commonly associated with a facial nerve palsy (**Figure 25.7**). This is the most common malignant tumour of the minor salivary gland.

**Mucoepidermoid carcinoma** (**Figures 25.8** and **25.9**) is the most common major salivary gland as well as parotid malignancy.

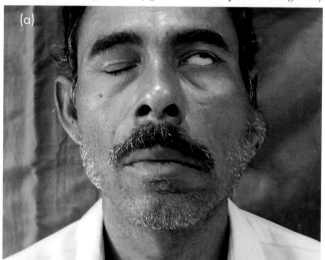

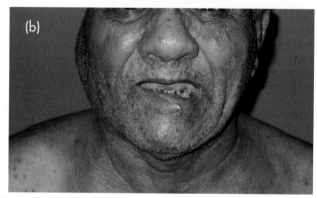

Figure 25.7 (a) A malignant tumour of the parotid causing a facial nerve palsy. (Courtesy of Shivkumar Thyagarajan MS, Assistant Professor, Malabar Cancer Center, Kerala, India.) (b) A mild mandibular nerve palsy.

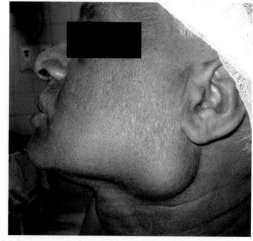

Figure 25.8 A mucoepidermoid carcinoma of the parotid.

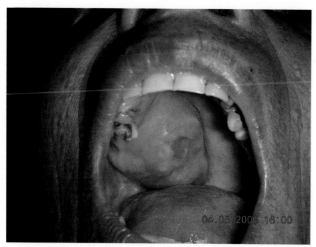

Figure 25.9 A mucoepidermoid tumour arising from a minor salivary gland in the hard palate. (Courtesy of Pankaj Chaturvedi MS, Professor of Surgical Oncology, Tata Memorial Hospital, Mumbai, India.)

It contains both mucus-secreting cells and epidermoid cells. The grade of the tumour is directly proportional to the epidermoid cell content.

**Acinic cell carcinomas** are low-grade malignant tumours that can affect the parotid glands bilaterally.

## SUBMANDIBULAR SALIVARY GLANDS

The submandibular gland lies near the inferior border of the mandible and has a deeper part that lies between the mylohyoid and hyoglossus muscles. The gland can therefore be palpated bimanually. This examination can also differentiate an enlarged submandibular salivary gland (**Figure 25.10**) from lymph nodes. As the lymph nodes are located superficial to the mylohyoid muscles, they are not palpable intraorally.

The submandibular glands are more prone to stone formation than the other salivary glands since they lie in a dependent position relative to the duct opening, encouraging stasis. Saliva from this gland also contains more mucus and calcium.

The sublingual glands lie just beneath the mucosa in the floor of the mouth and empty directly into the mouth or into the submandibular duct. These glands are not discretely palpable, nor are the duct openings usually visible.

**Mucoceles** are small cystic lesions that commonly occur after trauma and develop secondary to the blockage of a minor salivary gland duct.

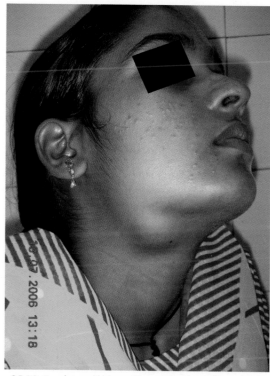

Figure 25.10 A submandibular salivary gland swelling. (Courtesy of Pankaj Chaturvedi MS, Professor of Surgical Oncology, Tata Memorial Hospital, Mumbai, India.)

### Key Points

- There are three pairs of major salivary gland and 300–400 minor salivary glands in the human body.
- The parotid is the largest salivary gland and the most commonly affected by the majority of pathological conditions.
- Sialolithiasis is more common in the submandibular gland.
- Malignant tumours of the parotid gland may involve the facial nerve and can lead to facial nerve palsy.
- Tumours arising in minor salivary glands are more often malignant.

PART 4 | HEAD AND NECK

## QUESTIONS

### SBAs

**1. Which one of the following parotid tumours commonly occurs in the lower portion (tail) of the parotid gland?:**
  a  Pleomorphic adenoma
  b  Mucoepidermoid tumour
  c  Warthin's tumour
  d  Lymphoma

**Answer**

*c Warthin's tumour. Warthin's tumour (papillary cystadenoma lymphomatosum) is a common benign tumor of the parotid gland with a very small malignant transformation rate. The tail of the parotid is the site most commonly involved.*

**2. A painful rapid enlargement with an appearance of facial nerve palsy in a long-standing parotid tumor is suggestive of which one of the following?:**
  a  Acute parotitis
  b  Carcinoma arising in a pleomorphic adenoma
  c  Retention cyst
  d  Lymphoma

**Answer**

*b Carcinoma arising in a pleomorphic adenoma. In this condition, malignant transformation causes a carcinoma to arise in the patient's long-standing pleomorphic adenoma. The appearance of a facial nerve palsy and rapid growth of the tumour are suggestive of this malignant transformation. Although acute parotitis can also cause sudden painful enlargement of the parotid gland, an associated facial nerve palsy is extremely rare. Parotid lymphomas are usually painless, progressively enlarging tumours with a very low incidence of facial nerve palsy.*

**3. All of the following statements regarding Frey's syndrome are true except which one?:**
  a  It is typically seen with malignant neoplasms of the parotid gland
  b  It is common after parotidectomy
  c  It occurs after trauma to the cervical sympathetic chain
  d  It can occur in diabetic neuropathy

**Answer**

*a It is typically seen with malignant neoplasms of the parotid gland, Frey's syndrome, also known as gustatory sweating, is commonly observed after parotidectomy or any trauma to the parotid region. It is believed to be due to aberrant regeneration of the injured parasympathetic fibres innervating the parotid gland.*

### EMQs

**1. For each of the following clinical conditions, select the site most commonly involved:**
  1  Minor salivary glands
  2  Sublingual gland
  3  Submandibular gland
  4  Parotid gland
  a  Calculus
  b  Tumour
  c  Retention cyst

**Answers**

*a  3 Submandibular gland.*

*b  4 Parotid gland.*

*c  2 Sublingual gland.*

**2. For each of the following glands, select the associated anatomical structure:**
  1  Wharton's duct
  2  Stensen's duct
  3  Hard palate
  4  Ducts of Rivinus
  a  Parotid gland
  b  Submandibular gland
  c  Sublingual gland
  d  Minor salivary glands

**Answers**

*a  2 Stensen's duct. The parotid duct (Stensen's duct) enters the oral cavity opposite the second upper molar tooth.*

*b  1 Wharton's duct. The submandibular duct (Wharton's duct) opens into floor of the mouth on both sides of lingual frenulum.*

*c  4 Ducts of Rivinus. The sublingual gland usually drains by multiple small ducts into the floor of mouth.*

*d  3 Hard palate. Minor salivary glands are present throughout the upper aerodigestive tract, with a greater concentration in the hard and soft palates.*

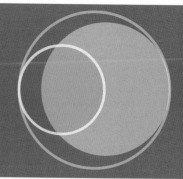

CHAPTER
26

# The Neck

Richa Vaish and Anil K. D'Cruz

## LEARNING OBJECTIVES

- To become familiar with common pathologies that occur in the neck
- To understand the relevance of the surgical triangles of the neck with respect to neck swelling
- To recognize the key features that will help in diagnosing neck swellings based on age at presentation, signs and symptoms

## INTRODUCTION

Swellings in the neck are a common surgical problem. As more than half the body's lymph nodes are located in this area, nodal enlargement is the most common pathology encountered in clinical practice. In addition, the neck contains many important anatomical structures and undergoes a complex embryological development, adding to the variety of swellings that may occur. The key to the diagnosis lies in differentiating nodal from non-nodal swellings. In addition, the neck is divided into well-established anatomical triangles (akin to the quadrants of the abdomen) that help the clinician form an accurate diagnosis.

The 'rule of 80' for neck swellings is that:

- 80 per cent of neck swellings are lateral;
- 80 per cent of lateral neck swellings are nodal;
- 80 per cent of swellings in those less than 40 years of age are inflammatory or congenital;
- 80 per cent of swellings in those over 40 years of age are malignant;
- 80 per cent of malignant swellings are squamous carcinoma.

## NODAL SWELLINGS

Nodes over 1 cm in size warrant investigation. Nodes smaller than this are rarely a cause for concern and are not investigated unless there is a high index of suspicion of pathology. The exception to this rule is supraclavicular nodes, which are investigated irrespective of size. In addition, the cut-off of size for jugulodigastric lymph nodes requiring evaluation is 1.5 cm.

The common and geographically specific important causes of lymphadenopathy are enumerated in **Table 26.1**.

Table 26.1 Causes of lymphadenopathy

| Causes | |
|---|---|
| **Inflammation** | |
| Acute | Infections of the upper respiratory tract |
| | Infections from other draining sites: scalp, lid, skin, parotid gland |
| | Specific infections: |
| | – Viral – infectious mononucleosis |
| | – Bacterial – diphtheria, actinomycosis |
| | – Parasitic – toxoplasmosis, leishmaniasis |
| | – Fungal – histoplasmosis |
| Chronic | Tuberculosis |
| | Sarcoidosis |
| | HIV |
| **Malignant** | |
| Haemopoietic and reticuloendothelial | Hodgkin's/non-Hodgkin's lymphoma |
| | Leukaemia |
| Metastatic | Upper aerodigestive tract |
| | Infraclavicular malignancy (usually the left supraclavicular node) |
| | Other draining sites: parotid, eye, scalp, skin, thyroid |
| **Immunological** | |
| | Rheumatoid arthritis |
| | Systemic lupus erythematosus |
| Miscellaneous | |
| | Kikuchi's disease |
| | Kimura's disease |
| | Rosai–Dorfman disease |
| | Castleman's disease |

PART 4 | HEAD AND NECK

## Diagnosis

The clinical history plays an important role in the diagnosis of neck swellings. A history of addiction to tobacco or alcohol suggests a malignancy of the upper aerodigestive tract. Constitutional symptoms are usually associated with chronic infections and lymphomas.

The consistency of the node aids in diagnosis. Inflammatory nodes are firm, malignant nodes are hard, lymphomatous nodes are rubbery, and cystic nodes are associated with caseation (tuberculosis, when the classical signs of inflammation are lacking) or abscess formation. Exceptions to this are large malignant nodes (secondary to necrosis), human papillomavirus-associated malignancies, and occasionally papillary thyroid cancer, which can be cystic (Figure 26.1).

Regional adenopathy (the involvement of a single anatomical area) is usually seen with localized pathologies, and generalized adenopathy (the involvement of three or more non-contiguous lymph node areas) is seen in chronic infections and reticuloendothelial malignancies.

## Acute Infective Lymphadenopathy

Lymph node enlargement is frequently associated with upper respiratory tract infections. **Tonsillitis** is a common paediatric condition that leads to enlargement of the jugulodigastric nodes with high-grade fever. It is caused by group A haemolytic streptococci.

**Infectious mononucleosis**, or glandular fever, presents as nodal enlargement in young adults that is associated with a sore throat, malaise and a membrane over the tonsil. It is also known as 'kissing disease' and is caused by Epstein–Barr virus.

**Diphtheria** is an important cause of cervical adenopathy in the paediatric age group. Although its incidence is decreasing with vaccination, the condition warrants timely diagnosis as advanced cases rapidly progress to respiratory distress and death. The classical presentation is a pseudomembrane over the tonsil with bull-neck lymphadenopathy.

**Actinomycosis** is an anaerobic infection caused by *Actinomyces israelii*, which is a commensal in the oral cavity. Infection usually occurs secondary to tooth extraction, trauma or poor oral hygiene. The common presentation is large abscess formation with lymphadenopathy.

**Toxoplasmosis** is caused by *Toxoplasma gondii*, an organism that infests via food contaminated with cat faeces or infested meat. **Leishmaniasis**, transmitted by the bite of the

sandfly, is characterized by skin ulcers with lymphadenopathy. **Histoplasmosis** is caused by *Histoplasma capsulatum*, which is found in soil contaminated with bird droppings. It is commonly associated with immunodeficiency syndrome. It may affect multiple organs and can mimic tuberculosis.

## Chronic Inflammatory Lymphadenopathy

**Tuberculosis** is the most common cause of chronic lymphadenopathy and is predominantly seen in the South-East Asian subcontinent. It is a granulomatous disease caused by *Mycobacterium tuberculosis*. Tuberculous adenopathy progresses through various stages associated with different clinical findings (Table 26.2 and Figure 26.2).

**HIV infection** may present with nodal enlargement in the chronic carrier phase. It may be associated with other head and neck manifestations such as oral candidiasis, hairy oral leukoplakia, multifocal parotid cysts and Kaposi's sarcoma.

**Sarcoidosis** presents as lymph node enlargement associated with non-caseating granulomas. It has an autoimmune aetiology

Table 26.2 Jones and Campbell classification of peripheral tuberculous lymphadenitis

| Stage | Description |
|-------|-------------|
| Stage 1 | Enlarged, firm, mobile, discrete nodes showing non-specific reactive hyperplasia |
| Stage 2 | Large rubbery nodes fixed to the surrounding tissue owing to periadenitis |
| Stage 3 | Central softening due to abscess formation |
| Stage 4 | Collar stud abscess formation |
| Stage 5 | Sinus tract formation |

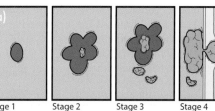

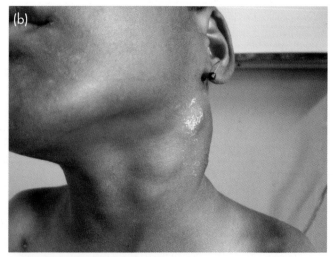

Figure 26.2 (a) The Jones and Campbell stages of tuberculous lymphadenitis. (b) Tuberculous lymphadenitis: the stage of periadenitis. (Courtesy of the Department of Paediatric Surgery, K.E.M. Hospital, Mumbai.)

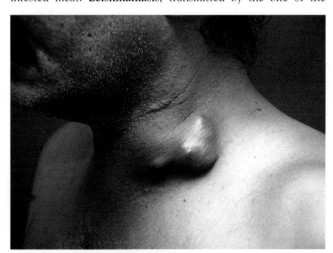

Figure 26.1 Necrotic malignant node mimicking suppuration.

that affects genetically predisposed individuals. Other associated manifestations include hilar lymphadenopathy, erythema nodosum, lupus pernio, arthropathy and uveitis. It usually affects young adults. High levels of serum angiotensin-converting enzyme are used to diagnose the condition.

## Neoplastic Lymphadenopathy

### Metastases

Enlarged nodes in patients over 40 years of age are frequently metastatic. Metastatic nodes are usually squamous and arise from an upper aerodigestive tract malignancy. There is a rising trend of human papillomavirus-related oropharyngeal malignancies in young adults.

The level of nodal involvement points towards the probable site of the primary (Table 26.3 and Figure 26.3). Involvement of the left supraclavicular node (**Virchow's node**) arises from infraclavicular pathologies of the gastrointestinal tract, bronchus, breast and testis (**Troiser's sign**) (Figures 26.4 and 26.5). In children, metastatic adenopathy is commonly seen from a primary in the nasopharynx or thyroid. Infiltration of the prevertebral fascia, manifested by restricted neck extension, and infiltration of platysma, shown by the platysma or fan sign (Figure 26.6), usually signify advanced disease. In about 5 per cent of cases, the primary site of the malignancy is not found despite a thorough clinical and radiological examination. This condition is known as metastasis of unknown origin (MUO).

### Reticuloendothelial Malignancies

Reticuloendothelial malignancies are usually associated with generalized adenopathy and constitutional symptoms. Examination in these patients should include the other lymph node areas (inguinal and axillary) as well as the liver and spleen. The most common reticular malignancies causing adenopathy are the lymphomas. These can be of Hodgkin's or non-Hodgkin's type.

Hodgkin's lymphoma shows (Table 26.4 and Figure 26.7) a bimodal distribution and usually affects patients in their second or third decade and fifth decade of life. Infradiaphragmatic presentation is unusual. It is also associated with mediastinal lymphadenopathy that sometimes presents as superior vena cava obstruction. Hodgkin's lymphoma occasionally involves extranodal sites, which in decreasing order of frequency are the spleen,

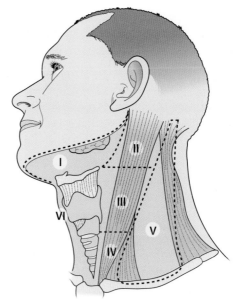

Figure 26.3 Lymph node levels.

liver and bone marrow. In a third of patients, it is associated with constitutional symptoms of fever, weight loss and night sweats. The presence of such symptoms is associated with a poor prognosis.

The pathological hallmark of Hodgkin's lymphoma is the presence of Reed–Sternberg cells. The Rye classification classifies Hodgkin's lymphoma into four types on the basis of the predominance of the cell types:

- lymphocyte predominant;
- nodular sclerosing;
- mixed cellularity;
- lymphocyte depleted.

Nodular sclerosing lymphoma is the most common type. Hodgkin's lymphoma is associated with chromosomal abnormalities and Epstein–Barr virus. Epstein–Barr virus DNA has been identified in the cells, although a causal association has not been established.

Table 26.3 Levels of lymph nodes and draining primaries

| Level of lymph nodes | Location | Usual site of primary |
|---|---|---|
| Level I | Submental/submandibular triangles | Upper and lower lip, buccal mucosa, alveolus |
| Level II (upper jugular) | Nodes between the skull base and carotid bifurcation | Tonsil, base of tongue, oral tongue, nasopharynx, scalp, parotid |
| Level III (mid-jugular) | Nodes between the carotid bifurcation and lower border of the cricoid | Hypopharynx, larynx, base of tongue, nasopharynx |
| Level IV (lower jugular) | Nodes between the lower border of the cricoid and clavicle | Larynx, hypopharynx, nasopharynx |
| Level V (posterior triangle) | Bounded by the posterior border of sternocleidomastoid and anterior border of trapezius | Nasopharynx, scalp, parotid |
| Level VI (central compartment) | Superiorly – hyoid<br>Inferiorly – innominate artery<br>Laterally – between the two carotid sheaths | Thyroid, larynx (glottis and subglottis) |

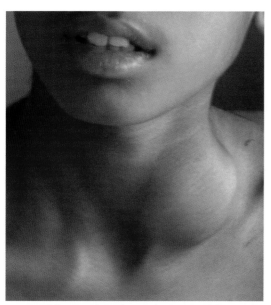

Figure 26.4 A left supraclavicular node in an adolescent boy. The common site of the primary is the testis. (Courtesy of P. A. Kurkure.)

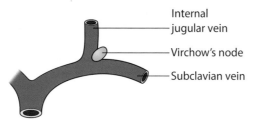

Internal
jugular vein

Virchow's node

Subclavian vein

Figure 26.5 A Virchow's node: showing the relationship to the junction of the internal jugular and subclavian veins.

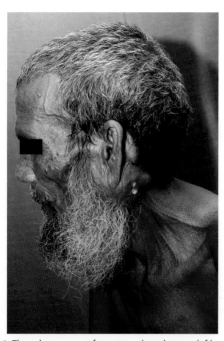

Figure 26.6 The platysma or fan sign: the platysmal fibres become prominent like a Japanese fan when stretched.

Table 26.4 Ann Arbor staging of Hodgkin's lymphoma

| Stage | Criteria |
| --- | --- |
| I | Single node region or extralymphatic site |
| II | Two or more node regions on the same side of the dia-phragm, or a single node region and one extra lymphatic site on one side of the diaphragm |
| III | Node regions on both sides of the diaphragm |
| IV | Diffuse involvement of one or more extralymphatic sites |

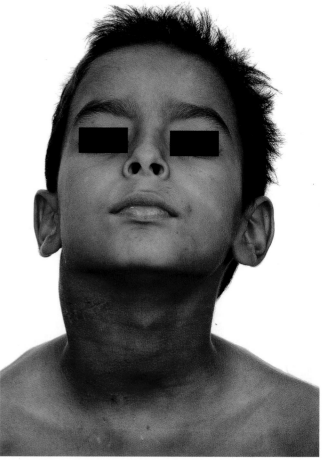

Figure 26.7 Lymphadenopathy in Hodgkin's lymphoma. (Courtesy S. D. Banavali and Girish Chinnaswamy.)

Non-Hodgkin's lymphoma occurs more commonly than Hodgkin's lymphoma. The differentiating features are outlined in Table 26.5. Multiple classification systems have been used for non-Hodgkin's lymphoma, such as the Rappaport, Kiel and Revised European–American Lymphoma classifications.

## Rare Causes of Lymphadenopathy

- *Kikuchi's disease* (histiocytic necrotizing lymphadenitis) is mainly seen in Japan with a few cases reported elsewhere. It is a self-limiting disease characterized by lymphadenitis, fever and skin rash.
- *Kimura's disease* is a chronic inflammatory disorder of unknown aetiology, characterized by painless inflammation of the nodes with subcutaneous lesions. Nephrotic syndrome occurs in a few cases.

- *Rosai–Dorfman disease* (sinus histiocytosis with massive lymphadenopathy) is characterized by an accumulation of histiocytes in the lymph nodes, leading to lymphadenopathy. Similar accumulations may also occur in the skin or paranasal sinuses.
- *Castleman's disease* (giant lymph node hyperplasia) is a rare lymphoproliferative disorder affecting the lymphoid tissue. It can be unicentric (affecting a single group of nodes) or multicentric (affecting more than one group of nodes or other lymphoid organs). It is sometimes associated with acquired immune deficiency syndrome. The disease is characterized by node enlargement with constitutional symptoms such as weight loss, malaise and fever.

**Table 26.5** Differences between Hodgkin's and Non-Hodgkin's lymphoma

| Hodgkin's | Non-Hodgkin's |
|---|---|
| Less common | More common |
| Bimodal distribution | Elderly |
| Contiguous involvement of nodes | Non-contiguous involvement of nodes |
| Extranodal involvement unlikely | Extranodal involvement common |
| Subdiaphragmatic presentation unusual | Subdiaphragmatic presentation common |

## NON-NODAL SWELLINGS

Non-nodal neck swellings are related to the triangles of the neck in which they arise (Table 26.6 and Figure 26.8).

## Congenital Neck Swellings
### Torticollis

Torticollis (wry neck) is usually the consequence of a difficult labour, most often associated with a breech presentation. The child develops a fusiform swelling involving the middle third of the sternocleidomastoid muscle that fibroses weeks later. This leads to shortening of the muscle, giving rise to the classical deformity of turning of the head to the opposite side, slightly upwards and with a tilt to the same side. Adults can also present with torticollis as a result of trauma to the muscle.

The differential diagnosis includes a tumour within the sternocleidomastoid (a rhabdomyosarcoma). The association with the muscle in this case is demonstrated as a loss of mobility of the lump when the sternomastoid is contracted. This is achieved by asking the patient to turn the head to the opposite side against resistance applied to the chin.

### Lymphatic Swellings

The most common site of a lymphangioma is the neck. A cystic hygroma is a congenital lymphangioma (Figure 26.9). It occurs due to sequestration of the lymphatics during development and usually arises in the lower neck and posterior triangle.

The pathognomonic features of a lymphatic cyst are that these are seen in the paediatric age group or young adults

**Table 26.6** Triangles of the neck

| Triangle | Boundaries | Contents | Common swellings |
|---|---|---|---|
| Submental triangle | Between the anterior bellies of the digastric, the base being formed by the body of the hyoid | Lymph nodes | Lymphadenopathy, sublingual dermoid, lipoma |
| Digastric triangle | Between the anterior and posterior bellies of the digastric, the base being the inferior border of the mandible | Submandibular gland, lymph nodes | Lymphadenopathy, salivary gland tumour, plunging ranula |
| Carotid triangle | Superiorly – the posterior belly of the digastric. Anteriorly – the superior belly of the omohyoid. Posteriorly – the anterior border of the sternocleidomastoid | Common carotid artery, carotid bulb and sinus, internal carotid artery, external carotid artery and its branches, internal jugular vein, vagus, spinal accessory and hypoglossal nerved, lymph nodes | Lymphadenopathy, carotid body tumour, vagal schwannoma, carotid artery aneurysm, branchial cyst |
| Muscular triangle | Anteriorly – midline of the neck. Posteriosuperiorly – superior belly of omohyoid. Posteroinferiorly – anterior border of sternomastoid | Strap muscles, lymph nodes | Lymphadenopathy |
| Posterior triangle | Anteriorly – posterior border of sternocleidomastoid. Posteriorly – anterior border of trapezius. Base – middle third of the clavicle | Lymph nodes, spinal accessory nerve, transverse cervical vessels | Lymphadenopathy, cystic hygroma, pharyngeal pouch, subclavian aneurysm, lipoma |

PART 4 | HEAD AND NECK

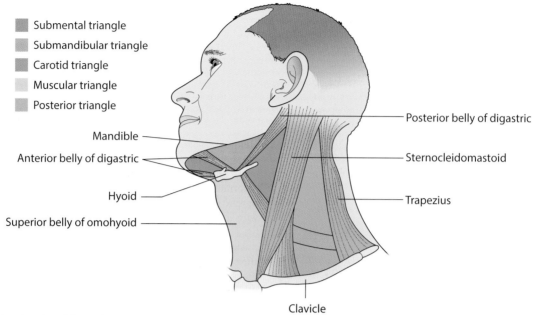

Submental triangle
Submandibular triangle
Carotid triangle
Muscular triangle
Posterior triangle

Mandible
Anterior belly of digastric
Hyoid
Superior belly of omohyoid

Posterior belly of digastric
Sternocleidomastoid
Trapezius

Clavicle

Figure 26.8 The triangles of the neck.

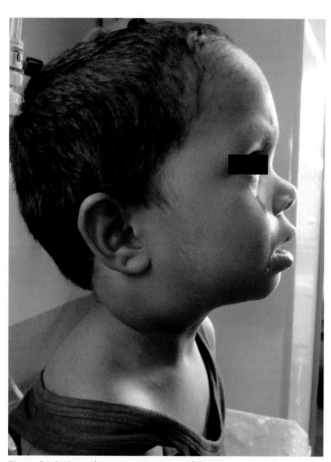

Figure 26.9 Cystic hygroma. (Courtesy of the Department of Paediatric Surgery, K.E.M. Hospital, Mumbai.)

and are compressible, fluctuant and brilliantly transilluminant (**Figure 26.10**). The swelling may be unilocular or multilocular. Large lesions and those located in the suprahyoid region are more likely to be associated with airway compromise.

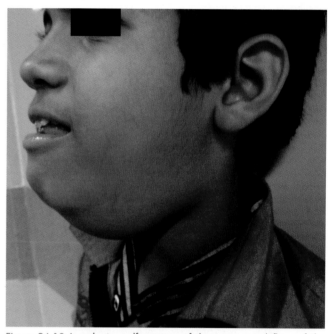

Figure 26.10 Lymphatic malformation of the tongue and floor of the mouth. (Courtesy of the Department of Paediatric Surgery, K.E.M. Hospital, Mumbai.)

### Branchial Swellings

The face and neck develop from six paired pharyngeal arches. The second ectodermal cleft overgrows to fuse with the sixth and is usually obliterated. Any defect in this process leads to the formation of a branchial cyst, sinus or fistula.

**Branchial cysts** most commonly arise from the second arch and less frequently from other arch defects. They present as painless cystic swellings related to the upper third of the sterno-cleidomastoid muscle, which lie between the sternocleidomastoid and the carotid sheath. The cyst is caused by persistence of the epithelial-lined cavity after fusion of the arches. Over a period of time, this accumulates fluid. The swelling contains cholesterol crystals and hence is not transilluminant.

The cyst may become infected and tender, and then rupture to give rise to a **branchial sinus**. This is a blind sac that discharges pus from its external opening, located at the anterior border of the sternocleidomastoid muscle.

**Branchial fistulae** are congenital openings that discharge secretions, with the external openings lying at the level of the lower third of the sternocleidomastoid. The tract passes between the internal and the external carotid arteries and lies superior to the hypoglossal nerve. It most commonly arises from the second arch, and in such cases the internal opening is at the level of the tonsillar fossa. On rare occasions, it may arise from the fourth arch, when the internal opening will be in the ipsilateral pyriform sinus.

## Lipomas

Lipomas are common benign swellings that occur in approximately 1 per cent of the population (**Figure 26.11**). The head and neck is a common site, lipomas having a predilection for the nape of the neck and the posterior triangle. They are usually located in the subcutaneous plane but can also be deep-seated and are characterized by a mobile, soft to rubbery, pseudofluctuant swelling whose edge slips under the palpating finger.

## Unusual Swellings

### Paragangliomas

Carotid body tumours or chemodectomas are the most common paraganglioma seen in the neck. They usually present as slow-growing tumours in the fourth or fifth decade of life. The pathognomonic findings are a pulsatile lesion located at the carotid bifurcation that is mobile horizontally but not vertically (Fontaine's sign). Large tumours may give rise to palsies of the IXth, Xth, XIth and XIIth cranial nerves. Carotid body tumours may be hereditary, occur bilaterally, be associated with paragangliomas elsewhere (jugulare, tympanicum or phaeochromocytoma) or be secretory in nature (<5 per cent).

### Schwannomas/Neurilemmomas

These are tumours arising from the Schwann cells surrounding the nerve. They present as a smooth, slowly growing swelling usually in the upper neck in relation to the parapharyngeal space, and commonly occur in relation to the IXth and Xth cranial nerves and the sympathetic nerve trunks (**Figure 26.12**). The nerve of origin is stretched by the tumour and patients may present with nerve dysfunction. The differential diagnosis is a carotid body tumour, which is pulsatile and brilliantly enhancing on MRI.

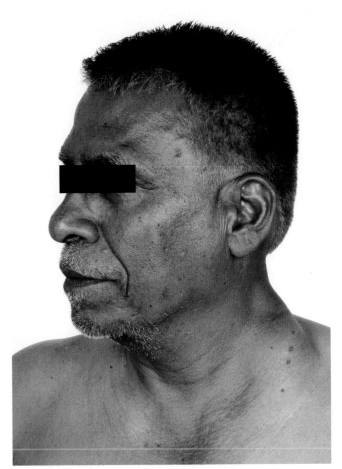

Figure 26.11 Lipoma of the posterior triangle of the neck.

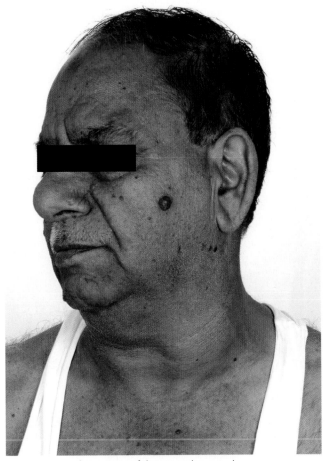

Figure 26.12 Schwannoma of the sympathetic trunk.

### Salivary Glands

Inflammation and neoplasms of the submandibular gland may present as neck swellings (**Figure 26.13**) (see Chapter 25). Ectopic salivary tumours and tumours of the deep lobe of the parotid occasionally present as deep-seated upper neck swellings in the parapharyngeal space, which are not clinically apparent but cause medial displacement of the tonsil (**Figure 26.14**).

### Diverticula and Laryngoceles

These may present as neck swellings and are covered in Chapter 24.

### Arteries and Aneurysms

The most common pulsatile swelling in the neck is a prominence and tortuosity of the common carotid artery, predominantly on the right side. This is caused by long-standing hypertension and atherosclerosis. The subclavian or innominate artery may occasionally be affected, which manifests as a pulsatile swelling in the lower neck or the suprasternal space of Burns.

Extracranial carotid aneurysms may also present as pulsatile neck swellings. Pseudoaneurysms may occur in relation to the carotid artery following surgery and trauma. These may be associated with neck pain or cerebral embolic symptomatology. Tender aneurysms of the extracranial carotid artery are associated with Takayasu's arteriopathy. Aneurysms have expansile pulsations and are associated with a bruit.

## Midline Neck Swellings

**Dermoid cysts** usually present along the line of fusion of the neck in young children. They are the result of an enclaving of

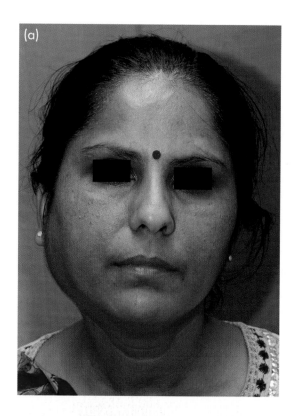

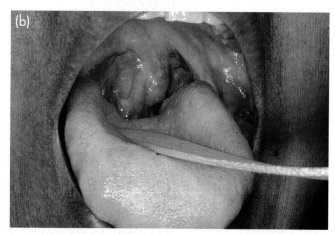

Figure 26.14 (a) A deep lobe parotid tumour that is not apparent clinically. (b) An apparent bulge in the tonsillar region.

epithelial cell rests during embryogenesis. The clinical presentation is a midline swelling occupying the upper or lower neck (**Figure 26.15**). The cyst is lined by squamous epithelium and filled with keratinaceous material and therefore it is not transilluminant. The cyst may show sebaceous or sweat appendages.

**Thyroglossal cysts, sinuses and fistulas** occur along the course of the thyroglossal duct and are described in more detail in Chapter 27.

A **ranula** is a cystic swelling in the floor of the mouth caused by mucous extravasation or a retention cyst due to blockage of the sublingual or less commonly the submandibular duct. Ranulas are of two types: simple and plunging. A plunging ranula (**Figure 26.16**) extends posterior to the mylohyoid and presents as a neck swelling. It is usually located lateral to the midline.

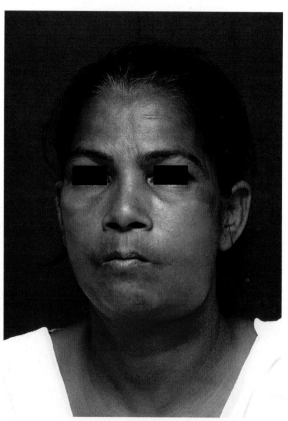

Figure 26.13 An enlarged submandibular gland.

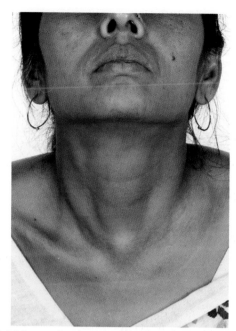

Figure 26.15 Dermoid at the root of the neck.

**Key Points**

- Swellings in the neck are common.
- It is important to differentiate between a nodal and non-nodal origin.
- Swellings in individuals under 40 years of age are usually benign, whereas those in individuals over 40 years of age are usually malignant.
- Diagnosis is helped by identifying the location of the non-nodal swelling in relation to the specific anatomical triangles of the neck.
- With malignancy, the level of the involved lymph nodes helps to establish the site of the primary.

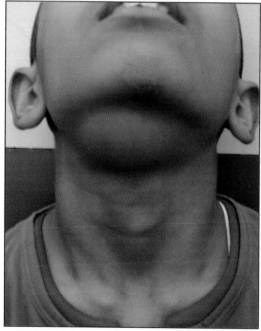

Figure 26.16 Plunging ranula.

PART 4 | HEAD AND NECK

## QUESTIONS

### SBAs

**1. All of the following are true about cystic hygromas except which?:**
a They transilluminate
b They are commonly located in the muscular triangle
c They fluctuate in size with upper respiratory tract infections
d They are common in the paediatric age group

**Answer**
b **They are commonly located in the muscular triangle i.e. this is incorrect.** A cystic hygroma is a congenital lymphangioma that affects the paediatric age group. It is a lymphatic sequestration manifesting as a swelling in the lower neck and posterior triangle. It is cystic in consistency and hence fluctuant and brilliantly transilluminant.

**2. Enlarged nodes usually warrant further investigation when the size of the node is:**
a ≤5 mm
b 5–10 mm
c ≥10 mm
d Any size

**Answer**
c **≥10 mm.** There are nearly 150 nodes on each side of the neck. The nodes in non-pathological lymphadenopathy rarely reach more than 1 cm in diameter. Nodes larger than 1 cm constitute significant lymphadenopathy and warrant further evaluation with fine needle aspiration cytology. The exception is the jugulodigastric node, which is not considered significant until it is larger than 1.5 cm, and a supraclavicular node of any size.

**3. A 'fan sign' is seen with which one of the following?:**
a Infectious mononucleosis
b Nodal metastasis with skin involvement
c Carotid body tumour
d Toxoplasmosis

**Answer**
b **Nodal metastasis with skin involvement.** The fan sign is also known as the platysma sign; its name is derived from its resemblance to the inverted Japanese fan. It is caused by the puckering of the platysma and overlying skin due to infiltration and is pathognomonic of neoplastic nodes. It is best demonstrated by stretching the platysma by rotating the patient's head to the opposite side.

### EMQ

**1. For the following case descriptions, select the most likely cause from the list below:**
1 Branchial cyst
2 Carotid body tumour
3 Human papillomavirus-associated malignancy
4 Lymphatic cyst
5 Chronic phase of HIV infection
6 Full-blown AIDS
a A 29-year-old man has presented with multiple neck nodes. Ultrasonography of his neck shows multiple neck nodes with bilateral parotid cysts. Fine needle aspiration cytology from the node shows reactive hyperplasia.
b A 15-year-old boy presents with a swelling in his upper neck that is located along the anterior border of the sternocleidomastoid. On examination, this measures 3 cm × 3 cm, is fluctuant and is brilliantly transilluminant.

**Answers**
a 5 **Chronic phase of HIV infection.** During the chronic phase of HIV, when patients are still immunocompetent, they develop a reactive lymphadenopathy. Full-blown AIDS is characterized by a drop in CD4 count and the development of opportunistic infections.

b 4 **Lymphatic cyst.** Even though this location is the classical site for a branchial cyst, these are not brilliantly transilluminant because of they contain cholesterol crystals. Therefore a brilliantly transilluminant fluctuant neck swelling is likely to be a lymphatic cyst.

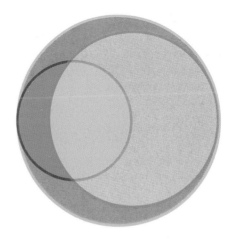

# PART
# 5

# Breast and endocrine

# The Thyroid and Parathyroids

Mitali Dandekar, S Kannan and Anil D'Cruz

## LEARNING OBJECTIVES

- To become conversant with the common causes of thyroid enlargement and the important clinical features that will aid in diagnosis and management

- To understand parathyroid dysfunction with respect to hyper- and hypoparathyroidism

## THE THYROID

**Goitre** is an enlargement of the thyroid gland. Thyroid enlargement may be due to a solitary nodule or enlargement of the entire gland, which could be diffuse or multinodular (Figure 27.1).

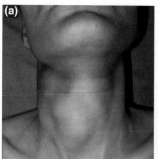
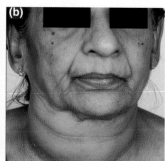
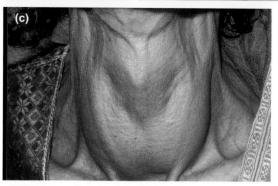

Figure 27.1 (a) A solitary nodule, (b) a multinodular goitre, and (c) diffuse enlargement of the thyroid. (Courtesy of Professor Nalini Shah, K.E.M Hospital, Mumbai.)

Thyroid nodules are common: clinically palpable solitary nodules are present in 4–8 per cent of the normal adult population. Most of these are benign, but in clinical practice up to 5–15 per cent of them may be malignant.

**Multinodular goitres** result from fluctuating levels of thyroid-stimulating hormone (TSH) as a consequence of iodine deficiency, goitrogens or dyshormonogenesis. If present in more than 10 per cent of the population in a region, they are known as endemic goitres. Long-standing multinodular goitres may undergo malignant transformation. The incidence of malignancy in a multinodular goitre is lower than in a solitary thyroid nodule in endemic areas.

**Diffuse enlargement** of the thyroid gland occurring at puberty is referred to as a physiological or simple goitre. These are usually not associated with hypo- or hyperfunctioning of the gland but are a response to increased metabolic demands. A similar enlargement may be seen in women during pregnancy.

Diffuse goitre in a middle-aged woman may be due to thyroiditis, most commonly chronic lymphocytic (Hashimoto's) thyroiditis. The gland may initially hyperfunction, but the process eventually leads to hypothyroidism. Hashimoto's thyroiditis can occasionally undergo malignant transformation into a lymphoma.

Thyroiditis may also present as subacute lymphocytic thyroiditis (postpartum or sporadic), subacute granulomatous (de Quervain's), drug- or radiation-induced, acute suppurative and invasive fibrous (Riedel's) thyroiditis. Riedel's thyroiditis is also known as 'woody' thyroiditis due to the replacement of the thyroid tissue with fibrosis.

The hallmark of a thyroid swelling is that the swelling moves on deglutition. Examination of the thyroid is best performed both from behind and in front of the patient with their neck in slight extension. The gland can be made more prominent

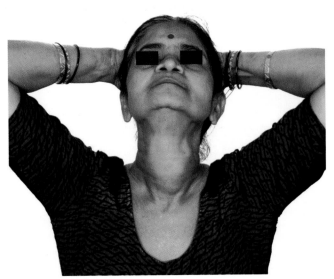

Figure 27.2 Pizillo's manoeuvre.

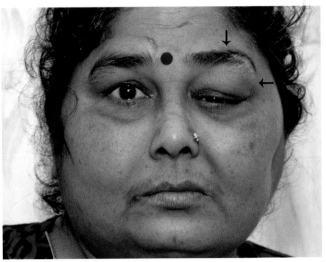

Figure 27.3 Orbital metastasis from follicular cancer thyroid. (Courtesy of S. Basu and G. Malhotra, Radiation Medicine Centre, Mumbai.)

by Pizillo's manoeuvre in which the patient's hands are placed behind their occiput and the head is pushed backwards against the clasped hands (Figure 27.2).

The lobes may be better examined by Lahey's method in which, for examination of the left lobe, the thyroid gland is pushed to the left from the right side by the examiner's left hand, and similarly to the right by the right hand. Smaller nodules within the substance of the gland are better appreciated by palpating the gland using the thumb while the patient swallows (Crile's method).

Nodules occurring at the extremes of age (younger than 15 and older than 45 years) and those associated with a prior history of radiotherapy, a family history of thyroid cancer, a recent onset or lymphadenopathy are more likely to be malignant.

Enlargement of the thyroid gland can be graded based on its presenting size using the World Health Organization (WHO) grading system:

- *Grade 0*: No goitre can be felt (it is impalpable and invisible).
- *Grade 1*: The thyroid is palpable, but it is not visible when the neck is in a normal position. A thickened mass moves upwards during swallowing.
- *Grade 2*: The neck swelling, which is visible when the neck is in a normal position, corresponds to the enlarged thyroid that is found on palpation.

Large goitres may result in deviation of the trachea, causing prominence of the ipsilateral sternocleidomastoid muscle (Trail's sign). They may also cause obliteration of the carotid pulsations due to displacement of the vessels (Berry's sign). These patients may develop stridor when pressure is applied to the lateral lobe of the thyroid (Kocher's test). Long-standing multinodular goitres may cause tracheomalacia due to persistent compression (a scabbard trachea).

Goitres have a tendency to extend to the mediastinum due to the negative intrathoracic pressure and lack of attachment of the deep layer of the cervical fascia inferiorly. The lower border of the goitre is not visualized or palpable in such cases on deglutition. Percussion over the manubrium elicits a dull note, although this test is not commonly used in practice today owing to the availability of better imaging.

Dilated veins may be visible over the neck and upper chest, and raising the arms above the shoulder may aggravate the prominent veins and induce facial flushing and stridor (Pemberton's sign). Hoarseness results from stretching of the recurrent laryngeal nerve, but this is more common with malignant infiltration. Patients with dysphagia need to be carefully evaluated as this symptom is rarely caused by a goitre.

A hard consistency in a nodule is not pathognomonic of malignancy as it may also arise from calcification in a long-standing multinodular goitre. Similarly, a rapid increase in size of a nodule is not indicative of malignancy as the majority of thyroid cancers are known to have an indolent growth rate. The rapid increase usually signifies an aggressive histology (poorly differentiated or anaplastic), lymphoma or haemorrhage into a nodule in a multinodular gland.

Papillary cancer of the thyroid gland is the most common thyroid malignancy (80 per cent of cases). It has a high propensity to metastasize to the cervical nodes. Follicular cancers occur less commonly (10–15 per cent of cases). Spread is usually via the haematogenous route to the lungs and bones (Figure 27.3). Follicular carcinomas have a lower propensity for cervical nodal metastasis.

Medullary cancers, arising from parafollicular C cells of neuroendocrine origin, are seen less commonly (5–10 per cent of cases). They are hereditary in about 20 per cent of cases and are of three types: familial, multiple endocrine neoplasia (MEN) type 2A and MEN type 2B (Table 27.1 and Figure 27.4). These are usually associated with RET proto-oncogene mutations (on chromosome 10q11.2).

Thyroid enlargement may be associated with the signs and symptoms of hyperthyroidism or hypothyroidism.

**Hyperthyroidism** occurs in diffuse toxic goitre (Graves' disease) (Figure 27.5), toxic nodular goitre (Plummer's syndrome) and toxic adenoma. Graves' disease is characterized by goitre, hyperthyroidism, ophthalmopathy and occasionally dermopathy (Table 27.2). The goitre in Graves' disease is diffuse and may be associated with a palpable thrill or bruit due to a hyperdynamic circulation. Neurological manifestations are more common in Graves' disease (primary hyperthyroidism). In contrast, secondary

Table 27.1 Syndromes of special interest

| Syndrome | Features |
| --- | --- |
| MEN 1 syndrome | An autosomal dominant condition associated with tumours of the parathyroid glands (90%), islet cell tumours of the pancreas (30–80%) and pituitary adenomas (15%) |
| MEN 2A syndrome | An autosomal dominant condition associated with medullary thyroid cancer (most common), phaeochromocytoma (30–50%) and primary hyperparathyroidism (5–20%) |
| MEN 2B syndrome | An aggressive type of MEN 2 syndrome that is autosomal dominant and characterized by medullary thyroid cancer, phaeochromocytoma (50%) with a marfanoid habitus and mucosal ganglioneuromas (see Figure 27.4) |
| Gardner's syndrome | An autosomal dominant condition associated with multiple colonic polyposis, papillary cancer thyroid, skull osteomas and desmoids with epidermoid cysts and fibromas |
| Cowden's syndrome | An autosomal dominant condition associated with intestinal hamartomatous polyps, macrocephaly, skin tumours such as trichilemmomas and other benign tumours, e.g. papillomatous papules and acral keratoses, with a predisposition to follicular thyroid cancer and endometrial and breast cancer |
| Pendred's syndrome | An autosomal recessive condition associated with dyshormonogenetic goitre and congenital sensorineural hearing loss with Mondini's deformity in the cochlea |
| Carney complex | Autosomal dominant condition characterized by spotty pigmentation, myxomas of the heart and endocrine tumours including tumours of the thyroid gland |

MEN, multiple endocrine neoplasia.

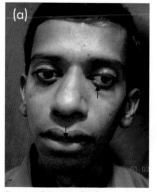
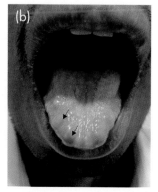

Figure 27.4 Multiple endocrine neoplasia 2B syndrome with a (a) marfanoid habitus, lip and eyelid neuromas and (b) tongue neuromas.

hyperthyroidism in a long-standing nodular goitre has a predominant effect on the cardiovascular symptoms.

**Hypothyroidism** is encountered 5–10 times more frequently in clinical practice than hyperthyroidism. Hypothyroidism is usually a medically treated condition for which surgery has a limited or no role. Severe hypothyroidism in infancy is known as cretinism and has hallmark features of mental and growth retardation with delayed milestones. The child suffers from failure to thrive, impairment of growth with dwarfism (the limbs being disproportionately shorter than the trunk), a delay in the onset of puberty, delayed tooth eruption, protruberance of the abdomen and dry skin, hair and nails.

Unrecognized and untreated hypo- or hyperfunction of the gland may result in life-threatening conditions.

**Myxoedema coma** is now uncommon but can result from prolonged, untreated hypothyroidism. It is usually precipitated by triggering factors such as hypothermia or infection. Patients present with hypothermia, hypotension, hyponatraemia, hypoventilation, hypoglycaemia, bradycardia, an altered sensorium, lethargy, stupor and delirium that progresses to coma.

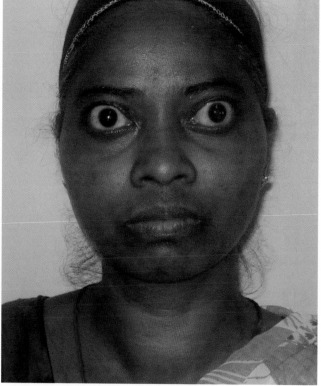

Figure 27.5 Exophthalmos in a patient with a diffuse toxic goitre. (Courtesy of Professor Nalini Shah, K.E.M Hospital, Mumbai.)

**Thyroid crisis or thyroid storm** is caused by an excessive release of thyroid hormones into the circulation. It manifests clinically with hyperpyrexia, tachycardia and hypertension that progresses to cardiac failure. It is commonly associated with neurological and gastrointestinal symptoms. It was formerly seen in patients inadequately prepared for surgery.

Table 27.2 The clinical features of hyper- and hypothyroidism

| System | Hyperthyroidism | Hypothyroidism |
|---|---|---|
| Skin | Moist, excessive sweating, palmar erythema, pretibial myxoedema | Non-pitting oedema, dryness, coarseness, capillary fragility resulting in a bleeding tendency |
| Hair | Fine, friable | Loss of hair, madarosis (Queen Anne sign) |
| Nails | Plummer's nails (onycholysis): separation of the distal margin of the nail from the nail bed | Brittle |
| Eyes | See **Tables 27.3** and **27.4** | Bogginess around the eye |
| Alimentary system | Increased appetite, weight loss, increased frequency of and ill-formed stools | Decreased appetite, weight gain, constipation |
| Cardiovascular system | Tachycardia, resting pulse >90/minute, atrial arrhythmias and fibrillation | Cardiomegaly, sinus bradycardia, pericardial effusion, heart block |
| Nervous system | Nervousness, restlessness, decreased attention span, emotional lability, fatigue<br>Fine tremors: hands, tongue, eyelid, eyeballs | Slowing of intellectual functions, lethargy |
| Musculoskeletal system | Muscles: weakness (proximal muscles), wasting, periodic paralysis<br>Osteoporosis, pathological fractures<br>Stimulation of bone maturation with growth acceleration | Stiffness, muscle aches, delayed muscle contraction and relaxation, macroglossia |
| Respiratory system | Weakness of the respiratory muscles causing a decrease in vital capacity and dyspnoea | Obstructive sleep apnoea, involvement of the respiratory muscles and depression of ventilatory drive |
| Reproductive system | Irregular menstruation, increased libido, decreased fertility<br>Gynaecomastia | Decreased libido, anovulation, amenorrhoea |
| Constitutional | Heat intolerance | Cold intolerance |

Table 27.3 Eye signs in hyperthyroidism

| Sign | Description |
|---|---|
| **Due to adrenergic overactivity** | |
| Lid retraction | Higher than normal position of the upper eyelid |
| von Graefe's | Lag of the upper eyelid on vertical movements of the eyeball |
| Dalrymple's | Visibility of the upper sclera due to upper eyelid retraction |
| Stellwag's | A staring look |
| **Due to infiltrative ophthalmopathy** | |
| Moebius | Inability to converge the eyeballs |
| Naffziger's | Visualization of the protruded eyeball from behind the patient |
| Joffroy's | Absence of wrinkling of the forehead on looking upwards |

## Development of the Thyroid

The thyroid develops from one median and two lateral anlagen in the region of the foramen caecum and descends to its final position in the neck. The thyroglossal tract, which represents this line of descent, usually atrophies. Abnormalities of descent of the thyroid or non-obliteration of the thyroglossal tract results in the following:

- *Ectopic thyroid*: This is a residual thyroid that occurs anywhere in the path of the embryological descent. The lingual thyroid is the most common location; this occurs at the junction of the anterior two-thirds and posterior one-third of the tongue.

It presents as a mass causing dysphagia, respiratory obstruction and haemorrhage. It is associated with cervical athyrosis in 70 per cent of cases. This can be suspected on palpation of bare tracheal rings.

- *Thyroglossal cyst* (**Figure 27.6**): This occurs due to non-obliteration of the thyroglossal tract. It presents, usually in the first decade of life, as a swelling that moves on protrusion of tongue. Around 70 per cent of thyroglossal cysts occur in the midline, with others lying laterally as far as the tip of the hyoid. The cysts may occasionally rupture and develop into a thyroglossal sinus. The opening of the sinus may be indrawn and overlaid by a fold of skin (the 'hood' sign).

Table 27.4  Classification of ophthalmopathy in thyrotoxicosis (American Thyroid Association): 'NOSPECS'

| Class | Signs |
| --- | --- |
| Class 0 | **N**o physical signs or symptoms |
| Class 1 | **O**nly signs, no symptoms (signs limited to upper lid retraction, stare, lid lag and proptosis ≤22 mm) |
| Class 2 | **S**oft tissue involvement (symptoms and signs) |
| Class 3 | **P**roptosis >22 mm |
| Class 4 | **E**xtraocular muscle involvement |
| Class 5 | **C**orneal involvement |
| Class 6 | **S**ight loss (optic nerve involvement) |

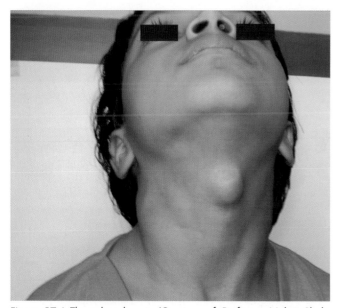

Figure 27.6 Thyroglossal cyst. (Courtesy of Professor Nalini Shah, K.E.M Hospital, Mumbai.)

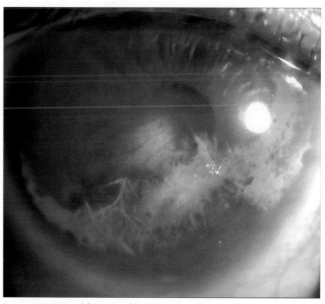

Figure 27.7 Band keratopathy. (Courtesy of Dr Vijay Kane, Bacchuali Hospital and Dr Nikhil Gokhale, Gokhale Eye Hospital.)

## THE PARATHYROIDS

The inferior parathyroids develop from the third pharyngeal pouch, and the superior parathyroids from the fourth. Thus, the inferior parathyroids have to migrate further than the superior glands and are more prone to anomalies of location.

The parathyroids may hyperfunction (resulting in hyperparathyroidism), hypofunction or be absent (most often from surgical misadventures); rarely, they give rise to carcinoma. Surgery is most often required for hyperparathyroidism.

## Hyperparathyroidism

Hyperfunction of parathyroid glands can be:

- *primary*: inappropriately high parathormone levels causing hypercalcaemia; the most common cause is an adenoma (75–90 per cent), followed by hyperplasia (20–24 per cent), double parathyroid adenoma (2–3 per cent) and rarely carcinoma (1 per cent). It can occur as part of MEN syndrome (see Table 27.1);

- *secondary*: parathyroid hyperplasia occurring secondary to chronic hypocalcaemia following renal failure, malabsorption or vitamin D deficiency;
- *tertiary*: long-standing secondary hyperparathyroidism resulting in autonomously functioning parathyroid glands.

The most common presentation is asymptomatic biochemical hypercalcaemia.

The classical features of hyperparathyroidism are summed up by the popular mnemonic 'stones, bones, abdominal groans and psychic moans'. Patients often present with brown tumours (osteitis fibrosa cystica) due to excessive osteoclastic bone resorption following hyperparathyroidism. This results in cyst-like pseudotumours and occasional fractures. Brown tumours initially affect the fingers, facial bones and ribs, but may eventually affect any bone (*bones*). The resulting hypercalcaemia leads to nephrolithiasis (*stones*) and hypergastrinaemic peptic ulcers (*abdominal groans*), as well as lethargy, fatigue and other neuropsychiatric symptoms (*psychic moans*). Other symptoms include polyuria, constipation, pseudogout and band keratopathy (Figure 27.7).

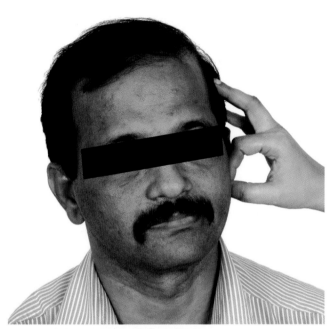

Figure 27.8 Demonstration of Chvostek's sign.

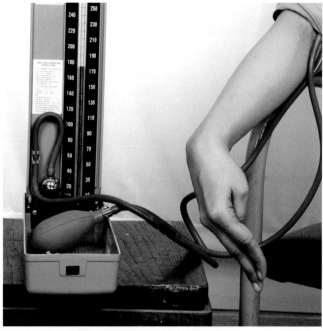

Figure 27.9 Trousseau's sign.

Carcinoma of a parathyroid gland is extremely rare and generally presents with hyperparathyroidism and malignant hypercalcaemia, and may be associated with a neck mass or metastasis.

## Hypoparathyroidism

This occurs primarily as a result of surgical trauma or inadvertent excision following thyroid surgery, and presents with the signs and symptoms of hypocalcaemia – circumoral tingling, numbness, paraesthesias, carpopedal spasm, laryngeal stridor, respiratory muscle spasm, arrhythmias, convulsions and blurred vision. Cataract is a late presentation. Dementia may occur following calcification in the basal ganglia.

Hypocalcaemia is clinically diagnosed by:

- *Chvostek's sign*: twitching of the facial muscle on stimulating the facial nerve in front of the tragus (Figure 27.8);
- *Trousseau's sign*: inflation of a sphygmomanometer above systolic blood pressure for 5 minutes induces carpal spasm, that is, muscular contraction with flexion of the wrist and metacarpophalangeal joints, hyperextension of the fingers and flexion of the thumb onto the palm (also known as obstetrician's hand) (Figure 27.9).

### Key Points

- It is important to differentiate goitre into either solitary, diffuse or multinodular.
- Malignancy occurs more frequently in solitary nodules. Nodules occurring at the extremes of age, with a prior history of radiotherapy, with a family history of thyroid cancer and of recent onset are more likely to be malignant.
- It is essential to recognize hypothyroidism or hyperthyroidism and compressive symptoms as this has a bearing on management.
- Hyperparathyroidism presents with symptoms of hypercalcaemia without gland enlargement. Hypocalcaemia generally occurs secondary to iatrogenic hypoparathyroidism.

## QUESTIONS

### SBAs

**1. Multinodular goitre is caused by all except which one of the following?:**
  a Dyshormongenesis
  b Iodine deficiency
  c Physiological changes
  d Consumption of goitrogens

**Answer**
c *Physiological changes. Physiological changes such as puberty and pregnancy cause a diffuse enlargement known as a simple goitre.*

**2. Which one of the following statements is true of the association between a lingual thyroid and cervical athyrosis?:**
  a There is an association in fewer than 50 per cent of cases
  b There is an association in more than 50 per cent of cases
  c It is not associated with cervical athyrosis
  d It is always associated with cervical athyrosis

**Answer**
b *There is an association in more than 50 per cent of cases. Lingual thyroid is associated with cervical athyrosis in about 70 per cent of cases.*

**3. All of the following are true except:**
  a Nephrolithiasis is commonly associated with hyperparathyroidism
  b Parathyroid adenoma is the most common cause of hyperparathyroidism
  c Cataract occurs in hypoparathyroidism while band keratopathy is seen in hypercalcaemia
  d Parathyroid carcinoma is associated with hypoparathyroidism

**Answer**
d *Parathyroid carcinoma is associated with hypoparathyroidism. This answer is untrue as parathyroid carcinoma causes hypercalcaemia secondary to hyperparathyroidism.*

### EMQ

**1. For each of the following cases, select the most likely diagnosis from the list below:**
  1 Physiological goitre
  2 Multinodular goitre
  3 Anaplastic cancer of the thyroid
  4 Papillary cancer of the thyroid
  5 Thyroglossal cyst
  6 Lingual thyroid
  a A 40-year-old woman presents with a midline neck swelling of 6 months' duration. On examination, the swelling moves with deglutition. Ipsilateral nodal enlargement is palpable, and the vocal cords are mobile. There is no similar family history, and the patient is not pregnant. She is euthyroid. Ultrasound scanning suggests a 4 cm thyroid nodule with microcalcification.
  b A 20-year-old man presents with a neck swelling of 4 months' duration. On examination, the swelling is in the midline and moves with deglutition as well as tongue protrusion. Ultrasound scanning suggests a 2 cm cystic swelling below the hyoid bone and above the thyroid, with a normal thyroid gland.

**Answers**
a 4 *Papillary cancer of the thyroid. Malignancy is more likely to occur in middle-aged woman who have a solitary nodule, a large nodule or microcalcification.*
b 5 *Thyroglossal cyst. A thyroglossal cyst occurs in the path of embryological descent, presents in younger age groups and moves with protrusion of the tongue.*

PART 5 | BREAST AND ENDOCRINE

# Breast and Axilla

Jesse Dirksen, Carol E. H. Scott-Conner and Ingrid Lizarraga

## LEARNING OBJECTIVES

- To know how to undertake a detailed history and physical examination of a patient presenting with a breast problem
- To be able to develop a differential diagnosis for a breast mass and describe the characteristics of both malignant and benign lesions

- To be able to describe the components of the 'triple test'
- To understand the various supportive diagnostic tools, which include imaging modalities and techniques for tissue diagnosis

## INTRODUCTION

With any woman presenting with a breast problem, the presence of breast carcinoma must first be excluded or confirmed. This diagnosis must be at the top of any list of possible diagnoses.

Breast complaints are common and in the vast majority of cases are due to benign alternations in the normal physiology. The difficulty for the clinician lies in distinguishing those relatively few women in whom underlying malignancy is the cause. In some instances, this is an easy process; in others, it becomes complex. In all cases, however, the use of the 'triple test' – clinical setting, radiological imaging studies and tissue sampling (Table 28.1) – provides the best assurance that nothing has been missed. There are of course other breast conditions that require diagnosis and treatment, but in these cases too the prudent clinician will first exclude carcinoma.

Men have a small amount of breast tissue that may hypertrophy and require treatment. Breast cancer is also (rarely) seen

Table 28.1 **The triple test**

| Clinical setting | History |
| | Physical examination |
| Imaging studies | Mammography |
| | Ultrasound |
| | MRI |
| Tissue sampling | Biopsy – tissue |
| |     Core (preferred) |
| |     Incisional |
| |     Excisional |
| | Fine needle aspiration – cytology |

in men. This chapter first reviews the general conduct of the breast-directed history and physical examination and then briefly discusses specific common diagnoses.

## PRESENTATION

Common symptoms of breast problems may include a mass or lump, pain and a nipple discharge. Women may also be referred for breast examination when a routine screening mammogram has shown an abnormality or because of a strong family history of breast cancer. These women may be otherwise asymptomatic.

## HISTORY

For any complaint, always ask how it began and whether it has changed (Table 28.2). Thus, for the woman presenting with a breast lump, enquire how she first noted it and whether the lump has grown or changed with her menstrual cycles. Seek associated symptoms such as pain or tenderness. Typically, breast cancers either grow or remain unchanged during a period of observation, whereas benign breast lumps wax and wane with hormonal influences. Pain and tenderness are more common with benign problems but are also seen with breast cancer.

Ask whether or not the woman has noted any nipple discharge. If so, is it spontaneous – that is, does it spot or stain her bra or nightwear – or elicited? Spontaneous discharge is more likely to be associated with a pathological process than is elicited discharge.

Pay attention to any previous history of breast problems; in particular, ascertain whether the woman has had a biopsy. This is important for two reasons: first, certain benign breast problems (lobular neoplasia, atypical ductal hyperplasia) are associated with an increased risk of breast cancer; and second, biopsy may produce some distortion and scarring in the breast contour and parenchyma.

A detailed gynaecological history is important. Ask the age of menarche, number of pregnancies, age at first pregnancy and whether or not the woman is still having periods. For menstruating women, ask the date of the last menses. In general, breast nodularity and tenderness associated with fibrocystic changes will be maximal between ovulation and menstruation; therefore re-examination after the onset of menses may help to demonstrate that a tender region is simply an exaggerated response to normal hormonal changes.

It is important to know if the woman is currently taking oral contraceptives or postmenopausal hormone therapy, and whether she has taken these in the past. Ask about treatment for infertility and prenatal exposure to diethylstilbestrol.

Finally, a personal history of cancer of the contralateral breast or other sites is important. Ovarian and endometrial carcinoma are each associated with an increased risk of breast cancer. Some malignancies can actually metastasize to the breast but this is rare and is usually associated with other manifestations of systemic spread. Radiation treatment to the head and neck or mantle irradiation (for Hodgkin's disease) substantially increases the risk of breast cancer.

**Table 28.2 The breast history**

| | Questions to ask |
|---|---|
| For any complaint | When did it start? Has it changed? |
| Lump | How was it discovered? Has there been a change in size? Is there any associated pain or tenderness? Does it change with menses? |
| Pain or tenderness | Is there an associated lump? Does it change with menses? |
| Nipple discharge | Duration? Spontaneous or elicited? Unilateral or bilateral? Colour? |
| Gynaecological history | Menarche? Number of pregnancies? Age at first pregnancy? Still menstruating? Last period? Exposure to exogenous hormones? |
| Family history | Breast cancer (including age at diagnosis) – bilateral? Ovarian cancer? Colon cancer? Melanoma? Other malignancies? |

## PHYSICAL EXAMINATION

Take care to ensure that the examining room is warm, comfortable and private. A mobile examining lamp provides extra illumination when examining the nipples for discharge or when looking for subtle signs of skin retraction. Begin the examination with the patient sitting upright facing you. A cape or other drape that can be elevated to reveal the breasts provides some warmth and comfort until the examination begins.

As with other parts of the body, start with inspection (Table 28.3). Expose both breasts and the entire anterior torso. A diagram or form on which to record abnormalities is useful (Figure 28.1). It is common for one breast to be slightly larger than the other. In some cases, this difference is exaggerated and unilateral hypoplasia or hypertrophy may be present (Figure 28.2).

Note the size and shape of the breasts and any recent change in size or shape. The breasts change during growth and development, and enlarge considerably during pregnancy. After the menopause, the glandular tissue involutes. The nipples typically point out, particularly when erect. In some women, this does not occur and nipple inversion is seen. It is important to distinguish this congenital nipple inversion (Figure 28.3) from inversion due to underlying pathology (Figure 28.4).

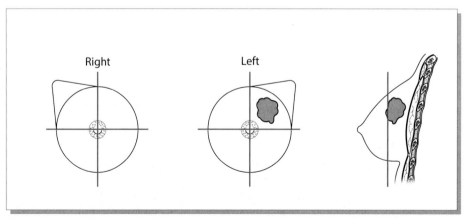

Figure 28.1 An example of a form on which abnormalities may be drawn. This form shows how a clinician has recorded the location, size and physical characteristics of a breast lump.

Table 28.3 Physical examination

| Inspection | Symmetry |
|---|---|
|  | Signs of retraction |
|  | Nipple retraction |
|  | Skin changes |
| Palpation | Masses |
|  | Axillae |

Have the woman raise her arms over her head and note how the breasts move. Skin retraction on one side suggests an underlying neoplasm (Figure 28.5). Similarly, ask her to lean forwards, and look for asymmetry. Then have her put her hands on her hips and push in to tense her pectoralis major muscles.

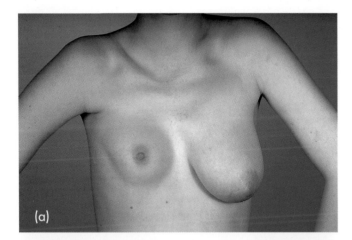

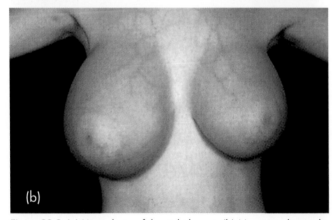

Figure 28.2 (a) Hypoplasia of the right breast. (b) Mammary hyperplasia in a 13-year-old girl.

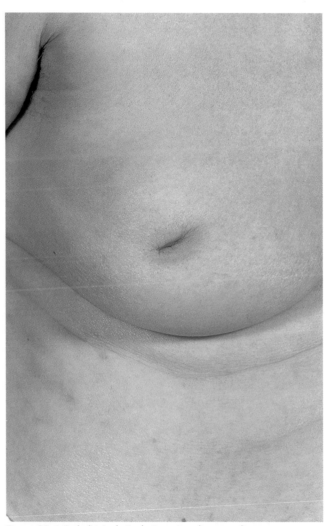

Figure 28.4 Pathological nipple inversion due to malignancy.

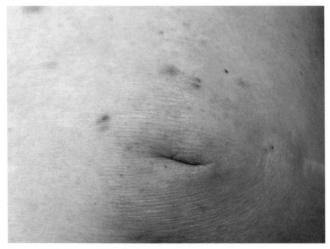

Figure 28.3 Congenital nipple inversion.

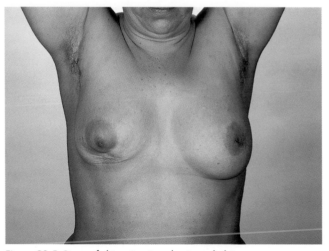

Figure 28.5 Signs of skin retraction due to underlying cancer.

PART 5 | BREAST AND ENDOCRINE

This may demonstrate skin retraction due to an underlying cancer adherent to these muscles (Figure 28.6).

Look for any skin abnormalities or indentations. In addition to the skin retraction noted with cancer, a vertical groove on the lateral aspect of the breast is sometimes seen in association with a benign condition, Mondor's disease, which is superficial phlebitis of a lateral thoracic vein (Figure 28.7). Locally advanced breast cancer may be associated with skin nodules (Figure 28.8) or ulceration (Figure 28.9). If the woman has received radiation treatment for breast cancer, telangiectases are common (Figure 28.10), but the sudden appearance of red or purple nodules suggests radiation-induced angiosarcoma. Oedema and reddening of the skin are seen with inflammatory breast cancer and with breast abscesses (Figure 28.11). The characteristic peau d'orange (French for 'orange peel') appearance results from subcutaneous oedema with associated tethering and retraction of the hair follicles and sweat glands (Figure 28.12).

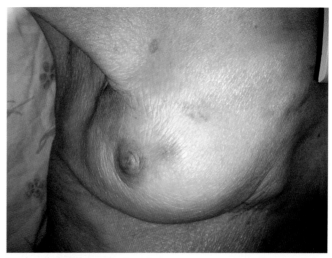

Figure 28.8 Skin nodules from breast cancer.

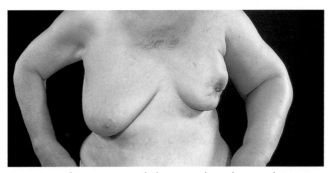

Figure 28.6 Skin retraction with the pectoral muscles tensed.

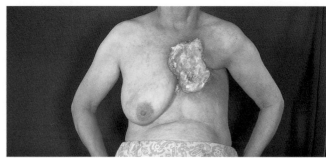

Figure 28.9 Extensive skin ulceration of the left breast from advanced breast cancer.

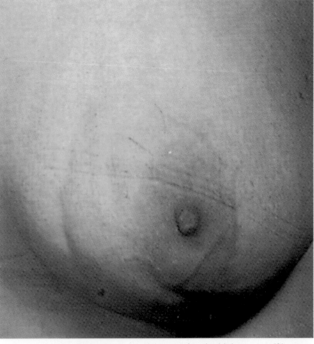

Figure 28.7 Mondor's disease. The superficial phlebitis is self-limiting and usually resolves within a few weeks.

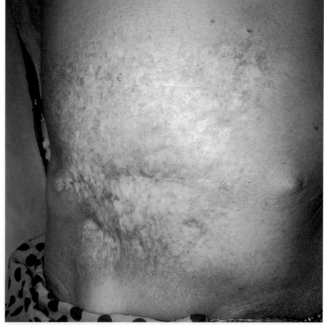

Figure 28.10 Radiation-induced telangiectases. (Courtesy of Dr D. N. Sharma, Department of Radiation Oncology, All India Institute of Medical Sciences.)

Use the examining lamp to bring extra light to bear, and look carefully at the surface of the nipples. Paget's disease, a form of breast cancer, is noted as a 'rash' extending radially out from the nipple surface (Figure 28.13). If the woman complains of nipple discharge, ask her to elicit it. Note where she presses and how firmly. Note the colour of the discharge (Table 28.4), and whether it comes from a single duct (and if so, which quadrant of the nipple surface it is in) or from multiple ducts (Figure 28.14). Test the discharge for the presence of blood. Smears may be made for cytological examination but this rarely yields useful information.

While the woman is still sitting up with her hands on her hips, feel the axillae for lumps. Have her relax her muscles. Lymph nodes associated with breast cancer are divided into three levels (Figure 28.15): level I nodes lie along the chest wall lateral to the pectoralis minor muscle; level II nodes lie under the pectoralis minor muscle; and level III nodes lie high at the apex of the axilla medial to pectoralis minor. Level I and II nodes are most easily felt by examining both sides simultaneously, placing a hand high up on each lateral chest wall and then sliding the fingers down. Small mobile nodes are often felt bilaterally in slender young women but the presence of unilateral enlarged nodes suggests underlying malignancy. Note the size, mobility and texture

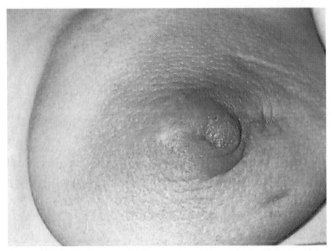

Figure 28.11 Oedema and inflammation of the right breast caused by an underlying abscess.

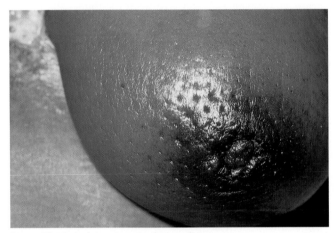

Figure 28.12 A close-up view of peau d'orange.

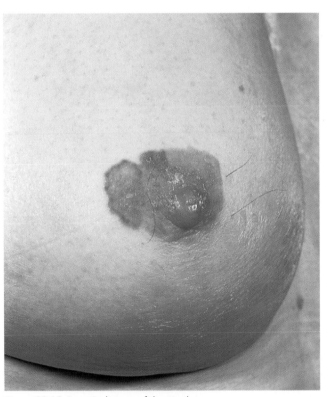

Figure 28.13 Paget's disease of the nipple.

Table 28.4 Types of nipple discharge

| Discharge | Causes |
| --- | --- |
| Bright red blood | The most common cause is a benign intraductal papilloma. Other causes include carcinoma. Bloody nipple discharge is sometimes seen during the third trimester of pregnancy and usually subsides once lactation begins |
| Dark, altered blood | As above, usually with an element of ductal obstruction |
| Slightly bloodstained fluid | Intraductal papilloma, intracystic carcinoma (especially with an associated mass) |
| Clear, yellow, serous fluid | May be due to malignancy but is usually due to underlying fibrocystic changes |
| Thick, green discharge | Ductal ectasia is the most common cause |
| Milky discharge | Usually due to insufficient suppression of lactation after weaning but is rarely the manifestation of a secreting prolactinoma of the pituitary gland |

PART 5 | BREAST AND ENDOCRINE

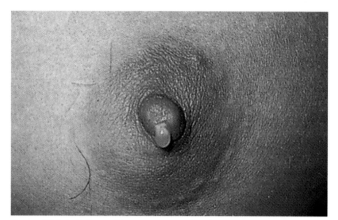

Figure 28.14 Galactorrhoea in a patient with a prolactinoma.

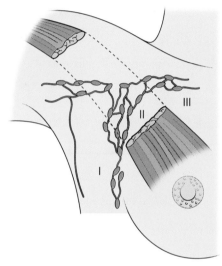

Figure 28.15 Drawing illustrating level I, II and III lymph nodes.

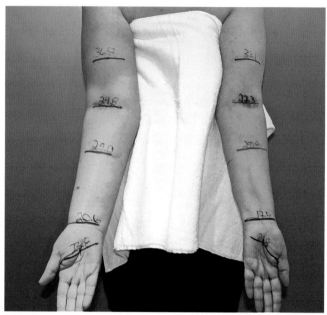

Figure 28.16 Lymphoedema of the right arm with measurements marked at standard points. (Courtesy of Wei F. Chen, MD.)

of any nodes. Similarly, feel the supraclavicular fossae for nodes, generally a sign of more advanced malignancy.

After examining the anterior part of the axilla and the level I and II nodes, gently introduce the hand further into the apex of each axilla. Nodes lying posteriorly around serratus anterior and latissimus dorsi, and the lateral group around the neck and shaft of the humerus, may most easily be felt with the examiner standing behind the woman. Obstructed lymphatics may cause arm oedema, as may previous axillary surgery (Figure 28.16). The presence of abnormal nodes should prompt a search for underlying malignancy. If no lump is palpable in the ipsilateral breast, additional imaging studies (see below) should be carried out. An MRI scan of the breast is sometimes required to find a small, clinically occult, breast cancer. Always consider other causes of isolated axillary adenopathy, such as melanoma (examine the arm and trunk for pigmented skin lesions) and lymphoma (check for enlarged nodes in other regions).

After the inspection is complete, palpate for lumps. If the woman has noted a lump, ask her to show you where it is and how it is most easily found. It is relatively common for women to note lumps while they are taking a shower, and in this case the lump may be most easily palpated with the woman sitting up

with the ipsilateral arm raised over her head. If the breasts are involuted and pendulous, feel the texture and thickness of both breasts by grasping each breast between the thumb and fingers. Use bimanual palpation for larger breasts. Diffuse and extensive involvement of the breast with lobular carcinoma is sometimes most easily found in this manner as the tumour may not form a discrete mass but rather replace a large amount of breast tissue in an insidious fashion.

Then have the patient lie down. Place a small pillow under her ipsilateral shoulder if necessary. Have her place her arm comfortably above her head. Use a systematic approach to feel the entire substance of the breast, either in a radial or a strip search pattern (Figure 28.17). Repeat this examination with three levels of pressure – light, medium and firm – so that nothing is missed.

Start with the normal or asymptomatic breast and compare one side with the other. Begin by getting a general sense for the texture and degree of nodularity of the unaffected breast parenchyma. If an abnormality is found, note the size, location (typically by clock face orientation and distance from nipple or areolar border), mobility and associated characteristics (Table 28.5). Do not neglect the axillary tails of the breast tissue where the breast feathers out along the upper outer quadrant (Figure 28.18). There are no physical characteristics that reliably distinguish benign from malignant masses; if a mass is detected, employ the triple test (see above).

If the presenting complaint is breast pain or tenderness, seek not only breast lumps, but also other causes for pain in the area. Tenderness of the costochondral junctions (Tietze's syndrome) is commonly perceived as having an origin in the breast. Any lump or area of tenderness should be further examined by imaging studies (see below) and freely employing the triple test cited above.

While the woman is lying supine, finish your examination by palpating the liver for metastatic deposits. Other signs of metastatic disease include localized skeletal pain and tenderness, and pleural effusion.

(a)

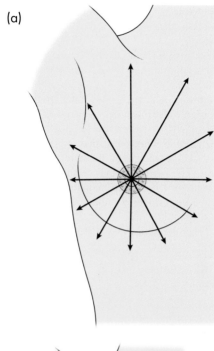

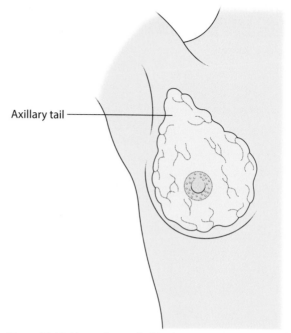

Axillary tail

Figure 28.18 The axillary tail of the breast.

(b)

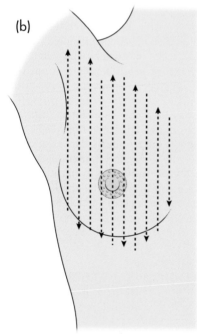

Figure 28.17 The (a) radial (sometimes called 'wedge') and (b) vertical strip patterns of breast examination.

Table 28.5 Characteristics of breast lumps

| Location | Clock face orientation |
| | Distance from nipple or areolar border |
| Size | |
| Mobility | Fixed to skin, underlying breast or muscle |
| Consistency | Firm |
| | Rubbery |
| | Hard |
| Edge | Well or poorly demarcated |
| Pain or tenderness | |

## DIFFERENTIAL DIAGNOSIS AND SPECIFIC PATHOLOGICAL ENTITIES

### Breast Cancer

Breast cancer vies with lung cancer as the most common type of cancer in women in the Western world today. After developing one breast cancer, a woman has an approximately five times greater risk of developing a second breast cancer. Around 1–2 per cent of breast cancers are diagnosed in men.

There is a strong genetic component, and testing is available for at least two genes (*BRCA1* and *BRCA2*) that are associated with a significantly increased genetic risk. Families that carry these genes typically include multiple women with early-onset breast cancer, bilateral breast cancer, ovarian cancer and male breast cancer. The genes are more common in certain populations (e.g. Ashkenazi Jews) than others. Several predictive models that can help to estimate the likelihood of a positive test are available online.

Links with hormonal activity (early menarche, late menopause, few or no pregnancies, exposure to exogenous hormones), radiation, smoking, alcohol intake and obesity have been noted in large epidemiological studies. Of these, the most clinically significant one is prior radiation to the region for Hodgkin's disease, as previously noted.

Breast cancer may be diagnosed as a lump on physical examination, or detected as an area of abnormality on screening mammography. The diagnosis is confirmed by obtaining a tissue sample by fine needle aspiration (FNA) cytology or core needle biopsy. These procedures may be performed under palpation or imaging (ultrasound or mammographic) guidance.

Cancer is staged according to the TNM system (Table 28.6), in which T refers to the tumour (by size in centimetres), N to regional node involvement and M to the presence or absence of metastatic disease. These gradings are then placed into stage groups, creating the overall stage I–IV, where I is the least and IV is the most advanced category of invasive disease. A clinical stage is assigned based upon the physical examination and imaging studies.

PART 5 | BREAST AND ENDOCRINE

Table 28.6 TNM classification (clinical)

| Stage | Description |
| --- | --- |
| **T = Primary tumour** | |
| Tis | Carcinoma *in situ* (ductal carcinoma *in situ* or Paget's disease of the nipple with no associated tumour mass) |
| T1 | Tumour less than 2 cm |
| T2 | Tumour 2–5 cm in greatest dimension |
| T3 | Tumour in excess of 5 cm |
| T4 | Tumour with direct extension to the chest wall or skin (oedema, ulceration, satellite skin nodules confined to the same breast), including inflammatory carcinoma |
| **N = Regional lymph nodes** | |
| NX | Cannot assess (i.e. previously removed) |
| N0 | No regional lymph node metastases |
| N1 | Metastasis to movable ipsilateral axillary lymph node(s) |
| N2 | Metastasis in ipsilateral axillary lymph nodes fixed to one another (matted) or to other structures (note: N2 subdivisions also include some cases of internal mammary node metastasis – see the TNM staging manual) |
| N3 | Other regional node involvement (see the TNM staging manual) |
| **M = Distant metastases** | |
| MX | Cannot assess |
| M0 | No distant metastases |
| M1 | Presence of distant metastases |

When surgical resection has been carried out, accurate pathological staging can be assigned. Additional tumour characteristics that are determined after biopsy include the presence or absence of oestrogen and progesterone receptors, and the presence or absence of HER2/neu positivity, as well as other markers. The stage is a strong predictor of the prognosis and helps to determine the treatment; therefore precise staging is essential, and the reader is advised to consult an up-to-date staging manual.

Malignant breast lumps tend to enlarge progressively and generally do not change with the menstrual cycle. If pain occurs, it is deep-seated and persistent. Nipple discharge if present is usually serous or serosanguinous, and the location of the duct may help to predict the quadrant in which the underlying tumour is found. Prompt diagnosis is essential for appropriate treatment. A delay in diagnosis is particularly common in young women (in whom the diagnosis may not be considered), during pregnancy or with rapidly growing tumours, which may simulate infection. The clinician must thus maintain a high index of suspicion for this common malignancy.

## Phyllodes Tumour

A phyllodes tumour (formerly called cystosarcoma phyllodes or Brodie's disease) is a stromal tumour with a spectrum of behaviour ranging from relatively benign through to malignant. It shares with sarcomas the tendency to recur locally if not adequately excised.

In populations where mammographic screening is common, many phyllodes tumours are found on mammography. These are often small and relatively low grade; they resemble the more benign fibroadenomas (see below) and simply require adequate excision. More aggressive tumours may cause progressive enlargement of either the lump or the whole breast and are often painful. The breast may be tense and firm with thin overlying skin (which may ulcerate) and enlarged veins (Figure 28.19). The treatment may require a total mastectomy. A phyllodes tumour, even when malignant, rarely metastasizes to the regional lymph nodes, so nodal staging is not commonly employed.

Although other sarcomas may arise in the breast, these are distinctly rare.

## Benign Breast Disease

Benign breast disease is extremely common, especially in women between the ages of 20 and 40. In the USA, it has been customary to refer to the spectrum of these conditions as fibrocystic changes. They may more accurately be termed aberrations of normal development and involution. Over the years, a series of terms have been used and abandoned, including fibroadenosis, chronic mastitis, cystic mastopathy and benign mammary dysplasia. The aetiology is poorly understood but is likely to involve the action of cyclical circulating hormone levels on breast tissue.

There is often a change in the nodularity of the breast tissue. This may be focal or diffuse, unilateral or bilateral. When focal, it may be perceived as a discrete lump. The most common site for lumps and nodularity is the upper outer quadrant and axillary tail (and unfortunately this is also the most common site of breast cancer because this quadrant has the largest volume of breast tissue). Lumps can be single or multiple and may grow suddenly or regress. They tend to enlarge and become more tender premenstrually.

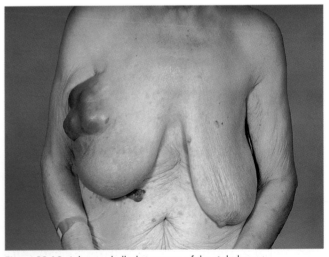

Figure 28.19 A large phyllodes tumour of the right breast.

## Simple Cysts

These present as tender masses and are fluid-filled collections (Figure 28.20). The diagnosis can be established by the aspiration of green or straw-coloured fluid and the disappearance of the mass, or by ultrasound (see below). There is no relationship between gross cystic disease and breast cancer.

## Fibroadenomas

Fibroadenomas are benign tumours of the breast that are common in women in their late teens to their early 30s. Most fibroadenomas grow to 1–2 cm in diameter, and their size can fluctuate due to the influence of hormones during the menstrual cycle. These benign masses usually present as a hard, painless lump that is freely mobile on palpation. An ultrasound of the mass can differentiate between a fibroadenoma and a cyst (Figure 28.21).

There is no clear consensus on whether a fibroadenoma should be surgically removed. If the triple test is consistent with a fibroadenoma, the lesion can be managed conservatively with a follow-up examination in 6 months.

## Trauma

After trauma to the breast, a woman may develop fat necrosis, which is the result of saponification of the adipose tissue. The major problem with fat necrosis is that it can be confused with breast cancer on imaging. There is often a characteristic oil cyst (a collection of lipids surrounded by a membrane) on mammography in the area of trauma, leading to the diagnosis of fat necrosis; however, the area of trauma may reveal fibrosis and calcifications that may mimic malignancy on mammography. If the patient does not recall trauma to the breast or imaging does not reveal an oil cyst, the area of concern should undergo a core or excisional biopsy to obtain a histological diagnosis.

## Galactoceles

These are milk-filled fluid collections most commonly seen during lactation or after the cessation of lactation. They are the result of ductal obstruction. Galactoceles routinely present as a slightly tender mass and can be multiple or bilateral. Ultrasound is routinely used to visualize the fluid-filled mass. Most galactoceles resolve after aspiration, and if the patient is asymptomatic the galactocele can also be simply observed.

## Abscesses

A subareolar abscess is often a recurring condition that is secondary to disease of the subareolar ducts. Patients are smokers in their late 20s to early 30s and present with a tender, palpable mass with associated erythema in the subareolar region (Figure 28.22).

Ultrasound examination can be used to identify an underlying abscess cavity. If the infection is early in its course and there is no underlying abscess cavity (induration with no fluctuance on palpation), a course of oral antibiotics should be prescribed. If an abscess cavity is present on sonography and the skin over the cavity is not thinned out or ulcerated, serial aspiration with a needle and syringe may be attempted, followed by antibiotics. If the skin is necrotic, surgical incision and drainage is warranted to drain the purulent fluid. Ideally, the skin incision should be made at the areolar border. It is important to remember that management of a subareolar abscess is only a temporizing measure as most of these patients will need definitive therapy that requires surgical removal of the diseased ducts.

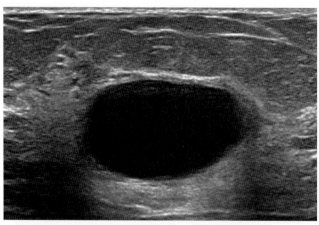

Figure 28.20 An ultrasound image of a cyst.

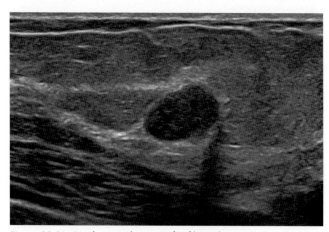

Figure 28.21 An ultrasound image of a fibroadenoma.

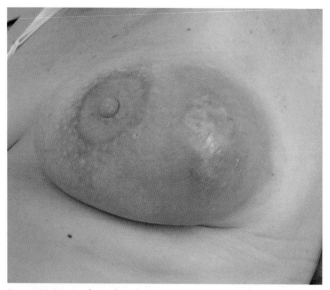

Figure 28.22 A subareolar abscess.

### Mammary Fistula

A mammary fistula is a consequence of a long-lasting or recurrent subareolar abscess that has spontaneously drained near the nipple–areolar complex on the skin (Figure 28.23). Surgical removal of the entire epithelialized tract is the mainstay of treatment.

### Gynaecomastia

Gynaecomastia is a benign proliferation of the glandular tissue of the male breast, and is the result of an imbalance in the oestrogen/androgen ratio that favours increased circulating oestrogen (Figure 28.24). Gynaecomastia is most often seen in infancy, during puberty and after the age of 50. Although physical pain can be associated with gynaecomastia, most men present for evaluation due to the psychological stress the condition can cause.

The list of causes of gynaecomastia is extensive and must be evaluated while taking a detailed history from the patient. Some of the more common aetiologies include physiological causes (puberty), obesity, malignancy (testicular cancer), genetic syndromes (Klinefelter's syndrome), liver failure, renal failure, anabolic steroids, marijuana use and medications (e.g. cimetidine, spironolactone, phenytoin).

The breast examination is performed while the patient is in the supine position with his hands behind his head. The examiner's thumb is placed on one side of the breast and the index finger on the other side of the breast. The two fingers are then brought together and the tissue behind the nipple is palpated. Patients with gynaecomastia have bilateral concentric, disk-like tissue that can often feel rubbery. Mammography and/or ultrasound has also been employed in patients with gynaecomastia to further delineate whether an underlying malignancy is present.

The treatment of gynaecomastia entails correction of the identifiable cause (e.g. the cessation of the causative medication), reassurance and observation (during puberty), medical therapy (tamoxifen) or surgical excision.

Male breast cancer accounts for approximately 1 per cent of all cases of breast cancer. Stage for stage, the prognosis is the same for men as it is for women with breast cancer, but men tend to present later than women and thus have a worse prognosis. Men have a reported average age at diagnosis from their late 60s to early 70s, which is approximately 10 years older than in women. Men with *BRCA1* or *BRCA2* mutations and those with Klinefelter's syndrome have an increased risk of developing breast cancer.

Most men with breast cancer will present with a painless mass in the subareolar area (Figure 28.25). It is not uncommon for the nipple to be retracted or ulcerated. Nipple discharge is less commonly seen. Fixation to the skin or to the underlying muscle may also be appreciated on physical examination.

As in women with a suspected breast malignancy, men must undergo the triple test, which includes a detailed history and physical examination, mammography and/or ultrasound, and tissue diagnosis with a core needle biopsy. A mastectomy with a sentinel lymph node biopsy is the preferred method of surgical treatment, as the relatively small amount of breast tissue in a man limits the use of breast conservation therapy.

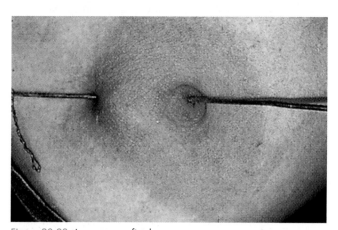

Figure 28.23 A mammary fistula.

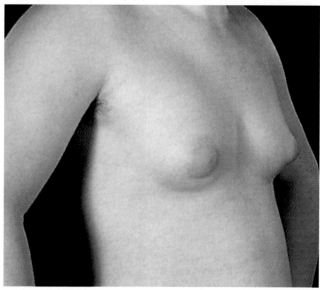

Figure 28.24 Gynaecomastia.

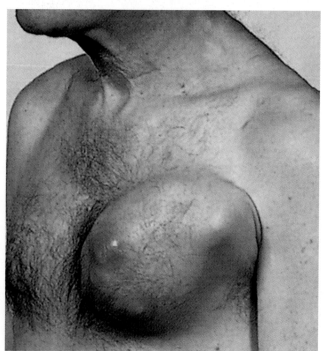

Figure 28.25 Male breast cancer.

## SUPPORTIVE DIAGNOSTIC TOOLS

### Ultrasound Examination

Because ultrasound is a targeted examination, it is ideally suited to the situation when a lump is felt by either the clinician or the woman herself. The transducer can be placed directly over the lump or region of tenderness, and careful scanning of the underlying area can confirm or exclude the presence of a mass. Cysts are typically anechoic or hypoechoic and smooth-walled, and exhibit edge effect and posterior enhancement (Figure 28.26). Solid masses contain internal echoes (Figure 28.27). While there are ultrasound characteristics that are more or less suggestive of malignancy, the safest course is to undertake tissue sampling for anything not definitively shown to be a cyst.

### Mammography

Ultrasound, while useful, does not supplant the need for mammography except perhaps in the very young patient. Two views are taken of each breast – craniocaudal (Figure 28.28) and mediolateral oblique (Figure 28.29). These are not strictly orthogonal views, and care must be taken in extrapolating the location of a mass from the region where it is seen on the mammogram.

Not all cancers can be seen on mammography. If a mass or abnormality is noted on physical examination but the mammograms are normal, this does not exclude cancer.

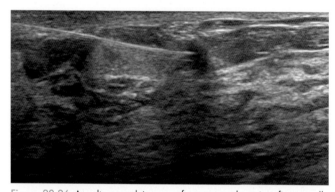

Figure 28.26 An ultrasound image of a cyst undergoing fine needle aspiration (note the needle entering obliquely from the upper left).

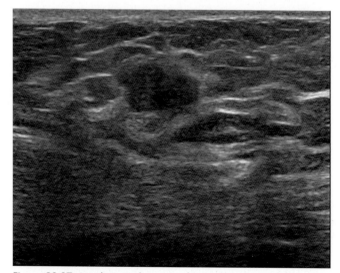

Figure 28.27 An ultrasound image of an indeterminate solid mass; a biopsy is now needed.

### MRI Scanning

MRI scans are the most sensitive and expensive imaging modalities currently available. They are used as screening modalities in women with an extremely high risk of breast cancer or during the search for an occult breast primary, most commonly one that has presented with enlarged axillary nodes. In the USA, they are increasingly used when lumpectomy (rather than mastectomy) is chosen for the treatment of the breast cancer and it is important to exclude multicentric disease.

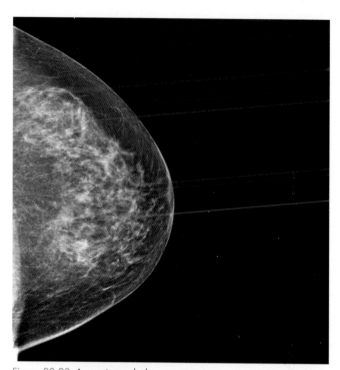

Figure 28.28 A craniocaudal mammogram.

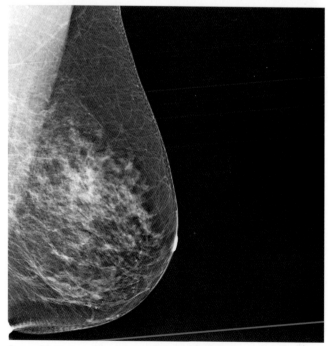

Figure 28.29 A mediolateral oblique mammogram.

PART 5 | BREAST AND ENDOCRINE

## Biopsies

Percutaneous biopsies such as FNA or core needle biopsy are preferred over open surgical biopsy to obtain tissue for pathological examination. Percutaneous biopsies can be carried out at the bedside, cost less and are less invasive than open surgical biopsies. Both FNA and core needle biopsies of palpable masses should be done under image guidance to decrease the risk of a sampling error.

## Fine Needle Aspiration Cytology

Fine needle aspiration is a quick and inexpensive biopsy that can be carried out at the bedside under ultrasound guidance. It can be used to sample a breast mass or an axillary lymph node using a hand-held syringe and a 22 or 25 gauge needle to aspirate cells for a cytology examination for pathological examination (Figure 28.30). Fine needle aspiration can also determine whether a breast mass is solid or cystic, and aspiration of a breast cyst can be not only diagnostic, but also therapeutic. The major limitation of FNA is that it does not provide any architecture and thus a cytopathologist cannot determine between *in situ* and invasive disease.

## Core Needle Biopsy

A core needle biopsy can also be carried out at the bedside under ultrasound guidance or in the radiology department with mammographic guidance (Figure 28.31) and has become the preferred method for tissue sampling in the USA, particularly when cancer is suspected. After a small incision has been made in the skin with a scalpel, a disposable, spring-loaded hand-held device with a 12–18 gauge needle is used to obtain at least three tissue samples from the lesion of concern. The main advantage of a core needle biopsy is that it provides tissue architecture and thus a cytopathologist can determine whether there is an invasive component to the specimen.

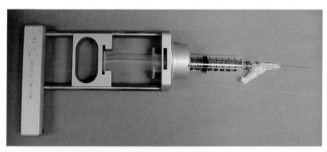

Figure 28.30 **Apparatus for fine needle aspiration cytology.**

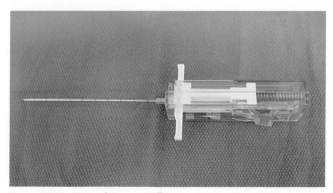

Figure 28.31 **A core biopsy needle.**

## TREATMENT

Isolated solid masses, such as large fibroadenomas, are commonly removed. Breast cancer may be treated by lumpectomy (removal of the tumour with a rim of surrounding tissue) followed by radiation therapy, or by mastectomy. With either lumpectomy or mastectomy, axillary staging is required. Further treatment with chemotherapy or hormone-blocking agents is commonly employed. Women who present with large or locally advanced breast cancer are generally treated with chemotherapy first; surgery is then performed after the tumour has shrunk. Radiation therapy is used after lumpectomy to decrease the risk of local recurrence. It is also used in selected situations after mastectomy. A very comprehensive set of guidelines is available from the National Comprehensive Cancer Network and may be accessed from their website after free registration as a medical professional.

Reconstructive surgery may be combined with mastectomy or performed at a later time. Reconstructive options include autologous tissue or prosthetics. Autologous tissue reconstruction techniques involve tissue flaps or transfers, and the most commonly utilized techniques include the transverse rectus abdominis myocutaneous flap and the latissimus dorsi myocutaneous flap. Prosthetic reconstruction involves the use of saline or silicone implants. Most patients who undergo prosthetic reconstruction have tissue expanders placed at the time of the mastectomy that are sequentially expanded over the next few weeks and then eventually replaced with a permanent implant.

### Key Points

- Common symptoms of breast problems may include a mass or lump, pain and nipple discharge.
- The 'triple test' includes the clinical examination, radiological imaging studies and tissue sampling.
- A detailed history must include a discussion of the presenting problem, any previous breast problems, a detailed gynaecological history and a family history.
- The physical examination includes a detailed inspection and palpation of the breasts and axilla, with the patient in both the sitting and supine positions.
- Breast cancer may be diagnosed as a lump on physical examination or detected as an area of abnormality on screening mammography, and the diagnosis is confirmed by obtaining a tissue sample by FNA cytology or core needle biopsy.
- Cancer is staged according to the TNM system, where T refers to the tumour (by size in centimetres), N to regional node involvement and M to the presence or absence of metastatic disease.
- Benign breast disease is a common entity in women aged 20–40 and covers a wide spectrum of conditions.
- Gynaecomastia is the result of an imbalance in the oestrogen/androgen ratio that favours increased circulating oestrogen, and the list of its causes is extensive.
- Male breast cancer accounts for approximately 1 per cent of all breast cancer cases.
- Men tend to present later than women, but stage for stage the prognosis is the same for men as it is for women with breast cancer.
- Supportive diagnostic tools for evaluating breast lesions include mammography, ultrasound, MRI, FNA and core needle biopsy.
- Breast cancer may be treated with lumpectomy, mastectomy, radiation, chemotherapy and/or hormonal blocking agents.

## QUESTIONS

### SBAs

**1. The 'triple test' does not include which of the following?:**
a History and physical examination
b Tissue diagnosis
c Genetic testing
d Radiological studies

Answer
c **Genetic testing.** *Genetic testing is not routinely performed on patients presenting with breast problems unless the patient is of a young age (less than 50 years old) or has a strong family history of breast or ovarian cancer.*

**2. Compared with women, men with breast cancer:**
a On average present at an earlier age
b Stage for stage have the same prognosis as women with breast cancer
c Are often hormone receptor-negative
d Account for 10 per cent of all breast cancers

Answer
b **Stage for stage have the same prognosis as women with breast cancer.** *Male breast cancer accounts for approximately 1 per cent of all breast cancer cases. Stage for stage, the prognosis is the same for men as it is women with breast cancer, but men tend to present later than women and thus have a worse prognosis. Men have a reported average age at diagnosis from their late 60s to early 70s, which is approximately 10 years older than in women. The majority of men are hormone receptor-positive.*

**3. Commonly employed imaging modalities used to evaluate patients presenting with breast lesions include all the following except:**
a Mammography
b MRI
c Ultrasound
d Positron emission tomography scanning

Answer:
d **Positron emission tomography scanning.** *Positron emission tomography scanning is not used to visualize a primary tumour of the breast. It is more commonly undertaken when a patient is suspected of having distant (metastatic) disease or recurrent breast cancer.*

### EMQ

**1. For each of the following descriptions, select the most likely matches for the presentations given below. Each option may be used once, more than once or not at all:**
1 Simple cyst
2 Fibroadenoma
3 Fat necrosis
4 Galactocele
5 Mammary fistula
6 Gynaecomastia
7 Subareolar abscess
a Often results from trauma to the breast and can be confused with breast cancer on imaging
b Most commonly seen during lactation and is the result of ductal obstruction

Answers
a 3 **Fat necrosis.** *After trauma to the breast, a woman may develop fat necrosis, which is the result of saponification of the adipose tissue. The major problem with fat necrosis is that it can be confused with breast cancer on imaging. If the patient does not recall trauma to the breast or imaging does not reveal a characteristic oil cyst, the area of concern should undergo a core or excisional biopsy to obtain a histological diagnosis.*

b 4 **Galactocele.** *Galactoceles are milk-filled fluid collections that are most commonly seen during lactation or after cessation of lactation. They are the result of ductal obstruction. Galactoceles routinely present as a slightly tender mass and can be multiple or bilateral. Ultrasound is routinely used to visualize the fluid-filled mass. Most galactoceles resolve after aspiration, and if the patient is asymptomatic the galactocele can also be simply observed.*

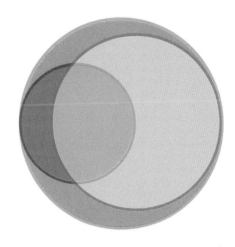

# PART

# 6

# Cardiothoracic

# The Thorax (Including the Oesophagus)

Fawwaz R. Shaw and Pierre M. Sfeir

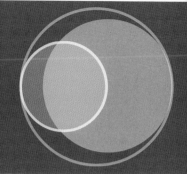

## LEARNING OBJECTIVES

- To identify the signs and symptoms of respiratory failure
- To recognize the signs and symptoms of lung tumours
- To identify the signs and symptoms of chest trauma
- To identify the signs and symptoms of oesophageal reflux and motility disorders
- To identify the signs and symptoms of oesophageal tumours
- To recognize the essential findings in a systematic physical examination of the lungs, chest wall and oesophagus

## EXAMINATION OF THE RESPIRATORY SYSTEM AND THORAX

### General Examination

Symptoms such as pleuritic chest pain, shortness of breath, dyspnoea, cough, cyanosis and the presence of respiratory embarrassment require a thorough examination of the respiratory system. This examination should include elements of inspection, percussion, auscultation and palpation, as the presence of clinical findings such as tachypnoea (an increased respiratory rate), the use of accessory respiratory muscles, poor air exchange, stridor and wheezing may offer clues as to the diagnosis.

#### Airway Obstruction

Obstruction of the respiratory airways is in many cases a medical emergency. The location of the airway obstruction may vary anatomically and can be supraglottic, laryngeal, tracheal or bronchial. A combination of anatomical airway segments is often involved, as in the presence of a tumour resulting in tracheobronchial obstruction.

**Stridor** is a harsh respiratory noise that is most often associated with an obstruction of the upper airways. It can be associated with tracheal or laryngeal obstructions, as in the presence of anaphylaxis with resultant vocal cord oedema.

Complete upper airway obstruction results in rapid respiratory embarrassment and additionally presents with dyspnoea, tachypnoea, diaphoresis (excessive sweating) and a subsequent loss of consciousness. There is also use of the accessory respiratory muscles (the abdominal and intercostal muscles) as an effort is made to re-establish the normal intrathoracic pressures. Examination of the thorax reveals deep retractions of the intercostal muscles, an exaggerated use of the abdominal wall musculature, nasal flaring and retraction of the supraclavicular fossa.

Productive **sputum** may be characteristic of an ongoing respiratory process, and information regarding the duration, character and associated symptoms should be obtained:

- *Mucoid sputum* is produced with acute or chronic bronchitis with viral upper respiratory infection.
- *White/pink frothy sputum* is seen in pulmonary oedema.
- *Yellow/green sputum* is typical of bacterial infection.
- *Rust-coloured sputum* is seen with pneumococcal pneumonia.
- *Blood-tinged sputum* occurs in lung cancer, tuberculosis and fungal infections with erosion into pulmonary vasculature.

#### Clubbing

This refers to the thickening of the distal aspect of the finger with an increase in the convex shape of the nail bed. It is associated with cigarette smoking and is associated with a number of cardiopulmonary pathologies including lung cancer, lung abscess, pulmonary fibrosis, chronic obstructive pulmonary disease, emphysema, pleural and mediastinal malignancies, cystic fibrosis and lung abscess.

### Examination of the Chest

The chest should be examined with the patient in both the supine and upright positions. This allows both the anterior and posterior chest as well as the symmetry to be evaluated.

#### Inspection

The thoracic spine should be examined for any abnormal curvature.

**Kyphosis** refers to an exaggerated anterior–posterior curvature of the spine, while **scoliosis** refers to an abnormal lateral curvature. Associate scoliosis is seen in up to 20 per cent of patients with pectus excavatum, which is a congenital sternal depression or concavity associated with the distal third of the sternum. Conversely, pectus carinatum is a outward bulge or convex deformity of the sternum.

The chest wall should be assessed for symmetry. Symmetry of the chest during inspiration and expiration should be evaluated. A failure of expansion of one side of the chest during a respiratory cycle indicates the presence of underlying pathology. The chest circumference can be measured at the level of the nipples during both the inspiratory and expiratory phases. The variation in diameter of the thoracic cavity is usually greater than 5 cm.

Counting the Ribs – The ribs can be counted using fixed landmarks on the rib cage:

- The sternal notch can be felt at the superiormost aspect of the manubrium.
- When palpating the manubrium from cranial to caudal, the sternomanubrial joint can be felt as a transverse convexity or ridge.
- Lateral to this is the second rib.
- Once this landmark has been identified, the interspaces and hence the ribs can be counted.
- The fourth rib usually correlates with the nipples in men and the inframammary crease in women.

Chest Wall Vasculature – Inspection of the chest wall may reveal abnormal dilated veins that are suggestive of a central venous occlusion, such as superior vena cava syndrome or venous involvement in thoracic outlet syndrome. Other venous chest wall changes are seen with chest wall irradiation. A reddish vascular-appearing mass on the chest wall in a patient who has had prior chest wall irradiation may represent an angiosarcoma.

A pulsatile mass in the supraclavicular fossa may be indicative of a post-obstructive aneurysm in the setting of thoracic outlet syndrome involving the axillary artery.

The Trachea – The trachea is usually found in the midline. Anteriorly, there are incomplete C-shaped cartilaginous rings, while posteriorly the trachea is membranous. Placing a finger in the suprasternal notch and palpating the location of these rings can confirm its position in the midline. Tension pneumothoraces, mediastinal tumours, cervical masses or volume loss from a hemithorax may result in tracheal deviation.

Auscultation of the chest may provide a clue as to the underlying pathology when tracheal deviation is present. For example, a loss of breath sounds in a hemithorax in conjunction with tracheal deviation is suggestive of a tension pneumothorax.

## Percussion

Percussion of the chest is usually performed on the posterior aspect of the thoracic cavity in the interspaces between the ribs. Consolidation of the underlying lung parenchyma, hydrothorax, haemothorax, chylothorax and lung- or pleural-based masses lead to decreased resonance or dullness to percussion. Hyperresonance is associated with pneumothoraces or air-trapping in the associated lung segments. As the examination of the right hemithorax proceeds caudally, dullness to percussion is experienced in the region of the liver.

## Auscultation

The lung should be examined by auscultation anteriorly and posteriorly as well as at multiple levels to evaluate all the lobes. The breath sounds heard over the normal lung parenchyma are softer and more even than those heard over the trachea and larynx, as the airway sounds are tempered by the chest wall and normal lung parenchyma.

Inspiratory breath sounds are heard throughout the inspiratory phase of respiration, while normal expiratory breath sounds are heard only during the first half to two-thirds of the expiratory cycle. The expiratory phase of respiration during normal ventilation is often twice as long as the inspiratory phase. This normal pattern on auscultation of the breath sounds is termed **vesicular breath sounds**.

Posteriorly, the lung should not be auscultated through the scapula. Instead, auscultation is performed medial to the medial borders of the scapula within the auscultatory triangle. Auscultation of the lung in the upright position may reveal the presence of an effusion and can provide useful information on the level and volume of such an effusion.

The breath sounds are difficult to auscultate or are diminished when the lung parenchyma no longer is in apposition to the chest wall, preventing the optimal conduction of the breath sounds. The underlying pathology includes pneumothorax, hydrothorax, haemothorax, chylothorax, pleural thickening, empyema and atelectasis. Obese patients with increased amounts of subcutaneous tissue may also present a challenge when auscultating the breath sounds.

**Bronchial breath sounds** are appreciated when the lung parenchyma becomes consolidated and the auscultatory qualities of the breath sounds heard in the main airway and over the consolidated parenchyma become similar.

**Wheezes** are coarse, high-pitched breath sounds that can be present during both the inspiratory and expiratory phases of the respiratory cycle. They imply bronchiectasis or narrowing of the airway and are present in reactive airway diseases such as asthma.

**Crackles** are breath sounds that most closely resemble the sound made by screwing up a sheet of paper. They vary in coarseness, and are uniformly present in patients with pulmonary oedema. Fine crackles are heard more in the early phases of pneumonia and alveolitis. Coarser crackles can also be heard in bronchiectasis. They represent the sound made by the opening and closing of the distal airways that are surrounded by diseased parenchyma. Crackles may be alternated with **rales**, but these terms are often used to refer to the same auscultatory finding.

**Pleural rubs** are present in inflammation of the pleural surfaces and are due to the visceral and parietal pleura sliding over each other.

## Palpation

Palpation of the chest wall may reveal sternal fractures, rib fractures, the presence of pathological lymphadenopathy or masses. Bony or cartilaginous tumours can be appreciated by palpating the surface of the chest wall and costochondral joints, as well as the sternum.

Supraclavicular lymphadenopathy may be indicative of malignancies of the lung or breast. Similarly, axillary lymphadenopathy may be present in breast cancer or other infectious pulmonary pathologies.

## THE CHEST

### Thoracic Trauma

#### Rib Fractures

The site of a rib fracture is usually easily determined due to the location of the chest wall pain. In some patients, the diagnosis can be made by palpation of the rib. In others with more substantial chest walls, radiographic imaging is most useful.

Inspection of the chest can reveal the presence of a **flail segment** of the rib cage. This occurs when fractures of multiple ribs in multiple locations creates a free segment of the rib cage that moves paradoxically with respiration. Flail segments may cause severe respiratory embarrassment, especially in the elderly, and can significantly alter the mechanics of respiration. Figure 29.1 demonstrates a flail segment of the rib cage from posteriorly.

Rib fractures often are associated with other traumatic injuries, and these should be investigated. Multiple lower left-sided rib fractures may be associated with concomitant splenic or renal injury, while lower right-sided rib fractures may be associated with right renal injuries. Left-sided complex rib fractures may also be associated with diaphragmatic injuries. It is not

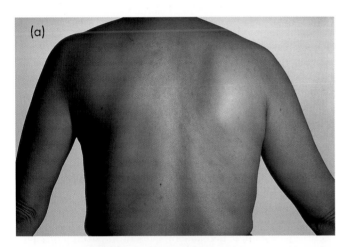

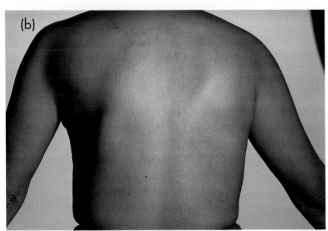

Figure 29.1 A flail section of the posterolateral aspect of the left chest. (a) At rest, there is slight asymmetry of the two sides of the chest. (b) On inspiration, the asymmetry is increased due to a drawing-in of the flail chest segment.

unusual for rib fractures to be associated with haemothoraces and pneumothoraces.

#### Sternal Fractures

Sternal fractures are associated with significant blunt force, and as such warrant an investigation for myocardial contusion and spinal injuries. Unstable sternal fractures may require surgical repair with plates or wires as these can significantly alter the mechanics of respiration. Severely displaced sternal fractures that are angulated towards the heart may also require reduction and stabilization to prevent subsequent cardiac injury.

#### Parenchymal Lung Injury

The lung is a fragile organ that, although protected in the bony framework of the rib cage, is still prone to injury. Any disruption of its protective housing can result in injury to the parenchyma. Parenchymal injuries should be suspected in patients who report a mechanism that is suggestive of trauma to the thorax and who present with clinical findings such as subcutaneous emphysema, decreased breath sounds, abnormal dullness to percussion of a hemithorax or a flail segment of the rib cage.

Subcutaneous Emphysema – This finding indicates that the parenchyma of the lung has been disrupted and air has been forced from the lung into the subcutaneous tissues. This condition is nearly always associated with a pneumothorax. Subcutaneous emphysema may be extensive, and can be associated with voice changes and extension into the face and abdominal soft tissues. It is best appreciated in the axillary soft tissues.

Subcutaneous emphysema is never life-threatening in isolation, but the cause must be quickly elucidated as it may pose a threat to life. The most impressive and rapidly developing subcutaneous emphysema is associated with major airway injuries such as tracheal injuries. In some cases, forceful exhalation against a closed glottis can result in subcutaneous emphysema.

Haemoptysis – In the setting of lung trauma, haemoptysis is indicative of disruption of the lung parenchyma with bleeding into an airway. Massive haemoptysis is usually a life-threatening finding, and can result in flooding of the contralateral airway and normal lung with blood, resulting in rapid decompensation.

A patient with a massive haemoptysis should be placed with the offending side downwards, and an airway should be established (usually with an endotracheal tube). A device such as a bronchial blocker can then be placed in the bronchus of the affected side, preventing the haemoptysis from filling the airways of the contralateral unaffected side. Massive haemoptysis may require surgical evaluation or angiographic evaluation and treatment.

#### Pulmonary Laceration

A laceration of the pulmonary parenchyma may result in a substantial **haemothorax** (blood in the pleural space) of the affected lung. This can usually be associated with dullness to percussion and distant breath sounds on the affected side. It is confirmed by chest X-ray.

Violation of the distal airways in a lung laceration may also produce a **pneumothorax** (air in the pleural space), which if untreated may result in a tension pneumothorax. **Tension pneumothoraces** are fatal if they are undiagnosed and untreated, as they result in a mediastinal shift and decreased venous return to the heart. This leads to pulmonary and cardiac decompensation. Figure 29.2 demonstrates a tension pneumothorax of the right lung with associated mediastinal shift and characteristic chest X-ray findings.

Treatment of a tension pneumothorax requires decompression of the affected pleural space. This can be accomplished by needle compression of the hemithorax in the second intercostal space at the midclavicular line.

Failure of a pulmonary laceration to heal may result in a chronic air leak, which characterizes an **alveolar-pleural fistula**. This is a communication between the alveoli and the pleural space that occurs when the parietal pleura in the region of a pulmonary laceration fail to heal. An injury to the distal bronchial airway that fails to heal leads to the formation of a **bronchopleural fistula**. Alveolar-pleural fistulae are more prone to healing over time than are bronchopleural fistulae. Bronchopleural fistulae may often require surgical intervention for closure.

If the chest wall is additionally violated, a **sucking chest wound** can be created. This occurs when the negative intrathoracic pressure created during respiration forces air into the thoracic cavity through the wound, creating a sucking noise. Similarly, air is forced through the wound during expiration. A sucking chest wound is managed by placement of a one-way valve over the wound, which prevents air entry during inspiration but allows air exit during expiration.

### Spontaneous Pneumothorax

Spontaneous pneumothoraces occur in the absence of chest trauma. They usually result from the rupture of a small bleb or bulla on the lung. Patients present with tachycardia, tachypnoea, absent breath sounds on the affected side, difficulty breathing, shortness of breath, increasing anxiety and chest pain.

Some pathological states may predispose a patient to spontaneous pneumothoraces; these include lymphangioleiomyomatosis, which predominantly affects women of childbearing age, and connective tissue disorders. They characteristically occur in tall slender adult males or females, are recurrent and can be bilateral. Pneumothoraces may also be iatrogenic and can occur with central venous access, thoracentesis, mediastinal biopsies and mechanical ventilation with high positive end-expiratory pressures.

## Chest Wall Deformities

### Pectus Excavatum

Pectus excavatum (Figure 29.3), or funnel chest, is a congenital abnormality that most frequently occurs in pubertal boys. It is due to an asymmetrical development of the costochondral cartilages along the distal one-third of the sternum. There are three types of pectus excavatum:

- a focal, cup-shaped deformity;
- a broad, shallow, saucer-type deformity;
- a long, furrowed, trench-like deformity.

The resultant deformity is a concavity in this region. It is characterized by an increased **Haller index**, which is the ratio between the lateral and anteroposterior dimensions of the thoracic cavity. A normal Haller index is 2.56. Patients with pectus excavatum most frequently present with decreased exercise tolerance, cardiac arrhythmias (due to compression of the right ventricle of the heart) and increased psychosocial awareness of the deformity.

### Pectus Carinatum

Pectus carinatum, or pigeon chest, is the opposite of pectus excavatum (Figure 29.4). It is characterized by a convex deformity of the chest wall due to an exaggerated asymmetrical development of the costochondral cartilages of the distal thoracic cavity. Like pectus excavatum, it is commonly present in pubertal and prepubertal boys who present with an increased psychosocial awareness of the deformity.

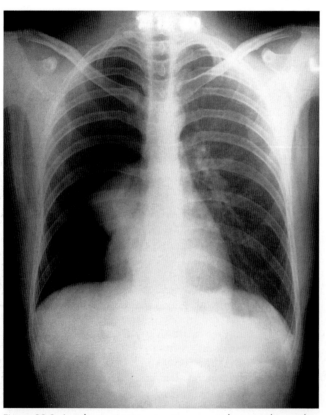

Figure 29.2 A right spontaneous tension pneumothorax with complete collapse of the right lung. The right pleural cavity is more lucent than the left, and there is an absence of any lung markings.

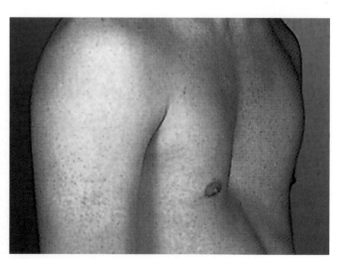

Figure 29.3 Pectus excavatum.

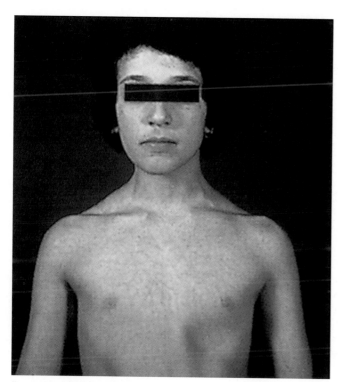

Figure 29.4 **Pectus carinatum.**

## Costochondritis

Costochondritis, or **Tietze's syndrome**, is inflammation and swelling of the costochondral cartilages. The most commonly affected is the second costochondral cartilage. The cartilage expands, creating the palpable mass that is often associated with this process. Costochondritis is usually treated with non-steroidal anti-inflammatory agents, with good results.

## Chest Wall Neoplasms

Chest wall neoplasms may be primary or metastatic.

The most common primary neoplasms of the rib are chondrosarcomas. These are usually anteriorly located and involve the constochondral joints. Patients present with symptoms of pain in the distribution of the affected intercostal nerve and may have a palpable mass on the affected costochondral joint. Chest CT scans or X-rays identify the lesion. Other primary neoplasms include chondromas, rhabdomyosarcomas, malignant fibrohistiocytomas and desmoid tumours.

Secondary neoplasms such as metastatic breast cancer, prostate cancer or multiple myeloma may also occur.

## Chest Wall Abscesses

These may arise as a result of any number or bacterial or mycobacterial pathogens. In the absence of concomitant pulmonary pathology, they may be associated with an infected lymph node or focus of infection in the underlying rib. These may also result in a chronic draining sinus of the chest wall. Underlying tuberculous disease may present in this fashion in an indolent yet persistent course.

## Notching of the Ribs

Aortic coarctation may result in notching of the ribs as a result of erosion of the inferior surface of the ribs in the region of the intercostal arteries, which become dilated as a result of collateralization. An aortic aneurysm is less likely to be diagnosed by physical findings on the chest wall.

## THE LUNGS

## Pulmonary Infection

Pulmonary infections are the source of much concern in the surgical as well as non-surgical patient. These infectious complications produce much morbidity and in some cases mortality in the hospitalized patient. Those more prone to pulmonary complications include active cigarette smokers, debilitated patients, patients requiring prolonged mechanical ventilation, individuals with altered mental status and those at risk of aspiration.

General endotracheal anaesthesia often results in a diminished ability to clear the airway secretions, leading to pooling in the airways. Failure to clear these secretions allows for a nidus of infection to be created, especially if aspiration, poor respiratory mechanics and a decreased ability to cough are present. Pre-existing microbial flora from the oropharynx and gastrointestinal tract or from nasopharyngeal colonization provide the inoculum for the subsequent pneumonia. Figure 29.5 demonstrates a left-sided pneumonia. Immunosuppressed patients or those in developing countries are at increased risk of mycobacterial infection (Figure 29.6).

If pneumonia goes undiagnosed or is unsuccessfully treated, this can result in the formation of a parapneumonic effusion. If this in turn becomes infected and goes untreated, an empyema can form. This complication, along with lung abscess, bronchiectasis, impaired oxygenation and ventilation and a persistent catabolic state, often leads to profound respiratory embarrassment.

Patients present with fever, chills, a productive cough or an inability to cough (as in the debilitated post-surgical patient), hypoxia, tachypnoea, tachycardia and pleuritic chest pain. Examination often demonstrates decreased breath sounds with crackles. Imaging of the chest reveals lobar consolidation, parapneumonic effusions, atelectasis and a loss of lung volume.

Bronchoscopy with bronchoalveolar lavage and culture allows a bacteriology result that will direct appropriate antibiotic therapy. Flexible fibreoptic bronchoscopy performed at the bedside in hospitalized patients has made diagnosis and treatment of this significant problem much more focused. Early parapneumonic effusions should be drained with a tube thoracostomy to prevent an empyema developing.

### Atelectasis

Atelectasis results when a portion of the lung parenchyma collapses around an occluded airway (Figure 29.7). This can be due to mucous plugging of the airway, or a neoplasm occluding the airway. In the post-surgical patient, this is often due to incomplete re-expansion of the lung after general anaesthesia. Splinting (rigidity of the chest muscles) due to pain during normal respiration also results in the development of atelectasis because of incomplete aeration of all the lung fields and a lack of re-expansion of the airways.

Failure of the atelectasis to resolve provides a nidus for bacteria and the subsequent development of a pneumonia, with the potential formation of a lung abscess. In young children, atelectasis can also occur after the inhalation of a foreign body that occludes a segment of the airway. In a similar manner, a tumour can occludes a segment of an airway. In this scenario, the subsequent pneumonia is referred to as post-obstructive.

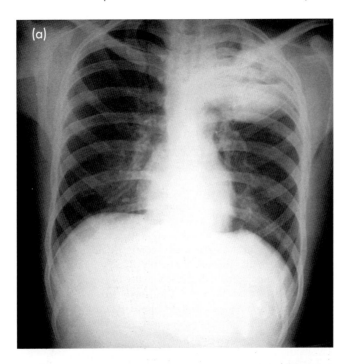

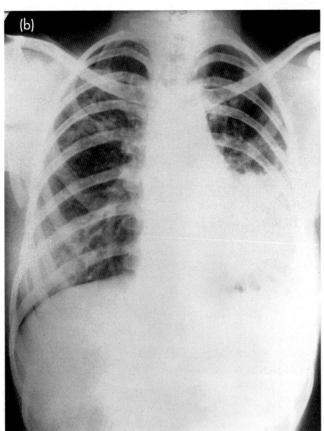

Figure 29.5 (a) Staphylococcal pneumonia. (b) Bronchopneumonia.

## Lung Abscess

A lung abscess (**Figure 29.8**) develops following a post-obstructive pneumonia that has been inadequately treated or an obstruction that has not been relieved. It may also follow an infection with a

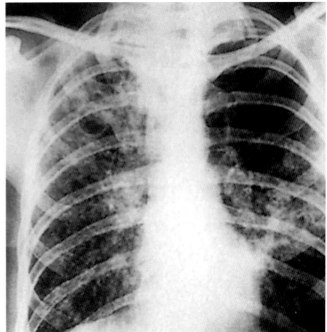

Figure 29.6 Post-tuberculosis lung infection, note the military involvement of the lung parenchyma.

particularly virulent strain of an organism such as *Mycobacterium tuberculosis*. Fungal or amoebic infections, or hydatid cysts, may also result in lung abscesses.

Lung abscesses are characterized by destruction of the pulmonary parenchyma and can be associated with bleeding as a result of erosion of the bronchial arteries. An air–fluid level often develops in the region of the pulmonary destruction and is pathognomonic of a lung abscess. In some cases, disruption of a surrounding airway leads to rupture of the abscess into the airway, and a bronchopleural fistula may arise. This can lead to seeding of the contralateral bronchial tree with the causative organism.

Due to the profound catabolic state that ensues, patients with lung abscesses are cachectic and severely ill. Surgery is almost never warranted in the setting of a lung abscess as there is too great a risk of severe complications.

## Bronchiectasis

Bronchiectasis is the destruction of medium-sized airways in the lung parenchyma. It may be seen in congenitally acquired pulmonary diseases, such as cystic fibrosis, or it may follow an acquired infectious process. This leads to inflammation of the involved airways with dilation of the airways and chronic infection.

Patients present with recurrent pulmonary infections, copious foul-smelling sputum, weight loss and cachexia (once again a sign of the profound catabolic state). Abnormal airway noises and wheezing are often present, indicative of the airway disease. The characteristic tram-track findings on a chest X-ray are diagnostic of the diseased airways involved.

Treatment of the underlying infection is key, but in some patients, such as those with cystic fibrosis, recurrent infection with multi-drug-resistant organisms are not unusual. Complete destruction of the lung can occur in states such as cystic fibrosis, ultimately requiring lung transplantation.

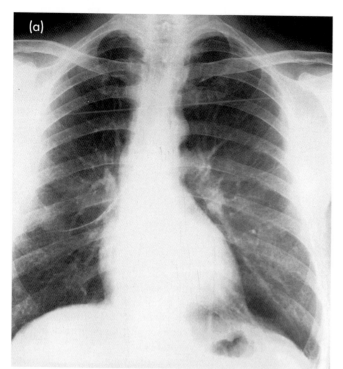

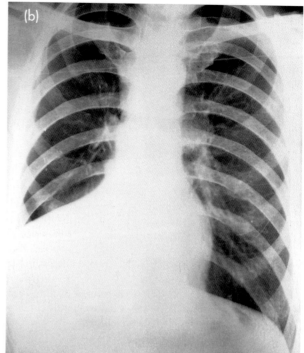

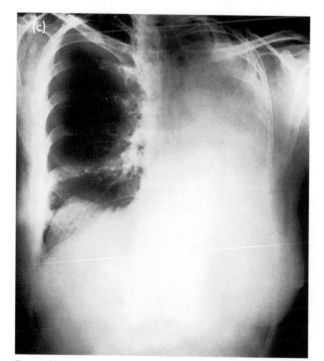

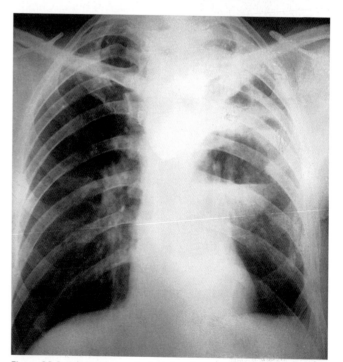

Figure 29.7 Atelectasis. (a) Right apical lower lobe. (b) Right lower lobe. (c) Left lung.

Figure 29.8 A lung abscess in the left mid-zone. Note the horizontal line at the pus–air interface.

## Pulmonary Embolism

Pulmonary emboli, found in the pulmonary arterial tree, usually originate in a distant source. Approximately one-third of pulmonary emboli derive from the lower extremities and pelvic veins.

The embolus usually travels from its site of origin through the right heart into the pulmonary artery, where it becomes lodged. This results in a filling defect and subsequent perfusion defect of that portion of the lung. The resultant physiological derangement is that of a ventilation–perfusion mismatch from the shunt that is created. A paradoxical embolus occurs when the passage of thrombus is from the left side of the heart via a congenital defect in the heart, such as a patent foramen ovale, into the right side of the heart and then into the pulmonary artery.

Pulmonary emboli classically develop subsequent to the formation of a deep venous thrombus that occurs as a result of Virchow's triad (stasis, endothelial injury, hypercoagulability). These are usually asymptomatic but may be associated with prolonged immobilization, the use of hormone replacement therapy or a family history of hypercoagulable states.

Tumours uncommonly embolize into the pulmonary arteries via the right side of the heart. The most common tumour to do so is an intracaval renal cell carcinoma, which may be dislodged during nephrectomy and embolize.

The characteristic clinical findings are tachycardia and tachypnoea in the setting of hypoxia. Investigations may show the following:

- ECG changes may demonstrate right heart strain or atrial fibrillation.
- Arterial blood gas measurements document the presence of a shunt.
- A chest X-ray may demonstrate wedge-shaped infarcts in the lung periphery.
- CT angiography or a pulmonary angiogram is diagnostic in most circumstances. Figure 29.9 demonstrates the filling defects associated with a pulmonary embolism.

Treatment in the acute setting involves anticoagulation, while acute tumour emboli may be removed by pulmonary artery embolectomy using cardiopulmonary bypass. Chronic pulmonary emboli with right heart dysfunction may be treated surgically with pulmonary thromboendarterectomy, using cardiopulmonary bypass and deep hypothermic circulatory arrest.

## Carcinoma of the Lung

Lung cancer (Figure 29.10) is the most common malignancy worldwide. It is predominantly associated with cigarette smoking, a minority of cases being associated with environmental exposure. Asbestos exposure is the most common occupational source of lung cancer.

There are many histological types of lung cancer. These can be divided into two large subgroups: non-small cell lung cancer and small cell lung cancer. They can further be identified histologically as:

- squamous cell cancer;
- adenocarcinoma;
- small cell lung cancer;
- bronchoalveolar carcinoma (now viewed as a variant of adenocarcinoma);
- pulmonary carcinoid.

The most common histological subtype is **squamous cell carcinoma**. These are centrally located tumours, unlike **adenocarcinomas**, which are more peripherally located. The small cell variant is highly aggressive, commonly presenting with early metastatic disease. The most common sites for metastases include the brain, adrenal glands, liver and bone.

Patients with lung cancer often are asymptomatic, the lesions often being found incidentally. More sinister clinical findings include weight loss, haemoptysis and the presence of paraneoplastic syndromes or symptoms associated with distant disease. These paraneoplastic syndromes include Cushing's syndrome, hypercalcaemia, hypertrophic pulmonary osteoarthropathy, ectopic antidiuretic hormone secretion and Horner's syndrome (miosis, ptosis and anhydrosis due to invasion and compression of the sympathetic chain at the level of the stellate ganglion, predominantly with superior sulcus tumours). Clubbing of the distal digits, tobacco staining of the fingernails and supraclavicular lymphadenopathy may also be present.

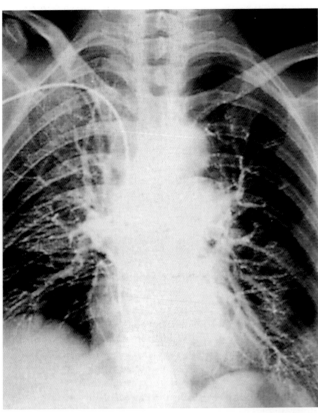

Figure 29.9 Pulmonary embolism (PE). Note the decreased pulmonary vasculature on the left. A PE may also occur with a completely normal chest xray.

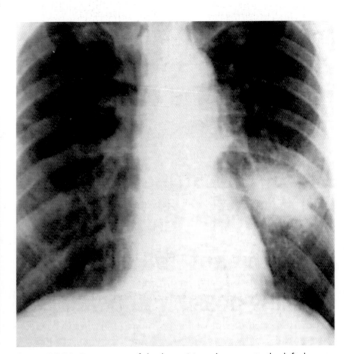

Figure 29.10 Carcinoma of the lung. Note the mass in the left lung.

Evaluation of the mediastinal lymph nodes is critical to the successful treatment of lung cancers. Extraparenchymal lymph node disease should be identified prior to planning surgical treatment as the presence of mediastinal or wider involvement warrants systemic therapy.

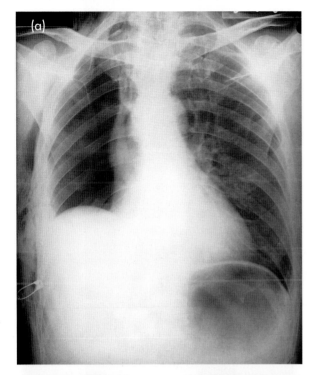

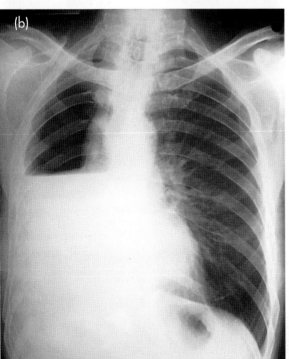

Figure 29.11 A right pneumonectomy undertaken for a carcinoma of the bronchus. (a) A first-day post-operation radiograph showing the air-filled right chest with no pulmonary markings. (b) A fifteenth-day radiograph showing a pleural effusion with an horizontal air–fluid interface and a mediastinal shift to the right.

Centrally located tumours may warrant pneumonectomy (Figure 29.11) if the patient's lung function will allow.

### Voice Changes

Involvement of the recurrent laryngeal nerve by the tumour results in hoarseness. This occurs particularly on the left side, where the recurrent laryngeal run in close proximity to the left main stem bronchus. Involvement of the recurrent laryngeal nerve is not, however, a frequent occurrence.

### Local Invasion

Rarely, carcinomas of the lung may result in an invasion of local structures such as the oesophagus. An oesophagobronchial fistula may be formed (Figure 29.12).

Superior sulcus tumours, also referred to as **Pancoast tumours**, may involve the brachial plexus and thoracic inlet, with neurological sequelae. **Horner's syndrome** may ensue, as may facial oedema from obstruction of the venous return (**superior vena cava syndrome**).

Lung cancers may also develop satellite lesions in the same or differing lobes, and may even show contralateral involvement. With multiple lung lesions, it is critical to determine whether these represent separate primary lung cancers or metastatic tumours.

The presence of a malignant pleural effusion (Figure 29.13) is also a poor prognostic factor and significantly alters the clinical stage, and therefore the treatment, of the disease.

### Lymphadenopathy

Lymph node involvement is most common in the mediastinum in the subcarinal region (level 7) and along the right and left main stem bronchi (level 4), as well as in the intraparenchymal

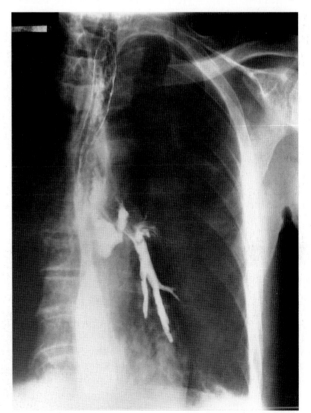

Figure 29.12 Invasion of carcinoma of the bronchus into the oesophagus. A barium swallow has demonstrated an oesophagobronchial fistula.

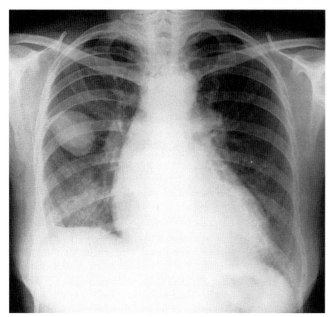

Figure 29.13 An interlobar right pleural effusion. Note its similarity to the appearance of the pulmonary metastasis in Figure 29.16a.

nodes (level 10). Palpable lymph nodes are a sinister sign as these represent distant nodal disease. The involved lymph nodes are firm and often fixed.

### Metastasis of the Lung Primary

Metastatic disease from the lungs can occur to anywhere in the axial skeleton, the most common sites being the long bones, ribs and spine. The presence of localized bone pain is often a poor prognostic finding and can offer clues as to the location of the disease. Pain may also occur at the ends of long bones due to hypertrophic pulmonary osteoarthropathy (Figure 29.14). This resolves after resection of the offending lesion.

**Pathological fractures** may occur in the long bones or spine. Figure 29.15 demonstrates a pathological fracture of the proximal right femur due to metastatic lung cancer.

The presence of hepatic enlargement, right upper quadrant pain or abdominal ascites portends a poor prognosis as this may represent hepatic metastatic disease from the lung primary.

### Metastases to the Lung

Metastatic disease may occur from primary cancers of, for example, the colon, breast, kidneys, sarcomas and prostate. Pulmonary metastases often appear as well-localized, circular 'cannon-ball' lesions and may be multiple (Figure 29.16). Complete removal of disease burden is usually sought in such cases, and parenchymal resection is pursued if this can be achieved.

### Unusual Bronchial Neoplasms

**Carcinoid tumours** occur much less frequently than other types of lung cancer and may present with carcinoid syndrome. **Cylindromas**, also referred to as **adenoid cystic carcinomas**, may result in airway obstruction and warrant bronchoscopy and coring-out of the tumour to restore airway patency. Other less common lesions include pulmonary hamartomas, fibromas, sarcomas and neurogenic tumours.

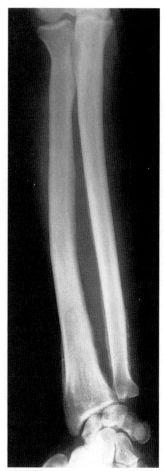

Figure 29.14 Hypertrophic osteoarthropathy of the distal right radius and ulna in a patient with carcinoma of the bronchus.

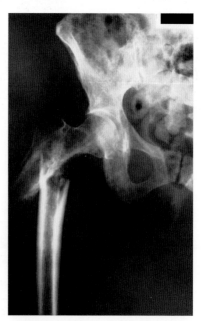

Figure 29.15 A pathological transverse fracture of the upper end of the shaft of the right femur through secondary metastatic disease from carcinoma of the bronchus.

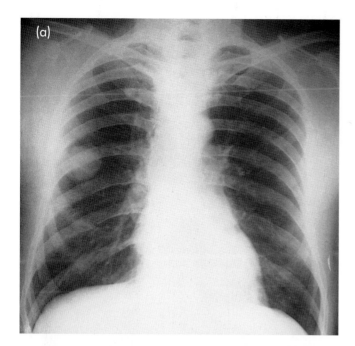

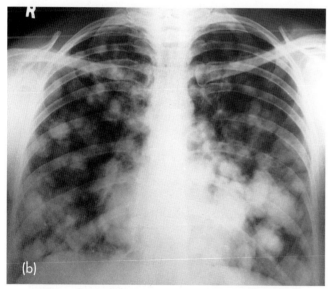

Figure 29.16 Lung metastases. (a) A cannon-ball secondary in the right mid-zone. (b) Multiple bilateral disc-like pulmonary secondary deposits.

## THE PLEURA

The pleura are the mesothelial lining of the thoracic cavity. There are two pleural surfaces: the visceral pleural is intimately associated with the lung parenchyma, and the parietal pleural covers the inner surface of the thoracic cavity.

The parietal pleura is innervated by the intercostal nerves, explaining the localized pain associated with pleural disease. Pleuritic pain or **pleurisy** occurs when there is inflammation of the pleural surfaces leading to pain on expiration, and less commonly on inspiration, as the pleural surfaces slide over each other.

The space between the pleural surfaces is lubricated by 10–15 mL of pleural fluid, which allows the pleural layers to slide over each other in normal respiration. In inflammatory states, the volume of pleural fluid can increase dramatically, sometimes up to several litres of effusion.

It is important to differentiate the aetiology of these effusions, as they may be exudative in the case of infections, or transudative in the case of heart failure. Bloody effusions may be present following traumatic injuries or recent thoracic surgery. Injury to the thoracic duct may result in a milky white, high-volume chylous effusion. Malignant effusions may also occur in lung cancer or other metastatic pulmonary diseases, including **Meigs' syndrome** (the triad of ascites, pleural effusion and ovarian cancer).

### Primary Pleural Tumours

**Mesotheliomas** are the most well-defined pleurally based tumours and are linked to asbestos exposure. Figure 29.17 demonstrates the characteristic pleural thickening associated with asbestosis. Mesotheliomas occur many years after exposure and are highly malignant, with only a small subset of patients being amenable to surgical resection. The epithelioid variant is the most commonly resected type; excision usually occurs after the patient has received trimodal therapy involving induction chemotherapy, extrapleural pneumonectomy and radiation therapy.

Benign fibrous tumours of the pleura may also occur and, due to their interference with respiratory dynamics and their large size, are usually resected. Resection is also advocated to ensure that they are not harbouring malignancy.

### Empyemas

Empyemas are bacterial infections of the pleural space. Less common sources of empyemas are tuberculosis, fungal infections, amoebic abscesses and malignant effusions that subsequently become infected.

Empyemas usually occurs in three phases:

- Initially, there is a parapneumonic effusion, which is a free-flowing effusion round the lungs that subsequently becomes infected.
- This is followed by a fibrinopurulent phase in which the effusion becomes loculated and internal septations develop.

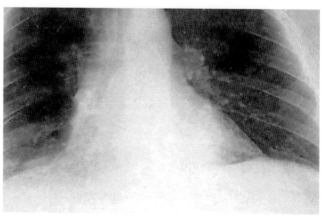

Figure 29.17 Thickening of the right lower mediastinal and diaphragmatic pleura in an individual previously exposed to asbestos.

- The final phase is one of fibrosis, in which a thick fibrous rind develops on the surface of the lung. This demands extensive decortication of the lung parenchyma as the lung becomes trapped.

The goals of treatment of an empyema are, first, evacuation of the purulent effusion, and second, elimination of the pleural space by restoring the ability of the lung parenchyma and diaphragm to expand. If it is not possible to eliminate an infected pleural space, external drainage of the pleural space is sometimes required via an **Eloesser flap** or **Clagett window**.

## THE MEDIASTINUM

The mediastinum is the space that is found between the medial surfaces of the left and right pleura. It is divided into three portions:

- The *anterior mediastinum* is the space anterior to the anterior pericardial reflection. Anterior mediastinal lesions include thymomas, thymic carcinomas, thyroid tumours, lymphomas, non-seminomatous germ cell tumours and germ cell tumours.

- The *middle mediastinum* is found between the anterior and posterior pericardial reflections. Middle mediastinal lesions include cysts, enteric duplication cysts and embryogenic remnants of bronchial and pericardial development.

- The *posterior mediastinum* lies posterior to the posterior pericardial reflection. Posterior mediastinal lesions are represented largely by neurogenic tumours such as ganglioneuromas, neuroblastomas and chemodectomas.

In all compartments, rare lesions such as angiosarcomas and leiomyoscarcomas may arise from the visceral structures. Figure 29.18 demonstrates the radiographic appearance of mediastinal lesions.

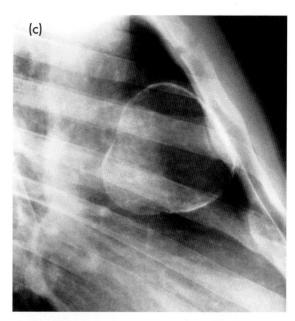

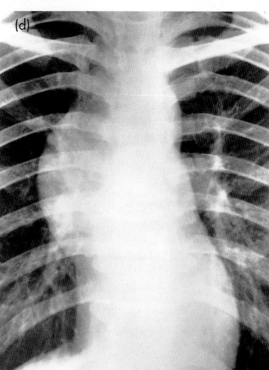

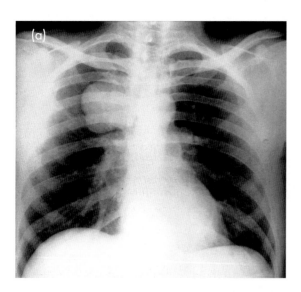

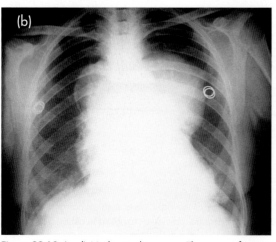

Figure 29.18 (a–d) Mediastinal tumours. These are often incidental radiological findings.

The mediastinal space may also become involved in descending infections from the oropharynx, for example Ludwig's angina. This can lead to **mediastinitis**, which carries a high morbidity and mortality.

## THE DIAPHRAGM

The diaphragm is the large dome-shaped muscular structure that separates the thorax from the abdominal cavity. Critical to the surgical anatomy of the diaphragm is an understanding of the location of the phrenic nerves, which innervate this important respiratory muscle.

The diaphragm has a large central tendon and attaches anteriorly to the xiphoid process, and posteriorly and laterally to the ribs and chest wall. The posterior aspect has diaphragmatic recesses that may extend as low as the 12th rib.

The diaphragm allows for passage of the inferior vena cava at T8, the oesophagus and vagus nerves at T10, and the aorta and thoracic duct at T12 via the diaphragmatic hiatus. As a result of these openings, diaphragmatic hernias may occur, which are broadly of two types: congenital and traumatic.

Congenital diaphragmatic hernias include the **Bochdalek** (posterolateral; Figure 29.19) and **Morgagni** (anterior and lateral to the xiphoid process) hernias. Hiatus hernias may occur through the oesophageal hiatus (see p. 447).

**Traumatic hernias** may occur as a result of fractures of the ribs corresponding to the insertion of the diaphragm, or from rapid exhalation against a closed glottis, for example during high-force abdominal trauma. They most commonly occur on the left (Figure 29.20) as the liver protects the right hemidiaphragm. The diagnosis is suggested by the pattern of injury and is best confirmed by diagnostic laparoscopy as these hernias are often missed on X-ray and CT evaluation.

Traumatic diaphragmatic hernias should be repaired at the time of diagnosis and can often be fixed primarily. Large defects or the presence of devitalized tissue may need the placement of a prosthetic mesh to repair the defect.

**Eventration** and paralysis of the diaphragm are also encountered (Figure 29.21). Eventration refers to an abnormal appearance or contour of the normally dome-shaped diaphragm due to protrusion of abdominal contents through a weakened diaphragmatic musculature. Diaphragmatic paralysis presents with cough, decreased exercise tolerance and a positive **sniff test** – a paradoxical movement of the diaphragm with normal respiration that is detected on fluoroscopy.

Excision of the diaphragm is sometimes required, for example with extrapleural pneumonectomy for epitheloid mesotheliomas. In such cases, a small rim of tissue is left circumferentially to allow for fixation of a neo-diaphragm composed of synthetic mesh. If it is not feasible to leave such a rim, for example if this will compromise the oncological resection, the neo-diaphragm is instead fixed to the chest wall circumferentially.

## THE OESOPHAGUS

Owing to its posterior location, the oesophagus does not lend itself to physical examination. It enters the chest at the thoracic inlet, running parallel to the vertebral column, and is most easily accessible on the left in its upper joint. It courses through the chest, then becoming more accessible on the right as it leaves the chest via the oesophageal hiatus at T10. Here it lies in close proximity to the thoracic duct and carries with it the left and right vagi. Throughout its course, it lies in close proximity to the aorta, and more cephalad it lies posterior to the membranous trachea.

The oesophagus is composed of a circular and a longitudinal muscle layer, with an inner mucosa; it lacks a true serosa.

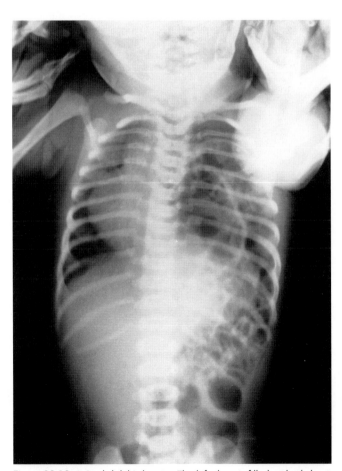

Figure 29.19 A Bochdalek's hernia. The left chest is filled with abdominal contents, with a mediastinal shift to the right.

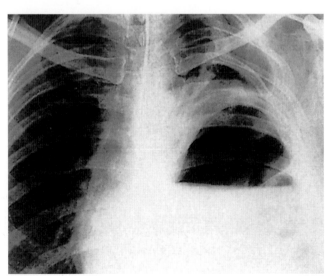

Figure 29.20 A ruptured left hemidiaphragm. The stomach and other viscera are sited in the left pleural cavity, and there is a mediastinal shift to the right.

PART 6 | CARDIOTHORACIC

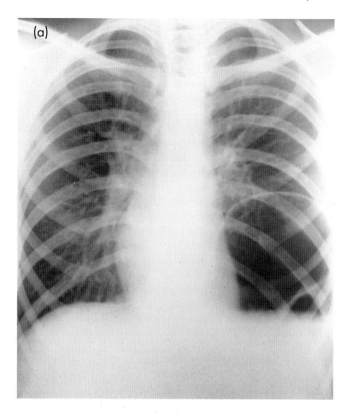

The blood supply arises from the thyroid arteries, bronchial arteries and aorta as it traverses the chest. These vessels are tiny and numerous, allowing for blunt dissection of the oesophagus without large-volume bleeding via the diaphragmatic hiatus, as during a transhiatal oesophagectomy.

## Oesophageal Rupture

Oesophageal rupture typically follows an episode of retching, resulting in an oesophageal tear. Patients complain of severe left-sided chest pain radiating to the back. Haematemesis is often also described. Imaging reveals the presence of a pleural effusion and may show a pneumomediastinum (Figure 29.22). Spontaneous oesophageal rupture carries with it a high morbidity and mortality – a failure to diagnose and treat this condition will result in death.

A **Mallory–Weiss tear** is a mucosal injury at the gastro-oesophageal junction that is associated with emesis. It often results in haematemesis but does not present as an oesophageal rupture. **Boerhaave's syndrome** refers to the oesophageal rupture that follows violent retching.

## Oesophageal Varices

Oesophageal varices often form at the gastro-oesophageal junction as this location provides one of the anostomotic sites for the portosystemic circulation (Figure 29.23). Portal hypertension leads to the development of varices of the oesophagus in conjunction with gastric varices. There is associated engorgement of the short gastric vessels. The presence of oesophageal varices without gastric varices is suggestive of splenic vein thrombosis and, unlike portal hypertension, the treatment is splenectomy.

In patients with cirrhosis, severe bleeding can occur from oesophageal varices and is often life-threatening.

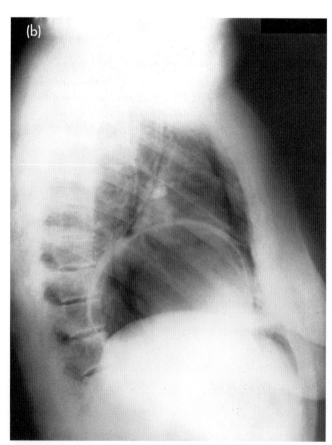

Figure 29.21 (a) Eventration of the diaphragm. (b) Segmental paralysis of the diaphragm.

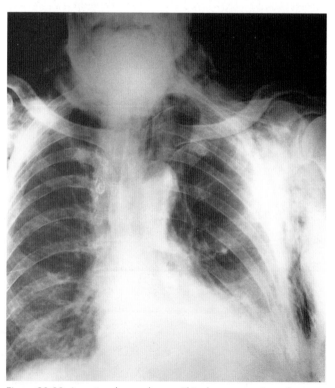

Figure 29.22 A ruptured oesophagus. This shows extensive subcutaneous emphysema and a left pleural effusion.

## Hiatus Hernias

There are four types of hiatus hernia:

- *Type 1*: The gastro-oesophageal junction lies above the oesophageal hiatus (a sliding hiatus hernia).
- *Type 2*: The gastro-oesophageal junction is below the hiatus, but the fundus is above the hiatus.
- *Type 3*: Both the gastro-oesophageal junction and a portion of the stomach are located above the hiatus (a true para-oesophageal hernia; Figure 29.24).
- *Type 4*: Additional viscera, for example the colon, can be found in the thoracic cavity.

Hiatus hernias present with symptoms of reflux and dysphagia. There is a sensation of early satiety and post-prandial fullness with an associated dull, aching chest pain. The symptoms may be relieved by emesis, belching or regurgitation of food.

Type 3 paraoesophageal hernias should be repaired as they are often associated with gastric volvulus. Volvulus of the stomach is of two types – organoaxial and atlantoaxial – and may compromise the blood, supply leading to gastric necrosis. Some patients may also present with a hypochromic, microcytic anaemia as a result of **Cameron's ulcers**. These are ring-like, mechanical ulcerations that form at the site where the stomach is compressed as it passes through the oesophageal hiatus.

Prior to the repair of a hiatus hernia, it is prudent to evaluate the oesophagus for motility disorders as these may occur concurrently and influence the operation performed.

## Dysphagia

Dysphagia is a broad term referring to difficulty swallowing and should be differentiated from **odynophagia**, which refers to painful swallowing. Table 29.1 depicts the variety of pathologies that may lead to dysphagia.

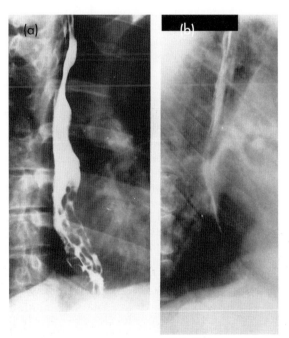

Figure 29.23 (a, b) Oesophageal varices. The barium is indented by the diffuse pattern of bulging varicosities at the lower end of the oesophagus.

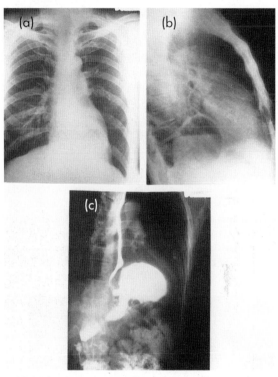

Figure 29.24 (a–c) A paraoesophageal hiatus hernia. The cardiac end of the stomach has passed through the oesophageal hiatus alongside the oesophagus and is sited above the diaphragm.

Table 29.1 Oesophageal obstruction

| Extrinsic pressure | Abnormalities of the wall | | Abnormalities within the lumen |
| --- | --- | --- | --- |
| | **Stricture** | **Abnormalities of oesophageal contraction** | |
| Thyroid | Post-traumatic | Achalasia | Foreign bodies |
| Pharyngeal pouch | Benign & malignant neoplasms | Failure of relaxation of the cricopharyngeus | Webs |
| Aortic aneurysm | Acute & chronic oesophagitis | Cerebrovascular accidents | Schatzki's rings |
| Abnormal aortic arch | Corrosives | Diffuse oesophgeal spasm | |
| Mediastinal tumours | Crohn's disease, post-radiotherapy | | |
| Paraoesophageal hiatus hernia | Oesophageal diverticulum Scleroderma | | |

Dysphagia to solids should be differentiated from dysphagia to liquids. In some situations, for example near-total oesophageal obstruction, there is dysphagia to both solids and liquids. Associated findings include a globus sensation, which refers to the feeling of a food bolus being stuck in the oesophagus. The location of this sensation is often reproducible and can offer an insight into the location of the pathological process.

Signs of cachexia and weight loss may also be present and can often be subtle. The presence of lyphadenopathy in the supraclavicular fossa is an ominous physical finding, as are hepatomegaly and abdominal ascites.

## Dysphagia Lusoria

In dysphagia lusoria, there is difficulty swallowing owing to a congenitally abnormal vascular ring or an anomalous origin of the right subclavian artery from the aorta that compresses the oesophagus, with the formation of a **Kommerell's diverticulum** – a bulbous configuration of the origin of an aberrant left subclavian artery in the presence of a right aortic arch. Neonates have difficulty feeding and preferentially lie with their necks hyperextended as flexion of the neck leads to dysphagia. The anomaly is corrected by ligation of the anomalous ring, transposition of the subclavian artery or carotid subclavian bypass.

## Oesophageal Strictures

Oesophageal strictures may be iatrogenic (as a result of mucosal injury during endoscopy) or acquired as a result of long-standing gastro-oesophageal reflux disease or lye ingestion (Figure 29.25).

The consumption of an alkaline agent results in a liquefaction necrosis of the oesophagus and is typically more destructive than an acidic agent. These chemical burns usually occur as a result of children ingesting household cleaning agents. The burns to the oesophagus usually require sequential dilatation. Alternate enteral access is required in the meantime, and conduits should be preserved with the expectation that oesophageal replacement might be necessary in the future.

When evaluating a stricture, it is important to identify whether a concurrent malignancy is present. This information can be obtained by a biopsy during oesophagogastroduodenoscopy. Balloon dilation of a benign oesophageal strictures may offer short-term relief.

Other less common causes of strictures include **oesophageal webs** (Figure 29.26) and **Schatzki's rings**. These congenital abnormalities are usually amenable to pneumatic dilatation of the oesophagus.

## Oesophageal Carcinoma

Oesophageal malignancy is a feared cause of dysphagia and oesophageal strictures (Figure 29.27). It is more common in older men. Over the last 10–15 years in developed countries, it has mostly been associated with long-standing gastro-oesophageal reflux disease that leads to Barrett's disease and subsequent adenocarcinoma. Risk factors include cigarette smoking, alcohol ingestion, lye ingestion and high levels of dietary nitrosamines.

Patients complain primarily of dysphagia and weight loss. Difficulty swallowing saliva and recurrent chest infections, due to aspiration, are a late finding suggestive of advanced disease. Pain occurs due to local invasion.

Evaluation of the oesophagus involves a barium oesophagram, typically followed by oesophagogastroduodenoscopy and biopsy. Once a diagnosis has been established, staging of the lesion is performed, usually by an endoscopic ultrasound. Chest and abdominal imaging are also undertaken as the majority of these tumours involve multiple layers of the oesophageal wall.

Treatment is initially with neoadjuvant (chemotherapy and radiation) therapy. Options for surgical resection include a transhiatal oesophagectomy, an Ivor-Lewis oesophagectomy or three-hole oesophagectomy. An Ivor-Lewis procedure involves an abdominal incision and right thoracotomy to resect the oesophagus; the bowel anastomosis is formed in the chest. The three-hole operation involves an abdominal incision, a right thoracotomy and a neck incision, with the bowel anastomosis in performed in the neck. Options for oesophageal conduits include the stomach, colon and jejunum.

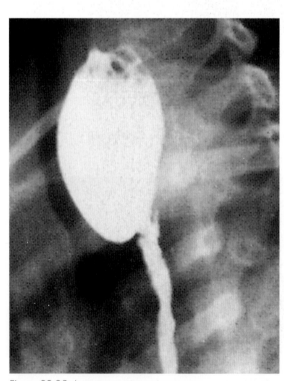

Figure 29.25 A post-corrosive stricture.

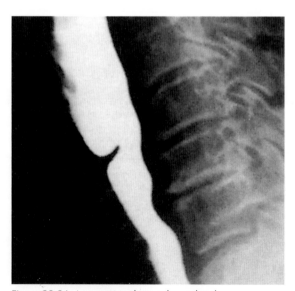

Figure 29.26 A post-cricoid oesophageal web.

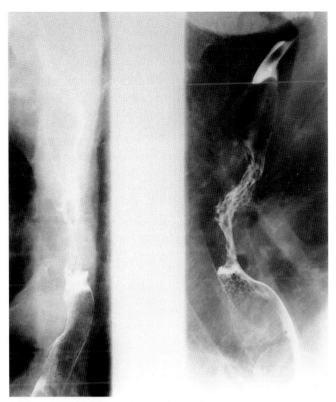

Figure 29.27 Carcinoma of the mid-oesophagus.

## Benign Oesophageal Lesions

Oesophageal leiomyomas and gastrointestinal stromal tumours are the most common benign oesophageal lesions. Leiomyomas are submucosal lesions and may present with oesophageal ulceration and bleeding. They are treated by enucleation. Biopsy is unsuccessful as the lesion is submucosal and rarely can it be biopsied. Attempts at biopsy result in biopsy of the mucosa only. Leiomyomas and stromal tumours may present with dysphagia.

Other benign lesions include lipomas, fibromas and papillomas (Figure 29.28).

## Oesophagitis

Oesophagitis may be chronic or acute. Acute oesophagitis may occur as a result of corrosive injuries as described earlier, or from fungal infections in immunocompromised or debilitated patients. Less commonly, gastro-oesophageal reflux disease may contribute to reflux oesophagitis.

Oesophagitis usually presents as odynophagia (painful swallowing). Chronic oesophagitis may occur in the presence of concurrent oesophageal pathology such as an oesophageal dysmotility disorder or hiatus hernia (Figure 29.29).

**Achalasia** (Figure 29.30) is a common dysmotility disorder characterized by aganglionosis of the Auerbach's plexus of nerves within the oesophagus. The presenting symptom is dysphagia, and the characteristic finding on imaging is a bird's beak tapering of the distal oesophagus on an oesophagram. Oesophageal manometry confirms the diagnosis by revealing a hypertensive lower oesophageal sphincter and absent oesophageal contractions. Mega-oesophagus can ensue. In developing countries, achalasia may be due to Chagas disease associated with *Trypanosoma cruzi* infection.

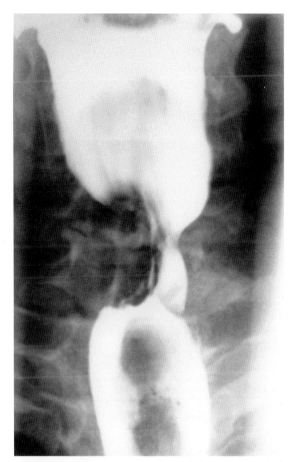

Figure 29.28 A hamartomatous polyp of the upper oesophagus indenting the barium column from the right side.

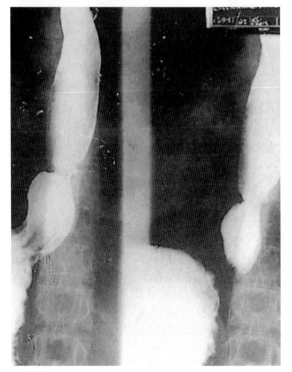

Figure 29.29 A hiatus hernia. The esophago-gastric junction in the posterior mediastinum.

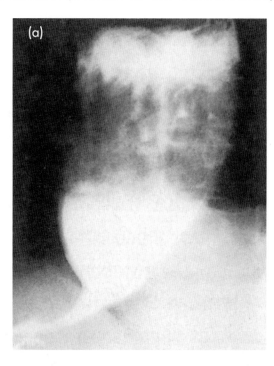

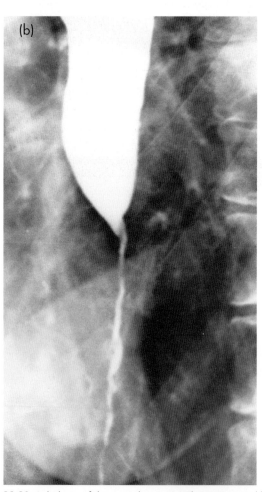

Treatment is with a Heller myotomy and partial fundoplication. In cases of burnt-out (end-stage) achalasia, oesophageal replacement may be necessary. Other oesophageal dysmotility disorders include nutcracker oesophagus, characterized by high-amplitude discoordinated oesophageal contractions, and diffuse oesophageal spasm.

## Oesophageal Diverticula

Diverticula can be divided into two main types:

- Traction diverticula occur as a result of surrounding inflammation.
- Pulsion diverticula occur as a result of high intraluminal pressures.

**Zenker's diverticulum** occurs as a result of cricopharyngeal hypertension and is treated by diverticulectomy in association with cricopharyngeal myotomy. Less commonly, enteric duplication cysts and other pseudodiverticula may occur. Pseudodiverticula usually do not contain all layers of the oesophageal wall and are most often incidentally detected on radiographic imaging (Figure 29.31).

Figure 29.30 Achalasia of the oesophagus. (a) There is gross dilatation of the oesophagus with smooth tapering at the lower end. The barium column is mixed with food residue. (b) Stricture of the distal part of the esophagus.

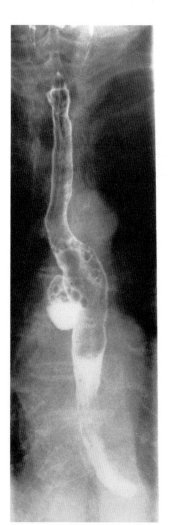
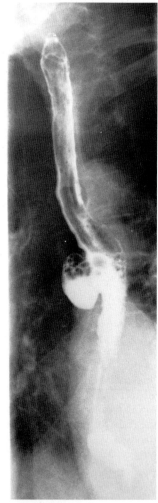

Figure 29.31 Oesophageal diverticula in the mid-oesophagus.

The classical presenting symptoms of a oesophageal diverticulum are the regurgitation of partially digested food and halitosis. Similar symptoms may be seen with oesophageal obstruction as a result of foreign body ingestion or a food bolus stuck in the oesophagus (Figure 29.32).

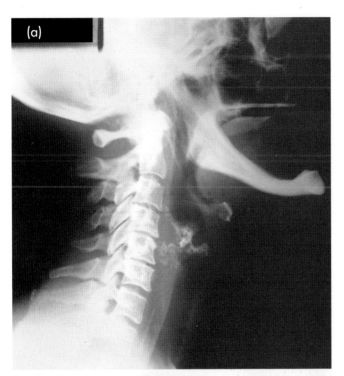

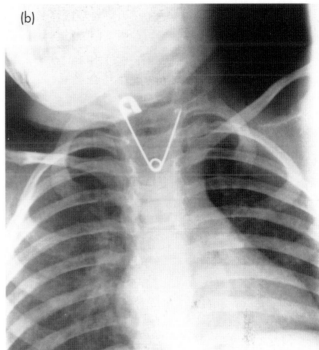

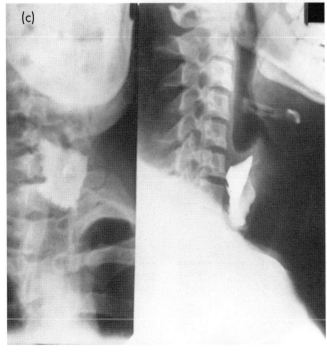

Figure 29.32 Foreign bodies in the oesophagus. (a). A chicken bone sited between the trachea and the C7 and T1 vertebral bodies. (b) An open safety pin. (c) A denture.

## Key Points

- Any patient presenting with respiratory complaints should undergo a comprehensive and complete physical examination including inspection, palpation, percussion and auscultation.
- Chest trauma may result in a range of thoracic organ injury from the trivial rib fracture to the life-threatening tension pneumothorax.
- Pulmonary infections present with fever and respiratory symptoms. Proper diagnosis with appropriate culture is paramount to guide adequate antibiotic therapy. Surgery, for drainage or resection, is reserved for very severe cases with lung tissue destruction.
- Lung cancer, the leading cause of cancer death in both men and women, is asymptomatic in its early stages. Symptoms including weight loss, haemoptysis and paraneoplastic syndromes are usually associated with advanced disease.
- The oesophagus is an entirely intrathoracic organ not amenable to physical examination.
- Any patient presenting with dysphagia or odynophagia should undergo a full comprehensive oesophageal evaluation including a contrast study, an oesophageal endoscopy and a manometric pressure study.

## QUESTIONS

### SBAs

**1.** 1. A 55-year-old gentleman presents to the emergency department with a sudden onset of pleuritic chest pain. His physical examination is unremarkable except for a swollen left lower extremity, which he has had for the past 2 days. He is tachycardic with an arterial oxygen saturation of 88% on room air. The most likely diagnosis is:
  a  Spontaneous pneumothorax
  b  Myocardial infarction
  c  Pulmonary embolism
  d  Pneumonia
  e  Atelectasis

Answer
*c  Pulmonary embolism.*

**2.** The most common symptom of lung carcinoma is:
  a  Haemoptysis
  b  Chest pain
  c  Dyspnoea
  d  Tachypnoea
  e  There are no symptoms

Answer
*e  There are no symptoms.*

**3.** Which of the following is true regarding the diaphragm?:
  a  It is a large dome-shaped muscle that separates the abdomen from the retroperitoneal space
  b  It is innervated by the vagus nerve
  c  Congenital diaphragmatic hernias include Bochdalek and sliding hernias
  d  Traumatic diaphragmatic hernias should be always repaired at diagnosis
  e  Eventration and paralysis of the diaphragm are always asymptomatic

Answer
*d  Traumatic diaphragmatic hernias should be always repaired at diagnosis.*

**4.** All the following are characteristics of achalasia except:
  a  Dysphagia
  b  Odynophagia
  c  Bird's beak appearance on an oesophagogram
  d  Hypertensive lower oesophageal sphincter on manometry
  e  Association with Trypanosoma cruzii infection

Answer
*b Odynophagia.*

**5.** A 70-year-old gentleman presents with a 10 year history of frequent episodes of regurgitation of partially digested food. The most likely diagnosis is:
  a  Oesophageal cancer
  b  Achalasia
  c  Hiatus hernia
  d  Zenker's diverticulum
  e  Schatzki's ring

Answer
*d  Zenker's diverticulum.*

CHAPTER
30

# Evaluation of the Cardiac Surgical Patient

Jamil Borgi and Pierre M. Sfeir

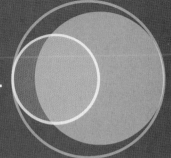

## LEARNING OBJECTIVES

- To identify the signs and symptoms of myocardial ischaemia
- To identify the signs and symptoms of valvular heart disease and heart failure
- To recognize the essential findings in a systematic physical examination of the cardiovascular system

## INTRODUCTION

Heart diseases are either acquired or congenital; this chapter describes the approach to diagnosing acquired diseases affecting the coronary arteries, heart valves, pericardium, myocardium and great vessels. A brief discussion of some congenital heart diseases is provided at the end.

The evaluation of heart conditions relies heavily on multiple diagnostic modalities including angiograms, echocardiograms, CT scans, MRI and other nuclear imaging techniques. However, astute clinicians should be able to identify and diagnose different disease processes. More importantly, they should be able to assess the severity of the disease, and the readiness of the patient to go through a corrective or a palliative procedure.

Heart diseases are dynamic so an assessment performed at a particular point in time may not hold true at a later time. This highlights the importance of continuous evaluation along with a focused history and physical examination. A knowledge of signs and symptoms may identify a clinical variation or deterioration and is imperative in evaluating the cardiac patient.

## HISTORY

Patients with cardiac disease can present with a variety of symptoms.

### Chest Pain

Chest pain is a common feature of heart disease. **Angina pectoris** is pain derived from the heart when a mismatch between the oxygen demand and the oxygen supply causes ischaemia of the myocardium.

Angina is usually a substernal pain, described as choking or crushing. It can radiate to the shoulders, arms or jaw. It is commonly exacerbated by exercise, cold weather or emotional distress. It can also occur after eating, or it can wake the patient from sleep. It is typically relieved by rest or sublingual nitrates. Atypical angina can be epigastric, mimicking peptic ulcer disease.

Stable angina is reproducible and lasts for minutes until the initiating factor ceases. If the pain lasts for longer than a few minutes or is associated with vomiting or nausea, this may indicate that the patient has unstable angina or is suffering an acute myocardial infarction.

Angina is most commonly a manifestation of stenotic lesions in the coronary arteries causing a limited blood flow to the area of myocardium they supply (Figure 30.1). It can also be the result of advanced valvular disease, typically aortic stenosis. In severe aortic stenosis, the mismatch between the supply and demand of oxygen, and therefore the resulting angina, is caused by a mismatch between the left ventricular hypertrophy and the

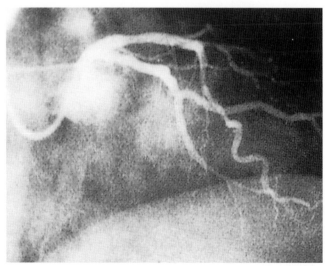

Figure 30.1 A left coronary arteriogram showing a bifurcation stenosis.

limited cardiac output. Right ventricular hypertrophy secondary to pulmonary stenosis or chronic pulmonary hypertension may occasionally present with angina.

Angina can be graded into four classes according to the classification of the Canadian Cardiovascular Society:

- *Class I*: Angina only during strenuous or prolonged physical activity.
- *Class II*: A slight limitation, with angina occurring only during vigorous physical activity.
- *Class III*: Symptoms with everyday living activities, i.e. a moderate limitation.
- *Class IV*: An inability to perform any activity without angina, or angina occurring at rest, i.e. a severe limitation.

Severe chest pain that is acute and radiates to the back may be secondary to **acute aortic dissection**. It is very important to differentiate this entity from acute coronary syndromes as the treatment strategies are completely different.

**Pleuritic chest pain** is associated with respiration and is usually unilateral. It is typically the result of pulmonary embolism or lung infarction. A pleural rub may be heard on auscultation secondary to local inflammation.

## Dyspnoea

Dyspnoea, or shortness of breath, is a common symptom of cardiac pathology. Most of the dyspnoea that results from cardiac disease is passive, meaning that it is the result of back-pressure from the left chambers of the heart. This can be caused by left ventricular failure, which may be acute or chronic (Figure 30.2). It may also be due to valvular stenosis or regurgitation, also on the left side of the heart. This contrasts with active congestion, which results from the increased pulmonary flow that is seen with a left-to-right shunt, for instance in some congenital heart diseases.

Dyspnoea may occur at rest or be associated with exertion. It can also be related to the patient's position or may wake the patient from sleep. **Orthopnoea** is dyspnoea that occurs when the patient is lying flat. This usually results in an increased venous return, which may overwhelm a left ventricle with borderline function or a dysfunctional valve. In addition, the increased abdominal pressure elevates the diaphragm, limits the expansion of the lungs and may worsen the breathlessness. Orthopnoea is usually quantified by the number of pillows the patient uses to breathe comfortably.

**Paroxysmal nocturnal dyspnoea** is orthopnoea that wakens the patient from sleep. It is the result of decreased dyspnoea awareness during sleep until the oedema and congestion is severe enough to waken the patient.

Acute left ventricular failure can present with severe dyspnoea and pulmonary oedema (Figure 30.3). This is characterized by frothy, blood-tinged sputum. Haemoptysis may also occur if a congested capillary ruptures.

Finally, it is useful to describe cardiac symptoms according to the New York Heart Association Functional classification (Table 30.1).

## Syncope

Syncope in cardiac disease is a cardinal sign of severe aortic stenosis, although it can have other cardiac causes. Patients with aortic stenosis have limited cardiac output and usually experience syncope during exercise because of the vasodilation

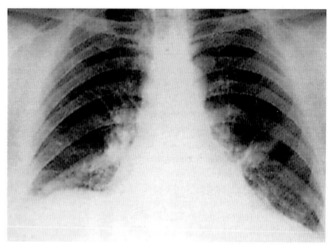

Figure 30.3 A radiograph of a patient with pulmonary oedema. This is most marked at the lung bases.

Table 30.1 New York Heart Association classification

| NYHA Class | Symptoms |
| --- | --- |
| I | Cardiac disease, but no symptoms and no limitation of ordinary physical activity, e.g. shortness of breath when walking or climbing stairs |
| II | Mild symptoms (mild shortness of breath and/or angina) and slight limitation during ordinary activity |
| III | Marked limitation of activity due to symptoms, even during less-than-ordinary activity, e.g. walking short distances (20–100 m). Comfortable only at rest |
| IV | Severe limitations. Experiences symptoms even while at rest. Mostly bedbound patients |

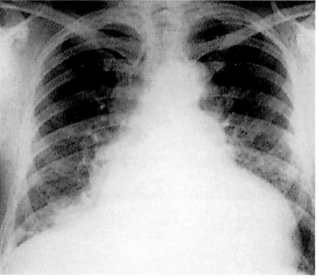

Figure 30.2 A radiograph of a patient in cardiac failure. This shows an enlarged heart, enlargement of the pulmonary conus (the left hilar marking between the aortic knuckle and the left ventricle) and increased pulmonary vascular markings.

associated with it. This is in contrast to syncope that occurs with hypertrophic cardiomyopathy, which occurs after the individual stops exercising; there is then a resultant pooling of blood and a decrease in venous return and left ventricular filling, which leads to an obstructed left ventricular outflow tract.

Pulmonary stenosis and mitral stenosis may also present with syncope due to a limited cardiac output. Other causes of cardiac syncope include heart block, arrhythmia and rarely a cardiac tumour (myxoma; Figure 30.4) causing obstruction of blood flow.

## Palpitations

This is an increased awareness of the heart beating. It may be the result of an extrasystole or tachyarrythmia. Supraventricular tachyarrhythmias are common. They can be completely benign or may be associated with valvular pathologies or ischaemic heart disease. Atrial fibrillation is a common supraventricular tachyarrythmia that is commonly related to an enlarged left atrium from mitral stenosis or regurgitation. Again, it may be one manifestation of ischaemic heart disease.

## Fatigue and Weight Loss

Fatigue is a non-specific symptom that is sometimes the result of advanced heart disease and decreased cardiac output. It is particularly important with right heart failure that lacks the more common symptoms of heart disease. Fatigue is explained by decreased peripheral perfusion, particularly cerebral perfusion. Weight loss can result from chronic heart failure, hence the term 'cardiac cachexia'.

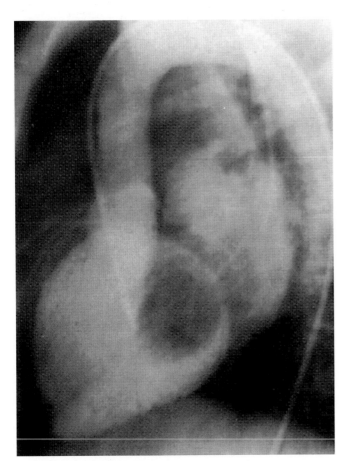

Figure 30.4 **An atrial myxoma.**

## Oedema

Cardiac oedema is a common feature of advanced heart disease. It starts at the ankles and extends upwards as it worsens in the ambulatory patient (Figure 30.5). It is usually better in the morning and worsens over the course of the day. Oedema may only occur over the sacrum and buttocks if the patient is bedridden.

Cardiac oedema is multifactorial. It is partly caused by salt and water retention that is the result of low peripheral perfusion. However, it is also caused by elevated venous pressure, particularly when the right heart is also involved.

(a)

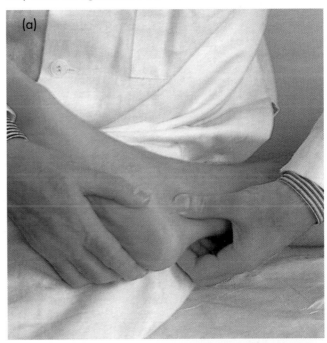

(b)

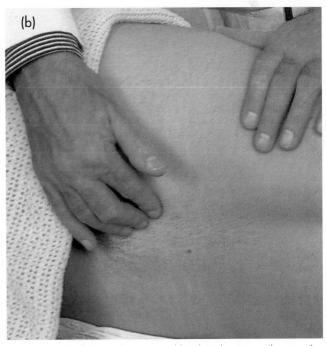

Figure 30.5 Oedema is demonstrated by digital pressure, leaving skin dents (pitting). Small amounts are first identified around the ankles, over the shins, on either side of the Achilles tendons and, after recumbency, over the sacrum.

PART 6 | CARDIOTHORACIC

## Risk Factors and Additional History

When assessing a cardiac patient, it is important to evaluate their risk factors. Common risk factors include:

- age;
- male gender;
- hypercholesterolaemia;
- diabetes mellitus;
- hypertension;
- smoking;
- peripheral vascular disease;
- a personal or family history of coronary, valvular or aneurysmal disease.

Cardiac surgery has witnessed a significant improvement in its overall mortality and morbidity over the last two decades. This is mostly attributed to the improvement in cardiopulmonary bypass techniques, myocardial protection and surgical intensive care. With this in mind, sicker patients are being referred for surgical treatment, and a proper evaluation of comorbid conditions and risk factors is crucial for stratifying the risk and anticipating the complications. The cardiac surgical patient should receive a full systems review as well as an evaluation of their functional status and social habits (Table 30.2).

## PHYSICAL EXAMINATION

As for any other surgical patient, the examination of the cardiac surgical patient should start with a general assessment followed by a focused cardiovascular examination. The general assessment starts by an appraisal of the patient's well-being, how sick they look and whether they appear anaemic, jaundiced, obese, malnourished or cachectic.

## Examination of the Cardiovascular System
### Cyanosis

This is the bluish or dusky discoloration of the skin or mucous membranes that results from the presence of unoxygenated haemoglobin (at least 5 g/dL [50 g/L]) in the blood. It is more often associated with polycythaemia and less evident when the patient is anaemic.

**Peripheral cyanosis** is a sign of shock, most commonly cardiogenic shock. It is observed in the extremities and results from stasis of the blood and an extraction of oxygen by the tissues. It can also be the result of vasoconstriction, for example with exposure to cold.

**Central cyanosis** is a better reflection of the mixing of arterial and venous blood. It commonly occurs with congenital heart disease and is observed in the mouth, lips, tongue and mucous membranes. It typically improves after oxygen has been given.

### Clubbing

Clubbing (Figure 30.6) is a common feature of congenital cyanotic heart disease, but also occurs with subacute endocarditis and conditions resulting in chronic hypoxia, such as end-stage lung disease. It first appears in the thumbs and big toes.

The mechanism leading to clubbing is not completely understood, but it may be related to blood factors that are usually cleared by the lungs but remain elevated in the circulation if there is a right-to-left shunt.

### Arterial Pulse

This is a key component of the cardiovascular examination. The following characteristics should be assessed:

- Rate.
- Rhythm.
- Character.
- Volume.
- Symmetry.
- Vessel wall.

The rate is considered to be bradycardic if it less than 60 beats per minute, and tachycardic if it is over 100 beats per minute. The pulse should be assessed for at least 30 seconds. In healthy and particularly young patients, the rate goes up with inspiration and down with expiration, a phenomenon referred to as **sinus arrhythmia**.

The rhythm should be described as regular or irregular. If it is irregular, the next step is to decide whether it is regularly irregular (commonly from dropped beats or extrasysole) or irregularly irregular, as in atrial fibrillation.

The pulse deficit is the difference between the pulses detected at the wrist and the apex of the heart. It is seen in, for example, atrial fibrillation, and occurs because not every ventricular contraction results in a transmitted pulse, due to the difference in filling time and filling volumes.

Table 30.2 Pertinent questions in the cardiac history

| | Examples |
| --- | --- |
| Respiratory system | History of cough, shortness of breath, dyspnoea, chronic obstructive pulmonary disease, emphysema |
| Renal system | History of renal failure, elevated creatinine, dialysis |
| Vascular system | History of peripheral vascular disease, aneurysmal disease, previous strokes or transient ischaemic attacks, deep vein thrombosis or pulmonary embolism |
| Gastrointestinal system | History of gastrointestinal bleeds, liver failure, oesophageal or gastric surgery |
| Infectious/ immune system | History of hepatitis B or C or HIV, history of a immunocompromised state |
| Surgical history | Particularly previous mediastinal or thoracic surgery or trauma, vein ablation |
| Personal history | Smoking, alcohol or other drug use |

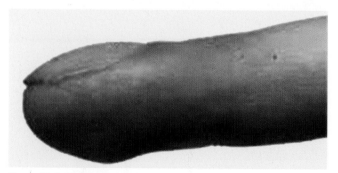

Figure 30.6 Clubbing

Symmetry of the pulse is assessed by comparing the right and left carotid, radial and femoral pulses. This is important in patients with aortic coarctation, aortic dissection or peripheral vascular disease.

The character of the pulse is best assessed at the carotid artery (Figure 30.7). The pulse usually rises moderately quickly, coinciding with ventricular ejection, and this is then followed by a gradual decrease to the diastolic level.

The detection of an abnormal character or volume requires knowledge and experience and may reveal the diagnosis in certain situations:

- *Corrigan's sign* is a large-volume pulse followed by a rapid collapse that is noted or seen in the carotid artery. It usually occurs with aortic regurgitation or when the patient has a high cardiac output and low peripheral resistance.
- A *slow-rising pulse* is noted when the stroke volume is ejected over a longer period, as in aortic stenosis.
- *Pulsus bisferiens* is a double or biphasic pulse that usually occurs with an obstructed ventricular outflow, for example in aortic stenosis or hypertrophic cardiomyopathy. The obstructed outflow results in a prolonged ejection time. The arterial elastic recoil that usually causes the dicrotic notch in diastole is now superimposed on systole and gives the double pulse impression.
- *Pulsus bigeminus* is the result of premature ventricular contraction that is usually followed by a pause. The premature ventricular contraction has a weaker pulse because of the short filling time. The following sinus beat is stronger because of the longer filling time.
- *Pulsus paradoxus* is an exaggerated decrease in blood pressure that is noted during inspiration. The normal decrease in blood pressure during inspiration is less than 10 mmHg. The paradox in pulsus paradoxus is that some beats are heard with a stethoscope over the heart but not felt over the arterial pulse during inspiration. It usually reflects severe heart disease such as cardiac tamponade, constrictive pericarditis or severe lung disease.
- *Pulsus alternans* is alternating strong and weak beats, and is a sign of left ventricular dysfunction.

Finally, the arterial wall should be assessed. This can provide information about the nature of the vascular bed. Healthy arteries are compressible and recoil easily. Atherosclerotic vessels and the vessels of patients with diabetes or renal failure show irregular calcification and in the worst instances feel like rigid pipes. The lack of compressibility can give rise to falsely elevated blood pressure readings.

## Jugular Venous Pulse

Assessment of the jugular venous pulse forms an indirect observation of the right atrial and venous pressure via visualization of the jugular vein. It is an indication of the level of filling and the level of competence of the right heart to receive and deliver blood. Three upward deflections and two downward deflections (Figure 30.8) are classically described:

- The 'a' wave corresponds to contraction of the right atrium and ends synchronously with the carotid artery pulse. The peak of the 'a' wave marks the end of atrial systole.
- The 'x' descent follows the 'a' wave and corresponds to atrial relaxation and rapid atrial filling due to the low pressure.
- The 'c' wave interrupts the 'x' descent and corresponds to right ventricular contraction, which causes the tricuspid valve to bulge towards the right atrium.
- The 'x″' descent then continues after the 'c' wave as the right ventricle pulls the tricuspid valve downwards during ventricular systole.
- The 'v' wave corresponds to venous filling when the tricuspid valve is closed and venous pressure increases from venous return. This occurs during and following the carotid pulse.
- The 'y' descent corresponds to the rapid emptying of the atrium into the ventricle following opening of the tricuspid valve.

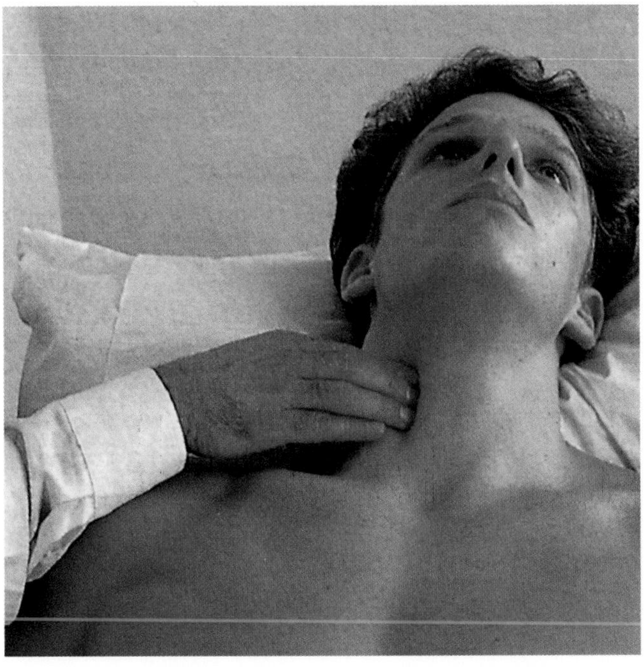

Figure 30.7 Assessment of the character of the carotid pulse.

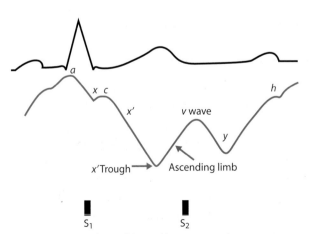

Figure 30.8 The waveform of the jugular venous pulse.

*Measurement of the Jugular Venous Pressure* – The patient should recline backwards at an angle of 45° with their head supported and turned to the side opposite to where the jugular venous pressure (JVP) is being measured (Figure 30.9). The JVP is the sum of the measured vertical height between the sternal angle of Louis and the point of maximal impulse over the jugular vein path, plus 5, which is the estimated height between the sternal angle and the right atrium. The normal JVP should be between 6 and 8 cmH$_2$O, or slightly above the sternal angle.

A low JVP (<5 cmH$_2$O) is observed in states of hypovolaemia. The absolute value cannot be measured clinically but can be transduced through a central venous line.

Many conditions can lead to an elevated JVP, including:

* cardiac tamponade;
* heart failure;
* volume overload;
* constrictive or restrictive pericarditis;
* compression of the superior vena cava.

**Kussmaul's sign** is a paradoxical rise of the JVP on inspiration. It can be seen in some forms of heart disease and is usually indicative of limited filling of the right ventricle due to right heart failure, cardiac tamponade or sometimes pericarditis.

Absent 'a' waves are noted with atrial fibrillation because of a lack of atrial contraction. Conversely, frequent 'a' waves are sometimes noted with atrial fibrillation.

Large 'a' waves are noted in conditions where the atrium is contracting against a higher resistance, as in tricuspid stenosis, or with pulmonary stenosis and associated right ventricular hypertrophy. Cannon 'a' waves occur when the atrium and ventricles contract at the same time, typically with atrioventricular dissociation or third-degree atrioventricular block.

On the other hand, if the tricuspid valve is regurgitant, the result is large 'v' waves as the ventricular contraction is transmitted to the right atrium and the jugular vein.

## Examination of the Precordium

The surface anatomy of the heart is shown in Figure 30.10.

### Inspection

The chest should be inspected for any musculoskeletal deformity that would affect surgical planning. Pectus excavatum, for example, may cause extrinsic compression on the heart. The morphology of the chest plays even a bigger role when planning minimally invasive cardiac surgery or surgery through a thoracotomy. Attention should be given to any scars that suggest previous surgery or trauma to the chest.

### Palpation

The cardiac impulse is the result of the heart striking against the chest wall during systole. The point of maximum impulse is the furthermost point laterally and inferiorly from the sternum at which the cardiac impulse can be felt. It is usually located in the midclavicular line in the fifth intercostal space. This location can vary with right and left ventricular hypertrophy or lung disease affecting the location of the heart in the chest.

The diameter of the palpated impulse should be less than 3 cm in both the supine and left lateral positions. A value greater than 3 cm is indicative of left ventricular hypertrophy or enlargement.

The nature of the impulse is also of importance. In aortic stenosis, the myocardium is hypertrophied. This is felt as a strong heaving impulse. In aortic regurgitation, the ventricle dilates and the resultant impulse is turbulent and hyperdynamic.

A parasternal impulse is palpated to the left of the sternum. A slight outward pulsation is occasionally present in children or thin adults with normal hearts. Generally, however, a left parasternal impulse is caused by a dilated or hypertrophied right ventricle, which can occur with pulmonary stenosis or pulmonary hypertension. The most common condition associated with right ventricular dilatation is functional tricuspid regurgitation. Other causes include atrial septal defect, pulmonary insufficiency and ventricular septal defect.

**Thrills** are cardiac murmurs that can be palpated by placing the palm of the hand over the precordium. A systolic thrill in the aortic area is felt with aortic stenosis. A systolic thrill at the apex

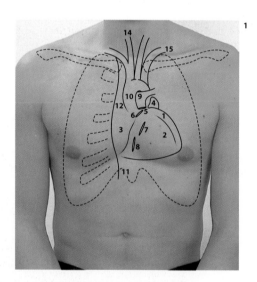

1 Anterior Thorax/Heart and Great Vessel

| | | | |
|---|---|---|---|
| 1 | Left ventricle | 9 | Pulmonary trunk |
| 2 | Right ventricle | 10 | Ascending aorta |
| 3 | Right atrium | 11 | Inferior vena cava |
| 4 | Left auricular appendage | 12 | Superior vena cava |
| 5 | Pulmonary valve | 13 | Left innominate vein |
| 6 | Aortic valve | 14 | Right common carotid |
| 7 | Mitral valve | | artery |
| 8 | Tricuspid valve | 15 | Left subclavian artery |

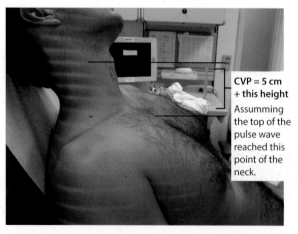

**CVP = 5 cm + this height**

Assuming the top of the pulse wave reached this point of the neck.

Figure 30.9 **Measurement of the jugular venous pressure.**

Figure 30.10 **The surface markings of the heart and great vessels.**

of the heart is felt with mitral regurgitation, whereas a diastolic thrill in the same location is due to mitral stenosis.

## Auscultation

Auscultation is an invaluable tool in the diagnosis of heart disease, particularly valvular pathologies. Once the examiner reaches the stage of auscultation, they should have a general idea of the disease process affecting the patient, and a stethoscope should be used to confirm the diagnosis.

Auscultation of four general areas is essential for the evaluation of heart sounds and murmurs:

- The aortic area over the second intercostal space to the right of the sternum.
- The pulmonary area over the second intercostal space to the left of the sternum.
- The tricuspid area over the fifth intercostal space to the left of the sternum.
- The mitral area over the fifth intercostal space in the midclavicular line or where the apex of the heart is located.

Heart Sounds – The first (S1) and second (S2) heart sounds are produced by closure of the atrioventricular and semilunar valves, respectively.

The first heart sound is caused by closure of the mitral (M1) and the tricuspid (T1) valves. Mitral closure slightly precedes tricuspid closure, but this may not be audible.

The second heart sound is caused by closure of the aortic (A2) and pulmonary (P2) valves. Again, a small gap usually exists, with A2 preceding P2. This physiological split is usually prominent on inspiration. A fixed split occurs with pathological states such as an atrial septal defect.

In addition to these normal sounds, a variety of other sounds may be present, including heart murmurs, adventitious sounds and gallop rhythms, also known as the S3 and S4 sounds.

The third heart sound (S3) closely follows the second heart sound and is the result of rapid filling of the left ventricle. It is normal in hyperdynamic states and in individuals younger than 30 years of age. Otherwise it is an indication of a dilated or failing left ventricle.

The fourth heart sound (S4), which is sometimes audible in an adult, is known as a presystolic gallop or atrial gallop. This gallop is produced by the sound of blood being forced into a stiff or hypertrophic ventricle. It is a sign of a pathological state, usually a failing or hypertrophic left ventricle, as in systemic hypertension, severe valvular aortic stenosis or hypertrophic cardiomyopathy.

Additional sounds may also be heard:

- The *opening snap* of mitral stenosis is a soft, low-pitched sound preceding the murmur of mitral stenosis. It is the noise caused by the calcified valve 'snapping' open but can be hard to detect.
- A *friction rub* is the sound produced when the parietal and visceral pericardia become inflamed, generating a creaky-scratchy noise as they rub together. This occurs with pericarditis or post-cardiotomy syndrome. It can be accentuated by asking the patient to sit up, lean forwards and exhale, bringing the two layers into closer communication.

Cardiac Murmurs – After listening for heart sounds, one should focus on the presence of murmurs (Figure 30.11). These are the result of turbulent flow. They may be secondary to a normal flow through an abnormal valve, or to an abnormal flow through a normal valve. In addition to the four areas of the heart,

the examiner should listen to referred murmurs over the carotid artery and left axilla.

The diaphragm of the stethoscope should be used for high-pitched sounds like S1, S2 and most murmurs. The bell of the stethoscope is used for low-pitched sounds such as S3, S4 and the murmur of mitral stenosis. Have the patient turned to left side when listening to the mitral valve and lean forwards when listening to the aortic valve.

Murmurs are graded from 1 to 6 (Table 30.3) but this is not a reflection of the degree of valvular pathology as the flow

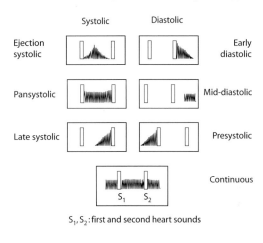

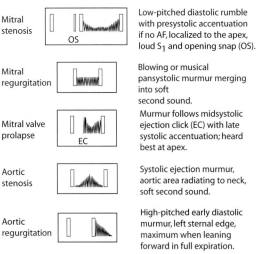

Figure 30.11 Cardiac murmurs. AF, atrial fibrillation.

Table 30.3 Grading of heart murmurs

| Grade | Description |
|---|---|
| Grade 1 | Very faint, heard only after the listener has 'tuned in'; may not be heard in all positions |
| Grade 2 | Quiet, but heard immediately after placing the stethoscope on the chest |
| Grade 3 | Moderately loud |
| Grade 4 | Loud, with a palpable thrill |
| Grade 5 | Very loud, with a thrill; may be heard when the stethoscope is partly off the chest |
| Grade 6 | Very loud, with a thrill; may be heard with the stethoscope entirely off the chest |

generating the murmur may become very low in, for example, severe stenosis of the valve.

**Systolic ejection murmurs** are seen in:

* aortic stenosis;
* pulmonary stenosis;
* atrial septal defects.

Aortic stenosis is associated with a harsh systolic ejection murmur that is heard over the aortic area but also radiates to the carotid arteries.

Pulmonary stenosis and the murmurs of an atrial septal defect are best heard at the left sternal edge on inspiration.

**Pansystolic murmurs** are seen in:

* mitral regurgitation;
* tricuspid regurgitation;
* ventricular septal defects.

Mitral regurgitation is best heard over the apex and radiates to the axilla, while the murmurs of ventricular septal defects and tricuspid regurgitation are best heard over the left sternal border.

**Mid-diastolic murmurs** occur with:

* mitral stenosis;
* tricuspid stenosis;
* aortic regurgitation (Austin Flint murmurs).

The murmur of mitral stenosis is best heard at the apex. It is a low-pitched diastolic rumble sometimes preceded by an opening snap. The murmur is accentuated on exertion. Tricuspid stenosis is best heard over the left sternal border. The Austin Flint murmur occurs when aortic regurgitation causes a backflow into the left ventricle that closes the mitral valve.

**Early diastolic murmurs** can be heard in:

* aortic regurgitation;
* pulmonary regurgitation.

Aortic regurgitation is best heard over the left edge of the sternum and the apex (in the direction of the regurgitant flow). Pulmonary regurgitation is best heard over the left edge of the sternum and on inspiration. A Graham Steell murmur results from a high-velocity regurgitant flow across the pulmonary valve; this is usually a consequence of pulmonary hypertension.

Finally, a **continuous or machinery murmur** is neither systolic nor diastolic. It is characteristic of a patent ductus arteriosus (**Figure 30.12**). Since the aortic pressure is higher than the pulmonary pressure, a continuous murmur occurs, which is best heard over the left axilla.

## CONGENITAL HEART DISEASES

Congenital heart diseases occur at a rate of approximately 10 per 1000 live births. Many are not compatible with life, although some (e.g. atrial septal defects) are asymptomatic and not detected until later in life. A high percentage of defects will require some form of medical intervention or surgical correction.

Abnormalities of development of the heart can affect the right chambers, the left chambers or the septum between the two sides (atrial and ventral septal defects). They can also affect the heart valves, the venous structures draining into the heart or any combination of these. The aorta can be affected by aberrant branches or rings or it may be tight, as in the case of coarctation (**Figure 30.13**).

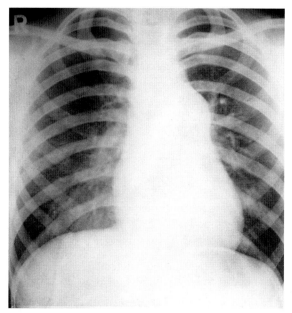

Figure 30.12 **A** patent ductus arteriosus. The pulmonary conus is enlarged, the aortic knuckle is reduced and there are prominent vascular markings.

Congenital heart diseases are best classified as cyanotic or non-cyanotic. Cyanotic heart diseases are associated with a right-to-left shunt and blood bypassing the pulmonary circulation. A classic and relatively common example is tetralogy of Fallot, which is characterized by pulmonary stenosis, a ventral septal defect, a hypertrophied right ventricle, and an aorta overriding the ventricles. A characteristic feature is that the child adopts a squatting position when tired.

Cardiac examination demonstrates palpable thrills, abnormal heart sounds and murmurs that are characteristic of each lesion.

## THE PERICARDIUM

The potential space between the visceral and parietal pericardia usually contains a thin film of fluid. Extra fluid can accumulate in this space for a variety of reasons and forms a **pericardial effusion** (**Figure 30.14**). When the volume of fluid reaches more than 1 L, it interferes with cardiac function, causing **cardiac tamponade**. This is characterized by vascular hypotension, an elevated JVP and pulsus paradoxus.

The pericardium may become inflamed, causing pericarditis. There are various causes of this, including infections with viruses or bacteria (e.g. *Mycobacterium tuberculosis*), idiopathic causes, uraemic pericarditis, post-infarction pericarditis and Dressler's syndrome (which occurs weeks to months after a heart attack or cardiac surgery). It may also be associated with a pericardial effusion. It is associated with a characteristic pain that is aggravated by inspiration and leaning forwards. Auscultation may reveal a friction rub.

Constrictive pericarditis is a late sequela of pericardial inflammation. It can be caused by infection (e.g. tuberculosis) but can also be secondary to radiation and at times idiopathic. It results in scarring and calcification of the pericardium (**Figure 30.15**) and results in impeded filling of the right heart. Patients have symptoms of right heart failure, with an elevated JVP, jaundice, ascites and peripheral oedema

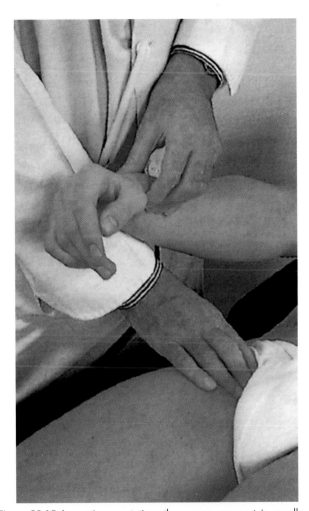

Figure 30.13 In aortic coarctation, the narrow segment is usually at the site of the primitive ductus arteriosus. Hypertension develops, and the collateral channels are particularly noted in the intercostal arteries, notching of the ribs being present on radiographs. A radiofemoral delay is detected by the simultaneous palpation of the radial and femoral arteries, the latter being attenuated.

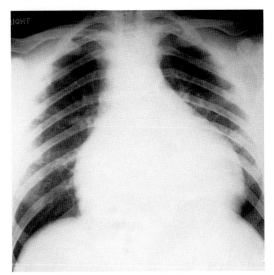

Figure 30.14 A pericardial effusion. There is a globular enlarged cardiac shadow with loss of the normal cardiac contour.

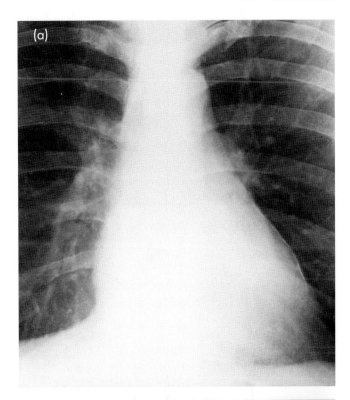

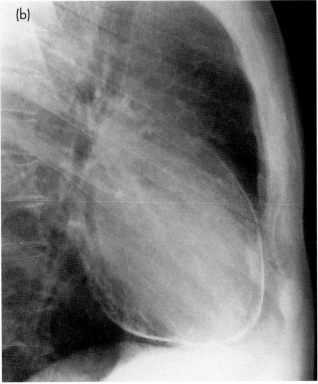

Figure 30.15 (a, b) A calcified pericardium.

**Key Points**

- A detailed history and a complete physical examination are essential in the evaluation of the cardiac surgical patient.
- Cardiac disease can have a variety of presentations. Dyspnoea, chest pain and syncope are the most common symptoms and should be investigated thoroughly.
- Cardiovascular examination requires proper assessment of the pulse and measurement of the jugular venous pressure.
- Cardiac examination includes inspection and palpation of the chest, but more importantly auscultation of the mediastinum for abnormalities in heart sounds and presence of murmurs.

## SBAs

**1. Which one of the following is *not* a sign or symptom of aortic stenosis?:**

a Chest pain at rest
b Lower extremity oedema
c Dyspnoea on exertion
d Syncope
e Chest pain on exertion

**Answer**

*a **Chest pain at rest.** Aortic stenosis has three main manifestations. First, it demonstrates angina that is induced by exertion and relieved by rest. This is related to a mismatch between blood supply and demand that is increased by wall stress during exercise. Aortic stenosis can also manifest with heart failure symptoms that include dyspnoea on exertion, paroxysmal nocturnal dyspnoea and lower extremity oedema. Finally, aortic stenosis can present with syncope that is caused by either low cardiac output or arrhythmia induced by wall stress and ischaemia. Chest pain at rest is not a usual manifestation of aortic stenosis and usually indicates acute myocardial infarction or aortic dissection.*

**2. Which of the following is not a usual cardiovascular cause of chest pain?:**

a Aortic dissection
b Aortic stenosis
c Coronary artery disease
d Mitral regurgitation
e Pericarditis

**Answer**

*d **Mitral regurgitation.** Aortic dissection usually presents with severe, acute-onset tearing chest pain. Aortic valve stenosis can give rise to chest pain with exertion. Coronary disease manifests with chest pain that is reproducible with exertion, as in stable angina. It can also present with acute chest pain at rest, as in unstable angina or myocardial infarction. Chest pain that is relieved by leaning forward is typical of pericarditis. Mitral disease does not typically present with chest pain, but rather with dyspnoea and symptoms of heart failure.*

## EMQs

**1. For each of the following patient histories, select the most likely diagnosis from the list below. Each option may be used once, more than once or not at all:**

1 Acute type A aortic dissection
2 Mitral regurgitation
3 Pericarditis
4 Aortic stenosis
5 Coronary artery disease

a A 63-year-old woman with dyspnoea on exertion, cough and a systolic murmur heard mostly over the apex
b A 55-year-old man with acute, tearing-type, mid-sternal chest pain and a cold left lower extremity
c A 66-year-old man with a history of diabetes mellitus, hypertension and hyperlipidaemia. He has chest pain that is induced by walking for half a mile and relieved by rest
d A 25-year-old man with chest pain that is relieved by leaning forward. A friction rub is heard on auscultation
e A 75-year-old man with progressive worsening of fatigue and dyspnoea on exertion. He also has occasional lightheadedness. Physical examination reveals a systolic murmur heard over the right upper sternal border

**Answers**

a 2 *Mitral regurgitation.*
b 1 *Acute type A aortic dissection.*
c 5 *Coronary artery disease.*
d 3 *Pericarditis.*
e 4 *Aortic stenosis.*

**2. For each of the following conditions, select the most likely matches for the presentations given below. Each option may be used once, more than once or not at all:**

**1** Mitral stenosis

**2** Mitral regurgitation

**3** Mitral valve prolapse

**4** Aortic stenosis

**5** Aortic regurgitation

**a** Murmur follows midsystolic ejection click (EC) with late systolic accentuation; heard best at apex.

**b** High-pitched early diastolic murmur, left sternal edge, maximum when leaning forward in full expiration.

**c** Systolic ejection murmur, aortic area radiating to neck, soft second sound.

**d** Low-pitched diastolic rumble with presystolic accentuation if no AF, localizing to the apex, loud S1 and opening snap (OS).

**e** Blowing or musical pansystolic murmur merging into soft second sound.

Answer

*a* *3*

*b* *5*

*c* *4*

*d* *1*

*e* *2*

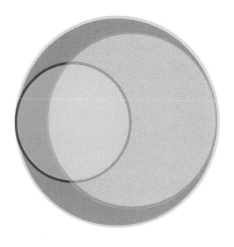

# PART

# 7

# Vascular

# Arterial Disorders

Jamal Jawad Hoballah, Maen Aboul Hosn

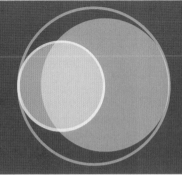

## LEARNING OBJECTIVES

- To identify the signs and symptoms of lower extremity occlusive disease
- To recognize the signs and symptoms of acute limb ischaemia
- To be aware of the signs and symptoms of carotid disease
- To identify the signs and symptoms of visceral arterial occlusive disease

- To know the signs and symptoms of aortic aneurysmal disease
- To identify the signs and symptoms of peripheral aneurysmal disease
- To recognize the physical examination findings in patients with peripheral arterial occlusive and aneurysmal disease
- To interpret the physical examination findings associated with diabetic foot pathology

## ANATOMY

The arterial wall is composed of three layers: the intima, media and adventitia:

- The *adventitia* is the outermost layer and is composed of connective tissue, neural fibres and small capillaries. As such, it is the main site for the nutrition and innervation of the vessel.
- The *media* is the thickest layer of the vessel wall. It is composed of smooth muscle cells and connective tissue bundles that provide its strength and elasticity.
- The innermost layer is the *intima*. This is lined with an endothelial cell layer that functions both as an interface between the circulating blood and the arterial wall, as well as a source of vasoactive products that prevent thrombosis and regulate the vascular tone by inducing vasoconstriction and vasodilation.

## ATHEROSCLEROSIS

Atherosclerosis is a systemic disease of the large and medium-sized arteries in which lipid and fibrous material accumulate between the intima and media of the vessel, eventually causing narrowing of the lumen. It is a degenerative process triggered by endothelial cell dysfunction followed by the adhesion and infiltration of inflammatory cells (macrophages and T lymphocytes), which leads to the formation of fibrocellular plaques. As these plaques continue to grow, they cause an inflammatory reaction that triggers smooth muscle proliferation in the affected area, resulting in luminal narrowing and a reduction of blood flow through the vessel.

In addition to genetic predisposition, the risk factors for the development of atherosclerosis include smoking, hypertension, dislipidaemia, diabetes mellitus and coagulation disorders. This process has been shown to start as early as childhood, with endothelial fat streaks being the first manifestations. This chronicity and gradual stenosis usually allows for the formation of collateral arterial channels to the affected organ. As such, the ischaemic symptoms vary depending on the vessel involved, the degree of narrowing and the presence or absence of collaterals. Examples include angina pectoris with diseased coronary arteries, intermittent claudication with diseased arteries in the extremities and renovascular hypertension with affected renal arteries.

Another complication of this inflammatory process is the ulceration and acute rupture of an unstable plaque, leading to either acute occlusion of the artery (thrombosis) or a distal showering of the plaque material (embolism). Acute occlusion does not allow for the development of collaterals and therefore leads to symptoms of acute ischaemia. Some manifestations of this process include acute myocardial infarctions, strokes and acute limb ischaemia.

Despite the fact that atherosclerosis is a systemic disease, the plaques tend to occur more in specific areas, mainly those with high turbulence, low shear stress and flow stagnation. As such, regions of arterial bifurcation are the most susceptible to the development of atherosclerotic disease. The most common site for these plaques are the coronary arteries, carotid bifurcation, aortic bifurcation and proximal iliac arteries, as well as the lower extremity arteries at the site of the adductor canal.

## CAROTID ARTERY OCCLUSIVE DISEASE

Stroke is the second leading cause of death worldwide and the fourth leading cause of death in the USA. Its incidence is highest among the ageing population. The impact of stroke is devastating, with a 20 per cent mortality from the acute event. Among those who survive, up to 20 per cent are unable to return to work. In addition, 25 per cent of those over 65 years of age require long-term institutional care after only a single event. Only a small fraction of those suffering an acute stroke actually benefit from thrombolytic therapy, especially if they present early on, while the majority will go on to suffer a completed stroke and sustain irreversible brain injury. As such, the greatest impact on this disease comes from stroke prevention through the management of modifiable risk factors or intervention on the carotid plaque. The major risk factors for stroke are:

- male sex;
- family history;
- advanced age;
- smoking;
- hypertension;
- dyslipidaemia;
- diabetes mellitus;
- a history of cerebrovascular accidents;
- coronary artery disease;
- cardiac dysrhythmias;
- carotid stenosis.

### Presentation

Patients with atherosclerotic carotid disease are classified as either symptomatic or asymptomatic. Patients are considered symptomatic if they have had transient or permanent focal neurological symptoms related to the affected artery, such as an ipsilateral partial or complete loss of vision, contralateral weakness or numbness of an extremity or the face, dysarthria or aphasia, within the previous 6 months.

A **transient ischaemic attack** (TIA) is defined as a transient episode of neurological dysfunction caused by focal brain, spinal cord or retinal ischaemia without acute infarction that resolves within 24 hours, an ischaemic stroke is defined as infarction of central nervous system tissue leading to neurological deficits that last more than 24 hours. Amaurosis fugax or transient mononuclear blindness is a transient loss of vision secondary to obstruction of a branch of the retinal artery.

Asymptomatic patients, on the other hand, are those with significant carotid stenosis that is discovered on physical examination or incidentally. In such patients, a carotid bruit, which is an audible sound arising from turbulent blood flow within the stenotic vessel, is sometimes heard on auscultation. Bruits, however, have a poor predictive value for cerebrovascular accidents and are considered markers of atherosclerotic disease in general rather than of stroke risk.

### Diagnosis

The work-up for carotid artery occlusive disease first begins with proper history-taking. This should focus on identifying previous episodes of neurological deficit and ocular symptoms as well as possible predisposing factors for stroke, such as hypertension, previous myocardial infarctions and a history of arrhythmias.

Next, a complete physical examination should be performed to determine the presence of cardiac or peripheral vascular disease. Carotid bruits discovered on auscultation may indicate carotid occlusive disease, but they can also represent a radiation of cardiac murmurs or denote the presence of mild carotid artery disease associated with calcification of the arterial wall. A carotid bruit may be related to a plaque extending into the external carotid artery. However, the absence of a carotid bruit does not indicate the absence of carotid disease as a carotid bruit may not be heard in patients with a totally occluded internal carotid artery.

A more focused neurological examination is then carried out to identify any focal and non-focal neurological deficits. This systematic approach allows clinicians to localize the area of cerebral ischaemia responsible for the neurological deficit and the possible aetiology behind it.

A number of imaging modalities are available for the assessment of carotid disease. These include colour-flow duplex scanning, CT and MRI scanning and angiography.

### Duplex Scanning

Duplex scanning uses real-time B-mode ultrasonography and colour-enhanced Doppler flow measurements to determine the extent of carotid stenosis as well as the presence or absence of calcifications within the plaque. Measurements of blood flow velocity within the vessel are also made, which directly correlate with the degree of intraluminal narrowing, an increase in velocity suggesting more significant stenosis (Table 31.1). Plaque heterogeneity and ulceration on duplex scanning have also been found to be predictive features of plaque instability and future neurological accidents.

Among the limitations of duplex scanning is the fact that it requires considerable expertise and skill in performing it and interpreting the results, and as such is operator-dependent. In addition, it does not allow the visualization of anatomically inaccessible areas in the neck, such as the proximal carotid artery and intracranial portions of the internal carotid artery.

### Computed Tomography Angiography and Magnetic Resonance Angiography

Computed tomography angiography (CT angiography) and magnetic resonance angiography (MR angiography) are contrast-based imaging modalities that are used when the results of duplex scanning are inconclusive or need further confirmation. They are also used when proximal or intracranial lesions are suspected. High-quality images are obtained that can be viewed

Table 31.1 Velocity measurements on Doppler scanning in relation to the degree of stenosis

| Stenosis (%) | Peak systolic velocity (cm/s) | End-diastolic velocity (cm/s) |
|---|---|---|
| <30 | <120 | <65 |
| 30–50 | 120–140 | <65 |
| 50–60 | >140 | <65 |
| 60–70 | >150 | <65 |
| 70–99 | >150 | >90 |

in multiple planes, allowing a better understanding of the arterial anatomy as well as plaque morphology, and therefore facilitating intervention-planning.

The limitations of these techniques remain their cost and availability, as well as the exposure to contrast and radiation. The presence of severe calcifications can affect the quality of images for both duplex ultrasonography and CT angiography. Magnetic resonance angiography studies tend to overestimate the degree of stenosis.

## Conventional Digital Subtraction Angiography

This technique used to be the gold standard for assessing carotid stenosis, but with the advent of CT angiography it is now rarely used as a primary imaging modality. This is because of the invasive nature of the procedure, the complications related to vascular access and the small but significant risk of stroke associated with it.

## Treatment

The management of carotid artery stenosis varies depending on a variety of factors including the degree of stenosis, whether the patient is symptomatic or asymptomatic, the presence and severity of medical comorbidities and local anatomical factors. Treatment options include medical therapy either alone or combined with open surgical intervention (carotid endarterectomy) or endovascular therapy (carotid artery angioplasty and stenting).

As most patients with carotid occlusive disease have associated cardiac and peripheral vascular disease, medical treatment aims to modify the risk factors so that the progression of the atherosclerotic disease can be halted. This includes the management of lipid disorders, the control of hypertension and diabetes, along with smoking cessation. As such, most at-risk patients are currently treated with antiplatelet therapy, statins, beta-blockers and angiotensin-converting enzyme (ACE) inhibitors.

**Carotid endarterectomy** involves surgically opening the internal carotid artery at the carotid bifurcation and excising the diseased arterial wall and plaque along with most of the media (Figure 31.1). The artery is then closed either primarily or using a patch to offset the luminal narrowing and reduce the risk of perioperative thrombosis and late re-stenosis. The patch can be prosthetic or autogenous, using a vein segment.

Based on major landmark trials, carotid endarterectomy combined with medical therapy has been shown to be superior to medical treatment alone in symptomatic patients with 50–99 per cent stenosis if the perioperative stroke or death rate is

less than 6 per cent. The greatest benefit was seen in those with severe stenosis (>70–99 per cent). Other factors were also noted to be associated with increased benefits in symptomatic patients, such as the severity of the presenting symptoms, the presence of ulcerated plaque and the status of the contralateral carotid. Patients with stroke benefited more than those with TIA, who in turn benefited more than those with transient monocular blindness. Similarly, patients with ulcerated plaques and contralateral occlusion benefited more than those without these factors.

In asymptomatic patients treated by surgery, the mortality and morbidity are close to 3 per cent, and carotid endarterectomy combined with medical therapy for stenosis exceeding 60 per cent has been found to be associated with an approximately 50 per cent reduction in the risk of stroke. The absolute risk reduction at 5 years was, however, approximately 6 per cent. The results are summarized in Table 31.2.

Most surgeons tend to use 80 per cent stenosis as the level of stenosis for intervention. It is worth mentioning, however, that medical management has changed significantly since the early carotid endarterectomy trials, indicating that the reduction in stroke risk from surgical therapy may be overstated, especially in women. Future studies will help to identify which asymptomatic plaques are more likely to progress to become symptomatic.

**Endovascular treatment** of carotid disease has emerged in recent years with the continued growth of minimally invasive surgery. This approach entails gaining access percutaneously into a distant artery and then advancing a thin wire through the stenotic area under fluoroscopic guidance. A balloon catheter is then advanced over the wire and inflated at the area of narrowing,

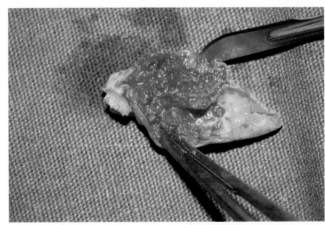

Figure 31.1 An ulcerated carotid plaque.

Table 31.2 Summary of the outcomes of medical therapy versus surgery in patients with symptomatic and asymptomatic carotid artery disease

| | Diameter of ICA stenosis (%) | BMT stroke or death at 5 years (%) | CEA and BMT stroke or death at 5 years (%) | Relative risk reduction at 5 years (%) | Absolute risk reduction at 5 years (%) | NNT to prevent one stroke |
|---|---|---|---|---|---|---|
| Asymptomatic | 60–99 | 11 | 5.1 | 54 | 5.9 | 19 |
| Symptomatic | 50–69 | 27.7 | 20 | 28 | 7.8 | 13 |
| | 70–99 | 32.7 | 17.1 | 48 | 15.6 | 6 |

BMT, best medical treatment; CEA, carotid endarterectomy; ICA, internal carotid artery; NNT, number needed to treat.

thus increasing the luminal diameter. In addition, a stent is deployed in the narrowed region in order to maintain the lumen and control the associated dissection.

Carotid artery stenting avoids some of the surgical risks associated with carotid endarterectomy, including cranial nerve injury, and wound problems. It also decreases the risk of cardiac events that could occur in the perioperative period. This makes it more appealing in high-risk patients. The procedure, however, still carries a risk of embolic stroke secondary to particle embolization while manoeuvring the wires and catheters. This risk is decreased with the use of embolic protection devices, whose function is to capture any dislodged embolic particles and prevent them from reaching the brain. These devices, nonetheless, have their own inherent risks and complications, such as an inability to cross the target lesion, a failure to capture the emboli and injury to the vessel wall.

A recent, large, randomized trial, Carotid Revascularization Endarterectomy Versus Stenting Trial (the CREST trial), comparing carotid endarterectomy with carotid artery stenting showed a comparable overall safety and efficacy for the two procedures. There were, however, higher rates of stroke in the stenting group (4.1 vs 2.3 per cent) and myocardial infarction in the surgical group (2.3 versus 1.1 per cent). In addition, the 30-day risk of stroke and death in patients undergoing carotid stenting was substantially higher in patients over the age of 80 compared with non-octogenarians (12.1 versus 3.2 per cent). These data, while validating the efficacy of carotid artery stenting, still pose questions pertaining to its long-term results and the subgroup of patients who can benefit the most from it.

For the time being, carotid artery stenting remains limited to patients with a symptomatic carotid artery stenosis of at least 70 per cent who are considered a high risk for open surgery. The definition of high risk is not limited to medical factors but can be related to local anatomical factors such as prior carotid endarterectomy, radical neck dissection, neck radiation or the presence of a tracheostomy. Asymptomatic patients with significant medical comorbidities may be better managed with best medical therapy since the stroke risk with stenting may exceed the stroke risk associated with best medical therapy.

## MESENTERIC OCCLUSIVE DISEASE

Mesenteric ischaemia is a rare life-threatening condition caused by a decreased blood flow to the bowel. Despite advances in diagnostic and treatment modalities over the last two decades, mesenteric ischaemia remains difficult to diagnose and has a high morbidity and mortality. It should be suspected in any patient presenting with abdominal pain out of proportion to the findings of the physical examination, especially in the presence of associated cardiovascular disease. Mesenteric ischaemia is categorized as acute or chronic depending on the extent and acuteness of intestinal blood flow compromise.

**Acute mesenteric ischaemia** refers to an acute severe drop in intestinal perfusion as a result of any of four distinct entities:

- embolic occlusion of the mesenteric circulation, usually from cardiac or aortic emboli (40 per cent);
- acute thrombosis of the mesenteric circulation, secondary to atherosclerotic disease (30 per cent);
- non-occlusive mesenteric ischaemia (NOMI) – a low-flow state or profound hypovolaemia or splanchnic vasoconstriction (20 per cent);
- mesenteric venous thrombosis (10 per cent).

**Chronic mesenteric ischaemia**, on the other hand, is usually due to progressive mesenteric atherosclerotic disease with episodic or persistent intestinal hypoperfusion. Symptoms occur as a result of insufficient splanchnic blood flow at times of increased intestinal demand, typically induced by food intake.

## Intestinal Vascular Supply

Blood to the intestines is supplied by the coeliac axis, the superior mesenteric artery (SMA), the inferior mesenteric artery (IMA) and the internal iliac arteries. The severity of intestinal ischaemia depends on the number of splanchnic vessels affected and the adequacy of the collateral circulations.

The **coeliac axis** originates from the abdominal aorta and gives off the splenic, hepatic and left gastric branches. The common hepatic artery usually gives rise to the right gastric artery and gastroduodenal artery, the latter in turn branching to give the right gastroepiploic artery and anterior and posterior superior pancreaticoduodenal arteries. The left gastroepiploic artery arises from the splenic artery and joins the right gastroepiploic artery along the greater curvature of the stomach. These gastroepiploic arteries, along with the gastric arteries, ensure an excellent gastric blood supply, making gastric ischaemia rare.

The **SMA** arises from the abdominal aorta distal to the coeliac artery and gives rise to the inferior pancreaticoduodenal artery, several jejunal and ileal branches, the right colic and the middle colic artery. It supplies the small intestines and ascending colon all the way to the proximal to mid-transverse colon.

The **IMA** arises from the abdominal aorta approximately half way between the renal arteries and the aortic bifurcation, and gives rise to the left colic artery, the sigmoid artery and the superior haemorrhoidal artery. It therefore supplies the distal transverse colon all the way to the rectum.

The internal iliac artery originates in the pelvis at the bifurcation of the common iliac artery. It provides a blood supply to the rectum through the middle and inferior haemorrhoidal arteries.

Collaterals exist between the four main vessels – the coeliac artery, SMA, IMA and internal iliac artery – ensuring a persistent and adequate intestinal flow if one vessel is compromised. These collaterals include the junction of the superior and inferior pancreaticoduodenal arteries between the coeliac axis and the SMA, the marginal artery of Drummond between the SMA and IMA and the junction of the superior and middle rectal vessels between the IMA and internal iliac arteries. Collaterals between these pelvic branches and the profunda femoris arteries also play a significant role in the presence of occlusive disease affecting the common femoral artery.

## Presentation

The clinical presentation of patients with mesenteric ischaemia varies depending on whether they are suffering from acute or chronic ischaemia.

Patients with acute mesenteric ischaemia typically present with sudden-onset mid-abdominal pain, usually associated with nausea, vomiting and rapid bowel evacuation. Fever and blood per rectum may also be present but to a lesser extent. Acute **embolic ischaemia** is seen mostly in patients with a history of cardiac events such as myocardial infarction, atrial fibrillation, mural thrombus, cardiac valve disease or thoracic aortic aneurysm, all of which carry a risk of dislodging thrombi. Patients with acute **mesenteric thrombosis** have a similar presentation, but unlike those with embolic occlusion, they typically have a history of chronic post-prandial abdominal pain and significant weight loss.

**Non-occlusive mesenteric ischaemia** is seen usually in severely ill elderly patients with atherosclerotic disease who are being treated in an intensive care setting. Examples are patients with severe aortic stenosis, sepsis or cardiac arrhythmias who are receiving drugs such as diuretics and pressors that cause hypotension or peripheral vasoconstriction. The pain is generally more diffuse and tends to wax and wane, making the diagnosis difficult. Some of these patients may be already in an intensive care unit setting on ventilator support and multiple vasoconstricting medications, making the diagnosis even harder.

In **mesenteric vein thrombosis**, the presentation may be more insidious, with patients reporting symptoms over weeks or months. These symptoms are usually non-specific and include vague abdominal pain, nausea, vomiting and malaise. Upper gastrointestinal bleeding secondary to gastroesophageal varices may also be a presenting symptom if the patient has associated portal or splenic vein thrombosis.

The physical examination of patients with acute mesenteric ischaemia varies depending on the phases of the disease. In the first few hours, the abdomen maybe soft and non-tender. The patient's pain is visceral in origin and is typically noted to be out of proportion to the physical findings. As the ischaemia progresses, the pain becomes parietal and associated with peritoneal signs of tenderness and rebound tenderness. In the late phases, the patient may present in shock with a board-like rigid abdomen. The physical examination may also reveal evidence of arrhythmias or peripheral arterial occlusive disease depending on the aetiology.

In patients with chronic mesenteric ischaemia, at least two or three of the visceral arteries are typically affected by the occlusive pathology. Patients usually complain of severe epigastric abdominal pain, mostly post-prandial, which is referred to as intestinal angina. The pain typically occurs within half an hour to an hour after eating, subsides after few hours and is worse with larger meals with a high fat content. Over time, patients develop food aversion, resulting in significant weight loss.

## Diagnosis

The diagnosis of mesenteric ischaemia requires a high index of suspicion and is based mostly on the patient's history and physical examination. Laboratory studies, including an elevated white blood cell count, elevated lactate level and abnormal base deficit, may aid in the diagnosis of acute mesenteric ischaemia, but are highly non-specific. Adjunctive imaging modalities are available in the work-up of mesenteric ischaemia, including abdominal X-rays, duplex ultrasound, CT angiography, MR angiography and contrast angiography.

**Abdominal X-ray films** are non-specific for mesenteric ischaemia and are normal in more than 25 per cent of patients with acute ischaemia. They may reveal indirect signs of bowel ischaemia such as bowel oedema and thickening referred to as thumbprinting, or gas in the bowel wall (pneumatosis intestinalis) or biliary tree. They are particularly helpful in excluding other identifiable causes of abdominal pain such as obstruction and perforation.

**Duplex ultrasound** is a useful tool in detecting mesenteric vessel stenosis in chronic mesenteric ischaemia; however, its role is restricted in acute mesenteric ischaemia. This is mainly due to the dilated air-filled bowel loops that are seen in the latter, and the significant abdominal pain that prevents the examination being conducted. In addition, duplex ultrasound has limited sensitivity for detecting emboli beyond the proximal portion of the vessel.

**Computed tomography angiography** is usually the preferred diagnostic imaging modality for mesenteric ischaemia. It allows a fast and accurate diagnosis and rules out any other intra-abdominal pathology. This is especially true of the multi-array helical CT scan, which provides a three-dimensional reconstruction of the aorta and the origins of the coeliac artery and SMA, as well as an accurate localization of the occlusion. It has been shown to have a sensitivity and specificity of 96.4 per cent and 97.9 per cent, respectively, in diagnosing acute mesenteric ischaemia.

Computed tomography angiography is also the imaging modality of choice for diagnosing mesenteric vein thrombosis and has a sensitivity close to 100 per cent. The efficacy of CT angiography drops, however, when defining the secondary, tertiary and smaller branches of the visceral circulation. In addition, the use of intravenous contrast carries the risk of nephrotoxicity and contrast allergy.

**Magnetic resonance angiography** also allows for a three-dimensional visualization of the visceral vessels. It has advantages over CT angiography in that gadolinium is significantly less nephrotoxic than the contrast agents used for CT scans and no ionizing radiation is used. However, like CT angiography, MR angiography does not adequately assess the distal branches of the mesenteric vessels. Furthermore, it is less readily available in an emergency setting.

**Contrast angiography** remains the gold standard for imaging the visceral vessels and diagnosing acute ischaemia. It provides images that are superior to those obtained with CT angiography or MR angiography and allows a visualization of the distal SMA and IMA and their branches. It is carried out by accessing the femoral or brachial artery percutaneously, advancing a catheter into the aorta over a guidewire and injecting contrast material under fluoroscopic vision. The origins of the coeliac artery and SMA are best seen on the lateral view, whereas the middle and distal SMA and the IMA are best seen on an anteroposterior view. In addition to its diagnostic role, angiography also has a therapeutic function by allowing selective catheterization of the target mesenteric vessels and the infusion of vasodilating agents and thrombolytic drugs.

Emboli are more likely to lodge in the SMA given its less acute take-off from the aorta compared with the coeliac axis and IMA. Depending on their size, emboli tend to travel through the SMA and lodge at bifurcations or in smaller branches with preservation of the blood supply to the jejunal branch. Thrombotic occlusion, on the other hand, involves the origin of the vessel where the atherosclerotic plaque is located. Thus, the entire vessel from its take-off is not seen on arteriography.

In patients with NOMI, contrast angiography reveals narrowing of the trunk of the SMA with progressive tapering of the branches, and decreased or absent flow in the smaller vessels. Contrast angiography is not the ideal modality to diagnose mesenteric vein thrombosis. However, venous thrombosis may be diagnosed during the venous phase of arteriography by visualizing the filling defect within the vein and sluggish or absent flow.

## Treatment

### Acute Mesenteric Ischaemia

The management of acute mesenteric ischaemia is aimed at promptly restoring the blood flow to the affected mesenteric vessel and its branches, and resecting non-viable bowel segments.

Prior to any intervention, patients should be aggressively managed to prevent hypovolaemia and haemodynamic instability, as these will worsen the bowel ischaemia. Antibiotics should be started early as well. Patients with diagnosed bowel ischaemia and peritoneal signs are taken directly to the operating room for exploratory laparotomy, while those with an unclear diagnosis may benefit from angiography, since, as mentioned earlier, this procedure can be diagnostic and therapeutic at the same time.

Embolic Mesenteric Occlusion – The standard treatment of an acute embolism in the SMA is exploratory laparotomy and surgical embolectomy. The SMA is localized intraoperatively. An arteriotomy is performed in the SMA proximal to the origin of the middle colic and other main branches. An embolectomy catheter is then used to extract the embolus and restore the blood flow. Once revascularization has been established, the bowels are carefully inspected and all grossly necrotic segments are resected. Segments of questionable viability are left to be reassessed in 24–48 hours in a 'second-look laparotomy' (Figure 31.2).

Endovascular intervention for SMA occlusion has been described but is reserved for patients in a stable condition with no peritoneal signs and only a partially occluding embolus. In such patients, angiography with catheter-directed thrombolysis may be contemplated. These patients should be monitored in an intensive care setting, with any signs of deterioration necessitating exploration.

Thrombotic Mesenteric Occlusion – Since thrombosis of the SMA usually occurs at its origin, the entire midgut becomes ischaemic. Unlike embolic occlusion of the SMA, revascularization is achieved by bypassing the occlusion in either an antegrade (from the supracoeliac aorta) or a retrograde (via the infrarenal aorta or iliac arteries) manner. Due to the high risk of bowel infarction and bacterial translocation, the preferred conduit is an autologous saphenous vein graft rather than a prosthetic graft. An infrarenal retrograde bypass is usually preferred since iliac exposure can be readily achieved while avoiding supracoeliac dissection and clamping. Compared with the antegrade approach, however, this approach carries a higher risk of graft kinking once the bowels are put back in their anatomical position.

A newer revascularization technique for acute mesenteric thrombosis that combines both an open and an endovascular approach has recently been popularized. This hybrid procedure involves an exploratory laparotomy to assess bowel viability and the SMA. Thrombectomy of the SMA is then performed, followed by retrograde angioplasty and stenting and patching of the vessel. As with embolic mesenteric ischaemia, a second-look laparotomy may be required after revascularization.

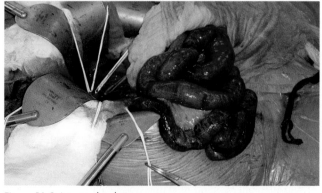

Figure 31.2 Intestinal ischaemia.

Non-occlusive Mesenteric Ischaemia – The management of NOMI is mainly non-operative and is directed at improving the visceral blood flow. This is done by providing adequate fluid resuscitation, improving cardiac output and avoiding drugs that cause vasoconstriction. A catheter-directed intra-arterial infusion of papaverine can also be initiated to induce dilatation of the small vessels, with repeat angiography carried out in 24 hours to confirm resolution of the vasoconstriction. Surgical exploration is reserved for patients with peritoneal signs.

Mesenteric Venous Thrombosis – The mainstay of therapy in mesenteric vein thrombosis is anticoagulation. Laparotomy is performed when the patient's condition deteriorates or fails to improve despite therapy, or when peritoneal signs are seen. A work-up for hypercoagulability should also be performed when the underlying cause of the thrombosis is not identified. Patients with a reversible cause should receive anticoagulation therapy for 3–6 months, while those with a hypercoagulable condition must stay on lifelong anticoagulation.

### Chronic Mesenteric Ischaemia

Given the extensive collaterals that exist between the different mesenteric vessels, high-grade stenosis in multiple mesenteric vessels must be demonstrated for the diagnosis of chronic mesenteric ischaemia, rather than single-vessel disease, to be made. After chronic mesenteric ischaemia has been diagnosed, the best treatment approach depends on the patient's age, the comorbidities, the number and severity of occluded vessels and the mesenteric vascular anatomy.

Therapeutic options involve surgical reconstruction and percutaneous transluminal interventions with angioplasty stenting. Surgical reconstruction includes bypass grafting, endarterectomy and re-implantation, with a perioperative mortality up to 11 per cent and an 80 per cent freedom from recurrence at 5 years. Percutaneous angioplasty, on the other hand, has been shown to provide clinical remission in up to 80 per cent of patients at 3 years. However, it has limited durability, with re-stenosis occurring in up to 50 per cent of patients within the first year. As such, percutaneous transluminal angioplasty is reserved for patients who are considered poor surgical candidates, while surgery is reserved for younger patients with fewer comorbid conditions.

## RENAL ARTERY OCCLUSIVE DISEASE

Renal artery occlusive disease is an important cause of secondary hypertension, accounting for 5 per cent of the total incidence of hypertension. It is seen in less than 1 per cent of patients with mild hypertension and up to 45 per cent of patients with severe or malignant hypertension.

Renal artery stenosis results in decreased kidney perfusion that stimulates the renin–angiotensin–aldosterone pathway, resulting in sodium retention, vasoconstriction and increased plasma volume. Among the surgically correctable causes of hypertension, renal artery stenosis is the most common.

Stenosis can occur due to atherosclerosis or fibromuscular dysplasia (Figure 31.3). Renal atherosclerotic disease is an extension of aortic atherosclerotic disease involving the proximal part of the renal artery and is seen in elderly patients with new-onset hypertension, while fibromuscular dysplasia represents a hyperplastic process in the layers of the distal segments of the artery and is more commonly seen in children and young women. Fibromuscular dysplasia is three times more common in men than

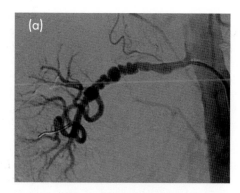

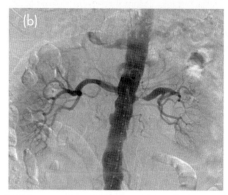

Figure 31.3 (a) Fibromuscular dysplasia of the renal artery. (b) Ostial stenosis in a renal artery.

women and has a peak incidence before the age of 40. Other less common surgically correctable causes of hypertension include phaeochromocytoma and coarctation of the aorta.

## Presentation

Renovascular hypertension should be suspected in all patients presenting with an unexplained acute rise of blood pressure or with resistant hypertension, which is defined as uncontrolled hypertension despite the concurrent use of three antihypertensive agents. Other clinical manifestations include severe hypertension (blood pressure ≥180 mmHg systolic and/or ≥120 mmHg diastolic), an unexplained deterioration of kidney function (a rise in serum creatinine of more than 30 per cent) after the initiation of antihypertensive therapy (mainly ACE inhibitors), unexplained kidney atrophy and severe hypertension with ensuing pulmonary oedema or heart failure. Clinical situations suggestive of an aetiology of renal artery occlusive disease therefore include:

- refractory resistant hypertension;
- malignant hypertension;
- worsening renal function while taking ACE inhibitors;
- unexplained kidney atrophy;
- flash pulmonary oedema;
- a late onset of hypertension (after the age of 55);
- unexplained renal failure.

On physical examination, fewer than 40 per cent of these patients have an audible bruit on abdominal auscultation. When this sign is present, however, it carries up to a 99 per cent specificity for renal artery stenosis. The physical examination may also show evidence of atherosclerotic disease elsewhere in the body,

such as diminished femoral or pedal pulses, the presence of carotid bruits, pulsatile masses and signs and symptoms of coronary artery disease.

## Diagnosis

Conventional angiography has traditionally been the gold standard for diagnosing renal artery stenosis. However, less invasive imaging modalities, including duplex ultrasonography, CT angiography and MR angiography, are now available to aid diagnosis.

### Renal Artery Duplex Ultrasonography

This is usually used as the first-line screening test for renal artery stenosis because of its easy accessibility and lack of ionizing radiation and nephrotoxicity. Images are taken from both the anterior and the oblique flank approach, allowing an assessment of renal blood flow as well as the size of both kidneys. The peak systolic and end-diastolic arterial velocities are measured, and the ratio between the velocities in the renal artery and those in the aorta is determined to detect any evidence of stenosis. The waveform obtained usually shows a continuous diastolic flow through the low-resistance vasculature. A significant discrepancy in size and mass between the two kidneys can also indicate significant renal artery stenosis.

Among the limitations of this procedure are that it is time-consuming and operator-dependent. In addition, the images are affected by the patient's body habitus and by proper preparation prior to the test.

### Computed Tomography Angiography

This is now preferred over formal catheter-based arteriography as a diagnostic test for renal artery stenosis due to its non-invasive nature and easily reproducible results. This imaging modality has excellent sensitivity and specificity for atherosclerotic renal artery stenosis, showing the aortic pathology spilling into the renal artery.

In patients with fibromuscular dysplasia, CT angiography will show the typical chain of lakes or string of beads appearance of the involved renal artery. It may also show associated aneurysms at the branching points of the renal arteries, although it may be less accurate for disease affecting the most distal segments of the renal arteries. Computed tomography angiography is also preferred for the diagnosis of renal artery stenosis when concomitant aortoiliac aneurysmal or occlusive disease is suspected. Among its obvious drawbacks are the use of nephrotoxic contrast agents and ionizing radiation.

### Magnetic Resonance Angiography

This is a highly sensitive imaging modality for detecting proximal renal artery stenosis. It provides three-dimensional anatomical detail of the renal vasculature that is superior to the results obtained with CT angiography. Although the gadolinium used during this procedure was once thought to be safer than iodine-based contrast media, recent studies have raised concerns about gadolinium-associated complications. These include nephrogenic systemic fibrosis, mainly in patients with reduced kidney function, and this has greatly reduced the use of gadolinium for renovascular disease.

### Other Diagnostic Tests

Other tests for renal artery stenosis are available, including captopril renal scintigraphy and the measurement of plasma renin activity or renal vein renin levels. These tests are, however, indirect tests with lower sensitivities and specificities than both CT angiography or MR angiography. Their results are also adversely affected by presence of significant renal dysfunction and bilateral renal artery stenosis, thus limiting their clinical use.

## Treatment

The management of renal artery occlusive disease varies depending on the patient's clinical condition and the aetiology behind the renal artery stenosis. In general, three therapeutic options are available:

- medical therapy;
- percutaneous angioplasty with or without stenting;
- surgical revascularization.

### Medical Treatment

In atherosclerotic renal artery stenosis, medical treatment is aimed at preventing further progression of systemic atherosclerosis and modifying cardiovascular risk factors. Measures include effective blood pressure control, weight reduction, smoking cessation, lipid-lowering therapy and antiplatelet therapy.

Angiotensin-converting enzyme inhibitors and angiotensin II receptor blockers can achieve excellent blood pressure control in patients with renovascular disease. They are, however, contraindicated in bilateral renal artery stenosis as they result in a worsening of renal function. This is attributed to their dilatory effects on the efferent arterioles, resulting decreased glomerular filtration. Furthermore, their use does not stop the progression of stenosis or the long-term renal ischaemic changes.

### Percutaneous Angioplasty with or without Stenting

Percutaneous transluminal renal angioplasty involves threading a wire through the stenotic lesion under fluoroscopic guidance and then introducing a balloon over it to dilate the area (Figure 31.4). The success rate of this procedure varies depending on the site of the lesion. In general, angioplasty works best for lesions that produce incomplete occlusion of the main renal artery. Due to elastic recoil and re-stenosis, total occlusions and ostial lesions generally do not respond well to angioplasty alone.

Angioplasty alone is successful in treating stenosis due to fibromuscular dysplasia in more than 80 per cent of the cases, with an improvement in blood pressure seen in more than two-thirds of patients. Angioplasty is, however, less successful for atherosclerotic stenosis, with a re-stenosis rate of up to 30 per cent between 6 months and 2 years. Ostial lesions are typically aortic plaques that spill into the renal ostium. As such, stent placement is performed for atherosclerotic renal artery stenosis following angioplasty; this results in a higher patency rate, a lower re-stenosis rate, more stable renal function and better blood pressure control compared with angioplasty alone.

The 2006 American College of Cardiology/American Heart Association guidelines on peripheral artery disease recommended stent placement in patients undergoing percutaneous angioplasty for atherosclerotic renal artery stenosis unless the anatomy precludes stenting, and balloon angioplasty alone for lesions

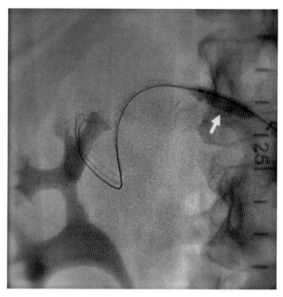

Figure 31.4 Percutaneous transluminal renal angioplasty.

due to fibromuscular dysplasia. The most recent study, the Cardiovascular Outcomes in Renal Atherosclerotic Lesions (CORAL) trial, showed that medical therapy was as effective as interventional therapy with angioplasty stenting in patients with hypertension and renal artery stenosis, resulting in a major decrease in the number of interventional procedures performed for atherosclerotic renal artery occlusive disease.

### Surgical Revascularization

Surgical options in unilateral atherosclerotic renal artery stenosis include endarterectomy of the atherosclerotic lesion, bypass of the stenotic segment from the aorta, hepatic or splenic arteries and removal of the atrophic kidney if there is nearly complete arterial occlusion. Although surgical bypass and angioplasty share similar technical success rates, surgery is associated with a markedly higher morbidity. The in-hospital mortality following renovascular surgery is estimated to be between 3 and 7 per cent, with an increased risk in patients with diffuse atherosclerosis, heart failure and bilateral renal artery stenosis. As such, surgical revascularization is reserved for the following:

- patients with failed angioplasty;
- arterial anatomy that is not amenable to percutaneous transluminal angioplasty;
- renal artery stenosis in the paediatric population;
- the presence of associated renal artery aneurysms;
- failed medical therapy with evidence of a significant loss of the renal parenchymal mass;
- rare cases of aortic reconstruction near the renal arteries for other indications (e.g. aneurysm repair).

Autologous saphenous vein grafts are usually used for renal artery bypass in adults, while internal iliac artery grafts are preferred in children as aneurysmal changes tend to occur with time in vein grafts constructed in paediatric patients. The patency rate at 3 years after surgical revascularization has been shown to exceed 80 per cent. Prosthetic grafts can be used as well but they are less compliant and more technically challenging when used on small dysplastic arteries.

## LOWER EXTREMITY OCCLUSIVE DISEASE

The prevalence of peripheral arterial occlusive disease is age-dependent, rarely being seen in individuals younger than 60 years of age. The prevalence steadily increases after the age of 70. It is estimated that there are about 8.5 million individuals aged over 40 years who are suffering from peripheral arterial occlusive disease.

The mortality of patients with peripheral arterial occlusive disease is increased compared with patients without it. This is due to the fact that it is a manifestation of a generalized diffuse pathology – atherosclerosis. Patients with peripheral arterial occlusive disease have a relative 5 year mortality rate of 28 per cent. The causes of death are coronary artery disease (60 per cent), cerebrovascular accidents (12 per cent) and other vascular pathologies (10 per cent). Risk factors include hyperhomocysteinaemia, diabetes, obesity, genetics, dyslipidaemia, hypertension, age and, most importantly, smoking.

Atherosclerosis may affect the carotid arteries resulting in TIAs or ischaemic strokes, the heart resulting in angina or myocardial infarctions, and the lower extremities resulting in lower extremity occlusive disease manifested by claudication or critical limb ischaemia.

### Presentation

Patients with peripheral arterial occlusive disease may be completely asymptomatic or may suffer from claudication, rest pain or tissue loss. Symptoms may occur abruptly due to a sudden drop in lower extremity perfusion, resulting in acute limb ischaemia. Rest pain and tissue loss are classified as critical limb ischaemia and are usually manifestations of chronic severe ischaemia. It is estimated that 50 per cent of patients with peripheral arterial occlusive disease are asymptomatic, 40 per cent have intermittent claudication, and the remaining 10 per cent have critical leg ischaemia.

### Intermittent Claudication

'Claudication' is a term used to describe limping from pain. Its origin lies in the Latin verb *claudicare*, to have a limp or be lame, exemplified by the Emperor Claudius. Hence the term 'claudicate' is preferably used for the lower extremity rather than for symptoms in other parts of the body such as hand or jaw claudication. Claudication can be due to an underlying arterial, neurogenic or venous pathology. It is not uncommon for a patient to have an element of both arterial and neurogenic claudication existing at the same time.

### Arterial Claudication

This is an exertional aching pain, cramping or fatigue that occurs in various muscle groups. It is not a joint pain. It usually resolves within 2–3 minutes after the exercise has ended. It tends to be reproducible at a similar distance of walking. It should be differentiated from neurogenic claudication, which is often associated with back pain, is not relieved by rest and is often relieved by bending the back. It should also be differentiated from venous claudication, which is usually only relieved by leg elevation and is due to a severe obstruction of venous outflow.

### Ischaemic Rest Pain

This represents a more advanced degree of limb ischaemia, which manifests itself as pain in the forefoot at the level of the metatarsal heads. At this stage, the metabolic demands of the foot at rest are not met (comparable to angina at rest for the heart).

Rest pain frequently occurs at night and typically requires narcotics to relieve it. The patient often learns to dangle the foot out of the side of the bed, thus improving the blood flow by dependency and gravity, and relieving the pain. Dependency and the effect of gravity also explains the associated oedema and rubor that is often seen in these patients. Once elevated, the leg turns cadaveric white, hence the phrase 'dependent rubor and elevation pallor'. Typically, the pressures at the ankle are less than 40 mmHg, which also reflects multi-level occlusive disease (such as iliac and femoral, or femoral and tibial, occlusive disease).

### Tissue Loss

Tissue loss presents either as gangrene or non-healing ulcers. These lesions tend to occur at the most distal aspect of the extremities (the tips of the toes) or the pressure points on the foot, and tend to be quite painful (Figure 31.5). They are often precipitated by some form of trauma (e.g. rubbing shoes or clipping of the toenails) (Figures 31.6–31.8).

Diabetic patients tend to have a peculiar form of ulceration due to the neuropathy that can affect the diabetic foot in addition to the vascular pathology that can develop in diabetic individuals (typically in the tibial vessels). Diabetic patients may develop ulcerations that are purely neuropathic, purely ischaemic or mixed, caused by a combination of both mechanisms. Purely neuropathic ulcerations are typically painless and arise on the plantar aspect of an insensate foot at pressure points around the level of the metatarsal heads (Figures 31.9 and 31.10).

The ulcerations should also be differentiated from venous stasis ulcerations, which tend to occur around the medial malleolus and at the level of the venous perforators. These ulcers develop as a result of venous hypertension. In these situations, the patient has brownish induration of the skin on the leg and usually has palpable pedal pulses. Venous stasis ulcers are typically treated with elevation and support compression stockings.

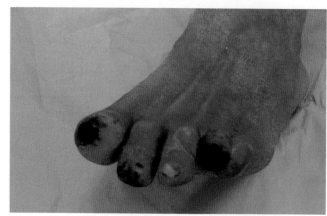

Figure 31.5 **Ischaemic toe ulcers.**

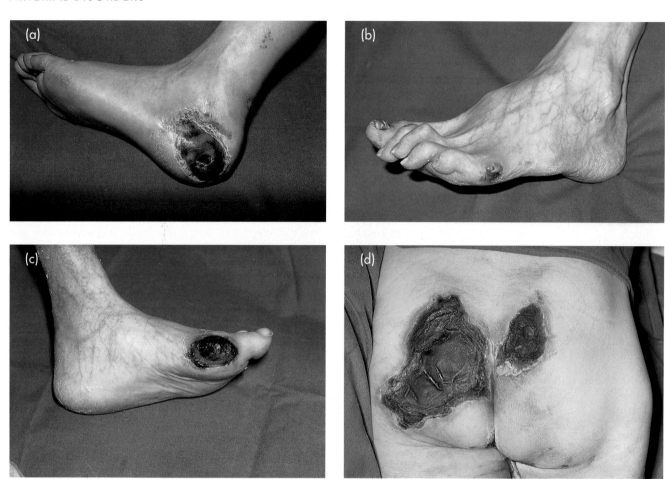

Figure 31.6 Cutaneous pressure necrosis in severe ischaemia. (a) An extensive ulcer over the heel. (b) Ischaemic changes over the lateral border of the foot after 24 hours of bed rest. (c) Ischaemic changes over the head of the first metatarsal. (d) Extensive sacral ischaemic changes.

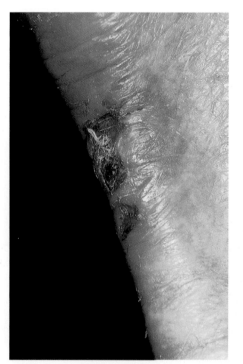

Figure 31.7 Pressure necrosis over the Achilles tendon following the application of a tight bandage.

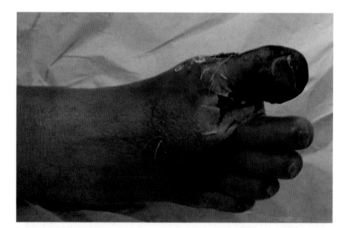

Figure 31.8 An ischaemic ulcer of the big toe.

Patients occasionally have a combination of arterial and venous ulcerations. In this situation, the patient has venous stasis ulceration in a leg with a poor arterial circulation. This should be suspected in patients with venous ulcers who have non-palpable pulses or are not responding to compression therapy. It is necessary to improve the arterial circulation before the ulcers can respond to compression therapy.

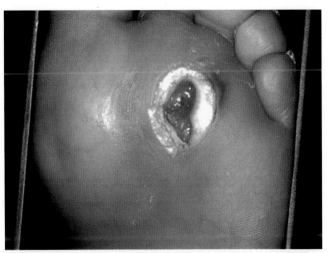

Figure 31.9 Mal perforans ulcer of a diabetic foot.

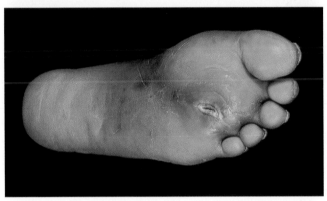

Figure 31.10 A perforating ulcer over the heads of the third and fourth metatarsals in a neuropathic diabetic foot.

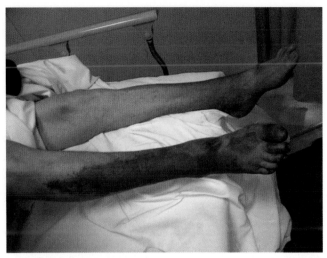

Figure 31.11 Advance limb ischaemia.

Table 31.3 Clinical categories of acute limb ischaemia

| Class | Category | Sensory loss | Muscle weakness | Arterial Doppler | Venous Doppler |
|---|---|---|---|---|---|
| I | Viable | None | None | Audible | Audible |
| IIA | Marginally threatened | Minimal to none | None | May or may not be audible | Audible |
| IIB | Immediately threatened | Moderate | Mild to moderate | None | Audible |
| III | Irreversible | Profound | Profound | None | None |

## Acute Limb Ischaemia

This usually occurs secondary to an embolus from a distant source lodging in a distal narrow arterial segment, or after the thrombosis of an existing atherosclerotic arterial segment. The classical signs of acute limb ischaemia are the '6 Ps':

- Pain;
- Paraesthesia;
- Pallor;
- Pulselessness;
- Poikilothermia (loss of core temperature);
- Paralysis.

Patients without underlying arterial occlusive disease usually have underdeveloped collateral vessels. An embolic occlusion in this setting leads to a rapid onset of symptoms of limb ischaemia (Figure 31.11). Conversely, patients with a history of peripheral arterial occlusive disease are more likely to develop ischaemia from arterial thrombosis, with a more gradual onset of symptoms due to the presence of existing collaterals.

Acute limb ischaemia can be classified into four categories – viable, marginally threatened, immediately threatened and non-viable – depending on the presence or absence of arterial and venous Doppler signals, as well as sensory loss and muscle weakness (Table 31.3). This classification helps to estimate the magnitude of ischaemia as well as dictate the plan of management.

## Diagnosis

The diagnosis of peripheral arterial occlusive disease is made by first obtaining a careful medical and social history. It is further confirmed by physical examination, which is essential to determine the quality of the pulses. The physical examination of the arterial system includes auscultation of the abdomen for the presence of a bruit, an evaluation of the presence of abdominal aortic aneurysms or other femoral or popliteal aneurysms, and palpation of the femoral, popliteal, posterior tibial and dorsalis pedis pulses. In addition, the feet, toes and web spaces should be inspected for ulcerations or fissures.

The physical examination is supplemented by non-invasive vascular laboratory evaluation. This includes pulse volume recordings, an ankle–brachial pressure index, segmental pressure measurement and duplex ultrasonography (Figure 31.12).

The **ankle–brachial index** is obtained by measuring the systolic pressure at the ankle and comparing it with the systolic pressure in the brachial artery:

- In a healthy individual, the ankle–brachial index is between 0.95 and 1.2.
- In patients with peripheral arterial occlusive disease, the value falls to less than 0.9.
- Patients with intermittent claudication tend to have single-level occlusive disease with an ankle–brachial index of 0.6–0.9.

PART 7 | VASCULAR

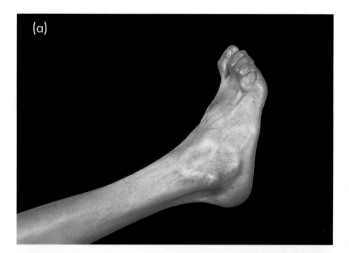

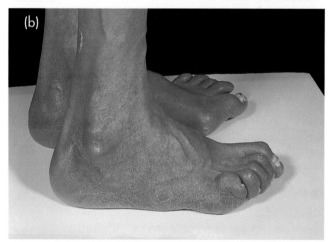

Figure 31.12 Postural changes. (a) Elevation of the limb has produced blanching and venous emptying. (b) The patient subsequently stood up for 3 minutes; the veins filling after 1 minute and hyperaemia developing.

- Individuals with rest pain and ulceration tend to have multilevel occlusive disease with an ankle–brachial index of less than 0.4.

Segmental pressure measurements determine the pressure at the high thigh, above-knee and below-knee levels in addition to the brachial and ankle pressures. A drop in pressure greater than 20 mmHg from one level to the next is usually indicative of significant occlusive pathology.

Measurement of the toe pressure is very useful with diabetic patients in whom the ankle–brachial index values are falsely elevated due to the calcified tibial vessels. Duplex ultrasonography is ideal for evaluating for the presence of aneurysms and for occlusive disease in localized arterial segments such as the carotid, visceral and renal arteries. The use of duplex ultrasonography is limited in lower extremity occlusive disease, especially below the knee.

**Arteriography** should only be performed when revascularization is contemplated. It should not be used as a plain diagnostic test since a great deal of information can be obtained by non-invasive testing. It is used mainly to determine the best methods of revascularization when intervention is deemed necessary. Conventional arteriography is now being replaced

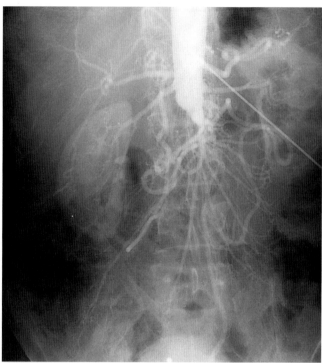

Figure 31.13 Occlusion of the infrarenal abdominal aorta. Chronic occlusion of this nature allows time for the development of extensive collaterals across the pelvis and through the mesenteric vessels, preventing acute ischaemic changes in the legs.

by MR angiography and CT angiography but can outline aortic (Figure 31.13) and iliofemoral (Figure 31.14) disease.

As a non-invasive test, MR angiography does not involve the need for percutaneous arterial punctures and the injection of nephrotoxic dye. Magnetic resonance angiography tends to overestimate the degree of occlusive disease. However, the accuracy of MR angiography continues to improve as the technology behind it continues to evolve.

Similarly, CT angiography is non-invasive and can be very useful when planning re-vascularization. However, it exposes the patient to radiation and nephrotoxic dye, and it may provide suboptimal visualization of the vessels below the knee.

### Treatment

Certain factors have been shown to improve the natural history of atherosclerosis and improve survival in patients with peripheral artery disease. These include smoking cessation, control of blood pressure and hyperlipidaemia, control of diabetes, antiplatelet therapy, exercise and achieving an ideal body weight. The indications for referral to a vascular specialist include the development of lifestyle-disabling claudication refractory to exercise or pharmacotherapy, rest pain or tissue loss.

#### Pharmacotherapy

Intermittent claudication is a benign process with respect to limb loss or the need for intervention. Over a period of 10 years, fewer than 25 per cent of patients will require intervention, and fewer than 10 per cent will require amputation. In general, claudication becomes fairly disabling when the walking distance falls to one city block or less, which is approximately 50–100 m. An exercise programme is very helpful in claudication to improve muscle

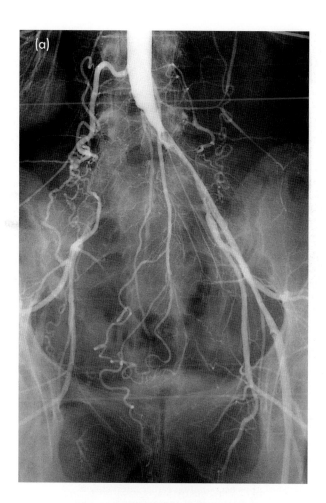

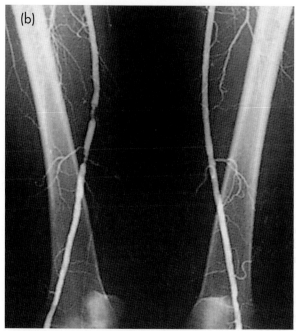

Figure 31.14 The typical radiological appearances of atheromatous disease. (a) Occlusion of the right common iliac artery with marked stenosis of the left common iliac vessel. (b) Stenotic disease of the superficial femoral artery (the continuation of the femoral artery after it has given off its deep branch). Such atheroma commonly starts at the level of the adductor hiatus.

efficiency, exercise performance, walking ability and physical functioning.

Pharmacological agents have also been developed to treat disabling intermittent claudication. Cilostazol, a quinolinone derivative, acts by inhibiting phosphodiesterase III, resulting in an increase in the level of cyclic AMP. This results in an inhibition of platelet aggregation and the production of vasodilatation. It also has a lipid-lowering effect and causes some improvement in blood lipid levels. It is thought that all of these factors contribute to its positive effects. Cilostazol seems to increase the maximal walking distance by 50 per cent, as well as increasing the pain-free walking distance.

## Revascularization

The main purpose of revascularization is to improve the blood supply prior to debridement or amputations for ischaemic ulcers, thus avoiding further ischaemia and non-healing of the amputation site. Even stubborn heel ulcers will heal once appropriately revascularized. The main objective is to prevent a major amputation such as a below-knee or above-knee amputation.

Contraindications to revascularization include non-ambulatory patients, very high-risk patients, an absence of target vessels and extensive tissue loss with a non-salvageable foot. In such situations, a primary amputation may be the most appropriate option. The presence of a popliteal arterial Doppler signal is associated with a 95 per cent incidence of healing for a below-knee amputation. In patients with knee contractures and those who are not candidates for rehabilitation, an above-knee amputation may be the most appropriate option.

Revascularization Options – Revascularization options vary depending on the location of the pathology. The occlusive disease may be in the aortoiliac segment, often referred to as inflow disease, or in the infrainguinal segment, often referred to as outflow disease. Some patients have a combination of inflow and outflow disease. When revascularization is planned in patients with combined inflow and outflow disease, the typical approach is first to address and improve the inflow disease, as it may be sufficient to restore adequate flow.

The treatment options for aortoiliac disease include the following:

- *Endovascular treatment* such as angioplasty or stenting is ideal for localized iliac stenoses. This endovascular approach has also been extended to more advanced aortoiliac disease, following the concept of 'endovascular first'.
- *Direct reconstruction*; in the form of endarterectomy or aortobifemoral bypass, can be used for diffuse aortoiliac disease. Endarterectomy is ideal for localized small segments in moderate to large arteries, such as at the carotid bifurcation. In the aortoiliac segment, endarterectomy requires extensive dissection, and its results are not superior to those of aortofemoral bypasses. Furthermore, the plaque may extend distally to levels that lead to challenging decisions of where to end the endarterectomy.
- *Indirect reconstruction* is also possible. Axillobifemoral bypass is usually used in patients with aortoiliac disease who also suffer from significant comorbidities such as cardiac failure, severe chronic obstructive pulmonary disease or ascites. Femorofemoral bypass is used for patients with a unilateral iliac occlusion.

In order to delineate the ideal revascularization approach (endovascular versus surgical) in treating peripheral occlusive disease, guidelines from the Inter-Society Consensus for the

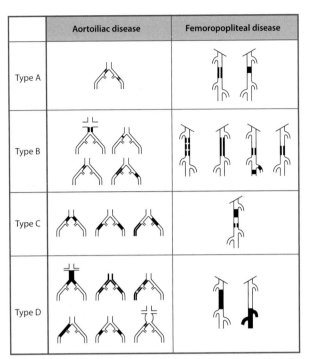

| | Aortoiliac disease | Femoropopliteal disease |
|---|---|---|
| Type A | | |
| Type B | | |
| Type C | | |
| Type D | | |

Figure 31.15 Inter-Society Consensus for the Management of Peripheral Artery Disease II classification of aortoiliac and femoropopliteal lesions.

Management of Peripheral Artery Disease (TASC II) classify arterial lesions into type A, B, C or D depending on the success rate of endovascular or surgical treatment; type A represents focal lesions of the iliac, femoral and popliteal arteries, and type D represents diffuse chronic disease occlusions. The classification is summarized in Figure 31.15.

In patients with infrainguinal pathology, endovascular interventions are not very durable procedures. Nevertheless, they are often used as a first modality of treatment if they do not interfere with potential future methods of revascularization. Despite their lack of durability, they may, however, last long enough to allow foot ulcerations to heal.

When endovascular procedures are not possible or fail, the treatment of choice is typically a bypass procedure. The conduit of choice is an autologous vein (greater saphenous, lesser saphenous or arm vein). The greater saphenous vein is the ideal conduit.

Because of the presence of valves, the vein must be reversed (a reversed vein bypass). Alternatively, the vein can be harvested and not reversed, the valves instead being destroyed using special instruments introduced through one end of the vein or through its side branches (a non-reversed translocated vein bypass). If the valves are disrupted without harvesting the vein, leaving the vein in its bed, the bypass is called an *in situ* vein bypass. In good size veins, all three forms of bypass are considered equivalent. In veins smaller than 3 mm in diameter, the reversed technique has inferior results compared with the other two methods.

Bypasses using autogenous veins usually result in an 85 per cent secondary patency rate and 90 per cent limb salvage rate over a 5 year period. It should be noted, however, that all vein bypasses have to be followed up indefinitely using ultrasound to identify any pathology that could lead to a graft failure.

## THORACIC AORTIC ANEURYSMS

A true aneurysm is defined as a permanent localized dilation of an artery that has a diameter at least 1.5 times the normal diameter of the respective arterial segment. Thoracic aortic aneurysms have an incidence of 10 cases per 100 000 persons per year, and they most commonly develop from cystic medial degeneration, which leads to weakening and subsequent expansion of the aortic wall.

The two most important risk factors for their development are hypertension and advanced age. As such, they are seen mostly in the sixth and seventh decades of life, although they can occur in younger patients with connective tissue diseases such as Marfan's syndrome and Ehlers–Danlos syndrome. Aneurysms can also develop several years after aortic dissection as a consequence of the weakened dissected aortic wall. Other less common aetiologies include infectious or inflammatory aortitis, a bicuspid aortic valve and coarctation of the aorta.

### Natural History

Patients with large untreated thoracic aneurysms are more likely to die from complications associated with their aneurysm as well as from their associated cardiovascular disease. The 5 year survival in such patients has been estimated to be as low as 20 per cent.

As with abdominal aortic aneurysms, the most important determinant of the rupture or dissection of an aneurysm is its size. Studies assessing the natural history of thoracic aneurysms have revealed that the complication rate increases significantly when the size of an ascending aneurysm reaches 6 cm and when one of the descending aorta reaches 7 cm. These diameters are used as guidelines for surgical intervention, keeping in mind the overall medical condition and risk factors. An essential guiding concept in the management is that the risk of the intervention should be lower than the risk of non-operative management, irrespective of the size of the aneurysm. However, in patients with Marfan's syndrome or other connective tissue disorders, aneurysm rupture has been shown to occur at smaller sizes, thus necessitating earlier intervention.

The rate of expansion of the aneurysm is another important factor affecting the prognosis. Thoracic aneurysms grow at a rate of 1–10 mm per year, and this rate has been shown to be directly related to the initial diameter, with larger aneurysms growing at a faster rate. A growth rate of more than 10 mm per year is considered to be accelerated growth and is usually an indication for intervention.

### Classification

Aneurysmal disease can involve the ascending aorta, aortic arch and descending thoracic aorta. As such, aneurysms of the thoracic aorta are classified into four general anatomical categories:

- Ascending thoracic aneurysms occupy the area between the aortic valve and the innominate artery; these comprise the majority of the thoracic aneurysms.
- Aortic arch aneurysms involve the brachiocephalic vessels.
- Descending thoracic aneurysms include the area distal to the subclavian artery.
- Thoracoabdominal aneurysms, as their name suggests, involve both the thoracic and the abdominal aorta.

Thoracoabdominal aneurysms are further divided according to the **Crawford classification** (Figure 31.16):

- *Type I* aneurysms begin above the sixth intercostal space at the level of the left subclavian artery, and extend down to the origins of the coeliac axis and SMAs. They may also involve the renal arteries.
- *Type II* aneurysms also arise at the level of the left subclavian artery, but extend distally into the infrarenal aorta down to the level of the aortic bifurcation.

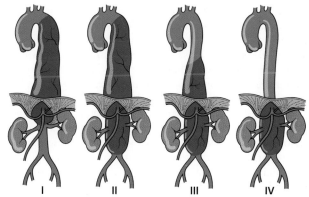

Figure 31.16 Crawford classification of thoracic aortic aneurysms.

- *Type III* aneurysms arise below the sixth intercostal space at the level of the distal descending thoracic aorta, and extend into the abdominal aorta.
- *Type IV* aneurysms generally involve the entire abdominal aorta from the level of the diaphragm to the bifurcation and are therefore considered to be primarily abdominal aortic aneurysms.

It should be noted that up to 30 per cent of patients with thoracic aneurysms have synchronous discontinuous abdominal aortic aneurysms, and these are considered to be a different entity from thoracoabdominal aneurysms.

## Presentation

The majority of patients with thoracic aortic aneurysms are asymptomatic at the time of presentation, the aneurysm being discovered incidentally on imaging that is performed to evaluate another disorder. When symptoms do occur, they are usually attributed to the compression or distortion of adjacent structures or vessels. As such, patients may present with chest, back, flank or abdominal pain. Ascending and arch aneurysms can also cause mediastinal compression. In such instances, patients can present with hoarseness if the left vagus nerve or left recurrent laryngeal nerve is involved, or hemidiaphragmatic paralysis if the phrenic nerve is compressed. Patients may also experience respiratory symptoms or dysphagia if there is compression of the tracheobronchial tree or oesophagus, respectively.

Ascending aneurysms in particular may also cause aortic root dilatation, resulting in aortic regurgitation and possible heart failure. Showering of emboli from the aneurysm is a feared complication as it can involve the coronary, cerebral, mesenteric and extremity vasculature.

The most dreaded complication is, however, rupture. The clinical manifestations of thoracic aneurysm rupture vary depending on the location of the aneurysm. Ascending aneurysms often rupture into the left pleural or pericardial space. A descending aneurysm, on the other hand, may erode into the oesophagus and may present as massive haematemesis. In cases of rupture, patients usually develop severe pain along with hypotension and shock, and the outcome is often catastrophic.

## Diagnosis

As already mentioned, the majority of thoracic aneurysms are discovered incidentally. In many instances, a **chest X-ray** may reveal mediastinal widening and tracheal deviation. Other suggestive findings include displaced calcifications and kinking of the aorta. These findings are, however, non-specific as a tortuous aorta may have similar X-ray features.

A thoracic aortic aneurysm may initially be diagnosed by **echocardiography**. A transthoracic echo scan is often useful in assessing the diameter of the aortic root and ascending aorta, while a transoesophageal echo scan is preferred for examining the entire aorta, mainly in an emergency setting. Transoesophageal echocardiography also helps to rule out any coexisting aortic dissection.

The gold standard, however, for diagnosing and assessing thoracic aneurysms remains **CT angiography** as it can accurately measure the diameter of the aneurysm, delineate vascular and anatomical features, and assist in planning future interventions. It is also useful in an emergency setting to rule out possible rupture or dissection.

## Treatment

The variable natural history of thoracic aneurysms implies that the proper timing for repair is often unclear. The current guidelines for the surgical repair of thoracic aneurysms include the following:

- symptomatic aneurysms;
- ascending thoracic aneurysms more than 6 cm in diameter;
- descending aneurysms more than 7 cm in diameter;
- accelerated growth of more than 10 mm per year;
- aortic regurgitation with an ascending aneurysm;
- aortic root disease and dissection.

Thoracic aneurysm repair can be carried out via an open surgical technique. A median sternotomy incision is usually performed for ascending aneurysms, while a left thoracotomy is employed for descending aneurysms. For thoracoabdominal repair, the thoracotomy incision is usually extended across the costal margins to allow access to the abdominal retroperitoneal space. As with the repair of an abdominal aneurysm, vascular control is achieved proximal and distal to the aneurysm sac, and the affected segment is replaced with a prosthetic graft. Arterial braches involved in the aneurysm are either ligated or re-implanted into the graft. If the aortic root is involved, the coronary arteries are re-implanted and the aortic valve may be replaced.

Another attractive treatment modality for descending and thoracoabdominal aneurysms is endovascular repair. **Thoracic endovascular aneurysm repair** (TEVAR) refers to the percutaneous placement of a stent graft in the aorta to exclude the aneurysm. The advantages of this minimally invasive procedure over open surgery include the absence of long incisions in the thorax or abdomen, the avoidance of aortic cross-clamping, a decreased blood loss, a decreased incidence of visceral and spinal cord ischaemia and a faster recovery. However, many factors have to be taken into consideration pre-operatively to allow for successful deployment of the graft. These include:

- the aortic diameter;
- the proximal and distal landing zones;
- the length of the graft used;
- anatomical considerations such as the angulation and tortuosity of the aorta.

TEVAR was initially developed to treat patients who were considered high risk for open surgical repair, but it has evolved to become a suitable alternative to open surgery in most cases. Recent advances and innovations in endovascular therapy have expanded its role. Hybrid approaches of open and endovascular therapy have paved the way to treating all segments of the aorta, including the ascending aorta and the aortic arch.

## ABDOMINAL AORTIC ANEURYSMS

The prevalence of abdominal aortic aneurysms appears to be increasing, involving 5 per cent of the population of individuals aged 60 years or older. This can be attributed to improved physician awareness and an increased utilization of imaging techniques. Approximately 75 per cent of abdominal aortic aneurysms are asymptomatic, being detected on routine physical examination or as incidental findings on imaging studies.

The cause of aortic aneurysm formation is multifactorial, with significant genetic, epidemiological and behavioural influences. This multifactorial aetiology ultimately results in the destruction of vital structural components of the aortic wall and aneurysm formation. With the loss of its structural integrity, the aortic wall becomes predisposed to rupture.

The consequences of such destruction are well recognized by surgeons, physicians and the family members of patients who have suffered from a ruptured abdominal aortic aneurysm. The overall 30 day mortality rate of patients presenting to hospital with a ruptured abdominal aortic aneurysm ranges between 50 and 70 per cent. The true mortality rate for all ruptured aneurysms, including patients who succumb before arriving at hospital, is undoubtedly higher and may be as high as 90 per cent. Thus, prevention of rupture is the primary goal of intervention in aneurysmal disease.

### Natural History of Abdominal Aortic Aneurysms

Although several factors may influence the risk of rupture of an abdominal aortic aneurysm, the size of the aneurysm remains the factor most commonly used to predict the risk of rupture. The true natural history of asymptomatic abdominal aortic aneurysms remains unknown. The ranges frequently quoted to predict the 5 year risk of rupture of these aneurysms are summarized in Table 31.4. Most surgeons agree that repair is indicated when, on balance, the risk of the operation is less than the risk of rupture for each size range.

Although the management of large aneurysms (greater than 6 cm) and very small aneurysms (less than 4 cm) is relatively well defined, the management of aneurysms ranging from 4 to 6 cm remains controversial. Some surgeons propose early repair for 'younger' patients and for patients who cannot follow a surveillance programme on a regular basis. Others consider that the risk of rupture of aneurysms measuring 4–6 cm is less than the risk of surgery, and that surgical intervention should be delayed until there is evidence of growth of the aneurysm. Although surgeons have tried to answer this question, there are only few prospective randomized trials comparing the results of surveillance versus early surgery in patients with small abdominal aortic aneurysms.

Table 31.4 Annual rupture risk according to abdominal aortic aneurysm diameter

| Size | <5 cm | 5–6 cm | 6–7cm | >7 cm |
|---|---|---|---|---|
| Risk of rupture (%) | 0–5 | 20–25 | 30–40 | >75 |

Two prospective randomized trials, the UK Small Aneurysm Trial and the VA small aneurysm trial, have shed some light on the situation. The annual rupture rate of aneurysms smaller than 5.5 cm was less than 1 per cent. Nevertheless, once the aneurysms were larger than 5 cm, a high percentage of patients ultimately converted into the surgical arm and ultimately underwent surgical treatment. These studies thus concluded that male patients with asymptomatic abdominal aortic aneurysms of 4.0–5.5 cm should undergo regular ultrasound surveillance accompanied by surgical intervention for aneurysms that grow rapidly, that is, more than 1.0 cm per year, or that reach 5.5 cm in diameter. In women, intervention is recommend when the abdominal aortic aneurysm reaches 5.0 cm in diameter. These guidelines are suitable assuming that the patient has an expected survival of at least 5 years and that there are no prohibitive risks for surgical intervention.

Over time, aneurysms do not get smaller and the patient's health does not get any better. Hence it is essential to identify the best window of opportunity to intervene before rupture occurs. Thus, once an aneurysm has reached 5 cm in size, it is no longer a matter of whether intervention is necessary but rather when the intervention will be carried out.

### Presentation

Most patients with an abdominal aortic aneurysms are asymptomatic, and of those who have a ruptured aneurysm, fewer than 50 per cent have the triad of abdominal pain, a pulsatile abdominal mass and hypotension. At some sites, aneurysms are visible and can be detected by the patient (Figures 31.17–31.20) before being confirmed by clinical examination; however, this is not a common presentation.

In symptomatic patients, **pain** is the most common symptom and is usually localized to the abdomen, back or flank area. These symptoms may not be related to the rupture of an abdominal aneurysm, but such symptoms in a patient with a known abdominal aneurysm are presumed to be due to the aneurysm until proven otherwise. Pain associated with aortic aneurysms can be attributed to the size of the aneurysm, its rapid expansion, inflammation of the surrounding structures in cases of an inflammatory aneurysm, or rupture of the aneurysm.

Pain from the rupture of an aneurysm is usually acute. Its location depends on the site of rupture, with back and flank pain being seen if there is a contained proximal rupture and

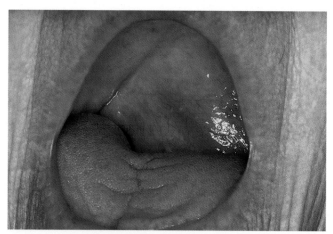

Figure 31.17 An aneurysm of the left common carotid artery deforming the posterior aspect of the oropharynx.

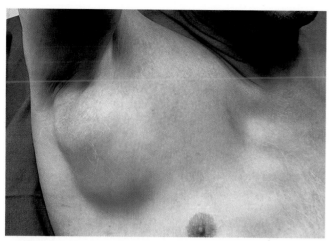

Figure 31.18 A congenital aneurysm of the right axillary artery. Similar changes were present on the left side.

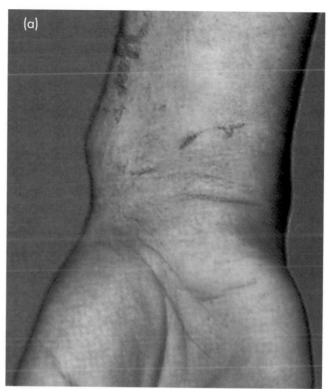

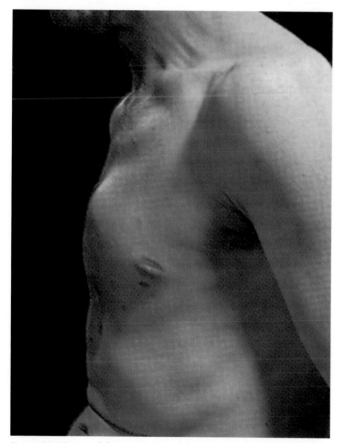

Figure 31.19 A syphilitic aneurysm of the ascending aorta eroding the sternum.

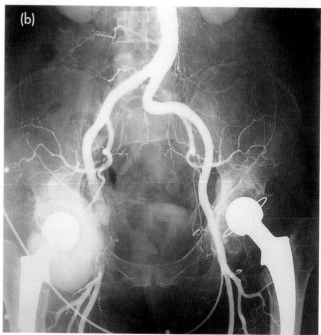

Figure 31.20 False aneurysms. (a) A false aneurysm of the right radial artery. (b) A false aneurysm of the right femoral artery following arthroplasty. The contrast medium has leaked into the aneurysmal sac anterior to the hip joint.

lower abdominal pain when the rupture occurs close to the iliac bifurcation. Free rupture into the abdominal cavity can present with sudden collapse and death.

**Limb ischaemia** may be another presenting feature of an abdominal aneurysm. It is usually caused by the embolization of atherosclerotic debris from the aneurysm. Depending on the size of the showered debris, embolisms may present acutely with painful, blue digits (blue toe syndrome) or with a painful, pulseless ischaemic extremity. Rarely, abdominal aneurysms present with acute aortic thrombosis leading to bilateral extremity ischaemia.

Other less common clinical features of abdominal aortic aneurysms include constitutional or systemic symptoms indicating the presence of an infected or inflammatory aneurysm or disseminated intravascular coagulation. In patients with an inflammatory aneurysm, the ureters may be entrapped by the

PART 7 | VASCULAR

inflammatory changes, resulting in ureteral obstruction. These patients may present with renal failure in addition to their constitutional symptoms. Very rarely, an aneurysm may erode into the gastrointestinal tract, resulting in an aortoduodenal fistula that typically presents with massive gastrointestinal bleeding.

## Diagnosis

The diagnostic approach to a patient with an abdominal aortic aneurysm depends on the symptoms and the haemodynamic status.

Many large asymptomatic abdominal aortic aneurysms can be detected by a thorough physical examination or incidentally on abdominal films. A pulsatile supraumbilical mass is usually palpated, although the accuracy of the clinical examination varies markedly depending on the patient's body habitus and the size of the aneurysm. In overweight patients, the detection of an aneurysm may be difficult even for the experienced physician. Examination should always include the lower extremity vessels to rule out any concomitant peripheral aneurysms or signs of limb ischaemia.

Once the diagnosis is suspected on physical examination, more objective methods are used to identify its exact size and location. The imaging modalities commonly used to diagnose and measure aneurysms include duplex ultrasonography, CT, MRI and aortography.

The advantages of duplex scanning include its widespread availability, the lack of radiation and its low cost and reproducible results. These advantages make this modality ideal for surveillance and follow-up to monitor aneurysmal growth. This modality, however, lacks access to the suprarenal and thoracic aorta, and the quality of its images is reduced in overweight patients and in the presence of large amounts of intestinal gas.

CT angiography allows an accurate determination of the size and extent of the aneurysm, as well visualization of the visceral and renal arteries and their relationship to the aneurysm. These measurements allow surgeons to decide on the best approach and treatment modality for the aneurysm. Intravenous contrast infusion also allows an assessment of the luminal size and the presence or absence of a retroperitoneal haematoma.

Magnetic resonance angiography has an advantage over CT angiography in that no ionizing radiation is given and no nephrotoxic agents are used. CT angiography, however, remains the most useful and most widely utilized imaging modality for the preoperative assessment of abdominal aortic aneurysms.

Aortography allows visualization of the aortic lumen and any associated arterial lesions in the visceral and renal arteries. However, its invasive nature, along with its risk of nephrotoxicity and of dislodging emboli while manipulating the catheters, significantly limit its use. In addition, it is inadequate for assessing the size of an aneurysm as it shows only the inner lumen rather than the entire diameter.

In a symptomatic patient with a pulsatile abdominal mass who is haemodynamically unstable, no further imaging studies are required, and the patient is sent directly to the operating room. Most operating rooms are equipped with hybrid rooms where an intraoperative angiogram can be obtained to determine suitability for endovascular repair. It can also allow for endovascular intra-aortic balloon inflation as a method for aortic control.

A bedside ultrasound examination may be carried out in the accident and emergency department to confirm the presence of an abdominal aneurysm, as long as it does not delay management. In symptomatic patients who are haemodynamically stable, an urgent CT scan is required and can be performed within a few minutes as the patient is being prepared for transfer to the operating room. This confirms the presence of a rupture or any other intra-abdominal pathology, as well as delineating the extent of the aneurysm; this provides important anatomical information with which to plan an urgent repair of an abdominal aortic aneurysm and determine whether it is suitable for endovascular repair.

## Treatment

The conventional surgical treatment of an abdominal aortic aneurysm involves replacing the aneurysmal segment with an in-line aortic graft. This procedure can be performed effectively using a transabdominal or retroperitoneal approach. A tube prosthesis is used when the disease is limited to the aorta, and a bifurcated prosthesis when the aneurysmal pathology extends into the iliac arteries.

An operative mortality rate of 3–5 per cent can be expected in properly selected individuals. The mortality and morbidity rate will, however, increase in the presence of comorbidities such as renal failure, coronary artery disease and chronic obstructive pulmonary disease. The average length of stay following such operations ranges from 5 to 12 days. The recovery following such procedures is relatively slow, and a full recovery occurs only weeks to months after surgery.

In line with the concept of minimally invasive procedures, endovascular aortic aneurysm repair has emerged as a viable treatment option and is now commonly performed. It is based on excluding the abdominal aortic aneurysm from within using a stent graft that is introduced through the femoral arteries. This endovascular approach allows for lower mortality and morbidity rates, a quicker recovery, decreased costs, a shorter hospital stay and even the possibility of outpatient aortic aneurysm repair.

However, this technology has its own set of limitations. Anatomical considerations are the main factors that will dictate whether an individual is a candidate for endovascular repair. The lack of a suitable infrarenal aortic neck is usually the most important limiting factor. A suitable neck may be defined as one longer than 1.5 cm and narrower than 30 mm, without severe angulation or circumferential intramural thrombus. As such, this technology is mostly limited to infrarenal aortic aneurysms with a suitable neck, isolated thoracic aneurysms and isolated peripheral traumatic and degenerative types. Special fenestrated endografts and branched grafts are now also available for juxtarenal and suprarenal aneurysms. Their use is not, however, widespread but is often limited to centres with special experience.

If an endovascular repair is not successful at excluding the aneurysm, blood will still flow into the aneurysm sac, resulting in an endoleak, which is classified into four types:

- *type I*: at the attachment site;
- *type II*: caused by retrograde flow into the sac through the IMA or lumbar branches;
- *type III*: at the junction between the main body of the graft and its other connection;
- *type IV*: through the graft material.

This can occur at the time of insertion or at any time later. Patients treated by endografts therefore require lifelong postoperative follow-up to rule out an endoleak, late graft migration or persistent growth of the aneurysm. Other complications such as stent fracture, metal fatigue and graft thrombosis have also been reported. The early perioperative benefits achieved by endovascular repair are often lost within 2 years by the need for reintervention to address endoleaks, graft migration or limb thrombosis.

Endovascular repair has also been successfully used in ruptured abdominal aneurysms. However, anatomical criteria for endovascular aneurysm repair and the need for a defined programme for emergency endovascular surgery that includes the appropriate team and inventory preclude it from currently being a feasible option in emergency cases at all centres.

## PERIPHERAL ARTERIAL ANEURYSMS

The detection of peripheral arterial aneurysms has been increasing, mainly due to improved surveillance and enhanced vascular imaging modalities. Femoral and popliteal aneurysms comprise the majority of peripheral arterial aneurysms. These aneurysms are classified as either true aneurysms involving all three layers of the arterial wall, or pseudoaneurysms secondary to trauma, anastomotic disruption or infection.

The aetiology behind the formation of these aneurysms remains unclear, although some anatomical and genetic factors have been proposed. One assumption is that relative stenosis at the level of the inguinal ligament and the heads of the gastrocnemius may result in turbulent flow with subsequent aneurysmal degeneration.

Genetic factors also appear to play a role in the pathogenesis of peripheral aneurysms, which is evident from the significant association between peripheral aneurysms and abdominal aortic aneurysms. Indeed, it is estimated that nearly 40 per cent of patients with popliteal aneurysms and 70 per cent of patients with femoral aneurysms have an associated abdominal aortic aneurysm. Conversely, around 15 per cent of those with an abdominal aortic aneurysm have an associated femoral or popliteal aneurysm.

### Presentation

Femoral and popliteal aneurysms can have a wide range of presentations. Most are asymptomatic and are discovered incidentally as a pulsating mass on examination or through radiological studies carried out for other indications. Others are discovered in patients with known aneurysmal disease who are being assessed for aneurysms elsewhere.

Symptoms from femoral and popliteal aneurysms are attributed to the compression of adjacent structures, thromboembolic events or rupture. Patients with compressive symptoms can present with neurological deficits, including sensorimotor weakness if the nerves are compressed. Alternatively, they can show leg swelling and phlebitis if the accompanying vein is involved and compressed.

Thromboembolic events may produce acute or chronic limb ischaemia depending on the rate of luminal narrowing, the extent of distal embolization and the presence or absence of collaterals. Symptoms of chronic ischaemia include claudication that may improve with the development of collaterals or can progress to rest pain and tissue loss if repeated embolization occludes the outflow vessels.

Another manifestation of repeated microembolizations affecting the distal circulation is 'blue toe syndrome', in which debris from the aneurysm dislodges and lands in the digital arteries, causing ischaemia despite the presence of palpable pedal pulses.

Acute thrombosis of the aneurysm follows a more dramatic course, the majority of patients presenting with signs and symptoms of acute limb ischaemia that necessitate emergency revascularization. In such instances, the rate of limb loss can reach up to 60 per cent. Rupture of the aneurysm is an uncommon but equally dreaded complication. It occurs in less than 5 per cent of patients, and these individuals usually present with severe pain rather than shock due to the relatively confined space of the limb.

### Diagnosis

A large portion of peripheral aneurysms are detected on routine vascular examination. The physical examination typically shows a pulsatile mass in the femoral area. The examination of the popliteal arteries is typically challenging. Prominent pulses in the popliteal space should trigger the suspicion of a popliteal aneurysm.

Adjunctive radiological tests are often required to confirm or assess the diameter and patency of the aneurysm as well as rule out other pathologies. In addition, a peripheral aneurysm may be missed on physical examination alone if it is small (<2 cm) or has already thrombosed.

Duplex ultrasonography is the first-line imaging modality for suspected peripheral aneurysms as it can provide information on the size of the aneurysm, its patency and the presence of a mural thrombus. It is also valuable in assessing the outflow vessels as well as detecting additional aneurysms.

In the absence of duplex ultrasonography, CT angiography and MR angiography are valid modalities to accurately assess the diameter of the aneurysm, identify the arterial anatomy in relation to the surrounding structures and detect other aneurysms. They are also helpful in delineating any contributing anatomical abnormalities.

Conventional arteriography is poor at estimating the actual size of the aneurysm, especially in the presence of an intraluminal thrombus. It may be useful, however, in the setting of acute ischaemia if thrombolytic therapy is contemplated. It can also provide a detailed evaluation of the outflow vessels if surgical revascularization in expected.

### Treatment

All symptomatic peripheral aneurysm should be treated expeditiously to minimize the risk of complications, mainly limb ischaemia. Management guidelines have not been clearly identified for asymptomatic aneurysms, especially smaller ones, mainly because the natural history of small femoral and popliteal aneurysms is poorly understood. The majority of surgeons would, however, agree that femoral aneurysms larger than 2.5 cm and popliteal aneurysms larger than 2 cm in diameter should be surgically repaired, especially in the setting of growth or enlargement.

Peripheral aneurysms can be managed by either endovascular or open surgical repair. **Endovascular repair** involves the percutaneous deployment of a stented graft across the aneurysm to exclude it. Its use in the setting of femoral aneurysms is, however, limited, mainly because the femoral artery is subject to repeated flexion and extension as it crosses the groin. Furthermore, the

PART 7 | VASCULAR

aneurysm typically extends to the level of the femoral bifurcation, limiting the availability of a distal zone without compromising the deep femoral artery. Similarly, with popliteal aneurysms, stent fracture and slippage in addition to aneurysm enlargement from retrograde perfusion by the geniculate branches of the artery also make endovascular repair less feasible as a treatment option, except when it is used for small localized aneurysms with a suitable anatomy.

The **open surgical repair** of femoral aneurysms involves resection of the aneurysm and the construction of an interposition graft. If the aneurysm involves either the superficial femoral artery or the profunda femoris, a bypass graft may be constructed between the common femoral artery and the profunda femoris with the superficial femoral artery re-vascularized by re-implantation or via a jump graft.

With popliteal aneurysms, proximal and distal ligation of the aneurysm along with a bypass graft may be sufficient if the aneurysm is small. Attention must be given to locating and ligating the geniculate branches to prevent continued aneurysmal growth from retrograde flow. With large popliteal aneurysms, on the other hand, it is recommended that the aneurysm should be opened after proximal and distal control has been obtained, the feeding branches are then ligated and a small interposition graft constructed. Autologous vein grafts are the preferred conduit for popliteal aneurysm surgical replacement.

## SMALL VESSEL DISEASE

A healthy individual handling snow or ice for any length of time develops white hands and, on re-warming, may have pain and reactive hyperaemia (Figure 31.21). White hands develop because normal arterioles and capillaries close down in response to cold, causing blood to be diverted from the capillary bed by proximal arteriovenous shunts. Such shunts are particularly prominent in the fingers, where two-hundred-fold blood flow changes have been recorded. This normal response is accentuated in individuals who have over-reactive (vasospastic) vessels, small vessel disease (vasculitis) or a reduced arterial inflow due to large vessel disease.

Cold sensitivity produces a characteristic set of colour changes in the hands and sometimes the feet that is known as **Raynaud's phenomenon**. The condition occurs in response to temperature change rather than extreme cold, and is influenced by autonomic activity and emotional changes. The sequence starts with paroxysmal blanching. The cold white changes to the blue of cyanosis on re-warming and finally the red of reactive hyperaemia. Re-warming is usually accompanied by pain, which can be severe – it is usually the patient's presenting complaint.

Everyone suffering from Raynaud's phenomenon is said to have **Raynaud's syndrome** regardless of its aetiology. The term **Raynaud's disease**, named after Maurice Raynaud, who first described the characteristic colour changes in 1865, is reserved for a group of individuals who have Raynaud's phenomenon with no associated vessel pathology.

Small vessel diseases comprise a wide variety of diverse abnormalities that differ markedly from the predominant atheroma of large arteries. They are considered under vasospastic and vasculitic disorders.

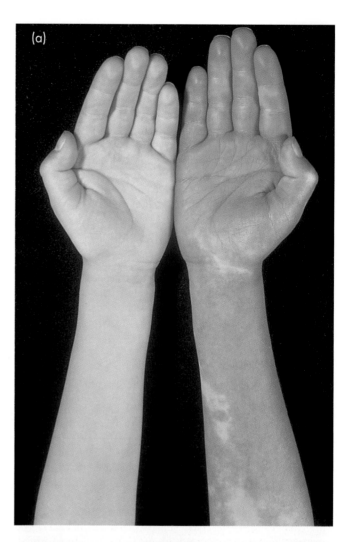

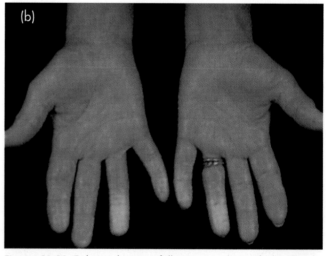

Figure 31.21 Colour changes following cooling of the hands. (a) Two sides of the body – the right side has been cooled before the left. (b) Delayed re-vascularization of the ring fingers following cold immersion.

## VASOSPASTIC DISORDERS

It has already been intimated that cold sensitivity is an extension of a normal response. What is not known, however, is whether the abnormality is in the autonomic supply, the receptor or over-sensitivity of smooth muscle or elastic tissue, or whether cold agglutinins, cryoglobulins or other mediators are involved in the response. Emotional and hormonal changes also play a role.

Damage of a small vessel, such as in vibration white finger disease, or the nerve supply, as in polio, can give rise to Raynaud's phenomenon (see above for a description of this and **Raynaud's disease**), and pathological changes occur in some of these conditions, thus blurring the division between vasospastic and vasculitic disorders. Drugs administered both systemically and intra-arterially can also have marked vasospastic effects and vas-culitic consequences due to endothelial damage and thrombosis. In addition, haemorrheological changes may produce spasm and promote endothelial damage and thrombosis.

**Chilblains (perniosis, erythema pernio**; Figure 31.22) are painful, often multiple localized swellings caused by cold injury. On exposure, the affected areas become cold and white due to vasospasm, but on warming they itch insatiably and are some-times accompanied by marked pain. They are common from childhood, are more frequent in women and may be familial. The swellings are usually 4–6 mm in size, sited over the toes, and may

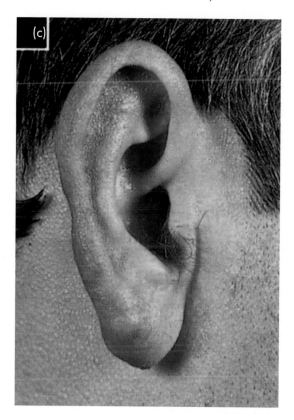

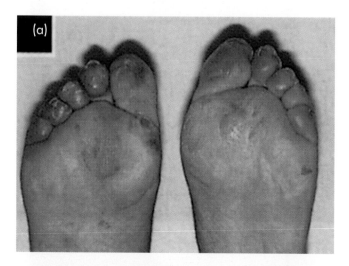

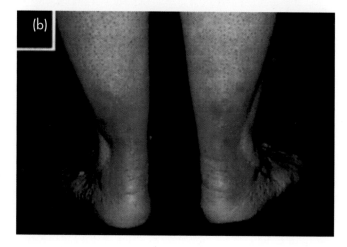

Figure 31.22 Chilblains: (a) toes, (b) legs, and (c) right ear.

be a few centimetres in diameter when on the legs. The oedema-tous nodules may weep fluid and ulcerate. Histological examina-tion demonstrates interstitial round cell infiltration.

**Bazin's disease (erythrocyanosis crurum puellarum frigida)** is a cold sensitivity, particularly over exposed areas. It is more common in women and found in the late teens and 20s. There is dusky purplish, blotchy swelling that may progress to induration, fatty necrosis and superficial ulceration. There may be associated chilblains.

**Paralysis** of a limb from polio or hemiparesis is accompa-nied by oedema and cyanosis of the limb, and there may be an enhanced response to vasomotor changes. Altered responses are also present after peripheral nerve injuries, in syringomyelia, post frostbite (see Figure 17.17a; p. 285) and after limb crush injuries. If a limb is not used and is left to hang dependent, there is pro-gressive oedema, cyanosis, muscle wasting and the development of a progressively useless appendage. This occurs in *oedem bleu*, a psychiatric problem that is very difficult to treat. The problem is complicated by the application of a proximal tourniquet. The line of application may be visible or palpable, although not admitted.

**Vibration white finger disease** is an occupational disorder caused by the use of chainsaws, grinders, pneumatic chipping tools and the swaging of copper pipes. Only tools of a specific frequency produce these effects, and each has a characteristic pattern of digital distribution. There is cold sensitivity with blanching, and there may be accompanying pain and loss of dexterity. Tissue damage, if present, is usually mild. However, the condition can interfere with work and recreational activity. Its severity is linked to the individual's susceptibility and the length of time of exposure. In the UK, vibration white finger disease is recognized for industrial compensation purposes.

Drugs and poisons may affect the small vessels, both by systemic administration and by inadvertent intra-arterial injection. **Ergot** (Figure 31.23) is a potent example of the former and can produce intense spasm followed by thrombosis and gangrene. It can occur from an overdosage of ergotamine tablets prescribed for migraine and is also produced by the fungus *Claviceps purpurea*, which contaminates grain. Nicotine and heavy metals also have vasospastic effects. Inadvertent intra-arterial injection of thiopentone into the brachial artery during anaesthesia produces intense spasm, and crystallization in small vessels, producing severe hand ischaemia. Similar effects can follow the introduction of a varicose vein sclerosant, inadvertently injected into an artery, and the intra-arterial injection of recreational drugs. Hypertonic solutions used for flushing intra-arterial lines may also produce focal spasm and ischaemia.

**Haemorrheological** changes give rise to hyperviscosity, capillary sludging and thrombosis. Hyperfibrinogenaemia, platelet abnormalities and the by-products of sickling episodes are examples producing these effects. The latter can cause diverse symptoms such as strokes and abdominal perforation, linked with cerebral and gut small vessel occlusion.

**Acrocyanosis** is a persistent, cold cyanosis of the hands, and occasionally the feet, due to arteriolar spasm, although the capillary bed remains perfused and dilated (Figure 31.24). It is usually but not invariably initiated by cold, and the palms are often moist. There is not usually any associated pain, and the diagnosis is based purely on the colour changes. It occurs mainly in young women and, once attacks wear off, the hands become red, warm and swollen. At this stage, there may be discomfort.

**Livido reticularis** (Figure 31.25) is a cyanotic blotching and mottling of the skin similar to a normal cold response but associated with autoimmune disease, in particular antiphospholipid syndrome.

**Erythromelalgia** (erythralgia; Figure 31.26) is a painful rubor affecting the feet and, more rarely, the hands. The skin is flushed with venous congestion, and distended veins are accentuated by dependency. There is hyperasthaesia, which may be extreme,

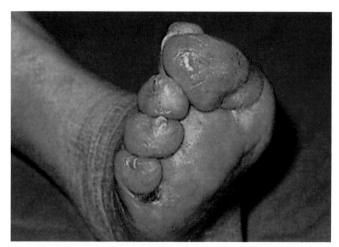

Figure 31.24 **Acrocyanosis of the toes.**

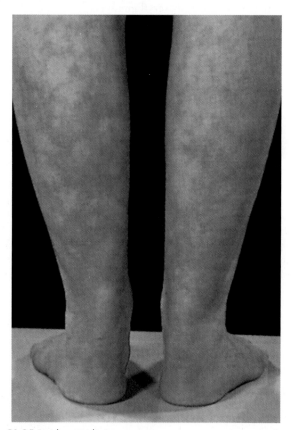

Figure 31.25 Livido reticularis.

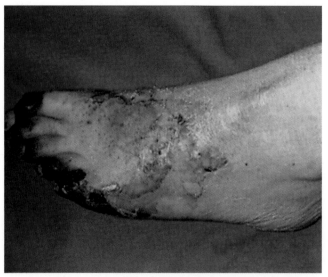

Figure 31.23 Ergot poisoning, demonstrating severe ischaemic changes of the left foot.

patients being unable to bear the touch of bed clothes and having to get out of bed to walk on a cold floor or immerse their feet in cold water. The condition occurs in older individuals, usually with no precipitating cause, but it may be associated with gout or polycythaemia, or it may follow frostbite or previous injury. Vitamins are sometimes prescribed but there is no evidence of vitamin deficiency.

Sweating is under sympathetic control and is increased in emotional states and high temperatures. **Hyperhidrosis** gives rise to disturbing social problems, for example palmar sweating making the individual avoid contact, and soiling of writing paper. Axillary sweating can spoil or ruin clothing, and the feet sweating

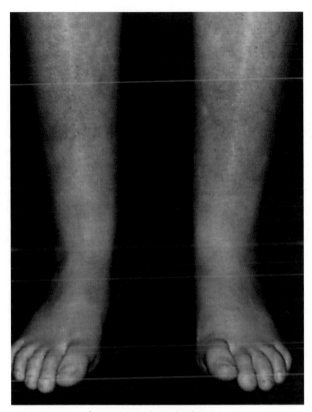

Figure 31.26 Legs of a patient with erythralgia.

can rot socks and shoes, as well as increasing the incidence of fungal infections. Autonomic denervation of affected limbs can increase sweating over the trunk. **Frey's syndrome** is increased sweating of the face, which can follow trauma or surgical incision due to cross-innervation between the facial and autonomic nerves of the face.

## VASCULITIC DISORDERS

Pathological changes of small vessels occur in a wide variety of diseases, including a number of primary skin disorders. Common changes comprise a periarticular cuff of inflammatory cells with fibrinoid degeneration within a thickened arterial wall. This gives rise to narrowing and occlusion of the vessel with consequent distal ischaemia. The organ involved in the process dictates the clinical picture, as evidenced by the different presentations of collagen diseases, those of surgical importance being related to cutaneous manifestations of scleroderma and temporal arteritis.

The term 'vasculitis' is also applied to occlusive disease of the medium and larger vessels, and the pattern of these diseases ranges worldwide; examples of such syndromes have already been referred to – thromboangiitis obliterans, Takayasu's disease and moyamoya – all of which are rare in the UK.

Proximal arterial disease may also give rise to distal vascular problems such as embolism (Figure 31.27), thoracic outlet syndrome (see p. 501) and compartment syndromes (see below), the latter giving rise to symptoms from vascular compression.

Acute digital thrombosis can occur in collagen diseases such as rheumatoid arthritis (Figure 31.28) and scleroderma, and is occasionally seen associated with malignancy, giving rise to gangrene of one or more fingers.

## Scleroderma (systemic sclerosis)

Collagen diseases are subject to inflammatory changes, thickened walls and narrowing of small arteries, with round cell infiltration and fibrinoid necrosis. Cutaneous involvement is most marked in scleroderma. Patients present with Raynaud's phenomenon, and this may, for many years or long term, be the only symptom. As subjects are usually female and in their 20s or 30s, the differential diagnosis from Raynaud's disease can be difficult.

In a few patients, the disease progresses, involving the skin, particularly of the fingers, where the established features are termed **sclerodactyly** (Figure 31.29). The skin and subcutaneous tissues become oedematous, thick, pale and rigid. There is reduced mobility and contractures, particularly of the interphalangeal joints. The skin cracks, and recurrent ulceration, necrosis and scarring produce pulp atrophy and finger tapering. The nails are brittle and ridged, and recurrent paronychia is common. Pain may be severe and is due to necrosis, infection and associated calcinosis, the latter being calcification of necrosed fat around the fingertips and over the dorsum of the fingers and hands.

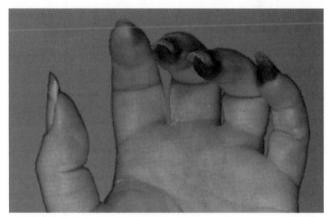

Figure 31.27 Acute ischaemia of the left hand. This followed an untreated brachial artery embolus.

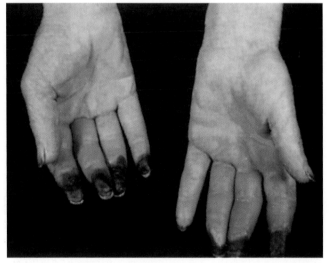

Figure 31.28 Late demarcation of gangrenous fingertips. This followed an episode of acute distal ischaemia in a patient with rheumatoid arthritis.

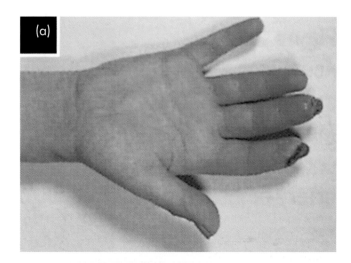

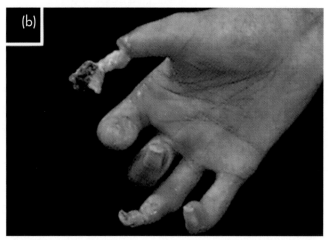

Figure 31.29   Scleroderma. (a) Distal ulceration. (b) Severe sclerodactyly with extensive tissue destruction.

Systemic involvement includes the small vessels of the heart, lungs and gastrointestinal tract. In the latter, there may be reduced motility, ulceration, sclerosis and stricture formation, producing dysphagia, constipation and abdominal colic. More rarely, there may be haemorrhage or perforation. **CREST syndrome** defines the advanced spectrum of the disease: calcinosis cutis, Raynaud's phenomenon, (o)esophageal involvement, scleroderma and telangiectasia. The latter is common around the mouth, on the skin and on the mucosa, and the mouth is often small and contracted (microstoma).

In **temporal arteritis** the inflammatory cell infiltrate includes giant cells. The patient complains of a severe headache and the temporal artery is palpable as a tender cord. The clinical importance of the condition is the associated disease of the ophthalmic artery, as occlusion of this vessel leads to blindness. Consequently, the superficial temporal artery may need to be biopsied to confirm the diagnosis.

## COMPARTMENT SYNDROMES

Muscle groups are contained within fascial or fascio-osseous compartments. An increase in the muscle bulk within a compartment, for whatever reason, can compromise muscle blood flow.

If this occurs, it is termed a muscle compartment syndrome; this may be an acute or a chronic event.

A muscle's contraction temporarily inhibits its arterial inflow but also empties its venous bed and this enhances inflow to the lowered resistant vessels during relaxation. An increase in compartment pressure can inhibit venous outflow, induce extracellular oedema and eventually inhibit the muscle's arterial supply.

**Acute compartment syndrome** usually follows injury. Bleeding may occur from muscle or other soft tissue damage and adjacent fractures. It may occur spontaneously in bleeding diatheses. Crushing and tearing of muscle produces oedema, which may be marked following reperfusion of a limb after arterial reconstruction, with trauma or on releasing a tourniquet or other external compression after some hours. Snake bites, prevalent in some countries, may give rise to severe local oedema within a muscle compartment. Late sequelae include Volkmann's ischaemic contracture (see Figure 7.7; p. 151).

The symptoms are severe muscle pain and tense, tender muscle compartments. These symptoms may be difficult to differentiate from the underlying injury. Pressure measurements are liable to sudden change and are therefore difficult to obtain and interpret, while the peripheral pulses may persist. Tense compartments should therefore be released whenever a compartment syndrome is considered as a possibility. In severe lower leg injury, and with major arterial reconstruction following a number of hours of ischaemia, all four vessel compartments should be released.

**Chronic compartment syndrome** occasionally complicates the overuse or overtraining of muscle groups. Characteristically, this is most common in the anterior compartment of the lower leg, although the other three compartments may also be involved. Such activity can increase muscle bulk by up to 20 per cent. Pain accompanies exercise and usually subsides on cessation, but may persist as an ache for some time afterwards. The age group and physical fitness help to differentiate the condition from chronic arterial occlusive disease, but popliteal entrapment syndrome and other musculoskeletal abnormalities have to be considered. Forearm compartment syndromes occur in rowers, canoeists and windsurfers.

### Key Points

- Carotid disease is often asymptomatic but can present with transient monocular blindness, transient ischaemic attacks or a stroke.
- Lower extremity occlusive disease is a manifestation of atherosclerosis. Most patients are asymptomatic. With progression of the disease, the patient may develop intermittent claudication, rest pain or tissue loss in the foot.
- Diabetic patients suffer from advanced atherosclerotic disease with involvement of the popliteal and proximal tibial vessels and sparing of the distal tibial and pedal vessels. This is amenable to endovascular or open surgical revascularization.
- Aortic aneurysms are due to a degenerative process in the aortic wall. Although typically asymptomatic, they can present with rupture, dissection or symptoms of distal embolization.
- Peripheral arterial aneurysms rarely rupture. Their symptoms are typically due to distal embolization, acute thrombosis or compression of adjacent vein.
- The symptoms of acute limb ischaemia include pain, pallor, pulselessness, poikilothermia, paraesthesia and paralysis.

## QUESTIONS

### SBAs

1. **A 55-year-old man presents with pain in his right calf muscles when he walks 100 m. The pain is relieved by rest. He denies back pain. He is not diabetic, smokes regularly and has a sedentary lifestyle. He has a family history of coronary artery disease. On physical examination, he has palpable femoral pulses bilaterally but no palpable pedal pulses. This patient is most likely to be suffering from which one of the following?:**
   a  Subacute embolic disease of his popliteal arteries
   b  Infrainguinal occlusive arterial disease affecting the superficial femoral arteries
   c  A herniated lumbar disc with nerve root impingement
   d  A ruptured popliteal Baker's cyst
   e  A gastrocnemius muscle tear

Answer
b  *Infrainguinal occlusive arterial disease affecting the superficial femoral arteries. This man's symptoms of calf pain that is relieved by rest are typical of claudication. This usually occurs with chronic arterial occlusive disease affecting the superficial femoral artery and/or popliteal artery.*

2. **A 72-year-old diabetic woman presents with a painful non-healing ulcer over her left fifth toe that is of 10 days' duration. The ulcer started after accidentally injuring the skin around the nail bed while she was clipping her toenails. On physical examination, the ulcer is 3 mm × 2 mm with a necrotic base and surrounding erythema. There are strong palpable femoral and popliteal pulses but no palpable pedal pulses. The Doppler examination of her pedal arteries reveals a monophasic signal. This patient is most likely to be suffering from which one of the following?:**
   a  Blue toe syndrome
   b  Arterial disease affecting the tibial arteries
   c  Leriche syndrome
   d  Popliteal artery thrombosis
   e  Occlusive disease of the superficial femoral artery

b  *Arterial disease affecting the tibial arteries. The location and description of the ulcer suggest an ischaemic toe ulcer. This usually occurs with tibial disease and is further confirmed by the presence of femoral and popliteal pulses and monophasic pedal signals.*

3. **A 51-year-old diabetic man presents with a 1 cm × 1 cm ulcer over the plantar aspect of his right great toe. The ulcer started as a blister after a prolonged walk wearing a new pair of shoes. The ulcer is not painful and has a pink base with good granulation tissue. The pedal pulses are strongly palpable bilaterally. This patient is suffering from which one of the following?:**
   a  Small vessel occlusive disease of the digital arteries
   b  Blue toe syndrome
   c  Diabetic neuropathic ulcer
   d  Buerger's disease
   e  Charcot foot

c  *Diabetic neuropathic ulcer. Diabetic foot ulcers occur as result of continuous pressure at one spot in the setting of diabetic neuropathy. This causes a painless ischaemic ulcer in the setting of normal foot circulation.*

4. **A 66-year-old man presents for a routine medical check-up. On physical examination, he has a palpable pulsatile abdominal mass at the level of the umbilicus. He denies abdominal pain or back pain. He stopped smoking 1 year ago, has well-controlled hypertension and is otherwise in good health. He has palpable femoral and pedal pulses with prominent popliteal pulses. The next step in the management of this patient is which one of the following?:**

   a  CT scan of the abdomen and pelvis with arterial and venous phases

   b  MR angiography of the abdomen and chest

   c  Abdominal X-ray looking for arterial wall calcification

   d  Ultrasound of the aorta and popliteal arteries

   e  Digital subtraction angiography

*d  **Ultrasound of the aorta and popliteal arteries.** The ideal initial imaging modality for diagnosing asymptomatic abdominal aortic and popliteal aneurysms is duplex ultrasonography, due to its widespread availability, lack of radiation, low cost and reproducible results.*

5. **A 59-year-old man presents with a history of a sudden onset of slurred speech associated with weakness in his right upper extremity 2 hours previously. The symptoms lasted for 3 minutes and slowly reverted to normal. He is a chronic smoker and is known to have stable coronary artery disease for which he receives medical therapy. His symptoms are most likely to be due to which one of the following?:**

   a  A brain tumor

   b  An intracranial arteriovenous malformation

   c  An ulcerated plaque at the carotid bifurcation

   d  A seizure disorder

   e  Intracranial arterial occlusive disease

*c  **An ulcerated plaque at the carotid bifurcation.** This patient's medical history is indicative of diffuse arterial occlusive disease, and his neurological symptoms are suggestive of a transient ischaemic attack. This makes an ulcerated carotid plaque high on the list of differential diagnoses.*

# Venous and Lymphatic Disorders

Maen Aboul Hosn and Jamal Jawad Hoballah

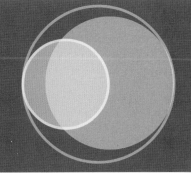

## LEARNING OBJECTIVES

- To identify the signs and symptoms of venous insufficiency
- To recognize the signs and symptoms of thrombophlebitis

- To be aware of the findings related to varicose veins, thrombophlebitis and lymphoedema

## CHRONIC VENOUS DISEASE

Chronic venous disease is the most common vascular disorder, being present in up to 50 per cent of individuals. It refers to morphological and functional venous disorders with clinical manifestations varying from simple superficial venous dilation to venous hypertension with chronic skin changes and ulceration.

Chronic venous disease usually starts as a result of venous valve dysfunction, venous pump failure or venous obstruction. Over time, a build-up of pressure within the venous system directs the blood flow abnormally from the deep to the superficial venous system, which in turn may result in skin fibrosis, local inflammation and ulceration. There are many risk factors for the development of venous disease, including advancing age, a family history of venous pathology, an increased body mass index, prolonged standing, smoking, prior venous thrombosis and pregnancy.

### Normal Venous Anatomy of the Lower Extremity

There are three major venous pathways in the lower extremity:

- The *deep system* forms from the confluence of the anterior, posterior and peroneal veins of the leg. These join to form the popliteal vein, which in turn becomes the femoral vein as it accompanies the superficial femoral artery. The femoral vein joins the deep femoral vein just below the saphenofemoral junction to become the common femoral vein.
- The *superficial venous system* (Figure 32.1) includes the great and small saphenous veins. These usually join the deep system at the saphenofemoral and saphenopopliteal junctions, respectively.
- The *perforating veins* connect the superficial and deep systems.

The venous flow in the veins of the lower extremity is normally directed from the superficial to the deep system, and this movement is controlled by the action of the venous valves and the pumping effect of the calf and thigh muscles. Competent valves prevent retrograde flow into the superficial venous circulation, and the venous pressure of the superficial circulation is maintained at between 20 and 30 mmHg during ambulation.

### Presentation

Chronic venous disease encompasses a wide spectrum of functional and morphological venous disorders, and as such its clinical manifestations vary significantly. The majority of patients present with leg pain, oedema and heaviness. Pain and oedema are typically worse when the patient is standing or when the feet are in a dependent position for prolonged periods of time; this usually improves with limb elevation. Nevertheless, the symptoms are often more prominent at night when the patient goes to bed.

Numbness and tingling may also be present but are difficult to differentiate from other causes of peripheral neuropathy in the leg. Some patients complain of cramping, itching and swelling, and this is usually associated with chronic skin changes. Skin ulceration and bleeding of varicose veins are usually late manifestations of severe venous reflux disease.

The physical findings are also variable and usually correlate with the severity of the symptoms. Telangiectasias, which are small dilated intradermal veins, are usually early manifestations of venous disease. Varicose veins, on the other hand, may represent a more advanced stage of venous disorders. These dilated long tortuous subcutaneous veins are usually associated with an underlying mild to moderate venous reflux and insufficiency (Figure 32.2). Long-standing venous insufficiency can result in venous hypertension with subsequent oedema and skin changes such as lipodermatosclerosis and ulceration (Figures 32.3–32.5).

Venous ulcers are usually located at the level of the medial aspect of the ankle or along the course of the great or small saphenous veins. They are usually tender and exudative with an

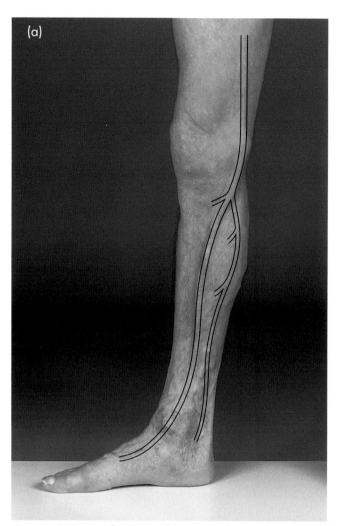

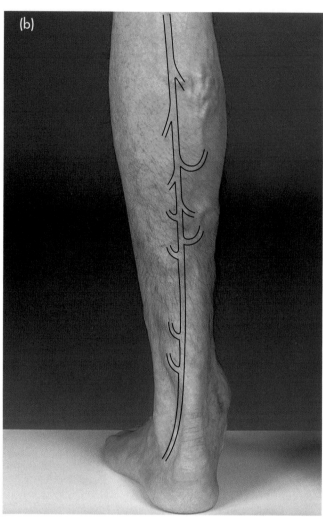

Figure 32.1 The superficial veins of the leg. (a) Great saphenous vein with the posterior arch vein, which connects with many perforators. (b) Lesser saphenous vein.

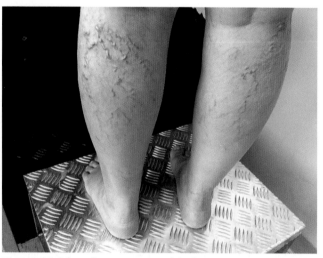

Figure 32.2 Bilateral varicose veins of the lower extremity.

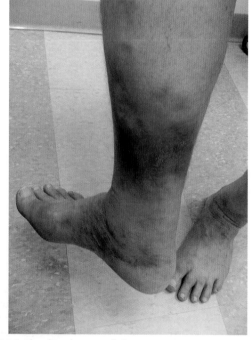

Figure 32.3 The skin changes of chronic venous stasis.

elevated base (Figure 32.5). These characteristics help to differentiate them from other types of leg ulcer, mainly neurogenic and arterial ulcers. A combination of these manifestations can be associated with marked disability and a diminished quality of life.

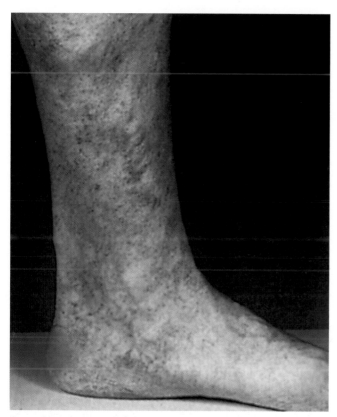

Figure 32.4 A great saphenous varicose vein. This shows prominent skin bulges over the varicosities of the posterior arch vein, together with widespread venular dilatation and loss of ankle contour in a postphlebitic leg.

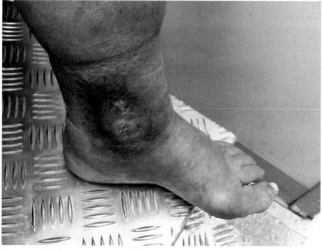

Figure 32.5 A venous stasis ulcer.

Because the association between the severity of the disease and its clinical signs and symptoms varies among patients, a clinical classification of the disease can be made using the Clinical–Etiology–Anatomy–Pathophysiology criteria (Table 32.1). This classification system allocates a different grade depending on the presence of certain findings on physical examination. Early disease is characterized by telangiectases or spider veins, which are 0.1–1 mm in diameter, superficial veins, reticular veins of 1–3 mm and varicose veins. Oedema, skin changes and healed or active ulcers signify more advanced

Table 32.1 The Clinical–Etiology–Anatomy–Pathophysiology classification

| Grade | Description |
| --- | --- |
| C0 | No evidence of venous disease |
| C1 | Superficial spider veins (reticular veins) only |
| C2 | Simple varicose veins only |
| C3 | Ankle oedema of venous origin (not foot oedema) |
| C4 | Skin pigmentation in the gaiter area (lipodermatosclerosis) |
| C5 | A healed venous ulcer |
| C6 | An open venous ulcer |

venous pathology. This classification system is important to stage the severity of the disease on presentation as well as to document changes over time.

## Diagnosis

The diagnosis of chronic venous disease is often a clinical one, established by taking an adequate medical history and performing a thorough physical examination. This approach is also helpful in ruling out any other systemic causes of venous hypertension such as heart failure or fluid overload.

The **Trendelenburg test** (also known as the Brodie–Trendelenburg test) can be used to assess for the presence of venous reflux. Typically, the patient is placed in a supine position and the leg in question is elevated. A tourniquet is placed around the proximal thigh and the patient is asked to stand up. The tourniquet should be tight enough to occlude only the superficial system while keeping the deep system unobstructed. The veins are then carefully inspected to assess the time taken for them to refill.

In individuals without venous insufficiency, the veins need 3–5 seconds to refill normally from the capillaries. Earlier refill is indicative of reflux below the tourniquet from the communicating perforator veins or the saphenous vein itself. If the veins do not refill after 20 seconds, the tourniquet is released and the vein is observed for refill. If it now refills in less than 20 seconds, this is indicative of reflux originating proximal to the level of the tourniquet. The level of the tourniquet can be changed to assess various levels of reflux.

**Perthes' test** is another test used to assess the patency of the deep venous system. With the patient supine, a compression bandage is applied to the leg tightly enough to occlude the superficial venous system. The patient is then asked to stand up and walk. If the patient develops severe pain upon walking, this indicates significant deep venous obstruction and suggests that the superficial venous system has been acting as an important collateral and contributor to the venous drainage of the lower extremity.

Although the Trendelenburg and Perthes tests can be useful, the inherent inaccuracies of applying the tourniquet or elastic bandages and the presence of other more direct objective testing modalities have led to a decrease in their use.

When a clinical diagnosis is difficult to establish but the patient's symptoms are suggestive of venous insufficiency, adjunctive tests can be utilized to assist in establishing the diagnosis.

### Duplex Ultrasonography

This has become the imaging modality of choice for assessing the superficial and deep venous circulation of the lower extremity.

By visualizing the blood vessels using B-mode ultrasonography and providing a blood flow analysis using colour Doppler scanning, duplex ultrasonography can confirm the presence of venous obstruction or valvular incompetence that could be precipitating venous hypertension.

Venous obstruction can present as deep vein thrombosis (DVT), which can be confirmed on duplex ultrasonography by the presence of non-compressible veins. Valvular incompetence and reflux can also be documented on duplex ultrasonography by demonstrating a reflux time of more than 0.5 seconds within the superficial and deep calf veins and longer than 1 second in the femoropopliteal veins. A normal venous duplex scan usually shows a compressible vein with changes in flow during the respiratory cycle, which is termed respiratory phasicity.

### Lower Extremity Arterial Doppler and Ankle–Brachial Index Studies

These studies can also be useful in patients with suspected concomitant peripheral arterial disease. This is usually the case in patients with diminished or absent pedal pulses or patients with skin ulcers in unusual locations, especially if the ulcers are not healing or not responding to conventional compression therapy. In such instances, a diagnosis of significant peripheral arterial disease will significantly alter the management.

### Venography

Venography was once the gold standard for diagnosing venous insufficiency and obstruction. However, it is no longer widely used due to its invasive nature and the associated nephrotoxicity that is seen with the administration of contrast material. In addition, the availability, reproducibility and low cost of duplex scanning has made the latter the imaging modality of choice for venous disorders.

### Management

The management of chronic venous disease depends on the severity and location of the underlying venous pathology. For less severe symptoms, conservative management is warranted, including elevation of the legs, weight loss, compressive stockings and lifestyle modifications.

In patients with varicose veins, the indication for treatment may be purely cosmetic. Alternatively, the symptoms may have been refractory to compression therapy and lifestyle modifications. Many patients live in hot climates and cannot tolerate wearing compression stockings, especially in the summer, or their job may demand prolonged standing and cannot be modified.

The interventions for varicose veins vary based on the affected segments. Spider and reticular veins are typically treated by sclerotherapy or ablation using external laser beams or radiofrequency applications. In patients with large varicosities, it is important to determine whether the disease is involving the trunk (the great or small saphenous vein) or whether it is limited to the tributaries of the saphenous veins.

The traditional treatment for great saphenous vein varicosities used to be surgical stripping of the saphenous vein from the ankle to the groin. This was then replaced by stripping from knee level to the groin to decrease the incidence of injury to the accompanying saphenous nerve. Similarly, the small saphenous vein used to be stripped from the ankle to the knee. Surgical stripping has now, however, been replaced with vein ablation that can be performed chemically or thermally as a same-day clinic procedure.

Sclerotherapy is a form of chemical ablation that involves the injection of sclerosing agents into the vein. The sclerosing agents can be mixed with air, resulting in a foam that can also be used for sclerotherapy and tends to accentuate the sclerosing effect.

Thermal ablation is delivered via a laser or radiofrequency catheter that is inserted percutaneously into the saphenous vein at knee level or below-knee level and advanced up to 2–3 cm below the level of the saphenofemoral junction. Prior to delivering the heating energy, tumescent fluid is typically injected between the vein and the skin to prevent transmission of the heat to the overlying skin, which could cause a burn injury. The heat is then delivered and the catheter withdrawn from the groin to the insertion level to fully ablate the saphenous vein. This approach is now preferred as it allows for a faster recovery and return to work and can be undertaken in the doctor's office without requiring hospitalization.

Varicosities affecting the tributaries can be treated by sclerotherapy or foam sclerotherapy. Alternatively, they can be removed using a stab phlebectomy approach that can also be performed as an office-based procedure.

Venous ulcers can also be treated conservatively with compressive bandages and frequent dressing changes. Leg elevation and the avoidance of prolonged standing are other essential components of the treatment. Ulcers refractory to medical management are often due to patients' non-compliance with compression therapy and elevation. However, patients with refractory ulcers should be reassessed for the possibility of an associated significant superficial venous disease or significant associated arterial insufficiency. The arterial insufficiency may need to be addressed first in order to allow for the use of compression therapy. The superficial venous insufficiency can be addressed by thermal ablation of the saphenous veins or perforators that are leading to the non-healing ulceration.

## VENOUS THROMBOEMBOLISM

Venous thromboembolism (VTE) includes both DVT and pulmonary embolism (PE). Its incidence is estimated to be around 2 per 1000 patients. The number of VTE-related deaths is, however, largely underestimated owing to the fact that up to 25 per cent of patients with an acute PE die suddenly before being diagnosed or treated. In the surviving patients, VTE also carries marked long-term complications and morbidities including recurrent VTE, bleeding complications and post-thrombotic syndrome.

The risk of developing VTE is higher in patients with hypercoagulability, stasis or injury to the vessel wall – factors known collectively as **Virchow's triad**. Other major risk factors include older age, malignancy, a prior history of VTE, inherited thrombophilia, obesity, prolonged hospitalization or immobilization, recent surgery, venous catheters, pregnancy and oral contraceptives. It should be noted, however, that no hereditary or acquired risk factors can be identified in up to 20 per cent of patients who develop VTE.

### Presentation

The majority of patients with DVT present with unilateral lower extremity oedema. Patients may also present with pain in the lower extremity, mainly in the calf area or in the thigh along the course of the major veins. Erythema and warmth of the lower extremity are frequently seen, and these can be mistaken for cellulitis (Figure 32.6).

Homans' sign, described as pain in the calf on dorsiflexion of the foot, was classically used to indicate the presence of a DVT. Most studies, however, have shown that this sign has very low sensitivity and specificity and can also be present with cellulitis, a haematoma or trauma. Its absence also does not rule out DVT, thus limiting its value.

Massive DVTs of the lower extremity can cause a complete obstruction of venous outflow (phlegmasia syndromes). In such instances, the patient initially presents with a severely swollen painful extremity. The extremity may initially be pale, and as a result this condition is termed **phlegmasia alba dolens** (Figure 32.7). As the thrombotic process extends into the branches of the veins and the capillaries, the arterial supply becomes also compromised, resulting in a cyanotic limb. The bluish, purplish discoloration of the lower extremity associated with pain and swelling is called **phlegmasia cerulea dolens**. Venous thromboembolism may also occur in the upper limb. This is a very serious condition that can result in venous gangrene (Figures 32.8 and 32.9) and amputation despite attempts with various therapeutic modalities.

The presenting signs and symptoms of a PE are equally variable and non-specific. Patients with PE can present with dyspnoea or tachypnoea, tachycardia, pleuritic pain, wheezing or cough. Massive PEs have a more dramatic presentation that may include hypotension, circulatory collapse and sudden death. Venous thrombosis can also affect the hepatic veins (**Budd–Chiari syndrome**), manifesting as generalized oedema, ascites and hepatomegaly, while thrombosis of the superior vena cava may produce upper body oedema, accentuated by lying down, and, if long-standing, varicose veins over the trunk (Figures 32.10 and 32.11).

## Diagnosis

The approach to a patient with suspected VTE starts with a thorough personal and medical history. Investigations should focus on identifying the risk factors that could predispose the patient to venous thrombosis, as mentioned above. A family history of DVT, particularly in relatives younger than

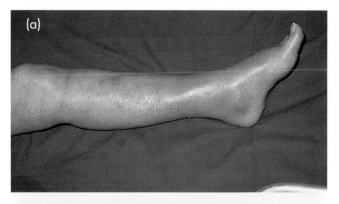

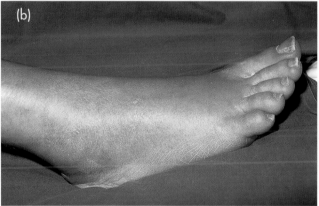

Figure 32.7 Phlegmasia alba dolens. (a) In pregnancy. (b) In a patient with an occult neoplasm of the bronchus.

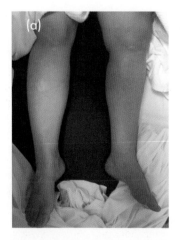

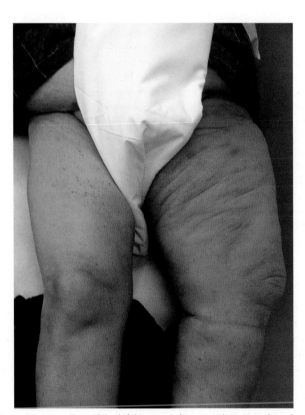

Figure 32.6 Swelling of the left leg secondary to a deep vein thrombosis of the ileofemoral vein.

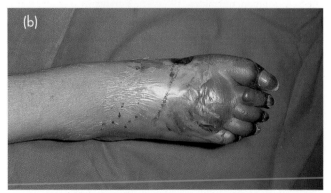

Figure 32.8 (a) Phlegmasia cerulea of the left leg. (b) Venous gangrene of the right foot.

50 years of age, is significant as it can point to a hereditary thrombophilia.

A comprehensive physical examination, with more focus on the vascular system, should follow. Physical signs such as unilateral swelling of a lower extremity, oedema, pain and erythema are suggestive of DVT but are non-specific. Other entities that may have similar presentations include a ruptured Baker's cyst, cellulitis, a muscle sprain, a thrombosed popliteal aneurysm and lymphoedema.

Adjunctive laboratory studies can be useful, particularly in low-risk patients. The D-dimer test has a negative predictive value of around 96 per cent. As such, a negative D-dimer result rules out the diagnosis of DVT in low-risk patients, with no additional testing needed. In high-risk patients, on the other hand, D-dimer levels are unreliable, with 10 per cent false-negative results. Other laboratory studies are important to rule out hypercoagulability; these include:

- partial thromboplastin time;
- prothrombin time;
- platelet count and antithrombin level;
- factor V Leiden;
- methylene tetrahydrofolate reductase level;
- homocysteine concentration;
- protein C and S levels.

Imaging studies play a pivotal role in diagnosing DVT and PE. Compression duplex ultasonography is the diagnostic modality of choice for diagnosing DVT of the extremities as it is non-invasive and readily available, with a sensitivity of approximately 96 per cent in moderate to high risk patients. Findings diagnostic of DVT include abnormal compressibility of the vein, impedance to flow and abnormal changes in the vein diameter on breathing and calf compression. Compression duplex ultrasonography is, however, less sensitive in low-risk patients and is often employed when the D-dimer assay is positive.

The diagnosis of PE requires additional imaging studies. CT angiography is the gold standard for making the diagnosis as it

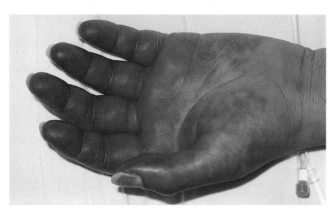

Figure 32.9 Venous gangrene of the left hand.

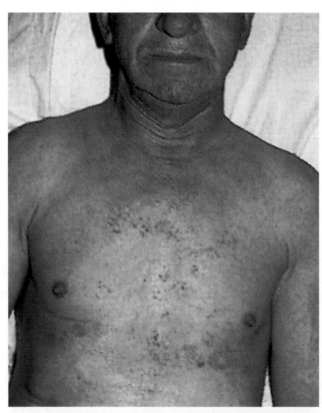

Figure 32.10 Oedema and plethora of the head and neck due to obstruction of the superior vena cava.

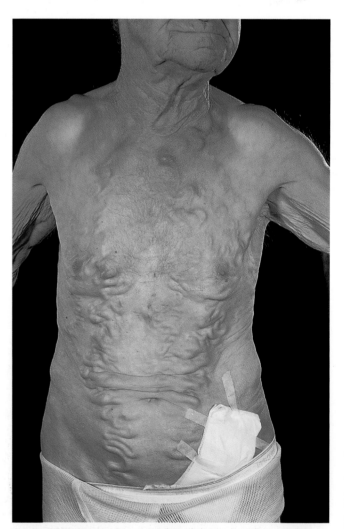

Figure 32.11 Varicosities over the abdominal wall secondary to obstruction of the superior vena cava.

has a sensitivity and specificity of 90 per cent and 95 per cent, respectively. It is also useful for detecting other abnormalities that could be contributing to the patient's signs and symptoms. An alternative non-invasive imaging modality is ventilation/perfusion lung scanning. Ventilation/perfusion scanning utilizes radionuclides and avoids ionizing radiation and nephrotoxic contrast material. However, it has a sensitivity of only around 40 per cent and is not useful in patients with existing lung disease.

Conventional angiography was once considered the gold standard for diagnosing DVT and PE. However, it has fallen out of favour due to its invasive nature and its complications, which are related mainly to vascular access, cardiac arrhythmias and exposure to contrast material, and the availability of CT angiography.

## Treatment

The management of a patient with a diagnosis of DVT or PE depends on the patient's clinical condition. In stable patients, treatment aims to prevent further propagation of the clot, preventing a recurrence of venous thrombosis and preventing the long-term complications of DVT.

Further thrombosis can be prevented by infusing unfractionated heparin and titrating it to reach a therapeutic activated partial thromboplastin time (1.5–2.5 times the control value). Heparin should also be started in high-risk patients suspected of PE even if the diagnosis has not yet been established. Low molecular weight heparin has emerged as a leading therapeutic option as it allows for outpatient management and does not require frequent blood tests to check the anticoagulation level. It is also reported to be associated with a lower incidence of heparin-induced thrombocytopenia.

Patients are also started on oral anticoagulation such as warfarin if their clinical condition permits, and this should be continued for at least 3 months. They are 'bridged' with unfractionated or low molecular weight heparins until they achieve adequate anticoagulation with warfarin. New oral anticoagulants (e.g. rivaroxaban) have now also been approved as treatment for VTE, avoiding the need to resort to the heparin family followed by warfarin.

Treatment also aims to manage risk factors for VTE as well as to test for hypercoagulability since high-risk patients may require anticoagulation for longer periods. Compression stockings are advised early on to mitigate post-thrombotic syndrome. In patients with phlegmasia or extensive iliofemoral DVT, thrombolytic therapy is also recommended. In patients who have a contraindication to anticoagulation, it may become necessary to insert an inferior vena cava filter.

In unstable patients who are in shock after a massive PE, more invasive options may be utilized. These include endovascular catheter-directed thrombolysis and mechanical thrombectomy. Open thrombectomy carries a high mortality rate and is only employed in unstable patients with contraindications to thrombolysis or in circumstances when the patient's condition does not allow a delay for pharmacological thrombolysis to take effect.

## MAY–THURNER SYNDROME

May–Thurner syndrome is a rare condition in which the left iliac vein is extrinsically compressed by the right iliac artery, causing venous outflow obstruction with subsequent pain, swelling or iliofemoral DVT. The diagnosis is made by CT venography or magnetic resonance venography, although a formal venogram is preferred when an iliofemoral DVT is suspected. The management depends on the severity of symptoms and can range from

compression therapy to angioplasty and stenting. Thrombolysis and mechanical thrombectomy may also be utilized in cases of extensive iliofemoral vein thrombosis.

## THORACIC OUTLET SYNDROME

Thoracic outlet syndrome (TOS) is a condition in which the neurovascular bundle reaching the upper extremity is compressed within the confined space of the thoracic outlet. It occurs in around 2 per cent of the general population. Thoracic outlet syndrome is divided into three distinct types depending on the structures being compressed:

- *Neurogenic TOS* is by far the most common type of TOS (95 per cent) and occurs when the brachial plexus is compressed. It usually leads to neck pain and numbness and weakness of the upper extremity.
- *Venous TOS* is the second most common type (4 per cent) and refers to subclavian vein compression. It may manifest as DVT and swelling of the upper extremity.
- *Arterial TOS* is the least common type (1 per cent) and is due to subclavian artery compression. Arterial compression may lead to distal embolization, arm pain or acute arterial thrombosis.

## Anatomy

The thoracic outlet is composed of two major spaces through which the neurovascular structures pass: the scalene triangle (Figure 32.12) and the costoclavicular space.

The **scalene triangle** is the most important anatomical space in the thoracic outlet. It is bounded anteriorly by the anterior scalene muscle, posteriorly by the middle scalene muscle and inferiorly by the superior border of the first rib. The anterior scalene muscle originates from the transverse processes of the C3–C6 vertebrae and inserts onto the anterior aspect of the first rib. The middle scalene muscle arises from the transverse processes of C2–C7 and inserts onto the posterior aspect of the first rib. The subclavian artery and brachial plexus pass through the scalene triangle while the subclavian vein courses anterior to it. These muscles can potentially hypertrophy or undergo fibrosis with repetitive motion or trauma, contributing to compression of the neurovascular structures.

The **costoclavicular space** comprises the area between the first rib and the clavicle through which the brachial plexus, subclavian artery and subclavian vein pass. The subclavius

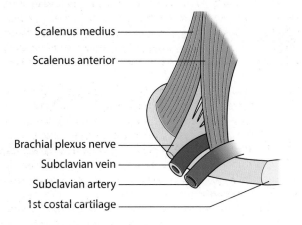

Figure 32.12 **The anatomy of the scalene triangle.**

muscle is also found within this space and may compress the neurovascular structures, mainly the subclavian vein, contributing to venous TOS.

Other congenital anatomical variations may contribute to the symptoms associated with TOS, including a cervical rib, a long transverse processes of C7 and congenital fibromuscular bands. Cervical ribs have an incidence of approximately 1 per cent in the general population, with 50 per cent of cases being bilateral (Figure 32.13). A long transverse process of C7 or a bifid first rib is even less common. Congenital fibrocartilaginous bands usually extend from the tip of the rudimentary cervical rib to the first rib and compress the brachial plexus trunk.

## Presentation

The presenting signs and symptoms of TOS vary significantly depending on its type. This reflects the compression of a specific structure, although more than one structure can be compressed, resulting in some overlap of the symptoms.

### Neurogenic Thoracic Outlet Syndrome

Patients with neurogenic TOS may present with pain in the neck and shoulder region along with weakness of the intrinsic muscles of the hand, mainly of the thenar aspect (Figure 32.14a). Examination reveals sensory abnormalities in the C8–T1 distribution, radiation of the pain or paraesthesias in the symptomatic arm upon deep palpation of the scalene muscles and reproduction of the patient's symptoms with elevation or sustained use of the arms or hands. These symptoms have, however, poor sensitivity and specificity, making the diagnosis of neurogenic TOS purely a clinical one.

### Venous Thoracic Outlet Syndrome

Venous TOS is mainly seen in athletic individuals who perform vigorous repetitive exertion of the upper extremities above shoulder level, such as swimmers and weightlifters. The most common presentation is acute thrombosis of the axillary subclavian vein, also known as **Paget–Schroetter syndrome**, which is characterized by a sudden onset of swelling, pain and discoloration of the upper extremity. Other manifestations include forearm fatigue,

finger paraesthesias secondary to swelling, and the development of collateral veins in the skin overlying the ipsilateral shoulder, neck and chest wall.

### Arterial Thoracic Outlet Syndrome

Arterial TOS is the least common of the three types of TOS and is almost always associated with a cervical or anomalous rib. Patients typically present with ischaemic symptoms in the hand, including pain, pallor, paraesthesia and coldness (Figure 32.14b). Ischaemia is usually the result of thromboembolization from a subclavian mural thrombus or post-stenotic subclavian aneurysm. In the Adson test (see below), the examiner feels the radial pulse while the patient is asked to rotate their head to the ipsilateral side with the neck extended and take a deep breath; a positive result, indicated by disappearance of the radial pulse, aids in the diagnosis but is non-specific.

## Diagnosis

The patient's presenting signs and symptoms dictate the diagnostic approach to be followed. Chest radiographs should always be taken to identify bony abnormalities such as a cervical rib or long transverse cervical process. Other imaging and electrophysiological tools may aid in the diagnosis, but in many instances the

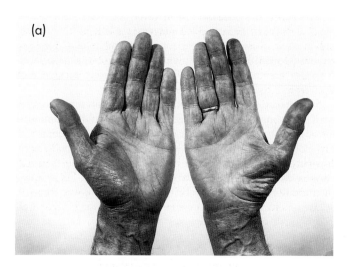

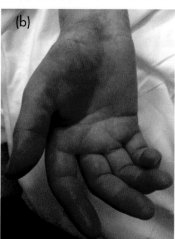

Figure 32.14 (a) Marked wasting of the right thenar eminence. This is due to a cervical rib pressing on the T1 root of the brachial plexus. (b) Ischaemia of the hand in the setting of arterial thoracic outlet syndrome.

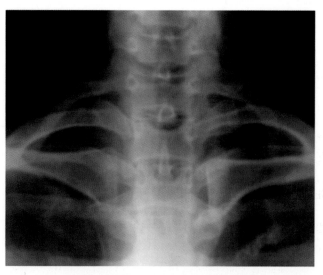

Figure 32.13 Radiograph showing bilateral cervical ribs.

diagnosis of TOS is purely a clinical one, emphasizing the role of proper history-taking and a thorough physical examination.

## Neurogenic Thoracic Outlet Syndrome

In neurogenic TOS, a good physical examination is essential as there are no definitive diagnostic tests to confirm the diagnosis. There may be tenderness over the scalene muscles or supraclavicular fossa on the involved side. Deep palpation of the scalene muscles may also elicit pain and paraesthesia in the affected limb.

The **Adson manoeuvre** used to be performed to assess for the presence of TOS. While the examiner is feeling the radial pulse, the patient is asked to rotate their head to the ipsilateral side with the neck extended and take a deep breath. The sign is positive if the radial pulse is lost. Loss of a radial pulse during this test is, however, not specific and may occur in the presence or absence of neurogenic compression. As such, the Adson manoeuvre is often unreliable.

The **90° abduction in external rotation stress test** is a modification of the Adson test and is sometimes referred to as the elevated arm stress test. It is performed by having the patient elevate the arms in a 'stick-'em-up' position. A positive test is reproduction of the patients' symptoms of pain and paraesthesia within 60 seconds but not necessarily with a reduction in the radial pulse.

The **upper limb tension test** involves abduction of the arms to 90° with the elbows extended and wrists dorsiflexed. The head is then tilted to each side, ear to shoulder. Each manoeuvre progressively increases the stretch on the brachial plexus; pain down the arm, especially around the elbow, and/or paraesthesia in the hand represents a positive response.

Nerve conduction studies can be useful and may reveal a significant reduction in the amplitude of the sensory as well as motor potentials in the ulnar nerve. The medial antebrachial cutaneous nerve, which runs in close proximity to the T1 root distribution and innervates the skin of the anterior and medial surfaces of forearm, is usually involved as well. Other tests need to also be performed to rule out the possibility of a carpal tunnel syndrome, ulnar nerve entrapment syndrome or cervical spine pathology.

## Venous Thoracic Outlet Syndrome

In venous TOS, the presence of acute-onset unilateral arm swelling and pain with non-pitting oedema in an otherwise healthy young individual is almost diagnostic. The diagnosis can be confirmed with duplex ultrasonography, which shows acute thrombosis of the axillary subclavian vein. Contrast venography is reserved for cases in which non-invasive tests are not conclusive or are unavailable. Although CT venography has largely replaced conventional venography, the advantage of conventional venography is that it serves both a diagnostic and a therapeutic role, mainly when the use of catheter-based thrombolytic therapy is contemplated.

## Arterial Thoracic Outlet Syndrome

In arterial TOS, examination may reveal varying degrees of arm or hand ischaemia including weakness, paraesthesias, pain and pallor. The pulses may diminish or disappear on positional changes, as is seen with the Adson test, but this sign is not pathognomonic as it lacks sensitivity and specificity.

Further investigations are also employed:

- A *chest X-ray* is essential in the work-up of arterial TOS since some patients with TOS have a bony abnormality.

- *Duplex ultrasonography* is useful in identifying subclavian artery stenosis or aneurysmal degeneration.
- *CT angiography* with three-dimensional reconstruction is now more commonly being used as it provides details of the vascular pathology along with the anatomical relationship between the vascular structures and the surrounding bone and muscle.
- *Arteriography* has a limited role in TOS. It is mainly employed when a patient has signs and symptoms suggestive of arterial insufficiency or ischaemia and when surgical intervention is being contemplated.

### Treatment

The management of TOS varies depending on its type, and intervention is only indicated in symptomatic patients.

## Neurogenic Thoracic Outlet Syndrome

With neurogenic TOS, management revolves around lifestyle modifications and physical therapy. This includes minimizing repetitive strenuous motion and following exercise regimens to promote relaxation of the neck muscles and increase their range of motion.

Anterior scalene block with local anaesthetic has been shown to relieve the symptoms by relaxing the anterior scalene muscle and alleviating tension on the brachial plexus. Surgical treatment such as resection of the first rib and anterior scalenectomy is reserved for patients who fail to improve or who develop progressive neurological weakness or disabling pain.

## Venous Thoracic Outlet Syndrome

The treatment of venous TOS is more aggressive and involves systemic anticoagulation and catheter-directed thrombolysis once the diagnosis has been made. Repeat venography is carried out after thrombolysis.

If there is compression and narrowing of the vein at the costoclavicular junction, patients should undergo thoracic outlet decompression via a first rib resection and anterior scalenectomy. Angioplasty and stenting are reserved for persistent stenosis following surgical decompression. In addition, a work-up for hypercoagulability should be undertaken in conjunction with this to decide on long-term anticoagulation and follow-up.

## Arterial Thoracic Outlet Syndrome

The treatment approach of arterial TOS depends on the severity and acuteness of the limb ischaemia. Severe ischaemia usually requires surgical embolectomy with or without thrombolysis. This is followed by thoracic outlet decompression and arterial reconstruction.

If the subclavian artery has a short affected segment, resection and primary anastomosis may be performed. If not, arterial reconstruction with an autologous vein is performed. Polytetrafluoroethylene and polyester grafts are also acceptable conduit options. Distal vascular occlusions due to chronic embolization may require a distal bypass.

# CONGENITAL VASCULAR DEFECTS

These defects may be either haemangiomas or vascular malformations, each with a different pathogenetic origin and outcome.

## HAEMANGIOMAS

Haemangiomas, although of vascular origin, result from cellular proliferation and differ from malformations that are embryonic developmental abnormalities representing errors of vascular morphogenesis. Table 32.2 illustrates the different characteristics of these two entities.

Haemangiomas usually become evident in the early neonatal period; approximately 80 per cent are single tumours and 20 per cent occur at multiple sites. The tumour proliferates in the superficial dermis, and the skin becomes raised, bosselated and a vivid crimson colour. If the haemangioma lies in the deeper dermis or the subcutaneous tissue, the overlying skin is slightly elevated with a bluish hue. The old terms cavernous haemangioma to describe a deep lesion and capillary haemangioma for a superficial one are confusing and best avoided.

Palpation makes it easier to differentiate a haemangioma from a venous malformation. A haemangioma is a fibrofatty structure and its contained blood cannot be completely evacuated by compression (Figure 32.15). By contrast, a venous malformation is soft and easily evacuated by compression; it enlarges with dependency and disappears with elevation of the involved limb.

A typical haemangioma grows rapidly over the first 6–8 months of life and reaches a plateau by 1 year. After this, signs of involution appear – the colour fades from vivid crimson to a dullish purple hue, the skin gradually gets paler, the tumour is less tense on palpation and its size slowly diminishes. Regression continues until the child reaches 5–10 years of age.

Infants with limb haemangiomas have a high risk of visceral lesions, mainly intrahepatic haemangiomas. These present with hepatomegaly, heart failure and anaemia.

Platelet trapping – **Kasabach–Merritt syndrome** – is another complication of cutaneous haemangiomas. The involved skin becomes deep reddish-purple, tense and shiny, and petechiae and ecchymoses are often seen overlying and adjacent to the haemangioma. Severe thrombocytopenia carries a risk of haemorrhage, either gastrointestinal, peritoneal, pleuropneumonic or intracranial. Other complications include local bleeding and ulceration. The bleeding, although frightening, can be controlled by 10 minutes' compression with a clean pad. Ulceration is rare and may be complicated by infection.

The site of the haemangioma may play an important role. For example, a small haemangioma in the eyelid can distort the growing cornea, producing astigmatism and amblyopia, and a subglottic haemangioma may be potentially life-threatening, presenting insidiously as biphasic stridor at 6–8 weeks of life. Large facial haemangiomas may grow to distort the normal anatomical structures.

## Vascular Malformations

Congenital vascular malformations are clinical syndromes that present with a variety of characteristics such as naevi (see p. 305), port wine stains (Figure 32.16), varicosities, hypertrophy or atrophy of the extremities and oedema. The majority of these malformations are recognizable in childhood, with an estimated

Table 32.2 Characteristics distinguishing haemangiomas from malformations

| Haemangioma | Vascular malformation |
| --- | --- |
| Usually not present at birth | All present at birth but not necessarily apparent |
| Rapid post-natal growth, slow evolution | Commensurate growth, may expand |
| Female to male ratio 3:1 to 5:1 | Female to male ratio 1:1 |
| Endothelial hyperplasia | Flat endothelium |
| Increased mast cells | Normal number of mast cells |
| Multi-laminated basement membrane | Thin, unlaminated basement membrane |
| Primary platelet trapping (Kasabach–Merritt syndrome) | Primary venous stasis Local/disseminated intravascular coagulopathy |
| Infrequent pressure on adjacent bone | Defects with arteriovenous fistula: hypertrophy |
| Rare overgrowth | Defects without arteriovenous fistula: atrophy |

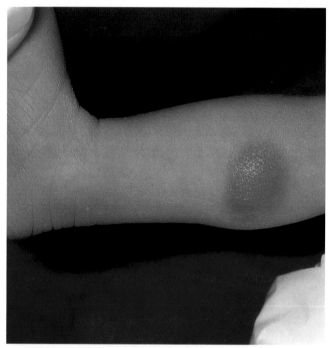

Figure 32.15 **Haemangioma of the right leg in an infant.**

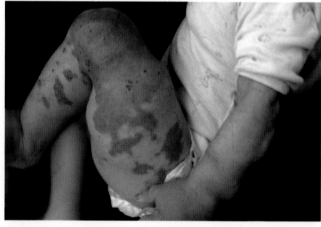

Figure 32.16 **Port wine stain of the lower extremity.**

prevalence of 1.2 per cent in all 3-year-old children routinely examined in hospital. They are the result of an interaction between genetic and environmental factors, and these factors are incorporated into the Hamburg classification (Table 32.3). This abandons less descriptive terms such as Klippel–Trenaunay and Parkes–Weber syndromes.

Although cutaneous vascular malformations are present at birth, not all are necessarily obvious:

*   A *capillary malformation*, or port wine stain, is visible in a neonate.
*   *Lymphatic malformations* (Figure 32.17) are usually seen in the nursery or become evident within the first year of life, only a small number appearing in childhood.
*   *Venous malformations* appear at birth or during childhood or adolescence.
*   *Arteriovenous fistulae* give rise to signs during childhood or adolescence.

These lesions grow in parallel with the child but sometimes suddenly expand, as seen, for example, with a lymphatic lesion complicated by a viral or bacterial infection. This also occurs when a venous lesion thromboses, or when venous and arteriovenous lesions are affected by hormonal changes.

In general, the lesions are macular and sharply demarcated, ranging from pale pink to deep red in colour. The overlying skin is normal in texture, and varicosities, ectasias or localized spongy masses may be evident. In the early stages, a pink stain and an increased temperature of the surrounding skin are the only signs suggestive of an arteriovenous malformation. Distended veins gradually appear, a thrill can be felt and an audible bruit can be heard (Figure 32.18). Eventually, local pain and dystrophic skin changes manifest an ischaemic state.

Limb hypertrophy or atrophy may occur. Malformations with arteriovenous fistulae are associated with hypertrophy, whereas atrophy is commonly seen with arteriovenous fistulae.

Pathophysiologically, the diversion of blood from the arterial to the venous circulation through the fistulae results in distal hypoxia. Hypoxia and venostasis increase the precipitation of calcium phosphate, enhancing osteoblastic activity. Bone atrophy can be explained by both mechanical (increased vascular pressure on the bone metaphysis in childhood) and haemodynamic

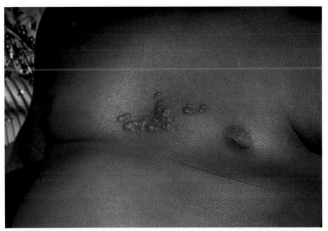

Figure 32.17 Lymphatic vesicles from a local lymphatic abnormality of the chest wall.

(a reduction in the distal circulation due to arterial and/or venous hypoplasia) factors.

In a **congenital arteriovenous fistula**, the lower extremity is the most common site, followed by the upper extremity, the head and the neck in decreasing order of frequency. Presentation at a young age is usual. Common signs include the following:

*   A *leg ulcer*. This is frequently the presenting lesion. This is sometimes known as a hot ulcer because the surrounding skin feels warmer than normal due to the diversion of blood. It is often extremely painful.
*   *Varicose veins and port wine discoloration* of the skin (Figure 32.19). This combination is always extremely suggestive of an arteriovenous fistula.
*   *Local gigantism*. If, as frequently occurs, the arteriovenous connections are widespread and the patient is young, an increased length and girth of the limb occurs (Figure 32.20). Care must be taken not to attribute the inequality of limb lengths – and the scoliosis that follows – to shortness of the unaffected leg.
*   *Increased local warmth*. The extremity is appreciably warmer and usually moister than that on the unaffected side.

Table 32.3 Hamburg classification of congenital vascular defects

| Type | Forms | |
| --- | --- | --- |
| | **Truncular** | **Extratruncular** |
| Predominantly arterial defects | Aplasia or obstructive Dilation | Infiltrating or limited |
| Predominantly venous defects | Aplasia or obstructive Dilation | Infiltrating or limited |
| Predominantly lymphatic defects | Aplasia or obstructive | Infiltrating or limited |
| Predominantly arteriovenous shunting defects | Deep or superficial | Infiltrating or limited |
| Combined/mixed vascular defects | Arterial and venous, no arteriovenous shunt Haemolymphatic, with or without an arterio-venous shunt | Infiltrating haemolymphatic or limited haemolymphatic |

PART 7 | VASCULAR

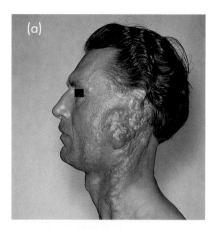

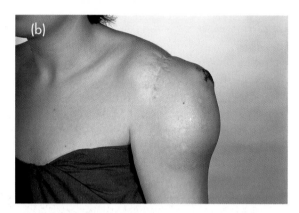

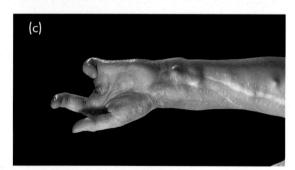

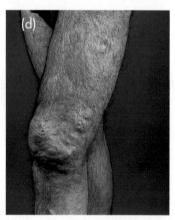

Figure 32.18 Arteriovenous malformations. (a) The left ear. (b) The shoulder. (c) The left hand. Proximal shunting has caused distal ischaemia requiring amputation of the middle and ring fingers. (d) The left leg.

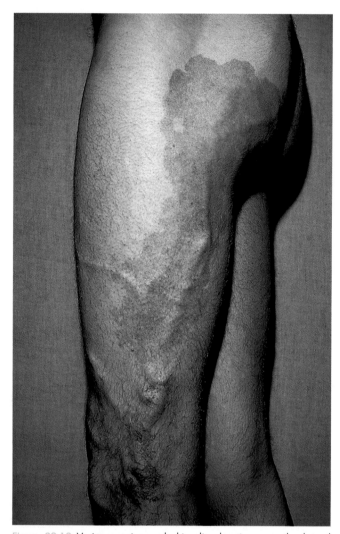

Figure 32.19 Varicose veins and skin discoloration over the lateral aspect of the left leg.

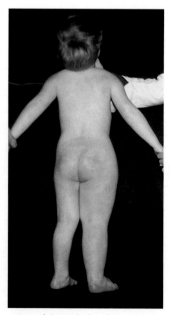

Figure 32.20 Gigantism of the right leg due to a vascular malformation.

- A *collapsing arterial pulse* (Corrigan's pulse). This can be demonstrated on the foot pulses of the affected limb.
- A *bradycardic reaction*. Digital occlusion of the main artery to the limb is followed by a slowing of the pulse rate, indicating that a considerable volume of blood is being short-circuited (**Branham's sign**).
- A *machinery murmur*. Using a stethoscope applied over the fistula, a continuous high-pitched bruit with systolic accentuation is pathognomonic.

There are two varieties of congenital arteriovenous fistula – localized and diffuse. In the diffuse variety, which is relatively common, the arteriovenous communications are deep and clinically indiscernible, probably being sited in the bone. In these, high-flow signs are absent.

Acquired arteriovenous fistulae result from injuries, usually stab wounds or through-and-through gun shot wounds. The superficial situation of the involved vessels often enables the clinician to palpate the resultant aneurysmal arterial dilatation (Figure 32.21). The signs of an aneurysm (see p. 482) may be present. The other signs of an arteriovenous fistula described above can also be observed. In addition, the fistula may have been surgically fashioned for access, for example in haemodialysis (Figure 32.22).

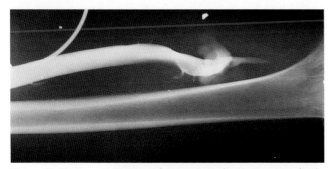

Figure 32.21 An arteriogram of an acquired arteriovenous fistula of the right femoral artery and vein. Note the arterial dilatation, the early venous filling and the residual metal fragments from the original shrapnel injury.

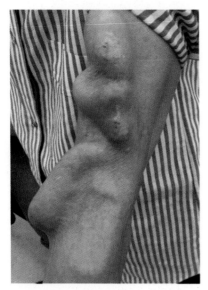

Figure 32.22 Venous dilatation following an arteriovenous fistula fashioned for haemodialysis.

## LEG ULCERS

Ulceration is a common lower limb pathology of diverse aetiology that often causes considerable disability (Figure 32.23). In general, the prevalence increase with age, from 0.5 per cent in patients over 40 to 2 per cent in those over 80, implying that an increase can be anticipated in developed countries as the proportion of elderly people rises. Pain, an offensive smell, time off work, loss of a job and social isolation are only some of the problems these patients encounter.

It is very important to take a detailed history as ulceration has a large variety of causes (Table 32.4). However, always bear in mind that 95 per cent of ulcers are of vascular origin. Previous deep venous thrombosis and/or the presence of varicose veins suggests primary or secondary chronic venous insufficiency and

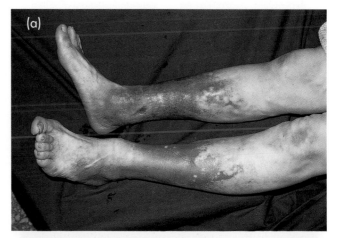

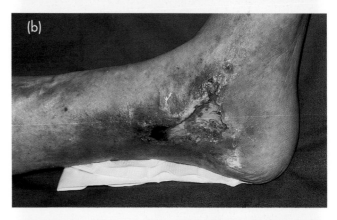

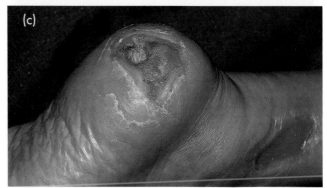

Figure 32.23 (See p. 510.)

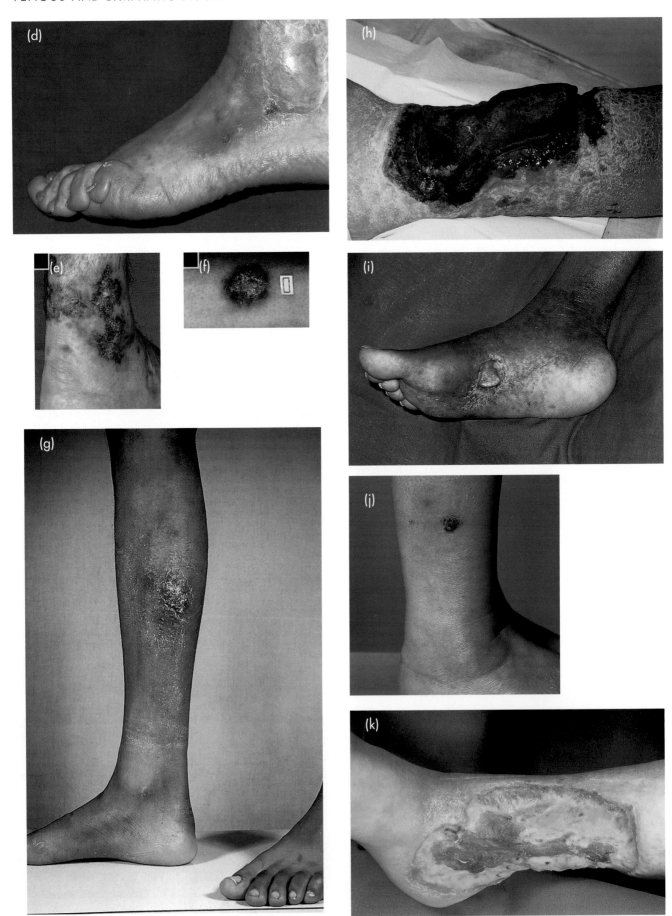

Figure 32.23 (See p. 510.)

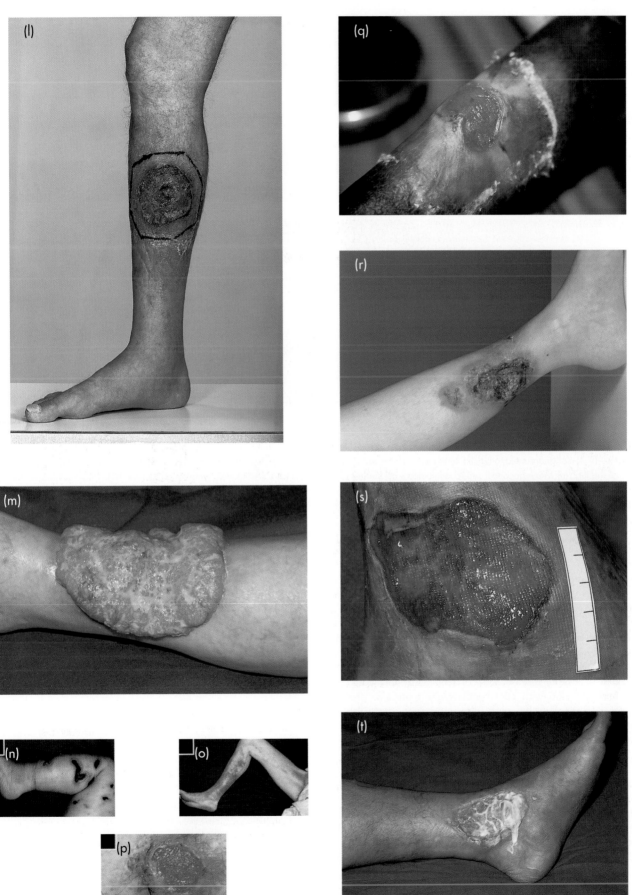

Figure 32.23 (See p. 510.)

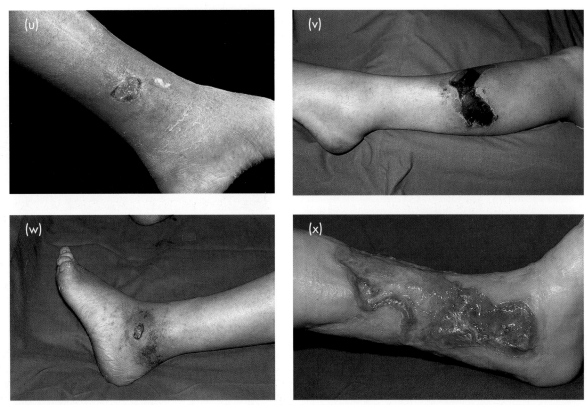

**Figure 32.23** Leg ulcers. (a) A healing venous ulcer on the right medial shin. (b) A mixed venous and arterial ulcer on the left malleolar region. (c) A typical ischaemic ulcer of the heel. (d) A vasculitic ulcer on the lateral aspect of the left foot. (e) Allergic vasculitis. (f) Necrobiosis lipoidica in a diabetic patient. (g) A healing ulcer in a patient with sickle cell disease. (h) A leukaemic ulcer following chemo- and radiotherapy. (i) Kaposi's sarcoma. (j) A malignant melanoma. (k) Malignant change in a chronic lower leg ulcer. (l) Squamous cell carcinoma. (m) A fungating malignant ulcer of the leg. (n) Meningococcal septicaemic ulcers on the leg of an infant. (o) Cellulitis with lymphangitis of the leg. (p) A gumma of the right leg. (q) A tropical ulcer. (r) A leg ulcer in a patient with inflammatory bowel disease. (s) An ulcer in a patient with rheumatoid arthritis. (t) An ulcer in a patient with scleroderma. (u) A healing ulcer following a cat bite. (v) An eschar following to the left shin. (w) An ulcer resulting from frostbite. (x) An artefactual ulcer of the left leg.

causes ulcers in the gaiter area, immediately above the medial (and far less commonly the lateral) malleolus. The ulcer is associated with swelling, skin pigmentation and induration, all suggestive of venous hypertension. The surrounding skin is warm and moist.

A history of intermittent claudication or rest pain, with an absence of palpable arterial pulses, is suggestive of ischaemic arterial disease. An ankle–brachial index of less than 0.9, as measured using a portable Doppler device, will confirm the presence of arterial disease. Loss of hair, dystrophic nails and pale and cold skin with poor capillary filling are also present. However, a swollen leg with skin induration may also be present if the patient keeps the leg dependent for pain relief in profound ischaemia.

Ischaemic ulcers tend to be dry, painful and deep, exposing tendons, fascia and bones. They more commonly develop on the foot but can also occur at any site on the leg, mainly the anterior aspect, where they can persist and enlarge following minor trauma. Mixed ulcers, with coexisting arterial and venous elements, make up 12 per cent of all ulcers and add to the difficulty of diagnosis.

**Diabetes mellitus** can cause neuropathic or neuroischaemic ulcers that result in an acute localized inflammatory condition affecting the deep soft tissues and bones, also known as a Charcot ulcer (Figure 32.24). Although it is difficult to exclude

**Table 32.4 Causes of leg ulcers**

| | |
|---|---|
| Vascular | Venous insufficiency (primary or secondary) |
| | Arterial obstructive disease |
| | Arteriovenous malformation |
| | Vasculitis |
| Neuropathic | Diabetes mellitus |
| | Alcohol |
| | Syringomyelia |
| | Paralysis |
| Haematological | Sickle cell disease |
| | Leukaemia |
| | Haemolytic jaundice |
| Malignant | Kaposi's sarcoma |
| | Melanoma |
| | Basal cell carcinoma |
| | Epithelioma |
| Miscellaneous | Infection |
| | Syphilis |
| | Tropical |
| | Pyoderma gangrenosum |
| | Skin diseases |
| | Rheumatoid arthritis |
| | Pressure sores |
| | Trauma/burns |
| | Artefactual |

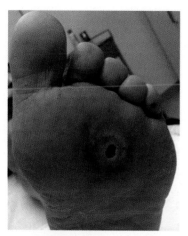

Figure 32.24 Charcot ulcer.

a neuropathic element in diabetic ulcers, there are differences between these two types of lesion. A painless ulcer located over the metatarsal heads on the sole of the foot with warm skin on the foot and palpable pedal pulses is more likely to be purely neuropathic in origin. Sensory impairment in the foot, mainly related to pain and temperature change, is very likely to be evident. Diabetic ulcers have a tendency to become infected. However, ischaemia should be suspected in ulcers that show no evidence of healing after 2 weeks of antibiotic therapy and local care.

**Skin cancer** may be the causative problem in long-standing ulcers without any tendency to heal, especially when they develop in the area of a previous burn or chronic ulceration (**Marjolin's ulcer**). Features that suggest this diagnosis are unusual or over-abundant granulation and rolled irregular edges. If there is any suspicion of cancer, the ulcer should be biopsied.

**Artefactual (fictitious) ulcers** are self-induced lesions from which the patient benefits, perhaps through increased attention or being the subject of litigation. They are usually produced on exposed sites by scratching with the nails or with various implements, or by cigarette burns. They should be suspected when ulcers are of unusual or artefactual shapes, show delayed healing or have a good healing edge and underlying granulation, or when unusual organisms are identified. Once suspected, an ulcer can be sealed and healing expected, provided continued trauma is not applied through or under the dressing.

## SWOLLEN LEG

Oedema represents an increase in tissue fluid and may affect any of the limbs or the whole body. When the oedema is generalized and symmetrical, the cause is a systemic abnormality, whereas in localized swelling a local cause should be suspected.

In general, oedema represents an imbalance between capillary filtration and lymphatic drainage. One function of the lymphatic system is to compensate for increases in capillary filtration; it therefore has a substantial role in the development of oedema. However, this does not mean that all oedemas are lymphoedemas, as the latter only occur when the lymphatic system fails to drain the tissue fluid produced by normal capillary filtration.

The pathophysiology of other forms of oedema is a redistribution of fluid from the arterial to the venous end of the capillaries (Starling's law). Venous hypertension and cardiac failure increase the pressure in the postcapillary venules, resulting in a back-diffusion of fluid into the interstitial tissues. When the permeability of the capillaries increases, for example in an allergic reaction, there is a exudation of protein-rich fluid into the tissues. Hypoproteinaemia reduces plasma osmolarity, with an increase in capillary diffusion.

The causes of swelling can be classified as:

- *General.* These are due to fluid retention and can cause either acute or chronic swelling. Examples are heart failure, renal failure and hypoproteinaemia (from liver failure or malnutrition).
- *Local.* These are due to venous or lymphatic insufficiency, inflammatory causes and a few uncommon conditions:
  - *Acute conditions* are DVT, allergy, cellulitis, snake and insect bites, trauma and rheumatoid arthritis.
  - *Chronic conditions* are venous insufficiency (primary or secondary), lymphoedema (primary or secondary), congenital vascular malformations, dependency of the limb and chronic oedema with cyanosis (*oedem bleu*).

### Clinical Signs

When oedema is widespread in the limb and body, it is likely to be due to a systemic cause (heart or renal failure, hypoproteinaemia). Swelling present in both lower limbs or in both upper limbs and the face indicates inferior or superior vena cava syndrome due to local disease in the abdomen or chest causing obstruction of the venous outflow. Unilateral swelling of a limb indicates local problems proximal to the upper limit of the swelling. If the feet are spared from the swelling, it is more likely to be venous than lymphatic. Lipoedema, that is, excess subcutaneous fat, also spares the feet.

Varicose veins, lipodermatosclerosis, skin pigmentation and ulcers in the gaiter area are suggestive of venous insufficiency. Hyperkeratosis, thickened skin and enhanced skin creases resembling elephant hide are characteristic of lymphoedema, hence the term elephantiasis for this condition.

**Pitting oedema** is usually systemic in origin. However, it is wrong to say that it cannot be lymphoedema because, in the early stages, lymphoedema does pit.

The **Kaposi–Stemmer sign** is the inability to pick up or pinch a fold of skin at the base of the second toe and is characteristic of lymphoedema.

## LYMPHOEDEMA

### Lymphatic Anatomy

The lymphatic drainage of the lower body, gastrointestinal tract and left upper body enters the venous circulation between the left subclavian vein and the left internal jugular vein through the left thoracic duct. Similarly, the right thoracic duct drains the right upper body and joins the venous circulation at the right subclavian vein or between this and the right internal jugular vein.

The upper and lower extremities possess both superficial and deep lymphatic channels. The superficial system drains the skin and subcutaneous tissue, while the deep system drains the muscles and bones. The two systems of the upper extremities merge in the axilla, and those of the lower extremities merge in the pelvis.

Lymph flow takes place in a low-pressure system that starts in lymphatic capillaries in the interstitial space and is facilitated by skeletal muscle contraction, unidirectional valves and smooth muscles. As such, lymphoedema occurs when the lymphatic load exceeds the transport capacity of the lymphatic system. This leads to the interstitial accumulation of protein-rich filtered fluid in the extravascular tissue, with subsequent water retention and swelling of the affected limb.

## Classification

Lymphoedema is classified as primary or secondary depending on the underlying aetiology.

**Primary lymphoedema** results from an inherited or congenital pathological development of the lymphatic vessels and is further classified according to the age of onset. Congenital lymphoedema occurs from birth and up to 2 years of age (Figure 32.25). Lymphoedema praecox occurs during puberty or pregnancy and up to 35 years of age. Late lymphoedema that presents after the age of 35 is termed lymphoedema tarda (Figure 32.26).

The incidence of primary lymphoedema is around 1 per 100 000 individuals, with unilateral involvement of the extremities seen in two-thirds of cases. The typical cause is dysplasia or hypoplasia of the lymphatic channels, most likely due to genetic mutations.

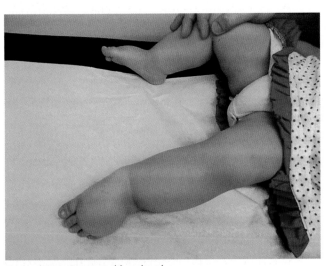

Figure 32.25 Congenital lymphoedema.

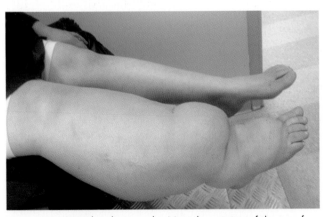

Figure 32.26 Lymphoedema tarda. Note the sparing of the toes from swelling.

**Secondary lymphoedema** (Figure 32.27) occurs as a result of acquired conditions that cause interruption, obstruction or infiltration of the lymphatic outflow channels. These include surgical ligation or excision combined with extensive nodal dissection and radiation therapy for cancer, compression of the lymphatic outflow channels by a tumour or nodes, tumour cell infiltration of the lymphatic vessels (lymphangitic carcinomatosis) or parasitic infections (filariasis). Other factors that have been associated with the development of lymphoedema are older age, obesity and inflammatory arthritis.

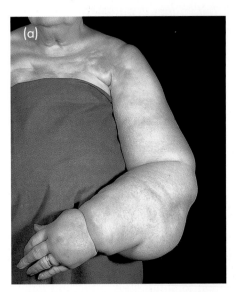

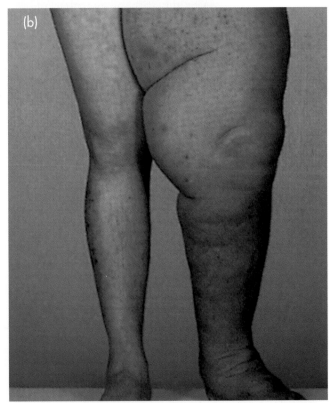

Figure 32.27 Secondary lymphoedema following the excision of regional lymph nodes and subsequent radiotherapy. (a) Malignant disease of the right breast. (b) Malignancy of the left ureter.

## Presentation

Lymphoedema affects the lower extremities in up to 80 per cent of patients with the condition. It usually follows an insidious course, with patients initially reporting pain, tightness and/or a sense of heaviness in the affected limb.

Swelling is first seen in the distal part of the extremity. It starts as pitting oedema, reflecting the accumulation of interstitial fluid in the early stages of lymphoedema. The toes are typically spared from the swelling. Over time, however, proximal involvement ensues and fibrosis and adipose tissue deposition take place, resulting in the characteristic non-pitting oedema. As the oedema progresses, patients may complain of restricted motion of the affected limb.

Skin changes are also seen in the later stages of lymphoedema secondary to dermal thickening, giving the characteristic peau d'orange appearance. Skin infections such as recurrent cellulitis, lymphangitis and ulceration are also seen with a higher prevalence with chronic lymphoedema. The development of ulceration or new changes in a limb after prolonged lymphoedema should raise a suspicion of transformation into lymphangiosarcoma.

## Diagnosis

The diagnosis of lymphoedema can most often be obtained by taking a through history and performing a focused physical examination targeting the vascular system, skin and lymph nodes. It can be confirmed by taking circumferential measurements of the affected limb at certain points and comparing them with the contralateral one. A difference of more than 2 cm is considered clinically significant.

In patients whose physical examinations are unreliable, such as obese patients, other methods can be used to confirm the diagnosis. These include optoelectronic volumetry, which measures the limb volume using infrared measurements, and bioimpedance spectroscopy, in which resistance measurements are used to compare the composition of the fluid compartments.

Imaging studies such as CT and MRI can be useful diagnostic tools in the work-up for lymphoedema. They can demonstrate accumulations of fluid within the soft tissue, skin thickening and the accumulation of subcutaneous oedema, in addition to delineating any obstructing lesions causing compression or occlusion of the lymphatic channels.

Lymphoscintigraphy is a technique in which subcutaneous or intradermal radioactive tracers are injected into the web space of the extremities, followed by repeated imaging to assess the flow of fluid from the skin to the lymph nodes and identify any impaired or delayed flow. However, this technique is not standardized, its results are not easily interpreted, and it rarely changes the management, thereby limiting its use.

## Treatment

There is no definitive cure for lymphoedema, and therapy is aimed at reducing pain, restoring the functionality of the affected extremity and preventing future infections. Treatment should be started as early as possible before fibrotic changes take place in the interstitium. Conservative measures include limb elevation, physical therapy, multilayer compression bandages, lymphatic massage and drainage, compression stockings and pneumatic pumps. In cases of secondary lymphoedema, the underlying cause should be addressed.

Surgical treatment is reserved for patients who do not improve with conservative measures or for cases in which the size of the extremity increases to such an extent that it impairs the patient's daily activities. One example is the Charles procedure, which involves the total excision of all skin and subcutaneous tissue from the affected extremity, followed by grafting of the underlying fascia using the skin that has been excised. Microsurgical techniques for lymphatic disorders can also be utilized in specific clinical scenarios.

### Key Points

- Venous insufficiency may affect the superficial venous system, the deep venous system or both.
- Venous thrombosis is precipitated by stasis, trauma or hypercoagulability, and may affect the superficial venous system, the deep venous system or both.
- Chronic venous insufficiency has a wide range of presentations, ranging from leg heaviness, swelling and itching to varicosities, skin thickening, hyperpigmentation and ulcerations.
- Varicose veins are a very common manifestation of chronic venous insufficiency. They vary in size from spider veins and telangiectasias to large varicosities affecting the saphenous veins and their branches.
- Anatomical compression of the venous system can cause chronic venous injury that leads to deep venous thrombosis. In the upper extremity, compression of the thoracic outlet by the anterior scalene muscle leads to axillary vein thrombosis. In the lower extremity, compression of the left common iliac vein by the right common iliac artery leads to iliofemoral DVT.
- Primary lymphoedema is due to dysplasia or hypoplasia of the lymphatic channels and can present at birth, in adolescence or in adulthood.
- Secondary lymphoedema is the most common form of lymphoedema and is due to either surgical interruption or infiltration and compression of the lymphatic channels.
- Vascular malformations can affect the capillaries, venous system or lymphatic system.

## SBAs

**1.** A 31-year-old woman presents with bulging veins in her left lower extremity. These veins became prominent during her first pregnancy and worsened after her second. She denies any history of deep venous thrombosis. On physical examination, she has enlarged veins along the distribution of the great saphenous vein and its branches below the knee. This patient is likely to be suffering from which one of the following?:

a  Subacute deep venous thrombosis
b  May–Thurner syndrome
c  Venous insufficiency affecting the great saphenous vein and saphenofemoral junction
d  Congenital arteriovenous fistula
e  Superficial venous thrombophlebitis

Answer
c  *Venous insufficiency affecting the great saphenous vein and saphenofemoral junction. The patient's symptoms and examination suggest venous insufficiency, which is typically exacerbated by pregnancy.*

**2.** A 53-year-old school teacher presents with an ulcer over his right medial malleolus. It started after he accidentally hit a sharp corner of a table a month ago. He has been suffering from swelling and discomfort in that leg for years following a fracture of his right leg sustained during a car crash. On physical examination, the skin over the medial aspect of his leg is brown and indurated. The leg is woody and swollen. He has palpable femoral, popliteal and pedal pulses. This patient is most likely to be suffering from which one of the following?:

a  Acute deep venous thrombosis
b  Superficial thrombophlebitis of the saphenous vein with ulcerated varicosity
c  Deep venous insufficiency with venous stasis ulcerations
d  Arterial insufficiency
e  Lymphoedema with superimposed cellulitis

Answer
c  *Deep venous insufficiency with venous stasis ulcerations. The location of the ulcer over the medial malleolus in the setting of chronic swelling and chronic skin changes points to venous stasis ulcerations with underlying deep venous insufficiency.*

**3.** A 47-year-old woman presents because of pain and redness over the medial aspect of her left thigh. She denies any trauma. She has recently been placed on hormone therapy for menopausal symptoms. On physical examination, an indurated cord-like structure is seen that is tender, hot and red. The patient also has several varicosities over the medial aspect of her thigh and below her knee. This patient is most likely to be suffering from which one of the following:?

a  Phlegmasia cerulea dolens
b  Acute superficial thrombophlebitis
c  Deep venous insufficiency
d  Acute cellulitis
e  Acute lymphangitis

Answer
b  *Acute superficial thrombophlebitis. The finding of an indurated cord-like structure that is tender, hot and red, in the setting of varicose veins and hormone therapy, is suggestive of acute superficial thrombophlebitis.*

# PART

# 8

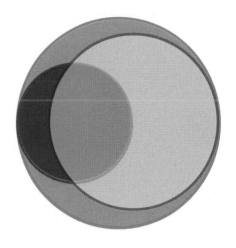

# Abdominal

# The Abdominal Wall, Umbilicus and Groin

Evgeny V. Arshava

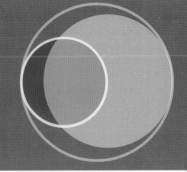

## LEARNING OBJECTIVES

- To understand the anatomy of the abdominal wall, umbilicus and groin
- To be able to describe the common pathological processes found in these regions

## INTRODUCTION

The abdominal wall has several important functions, which are reflected in its anatomy. It accounts for approximately 10 per cent of the total body surface area. It provides protection and support for the underlying organs, allows complex movements of the trunk, and participates in the respiratory cycle and functions of the intra-abdominal organs.

The umbilicus is a scar formed when the umbilical cord heals. It is a point at which the skin is adherent to the underlying fascia, without any intervening fatty tissue. The groins are sites of hernia formation (see Chapter 34) and pathological enlargement of the lymph nodes.

This chapter provides an introduction to the anatomy and pathology of these areas. It should be read in preparation for reading Chapter 34.

## THE ABDOMINAL WALL

The anatomical nomenclature of the skin and subcutaneous tissues is confusing. Under the skin is a fatty layer of subcutaneous fibroadipose tissue. This is traditionally divided into the superficial and deep layers because they possess different morphological and mechanical characteristics. They are separated by a membranous superficial fascia (commonly called Scarpa's) that stretches across the entire abdomen, but is less prominent in the upper and midline areas. The superficial fatty layer is thicker in most subjects, while the deep layer is more metabolically active and undergoes greater changes with weight loss and gain (**Figure 33.1**).

The paired rectus muscles, and laterally the three layers of the oblique abdominal muscles and their aponeuroses, provide complex motor function. In the lower abdomen, the posterior rectus sheath ends at the arcuate line. The transversalis fascia and peritoneum further cover the underlying organs.

While the nerve supply of the abdominal wall has a segmental dermatome pattern, the vascular supply has extensive collaterals.

The lymphatic drainage of the anterior abdominal wall is divided into the infraumbilical and supraumbilical networks. The

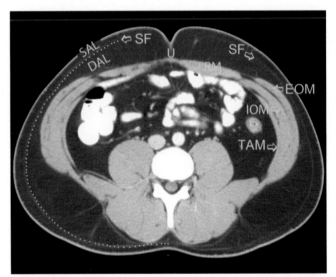

Figure 33.1 Anatomy of the abdominal wall SF, superficial fascia; SAL, superficial adipose layer; DAL, deep adipose layer; U, umbilicus; RM, rectus abdominis muscle; EOM, external oblique muscle; IOM, internal oblique muscle; TAM, transversus abdominis muscle.

superficial lymphatics of the infraumbilical region drain to the superficial inguinal lymph nodes, while the deeper layers may drain into the aortic nodes. The superficial supraumbilical lymphatics drain into the axillary, pectoral and infraclavicular lymph nodes, and the deep network drains to the internal mammary nodes.

A thorough examination of the abdomen should begin with visual inspection and auscultation, followed by palpation and percussion.

**Carnett's sign** may help to localize the origin of chronic abdominal pain. Ask the patient to tense their abdominal muscles (either by lifting their head and shoulders, or by raising both their legs with straight knees from the examination table). A positive test (no change or an increase in pain) suggests that the abdominal wall is the origin of the pain, for example from a rectus sheath haematoma, muscle strain or tumour, pathology of the sensory nerves or an abdominal wall hernia. A negative test (a decrease in abdominal pain) indicates intra-abdominal pathology. Acute pathology of the intra-abdominal organs resulting in inflammation of the parietal peritoneum (see the signs of peritoneal inflammation in Chapter 36) may give false-positive results, so Carnett's sign is more helpful in the differential diagnosis of chronic abdominal pain.

The entire spectrum of dermatological pathology, including any neoplastic or immune-mediated conditions, infections and other skin diseases, can affect the abdomen. Most of these entities are beyond the scope of this chapter (see Chapter 18).

## Striae

Abdominal striae, or stretch marks, are a form of skin scarring secondary to disruption of the dermis. They occur when the tensile force on the skin exceeds its elasticity. Striae develop during the periods of rapid stretching of the skin and are of cosmetic significance only. Dermal structure and elasticity are affected by multiple factors, including hormonal changes and genetics. Teenagers are at increased risk of developing prominent striae. Striae are commonly seen in pregnancy (striae gravidarum), but may be seen in a number of other conditions, including obesity and the use of glucocorticoid hormones. They are usually pink (pregnancy) or purplish (Cushing's disease) in colour and fade with time to a whitish hue.

## Scars

Abdominal scars are the permanent marks of a previous operation or injury. Their prominence varies from subtle small lines after laparoscopic operations to unsightly keloids. The size and location of scars vary, but they may provide some insight into the nature of the intervention that was performed (Figures 33.2 and 33.3).

## Infection

Infection in the soft tissue of the abdominal wall can vary from furuncles and superficial cellulitis, to localized abscesses and life-threatening necrotizing acute soft tissue infection (NASTI). NASTI presents with severe sepsis and pronounced tenderness of the abdominal wall.

In the postoperative or trauma patient, spreading infection across the abdominal wall may be a grave sentinel sign of underlying polymicrobial necrotizing soft tissue infection (type I) involving the deep muscle and fascia, secondary to intra-abdominal sepsis or enteric leak. Necrotizing soft tissue infection affecting the perineal area (Fournier's gangrene) may also extend onto the abdominal wall (Figure 33.4). Thus, careful examination of the perineum is mandatory in such patients. Like other infections caused by coliforms and anaerobes, Fournier's gangrene has a very characteristic strong foul odour and may show subcutaneous crepitus.

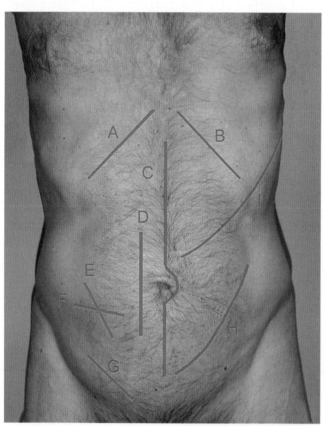

Figure 33.2 Common vertical and oblique abdominal incisions: A, right subcostal (cholecystectomy and bile duct surgery); B, left subcostal (splenectomy); C, midline laparotomy; D, right paramedian; E and F, right lower quadrant (appendectomy); G, right inguinal (groin hernia repair); H, left lower quadrant oblique (kidney transplant or pelvic surgery); I, left thoracoabdominal.

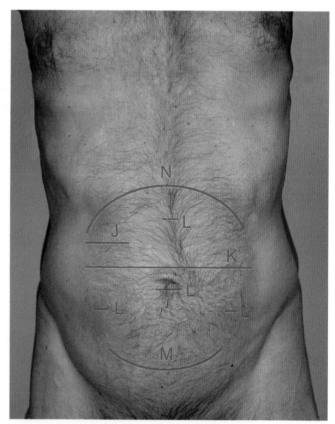

Figure 33.3 Common transverse abdominal incisions: J, right upper quadrant (ventriculoperitoneal shunt); K, transverse; L, examples of laparoscopic incisions; M, Pfannenstiel incision (common in gynaecology); N, bilateral subcostal (roof top).

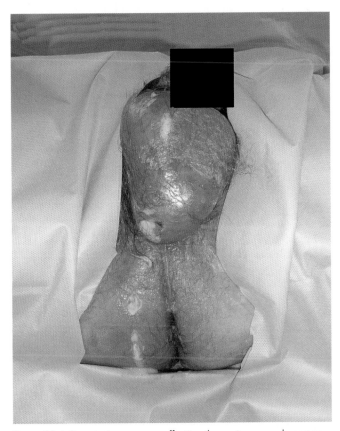

Figure 33.4 Fournier's gangrene affecting the perineum and scrotum.

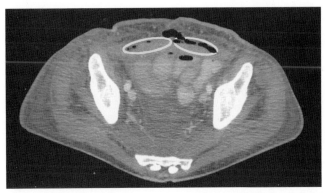

Figure 33.5 Polymicrobial necrotizing soft tissue infection of the abdominal wall in a patient with fistulizing Crohn's disease. The contours of the rectus abdominis muscle sheaths are outlined. Air is present in both the subcutaneous and subfascial plains.

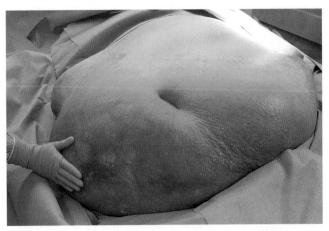

Figure 33.6 Group A streptococcal acute necrotizing soft tissue infection of the right abdominal wall, with characteristic oedema and epidermolysis in a morbidly obese patient.

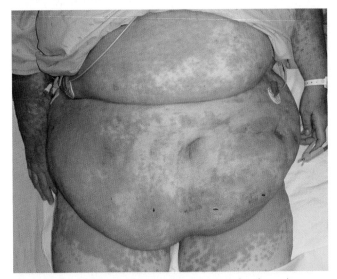

Figure 33.7 Example of a benign rash (acute generalized exanthematous pustulosis) involving the abdomen as a reaction to a course of antibiotics. Note the lack of oedema and the discontinuous pattern of a non-tender rash.

Clostridial and other anaerobic organisms (**gas gangrene**) may affect the superficial and deep fascia and the muscle layers, or the entire wall. This is most commonly part of a polymicrobial infection, but it may also present as a monomicrobial infection. On physical examination, crepitus secondary to gas bubbles within the abdominal wall, along with the tissue necrosis, is characteristically present (**Figure 33.5**). It should be noted that after abdominal operations, especially laparoscopic surgery, air may be present within the abdominal wall during the early post-operative period. Such crepitus is of no clinical significance.

Limited NASTI of the superficial fascia, fatty layer and skin is commonly monomicrobial (type II), and occurs in immunocompromised or morbidly obese patients (**Figure 33.6**). This type is less common on the torso than that found on the extremities, but it has the same characteristics. The entry point for the infection may be minimal or occult. Depending on the stage, skin changes can vary from erythema to purple discoloration.

Distinguishing NASTI from cellulitis in the early stages is of paramount importance, but may be very difficult. Characteristic oedema, induration of the tissues and severe pain are the hallmarks of this morbid disease. With advanced disease, blistering develops secondary to inflammatory changes within the subcutaneous plane and thrombosis of the vascular network. A positive **Nikolsky's sign** (separation of the epidermis at the basal layer with rubbing of the skin) precedes spontaneous blistering. Epidermolysis signifies an irreversible stage of disease requiring surgical intervention.

Other dermatological conditions may affect the abdominal wall and also have a dramatic appearance, but these can be distinguished from NASTI based on their lack of physical characteristics and signs of sepsis (**Figure 33.7**).

## Bleeding

**Bruising (ecchymosis)** or **haematomas** of the abdominal wall develop due to trauma or the use of prophylactic and therapeutic anticoagulation or illicit drug injection.

Bruising of a surgical site is not rare. Bruising around a post-operative incision evolves in a pattern of colour changes from erythema to greenish and yellowish hues. Bruising in the early stages may have the same colour as cellulitis, but will not have the oedema and the characteristic tenderness of infection. Superficial rubbing with the finger usually produces pain in cellulitis, and is generally painless in patients with bruising.

**Rectus sheath haematomas** develop acutely secondary to rupture of the inferior and, less commonly, superior epigastric arteries. Haematomas may occur in young individuals due to vigorous exercise, and may be also seen in pregnancy. Most commonly, they are spontaneous in nature and occur in patients with a coagulopathy. Such haematomas cause tenderness and fullness of the abdominal wall. There may or may not be visible changes in the overlying skin. Unless they are expanding or causing pressure changes in the skin, observation and the reversal of coagulopathy are sufficient. This condition may mimic acute intra-abdominal pathology (appendicitis, cholecystitis, incarcerated spigelian hernia and other conditions), and imaging may be essential for an accurate diagnosis (**Figure 33.8**).

Flank bruising secondary to a dissection of blood along the retroperitoneal plane can be seen in haemorrhagic pancreatitis (**Grey Turner's sign; Figure 33.9a**) or the rupture of an aortic or iliac artery aneurysm (**Figure 33.9b**). Similarly, periumbilical bruising may result from haemorrhagic pancreatitis (**Cullen's sign; Figure 33.10**), ruptured ectopic pregnancy or any other cause of haemoperitoneum.

## Masses

A variety of benign and malignant lesions can present as abdominal masses. It is important to determine whether the mass is intra-abdominal or located within the abdominal wall. An intra-abdominal mass may be palpable through relaxed abdominal muscles, but impalpable when the musculature is tense while

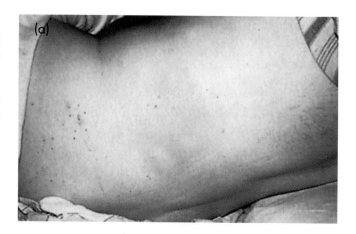

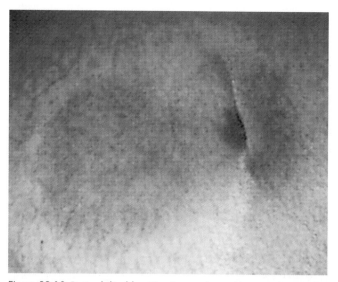

Figure 33.9 (a) Flank bruising in a patient with a haemorrhagic pancreatitis (Grey Turner's sign). (b) Flank bruising following the rupture of an abdominal aortic aneurysm.

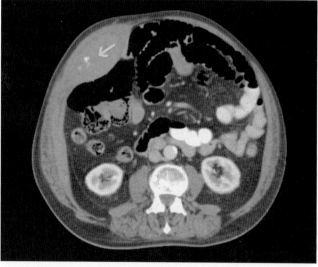

Figure 33.8 Right rectus sheath haematoma in a patient on anticoagulation, with an arrow pointing to the active extravasation of a contrast ('blush') from the inferior epigastric artery.

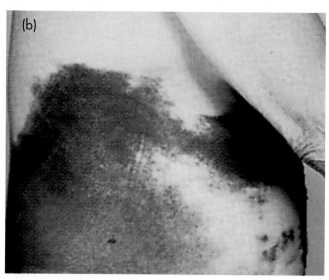

Figure 33.10 Periumbilical bruising in a patient with acute pancreatitis (Cullen's sign).

the legs are raised. An abdominal wall mass generally remains palpable with leg-raising.

Any soft tissue mass, benign or malignant, that is seen in other areas of the body may be encountered on the abdominal wall. Most benign lesions (inclusion cysts, lipomas, fibromas) are subcutaneous and are easily mobile (**Figure 33.11**). Benign subfascial masses on the other hand, and locally aggressive neoplasms such as sarcomas or desmoid tumours, can be suspected based on their lack of mobility relative to the surrounding tissues (**Figure 33.12**). Similarly, very rare mesotheliomas arising from the parietal peritoneum have the clinical signs of an intraperitoneal mass. Both subcutaneous and deep subfascial tumours may reach an impressive size before diagnosis.

**Endometriosis** of the abdominal wall is a rare condition in which endometrial implants develop in the umbilicus and other locations where there have been abdominal incisions. The principal manifestations of this condition are pain, swelling and bloody discharge if the lesion is superficial. The symptoms usually, but not always, follow the pattern of the patient's menstrual cycle.

Both hernias and lymphadenopathy should be part of a differential diagnosis when examining any patients with an abdominal wall mass. Groin and ventral hernias represent an important group of abdominal wall pathology and are discussed in Chapter 34. In the obese person, a large pannus (**Figure 33.13**) may easily cover and hide any groin pathology, including symptomatic incisional, inguinal or femoral hernias.

## INGUINAL LYMPH NODES

The number of superficial inguinal lymph nodes is variable, averaging between 10 and 20. They are located in the subcutaneous plane, and some may be easily palpated. The deep inguinal lymph nodes are fewer in number, and are located below the fascia lata along the femoral vein. They are not palpable unless enlarged.

Normal lymph nodes are no larger than 1.5 cm, mobile, soft and non-tender. Abnormal changes may be part of a generalized lymphadenopathy or represent a local reaction to pathology (inflammation or neoplasm) in regions whose lymphatic drainage is to the groin.

An assessment of inguinal lymphadenopathy must therefore include a review of constitutional symptoms and a thorough examination of the drainage basins of the inguinal lymph nodes (lower torso, lower extremity, perineum, anus, external genitalia) as well as other lymph node groups (neck, axillae). Imaging studies may also be indicated. If no primary source is found during the evaluation, one should also consider specific pathogens: cat-scratch disease, tuberculosis and sexually transmitted diseases

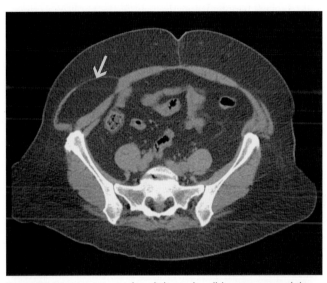

Figure 33.12 An intermuscular abdominal wall lipoma, not mobile on palpation.

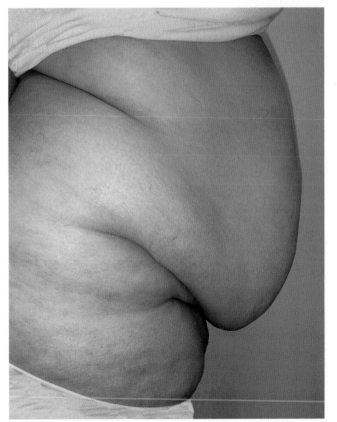

Figure 33.13 A large pannus may cover unsuspected groin pathology.

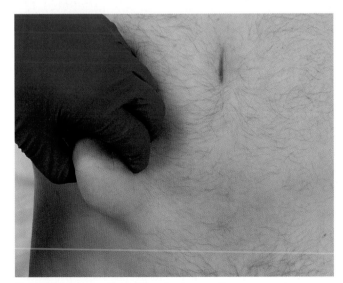

Figure 33.11 An easily mobile subcutaneous lipoma.

(HIV, syphilis, chancroid, lymphogranuloma venereum, granuloma inguinale).

The ongoing inflammation in cases of bacterial lymphadenitis may result in the formation of an abscess. Signs of a purulent lymphadenitis are erythema, oedema, tenderness and, if superficially located, fluctuation (**Figure 33.14a**). In rare cases, the retroperitoneal purulent process may dissect along the tissue planes into the groin, and mimic primary groin pathology or even a perirectal abscess.

**Malignant lymphadenopathy** may be the result of a primary lymphoma or of various metastatic lesions from regions draining to the inguinal lymph nodes (**Figure 33.14b**). Advanced cases may present with erosion of the affected lymph nodes through the skin (**Figure 33.14c**). On rare occasions, the primary lesion may not be identified (e.g. a metastatic melanoma with an unknown primary site).

## THE UMBILICUS

The umbilicus is the scar that forms during closure of the umbilical ring after the umbilical cord has separated. Inadequate healing and closure of the umbilical ring leads to hernia formation, which represents the most common umbilical pathology.

Umbilical hernias and conditions that occur in neonates, including omphalocele (exomphalos) and neonatal omphalitis, are discussed elsewhere in the text.

The umbilicus is an important anatomical landmark and is normally situated almost halfway between the xiphoid process

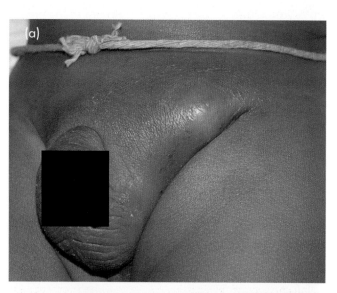

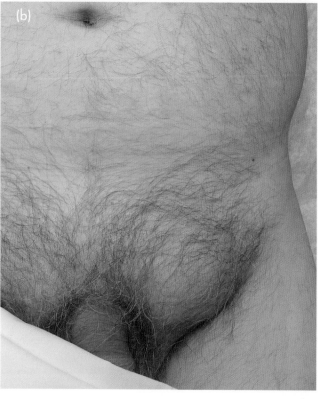

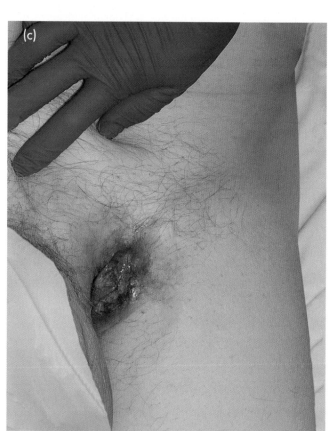

Figure 33.14 (a) Left inguinal purulent lymphadenitis in a child (courtesy of Graeme Pitcher, MD). (b) Squamous cell carcinoma of the anus with metastases in the left inguinal lymph nodes. (c) Erosion of inguinal lymphadenopathy through the skin in a patient with a B-cell lymphoma.

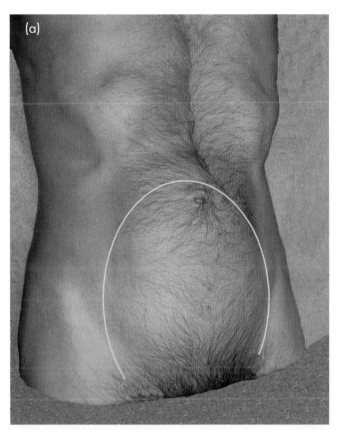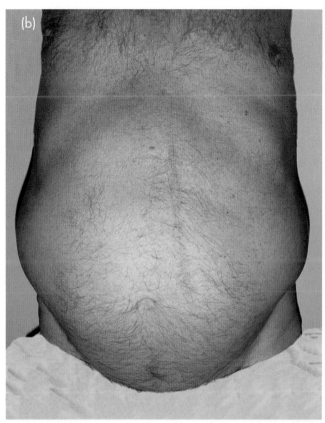

Figure 33.15 (a) Cephalad displacement of the umbilicus in a patient with a bladder outlet obstruction and distention (bladder contour outlined). (b) Caudad displacement of the umbilicus in a patient with bowel obstruction.

Table 33.1 Abnormalities of the umbilicus

| Aetiology | Example |
|---|---|
| Congenital | Omphalocele |
| | Patent omphalomesenteric (vitellointestinal) duct |
| | Urachal cyst, patent urachus and related polyps |
| Hernias | Congenital and acquired |
| Inflammation | Neonatal omphalitis |
| | Granuloma |
| | Infection of the umbilical skin |
| Neoplasms | Benign |
| | Primary umbilical malignant |
| | Metastatic intra-abdominal malignancy |

Varicose veins (caput medusae)

and the symphysis pubis. Its position can be altered by both the patient's body habitus and intra-abdominal pathology. The umbilicus may be displaced upwards by a pelvic mass or bladder distension, and downwards by bowel distension, ascites or an upper abdominal mass (**Figure 33.15**). The umbilicus is subject to a wide range of congenital and acquired lesions (**Table 33.1**).

## Umbilical Concretions and Inflammation

Umbilical concretions are common in those who are obese or elderly. They are typically composed of dirt and desquamated epithelium, and their extent varies. They are usually asymptomatic, but at times they may give rise to inflammation and bloody discharge.

Inflammation of the umbilicus occurs in the setting of obesity, dermatitis, intertrigo, bacterial or fungal infections. It is primarily due to poor hygiene, but may occasionally be caused by excessive manipulation and cleansing of the umbilicus.

## Umbilical Fistulas and Related Conditions

Both congenital and acquired conditions can present with umbilical drainage or infection.

Embryologically, the omphalomesenteric duct, connected to the midgut, and the urachus, connected to the bladder, are the elements of the umbilical cord. During normal embryogenesis, these structures involute. Rare cases of a **patent omphalomesenteric duct (vitelline duct)** manifest with drainage of the ileal contents from the umbilicus (**Figure 33.16a**). An omphalomesenteric duct cyst or cord connected to the umbilicus, while not detectable on physical examination, may present with small bowel obstruction (**Figure 33.16b**).

**Urachal anomalies** may not manifest until early adulthood. A patent urachus presents with intermittent drainage and occasionally urinary tract infections. Underlying urachal cysts may manifest with acute or recurrent umbilical infections (**Figure 33.17**).

The umbilicus is a weaker area of the abdominal wall through which various inflammatory processes can drain and give rise to **acquired fistulas**. Aetiologies described include gallstones, retained foreign bodies, fistulas from a perforated viscus and tuberculous peritonitis. Apart from post-operative enterocutaneous fistulas, this pathology is now rarely seen.

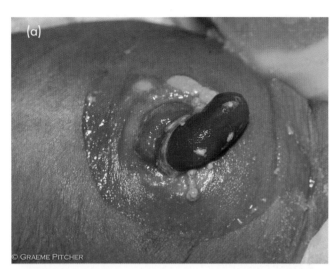

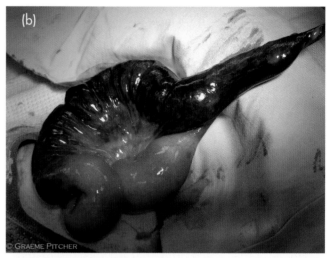

Figure 33.16 (a) Patent omphalomesenteric duct (vitelline duct). (b) Volvulus and gangrene of the small bowel around a Meckel's diverticulum attached to the umbilicus with a cord. (Both courtesy of Graeme Pitcher, MD.)

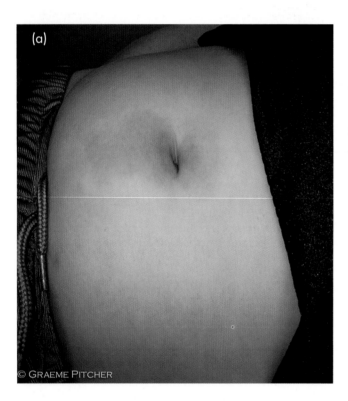

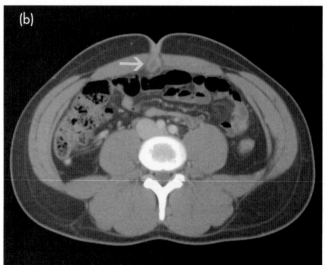

Figure 33.17 (a) Periumbilical cellulitis secondary to an infected urachal cyst in a 10-year-old boy (courtesy of Graeme Pitcher, MD). (b) A CT scan of an infected urachal cyst in an adult.

Although much less common than in the sacrococcygeal region, **pilonidal disease** can affect the umbilicus and manifest with hair protruding from the sinus tract. Similar to the more common sacrococcygeal disease, the typical patient is a hirsute young man. Recurrent infections can potentially lead to peritoneal extension.

## Umbilical Tumours

A wide variety of benign lesions, seen anywhere on the body, may involve the umbilicus (**Figure 33.18**).

Umbilical granuloma (**Figure 33.19**) is a common abnormality and is the most common aetiology for an umbilical mass. Granulation tissue forms at the site of cord separation secondary to inflammation and usually responds to topical silver nitrate treatment.

Umbilical polyps are much less common. These benign lesions are firm nodules composed of residual omphalomesenteric duct epithelium and, less commonly, urachal uroepithelium; they can be diagnosed by a biopsy.

Primary malignant tumours of the umbilicus are very rare and include malignant melanoma, basal or squamous carcinoma, and urachal carcinomas (**Figure 33.20**).

Advanced intra-abdominal malignancy (e.g. adenocarcinoma of the stomach, colon and pancreas, and gynaecological cancers) may spread to the umbilicus, where such a lesion is known as Sister Mary Joseph's nodule.

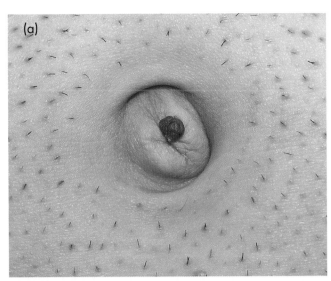
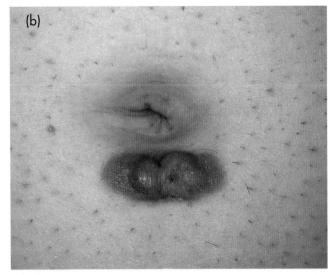

Figure 33.18 (a) A dermal naevus. (b) A keloid scar at the site of a periumbilical piercing.

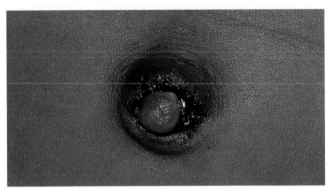

Figure 33.19 An umbilical granuloma (courtesy of Graeme Pitcher, MD).

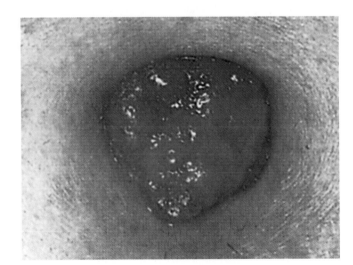

Figure 33.20 Carcinoma of the urachus. (Courtesy of John Lumley, MD.)

## VARICOSE VEINS OF THE ABDOMINAL WALL

The normal venous flow of the abdominal wall below the umbilicus is caudate towards the iliofemoral venous system. Veins above the umbilicus drain towards venous plexuses on the chest wall and axillae. The normal venous network is not prominent.

Superior vena cava syndrome is accompanied by dyspnoea, oedema of the face and head fullness, which is worse in the dependent position. In rare cases when the venous collaterals become prominent on the torso, they are located on the chest and the upper abdomen, and drain inferiorly.

In inferior vena cava syndrome, varicosities develop on the lateral and middle abdomen and drain superiorly (**Figure 33.21**).

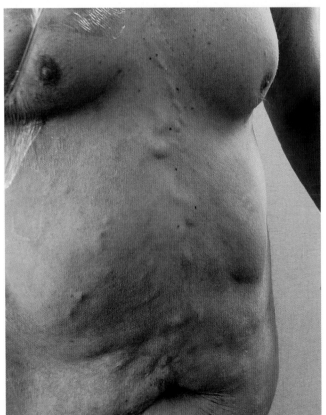

Figure 33.21 Upper abdominal wall varicosities with sparing of the chest wall in a patient with inferior vena cava obstruction.

If only one side of the iliofemoral system is obstructed, varicosities affect only the ipsilateral side. Oedema of the lower extremities is usually present as well.

In cases of portal venous hypertension, the blood flow is directed into the normally obliterated umbilical vein, leading to a radial engorgement of the periumbilical venous plexus (caput medusae). In portal hypertension, the direction of the venous flow on the abdomen is typically otherwise unchanged.

Although it is not always accurate in mixed conditions, determining the direction of flow in a dilated vein located below the umbilicus can frequently help with the differential diagnosis: away and inferiorly from umbilicus in portal hypertension, and superiorly in inferior vena cava syndrome. A simple technique is to compress the vein with the index fingers of both hands and slide the fingers apart to empty the segment. One finger is then released to determine whether the segment refills. The segment is emptied again before releasing the other finger. The direction of the venous flow corresponds to the direction of the faster refill.

### Key Points

- The abdominal wall has a complex anatomy and an important physiological function.
- It may be affected by a variety of local and systemic pathological processes.
- The differential diagnosis of abdominal wall lesions should include infections, hernias, haematomas, tumours and varicose veins.

# QUESTIONS

## SBAs

**1. Which of the following statements regarding the abdominal wall is correct?:**

a   Abdominal wall tumours arising from muscles are mobile on palpation

b   Having the patient raise their legs to tense the abdominal musculature may help to differentiate abdominal wall masses from intra-abdominal masses

c   Abdominal wall varices only occur secondary to advanced portal hypertension

d   Malignant melanoma of the supraumbilical area is expected to metastasize to the inguinal lymph nodes

e   Squamous cell carcinoma of the anus metastasizes primarily to the periaortic lymph nodes

**Answer**

*b Having the patient raise their legs to tense the abdominal musculature may help to differentiate abdominal wall masses from intra-abdominal masses.*

*An intra-abdominal mass, while palpable through relaxed abdominal muscles, may be less prominent or impalpable when the abdominal wall is tense during raising of the legs (Carnett's sign).*

*Benign subcutaneous tumours are typically well circumscribed and mobile relative to the underlying abdominal wall musculature and deep fascia. Malignant tumours and tumours arising from the musculoaponeurotic layers appear fixed to the abdominal wall.*

*While periumbilical varices (caput medusae) are pathognomonic of portal hypertension, varicosities of the abdominal wall may develop secondary to occlusion of the superior or inferior vena cava.*

*The lymphatics of the supraumbilical skin drain primarily to the axillary lymph nodes, and those of the infraumbilical regions drain to the superficial inguinal lymph nodes. The periumbilical lymphatics may drain in either direction. Cancer of the anorectal region below the dentate line metastasizes to the superficial inguinal lymph nodes. Thus, the lower extremities, torso, anorectal area and external genitalia must be examined in cases of inguinal lymphadenopathy.*

**2. Which of the following statements is correct?:**

a   Rectus sheath haematomas usually occur spontaneously without predisposing factors

b   Unless skin changes are obvious, a rectus sheath hematoma is not considered significant

c   Groin hernias and inguinal lymphadenopathy can always be easily differentiated by an attempt to reduce the mass

d   Skin erythema over an areas of groin lymphadenopathy indicates a purulent process requiring drainage

e   Infectious and malignant lymphadenopathy cannot be differentiated based on the size and mobility of the enlarged lymph nodes

**Answer**

*e Infectious and malignant lymphadenopathy cannot be differentiated based on the size and mobility of the enlarged lymph nodes. Both infectious and neoplastic diseases may cause lymphadenopathy. Only examination in a pathology laboratory can rule out cancer.*

*Although most rectus sheath haematomas develop in the absence of a traumatic episode, the vast majority of such patients receive some form of anticoagulation or antiplatelet therapy. Given the location under the anterior rectus sheath, bleeding may be physiologically significant and haematomas may reach a significant size even without any obvious overlying skin discoloration.*

*While an uncomplicated groin hernia can be reduced into the abdomen, both incarcerated hernias and prominent lymphadenopathy may present as irreducible bulges.*

*Acute inflammation of the inguinal lymph nodes presents with pain and swelling. Purulent lymphadenitis may be present without overlying cellulitis, but the development of overlying skin erythema and induration certainly indicates an underlying collection.*

**3. Which of the following statements is not correct?:**
a Unfolding of the umbilicus indicates an underlying fascial defect
b Umbilical infections are usually due to an underlying fistula
c Umbilical hernias in obese patients typically contain fatty tissue
d Urachal anomalies may not present until adulthood
e Pilonidal disease may affect the umbilicus

**Answer**

*b Umbilical infections are usually due to an underlying fistula.*

*Unfolding of the umbilicus indicates a small underlying hernia and may occur with increased intra-abdominal pressure (ascites, pregnancy).*

*Umbilical hernias in obese individuals, especially if the defect is small, usually contain fatty tissue (omentum or preperitoneal fat). With time, the hernia contents often become irreducible owing to adhesions.*

*Most umbilical infections are due to poor hygiene and other benign skin conditions. In young adults, especially those with recurrent infections, an underlying congenital anomaly should be considered. For example, urachal anomalies may not present until young adulthood and manifest as drainage or infections.*

*Pilonidal disease of the umbilicus is very rare, develops in individuals with abundant trunk hair and manifests similarly to the much more common sacrococcygeal disease, with hair poking out of the sinus tract and recurrent infections.*

## MCQs

**1. All of the following regarding necrotizing acute soft tissue infection are true except for which?:**
a Monomicrobial acute necrotizing soft tissue infections are less severe than polymicrobial ones
b Perineal infections are typically polymicrobial
c A decreased white blood cell count is characteristic
d Severe pain and oedema of the tissues are the hallmark presenting signs
e Underlying necrosis can be ruled out if epidermal blistering is not present
f Crepitus is diagnostic

**Answer**

*a, c, e, f. Necrotizing acute soft tissue infection is a life-threatening condition so its early recognition is vital. The prognosis depends on multiple factors, including patient factors, the virulence of the bacteria and the duration of illness, rather than on simply the monomicrobial versus polymicrobial nature of the infection.*

*Physical examination rather than imaging or laboratory analysis is the key to making the diagnosis. Severe pain and oedema of the tissues are the hallmark presenting signs. Skin blistering secondary to underlying necrosis and thrombosis occur late and signify irreversible damage to the underlying soft tissues. Crepitus is diagnostic but is present only in cases of clostridial infection (gas gangrene). The white blood cell count is usually elevated but may be normal or low.*

*The extremities are more commonly affected by monomicrobial (streptococcal or staphylococcal) infection, while the perineum tends to be affected by polymicrobial infections (gram-negative and gram-positive organisms and anaerobes). Abdominal wall infections secondary to an intra-abdominal source are polymicrobial, while cryptogenic ones are usually monomicrobial.*

**2. Which associations are not correct?:**
  a Sister Mary Joseph's nodule and endometriosis of the abdominal wall
  b Grey Turner's sign and haemorrhagic pancreatitis
  c A patent urachus and drainage of the small bowel contents
  d A urachal cyst and umbilical infections
  e Cullen's sign and intra-abdominal bleeding
  f A patent omphalomesenteric duct with non-enteric drainage and urinary tract infections

**Answer**

*a, c, f.* Sister Mary Joseph's nodule is an umbilical lesion secondary to metastatic intra-abdominal adenocarcinoma. Grey Turner's sign is flank bruising secondary to retroperitoneal bleeding (from haemorrhagic pancreatitis or a ruptured vascular aneurysm).
A patent urachus connects the urinary bladder to the umbilicus and presents with intermittent drainage and urinary infections.
Urachal cysts usually present as an umbilical infection.
Cullen's sign is periumbilical bruising secondary to intra-abdominal or retroperitoneal bleeding.
A patent omphalomesenteric (vitelline duct) manifests with drainage of the enteric contents.

# Abdominal Hernias

Evgeny V. Arshava

## LEARNING OBJECTIVES

- To recognize the wide variety of hernias and the symptoms that they cause
- To understand the key anatomy of the muscular and aponeurotic layers through which common hernias form

- To be able to perform a groin examination for a hernia
- To understand how to reduce an incarcerated hernia
- To be able to examine the anterior abdominal wall for hernias

## INTRODUCTION

An abdominal wall hernia is a protrusion of an underlying structure or organ (the **contents of the hernia**) through a **hernial defect** (hernial orrifice) in the musculoaponeurotic or fascial layer that normally would contain it. A **hernial sac**, formed by peritoneum, is usually but not always present and envelops the hernia contents. The sac consists of a neck (the part located within the defect), a wider body and the apex (fundus). A hernia with a narrow neck and a rigid defect is more likely to become incarcerated and strangulated.

Rare internal hernias, which usually present with intestinal obstruction, and hiatus hernias that do not meet this definition, usually present with bowel obstruction and are discussed in Chapter 36.

Hernias affect both males and females, can be congenital or acquired and affect all age groups. Abdominal wall hernias are an important cause of morbidity and mortality, and their repairs are the most common procedures performed in general surgery today.

Conditions that chronically increase intra-abdominal pressure (obesity, chronic obstructive pulmonary disease, ascites, constipation, benign prostatic hypertrophy) are associated with the development and progression of hernias. Single or repeated strenuous bouts of physical activity are frequently reported by patients as a first precipitating event. Patient may be asymptomatic or present with a variety of symptoms, ranging from cosmetic concerns and a sensation of fullness and pain, to intestinal obstruction and bowel necrosis.

## CLASSIFICATION AND GENERAL CHARACTERISTICS

Abdominal wall hernias are classified by location into either groin or ventral hernias. Around 75 per cent of all abdominal wall hernias are found in the groin (inguinal and femoral). A ventral hernia is any spontaneous (epigastric, umbilical, spigelian, lumbar) or post-operative (incisional) herniation of the abdominal wall.

Hernias are additionally classified into reducible and irreducible. In the case of **reducible hernias**, the contents of the hernia can be completely returned to the abdomen. This may require lying the patient down, manual manipulation or both.

**Irreducible (incarcerated) hernias** cannot be completely returned to the abdomen, due to either existing adhesions or a discrepancy between the volume of the herniating structures and the size of the defect. Incarceration can be acute or chronic. If the bowel is involved, incarceration may produce intestinal obstruction, manifested by colicky abdominal pain, abdominal distension, vomiting and constipation, depending on the level of the obstruction.

**Strangulation** is an acute compromise of blood flow to the irreducible hernial contents. It can develop acutely in previously reducible or chronically incarcerated hernias. Without prompt intervention, strangulation leads to bowel wall necrosis and perforation. New or unusually severe pain over the hernia or symptoms of bowel obstruction, regardless of the prior existence of a hernia, should be regarded as impending strangulation of the bowel until proven otherwise.

Bowel necrosis may be accompanied by inflammatory changes in the overlying skin with or without signs of systemic toxicity (see Figures 34.10b and 34.13c, later in the chapter). Such local skin changes must be differentiated from skin changes caused by external factors (e.g. contact dermatitis from an ill-fitting truss, or fungal infection).

Strangulation of the bowel is almost invariably associated with intestinal obstruction. A rare potential diagnostic pitfall is **Richter's hernia**, in which only one side of the bowel wall is trapped in a small hernial defect, such as the femoral canal or a small incisional hernia (see Figure 34.16c, below). Strangulation in this case occurs without obstruction of the entire lumen and with no symptoms of bowel obstruction. Local signs of strangulation may also be minimal, but if this condition is not diagnosed early, the incarceration may lead to perforation and peritonitis.

## Physical Examination

Abdominal hernias have following important characteristics:

- They occur at well-recognized sites of congenital or acquired structural weakness.
- Most have a visible or palpable expansile impulse.
- Most can be completely or partially reduced.
- An acutely incarcerated hernia requires prompt surgical evaluation.

Examination of the patient begins with a visual inspection looking for surgical scars (see Figures 33.2 and 33.3) and bulging. Assess the symmetry of the abdomen as patients do not always notice they have a hernia. Many hernias present as an obvious bulge, but smaller and occult hernias may be missed if physical examination is not thorough or the patient has a difficult anatomy (see Figure 33.13).

Carefully evaluate the entire abdominal wall during relaxation and strain in both the supine and the upright position. Search for a visible or palpable impulse. With the patient in the supine position, ask them to increase their intra-abdominal pressure by lifting the upper torso or the legs off of the bed (depending on the patient's strength). In the upright position, ask the patient to cough or perform a Valsalva manoeuvre. Note that a palpable incarcerated hernia may not have much of an impulse.

Visual inspection and careful palpation are performed to better assess reducibility and the volume of the herniating contents. In reducible ventral hernias, fascial defects can be easily palpated in thin individuals, and the size of the hernial defect can be measured.

## Groin Hernias

Groin hernias are located in the anatomically weak myopectineal orifice (**Figure 34.1**). Over 95 per cent of groin hernias are inguinal and the rest are femoral. Inguinal hernias are the most common types in both males and females, but femoral hernias are more common in women than they are in men.

### Inguinal Hernias

Inguinal hernias are very common – every fourth male develops a hernia during his lifespan. Anatomically, inguinal hernias are classified as indirect, direct or combined (pantaloon hernias). Inguinal hernias may be asymptomatic or cause bothersome bulging and pain. Minimally symptomatic inguinal hernias may be safely observed, with a very low long-term risk of serious complications (strangulation).

**Indirect inguinal hernias** are the most common type in both males and females. This type of hernia always has a true hernial sac since it results from a failure of peritoneal extension (the processus vaginalis in males and the corresponding canal of Nuck in females) to obliterate after embryological descent of the testicle into the scrotum, or the round ligament into the labium majus. The right testicle descends last, and hence indirect hernias are more common on the right.

Hernias in infancy are exclusively indirect and manifest early in life (**congenital indirect hernia**). Although all indirect hernias

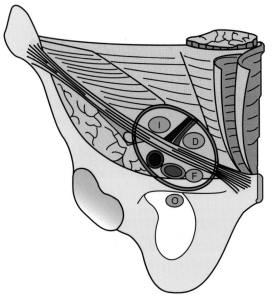

Figure 34.1 Diagram of a right myopectineal orifice with the aponeuroses of the oblique muscles reflected, exposing the transversus abdominis muscle. The sites of groin and obturator hernias are shaded in green. I, indirect inguinal hernia (through the internal inguinal ring); D, direct inguinal hernia (Hesselbach's triangle); F, femoral hernia (in the femoral canal below the inguinal ligament); O, obturator hernia, in the obturator canal (outside the myopectineal orifice).

are congenital, a small or partially obliterated partial processus vaginalis sometimes does not enlarge, in childhood, only manifesting in adulthood as a result of increasing intra-abdominal pressure and wearing of the inguinal floor structures (and thus occasionally being termed an **acquired indirect hernia**).

The indirect hernia and sac pass through the internal inguinal ring lateral to the inferior epigastric vessels. As the hernia enlarges, it typically descends through the external ring obliquely into the scrotum or labium majus (**Figure 34.2**). This does not occur with other groin hernias. Neglected hernias occasionally reach very large sizes and become chronically incarcerated and difficult to repair. Even giant hernias, however, may not necessarily be associated with obstructive symptoms (**Figure 34.3**). Atypical cephalad extension of the inguinal hernia represents an uncommon interparietal variant (**Figure 34.4**).

Occasionally, the peritoneal sac contains only fluid. When the sac extends to the tunica vaginalis of the testicle, it is called a **communicating hydrocele**. This is common in children. In patients with cirrhosis, the entire hernial sac may be filled with ascitic fluid. In cases in which the processus vaginalis becomes obliterated both proximally and distally but persists within the inguinal canal, an isolated cyst can form that is associated with the cord or round ligament (a **cyst of the canal of Nuck in females** or a **cord hydrocele in males**; see Figure 34.9c). Proximal obliteration of the peritoneum with the persistence of a large distal processus vaginalis forms a **non-communicating hydrocele** in adults and children.

**Direct inguinal hernias** develop through the posterior wall of the inguinal canal medial to the inferior epigastric vessels (Hesselbach's triangle). A clinical distinction between the two types of inguinal hernia may be very difficult even for an experienced examiner. In general, direct hernias rarely descend into the scrotum or labium majus. They are located next to the pubic

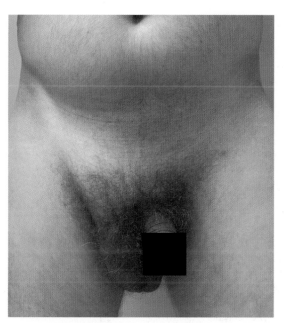

Figure 34.2 An indirect inguinal hernia extending along the cord into the right hemiscrotum with marked asymmetry of the groin creases.

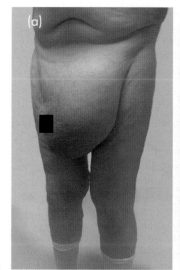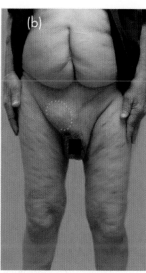

Figure 34.3 (a) A giant left indirect inguinal hernia extending below the middle of the thigh and completely distorting scrotal and groin anatomy. It contained large segments of colon and most of the small bowel. (b) After its repair, coexisting right inguinal hernia becomes apparent (bulge outlined).

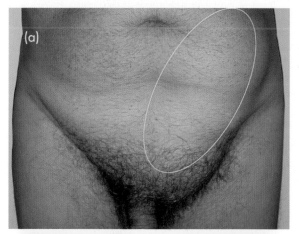

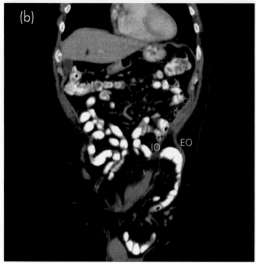

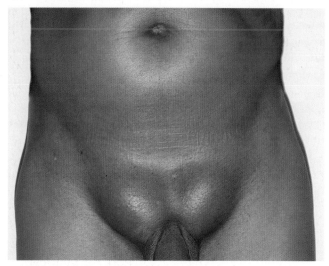

Figure 34.5 Bilateral direct inguinal hernias. The course of the symmetrical bulges is more straight than oblique.

Figure 34.4 (a) A large irreducible left indirect inguinal interstitial hernia with an unusual extension towards the umbilicus rather than into the scrotum. (b) Computed tomography demonstrates that most of the bowel is incarcerated between the internal (IO) and external oblique (EO) muscles.

tubercle and have a wide defect. They have a straighter orientation and usually reduce instantly in the supine position, or require more direct rather than oblique pressure to encourage their reduction (**Figure 34.5**). Both indirect and direct inguinal hernias are commonly bilateral, but direct hernias tend to occur later in life, are very rare in women, do not occur in children and rarely strangulate.

A **sliding hernia** is an uncommon form of inguinal hernia in which an extraperitoneal structure, such as the sigmoid colon, ileocaecum or bladder, slides into the hernia alongside the true peritoneal sac. These hernias tend to be larger, occur in older patients and are more frequently associated with obstructive or urinary symptoms.

## Femoral Hernias

The femoral canal is located posterior to the inguinal ligament, above the superior pubic rami, medial to the femoral vein and lateral to the pubic tubercle (**Figure 34.6a**). As the hernia enlarges, it descends along the vein through the saphenous opening into the femoral triangle on the medial thigh. Any further downward expansion is prevented by the confluence of the fasciae. With ongoing enlargement, a large femoral hernia may ascend over the inguinal ligament and at this stage usually becomes irreducible.

Femoral hernias are very rarely seen before the adult years and are much more common in females. They are ten times more likely to incarcerate and strangulate than inguinal hernias because the femoral canal is narrow and semi-rigid. Intestinal obstruction, especially in obese females, may occur without an obvious groin bulge (**Figure 34.6b**). In such cases, a misdiagnosis of the pathology may occur unless an incarcerated hernia is considered in the differential diagnosis and a thorough examination is performed.

Very rarely, femoral hernias are located more lateral to and in front of the femoral vessels (**pre-vascular femoral hernia**). This variant has a wider and softer neck, descends onto the anterior thigh and rarely strangulates.

## Examination of the Groin

Examination of groin is best begun with the patient standing in front of the seated examiner. The entire abdomen, scrotum and upper thighs should be exposed. The following characteristics should be determined during examination:

- The anatomical location.
- The colour and temperature of the overlying skin.
- Any tenderness.
- The size and shape.
- The presence of a cough impulse.
- The contents.
- The reducibility.

**Inspection** – Look carefully for any asymmetry and abnormal colour or overlying skin changes. Look for old scars. Many groin hernias are obvious. Up to 10 per cent are bilateral. Establish the relationship of the mass relative to the inguinal ligament, pubic tubercle and inguinal crease (**Figure 34.7a**). If the hernia extends into the scrotum or labium majus, it is more likely to be an indirect inguinal hernia. An elongated bilateral muscular bulge along the inguinal ligament (**Malgaigne's bulge**) can be seen in thin individuals during straining and is not a hernia. If no hernia is seen, ask the patient to perform a Valsalva manoeuvre by holding their nose and blowing, or by bearing down as if having a bowel movement. Alternatively the ask patient to cover their mouth with a hand, turn their head away and cough. This may produce a visible bulge (**Figure 34.7b**).

**Palpation** – Examine the patient carefully, taking into account the location of any active pain and tenderness. If the patient has had a previous operation, assess sensation and areas of hyperaesthesia in the distribution of the ilioinguinal and iliohypogastric nerves and branches of the genitofemoral nerves.

First, in a male, simultaneously palpate the spermatic cords, epididymides and testes bilaterally to assess these structures for symmetry, masses, tenderness and varicosities (**Figure 34.8**). If you can circumferentially palpate the spermatic cord *above* the scrotal mass, it is not an inguinal hernia (**Figure 34.9a**). In this case, suspect a testicular tumor or non-communicating hydrocele. If no mass is visible, ask the patient to perform a Valsalva manoeuvre and watch for the appearance of a bulge.

Palpate the groin above and below the inguinal ligament. For convenience, move the examiner's chair slightly towards the side to be examined and use the hand corresponding to the side of examination. Palpate both groins, but start with the asymptomatic side.

Assess the inguinal canal. Depending on the size of the patient, use either the little or the index finger. Invaginate the base of the scrotum along the cord. Rotate the finger so that the nail lies against the cord, and advance it through the external ring. Ask the patient to cough. A palpable impulse against the tip of the finger suggests an indirect hernia, whereas an impulse against the side of the finger suggests a direct hernia. It is not, however, always possible to make this distinction. Keep in mind that the important thing is to diagnose the presence or absence of a hernia; determining the specific type is secondary.

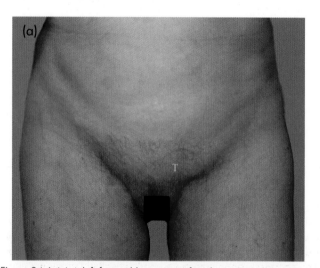
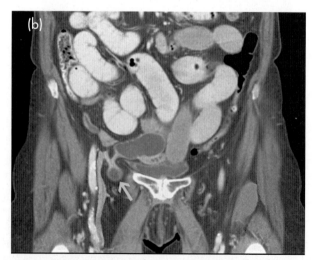

Figure 34.6 (a) A left femoral hernia in a female containing incarcerated fat. Note its lateral position to the pubic tubercle (T). An inguinal hernia would be located more superiorly. (b) A right femoral hernia (arrow) with incarcerated small bowel, causing bowel obstruction but producing only a minimal bulge and tenderness in the groin. Note the location of the hernial sack along the femoral vessels.

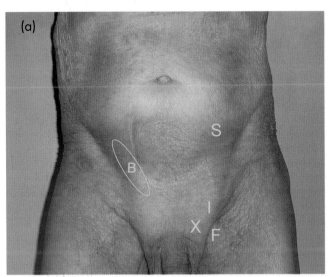

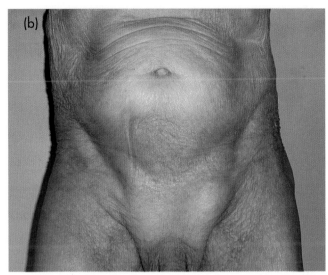

Figure 34.7 (a) X marks the location of the pubic tubercle. The expected projections of an inguinal (I), femoral (F) and spigelian (S) hernia and a Malgaigne's bulge (B) are shown. (b) Malgaigne's bulges and a left inguinal hernia become obvious during straining in the upright position. Note the well-healed right paramedian scar from a prior appendicectomy.

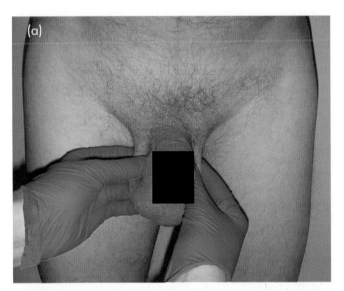

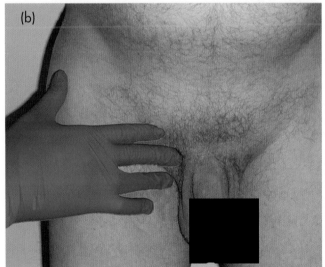

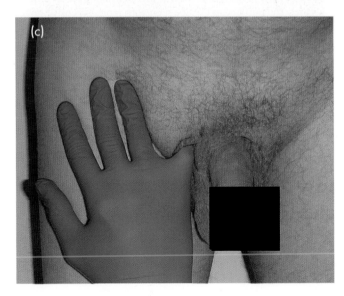

Figure 34.8 (a) Bilateral palpation of the scrotal structures for symmetry and masses. (b) Palpation of the groin with the patient in an upright position. Position the index finger over the expected projection of an indirect hernia, the middle finger over an expected direct hernia, and the ring finger over an expected femoral hernia and ask the patient to cough. Alternatively, hold the fingers together and palpate one location at a time. (c) Explore the inguinal canal. The finger is passed through the scrotal skin under the subcutaneous tissue of the groin.

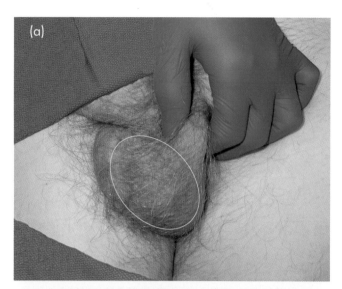

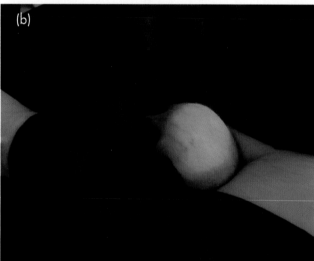

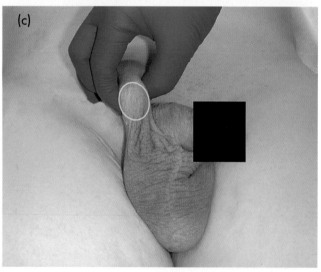

Figure 34.9 (a) The cord can be palpated above the left scrotal mass (outlined), ruling out an inguinal hernia. (b) Transillumination of this mass demonstrates that it is fluid-filled (a spermatocele in this case). (c) A right cord cyst (contour outlined) that does not extend into the inguinal canal.

In females, unless the patient is extremely thin, it may be difficult to palpate the inguinal canal, and it is essentially impossible to invaginate it. Examination is usually limited to direct palpation of the groin and the base of the labium majus.

**Assessing Reducibility of the Groin Hernia** – Next, examine the patient with them lying supine. Assess the hernia for reducibility. In some cases, the hernia will reduce spontaneously. Have the patient flex their hips and adduct them to relax the abdominal muscles. If the hernia does not reduce spontaneously, ask the patient to reduce it.

If the patient cannot reduce the hernia, attempt manual reduction. Simply pressing straight down on top of the hernia pushes the entire contents onto the neck, occluding it, and is unlikely to result in a successful reduction (the 'mushroom' effect). Instead, grasp the neck of the hernia with the fingers of the non-dominant hand, elongating and straightening the hernia while using the fingers of the dominant hand to gently milk the contents of the hernial sac back through the neck. It is often necessary to first milk the bowel contents back into the proximal and distal bowel before attempting to push the bowel itself back inside.

In cases of bowel obstruction, hernia reduction must be performed with great care. Do not attempt reduction if skin redness or oedema is present overlying the mass. These advanced changes suggest the possibility of underlying bowel necrosis. In these cases, urgent surgical attention is mandatory since further manipulation may cause bowel perforation.

It is not always possible to accurately determine the contents of the hernia. If the hernia contains bowel loops, initial difficulty in reduction is usually followed by prompt reduction associated with a characteristic gurgling sound. Omentum has a more doughy consistency with absent bowel sounds on auscultation and frequently does not completely reduce. Transillumination may help to differentiate a hernia from a hydrocele, epididymal cysts and spermatoceles (**Figure 34.9b**). Percussion has a very limited role.

In most patients careful physical examination is all that is required to diagnose or exclude the presence of a groin hernia. Physical examination may be difficult in obese or very thin patients and those who have previously undergone surgery. It is not uncommon to feel a subtle impulse in the inguinal floor in a very thin asymptomatic patient, which is not a hernia. On the other hand, hernias in patients with a prominent pannus may be missed.

Real-time ultrasound is a cost-effective way to delineate the anatomy of the groin and exclude a hernia in some cases. In very few cases, the hernia can only be seen with more expensive imaging technologies such as CT or MRI scanning.

## Groin Hernias in Children

Groin hernias in infants and children are virtually always indirect inguinal hernias. Most patients are boys. Patients frequently report typical episodes of bulging of the groin during crying or physical activity that disappear spontaneously or with manipulation. The bulge may not be present during evaluation. Encourage older children to run around or jump up and down in order to allow descent of the hernia.

Physical examination may be difficult, especially in infants, due to a lack of cooperation and a frequently prominent fat pad in the groin. Asymmetry of the groin crease may provide a hint to the presence of an inguinal hernia (but remember that this test will fail in the common situation of bilateral hernias). A small hydrocele may indicate the existence of a patent processus vaginalis.

In young children, digital palpation of the inguinal canal through the scrotum may be difficult, and it is impractical to attempt it. Gently palpate the cord just outside the external ring between the index finger and thumb, and compare its thickness with that of the opposite side. Alternatively, with the index finger, gently roll the cord back and forth over the pubic tubercle. A thickened cord indicates the presence of a hernial sac even if it is empty. Remember to examine both sides since 15 per cent of cases are bilateral.

Reduction of an incarcerated hernia in a child should be carried out extremely delicately. Have an assistant flex and adduct both the child's thighs and slightly elevate the pelvis. It is important to mention that the ovary is the most commonly incarcerated structure in the inguinal hernia in pre-pubertal girls.

## Differential Diagnosis of Groin Masses and Pain

The differential diagnosis will include the following:

- *Inguinal hernia versus femoral hernia.* These are distinguished based on their location relative to the pubic tubercle and the inguinal ligament. Inguinal hernias originate above and over the pubic tubercle. Femoral hernias are located below and lateral to the pubic tubercle, and below the inguinal ligament (see **Figure 34.7a**). If the hernia is present but the inguinal canal is empty on simultaneous palpation, it is a femoral hernia (or a scrotal or subcutaneous mass).
- A *communicating hydrocele* can be transilluminated and, if it is large, it cannot be reduced and may obscure palpation of the testis on that side.
- *Hydrocele of the cord (males) or the canal of Nuck (females)* may be difficult to diagnose on palpation. A hydrocele of the canal of Nuck is fixed, smooth and translucent. A hydrocele of the cord may be differentiated from an incarcerated hernia if it moves with the cord when the testis is gently pulled down. Uncommonly, it can be brought down with the cord sufficiently to palpate the cord above the mass.
- A *hydrocele of a femoral hernial sac* is rare and always translucent.
- A *scrotal mass* or other pathology can be differentiated from a groin hernia if it is possible to palpate normal structure proximal to the mass.
- A *Bartholin's gland cyst* is confined to the labium majus. It is easy to palpate above the cyst as it does not extend to the pubic tubercle. It is not usually translucent.
- An *ectopic testis* is usually diagnosed early in life and should be considered if an ipsilateral testis is not palpable in the scrotum.
- A *cord lipoma* is a common extension of normal pre-peritoneal fat along the cord structures through the internal inguinal ring. This is not a true hernia, although it commonly coexists with inguinal hernias. The lump has no impulse on straining. It may be the only abnormality in the inguinal canal found during surgical exploration for a symptomatic mass.
- *Enlarged lymph nodes* may be inflammatory or neoplastic in nature. Enlarged inflammatory lymph nodes are usually well circumscribed and mobile unless they are infected. Large malignant lymph nodes may mimic an incarcerated inguinal hernia but can be differentiated on palpation of the inguinal canal (**Figure 34.10a**). Differentiation from an incarcerated femoral hernia may be especially difficult when a solitary enlarged lymph node is located in the femoral canal (Cloquet's node). Areas draining to the groins must be carefully examined: the lower limbs, anterior and posterior lower torso, perineum, anus and genitalia.
- An *abscess* is typically accompanied by overlying erythema and warmth, and usually develops secondary to purulent lymphadenitis or occasionally may represent extension of a retroperitoneal purulent process (see Figure 33.14a). It must be differentiated from a strangulated hernia with necrotic bowel (**Figure 34.10b**).
- A *saphenous vein varix* may be visible in thin subjects as a lump with a blue discoloration. It may resemble a reducible femoral hernia since both may produce a cough impulse and disappear in the supine position. A varix is usually softer than a hernia and has a fluid thrill when the patient coughs (Cruveilhier's sign). A varix is usually associated with pronounced varicose changes of the greater saphenous vein and may demonstrate

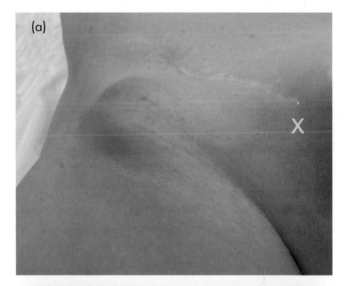

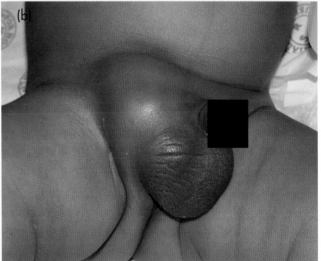

Figure 34.10 (a) Right inguinal lymphadenopathy secondary to a metastatic malignant melanoma. Note the discoloration of the thin overlying skin, the lymphoedema of the thigh and the scar from the previous inguinal hernia repair. Such a lateral and low location is unusual for a recurrent groin hernia. X, pubic tubercle. (b) A strangulated right inguinal hernia in a child with necrotic bowel and overlying skin erythema (courtesy of Graeme Pitcher, MD).

a transmitted impulse on percussion of the dilated distal portion of the vein.

- An iliopsoas bursa, when enlarged, may occasionally present as a bulge in the groin.
- A *femoral artery aneurysm* has an arterial pulse and is located below the midportion of the inguinal ligament.
- A subcutaneous inclusion cyst or lipoma is usually mobile relative to the surrounding tissues.
- *Myofascial or musculoaponeurotic pain* (a 'muscle strain') is common given the complexity of the anatomy and functions of the groin. Patients present with persistent groin pain, frequently with a history of a strenuous event. Physical examination is negative for a hernia but reveals focal tenderness of the lower abdominal muscles, adductor thigh muscles or pubic symphysis ('osteitis pubis'). Most strains resolve with conservative management over a period of weeks to months.
- *'Sports hernia'* is a popular but misleading misnomer recently encountered in the literature. It is used to describe persistent groin pain secondary to repeated vigorous physical exertion. Most of these cases represent musculoaponeurotic strain. Those few patients who fail conservative management may have tears or an attenuation of the musculofascial layers. This is not a true hernia since there are no 'hernia contents'.
- *Chronic post-operative groin pain* is a not uncommon but frequently disabling condition that occurs after hernia repair. The somatic pain is described as dull and pounding. Similar to the pain of a musculoaponeurotic strain, it is precipitated by physical activity and easily reproduced on palpation. Neuropathic pain, which is sharp, stabbing or burning, typically has specific trigger points and is localized to the distribution of the affected nerves: the ilioinguinal, iliohypogastric or lateral femoral cutaneous nerve, or the genital branch of the genitofemoral nerve. Recurrence of the hernia must be ruled out in each case with a thorough physical examination.
- *Referred groin pain* is caused by different aetiologies – lumbar radiculopathy, ureteral stones, chronic prostatitis, testicular pathology, endometriosis and hip joint pathology among others.

A patient may describe symptoms suggestive of hernia, but sometimes no hernia is found on a thorough examination. Ask the patient to walk up- and downstairs or remain in a squatting position for a period of time and repeat the examination. Rule out other differential diagnoses. If a hernia still cannot be detected, repeat the examination at a different visit or ask the patient to return when the bulge is obvious. In difficult cases, imaging (real-time ultrasound, or even an MRI or CT scan) may be considered.

## Ventral Hernias
### Diastasis Recti

Diastasis recti is a noticeable separation of the medial edges of the rectus abdominis muscles, usually in the upper abdomen. It is not a true hernia since the fascial layer is intact, albeit thinned out and stretched. This widening of the linea alba results in a ridge-like bulging of the underlying structures during straining (**Figure 34.11**). During relaxation, the medial edges of the muscles can be palpated with the fingertips in a thin individual.

This condition is seen in children, but as they grow it usually disappears. In the adult years, it is typically a result of a chronically increased intra-abdominal pressure that separates the muscles (multiparous females or patients with central obesity).

Diastasis recti has some cosmetic implications but is otherwise asymptomatic.

### Epigastric Hernia

An epigastric hernia protrudes through a midline defect of the linea alba in the upper abdomen. It is more common in men. The defect is usually less than 1 cm in size. This is typically a protrusion of extraperitoneal fat only. Larger hernias are frequently irreducible (**Figure 34.12a**). Less commonly, there is a larger defect with a true peritoneal sac, which typically contains only the greater omentum with no bowel involvement (**Figure 34.12b**). The hernia is palpable as a firm, tender nodule that typically has no cough impulse. Frequently, the smaller the hernia, the less obvious it is and the greater are the symptoms. Pain from a non-palpable hernia may mimic the symptoms of a peptic ulcer and result in post-prandial dyspepsia, possibly due to the gastric distension pushing on the hernia.

### Umbilical Hernia

The umbilical plate develops at the site of healing of the umbilical cord. Inadequate scar formation results in the development of umbilical hernias.

**Congenital umbilical hernias** are usually apparent shortly after birth and are more noticeable during crying. The defect is located at the centre of the umbilical plate and is completely covered by the umbilical skin. The size of hernial defect varies but is usually 1–2 cm. In most babies, the hernia closes spontaneously by 5 years of age, but in some persists into adult years (**Figure 34.13a**). Complications are very rare. This condition is more common in babies of African descent.

**Acquired umbilical hernias** develop secondary to a progressive stretching of the umbilical scar or to a small subclinical defect in the adult years due to a chronic increase in intra-abdominal pressure (obesity, cirrhotic or malignant ascites, chronic obstructive pulmonary disease). Most adult umbilical hernias are actually periumbilical, protruding to the side of the umbilical plate, typically superior to it. Only part of the hernia is covered by the umbilical skin, and the rest by the adjacent subcutaneous fat and abdominal skin (**Figure 34.13b**). Periumbilical hernias may not have a peritoneal sac and may contain only pre-peritoneal fat. Umbilical hernias may progressively enlarge and become irreducible (**Figure 34.13c**).

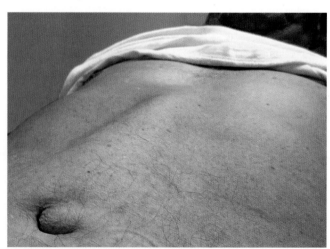

Figure 34.11 The bulge from the diastasis recti becomes prominent as the patient lifts the upper torso off the examination table. Note the frequently coexisting periumbilical hernia.

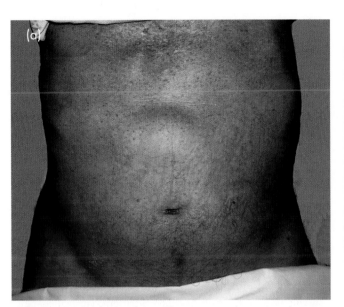

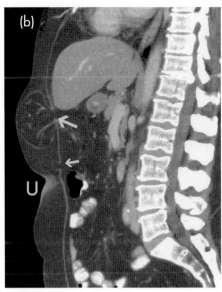

Figure 34.12 (a) A large, chronically incarcerated epigastric hernia containing pre-peritoneal fat. (b) An uncommon case of two separate epigastric hernias (marked with arrows). The smaller hernia contains pre-peritoneal fat, and the larger one an incarcerated greater omentum. U, umbilicus.

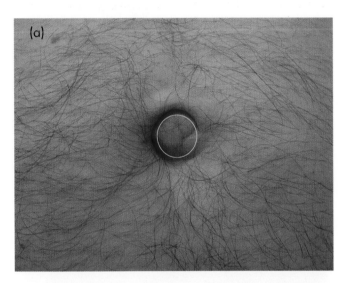

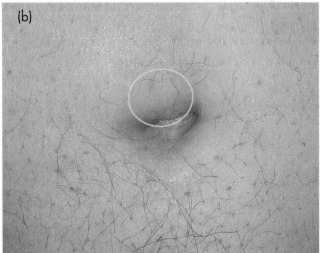

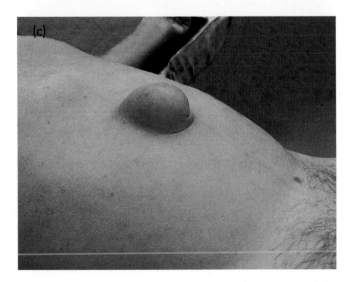

Figure 34.13 (a) A small umbilical hernia containing omentum, with the defect centred on the umbilical plate and is completely covered by umbilical skin. (b) A periumbilical hernia containing chronically incarcerated pre-peritoneal fat, located in the upper umbilical plate and partly covered by abdominal wall skin and subcutaneous fat. (c) An acutely incarcerated umbilical hernia in a patient with cirrhosis. Note the overlying skin discoloration secondary to an advanced ischaemia of the strangulated bowel.

**Omphalocele (exomphalos)** is a severe form of incomplete closure of the abdominal wall during embryogenesis. The herniating intra-abdominal organs are covered by a thin membrane attached to the umbilical cord, with no skin coverage. Most children have associated other organ systems anomalies (**Figure 34.14a**).

An omphalocele should be differentiated from **gastroschisis**, which has no protective membrane, typically has a smaller defect, is almost always located to the right of the umbilicus and is only rarely associated with other congenital pathology (**Figure 34.14b**).

### Evisceration

Evisceration is a rare but a dreaded complication of fresh abdominal incisions. It may be related to poor closure techniques or materials, or to underlying disease processes such as continuing sepsis, malnutrition, immunosuppression or obesity. Violent coughing, vomiting and abdominal distension may also contribute.

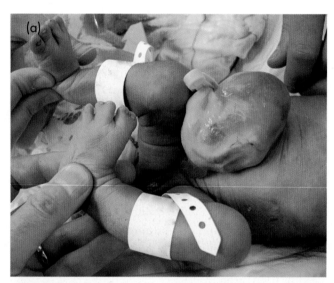

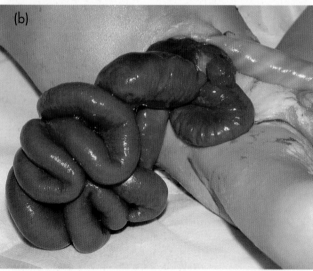

Figure 34.14 (a) An omphalocele. Note the associated anomalies of the feet. (b) Gastroschisis. Note the oedematous and inflamed bowel secondary to a lack of protective coverage. (Photographs courtesy of Graeme Pitcher, MD.)

This morbid complication typically occurs during the first post-operative week. It begins with drainage of serosanguineous fluid from the incision due to dehiscence of the fascial closure. As the dehiscence increases, a gush of larger volume heralds an impending disruption of the skin and evisceration of the intestines (**Figure 34.15**). Immediate surgical attention is necessary. Minor degrees of fascial dehiscence may go unnoticed and present later as incisional hernias.

### Incisional Hernia

This type of ventral hernia occurs when part or all of the musculoaponeurotic layer of a laparotomy incision fails to heal properly. Multiple factors contribute to the development of incisional hernias, including surgical technique, post-operative wound infections and the patient's comorbidities.

Incisional hernias vary greatly in size and the actual fascial defect is usually smaller than expected (**Figure 34.16a**). Hernias may reach large sizes with a complete loss of the abdominal domain (**Figure 34.16b**). There are commonly multiple small contiguous defects in a 'Swiss cheese' pattern. During examination, define the fascial edges if the hernia is reducible.

The clinical manifestations vary. Most hernias are minimally symptomatic, some produce intermittent episodes of pain or obstruction, and others present with acute incarceration. Hernias with larger fascial defects are generally at a lower risk of incarceration and strangulation. The smaller the hernial defect, the greater the possibility of complications (**Figure 34.16c**).

### Parastomal Hernia

This is a type of incisional hernia that occurs at the site of stoma formation. These hernias may reach considerable size, and patients may encounter difficulty with fitting their stomal

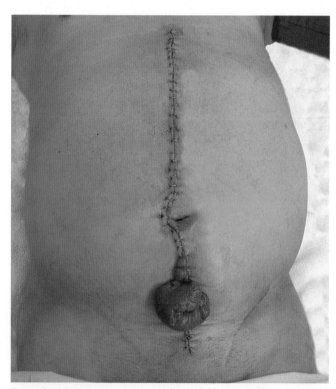

Figure 34.15 Evisceration in a malnourished patient after emergency aortic surgery.

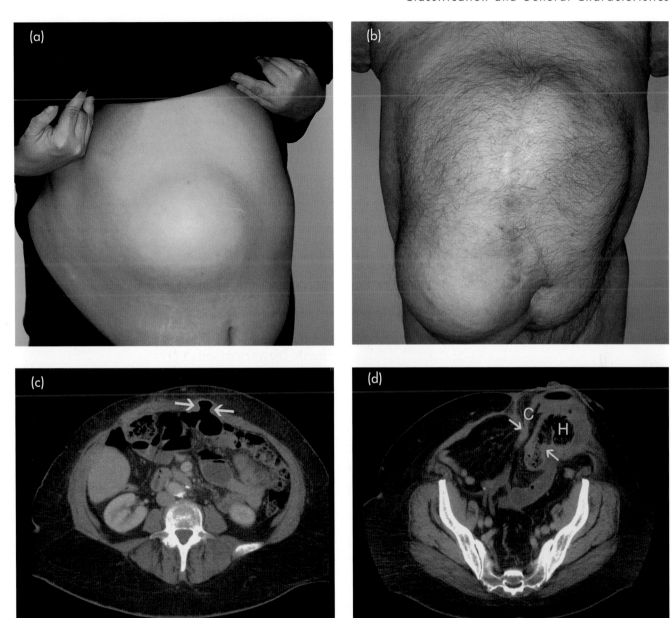

Figure 34.16 (a) A prominent incisional hernia at the site of a laparoscopic incision with only a 3 cm fascial defect and large subcutaneous hernia. (b) Complex chronically incarcerated incisional hernias with intermittent obstructive symptoms in a patient with a history of multiple abdominal operations. (c) A CT scan of an uncommon type of incisional hernia, when only a part of the colonic wall is incarcerated in the small fascial defect (arrows). In this type of incarceration (Richter's hernia), strangulation and perforation may occur without symptoms of bowel obstruction. (d) An acutely incarcerated parastomal hernia (H) presenting with complete bowel obstruction. Note the narrow fascial defect (marked with arrows) around the urinary conduit (C) and an incarcerated obstructed small bowel loop.

appliance over the bulge. Bowel obstruction and strangulation are rare but must always be considered as a possible cause of pain at the ostomy site (**Figure 34.16d**).

## Spigelian Hernia

A spigelian hernia develops at the intersection of the linea semilunaris (the lateral edge of the rectus abdominis muscle) and the arcuate line (usually a few centimetres below the umbilicus), below which the posterior rectus sheath is deficient (**Figure 34.17**; see also Figure 34.7a). In the early stages, a spigelian hernia remains contained under the external oblique aponeurosis (as an interparietal hernia) and may thus not be

easily palpable, especially in obese patients (**Figure 34.17b**). Real-time ultrasound or other imaging modalities may assist in the diagnosis.

## Obturator Hernia

This uncommon hernia occurs through the obturator canal, under the superior pubic rami along the obturator vessels and nerve. It is typically seen in elderly women due to laxity of the pelvic floor. These hernias frequently present as intestinal obstruction and may be difficult to diagnose. The strangulation of a Richter's-type hernia may also occur.

The other manifestation is intermittent pain along the medial thigh. Occasionally, the patient complains of pain referred to the knee along the genicular branch of the obturator nerve.

A larger hernia may be palpated in the upper medial thigh while the hip is flexed, abducted and externally rotated or during vaginal examination.

## Lumbar Hernia

Lumbar hernias are very rarely encountered. Inferior lumbar hernias arise on the posterolateral abdominal wall through a potential site of weakness in the triangle of Petit, formed by the iliac crest inferiorly, the latissimus dorsi muscle medially and the posterior edge of the external oblique muscle. The superior lumbar hernia originates through the triangle of Grynfeltt, which is bounded by the 12th rib superiorly, the posterior border of the internal oblique muscle inferiorly and the erector spinae and quadratus lumborum muscles medially. Since the predominantly

muscular boundaries are soft, these hernias are usually easily reducible during examination and rarely incarcerate.

## Recurrent Hernia

When a hernia develops at the same site after a surgical repair, it is termed 'recurrent'. With groin hernias, recurrence may result not only from an inadequate technique, but also from a failure to recognize a second coexisting type of groin hernia during the initial operation. Large incisional hernias have an increased risk of recurrence.

## Interparietal Hernia

Most hernias herniate through the musculoaponeurotic layers of the abdominal wall to present directly under the skin. Less common variants are interparietal hernias, located between the layers of the abdominal wall; these are either pre-peritoneal (between the transversalis fascia and peritoneum) or interstitial (between the muscle layers; see Figure 34.4). This deep location may create difficulties with physical diagnosis, and imaging may be needed. Some incisional, spigelian and inguinal hernias may be of this type.

## Flank Denervation

A bothersome bulge may occur from denervation and atrophy of the abdominal muscles (typically after flank incisions that divide the lower intercostal nerves). This is not a hernia since the integrity of the musculoaponeurotic layers is preserved, and it is only of cosmetic significance. Such denervations should, however, be distinguished from incisional hernias with the fascial defect in the same location, which can be palpated or visualized on imaging (**Figure 34.18**).

Flank denervation may also develop in the absence of surgical incisions and be secondary to intrinsic pathology of the nerves, such as an underlying neuropathy or herpes zoster paralysis (**Figure 34.19**).

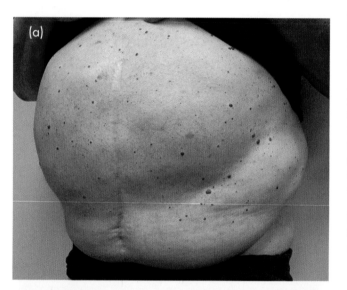

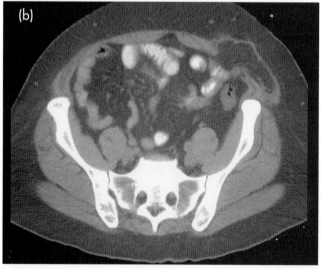

Figure 34.17 (a) An uncommonly large, chronically incarcerated left spigelian hernia containing colon. (b) A CT scan of a non-palpable left spigelian hernia contained under the stretched external oblique aponeurosis in a morbidly obese patient containing fat.

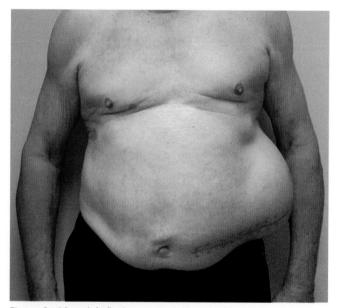

Figure 34.18 A left flank incisional hernia after the retroperitoneal repair of an abdominal aortic aneurysm.

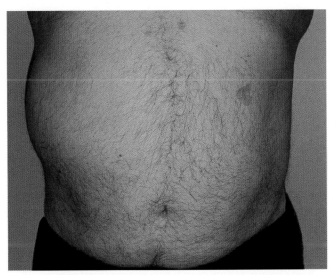

Figure 34.19 Right abdominal wall denervation secondary to a neuropathy of the intercostal nerves.

**Key Points**

- Abdominal hernias must be a part of the differential diagnosis in any patient presenting with abdominal pain, bowel obstruction or mass.
- Hernias can be classified as ventral or groin.
- Assess hernias of the abdominal wall for their reducibility.
- Groin hernias are best examined with the patient in an upright position and should be characterized as inguinal or femoral.
- While minimally symptomatic inguinal hernias may be observed, femoral hernias are much more likely to cause incarceration or strangulation and should be repaired.
- Assess incarcerated hernias (both acute and chronic) for the presence of strangulation.
- Symptoms and signs of strangulation imply a surgical emergency.
- The differential diagnosis of groin pain is wide and includes hernias, genital pathology, musculoaponeurotic pain, abnormalities of the lymph nodes and femoral vessels, and referred pain.

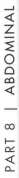

## QUESTIONS

### SBAs

1. **The pathophysiological mechanism responsible for the most severe complication of incarcerated hernias is:**
   a  Gastrointestinal bleeding
   b  Ischaemia
   c  Intestinal obstruction
   d  Pain
   e  Urinary difficulty

**Answer**

**b  *Ischaemia.*** *In any patient presenting with acute hernia, incarceration, compromise of perfusion (strangulation) and viability of the hernia contents should be the principal concern. Various visceral organs, including the intestines, omentum and ovaries, can be incarcerated in a hernia. Strangulation of the bowel results in ischaemia of its wall that may result in perforation and sepsis. Strangulation is usually associated with obstructive symptoms (unless it is the rare Richter's type of hernia). Intestinal obstruction, on the other hand, may initially occur with or without strangulation and compromise of blood flow.*

*Pain can accompany even a non-strangulated hernia and by itself is a symptom and not a pathophysiological mechanism. Bleeding is not a sign of an incarcerated hernia. Incarceration of the omentum can cause significant pain but is otherwise not associated with serious adverse sequelae.*

2. **Which patient requires more urgent surgical intervention?:**
   a  A patient with large long-standing incisional hernia presenting with an acute exacerbation of pain
   b  A woman with a reducible femoral hernia
   c  A 1-year-old child with an inguinal hernia
   d  An older patient with bilateral groin hernias
   e  A patient with an acutely tender irreducible inguinal hernia

**Answer**

**e  *A patient with an acutely tender irreducible inguinal hernia.*** *In any patient presenting with an acutely incarcerated groin hernia (inguinal or femoral), an attempt at gentle reduction should be made. If the hernia is irreducible and contains bowel or ovary, urgent surgical intervention must be instigated.*

*Patients presenting with symptomatic hernias should be questioned about the duration and nature of their symptoms, looking specifically for evidence of intestinal obstruction. The size of the hernia contents is by itself not the criterion for urgency of intervention.*

*Incisional hernias, especially those with a large hernial defect in the absence of obstructive symptoms and with a benign abdominal examination (no concern for strangulation), may be observed.*

*Asymptomatic and minimally symptomatic inguinal hernias in adults, even if bilateral, may be observed. Due to the relatively small and rigid hernial ring of femoral hernias, they are more likely to cause incarceration and strangulation and should be repaired electively even if they are reducible.*

*Inguinal hernias in children should always be repaired, but this can also be done electively if the hernia is reducible.*

**3.** Which of the following statements regarding umbilical hernias is correct?:

**a** Umbilical hernias in infants should be promptly repaired to prevent complications

**b** Symptomatic hernias in adults should be repaired

**c** Umbilical hernias in children are the equivalent of a small omphalocele

**d** Umbilical hernias are less common in babies of African descent

**e** They are usually associated with a patent urachus or omphalomesenteric duct

**Answer**

**b  *Symptomatic hernias in adults should be repaired.***

*Acquired umbilical hernias develop in adults due to progressive stretching of the umbilical scar (typically in its weaker upper portion) due to chronically increased intra-abdominal pressure. Symptomatic hernias should be considered for repair to improve the quality of life and avoid complications.*

*Congenital umbilical hernias result from a failure of the umbilical ring to heal and are completely covered by umbilical skin. They rarely incarcerate, resolve spontaneously in most patients and need repair in only a minority of patients.*

*An omphalocele is incomplete closure of the abdominal wall during embryogenesis. The herniating viscera have a thin membranous, but no skin, coverage.*

*Congenital umbilical hernias are more common in children of African descent.*

*A patent urachus and omphalomesenteric (vitelline) duct are congenital abnormalities that communicate with the umbilicus but are not directly associated with development of an umbilical hernia.*

## MCQs

**1.** The examination of a painful groin mass of pain should include which of the following?:

**a** Inspection and palpation of the abdomen and inguinal regions

**b** Examination of the scrotum in males and labia majora in females

**c** An assessment of the reducibility of the hernia

**d** An attempt to reduce a groin hernia if there are inflammatory changes in the overlying skin

**e** Evaluation of the anus and rectum if inguinal lymphadenopathy is found

**Answer**

***a, b, c, e.*** *Examination of the groins should be performed with the patient in the upright and supine positions. The abdomen, groins and upper thighs should be examined using visual inspection and palpation. The location of the hernia, mass or area of tenderness should be noted in relation to the anatomical landmarks (specifically the umbilicus, pubic tubercle and inguinal ligament).*

*Examine the testicles and spermatic cords in males and the labia majora in females. Digitally palpate the inguinal canal. A differentiation should be made between a hernia, lymphadenopathy and a scrotal mass. The presence of inguinal lymphadenopathy mandates an examination of the extremities, lower torso, external genitalia and anorectal region.*

*Hernias should be assessed for their reducibility.*

*Avoid repeated and aggressive attempts to reduce an incarcerated groin hernia; prompt surgical consultation should be obtained.*

*No attempt should be made to reduce a hernia with overlying inflammatory changes that suggest an underlying strangulated hernia.*

PART 8  |  ABDOMINAL

**2. Which associations are correct?:**

**a** Epigastric hernia – a protrusion of extraperitoneal fat devoid of a peritoneal hernial sac

**b** Obturator hernia – may initially present with bowel obstruction, pain or thigh paresthesias

**c** Direct inguinal hernia – usually descends into the scrotum or labia major

**d** Indirect inguinal hernia – herniation through the posterior wall of the inguinal canal, just lateral to the pubic tubercle

**e** Spigelian hernia – found at the lateral border of the rectus abdominis muscle

**f** Sliding hernia – may be associated with urinary symptoms

**Answer**

***a, b, e, f.*** *Epigastric hernias are painful midline protrusions above the umbilicus, almost always involving only extraperitoneal fat, that do not contain intra-abdominal viscera.*

*Obturator hernias may be difficult to diagnose unless they extend onto the thigh or can be palpated through the vagina. They may present as an acute intestinal obstruction. Alternatively, they may manifest with intermittent symptoms of pain and thigh paraesthesias.*

*Direct inguinal hernias protrude through the wide posterior wall of the inguinal canal (Hesselbach's triangle) and rarely become incarcerated. The peritoneal sac of an indirect inguinal hernia emerges lateral to the epigastric vessels via the internal inguinal ring (where they may become incarcerated) and travels along the testicular vessels or round ligament.*

*Spigelian hernias originate a few centimetres below the umbilicus along the lateral edge of the rectus abdominis muscle at the site of its intersection with the arcuate line. They are initially interparietal hernias and may be not easy to palpate.*

*Sliding inguinal hernias contain viscera as part of their wall and may involve the caecum, sigmoid colon or urinary bladder. Involvement of the bladder may be associated with urinary urgency or frequency.*

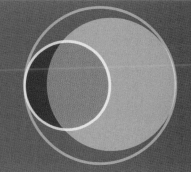

# CHAPTER 35

# Non-acute Abdominal Conditions

Malini D. Sur and Celia M. Divino

## LEARNING OBJECTIVES

- To review the techniques of abdominal examination through inspection, auscultation, percussion and palpation
- To understand symptoms and signs of major non-acute abdominal conditions

- To be able to create a differential diagnosis for common presenting symptoms of non-acute abdominal conditions

## INTRODUCTION

Despite the widespread use of laboratory and radiographic tests for patients with abdominal pain, a detailed history and physical examination remain crucial to formulating a presumptive diagnosis on which to base further investigations. Costly imaging is sometimes reflexively ordered for these patients only to reveal – several hours later – a diagnosis that could have been elucidated with proper clinical assessment, such as an incarcerated hernia. On the other hand, when abdominal pathology is identified early, steps for further treatment can be expedited. For example, a patient can be referred to a surgeon more urgently and, if needed, the appropriate radiographic test can be ordered and prioritized over elective studies.

Thus, strong history and physical examination skills are essential in the outpatient as well as the emergency room setting. The aim of this chapter is to review the symptoms and physical signs associated with major non-acute abdominal conditions that all healthcare providers should be able to appreciate.

## EXAMINATION OF THE ABDOMEN

### Inspection

A complete abdominal examination begins with careful inspection (**Figure 35.1**). It is important that the patient is as comfortable as possible. The examination should take place in a private location that is relatively quiet. Family members can be asked to step away. The clinician should wash their hands or wear gloves. The patient is asked to lie in the supine position with the knees extended and the head of the bed as flat as can be tolerated. A sheet can be used to temporarily cover the lower extremities and genitalia, and the anterior abdominal wall should be completely exposed.

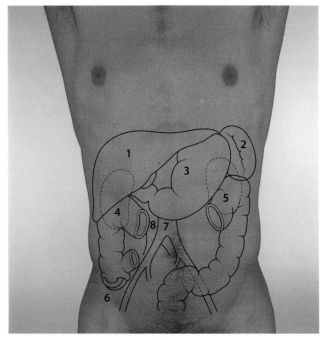

Figure 35.1 The positions of the abdominal viscera. 1, Liver; 2, Spleen; 3, Stomach; 4, Hepatic flexure of colon; 5, Splenic flexure of colon; 6, Appendix; 7, Aortic bifurcation; 8, Inferior vena cava.

Note the size and contour of the abdomen. A scaphoid (concave) abdomen may be present in an emaciated patient with a poor nutritional status resulting from an advanced malignancy or inflammatory bowel disease (IBD). A large or protuberant abdomen may reflect marked obesity or abdominal distension from a dilated bowel, a large intra-abdominal mass or ascites.

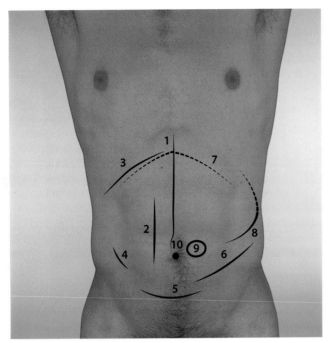

Figure 35.2 Scars that may be present on the abdomen. 1, Mid line; 2, Paramedian; 3, Right subcostal; 4, Appendectomy; 5, Supra pubic; 6, Left iliac; 7, Roof top; 8, Nephrectomy; 9, Left paraumbilical endoscoptic port; 10, Umbilical port.

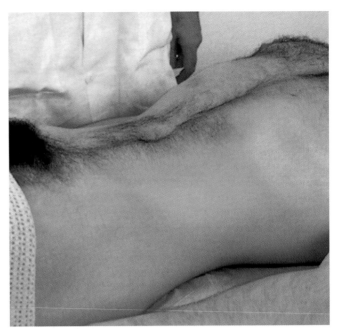

Figure 35.3 Observe the abdomen for respiratory movements and abnormalities.

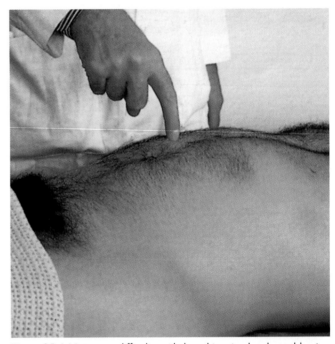

Figure 35.4 Note any difficulty with breathing in deeply or blowing the belly out. Blowing out the abdomen demonstrates any limitation of movement due to tenderness and provides a good deal of information without any manual contact.

Next, carefully inspect the skin for any scars (**Figure 35.2**) and simultaneously question the patient to confirm the surgical history. A lower midline laparotomy scar in a woman may suggest a past hysterectomy or caesarean section, particularly if she has lived in a developing nation. A transverse or subcostal incision in the right upper quadrant (RUQ) typically implies a past open cholecystectomy. A right lower quadrant (RLQ) scar typically reflects a past open appendectomy. Inspect the groins for scars from a previous hernia repair. Given the increasing use of laparoscopy, it is important to actively search for any small, 1–2 cm scars that may be hidden in the umbilicus, bikini line or elsewhere on the abdomen.

Identify any skin lesions or areas of discoloration. A vesicular rash in a dermatomal distribution suggests herpes zoster infection. Dilated superficial veins coursing along a protuberant abdomen are likely to represent a caput medusae, a mark of portosystemic venous shunting in response to portal hypertension.

Skin erythema should be identified as this can be an ominous marker of necrotic underlying bowel. Indeed, erythema over an incarcerated inguinal or ventral hernia is an indication for immediate operative intervention without attempts at reduction. A patient with faecal peritonitis may have extensive flank erythema bilaterally.

Observe how the abdomen moves during respiration and coughing, and on drawing in and blowing out the abdominal wall (**Figures 35.3** and **35.4**).

## Auscultation

During auscultation, place the stethoscope gently on each of the four quadrants. It is useful to simply place the bell on the abdomen and release the hand so that only abdominal sounds are transmitted.

Patients with non-acute abdominal pain may be found to have normal bowel sounds in all quadrants. High-pitched sounds may be heard in the presence of a small bowel obstruction, whereas low-pitched sounds are more common in impending large bowel obstruction. A paucity of sounds is typical of a postoperative ileus. A patient who presents with new, severe abdominal pain and a truly silent abdomen in which no sounds are heard over 10 minutes raises concerns of a surgical emergency such as a perforated viscus.

Listen carefully for vascular bruits, indicating the presence of turbulent blood flow. Such bruits are clues to vascular pathology such as renal artery stenosis or aortic disease, or large vascular abdominal tumours.

## Percussion

Percussion is a useful tool to detect the presence of air, fluid and solid organs within the abdomen, and to identify areas of tenderness (**Figure 35.5**). In patients with acute abdominal pain, loss of dullness over the liver suggests pneumoperitoneum from a perforated viscus. In individuals with obstructive symptoms, drum-like tympanic sounds over a distended abdomen suggests a high-grade small or large bowel obstruction.

A full or protuberant abdomen with diffuse dullness to percussion suggests the presence of ascites (**Figure 35.6**). To further assess for ascites, ask the patient to roll slightly onto to their left side, and percuss the left side of the abdomen laterally from the umbilicus. Note the point at which the percussion note changes from resonant to ascitic. Then have the patient turn to the supine position and repeat the percussion manoeuvre. If ascitic fluid is present, the change from resonant to dull occurs more anteriorly and/or medially as the fluid level changes. This is called shifting dullness (**Figure 35.7**).

Alternatively, have an assistant examiner or the patient place the side of their hand vertically over the umbilicus and apply gentle pressure towards the spine. Place your hand on one flank and tap gently and firmly on the other side. If copious fluid is present, a vibration (transmitted by the fluid) will be felt by the stationary hand (**Figure 35.8**).

Finally, estimate the size of the liver by first percussing over the right anterior chest wall, where there should be resonance from air in the lungs. As the percussing hand is moved downwards, the

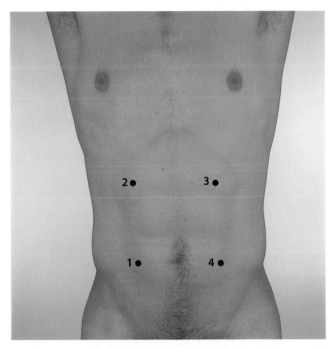

Figure 35.5 Gently percuss over the four quadrants, leaving any tender areas until last.

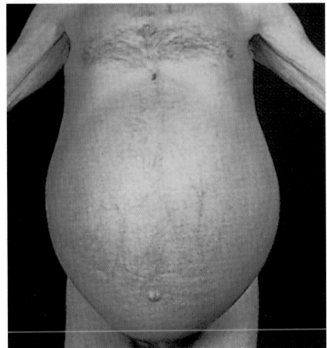

Figure 35.6 Acites.

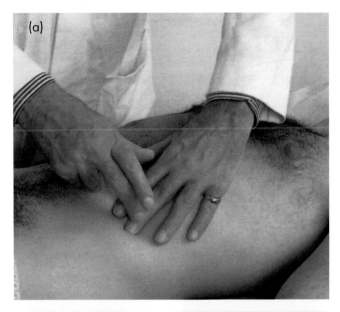

(a)

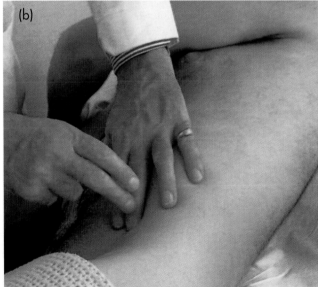

(b)

Figure 35.7 (a) Continue light percussion to outline the organs and check for ascites. Percuss away from the midline until a change in the percussion note is located. Mark this point and (b) roll the patient through 30°: when fluid is present, the percussion note changes at a different location due to fluid movement.

solid liver sounds dull. At the interface between the lower edge of the liver and the bowel, resonance will be heard again.

Patients with peritonitis may not tolerate percussion; gentle percussion is one way to elucidate peritoneal signs (see below and Chapter 36).

## Palpation

Palpation is the most informative part of the abdominal examination. Palpation is started by the patient (**Figure 35.9**), providing an indication of how the clinician's palpation should proceed (**Figures 35.10** and **35.11**). Take care not to frighten the patient with cold hands, poking movements or sudden, deep palpation. Gentle movements avoid voluntary muscle guarding, which can be confused with signs of peritonitis or make it difficult to detect intra-abdominal masses. Examine the area of reported pain last to avoid putting the patient in distress for the majority of the examination.

Asking a few casual questions during the examination may help with distraction. Keep in mind that the purpose of the examination is to detect *signs* of intra-abdominal pathology. Patient-reported complaints of pain during the examination should be noted but always compared with the objective findings.

Begin with light palpation and assess each of the four quadrants. Take note of any pained facial expressions or 'guarding' (abdominal wall muscle contraction during the application or release of manual pressure). Document objective signs of pain during the application of minimal pressure as 'tenderness to light palpation with (or without) guarding' for the relevant quadrant. 'Voluntary guarding' denotes purposeful contractions initiated by the patient, usually in response to fear or startle, while 'involuntary guarding' reflects reflexive contractions upon palpation that are more indicative of peritoneal irritation. Use clinical judgement to distinguish between the two. 'Rigidity' describes diffuse board-like guarding of the abdominal wall due to inflammation of the parietal peritoneum.

Pained expressions or involuntary guarding upon release of the examiner's hands constitute rebound tenderness, which is a sign of peritonitis. When these signs are limited to one quadrant, they reflect localized peritonitis, as in cases of uncomplicated appendicitis or diverticulitis. When these signs are elicited over the whole anterior abdominal wall, diffuse peritonitis is present. Diffuse involuntary guarding to light palpation with associated diffuse rebound tenderness raises the suspicion of a perforated viscus or bowel ischaemia, although non-surgical conditions such as acute pancreatitis can mimic these findings. Diffuse rebound tenderness without significant guarding is more often seen in the presence of irritating peritoneal fluid with a relatively lower

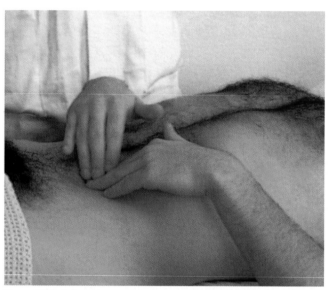

Figure 35.9 Asking the patient to point out tender spots and examining them personally indicates the degree of local tenderness and is particularly useful in children.

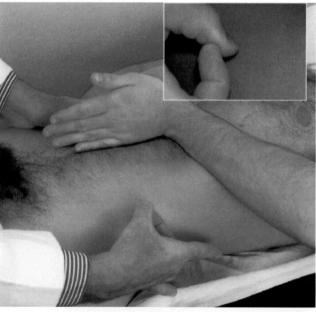

Figure 35.8 When much fluid is present (as in Figure 35.6), vibration initiated on one side of the abdomen can be felt on the other.

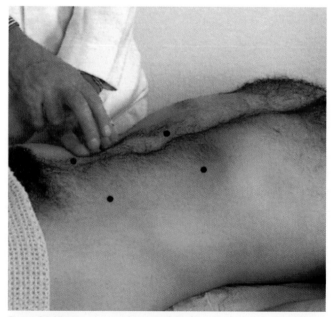

Figure 35.10 Start your palpation of the four quadrants very gently and in the quadrant away from any tender area.

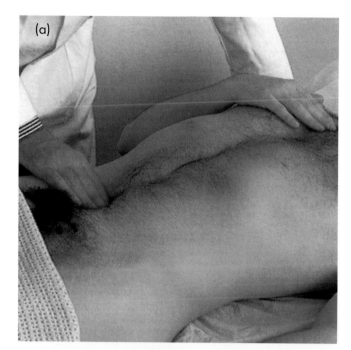

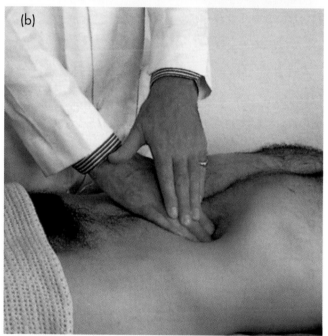

Figure 35.11 Once the amount of tenderness has been assessed, deeper palpation is undertaken over the whole abdomen.

bacterial content, which can be due to a ruptured haemorrhagic ovarian cyst, spontaneous bacterial peritonitis, peritoneal catheter infection or ruptured bladder. A full discussion of acute surgical conditions is available elsewhere in this book.

After an initial evaluation for abdominal tenderness, direct your attention to assessing the size of the major abdominal organs (**Figure 35.12**). To palpate the inferior edge of the **liver**, place your examining hand first in the RLQ, lateral to the rectus sheath, with the fingers pointing towards the left axilla. As the patient inhales deeply, the edge of an enlarged liver will move down to touch the examining hand. Repeat the manoeuvre, progressing up to the costal margin. The edge of a

normal-sized liver will usually not move below the right costal margin on inspiration. An enlarged liver may reflect early cirrhosis, bulky metastatic disease or other liver disorders. In late cirrhosis, the liver is shrunken and not palpable.

Palpation of the RUQ during deep inspiration may also reveal an enlarged or inflamed **gallbladder**. In the presence of RUQ pain, this is called a positive Murphy's sign. In the presence of jaundice, a palpable, distended gallbladder is termed Courvoisier's sign and is suggestive of periampullary malignancy.

The **spleen** and kidneys are normally palpable only when pathologically enlarged. Palpate an enlarged spleen by placing the examining hand initially in the left mid-abdomen (**Figure 35.13**). On deep inspiration, the lower edge of an enlarged spleen can be detected below the left costal margin.

In thin patients, the inferior pole of the right **kidney** is sometimes palpable using the ballottement method (**Figure 35.14**). The anterior hand applies firm pressure in the RUQ lateral to the rectus muscle, while the other hand gently presses the kidney in the costophrenic angle towards the anterior hand. This method can also be used to palpate enlarged kidneys or assess for tenderness.

Always assess the **abdominal aorta** in patients with acute or chronic abdominal pain. Gently press down in the centre of the abdomen until the aortic pulsation is felt. Estimate the width of the aorta by placing a hand on either side. An expansile mass indicates an aneurysm. Aneurysms are not always palpable in obese patients, and conversely, a prominent aortic pulsation may be normal in a slender individual. Ultrasound is a convenient way to assess the abdominal aorta. Immediately refer patients with an enlarging aortic width or tenderness over a known aortic aneurysm to a vascular surgeon.

The **stomach** and **colon** can also be appreciated on physical examination in some patients. A firm, palpable mass in the epigastrium may represent a transverse colon or gastric malignancy. Hard stool may be palpated within the transverse or sigmoid colon in patients with severe constipation. Finally, always perform a **rectal examination** in any patient with abdominal pain to evaluate for rectal masses and occult blood. In women, a dedicated pelvic examination can exclude a **gynaecological cause** of non-acute abdominal pain.

Combined inspection and palpation of the abdominal wall surface and both groins allows for the detection of any **hernias**, abscesses or other masses. Hernias may cause intermittent pain or obstructive symptoms; they are considered in Chapter 34:

- An epigastric bulge without an associated scar reflects a *congenital or acquired epigastric hernia*.
- Bulges over prior scars typically represent *incisional hernias*, although a benign postoperative fluid collection or asymmetrical fat distribution may also appear as a bulge.
- An *inguinal hernia* is detected as a bulge over the inguinal ligament that can be increased in size by coughing or the Valsalva manoeuvre.
- A bulge inferior to the inguinal ligament suggests a *femoral hernia*.
- If present, intestinal stomas should be examined for the presence of *parastomal hernias*, which may be chronically or acutely incarcerated with bowel.

In the outpatient setting, any hernia should be reducible with gentle pressure over the hernia with the patient in the

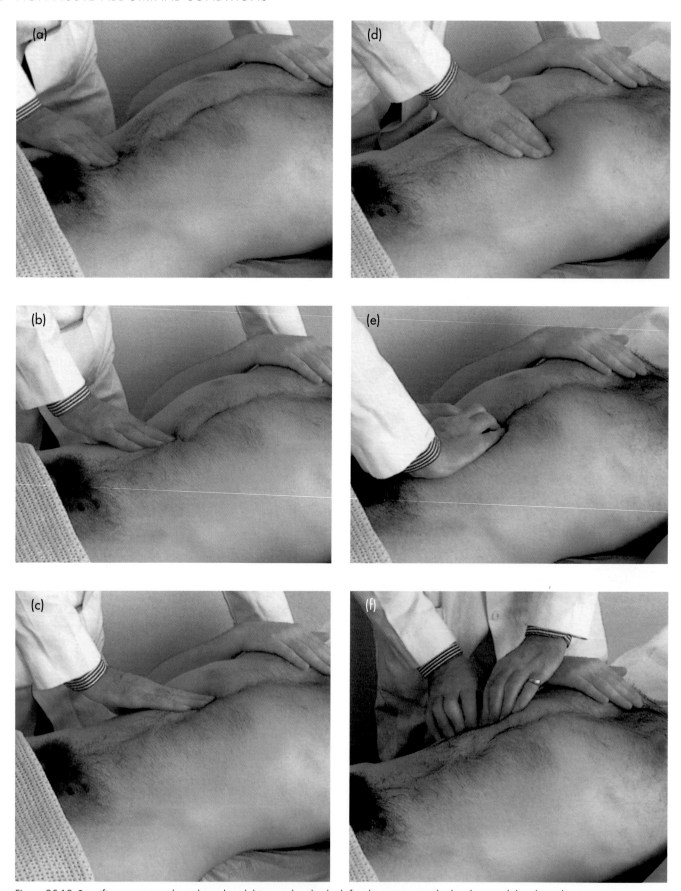

Figure 35.12 Specific organs may be enlarged and this must be checked, first by percussing the borders, and then by palpating target areas, as in this search for the liver.

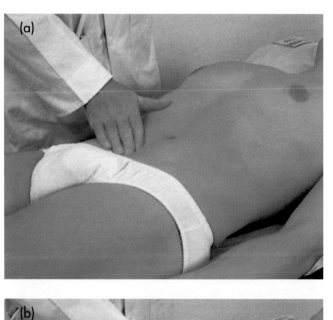

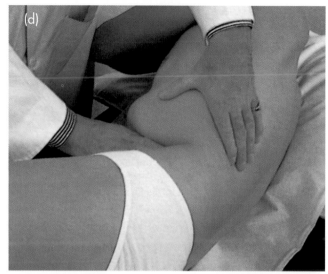

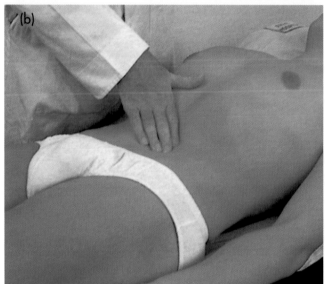

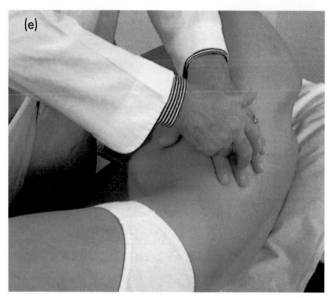

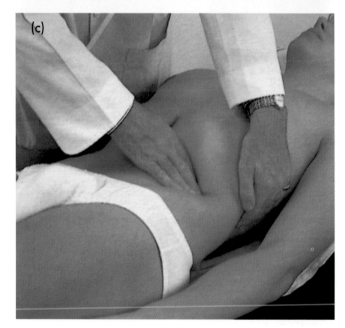

Figure 35.13 Palpating the spleen.

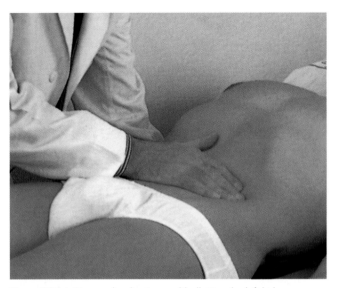

Figure 35.14 Bimanual palpation and ballotting the left kidney.

supine position. Non-reducible or incarcerated hernias have a higher risk of strangulation or ischaemia of the contents of the hernial sac, such as bowel or omentum.

An abdominal wall **mass** that is tender, fluctuant and erythematous suggests an abscess. Abdominal wall abscesses may be more commonly seen in obese, diabetic patients or immunocompromised individuals.

## EVALUATION OF PATIENTS WITH ABDOMINAL PAIN

The chief complaint of the vast majority of patients with underlying abdominal conditions is abdominal pain or discomfort. The presence or absence of associated symptoms such as nausea, vomiting, diarrhoea, constipation and abdominal distension should be noted. It is important to be able to generate a list of possible diagnoses based on the location of the patient's discomfort. The physical examination should identify disease-specific signs to assess for the likelihood of each possible diagnosis.

Upper gastrointestinal endoscopy is the primary diagnostic modality for non-acute conditions of the upper gastrointestinal tract. In many patients, preliminary upper gastrointestinal contrast studies or CT scans are performed.

### Epigastric Pain

In the differential diagnosis, remember:

- gastro-oesophageal reflux disease;
- hiatus hernia;
- gastritis;
- gastric ulcer;
- duodenal ulcer;
- gastric neoplasm;
- pyloric outflow obstruction;
- biliary colic;
- pancreatitis;
- pancreatic neoplasm;
- endocrine causes;
- abdominal aortic aneurysm;
- cardiac pathology.

### Gastro-oesophageal Reflux Disease

Many gastric conditions result in chronic epigastric pain or discomfort, including gastro-oesophageal reflux disease, hiatus hernia, gastritis and peptic ulcer disease. Patients with gastro-oesophageal reflux disease may describe a burning sensation in the chest and epigastric area that is worse with meals, bending over or lying flat. Dysphagia and coughing may also be reported.

### Hiatus Hernia

Symptomatic hiatus hernia should be considered in patients who report vague, intermittent epigastric or substernal pain, postprandial fullness, nausea or retching. Gastro-oesophageal reflux disease is frequently present, and sliding hernias account for the vast majority of cases. Paraoesophageal hernias (**Figures 35.15** and **35.16**) are rarer and can also present with gastric volvulus, bleeding and respiratory symptoms. The physical examination findings are typically normal in patients with gastro-oesophageal reflux disease and hiatus hernia, although patients with concomitant laryngopharyngeal reflux may have pharyngeal erythema and oedema.

### Gastritis and Peptic Ulcer Disease

Patients with gastritis and peptic ulcer disease (**Figure 35.17**) typically report non-radiating, burning epigastric pain. The pain of a duodenal ulcer is usually experienced 2–3 hours after meals and may wake the patient during the night. Pain from a gastric ulcer usually occurs during meals. Nausea, bloating, weight loss or anaemia may also be present. The physical examination findings are typically normal in patients with gastritis and peptic ulcer disease unless there is significant anaemia leading to pallor of the conjunctivae, nail beds, palmar creases and face, and a positive stool guaiac test.

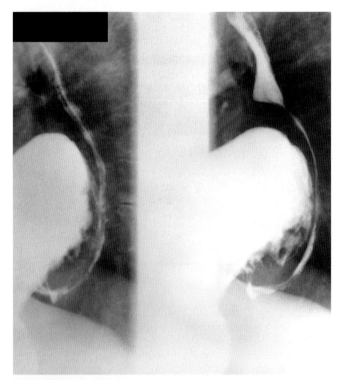

Figure 35.15 A rolling hiatus hernia.

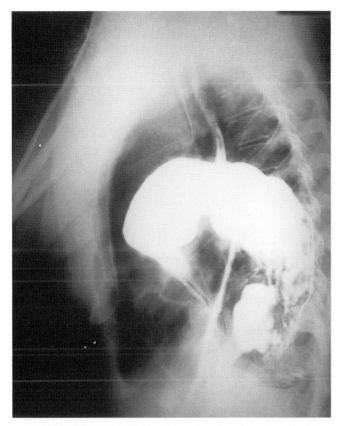

Figure 35.16 Relocation of the gut into the chest through a diaphragmatic defect.

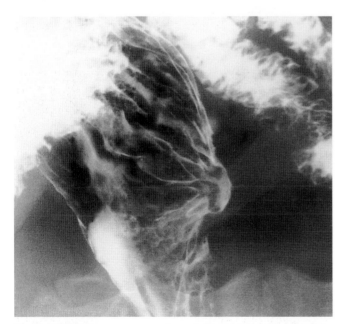

Figure 35.17 A benign gastric ulcer of the greater curvature of the stomach.

The majority of ulcers are caused by *Helicobacter pylori* infection or use of non-steroidal anti-inflammatory agents, but alcohol abuse, smoking, trauma from burns or head injury, and other sources of stress have also been implicated. In **Zollinger–Ellison syndrome**, gastric ulcers are caused by increased gastrin production from a gastrin-secreting tumour, usually located within the pancreatic head.

## Gastric Neoplasms

Vague but persistent epigastric discomfort may be an early sign of a gastric neoplasm. Early satiety and anaemia from gastrointestinal bleeding may also be found in large or ulcerated lesions. Nausea and vomiting is present in patients with gastric outlet obstruction from a large antral or pyloric tumour. Benign gastric tumours include gastrointestinal stromal tumours, leiomyomas (**Figure 35.18**) and adenomatous polyps. Gastric adenocarcinomas (**Figures 35.19** and **35.20**) are more frequent in smokers and nitrosamine consumers.

Weight loss, fatigue and night sweats may be found in patients with malignancy. Advanced malignancy may be associated with cachexia or temporal muscle wasting on physical examination. Abdominal examination may reveal a firm epigastric mass that moves with respiration. Hepatomegaly may be identified if bulky liver metastases are present. Ascites occurs with carcinomatosis.

The classic distribution of metastatic nodal deposits includes Virchow's node in the supraclavicular region, Sister Mary Joseph's node in the umbilicus and Blumer's shelf of nodes in the

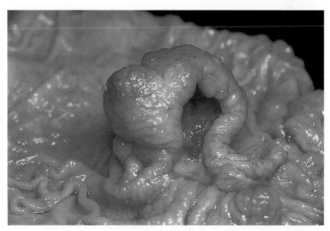

Figure 35.18 A leiomyoma of the stomach with associated ulceration.

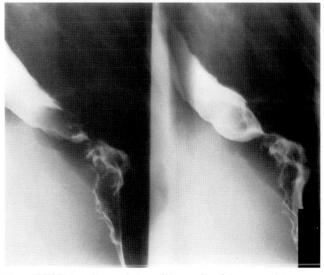

Figure 35.19 A malignant lesion of the cardia of the stomach.

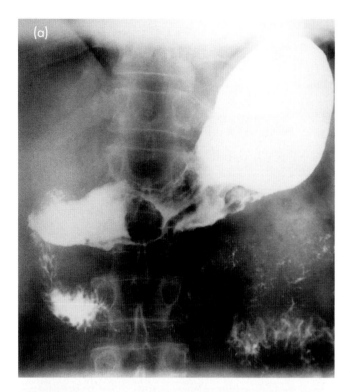

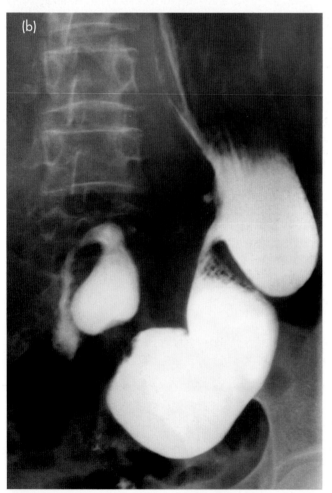

Figure 35.20 (a) A carcinomatous polyp and mural plaque. (b) An hour-glass stomach.

rectovesical pouch or the pouch of Douglas. The latter can be palpated on rectal examination. Pelvic examination may reveal metastatic deposits in the ovaries (**Krukenberg tumours**).

## Pyloric Obstruction

Pyloric outflow obstruction results from a variety of causes and occurs over a wide age range from birth onwards (**Figures 35.21–35.23**).

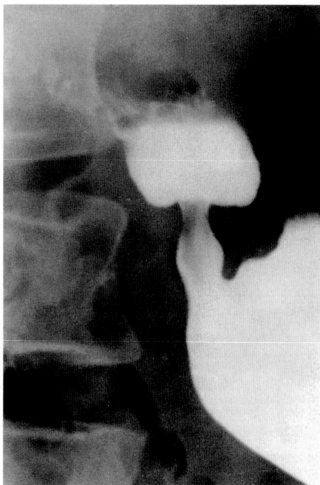

Figure 35.21 Hypertrophic pyloric stenosis.

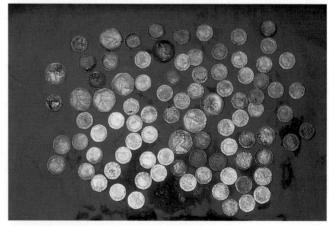

Figure 35.22 Loose change from a collector's stomach.

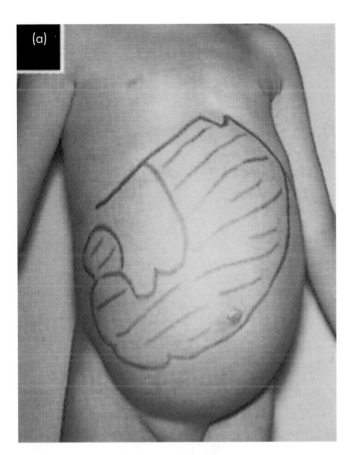

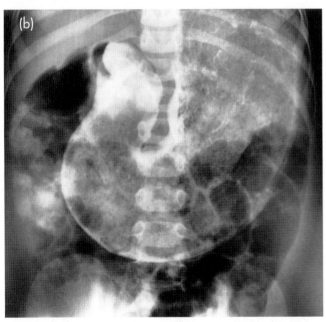

Figure 35.23 (a) Pyloric obstruction due to a trichobezoar. (b) The radiological appearance in this patient.

## Biliary Colic

Biliary colic occasionally results in epigastric pain, although there is usually a right-sided component. It is discussed below.

### Pancreatitis

Pancreatitis should be considered as a source of acute or chronic epigastric pain radiating to the back or chest in patients with a history of gallstones or alcohol abuse. Common medications that can cause pancreatitis include corticosteroids, furosemide, valproic acid, oestrogen, tetracycline, trimethoprim/sulfamethoxazole, opiates and anti-inflammatory medications.

In the acute setting, patients may demonstrate fever, tachycardia, tachypnoea or hypotension if a systemic inflammatory response is present. The examination findings range from minimal epigastric tenderness to diffuse guarding from chemical peritonitis and bowel oedema. Retroperitoneal haemorrhage from necrotizing pancreatitis is manifested by flank ecchymosis, known as **Grey Turner's sign**, and periumbilical ecchymosis, known as **Cullen's sign (Figure 35.24)**. Both are predictive of a high risk of death.

Patients with chronic pancreatitis do not have signs of systemic toxicity, but their pain is often debilitating and either constant or worse with meals. A history of long-term alcohol abuse is typically present. Steatorrhoea, weight loss and new-onset diabetes occur with pancreatic endocrine and exocrine insufficiency. Physical examination may only be significant for generalized wasting in these cases. Patients with a large pancreatic pseudocyst **(Figure 35.25)** may have a mildly tender epigastric mass.

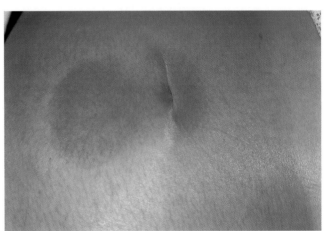

Figure 35.24 Cullen's sign.

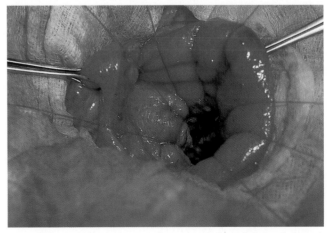

Figure 35.25 A pancreatic pseudocyst opened, and drained, through the back wall of the stomach, the communication being left open.

## Pancreatic Neoplasms

Patients with a history of smoking, obesity and diabetes have a higher risk of pancreatic cancer. The classic presentation of a pancreatic head or periampullary neoplasm is painless obstructive jaundice accompanied by dark urine, clay-coloured stools and pruritis. However, persistent dull epigastric pain may be reported in some cases of pancreatic neoplasm. The pain may be exacerbated by meals or supine positioning. Pancreatic body and tail lesions tend to present later and do not cause jaundice. Constitutional symptoms such as weight loss, fatigue and night sweats with associated cachexia may be present with malignant neoplasms.

The conjunctivae and tongue should be examined for early jaundice. **Courvoisier's sign** denotes a non-tender but palpable, distended gallbladder that results from back-pressure in the biliary tree. Pancreatic masses are usually not palpable. Liver metastases may cause hepatomegaly in advanced cases. Ascites may be present. As with gastric cancer, nodal metastases may be detected in the supraclavicular or umbilical region. **Trousseau's sign** is present when there are areas of superficial thrombophlebitis.

## Endocrine Causes

The adrenal glands are retroperitoneal and are therefore rarely large enough to produce abdominal examination findings. However, any malfunction of their hormone secretion has profound systemic effects.

Acute destruction of the gland usually results from haemorrhage or sepsis. Haemorrhage may occur at birth and is usually fatal. In later life, it may follow meningococcal septicaemia and is followed by hyperpyrexia and profound shock – **Waterhouse–Friderichsen syndrome**. Chronic destruction of the glands may follow tuberculosis infection or replacement by metastatic deposits. The clinical effect of chronic hyposecretion of corticosteroids is **Addison's disease** (see p. 42).

Hypersecretion of corticosteroids may result from tumours of the adrenal cortex or pituitary gland. **Cushing's syndrome** (see p. 41) may result from a pituitary tumour that overproduces adrenocorticotrophic hormone, or an adrenal cortical tumour that oversecretes glucocorticoids. An aldosteronoma is a tumour of the adrenal cortex that oversecretes aldosterone. The resulting sodium retention and loss of potassium leads to **Conn's syndrome**, which is marked by hypertension that is difficult to control, muscle weakness and polyuria. Bilateral adrenal hyperplasia may also result in primary hyperaldosteronism. Finally, adrenal cortical carcinomas may produce multiple symptoms based on excess steroid hormone production, including Cushing's syndrome, Conn's syndrome, and feminization or virilization if sex hormones are oversecreted.

Tumours of the adrenal medulla may be neurogenic or neoplasms of chromaffin cells. **Neurogenic tumours** include benign ganglioneuromas and malignant neuroblastomas. The latter occur in children, grow rapidly to a large size and metastasize early. They may secrete vasoactive intestinal polypeptide, but the clinical picture usually features weight loss, abdominal pain, distension, ascites, fever and anaemia.

**Chromaffin tumours** are phaeochromocytomas (**Figures 35.26** and **35.27**). The tumours secrete catecholamines, producing sustained marked hypertension that can give

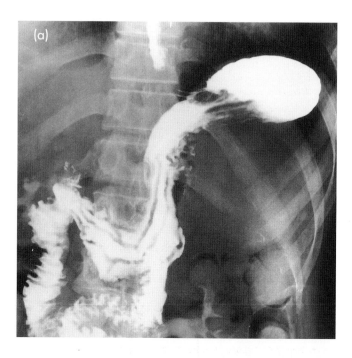

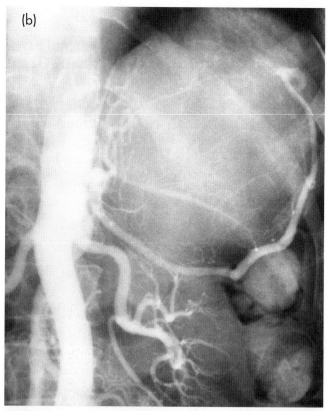

**Figure 35.26** A large left phaeochromocytoma. (a) Displacement of the stomach. (b) The blood supply to the tumour.

rise to fatal cerebral haemorrhage and cardiac dysrhythmias. The patient may complain of headaches, palpitations, excess sweating and shortness of breath.

A diagnosis of phaeochromocytoma should lead to an immediate consideration of a hereditary predisposition such as a multiple endocrine neoplasia (MEN) syndrome. The most common variant is MEN type 1, which involves:

- parathyroid tumours (80 per cent);
- islet tumours of the pancreas, producing gastrin (**Zollinger–Ellison syndrome**), insulin (**Figure 35.27**), glucagon, somatostatin and vasoactive intestinal polypeptide;
- pituitary chromaffin adenomas (65 per cent), which produce prolactin or give rise to acromegaly;
- thyroid and adrenocortical tumours.

In MEN type 2a, there is a 50 per cent incidence of parathyroid tumours, together with medullary carcinoma of the thyroid, producing calcitonin, and phaeochromocytomas. Type 2b disease has, in addition, neurological components, with neuromas of the eyelids and lips, and ganglioneuromatosis, together with marfanoid facial appearances and megacolon.

## Vascular and Cardiac Pathology

**Vascular aetiologies** must be considered in all patients with abdominal pain, particularly those with coronary artery disease, peripheral arterial disease, carotid artery disease or diabetes, and those who smoke.

A slowly enlarging abdominal aortic aneurysm does not usually cause symptoms but may occasionally cause progressive vague epigastric or central abdominal pain radiating to the back. A pulsatile mass may be present on abdominal examination. Patients with acute rupture report severe abdominal and back pain and are typically hypotensive with obvious diaphoresis and pallor. A palpable abdominal mass may be detected when there is a contained rupture. A free intraperitoneal rupture will quickly lead to peritonitis and death.

**Cardiac pathology** must be considered in patients with chronic epigastric complaints without definitive findings on abdominal examination or a related work-up.

## Right Upper Quadrant Pain

The differential diagnosis includes:

- gastritis;
- gastric ulcer;
- biliary colic;
- cholecystitis;
- cholangitis;

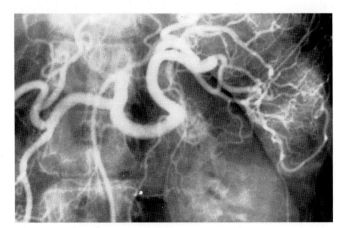

Figure 35.27 An arteriogram of an insulinoma.

- hepatitis;
- hepatic neoplasm;
- hepatic abscess.

Right upper quadrant pain is a common presenting complaint. Ultrasound of the liver, gallbladder and pancreas (supplemented by blood tests) is the primary diagnostic modality for this region, once gastric and duodenal pathology has been excluded.

### Gastritis and Gastric Ulcers

Gastritis and gastric ulcers, especially those in the antrum and pylorus, may cause vague RUQ and epigastric pain. Patients with these conditions do not typically have significant tenderness on examination.

### Biliary Colic

Biliary colic is the most common aetiology of isolated RUQ pain, particularly in multiparous or obese women. Sickle cell disease, Crohn's disease and dependence on total parenteral nutrition are also risk factors for gallstone formation (**Figure 35.28**).

The pain of biliary colic is thought to result from the gallbladder contracting against gallstones transiently blocking the gallbladder neck. It typically originates in the RUQ or epigastrium and radiates to the back or right shoulder blade. It is brought on by fatty meals, lasts for a few hours and generally regresses spontaneously. Nausea and vomiting are usually present. Some patients may experience intermittent postprandial pain for years before reporting their symptoms to a healthcare provider.

There are no signs of systemic toxicity or jaundice on physical examination. There may be mild RUQ tenderness but no rebound, guarding or palpable masses.

### Cholecystitis

Prolonged cystic duct obstruction from gallstones leads to stasis of the bile and bacterial overgrowth, causing symptoms of cholecystitis. These include unrelenting RUQ pain, nausea, vomiting and signs of systemic toxicity such as fever and tachycardia. Patients with gangrenous cholecystitis may have an altered mental status or signs of shock. Jaundice is classically absent but can be present in rare cases of **Mirizzi syndrome**, in which an inflammatory mass at the neck of the gallbladder may compress the adjacent common bile duct.

In most cases, the abdomen is soft with localized guarding in the RUQ. A tender, palpable gallbladder may be present, particularly with complete cystic duct obstruction leading to hydrops. **Murphy's sign** can be elicited by applying pressure with one hand just below the right costal margin in the midclavicular line and asking the patient to inhale deeply. As the inflamed gallbladder moves down towards the area of pressure, the patient will suddenly stop inhaling due to discomfort. Note that elderly diabetic and immunocompromised patients with severe or gangrenous cholecystitis frequently have minimal symptoms and examination findings. A high index of suspicion is required in such patients.

### Cholangitis

Cholangitis is an acute ascending bacterial infection of the intrahepatic biliary tree that results from common bile duct or common hepatic duct obstruction. The usual aetiology is a gallstone that has passed into the common bile duct, causing

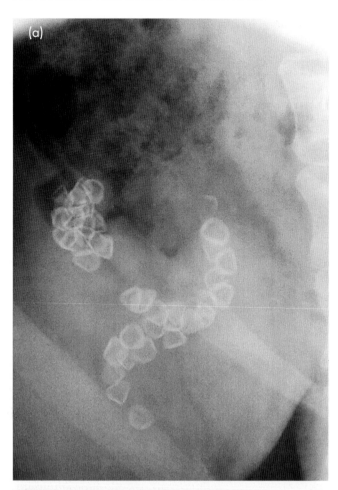

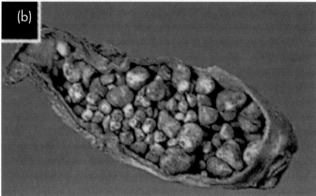

Figure 35.28 (a) A plain radiograph demonstrating stones in the gallbladder and throughout the length of the common bile and hepatic ducts. (b) An operative specimen following cholecystectomy for cholelithiasis.

choledocholithiasis and ascending cholangitis. Less frequently, an obstructing cancer at the pancreatic head or a **Klatskin tumour** at the hepatic duct confluence is the culprit. In East-Asian patients with oriental cholangiohepatitis, an underlying bacterial or parasitic infection that leads to intrahepatic stone formation, should be considered.

Regardless of the cause, **Charcot's triad** of RUQ pain, high fever and jaundice is the classic presentation of acute cholangitis.

**Reynolds' pentad** describes the addition of shock and altered mental status in severe cases. Vital signs may demonstrate fever, tachycardia and hypotension. Examination findings include jaundice, scleral icterus and mild to moderate tenderness in the RUQ without peritonitis.

### Hepatitis

Liver pathology often results in RUQ pain or discomfort. A thorough history will reveal any risk factors for acute infection with hepatitis A (HAV), B (HBV) or C (HCV) virus:

- Individuals who have recently travelled to areas with poor sanitation and been in contact with contaminated food are at risk of a self-limiting infection with HAV.
- Those with a history of blood transfusion, intravenous drug use and exposure to contaminated needles are at risk of HBV and HCV infection.
- A history of unprotected sex or contact with the bodily fluids of infected persons increases the risk of HBV infection. Sexual transmission of HCV is rare but has been reported in patients with high viral loads.

Patients with acute viral hepatitis sometimes report prodromal symptoms of anorexia, nausea, vomiting, malaise, arthralgia and headache. Jaundice (**Figure 35.29**) may develop 1–2 weeks after these symptoms, along with RUQ pain. Low-grade fevers are more often reported with HAV infection. Abdominal examination often reveals a tender, enlarged liver and, less commonly, splenomegaly. Cervical and epitrochlear lymphadenopathy may also be present.

Chronic infection with HBV or HCV may lead to signs and symptoms of cirrhosis and portal hypertension (**Figure 35.30**). Other intrahepatic aetiologies of portal hypertension include chronic alcoholism, the most common cause in the USA, as well as Wilson's disease, haemochromatosis, sarcoidosis and schistosomiasis. Post hepatic portal obstruction is rare and is associated with Budd–Chiari syndrome, constrictive pericarditis and right heart failure. Presenting symptoms include increasing abdominal girth, oesophageal variceal bleeding, portosystemic encephalopathy and spontaneous bacterial

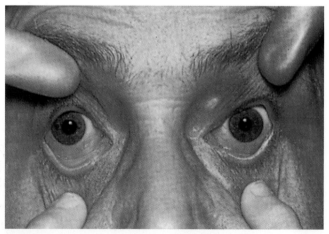

Figure 35.29 The yellow scleral discoloration of jaundice.

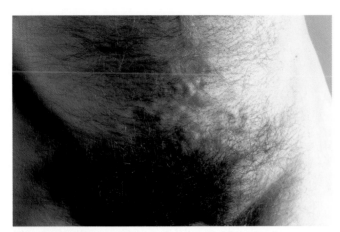

Figure 35.30 Varicose veins over the lower abdominal wall in a patient with inferior vena cava obstruction.

peritonitis. Incidental findings of thrombocytopenia or splenomegaly may also lead to a diagnosis of portal hypertension. Patients may have mild chronic systemic hypotension from splanchnic vasodilatation.

Physical examination may reveal temporal wasting with a protuberant abdomen and jaundice in advanced cases. Hair loss, palmar erythema, clubbing, gynaecomastia, telangiectasias, testicular atrophy and distended paraumbilical veins (caput medusae) may be seen (**Figure 35.31**). Encephalopathy may manifest as mild drowsiness or lethargy.

A fibrotic and enlarged liver may be palpable below the costal margin, but in advanced cirrhosis the liver shrinks and hepatomegaly is absent. A palpable liver in a patient with chronic liver disease should raise a suspicion of hepatocellular carcinoma. Occasionally, a bruit may be auscultated over this hypervascular tumour. Splenomegaly results from back-pressure in the portal system and is common. Ascites may be appreciated on examination when the total volume exceeds 1.5 L.

## Hepatic Neoplasms

Benign and malignant hepatic neoplasms should be considered in patients who report vague RUQ discomfort. Symptoms typically exist only when the lesion is fairly large.

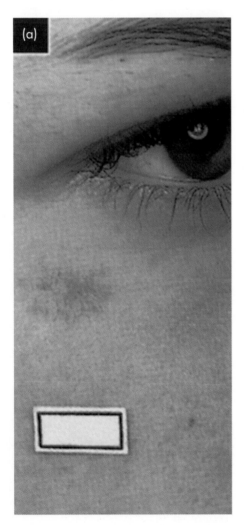

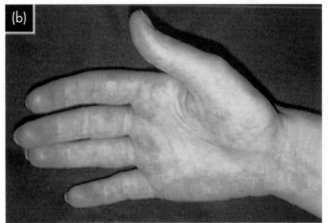

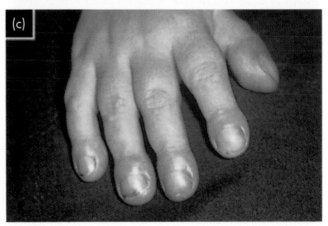

Figure 35.31 Signs of liver failure. (a) Spider naevi. (b) Liver palms. (c) Clubbing.

Women with a history of oral contraceptive use may have hepatic adenomas or fibronodular hyperplasia. The former are at risk of rupture and malignant degeneration, particularly when the diameter exceeds 5 cm. Haemangiomas are usually asymptomatic and found incidentally on imaging. Liver metastases must be considered in a patient with a history of extrahepatic cancer with RUQ discomfort or hepatomegaly. Rarely, hepatocellular carcinoma arises spontaneously and may invade adjacent organs including the diaphragm, stomach and spleen. A firm mass in the RUQ may also represent a primary gallbladder cancer.

## Left Upper Quadrant Pain

The differential diagnosis of left upper quadrant (LUQ) pain includes:

- splenomegaly;
- splenic cyst;
- splenic abscess;
- splenic neoplasm;
- splenic artery aneurysm;
- subphrenic abscess;
- gastric–colitis;
- colonic neoplasm;
- pancreatic neoplasm;
- left renal pathology.

Pain in the LUQ is rare and usually reflects splenic pathology. The physical examination of patients with LUQ pain should focus on identifying splenomegaly and excluding extra-abdominal signs of systemic disease. Although ultrasound may be helpful when the spleen is grossly enlarged, CT scanning is the primary diagnostic modality for pathology in this region.

Massive **splenomegaly (Figure 35.32)** can cause discomfort from diaphragmatic irritation. It is seen in patients with sickle cell anaemia, polycythaemia vera, portal hypertension and splenic lesions, such as cysts, tumours and abscesses.

Parasitic **cysts** are typically echinococcal. Non-infected cysts **(Figure 35.33)** include dermoid, epidermoid, endothelial and pseudocysts, which usually result from trauma or infarction.

**Splenic abscess** should be considered in patients with LUQ pain and a history of intravenous drug use, endocarditis, blunt abdominal trauma or human immunodeficiency virus (HIV) infection. Malaise, weight loss and fever may also be reported.

Rare primary **splenic neoplasms** include lymphomas, sarcomas, haemangiomas, lymphangiosarcomas and hamartomas. Splenic metastases are rare but may occur with melanoma or lung and breast cancer.

The spontaneous rupture of a **splenic angioma** with massive haemoperitoneum and resulting peritonitis has been reported.

Rarely, locally advanced colonic, gastric, pancreatic or hepatic malignant **neoplasms** may produce LUQ discomfort and constitutional symptoms. Physical examination may reveal a palpable mass in the epigastrium or LUQ. Patients with colitis may present with LUQ pain with associated diarrhoea or blood per rectum.

**Left renal pathology** such as nephrolithiasis, pyelonephritis or neoplasm should also be considered in patients with LUQ complaints, especially if there is associated dysuria or haematuria.

## Right Lower Quadrant Pain

The differential diagnosis of RLQ pain is:

- appendicitis;
- Crohn's disease;

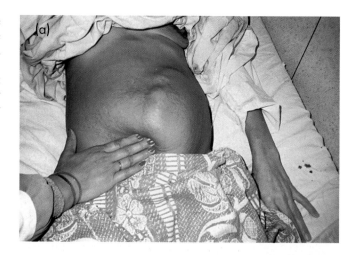

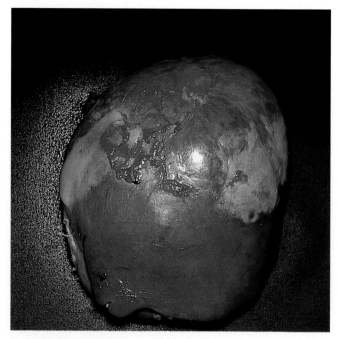

Figure 35.32 Splenic enlargement. (a) Egyptian splenomegaly due to schistosomiasis. (b) A splenic cyst.

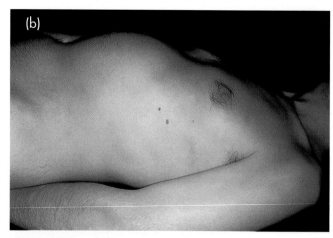

Figure 35.33 An operative specimen of splenic cyst.

- right-sided diverticulitis;
- right-sided colitis;
- typhilitis;
- right renal pathology;
- right ovarian pathology;
- ectopic pregnancy.

Asking the patient about specific symptoms of a change in bowel habits, dysuria and vaginal discharge will help to distinguish between the possible organ systems affected. A menstrual and sexual history is mandatory in all female patients. Abdominal or transvaginal ultrasound may reveal appendiceal or gynaecological pathology, but CT and colonoscopy are the primary diagnostic modalities for this quadrant.

**Acute RLQ pain** should raise a suspicion of acute appendicitis, right-sided colitis, acute terminal ileitis from Crohn's disease, a right-sided renal stone, an ectopic pregnancy or right ovarian pathology such as torsion, a ruptured cyst or a tubo-ovarian abscess. Immunocompromised patients with RLQ pain and fever may have typhlitis, an enterocolitis of the ileocaecal region that is poorly understood.

With acute conditions, the examination may reveal localized RLQ peritonitis with rebound and guarding. An RLQ mass may be appreciated in patients with an underlying appendiceal abscess or inflammatory mass (**phlegmon**) (**Figures 35.34–35.36**).

Diffuse peritonitis with complaints of RLQ pain may reflect perforated appendicitis. Classically, a patient with renal colic from an obstructing renal stone is found writhing on the examination table whereas a patient with peritonitis from a gastrointestinal source lies still as any movement exacerbates the pain. Patients with renal pathology are also more likely to have flank tenderness at the costovertebral angle than anterior abdominal tenderness.

A pelvic examination should be performed in all women with lower abdominal pain to exclude adnexal tenderness from ovarian pathology. A pregnancy test should always be performed.

Patients with **non-acute or recurring RLQ pain** may have a mild chronic appendicitis. Crohn's disease must be considered, particularly in patients with an Ashkenazi Jewish background or a family history of IBD. Diverticulitis of the caecum or a redundant

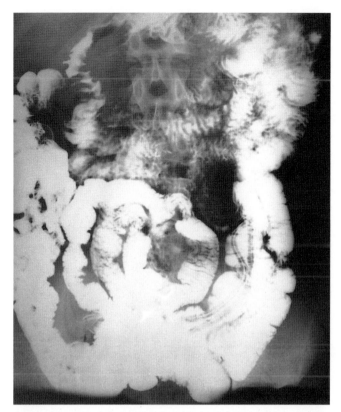

Figure 35.35 *Ascaris* worms within the ileum, outlined by a barium study.

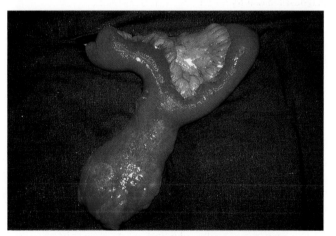

Figure 35.36 An operative specimen of a Mekel's diverticulum.

RLQ sigmoid colon is another possibility. Chronic right ovarian pathology such as an enlarging cyst or neoplasm should be considered in women. In non-acute conditions, the abdominal examination may show only mild RLQ tenderness.

Patients with Crohn's disease (**Figure 35.37** and **35.38**) usually report a waxing and waning of their symptoms, including abdominal pain, diarrhoea and weight loss. They may have generalized wasting from chronic malnutrition and a palpable RLQ mass reflecting a chronic inflammatory process due to active Crohn's disease. The perianal examination may reveal characteristic fissures and fistulas (**Figure 35.39**).

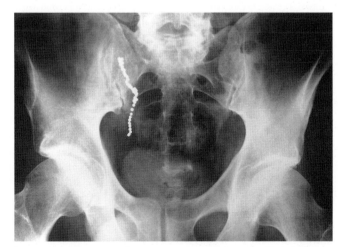

Figure 35.34 An appendix containing radio-opaque pellets that show its pelvic position.

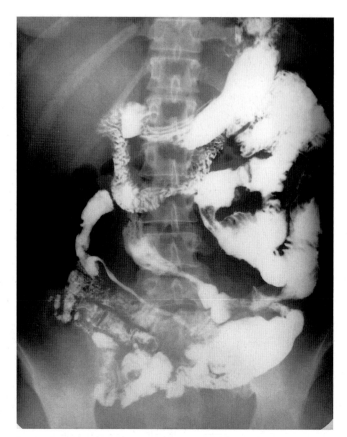

Figure 35.37 Crohn's disease of the terminal ileum demonstrating the string sign of Cantor.

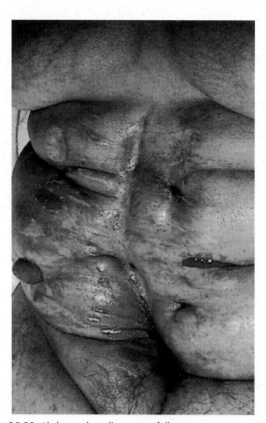

Figure 35.38 Abdominal wall sinuses following surgery in Crohn's disease.

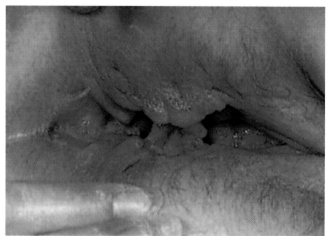

Figure 35.39 Perianal Crohn's disease.

Patients with long-standing Crohn's disease may show cutaneous manifestations such as erythema nodosum or pyoderma gangrenosum (**Figure 35.40**). Erythema nodosum presents as tender, subcutaneous nodules on the extensor surfaces and is more prevalent during Crohn's flares. Pyoderma gangrenosum appears as ulcerated skin lesions and may occur independent of disease activity.

In some regions, tuberculosis remains an important differential diagnosis (**Figure 35.41**).

## Left Lower Quadrant Pain

The differential diagnosis involves:

- diverticulitis;
- left-sided colitis;
- appendicitis with malrotation;
- left renal pathology;
- left ovarian pathology;
- ectopic pregnancy.

Left lower quadrant (LLQ) pain associated with anorexia, nausea and fever is the typical presentation of diverticulitis. **Diverticulosis**, the presence of colonic mucosal outpouchings (**Figure 35.42**), is widespread in Western adults, but infectious complications affect only a subset of patients. The range of clinical presentation varies from acute, severe symptoms with sepsis and peritonitis, to chronic, low-grade symptoms with more benign findings on examination.

All patients with possible **diverticulitis** should be questioned about prior colonoscopy and any symptoms of a colovesicular fistula such as chronic pneumaturia or faecaluria. Patients with mild pain, normal vital signs and mild LLQ tenderness without marked guarding are likely to have uncomplicated diverticulitis. Those with fever, tachycardia or hypotension along with localized peritonitis may have a diverticular abscess from a small, contained perforation. A palpable LLQ mass may be appreciated in patients with a large, dense inflammatory reaction or mass. Those with shock and diffuse peritonitis are likely to have free colonic perforation with faecal peritonitis.

Colonic ischaemia with pneumatosis coli (**Figure 35.43**), perforation after removal of a colonoscopic polyp (**Figure 35.44**), perforated colon cancers (**Figures 35.45** and **35.46**) and fulminant ulcerative colitis or *Clostridium difficile*-associated colitis should also be considered in patients with LLQ pain, peritonitis and shock.

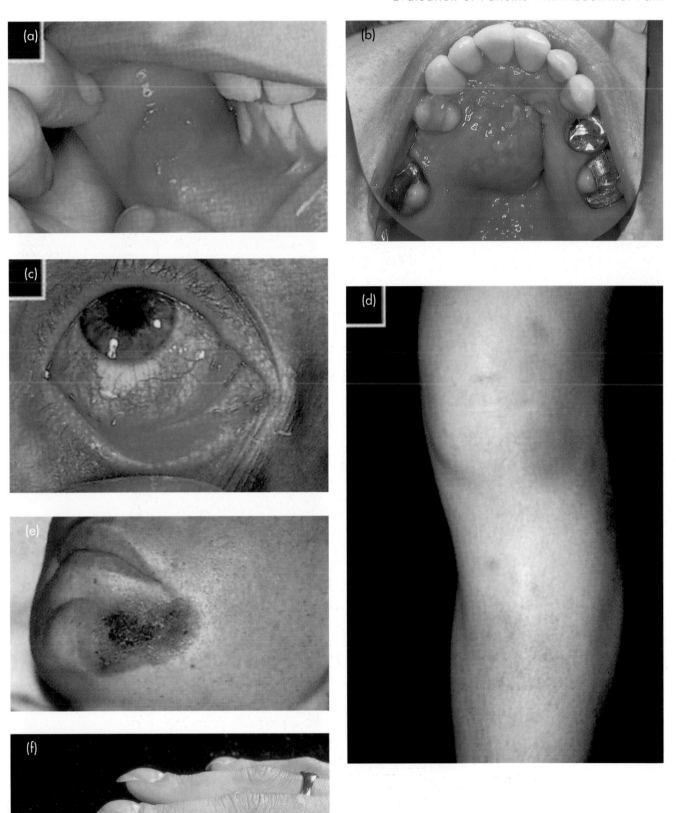

Figure 35.40 Extraintestinal manifestations of inflammatory bowel disease. (a) A Crohn's lesion on the lip. (b) Palatal Crohn's disease. (c) Episcleritis. (d) Erythema nodosum. (e) Pyoderma gangrenosum. (f) Finger clubbing.

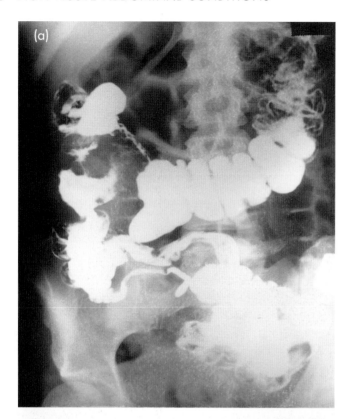

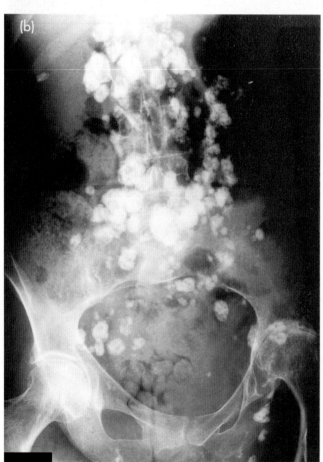

Figure 35.41 Abdominal tuberculosis. (a) Stricture of the hepatic flexure of the colon. (b) Calcification in tuberculous lymphadenitis.

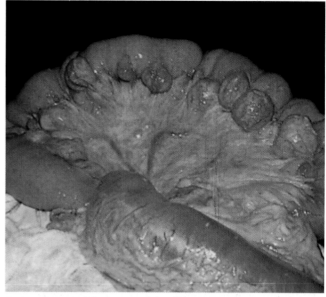

Figure 35.42 An operative specimen demonstrating multiple diverticula of the colon.

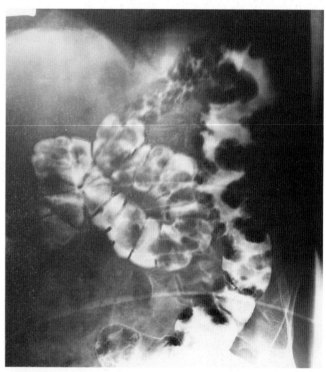

Figure 35.43 Pneumatosis coli. Note the multiple lucent gas shadows indenting the barium columns.

Patients complaining of LLQ pain in association with watery or bloody diarrhoea may be suffering from left colonic irritation from an infectious, inflammatory or ischaemic aetiology. Recent travel or contact with contaminated food should raise a suspicion of *Salmonella* or *Shigella* infection or amoebiasis. Patients who have had recent antibiotic use or hospitalization may have *Clostridium difficile* infection. Those with HIV or on chemotherapy are susceptible to the usual organisms as well as cytomegalovirus (CMV) colitis or HIV-associated colitis.

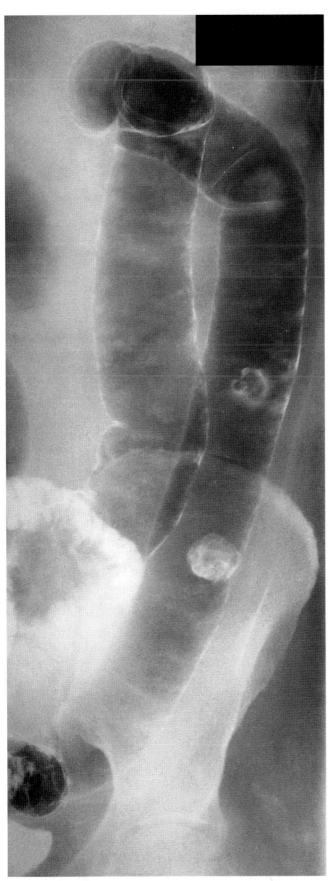

Figure 35.44 Colonic polyps outlined by a barium enema with air insufflation.

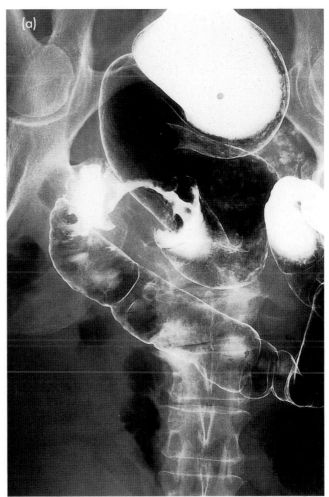

(a)

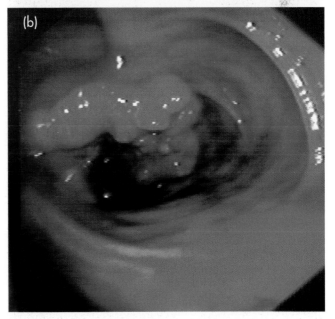

(b)

Figure 35.45 (a) The typical 'apple core' appearance of barium indentation by a colonic carcinoma with a thin stream of contrast medium passing through the stenosed lumen. (b) A colonic neoplasm as viewed through a colonoscope, showing the elevated rolled edge and adjacent normal mucosa.

PART 8 | ABDOMINAL

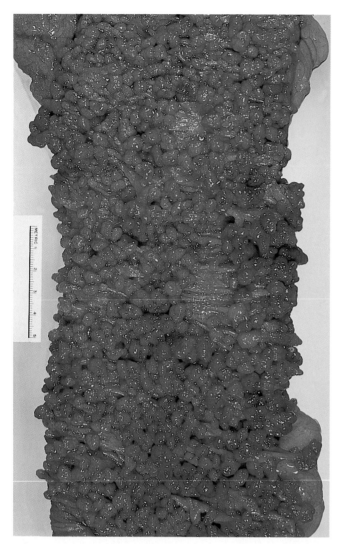

Figure 35.46 An operative specimen from a patient with multiple polyposis coli. Although malignant change in a polyp occurs in only 1 in 100 patients, it is usually inevitable with this number of polyps.

Inflammatory diseases such as Crohn's colitis or ulcerative colitis (**Figure 35.47**) should be considered in patients with a long-standing history of diarrhoea. Ischaemic colitis should be considered in older patients with known coronary or peripheral vascular disease. LLQ pain may also be seen in patients with acute appendicitis and congenital malrotation.

Abdominal examination may show mild to moderate tenderness in the LLQ with or without guarding. Left costovertebral angle tenderness makes left renal pathology more likely. Rectal examination should be performed to exclude gross or occult blood or signs of IBD.

Pelvic examination will exclude left adnexal tenderness or masses that may be seen in cases of left ovarian torsion, tuboovarian abscess, left-sided ectopic pregnancy or left ovarian malignancy.

CT and colonoscopy are the primary diagnostic modalities for this region.

## STOMAS

Stomas may be temporary or permanent. A **temporary stoma** may be required to protect a distal anastomosis. A loop ileostomy or colostomy facilitates closure.

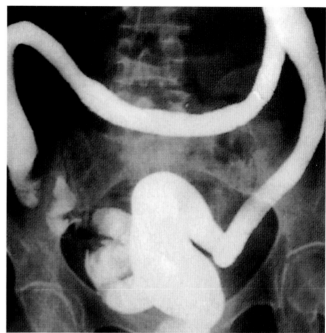

Figure 35.47 Barium enema of a patient with ulcerative colitis showing the featureless 'pipestem' bowel wall with loss of the normal colonic haustral pattern.

**Permanent colostomies** (**Figure 35.48**) involve a single end of bowel that is circumferentially sutured to the skin, for example after an excision of the rectum in an abdominoperineal resection. These are usually placed along a line joining the umbilicus to the left anterior superior iliac spine at the lateral border of the rectus sheath. Complications of colostomies include oedematous stomas, haemorrhage and ulceration from the divided end, ischaemic stenoses, detachment of the cutaneous suture line, prolapse and paracolic hernias.

**Ileostomies** (**Figure 35.49**) may be loop or end stomas placed to the right of the umbilicus and fashioned after proctocolectomy for IBD. Because of the acidic nature of the efflux, a spout is often fashioned to prevent skin excoriation (a Brooke ileostomy). The technical complications of an ileostomy are similar to those of a colostomy, but in addition high output may lead to dehydration and electrolyte disturbance.

## Pelvic Pain

The differential diagnosis of pelvic pain includes:

- diverticulitis;
- cystitis;
- ruptured bladder;
- ruptured haemorrhagic ovarian cyst;
- pelvic inflammatory disease;
- endometriosis;
- ovarian neoplasm;
- uterine neoplasm.

Pelvic or suprapubic pain may be the initial presentation of a host of conditions affecting the lower abdominal viscera. Patients with diverticulitis in a redundant or distal sigmoid colon may identify the suprapubic region instead of the LLQ as their site of maximal pain.

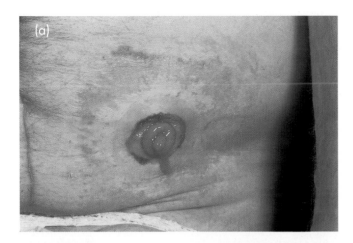

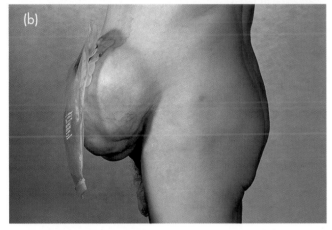

Figure 35.48 (a) An end colostomy. (b) A parastomal hernia in a patient with an end colostomy.

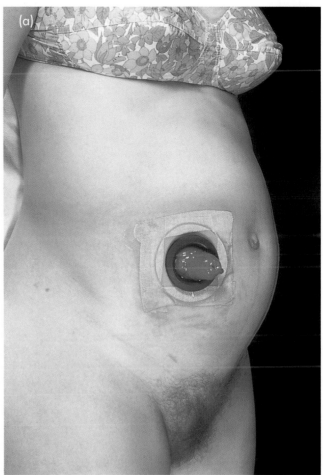

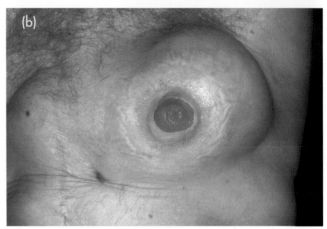

Figure 35.49 (a) A typical ileostomy showing the ileal spout. This is fashioned to divert the small bowel contents into a bag and away from the adjacent skin. (b) A parastomal hernia in an ileostomy.

Patients with cystitis usually report pelvic discomfort, a burning sensation while urinating, a persistent urge to urinate and low-grade fever. The urine may be bloody, cloudy or foul-smelling. Although rare, a ruptured bladder may present with suprapubic pain in a patient with a history of recent alcohol intoxication with blunt trauma. With intraperitoneal rupture, irritation of the parietal peritoneum by urine produces diffuse rebound tenderness. Given the relative sterility of urine, the abdomen may be soft without rigid guarding upon early presentation.

Women with pelvic pain may be suffering from one of many possible gynaecological conditions. Pregnancy must always be excluded. A history of unprotected sex or multiple sex partners along with adnexal tenderness or a purulent cervical discharge raises concerns of pelvic inflammatory disease. A ruptured haemorrhagic cyst may produce suprapubic, RLQ or LLQ pain. If there is a large amount of blood in the free peritoneal cavity, irritation of the parietal peritoneum also produces diffuse rebound with or without significant guarding. Young women with chronic cyclical pelvic pain, painful menstrual cycles, pain during sexual intercourse, pain with bowel movements or irregular bleeding may be suffering from endometriosis. Endometrial implants are sometimes palpable on pelvic examination.

Finally, progressive pelvic pain may be the first symptom of an enlarging ovarian or uterine neoplasm (**Figure 35.50**). Benign

uterine fibroids are common and may be massive and painful. Vaginal bleeding, an increasing abdominal girth, weight loss and fatigue raise a suspicion of malignancy. Abdominal examination may reveal ascites and hepatomegaly if bulky liver metastases are present. A firm adnexal or uterine mass may be appreciated on pelvic examination.

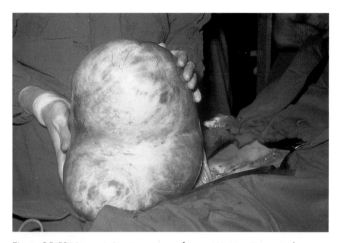

Figure 35.50 An operative specimen of a massive ovarian cystadenoma.

Transvaginal ultrasound is an excellent way to visualize the uterus and adnexae. Laparoscopy is sometimes used.

## Generalized Abdominal Pain

Many patients report abdominal pain that cannot be easily localized to a particular region. Although the conditions discussed above should remain in the differential diagnosis for patients with this kind of generalized abdominal pain, the following conditions must be given special consideration:

- perforated viscus;
- haemoperitoneum;
- pancreatitis;
- mesenteric ischaemia;
- small bowel obstruction;
- intramural haematoma;
- large bowel obstruction;
- pseudo-obstruction;
- spontaneous bacterial peritonitis;
- peritoneal dialysis catheter-associated peritonitis;
- right heart failure;
- carcinomatosis;
- gastroenteritis;
- constipation;
- urinary retention;
- medical conditions.

Severe and sudden-onset generalized abdominal pain is the initial complaint in many surgical abdominal conditions. Fever, tachycardia or hypotension, and a firm abdomen with diffuse board-like guarding and absent bowel sounds raises concerns of peritonitis from bowel **perforation**. Perforated duodenal ulcer, diverticulitis and colon cancer are the most likely possibilities in elderly patients. An anastomotic leak is likely in patients with recent intestinal surgery. Less frequently, appendicitis may result in the spread of purulent content in the abdomen, leading to diffuse guarding.

Patients with **haemoperitoneum** from blunt or penetrating trauma or ruptured vascular tumours such as hepatocellular carcinoma or hepatic adenoma, may also exhibit board-like abdominal wall rigidity.

Finally, severe **pancreatitis** causing mesenteric and intestinal oedema may produce an abdominal examination consistent with diffuse peritonitis.

### Mesenteric Ischaemia

Mesenteric ischaemia must be considered in all patients with known cardiovascular disease and complaints of severe abdominal pain. Acute ischaemia from an arterial embolus in patients with atrial or ventricular thrombi or valvular lesions presents with sudden, severe colicky mid-abdominal pain. Acute mesenteric venous thrombosis is seen in patients with an underlying hypercoagulable state or chronic pancreatitis.

Classically, patients with acute ischaemia initially have pain out of proportion to the actual tenderness found on examination. Peritonitis and the passage of bloody stools are late findings. By contrast, patients with atherosclerotic lesions in at least two of the three main mesenteric arteries are more likely to experience chronic symptoms of postprandial pain leading to food aversion, diarrhoea and weight loss. The abdominal examination may be relatively benign.

### Bowel Obstruction

Patients with diffuse abdominal pain in association with abdominal distension, nausea, vomiting and constipation may have an underlying small or large bowel obstruction. Faeculent-smelling emesis suggests a prolonged stasis of enteric fluid within dilated loops of bowel. Fluid loss through emesis and intraluminal secretions can lead to profound dehydration manifested by tachycardia, hypotension, lethargy and skin tenting. Fever is a marker of possible bacterial translocation.

Patients with bowel obstruction usually have a clearly distended abdomen with hyperactive or hypoactive bowel sounds, but it may be difficult to assess for distension in obese patients. There may be diffuse mild to moderate tenderness. Pronounced guarding raises concerns of bowel ischaemia. Rectal examination excludes an obstructing rectal mass or faecal impaction.

**Small bowel obstruction** is most often due to adhesions from prior abdominal surgery or incarcerated hernias. Gallstone ileus occurs when a gallstone passes through a cholecystoenteric fistula (**Figure 35.51**) caused by chronic cholecystitis and lodges in the ileum. Strictures are likely to be found in patients with Crohn's disease and small bowel obstruction. Carcinomatosis should be considered in patients with known advanced malignancy. Patients without clear risk factors are presumed to have primary small bowel obstruction from congenital bands, internal hernias or primary small bowel tumours.

A **closed-loop obstruction** occurs with the mechanical occlusion of two ends of a segment of bowel so that there is no route of decompression for the involved segment (**Figure 35.52**). Patients tend to report severe pain with nausea but no copious vomiting. There is marked tenderness over the loop while the remainder of the abdomen is usually soft and not particularly distended.

**Intussusception** – the invagination of one segment of intestine into another – is more common in children than adults due to hypertrophy of the Peyer's patches. Adult intussusception is usually caused by a neoplasm serving as a lead point. Adenomatous polyps in patients with Peutz–Jeghers syndrome may cause intussusception or bleeding. These patients have trademark pigmentation of the vermillion surfaces of the lips (**Figure 35.53**). Patients on anticoagulation may develop spontaneous **intramural haematomas** that can also cause intussusception. A tender, palpable abdominal mass may be appreciated.

Infectious intra-abdominal processes such as diverticulitis or appendiceal abscesses may lead to hypomotility of the adjacent small bowel leading to a segmental **paralytic ileus**. Diffuse

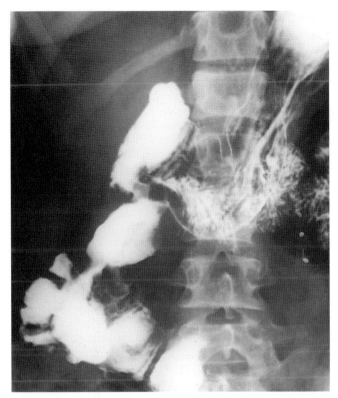

Figure 35.51 A duodeno-colic fistula resulting from the abscess and erosion of a large gallstone.

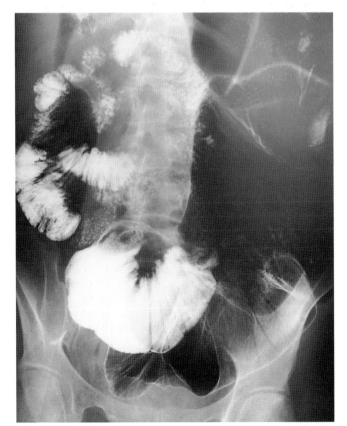

Figure 35.52 A dilated loop of obstructed ileum filling the left side of the abdomen.

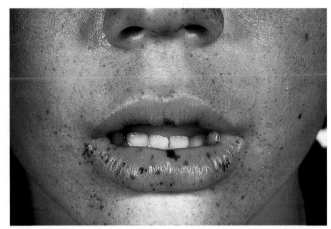

Figure 35.53 Perioral pigmentation in a patient with Peutz–Jeghers syndrome.

dysmotility or ileus is often seen in patients with gastroenteritis or recent intestinal surgery, and the abdominal examination may mimic that of small bowel obstruction. Primary intestinal dysmotility disorders are rare but should be considered in patients with chronic nausea, vomiting, abdominal distension and constipation without a clear aetiology.

Most patients with **large bowel obstruction** have an incompetent ileocaecal valve that allows the colon to be somewhat decompressed as pressure is transmitted to the small bowel. These patients have a presentation similar to those with small bowel obstruction. Patients with a competent ileocaecal valve effectively have a closed-loop large bowel obstruction leading to severe pain and progressive abdominal distension with localized peritonitis over the colonic segment involved.

The most common causes of large bowel obstruction are colon cancer, incarcerated hernia, sigmoid or caecal volvulus, faecal impaction and diverticular strictures. Classically, left-sided colon cancers tend to present with obstruction while right-sided cancers produce bleeding. Obstructing cancers or impacted faeces may paradoxically produce diarrhoea as liquid stool leaks through the mass. In toxic patients with abdominal distension and diarrhoea, toxic megacolon from overwhelming *Clostridium difficile* infection must be considered.

**Pseudo-obstruction** describes colonic dysmotility that may be triggered by medications, stress and infection. Patients with pseudo-obstruction usually continue to pass stool and flatus intermittently. In any large bowel obstruction, localized peritonitis in the RLQ raises a suspicion of progressive caecal dilation and ischaemia. Rectal examination is essential.

## Ascites

Progressive, vague, non-acute and poorly localized abdominal pain in association with a sense of increasing abdominal girth raises a suspicion of new-onset ascites. Patients with advanced liver disease have the stigmata of portal hypertension discussed above. New or progressive ascites in these patients may reflect a new insult to an already failing liver, such as a portal vein thrombosis or hepatocellular carcinoma. In a patient with known ascites, new-onset abdominal pain may be the first symptom of **spontaneous bacterial peritonitis**. The abdomen is generally soft but distended with ascites, and mildly tender.

## Peritoneal Dialysis

Patients with end-stage renal failure receiving peritoneal dialysis may also develop primary bacterial peritonitis. Abdominal examination usually reveals a soft abdomen with diffuse mild rebound tenderness without significant guarding. The catheter insertion site should be inspected for erythema or purulent drainage, although these signs may be absent.

## Right Heart Failure

Chronic right heart failure may cause hepatic congestion resulting in ascites, hepatomegaly and even splenomegaly. Patients may complain of mild, diffuse or epigastric abdominal pain with associated nausea.

**Rosenbach's sign** refers to pulsations that are transmitted to the examiner's hand on gentle palpation of the liver. Tricuspid stenosis is likely to be present if the pulsations occur just before ventricular systole, while tricuspid regurgitation is more likely if the pulsations occur during systole. A thorough cardiopulmonary examination will clarify the diagnosis.

## Carcinomatosis

Peritoneal carcinomatosis from advanced gastrointestinal or gynaecological malignancy should be considered in patients with new-onset ascites (**Figure 35.54**). The history may reveal worrisome symptoms such as a change in bowel habit, chronic blood-tinged stools or postmenopausal vaginal bleeding coupled with weight loss, night sweats and fatigue.

A firm, palpable mass may be appreciated on abdominal examination if the underlying cancer is sufficiently large. If a rectal cancer is palpated on digital rectal examination, the sphincter tone should be assessed to identify involvement of the sphincter muscles. All major lymph node basins should be assessed. Ruptured mucoceles of the appendix or ovaries may lead to pseudomyxoma peritonei, in which extensive gelatinous fluid fills the abdomen. The disease is slow to progress, but the presentation is often similar to that of a gynaecological malignancy.

## Gastroenteritis

Fortunately, there are many benign, self-limiting conditions that cause non-acute, generalized abdominal pain. Bacterial or viral gastroenteritis presents with vague, crampy abdominal pain, nausea, vomiting and diarrhoea. Recent travel or contact with contaminated food is typically present. The patient may be pale and ill-appearing with a low-grade fever. The abdominal examination is usually relatively benign. There may be mild distension and mild diffuse tenderness, but rebound and guarding are unusual.

## Constipation

Chronic constipation causes significant diffuse abdominal pain in elderly patients. In thin patients, dense stool can be palpated in the transverse and sigmoid colon. Rectal examination may typically reveal pellet-like firm stool in the vault. Rarely, faecal impaction produces the clinical picture of bowel obstruction with nausea, vomiting, abdominal distension and abdominal tenderness. An underlying neoplasm must be excluded in these patients.

## Urinary Retention

Older patients are also prone to developing acute or chronic urinary retention. Benign prostatic hyperplasia is the most common cause in men, while pelvic floor laxity with the development of a cystocele or rectocele is a common aetiology in women. In both sexes, urinary tract infection and medications may trigger retention.

Patients report may report diffuse or lower abdominal pain. Some may only report urinary frequency and overflow on questioning as they become accustomed to their chronic symptoms. Physical examination will reveal suprapubic fullness, and palpating the dome of the bladder will make the patient feel an urge to urinate. When the bladder is massively distended, there may be significant tenderness, mimicking peritonitis in some cases.

## Medical Conditions

Medical conditions occasionally give rise to abdominal pain. These include:

- nerve root lesions such as pre-eruption herpes zoster;
- diabetes;
- hyperparathyroidism;
- porphyria;
- tabes dorsalis, which is a form of syphilis.

CT scanning is the primary diagnostic modality in patients who do not have localizing signs or symptoms and who do not require immediate laparotomy for an 'acute surgical abdomen'.

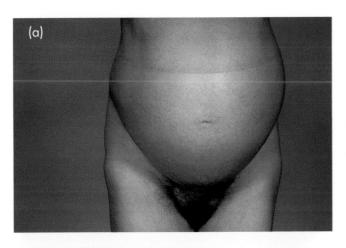

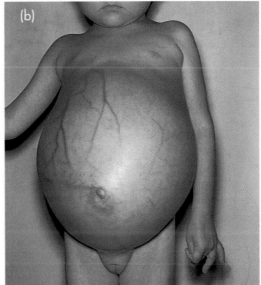

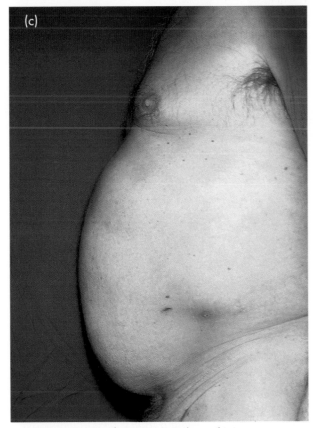

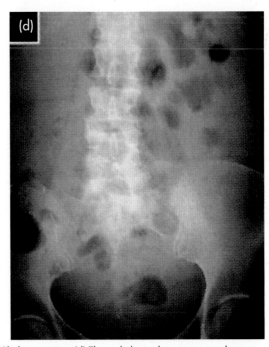

Figure 35.54 Causes of ascites. (a) Cirrhosis. (b) Ovarian carcinoma. (c) Chylous ascites. (d) The radiological appearance, the generalized opacity obscuring and separating the gut gas shadows.

**Key Points**

- A thorough history and physical examination allow the healthcare provider to formulate a differential diagnosis upon which to base further testing and interventions if necessary.
- When a patient localizes their abdominal pain to a particular region, the history and physical examination should be tailored to distinguish between the conditions that commonly affect the identified region.
- Generalized abdominal pain has a vast differential diagnosis, but it is still possible to identify the most likely condition present using detailed history and physical examination skills.

## SBAs

1. **A 65-year-old woman presents with complaints of vague, poorly localized abdominal pain over the last 3 weeks. She has also noted some abdominal distension and thin, blood-tinged stools over the last 3 months. She has no appetite and has lost 20 kg. She has no medical problems and has never had surgery or a colonoscopy. She denies abnormal vaginal bleeding. On examination, she is cachectic and pale. Her abdomen is distended and mildly tender without peritonitis. The liver is prominent. There are no abdominal masses and no adnexal masses on pelvic examination. The rectal vault is empty. Which of the following are you most concerned about?**
   a  Chronic mesenteric ischaemia
   b  Small bowel obstruction
   c  Colon cancer
   d  Ovarian cancer
   e  Liver failure

**Answer**

c  *Colon cancer. The patient has constitutional symptoms suggestive of malignancy and progressive obstructive symptoms without a prior screening colonoscopy. An obstructing colon cancer is the most likely diagnosis.*

2. **A 19-year-old woman complains of progressive right lower quadrant pain over the last 5 days. She has had low-grade fevers, nausea and diarrhoea. She thinks her urine is darker than usual but not grossly bloody. She is otherwise healthy. Her last menstrual period was 3 weeks ago. She has a sister with ulcerative colitis. On examination, she is anxious. The abdomen is soft, with tenderness to deep palpation of the right lower quadrant. Which of the following is the least likely diagnosis?**
   a  Appendicitis
   b  Nephrolithiasis
   c  Crohn's disease
   d  Typhlitis
   e  Ectopic pregnancy

**Answer**

d  *Typhlitis. This patient has no history to suggest an immunocompromised state. Typhlitis would not be expected to occur in an otherwise healthy patient.*

3. **A 57-year-old man with hypertension and diabetes reports 4 days of right upper quadrant and epigastric pain. He reports low-grade fevers, nausea and intermittent vomiting. He has a history of an appendicectomy at age 15. On examination, his pulse is 100 bpm and he is slightly hypertensive. There is no jaundice. The abdomen is soft but obese and tender to deep palpation of the right upper quadrant, with a positive Murphy's sign. Which is of the following is the most likely diagnosis?**
   a  Cholangitis
   b  Choledocholithiasis
   c  Cholecystitis
   d  Gallstone ileus
   e  Cholangiocarcinoma

**Answer**

c  *Cholecystitis. The patient is acutely ill with a positive Murphy's sign, which suggests cholecystitis. There is no jaundice to suggest cholangitis from choledocholithiasis or cholangiocarcinoma. Gallstone ileus typically presents as a small bowel obstruction, and not with right upper quadrant pain.*

## EMQs

**1.** For each of the following eponyms, select the correct site of the metastatic deposit. Each option may be used once, more than once or not at all:

- **1** Ovaries
- **2** Supraclavicular lymph node
- **3** Rectovesical pouch
- **4** Periumbilical lymph node
- **a** Blumer
- **b** Virchow
- **c** Sister Mary Joseph
- **d** Krukenberg

**Answers**

**a** **3 Rectovesical pouch.** *Blumer's shelf refers to disease within the rectovesical pouch.*

**b** **2 Supraclavicular lymph node.** *Virchow's node refers to a supraclavicular lymph node, typically on the left.*

**c** **4 Periumbilical lymph node.** *A palpable periumbilical lymph node metastasis is termed a Sister Mary Joseph's nodule.*

**d** **1 Ovaries.** *Drop metastases to the ovaries are termed Krukenberg tumours.*

*It should be remembered that nodal or peritoneal metastases from gastrointestinal malignancies may be palpable on physical examination.*

**2.** For each of following list of patient traits, select the most likely diagnosis. Each option may be used once, more than once or not at all:

- **1** Right heart failure
- **2** Ovarian cancer
- **3** Liver failure
- **4** Colon cancer
- **a** Ascites, gynaecomastia, caput medusae
- **b** Ascites, a firm palpable left lower quadrant mass, bloody stools
- **c** Ascites, a pulsatile liver
- **d** Ascites, and a firm adnexal mass

**Answers**

**a** **3 Liver failure.** *Patients with liver failure due to cirrhosis may demonstrate ascites, gynaecomastia and caput medusae.*

**b** **4 Colon cancer.** *Patients with advanced colon cancer may have ascites, a palpable mass in the lower left quadrant and bloody stools on rectal examination.*

**c** **1 Right heart failure.** *Patients with right heart failure may demonstrate ascites and a pulsatile liver.*

**d** **2 Ovarian cancer.** *Patients with ovarian cancer may have ascites and a firm adnexal mass.*

*Ascites may be due to advanced malignancy or end-stage organ failure.*

# The Acute Abdomen

Evgeny V. Arshava

*"Knowledge is a hard won gift, but it will lead to diagnostic wisdom."* G.P. Kealey, MD.

## LEARNING OBJECTIVES

- To understand the characteristics and pathophysiology of abdominal pain
- To be able to examine the patient with an acute abdomen

- To know the disease processes that present with acute abdominal pain and be able to develop an appropriate differential diagnosis
- To be able to identify patients with acute surgical abdomen who need surgical intervention

## INTRODUCTION

Abdominal pain (whether a new pain or an exacerbation of a chronic pain) is one of the most common reasons why patients seek medical attention. The main questions that the clinician needs to answer when evaluating a patient with abdominal pain are 'Does the patient have an acute abdomen or not?' and 'Does the patient need an operation?' Without prompt diagnosis and treatment, an 'acute abdomen' may lead to serious complications and possibly the patient's death.

'Acute abdomen' is a general term used to describe a variety of serious intra-abdominal pathologies that mandate emergency or urgent surgical ('surgical abdomen') or major medical intervention. The aetiologies of this condition are very diverse (**Table 36.1**). Their prevalence varies by age, gender and geography.

Table 36.1 The differential diagnosis of acute abdominal pain (in order of anatomical location rather than relative incidence)

| System | Condition |
|---|---|
| Gastrointestinal system | Oesophageal, gastric and duodenal ulceration or perforation |
| | Cholelithiasis (acute cholecystitis, choledocholithiasis) |
| | Pancreatitis |
| | Inflammatory bowel disease |
| | Mesenteric adenitis |
| | Meckel's diverticulum |
| | Intussusception |
| | Appendicitis |
| | Diverticulitis |
| | Small and large bowel obstruction or perforation |
| | Constipation |

*contd...*

| System | Condition |
|---|---|
| Vascular conditions | Mesenteric ischaemia |
| | Ruptured abdominal aortic or visceral artery aneurysm |
| Abdominal wall | Rectus sheath haematoma |
| | Abdominal wall hernia |
| Urinary system | Pyelonephritis |
| | Nephrolithiasis |
| Reproductive system | Torsion or rupture of an ovarian cyst |
| | Ectopic pregnancy |
| | Pelvic inflammatory disease |
| Intra-abdominal trauma | Bleeding |
| | Peritonitis |
| Conditions that may mimic an acute abdomen | Myocardial infarction |
| | Pneumonia and empyema |
| | Neurogenic and musculoskeletal pain |
| | Various metabolic and infectious diseases |

A detailed medical and surgical history and a thorough physical examination help to narrow the differential diagnosis. An knowledge of anatomy and an understanding of the nature of the patient's symptoms are essential.

During the interview, specific characteristics of the pain need to be evaluated (**Table 36.2**).

## Characteristics of the Abdominal Pain

The embryology and innervation of the abdominal organs determine the type and location of the pain:

- **Visceral pain** is described as dull, cramping and poorly localized. It may be colicky (beginning rapidly, increasing and then resolving). Pain in the foregut (oesophagus, stomach,

Table 36.2 Significant characteristics of abdominal pain, to be elicited as the history is taken

Onset of pain and history of prior episodes
Character (constant or intermittent, sharp or dull)
Location and radiation
Severity
Changes in severity and nature over time
Alleviating and exacerbating factors (oral intake, bowel movements, position, activity, analgesics)
Associated symptoms (constitutional, gastrointestinal, genitourinary)

duodenum, pancreatobiliary system) is perceived in the epigastrium, pain in the midgut (small bowel to right colon) in the periumbilical area, and pain from the hindgut (the rest of the colon) in the lower abdomen. Visceral pain is associated with nausea and perspiration.

- **Somatic (parietal) pain** is distinctly sharp, constant and generally more severe. It is felt in a precise location corresponding to the somatic innervation of the overlying muscle group and corresponds to the organs that underlie the area anatomically.
- **Referred pain** is a type of pain in which pain is perceived in a location remote from the diseased organ, based upon its embryological origin rather than its adult location. For example, ipsilateral subscapular or shoulder pain may be felt with diaphragmatic irritation, or pain in the groin or genitalia with the passage of a ureteral stone.

Several pathophysiological mechanisms can produce an acute abdomen. These may overlap and merge into each other.

**Perforation** is a disruption of the integrity of a hollow viscus. The gastrointestinal contents leak into the peritoneal cavity, causing first chemical, then inflammatory and finally infectious peritoneal irritation. The perforation usually develops acutely and presents with a sudden onset of pain that rapidly builds up to maximal intensity. The rupture of other structures (e.g. from trauma to a solid organ, rupture of a hepatic adenoma or an ovarian cyst) also results in acute pain and may be associated with intra-abdominal bleeding.

**Inflammation** may result from infectious (purulent, faeculent) or chemical (bilious) irritation of the peritoneal cavity. It usually presents with signs of peritoneal irritation and of systemic toxicity. Depending on the disease, the peritonitis may be diffuse (from a perforated viscus) or focal (with cholecystitis or an intra-abdominal abscess).

**Torsion** is an acute twist of the organ (such as the bowel or ovary) around its axis, usually the vascular pedicle. The pain is typically sudden and severe. Initially, the abdomen is soft and the tenderness is localized to the affected organ. Torsion of a segment of the gastrointestinal tract (volvulus) typically results in bowel obstruction. Whereas a rotation of less than 180° around the axis may result in partial obstruction, a rotation of over 360° results in complete visceral obstruction and interruption of the blood supply (one of the causes of ischaemia).

**Bowel obstruction** is associated with nausea, vomiting, constipation and distension as material fails to pass normally through the gastrointestinal tract. The abdominal pain is of a visceral type and is due to intestinal distension and peristalsis. With overdistension of the bowel, pain and abdominal tenderness may become severe and constant. With ongoing distension (as in complete bowel obstruction), bowel wall ischaemia may develop.

Thus, the most important question the clinician needs to answer when examining a patient with bowel obstruction is 'Is bowel ischaemia present or impending?'

**Ischaemia** of a hollow or solid organ develops from an interruption of its blood supply (arterial or venous thrombosis), inadequate blood flow within the bowel wall (a 'low-flow state') or extrinsic compression of the vessels (volvulus or strangulation in a hernia). The pain is initially visceral (commonly described by the patient as very severe, and classically 'out of proportion to the physical findings'). With advancing ischaemia, signs of parietal peritoneal irritation and physical findings of guarding develop. Full-thickness ischaemia of the bowel wall may lead to its necrosis and perforation.

During the period of observation, a change from a previously vague pain to a sharp, constant, parietal peritoneum irritation pain implies a surgical emergency unless proven otherwise.

Any associated symptoms are usually non-specific but may be helpful in determining the severity of the illness and the differential diagnosis. Constitutional symptoms, including fever, chills, malaise and anorexia, may accompany any inflammatory process. Gastrointestinal symptoms such as nausea, vomiting and alterations in bowel habit may accompany various surgical and medical conditions. Certain clinical characteristics (bilious vomiting, haematemesis, melaena) may help to narrow the differential diagnosis. Always ask about genitourinary symptoms of dysuria, pyuria and haematuria, and obtain a careful menstrual history in women.

### Examination

The patient's general condition is determined by the stage of the disease and may vary from normal to septic or hypovolaemic shock with multiple organ system failure. Therefore always assess haemodynamic and respiratory stability early and continue to monitor it.

In the early stages of an acute surgical condition, systemic signs may be minimal and abdominal symptoms predominate. As the pathological process evolves, the systemic inflammatory response and sepsis develop. Fever may accompany any inflammatory process. Patients with a delayed presentation have obvious signs of peritoneal irritation and signs of progressing shock. Classically, patients with advanced peritonitis or bowel ischaemia, regardless of its aetiology, are tachycardic and have a thready pulse and labile blood pressure. They are tachypnoeic and may have altered mental status and poor tissue perfusion, manifested by a low urine output and cool and cyanotic skin.

Tachycardia is a very important sign of an early physiological response to the acute illness. In morbidly obese patients, it may be the earliest sign of an intra-abdominal catastrophe. Always remember that patients receiving beta-blockers may not manifest changes in heart rate. As the intra-abdominal process progresses, the abdomen becomes more distended secondary to paralytic ileus.

During evaluation, pay attention to the position of the patient, their facial expression and their overall comfort level. Patients with intra-abdominal sepsis look unwell and lie still in order to protect a tender abdomen. They may flex their hips and in extreme cases refuse examination.

Ask the patient to lie flat in the most comfortable position with their head supported on a pillow (as one cannot reliably assess the abdomen in any position other than supine). Inspect the entire abdomen from the rib cage to below the inguinal ligaments for skin colour, bruising and the presence of surgical scars and underlying masses (see Chapter 33). Note the respiratory movements, and whether the patient can draw in or blow out the abdominal wall without discomfort.

A degree of abdominal distension may be arbitrarily assigned relative to the level of the costal margin. In a non-obese patient in the supine position, the abdomen is described as scaphoid, mildly distended (distension at the level of the costal margin) or significantly distended (the distension protrudes above the costal margin). Always consider the possibility of ascites.

On auscultation, bowel sounds may be diminished or absent in peritonitis or ileus from other causes, or hyperactive and high-pitched in early mechanical bowel obstruction. Auscultation of the chest may reveal consolidation of the lower lobe mimicking an acute abdomen.

Gentle palpation is performed next. Ask the patient to outline the tender areas. Start palpation away from these areas, thus creating the least discomfort and obtaining a more accurate evaluation. Observe the patient's face throughout the examination. Assess the abdominal wall for asymmetry, and always check for hernias, especially when bowel obstruction is present.

**Voluntary guarding** is contraction of the abdominal wall muscles by the patient due to fear, an anticipation of feeling pain or the cold hands of the examiner. It should be differentiated from involuntary guarding.

**Involuntary guarding** is reflex rigidity of the abdominal wall muscle due to inflammation of the underlying peritoneum. It is a cardinal sign of peritoneal irritation produced by abdominal wall movement. It is best detected with superficial palpation and percussion. A rough examination may scare the patient, cause voluntary guarding and make subsequent evaluation difficult. Deep palpation, while occasionally useful in patients with chronic pain and abdominal masses, is usually not possible in patients with an acute abdomen.

An examination may be very difficult in children, and the clinician must be particularly patient and careful. Attempt to distract the child with conversation and questions, while simultaneously gently palpating to differentiate voluntary from involuntary guarding. Using the child's own hand and palpating over is frequently helpful.

Several signs may be of use in evaluating patient with an acute abdomen:

• The skin hypersensitivity test – rapid superficial rubbing of the patient's skin with an open palm may detect areas of skin hyperaesthesia, suggestive of underlining peritoneal irritation (Voskresensky sign).
• The pointing sign. Ask the patient to point the area of maximum pain, and start palpation away from this. If the area pointed to is also the site of maximum tenderness, the underling viscus is highly likely to be the culprit.
• The 'cough test'. Localization of pain to the abdomen during coughing indicates irritation of the parietal peritoneum. Localization of pain to the chest indicates irritation of the parietal pleura.
• The 'bed-shaking sign' and the 'heel-tapping sign'. As their names imply, these manoeuvres may reproduce pain in the areas of peritoneal irritation.
• Percussion rebound. Tenderness upon gentle percussion suggests irritation of the undying peritoneum and may avoid the need for distressing palpation. This approach is particularly useful in children. Percussion may also help to differentiate gaseous distension (tympanic) from ascites (dull).

• Rebound tenderness (Blumberg's sign, or the release sign). A sudden release of a deeply palpating hand produces pain in cases of peritoneal irritation. It is unnecessary to perform this test in cases with obvious peritoneal irritation noted on percussion and is very distressing for patients.
• Irritation of the parietal peritoneum overlying the muscles of the posterior abdominal wall and pelvis may be elicited with additional manoeuvres such as the obturator sign (rotating the flexed hip internally with the knee flexed) and psoas sign (hyperextension of the thigh while the patient is lying on the opposite side).
• Simultaneous palpation of symmetrical areas of the abdomen with both hands (the Butov manoeuvre) helps the clinician to appreciate subtle differences in muscle tone. It may also be helpful in examining children and patients with factitious disorders.

Never omit examining the groins for a hernia (see Chapter 34).

Rectal examination may reveal blood within the gastrointestinal tract or focal tenderness secondary to pelvic inflammation (appendicitis or a pelvic abscess). In women, bimanual examination (with one hand on the abdomen and the other on the cervix) may be diagnostic of pelvic inflammatory disease or other gynaecological pathology. Perform a scrotal examination in males since torsion of the testicle may present initially as lower abdominal pain.

Physical findings in acute abdominal conditions vary depending upon the stage of the disease and the particular patient. Abdominal examination of elderly, immunosuppressed or morbidly obese patients is notoriously unreliable: they may initially have diminished signs of a systemic inflammatory response. Children, on the other hand, frequently have accentuated systemic symptoms and signs. It is difficult to examine morbidly obese individuals owing the thickness of their abdominal wall and altered surface anatomy.

Very commonly, the exact aetiology of an acute abdominal condition cannot be determined from the history and physical examination alone. Imaging and laboratory studies may be necessary for appropriate decision-making. Leukocytosis with a 'left shift' in the ratio of immature to mature neutrophils, an elevated C-reactive protein and a raised erythrocyte sedimentation rate are non-specific markers of an inflammatory state. In critically ill patients, the development of lymphopenia may be a marker of an advanced septic process. Lactic acidosis may indicate intestinal ischaemia or be a marker of global tissue hypoperfusion. Liver function tests, pancreatic enzyme levels, cardiac markers and urinalysis may be needed for the differential diagnosis. No test should, however, replace a conscientious physical examination.

The adjunctive use of radiographic studies including an upright chest X-ray, abdominal films and ultrasound or CT scans of the abdomen may be extremely helpful. Repeated examinations are commonly required to make a diagnosis and formulate the optimal treatment plan.

## ACUTE CONDITIONS OF THE OESOPHAGUS, STOMACH AND DUODENUM

### Acute Gastritis

Patients with acute mucosal inflammation present with variable degrees of acute upper abdominal pain, nausea and vomiting. A variety of infectious and chemical agents may cause acute inflammation of the upper gastrointestinal tract. Depending on the specific bacterial or viral pathogen, an infection may continue as gastroenteritis and cause diarrhoea shortly after the onset of upper abdominal symptoms. Fever and anorexia may be present. Epigastric tenderness is present, with no signs of peritoneal irritation.

Although the symptoms are usually mild, severe conditions may in some patients mimic an acute abdomen. Acute infectious or chemical (alcohol, non-steroidal inflammatory drugs [NSAIDs]) gastritis is usually self-limiting as the gastric mucosa is replaced every few days. In cases involving more severe offending agents (caustic ingestion), higher amounts of toxic substances (NSAID overdose) or chronic bacterial exposure (*Helicobacter pylori* infection), mucosal changes may progress to erosions and more severe consequences.

## Acute Gastric Erosions

Acute multiple gastric erosions may occur with an excessive use of NSAIDs. They may occur following any type of shock, resulting from reduced tissue perfusion and mucosal ischaemia. Stress ulcers, secondary to a raised gastrin level, can develop following traumatic brain injury, neurosurgical procedures and extensive burns. These acute ulcerations typically present with epigastric pain and signs of, occasionally massive, upper gastrointestinal bleeding.

## Peptic Ulcer Disease

Peptic ulcer disease of the stomach and duodenum remains an important cause of morbidity worldwide. The pathophysiology of this multifactorial disease is complex and is related to an imbalance between gastroduodenal secretory mechanisms and the mucosal defence system. *Helicobacter pylori* infection and NSAIDs are the most common causes of mucosal function injury. Gastric acid hypersecretion and decreased duodenal bicarbonate secretion are additionally affected by other factors that play a role in the development of peptic ulcer disease: smoking, alcohol, a genetic predisposition, psychosocial factors and diet. Specific hypersecretory conditions that are independent of *H. pylori* and should also be on the list of differential diagnoses include gastrinoma (Zollinger–Ellison syndrome), hyperparathyroidism and a retained antrum following partial gastrectomy.

### Peptic Ulceration

The location and duration of the peptic ulcer determine the symptoms. Dyspepsia, vague crampy discomfort and burning, hunger-like pain are the most common symptoms. The pain is usually centred in the epigastric region but may be located in the right or left upper quadrant. Radiation to the back is unusual unless there is perforation into the retroperitoneum.

In the untreated patient with gastric peptic ulcer disease, chronic symptoms occur in clusters with alternating periods of exacerbation and remission lasting weeks or months. There is less periodicity with duodenal ulcers. Such a classic presentation is, however, rarely encountered in modern medicine.

When an ulcer is located in the stomach and the pyloric channel, the pain is frequently precipitated by eating and may be relieved by vomiting and lying down. Non-bilious vomiting may occur as a result of pyloric obstruction secondary to oedema or fibrosis. The patient may avoid eating and may lose weight.

Pain from a duodenal ulcer is precipitated by acid secretion in the absence of a food buffer, while a meal alleviates the pain. The stomach empties 2–3 hours after a meal, but the acid secretion persists for several hours longer. Consequently, the pain of a 'classic' duodenal ulcer reoccurs 2–5 hours after meals and frequently around midnight, at the peak of the circadian acid secretion.

When peptic ulcer disease progresses, the symptoms may become mixed and non-classical. Imaging studies, once mandatory in the diagnosis of peptic ulcers, have been replaced by upper gastrointestinal endoscopy.

Peptic ulcer disease may result in severe complications causing perforation (if the ulcer erodes through the wall of the viscus), haemorrhage (if the ulceration erodes into a blood vessel) or pyloric obstruction. Peptic ulcer disease is one of the most common causes of upper gastrointestinal bleeding.

### Perforated Peptic Ulcer

Perforated peptic ulcer is a classic example of an acute perforation of the gastrointestinal tract with resulting peritonitis. A history of peptic ulcer disease is not always present. Perforation results in the leak of gastric or duodenal contents into the peritoneal cavity and peritonitis. The location of the ulcer, its size, the presence of adhesions from previous abdominal operations and the anatomy of the adjacent organs may affect the clinical picture at presentation. Perforated duodenal ulcers – the most frequent type of peptic ulcer – are usually indistinguishable from perforated gastric ulcers on examination.

The patient commonly presents with a sudden onset of severe upper abdominal pain and occasionally vomiting. Massive and ongoing contamination throughout the abdomen results in diffuse peritonitis. On abdominal examination, there are no bowel sounds, and a very characteristic diffuse 'board-like' abdominal rigidity is present due to generalized peritonitis.

As the condition progresses, tachycardia and other systemic signs of shock develop, signifying a life-threatening condition. The abdomen may become more distended, and the pain may diminish. Free intra-abdominal air and gaseous distension of bowel may lead to a tympanic abdomen on percussion. Rectal examination can occasionally elicit tenderness in the rectovesical pouch.

The perforation of a hollow viscus can be confirmed by the presence of intraperitoneal gas under the diaphragm on an upright chest or left lateral decubitus abdominal radiograph (**Figures 36.1** and **36.2**). Plain radiography may not be sensitive enough in morbidly obese patients, especially if smaller volumes of gas are present (**Figure 36.3**). The pitfall of finding free gas under the right hemidiaphragm on a radiograph taken for other reasons in an asymptomatic patient could be an instance of the uncommon Chilaiditi's syndrome – the asymptomatic location of the hepatic flexure of the colon above the liver (**Figure 36.4**).

The omentum or overhanging liver will frequently seal the perforation, leading to focal and possibly self-limited peritonitis. In such cases, signs of peritoneal irritation may be present only in the epigastrium, and signs of systemic toxicity may be less pronounced. The right colon occasionally acts as a watershed, diverting the leak out of the perforated duodenal ulcer and along the right paracolic gutter in the iliac fossa, mimicking perforated appendicitis. The tenderness elicited in such a condition tends to be more generalized and slightly higher than in 'classic' appendicitis. The perforation of a posterior gastric ulcer into the lesser sac may similarly limit the abdominal signs. A retroperitoneal perforation of the duodenal ulcer may result in attenuated abdominal symptoms. The patient complains predominantly of back pain.

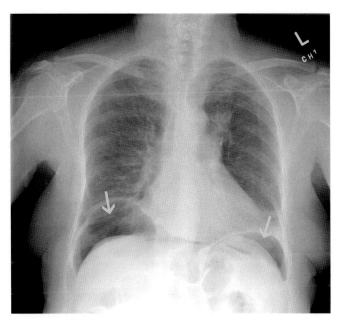

Figure 36.1 Free intraperitoneal gas under both hemidiaphragms (arrows) on an upright chest radiograph in patient with a perforated peptic ulcer.

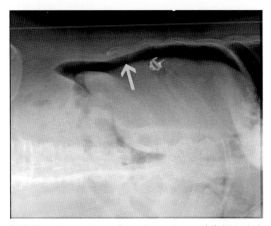

Figure 36.2 Free intraperitoneal gas (arrow) on a left lateral decubitus abdominal radiograph.

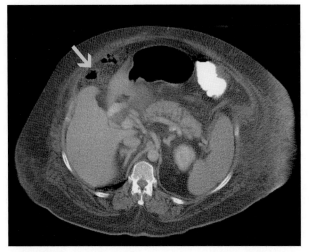

Figure 36.3 Free intraperitoneal gas (arrow) in a morbidly obese patient with an equivocal physical examination and negative plain radiographs.

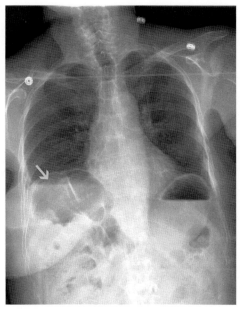

Figure 36.4 Chilaiditi's syndrome (an uncommon location of the colonic loop between the liver and the diaphragm that mimics free subdiaphragmatic air, arrowed, on an upright chest radiograph) in a patient with an unremarkable abdominal examination.

In any of the above situations, once the diagnosis has been made, there should be prompt and aggressive fluid resuscitation followed by surgical intervention.

A perforated gastric or duodenal ulcer may at times be confused with a myocardial infarction or other thoracic problem that causes diaphragmatic and pleural irritation. Posterior and retroperitoneal perforation may mimic both pancreatitis and a dissecting aortic aneurysm. A neoplasm should always be considered as an aetiology for perforation of the gastroduodenal complex.

## Oesophageal Perforation

Perforation of the oesophagus is another life-threatening condition. It may occur secondary to iatrogenic causes, trauma, tumours, foreign bodies, caustic injuries or forceful vomiting. The clinical presentation depends on the location and size of the injury and may mimic various pathologies, including myocardial infarction, aortic dissection, pancreatitis and pneumonia.

Perforation of the cervical oesophagus manifests with dysphagia, neck pain aggravated by movement and subcutaneous emphysema (**Figure 36.5**). These symptoms develop gradually compared with distal sites. Thoracic and abdominal perforations result in more acute symptoms. Thoracic perforations are more common and present with chest pain, tachycardia, tachypnoea and fever secondary to mediastinitis. Abdominal perforations present with symptoms of an acute abdomen, similar to a perforated peptic ulcer.

A rapid increase in intraluminal pressure in the stomach and oesophagus may produce barotrauma of the distal oesophagus. This most commonly occurs with forceful retching and vomiting; a history of alcohol abuse is present in many patients. It may also develop with heavy lifting and straining during childbirth. The resulting longitudinal lacerations of the mucosal may result in upper gastrointestinal bleeding from the submucosal arteries (Mallory–Weiss syndrome). If the injury is full thickness, intrathoracic or intra-abdominal, perforation occurs (Boerhaave's syndrome). This is a surgical emergency.

PART 8 | ABDOMINAL

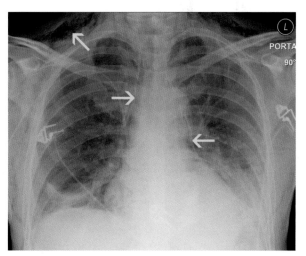

Figure 36.5 Pneumomediastinum and subcutaneous emphysema of the neck (sites arrowed) in a patient with a caustic injury and perforation of the distal oesophagus.

Severe reflux or infectious (e.g. candidal) oesophagitis, or abnormalities of oesophageal motility, may occasionally present with severe pain and dysphagia, but they generally do not produce the same intensity of symptoms as perforation.

## Hiatus Hernia

A hiatus hernia is a protrusion of intra-abdominal organs through the oesophageal hiatus of the diaphragm. These hernias may be spontaneous or post-operative. Around 95 per cent of them are sliding hernias, in which only the gastro-oesophageal junction and part of the cardia herniates though the oesophageal hiatus into the posterior mediastinum. In the remaining 5 per cent (paraoesophageal hernias), the gastric fundus, other parts of the stomach and, in advanced cases, other intra-abdominal organs may be involved.

Many patients are asymptomatic. Others have intermittent vague pain, fullness, nausea and retching. The dominant symptoms are epigastric, substernal and occasionally back pain. Attacks of substernal pain may occasionally be severe enough to simulate myocardial ischaemia or aortic dissection. Complications are rare but include life-threatening gastric volvulus, bleeding, intra-abdominal or intrathoracic perforations and respiratory complications.

## Gastric Volvulus

Anatomically, the stomach is fixed proximally by the gastrophrenic ligaments, and distally by the retroperitoneal attachments of the duodenum. If the stomach rotates between these points, volvulus occurs. Volvulus typically occurs in adults over the age of 50 years but may also be seen in infancy. Rotation usually occurs along the long axis of the stomach (organoaxial; **Figure 36.6a**). In adults, this type is usually associated with a large paraoesophageal hiatus hernia and congenital or traumatic diaphragmatic defects. Much less commonly, the volvulus may occur due to abnormal fixation of the stomach and duodenum, either from insufficiency of the supporting ligaments or secondary to the adhesions from previous surgery that form the axis for rotation. This results in partial volvulus around the short perpendicular axis (mesenterioaxial) and is usually not associated with a diaphragmatic defect. Combined types may also occur.

Patients with chronic partial volvulus present with postprandial pain, bloating, vomiting and early satiety. In contrast, acute complete gastric volvulus (a twist greater than 180°) is a life-threatening emergency. Patients present with acute gastric obstruction. Depending on the location of the stomach, patients may complain of abdominal or lower thoracic pain, with radiation to the back or neck. Early vomiting may be followed by unproductive retching due to cardial obstruction. Prominent upper abdominal distension may be accompanied by minimal abdominal tenderness. The abdominal findings may be minimal if a stomach that has undergone volvulus is located above the diaphragm. The classic Borchardt's triad consists of a sudden epigastric pain, intractable retching (with an inability to vomit) and an inability to pass a nasogastric tube into the stomach.

Plain radiographs usually demonstrate the distended gastric shadow in the chest or upper abdomen, and an elevated colon. Acute gastric volvulus may progress to ischaemia and perforation (**Figure 36.6b**).

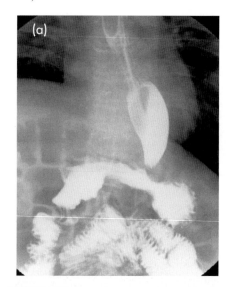

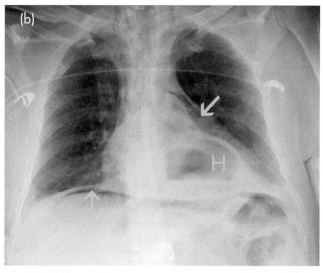

Figure 36.6 (a) Partial organoaxial volvulus along the long axis of the stomach, with upward rotation of the greater curvature in front of the lesser curvature. (b) Perforation of the gastric volvulus, associated with a hiatus hernia (H) with a pneumomediastinum and pneumoperitoneum (arrows).

## Acute Gastric Dilatation

This uncommon but serious condition usually occurs after upper abdominal surgery. It may also be encountered after trauma and in patients with spinal pathology, gastric outlet obstruction, anorexia nervosa and bulimia, electrolyte disturbances or other major medical illnesses. It may be isolated or seen in association with small bowel obstruction and post-operative ileus. The pathogenesis is unknown. It is thought to be related to various disturbances of gastric autonomic innervation secondary to regional or systemic disease. Gastric atony may develop during starvation, and the sudden ingestion of a meal may precipitate acute dilatation. Pathological eating and drinking habits and aerophagia are also associated with it.

The stomach may distend to very large dimensions, contain several litres of fluid and air and extend into the pelvis. When the intraluminal pressure exceeds the normal tissue perfusion pressure, ischaemia of the gastric wall occurs. If left untreated, necrosis and perforation will result.

An accurate history is essential in these patients. They complain of nausea and abdominal distension. Emesis is present in most patients. An occasional patient is unable to vomit due to the resulting kinking of the gastro-oesophageal junction. On physical examination, the abdomen is distended, tympanic and tender to palpation. A characteristic sloshing sound (a succussion splash) over the stomach may be heard with sudden movement of the patient. Patients may displays signs of respiratory distress secondary to compression on the diaphragm, and signs of hypovolaemic shock due to fluid sequestration in the stomach.

Abdominal imaging is diagnostic (**Figure 36.7**). The prompt placement of a nasogastric tube empties the stomach and prevents aspiration. If the abdominal tenderness persists after decompression or the patient has signs of systemic toxicity, gastric ischaemia and necrosis may be present.

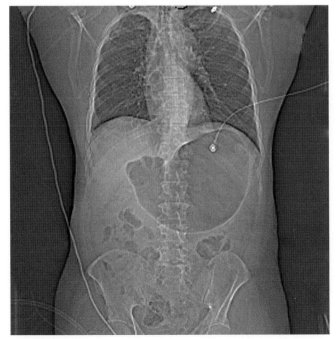

Figure 36.7 Acute gastric dilatation in a patient after splenectomy for splenomegaly.

## Acute Gastrointestinal Bleeding

Gastrointestinal bleeding may present with anaemia, haematemesis (vomiting of blood or coffee-ground-like material), melaena (black, tarry stools with a characteristic smell, caused by the digestion of blood) and haematochezia (maroon, bright red blood or blood clots in the stool).

Gastrointestinal bleeding is classified into upper and lower on the basis of the anatomical location of the source relative to the duodenojejunal junction. Upper gastrointestinal bleeding usually presents with haematemesis and melaena. Lower gastrointestinal bleeding should be suspected in patients with haematochezia. This distinction is not absolute: melaena can be seen in patients with proximal lower gastrointestinal bleeding, while haematochezia may occur with a massive ongoing upper gastrointestinal bleeding.

Nasogastric tube lavage may be helpful in constructing the differential diagnosis. The presence of both bile and blood in the nasogastric tube fluid is diagnostic of upper gastrointestinal bleeding, whereas the presence of clear bilious fluid rules out an active upper gastrointestinal bleed. The pitfall of gastric lavage is that clear lavage fluid may be non-diagnostic if the source is located distal to the closed pylorus.

Peptic ulcer disease is the leading cause of upper gastrointestinal bleeding. Gastric ulcers have a higher incidence of haematemesis and a lower incidence of melaena compared with duodenal ulcers. Oesophagogastric varices, arteriovenous malformations, tumours, Mallory–Weiss tears and Dieulafoy's lesions (bleeding superficial arteries) are the other important causes of upper gastrointestinal tract bleeding.

Lower gastrointestinal bleeding may be caused by diverticulosis, ischaemia, tumours, anorectal pathology, angiodysplasia, inflammatory bowel disease, radiation-induced and infectious colitis, and a Meckel's diverticulum.

Patients presenting with gastrointestinal bleeding should be evaluated for signs of liver disease, portal hypertension and gastrointestinal malignancy. The abdominal examination is usually unremarkable. Digital rectal examination and anoscopy should be performed to evaluate to presence of rectal masses and other anorectal pathology. The stools should be tested for blood.

Gastrointestinal bleeding results in hypovolaemia. The physical examination is also focused on an assessment of haemodynamic stability. Compensatory mechanisms for acute bleeding include an increase in the heart rate and vasospasm.

Ongoing bleeding results in tachycardia and hypotension. The pulse and blood pressure should be noted and recorded at regular intervals depending on the acuteness of the case. If the rate and volume of bleeding are significant, the patient will be in shock and will have organ malperfusion, as evidenced by a deteriorating mental status, pallor, peripheral vasoconstriction, sweating, dry mucous membranes and oliguria. A classification of haemorrhagic shock is discussed in the section on abdominal trauma later in the chapter. Massive uncontrolled gastrointestinal bleeding can result in exsanguination and death.

Compensatory mechanisms may be insufficient in the elderly and in patients with cardiovascular and other medical comorbidities, in whom deterioration occurs rapidly. Beta-blockers and other medications may also alter the usual clinical signs.

The management of gastrointestinal bleeding is determined by its aetiology and the location of its source. Early endoscopy can be useful for diagnosis and therapy. This may be supplemented with angiography and a tagged red blood cell scan.

## Cholelithiasis

Most gallstones are of the cholesterol type and result from lithogenic changes in the bile. Their prevalence increases steadily with age. Predisposing factors include obesity, female gender, parity and a diet high in animal fat. Black stones are formed most commonly in the setting of haemolysis. Brown stones develop secondary to bacterial colonization of the biliary tract and may develop in either the bile ducts or the gallbladder.

Most gallstones are asymptomatic. The most common symptom is an attack of biliary colic, which usually develops 1–2 hours after a fatty meal. Gallbladder contractions force the stone against the orifice of the cystic duct, causing a rise in intraluminal pressure and pain. When the stone falls back, the gallbladder relaxes and the pain subsides. The term 'colic' is misleading since the pain is usually constant.

The pain is generally severe and described as a dull pressure-like discomfort in the right upper quadrant or epigastrium that may radiate to the back and right shoulder. The attack may be associated with nausea and vomiting. In some patients, the pain may be unrelated to meals and have a circadian pattern, peaking in the evening. Similar symptoms may develop in patients with biliary dyskinesia in the absence of stones. The pain of biliary colic is visceral, and the physical findings are minimal and limited to mild right upper quadrant tenderness.

### Acute Cholecystitis

The persistence of biliary colic for over a few hours may be a manifestation of the development of acute cholecystitis. If obstruction of the gallbladder persists, inflammation and oedema develop, with or without bacterial infection (**Figure 36.8a**). The symptoms of acute cholecystitis are unremitting and more severe than those of colic. Fever develops with the onset of infection. As transmural inflammation develops, the pain becomes duller and more localized.

During palpation, signs of peritoneal irritation may be elicited. A positive Murphy's sign is indicative of gallbladder inflammation: ask the patient to take a deep breath while you palpate just below the right costal margin. With inspiration, the gallbladder moves downwards, and if it is inflamed the resulting contact with your hand will cause pain and the patient will generally hold their breath. A positive test requires a negative result when the test is repeated on the left.

Inflammation may progress to necrosis and perforation of the gallbladder. The omentum often seals off the area of inflammation, causing a tender and commonly palpable mass in the right upper quadrant. On the other hand, if the inflammation resolves but the obstruction persists, old bile may be absorbed and the gallbladder will fill with clear fluid (hydrops of the gallbladder), producing chronic right upper quadrant tenderness.

Emphysematous (secondary to infection with gas-forming organisms) and gangrenous forms of cholecystitis tend to occur in elderly, diabetic and immunosuppressed patients, and may result in gallbladder perforation and increased morbidity (**Figure 36.8b**).

Acute acalculous cholecystitis may develop in the absence of gallstones in some critically ill patients. It is associated with the use of central venous nutrition.

The differential diagnosis of acute right upper abdominal pain also includes acute appendicitis, hepatitis, hepatomegaly, pyelonephritis, nephrolithiasis and the perforation of a peptic ulcer. The pain in acute gastritis and pancreatitis is located more centrally. Intrathoracic conditions include myocardial infarction and right lower lobe pneumonia. Right-sided heart failure may result in symptomatic enlargement of the liver and dyspnoea. It is associated with an elevation of central venous pressure and is not accompanied by systemic inflammation.

### Choledocholithiasis

Stones may pass from the gallbladder into the common bile duct or develop there *de novo*. Small stones can pass through the ampulla into the duodenum, causing self-limiting symptoms of biliary colic. However, passage of the stone may also trigger the onset of acute pancreatitis. Impaction of the stone in the common bile duct produces persistent symptoms and obstructive jaundice. Obstruction may also result from a large stone lodged in the gallbladder that compresses the biliary tree through the

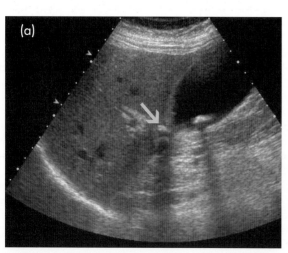
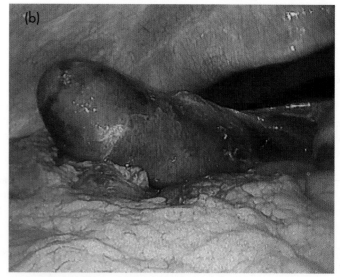

Figure 36.8 (a) Ultrasonography in a patient with acute cholecystitis, demonstrating thickening of the gallbladder wall (>3 mm is considered abnormal) and one of the stones with an acoustic shadow lodged in the neck (arrow). (b) Intraoperative photograph of gangrenous cholecystitis in a diabetic patient.

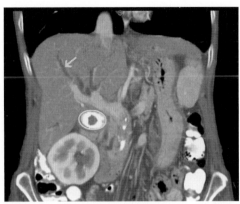

Figure 36.9 Computed tomography demonstrating intrahepatic biliary dilatation (arrow), secondary to a large stone (outlined) causing Mirizzi's syndrome with a concomitant cholecystocholedochal fistula (type II).

gallbladder wall (Mirizzi's syndrome, type I) or erodes into it (type II; **Figure 36.9**).

Obstruction of the bile ducts often causes ascending cholangitis and systemic sepsis. Charcot's triad (right upper quadrant abdominal pain, jaundice and fever) is the cardinal sign of cholangitis. Septic shock may develop very rapidly and manifests with the addition of hypotension and changes in mental status (to make up Reynolds' pentad). Urgent decompression, by either endoscopy or surgery, is mandatory.

## Acute Pancreatitis

The most common causes of acute pancreatitis are gallstones and alcohol. Other aetiologies are less common and include medications, metabolic causes (hyperlipidaemia and hypocalcaemia), trauma, endoscopic retrograde cholangiopancreatography, pancreas divisum, viral infections, vascular causes (ischaemia and vasculitis) and tumours. The degree of the resulting inflammatory process ranges from mild oedema to haemorrhage, necrosis and infection (**Figure 36.10**). Most patients do not require surgery; thus, the clinician's task is to make the diagnosis and differentiate acute pancreatitis from other causes of an acute abdomen that need operative intervention.

Pancreatitis typically presents with severe acute upper abdominal pain with radiation to the back. The pain is constant and slowly increases. Sitting up and leaning forwards, or lying on the side in the knee–chest position, may bring some relief. The pain is frequently accompanied by nausea and vomiting.

Low-grade fever is common. Tenderness is limited to the upper abdomen and is usually not associated with signs of peritoneal irritation. Concomitant cholecystitis or cholangitis may result in mixed findings. Biliary pancreatitis usually resolves rapidly. In cases of severe pancreatitis, tachycardia, hypotension and oliguria may occur secondary to hypovolaemia. Abdominal distension may develop due to ileus, resulting in hyperresonance, and later be augmented by ascites, resulting in dullness on percussion. A reactive left-sided pleural effusion is common.

Retroperitoneal haemorrhage may lead to bruising of the flanks (Grey Turner's sign) or in the periumbilical region (Cullen's sign). Ongoing inflammation and necrosis may result in a palpable epigastric mass. Pancreatic pseudocysts may reach a large size and lead to severe bleeding, gastric outlet obstruction or adjacent organ erosion (**Figure 36.10c**).

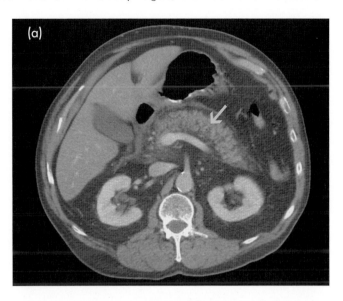

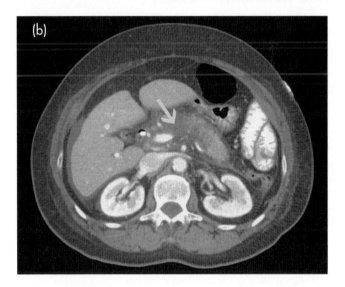

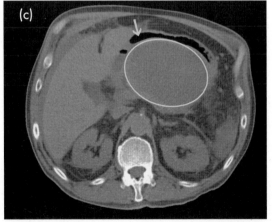

Figure 36.10 (a) Mild acute pancreatitis. Computed tomography demonstrates oedema of the pancreas and surrounding tissues (arrow). (b) Acute necrotizing gallstone pancreatitis with a lack of perfusion (arrow) of the proximal half of the gland. (c) A pancreatic pseudocyst (outlined) compressing the stomach (arrow).

PART 8 | ABDOMINAL

The management of acute pancreatitis is usually conservative. The management of the other severe pathologies that may mimic pancreatitis (gastrointestinal perforation, rupture of an abdominal aortic aneurysm, acute mesenteric ischaemia) is an emergency operation. Serum amylase and lipase levels are useful tests in the differential diagnosis. Ultrasonography and CT scanning may help to diagnose pancreatitis and its complications.

## Chronic Pancreatitis

Unless necrosis develops, the inflammation and the damage to the gland caused by acute pancreatitis are reversible. Chronic pancreatitis, secondary to repeated insults (usually alcohol), results in atrophy of the pancreatic parenchyma and stricturing of the ducts. Patients complain of recurrent abdominal and back pain. Weight loss accompanies anorexia and steatorrhoea. Diabetes occurs in the later stage. Jaundice occasionally develops secondary to a stricture of the ampulla of Vater.

## Intra-abdominal Abscess

Intra-abdominal abscesses may develop as the result of an infectious process (e.g. perforation of the gastrointestinal tract, pelvic inflammatory disease) or as a post-operative complication. Patients have non-specific signs of systemic inflammatory response with variable degrees of sepsis, including an intermittent spiking fever. Examination of the abdomen usually elicits tenderness in the area where the abscess is located. With an intraperitoneal abscess, the severity of guarding and rebound tenderness depends on the size of the abscess and its relation to the abdominal wall. Abscesses underlying the abdominal wall are accompanied by signs of local peritoneal irritation. Occasionally, a large gas-filled abscess may produce hyperresonance on percussion.

Patients with a subphrenic abscess usually complain of upper abdominal or back pain, which may radiate to the ipsilateral shoulder. Diaphragmatic irritation may cause hiccups: subcostal and lower thoracic wall tenderness is present. On examination and imaging, the signs of pleural effusion and atelectasis are characteristic.

A pelvic abscess (**Figure 36.11**) irritates the adjacent organs and may present with urinary frequency or retention, rectal urgency or diarrhoea. Lower abdominal tenderness is present. Exquisite tenderness may be present on rectal and vaginal examination, where the bulging, fluctuant area may be palpated.

Retroperitoneal abscesses (**Figure 36.12**) may develop secondary to extraperitoneal posterior perforation of the duodenum or colon, retrocaecal appendicitis or pyelonephritis. In these cases, abdominal tenderness may be minimal, with flank and costovertebral angle tenderness predominating. These abscesses are best diagnosed on a CT scan.

## Acute Pyogenic Liver Abscess

An intrahepatic abscess may mimic a subphrenic abscess. Intrahepatic abscesses are multiple in half of the patients. The two main sources are direct spread from a biliary infection and portal vein spread from any intra-abdominal infection (e.g. pylephlebitis, diverticulitis, appendicitis). Haematogenous spread is possible from distant sources (endocarditis, pyelonephritis). Local spread may result from penetrating injuries, a subphrenic abscess or an empyema. Abscesses with no identifiable source are termed cryptogenic abscesses (**Figure 36.13a**).

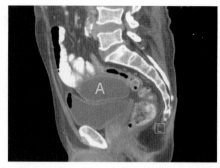

Figure 36.11 A pelvic abscess, secondary to complicated diverticulitis, located in the rectovesical pouch (A) in patient with a rectal urgency and urinary retention.

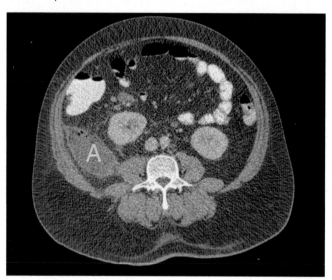

Figure 36.12 Retroperitoneal abscesses (A) secondary to a perforated appendiceal adenocarcinoma.

Patients present with intermittent spiking fever, rigors, malaise, pain and fullness in the right upper quadrant, which is due to hepatomegaly. Jaundice may be present with concomitant biliary tract disease. There may be tenderness in the right upper quadrant and costovertebral angle. Pyogenic liver abscesses may promptly progress to a fulminate sepsis.

Splenic abscesses most commonly develop secondary to haematogenous spread and present with similar symptoms in the left upper quadrant of the abdomen (**Figure 36.13b**).

## Amoebic Liver Abscess

*Entamoeba histolyticum* occurs worldwide, with an increased prevalence in counties with low sanitation levels. Primary intestinal infection may result in the spread of parasites via the portal circulation into the liver. The abscess is usually solitary and contains pasty fluid and necrotic debris. The signs and symptoms are similar to those of a pyogenic liver abscess but are less prominent and may be present for a longer period of time.

Effective systemic antiparasitic agents are available. If inadequately treated, the abscess may rupture into the peritoneal cavity or erode into adjacent organs. The granulomatous reaction from colonic infection may produce a focal mass lesion. Such an amoeboma may mimic a colorectal carcinoma or appendiceal mass.

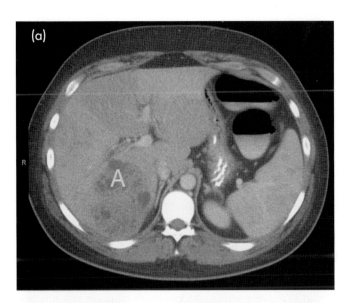

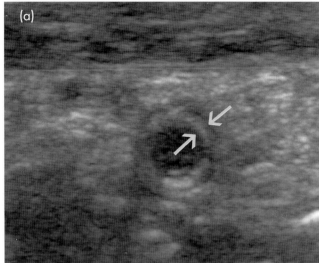

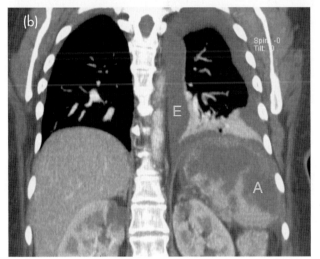

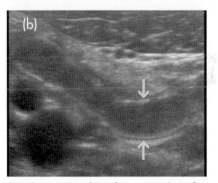

Figure 36.14 Ultrasonography of an acutely inflamed appendix (arrows) (the diagnostic criteria are a diameter >7 mm and concentric wall thickening >2 mm): (a) transverse, and (b) longitudinal.

Figure 36.13 (a) A cryptogenic liver abscess (A) in a 22-year-old man with a recent episode of bronchitis. (b) A multiloculated splenic abscess (A) in a patient with infective endocarditis. A large reactive left pleural effusion (E) is present.

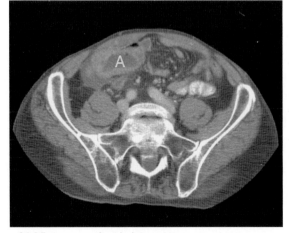

Figure 36.15 An appendiceal abscess (A).

## PATHOLOGY OF THE APPENDIX

### Acute Appendicitis

Acute appendicitis is one of the most common acute abdominal surgical pathologies. It usually affects teenagers and young adults but may occur at any age. The underlying cause is obstruction of the lumen by hyperplasia of the lymphoid follicles, faecoliths, parasites or tumour. The ensuing rise in intraluminal pressure is followed by oedema, circulatory disturbances and infection (**Figure 36.14**).

Contamination of the peritoneal cavity may result in peritonitis. If the perforation is walled off by the omentum and adjacent organs, the appendiceal mass (phlegmon [an inflammatory masses] or an actual abscess; **Figure 36.15**) may form in about 5 days. The omentum is underdeveloped in young children, resulting in a higher morbidity in this group.

The classic presentation is the gradual development of mid-abdominal visceral pain over a period of less than 24 hours.

The onset of vague colicky pain is followed by anorexia and, in most patients, nausea and vomiting. Patients may or may not have a change in bowel habit. As transmural inflammation develops and irritation of the parietal peritoneum occurs, the constant pain localizes to the right lower quadrant and is exacerbated by movement and coughing.

The findings on physical examination depend on the stage of the disease. In the early stages, the patient looks well but may have low-grade fever or leukocytosis. Ask the patient to point to the site of maximal pain. In typical appendicitis, this should correspond to the McBurney's point (two-thirds of the way along the line from the umbilicus to the right anterior superior iliac spine). Cutaneous hyperaesthesia may be present.

Classically, there is right lower quadrant tenderness and guarding, maximal at McBurney's point. If these signs are absent or equivocal, rebound tenderness can be assessed. Additionally, palpation in the left lower quadrant resulting in pain in the right lower quadrant may confirm peritoneal irritation in the right iliac fossa (**Rovsing's sign**). This is due to a displacement of bowel loops and movement of the inflamed appendix. Simultaneous palpation of the right lower quadrant with the left hand and of the left lower quadrant with the right hand may help to better identify subtle differences and the involuntary guarding of early disease (the **Butov manoeuvre**).

The tenderness may be higher and simulate acute cholecystitis if the anatomical position of the caecum is unusually high. This is typical of acute appendicitis during pregnancy (see below).

A retrocaecal appendix may produce few abdominal findings. In these cases, tenderness may be predominantly on the lateral and posterior abdominal wall. A positive psoas sign (an exacerbation of pain on passive hyperextension of the right thigh with the patient lying on left side) may be present. The constellation of findings may mimic urinary pathology.

Pelvic appendicitis may produce tenderness that is lower in position than is typical for appendicitis and may be confirmed by rectal examination and a positive obturator sign (exacerbation of the pain with passive hip rotation). To demonstrate this, ask the patient to lie supine, and lift their right leg so that the hip and knee are flexed to a right angle. Then, while supporting the calf, move the ankle outwards, watching the patient's face for signs of discomfort.

With advanced disease, patients may look unwell, with signs of a systemic inflammatory response. Diffuse peritonitis may be present, or a tender right iliac fossa mass may be palpated.

Only half of the patients have a typical presentation. One-quarter of patients report no preceding visceral pain. Vomiting may be absent and diarrhoea may occur in some patients. Some cases may have a delayed presentation. An atypical presentation is more common in very young, elderly, pregnant and immunosuppressed patients.

## Appendicitis in the Elderly

The diagnosis of acute appendicitis may be difficult. The differential diagnosis in this age group is much broader, and patients have frequently undergone previous abdominal operations and have antecedent medical conditions. These patients may be more obese, have lax abdominal musculature and manifest less prominent rigidity.

## Acute Appendicitis in Pregnancy

Acute appendicitis occurs in 1 in 1500 pregnancies and is the most common general surgical pathology seen during pregnancy. It carries an additional risk of fetal loss and preterm labour.

The presentation of the appendicitis is similar to that seen in patients who are not pregnant. A large number of common pregnancy-related complications (morning sickness, urinary tract infections) may obscure the clinical picture. Perforation occurs more frequently in the third trimester. Right lower quadrant pain remains the most common symptom of the appendicitis.

The appendix is located further away from parietal peritoneum, resulting in decreased somatic pain. The gravid uterus displaces the appendix several centimetres cephalad as well, but the abdominal tenderness in most patients is usually present close to McBurney's point regardless of the stage of pregnancy.

To differentiate between uterine and appendiceal sources of pain, note or mark the point of maximal tenderness with the patient in the supine position. Ask the patient to roll onto her left side and wait for a minute. With a uterine cause of pain, such as tension on the round ligament, the point of maximal tenderness will shift to the left along with the uterus.

## The Differential Diagnosis of Acute Appendicitis

Virtually any pain caused by the diseased organs on the right side of the trunk can mimic the symptoms of acute appendicitis. In most patients, a detailed history, a careful physical examination and observation are sufficient to make the correct diagnosis of uncomplicated appendicitis. Computed tomography is unnecessary in most cases and is associated with radiation exposure and the risks of intravenous contrast administration. The following points may be helpful:

- A duration of abdominal pain longer than 36 hours implies appendiceal perforation and is associated with obvious signs of peritoneal irritation and invariable leukocytosis.
- Submitting a patient to a general anaesthetic if they actually have pleuritic pain secondary to right lower lobe pneumonia or empyema would be dangerous for patient and embarrassing for the surgeon. Such changes should be obvious on auscultation and percussion of the chest. The Dott test consists of compression of the lower thorax to exacerbate the pain and could be especially helpful in children. If doubt still exists, chest radiography confirms the diagnosis of pneumonia.
- Gastroenteritis can be distinguished by the onset of nausea and vomiting before the abdominal pain. Abdominal pain is more diffuse and leukocytosis is usually absent. Diarrhoea is uncommon in appendicitis.
- Streptococcal pharyngitis in young children may cause vomiting and abdominal pain. Inflammation of the pharyngeal mucosa, cervical lymphadenopathy and a rapid antigen test of the throat for group A *Streptococcus* usually confirms the diagnosis.
- Mesenteric adenitis is usually seen in children and usually occurs secondary to a viral infection. Inflammation and enlargement of the mesenteric lymph nodes to larger than 1 cm on ultrasonography may be associated with upper respiratory and gastrointestinal symptoms. The abdomen remains soft, and the tenderness is localized along the projection of the root of the mesentery, closer to the umbilicus than McBurney's point.
- Diseases of the right kidney and ureter may simulate symptoms of retrocaecal appendicitis (**Figure 36.16**). Although microscopic leukocyturia and haematuria may occasionally result from appendiceal inflammation irritating the urinary tract, significant changes in urinalysis are not typical. Pyelonephritis is associated with high fever and rigors. During the passage of a ureteral stone, pain radiating to the groin or genitalia is intense and intermittent, often causing the patient to be restless. In both conditions, the abdomen is soft without localized involuntary guarding.

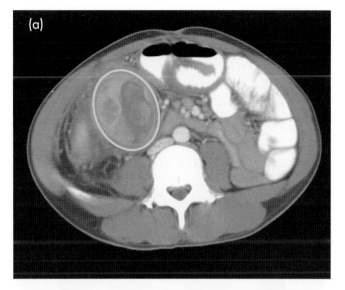

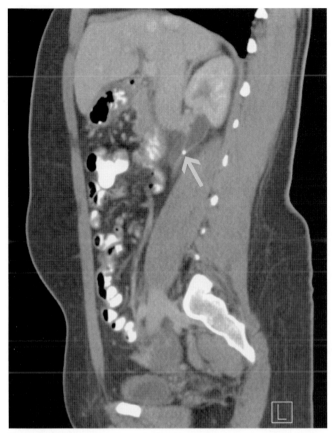

Figure 36.16 An stone (arrow) obstructing the right ureteropelvic junction, causing acute right flank and abdominal pain in a 24-year-old patient.

- Gynaecological pathology is a frequent culprit for a misdiagnosis and will be discussed later in the chapter. This is a rare situation in which advanced imaging may be needed after an equivocal abdominal and pelvic examination.

## Appendiceal Mass

In cases of the delayed presentation of a perforated appendicitis, a right lower quadrant phlegmon (inflammatory mass) or an abscess may be present (see Figure 36.15). In these cases, the inflammatory process is walled off by the greater omentum (the 'abdominal policeman') and adjacent structures over the course of a few days. The patient has systemic signs of inflammation. There is a tender palpable mass, and manipulation elicits signs of peritoneal irritation. This may extend into the pelvis and be palpable on rectal or pelvic examination. These patients frequently have variable degrees of ileus. Non-operative management is the best approach for these patients.

The differential diagnosis of a mass in the right iliac fossa includes:

- caecal carcinoma (there will be no signs of systemic inflammation and peritoneal irritation unless perforation is present) (**Figure 36.17**);
- inflammatory bowel disease;
- an infectious process of the caecum (e.g. tuberculosis, amoebiasis, actinomycosis);
- diverticulitis of the right colon (**Figure 36.18**);

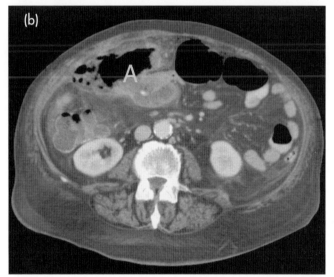

Figure 36.17 (a) A poorly differentiated ileocaecal adenocarcinoma (outlined) in a 37-year-old man presenting with an exacerbation of a several week long history of right lower quadrant pain. (b) A perforated right colon cancer resulting in a right lower quadrant abscess (A) and sepsis in a 78-year-old patient who had had anorexia and abdominal pain for several months.

- a tubo-ovarian abscess (**Figure 36.19**);
- cysts, torsion or neoplasms of the ovary (**Figure 36.20**).

Computed tomography and additional tests are frequently necessary to make an accurate diagnosis in these cases.

## Tumours of the Appendix

Tumours of the appendix are rare and are most commonly of neuroendocrine origin. Most tumours are small and asymptomatic. A few tumours are located at the base of the appendix, where they may cause luminal obstruction and symptoms of acute appendicitis. Both neuroendocrine and other epithelial tumours may occur. These are often encountered as incidental findings during appendicectomy for presumed acute appendicitis. Carcinoid tumours rarely present with the full syndrome of flushing, diarrhoea, bronchoconstriction and right-sided cardiac valve disease.

PART 8 | ABDOMINAL

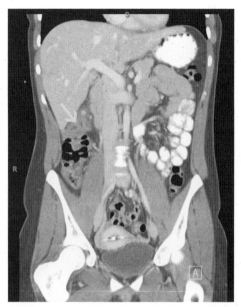

Figure 36.18 An uncommon case of acute diverticulitis of the right colon (arrow) in a 19-year-old Caucasian woman.

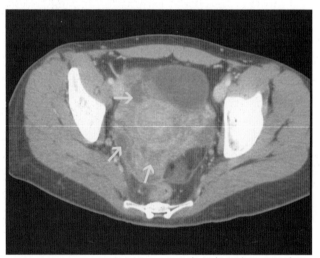

Figure 36.19 Pelvic inflammatory disease mimicking perforated appendicitis (the arrows mark multiple abscesses) in a young woman.

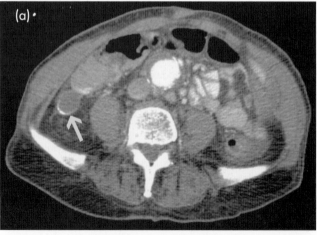

Figure 36.21 (a) A low-grade mucinous neoplasm of the appendix (arrow), with calcification of the wall and a lack of surrounding inflammation on CT scanning. (b) The removed specimen, showing a non-inflamed wall.

Mucinous neoplasms secrete mucus that may fill the lumen of appendix, resulting in a prominent mucocele that causes right lower quadrant pain. The duration of the symptoms, the large diameter and the lack of periappendicular inflammation on imaging distinguishes them from acute appendicitis (**Figure 36.21**).

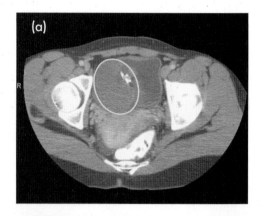

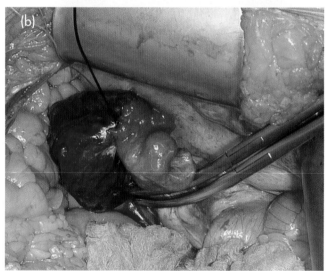

Figure 36.20 (a) A right ovarian teratoma (outlined) presenting with torsion and mimicking appendicitis in a 22-year-old woman. (b) A ruptured haemorrhagic ovarian cyst presenting as an acute abdomen in a 43-year-old woman.

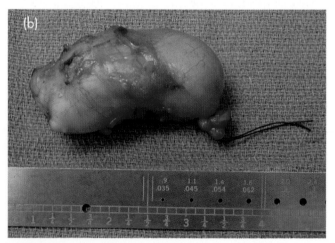

Perforation of lesions with a malignant potential results in pseudomyxoma peritonei – a gradual filling of the peritoneal cavity with mucinous fluid ('jelly belly') – which is similar to intraperitoneal mucinous dissemination from other organ tumours, resulting in a subacute presentation (**Figure 36.22**). Adenocarcinomas of the appendix do occur and are associated with a worse prognosis than other colorectal cancers (**Figure 36.23**).

## SMALL BOWEL AND ASSOCIATED PATHOLOGY

A single diverticulum very occasionally occurs in the second or third portion of the duodenum. It may rarely be symptomatic due to its large size. Multiple jejunoileal diverticula are a rare entity that may cause symptoms of bacterial overgrowth and only in minority of cases result in inflammation, bleeding or perforation (**Figure 36.24**).

Tumours of the small bowel are uncommon and can be either malignant (neuroendocrine tumours, adenocarcinomas, gastrointestinal stromal tumours, lymphomas, metastatic tumours) or benign (adenomas). Patient with rare hereditary cancer syndromes (familial adenomatous polyposis, hereditary non-polyposis colorectal cancer, familial intestinal hamartomatous polyposis [Peutz–Jeghers syndrome]) have an increased risk of malignant change. Patients with Peutz–Jeghers syndrome have characteristic pigmented macules on the oral mucosa. Small bowel tumours present with abdominal pain, bleeding, obstruction and, less commonly, perforation (**Figure 36.25**).

Mesenteric panniculitis (sclerosing mesenteritis) is an idiopathic disease of inflammation and fibrosis that affects the mesenteric fat. It presents with fever, abdominal pain, obstructive symptoms, diarrhoea and anorexia. An abdominal mass can be palpated in many patients. The symptoms are usually chronic but patients may present with acute exacerbations. Imaging and biopsy are diagnostic (**Figure 36.26**).

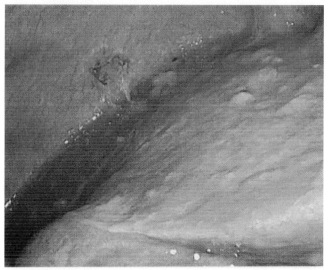

Figure 36.22 Pseudomyxoma peritonei filling the right subdiaphragmatic space with multiple liver lesions.

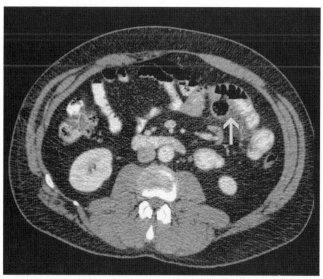

Figure 36.24 Jejunal diverticulitis with microperforation into the mesentery (arrow), presenting as an acute abdomen.

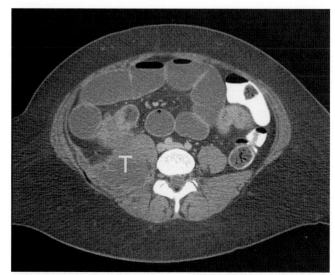

Figure 36.23 Locally advanced mucinous adenocarcinoma of the appendix (T) invading the retroperitoneum in a 32-year-old woman and presenting with acute pain secondary to perforation.

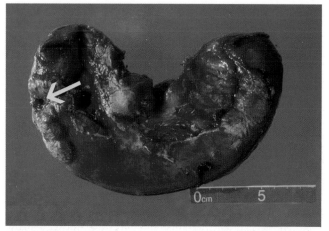

Figure 36.25 Metastatic laryngeal squamous cell carcinoma of the head and neck, thought to be in remission, presenting with carcinomatosis and peritonitis secondary to small bowel perforation at the site of a metastatic implant (arrow).

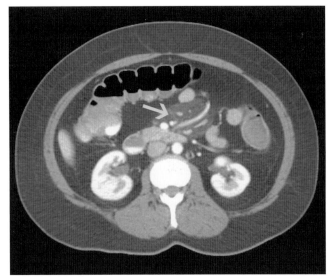

Figure 36.26 Computed tomography is a very sensitive tool for the diagnosis of sclerosing mesenteritis and demonstrates fat stranding along the mesenteric vessels (arrow). Lymphoma, peritoneal carcinomatosis and carcinoid tumours may have a similar appearance and need to be ruled out.

Various anomalies, such as mesenteric cysts and enteric duplications, may present with acute and chronic symptoms of abdominal pain and obstruction (**Figure 36.27**).

## Meckel's Diverticulum

A Meckel's diverticulum is a remnant of the vitellointestinal duct and occurs in 2 per cent of patients. It is located approximately 60 cm from the ileocaecal valve and is usually about 5 cm long. In most patients, it is asymptomatic. It can be subject to acute inflammation and mimic the symptoms of an acute appendicitis. If the appendix is found during surgery to be normal in a patient with suspected appendicitis, examine the terminal ileum for the presence of a Meckel's diverticulum.

A Meckel's diverticulum may serve as a lead point for intussusception or small bowel volvulus, which both present with symptoms of small bowel obstruction (**Figure 36.28**). A fibrous band may occasionally connect it to the umbilicus and further contribute to the development of bowel obstruction. A Meckel's diverticulum occasionally contains ectopic gastric mucosa, and bleeding may develop from peptic ulceration of the adjacent ileal wall. This usually produces painless episodic lower gastrointestinal bleeding that is not massive.

Groin hernias containing a Meckel's diverticulum can occur and are called Littre's hernias.

## Pathology of the Ileocaecum

The ileocaecum contains abundant lymphoid tissue and can be subject to a variety of infections. Acute inflammation of the terminal ileum (ileitis) and caecum (typhlitis) occurs close to the appendix, and may present with symptoms of an acute abdomen and mimic appendicitis.

Infection with *Yersinia* and *Campylobacter* spp. may present with symptoms very similar to those of acute appendicitis. In some patients, prodromal symptoms preceding the abdominal pain, the presence of diarrhoea and pharyngitis (*Yersinia* pharyngitis) may be clues to the diagnosis.

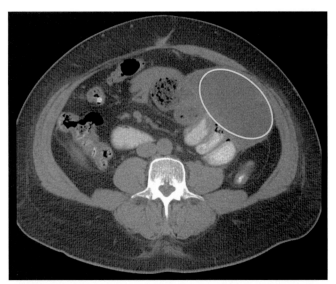

Figure 36.27 A mesenteric cyst (outlined) in a patient presenting with a small bowel obstruction.

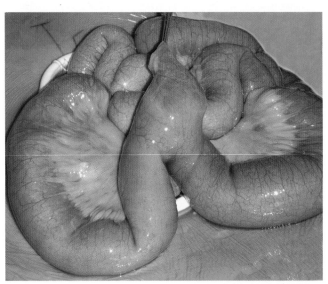

Figure 36.28 A Meckel's diverticulum presenting as an acute small bowel obstruction.

In immunosuppressed patients, the life-threatening neutropenic enterocolitis preferentially involves the caecum and may extend into the terminal ileum and ascending colon. These patients commonly present with fever and right lower quadrant pain 10–14 days after a cycle of cytotoxic chemotherapy.

Typhoid fever is a systemic disease, preventable with appropriate vaccinations prior to travel to endemic regions. Classically, the first week of illness manifests with rising fever and bacteraemia. Abdominal pain and macular 'rose spots' develop on the trunk and abdomen during the second week. During the third week, intestinal bleeding, perforation and peritonitis develop in areas where there is lymphatic hyperplasia of the Peyer's patches in the ileocaecum.

*Mycobacterium tuberculosis* also has an affinity for the ileocaecum. Gastrointestinal tuberculosis can have an acute or a chronic presentation with non-specific abdominal pain and constitutional and gastrointestinal symptoms. The inflammatory reaction may result in ileitis, bowel obstruction, a mass and perforation. The presence of ascites secondary to subclinical peritoneal involvement may help to differentiate intestinal tuberculosis from Crohn's disease.

## Crohn's Disease

Crohn's disease is a transmural inflammation of the gastrointestinal tract of unknown aetiology. It may affect any part of gastrointestinal tract from the mouth to the perineal area (**Figure 36.29**). The inflammation and ulceration involves the distal ileum and colon, frequently in a discontinuous pattern, with normal 'skip areas' present in between. In contrast to ulcerative colitis, the rectum is usually spared.

This chronic, incurable disease may present acutely and has a tendency for recurrent exacerbations. Patients with Crohn's disease may have extraintestinal involvement of the joints, eyes, skin and biliary tree. Abdominal pain, diarrhoea, malabsorption, anorexia and fatigue are the typical symptoms and may lead to substantial weight loss.

The acute flare-up typically presents with abdominal pain and fever and may mimic acute appendicitis and other pathology. Severe inflammation may result in the formation of intra-abdominal and retroperitoneal abscesses, enteroenteric and enterovesical fistulas and, uncommonly, free perforation. Chronic inflammation and fibrosis may lead to stricture formation and obstruction.

## Appendicitis Epiploicae and Omental Infarct

An abnormally long or large appendix epiploica may twist around its base. Such torsion, although benign and self-limiting, usually presents with acute abdominal pain and may be confused with acute appendicitis or diverticulitis. Constitutional and gastrointestinal symptoms are rare.

An omental infarct is due to the torsion of a segment of the greater omentum. It has a very similar presentation. Computed tomography is usually diagnostic (**Figure 36.30**).

### ACUTE COLONIC DIVERTICULITIS

Colonic diverticula are false diverticula consisting of mucosal protrusion outside the bowel wall along the penetrating arteries. They primarily develop in the left colon and are related to abnormal colonic motility and increased intraluminal pressure. The prevalence is high in countries with a low intake of dietary fibre (a Western-type duet) and increases with age (reaching approximately 60 per cent of the population by the age of 80 in the USA). Most patients remain asymptomatic, and only a quarter develop complications of inflammation or bleeding.

Acute diverticulitis, resulting from microperforation, manifests with signs and symptoms resembling those of acute appendicitis. Low-grade fever is common. Since most diverticula are concentrated in the sigmoid colon, the abdominal tenderness and accompanying signs are located in the left lower quadrant (hence the

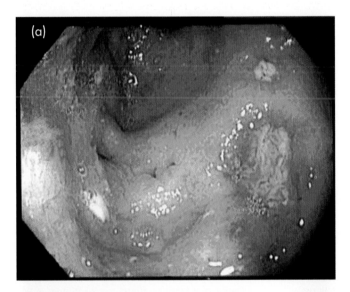

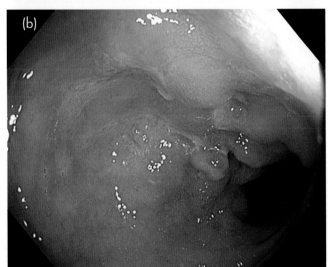

Figure 36.29 Endoscopic appearance of active Crohn's disease. (a) Inflammation of the terminal ileum with superficial aphthous ulcers and deep ulceration. (b) Sigmoid Crohn's colitis with cobblestoning (courtesy of Dr Rami El Abiad).

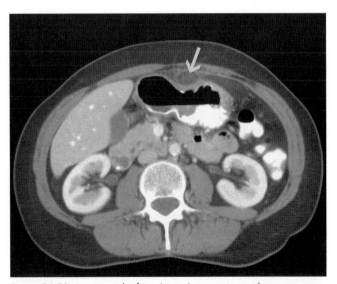

Figure 36.30 An omental infarct (arrow) presenting with acute epigastric pain, guarding and rebound tenderness.

term 'left-sided appendicitis') (**Figure 36.31**). The affected loop of a long 'S-shaped' left colon may indeed extend across the midline to the right, simulating appendicitis. Right-sided diverticula, usually single and unrelated to the consumption of refined food, are prevalent in Asian countries. Their inflammation will also present with right abdominal symptoms.

Only a minority of patients present within the first day of symptoms. Many patients report a history of previous attacks. Up to one-third may have a normal white blood cell count. Inflammation lasting for several days results in a palpable left lower quadrant mass at the time of presentation – either a phlegmon or an abscess (**Figure 36.32**). Depending on the location of the perforation, an intra-abdominal or retroperitoneal abscess may result. Severe inflammation and mass lesions may cause acute bowel obstruction.

The inflamed colon may also erode into an adjacent viscus. Colovesical fistulas present with recurrent urinary tract infections and characteristic pneumaturia (the passage of air during urination) (**Figure 36.33**). The passage of gross faeculent matter is rare. A colovaginal fistula may develop in women who have undergone hysterectomy and manifests with a debilitating passage of stools and flatus through the vagina. Colocutaneous and coloenteric fistulas are rare.

When the acute diverticular perforation is sizeable and not walled off by the adjacent structures, there may be a rapid development of diffuse purulent or faeculent peritonitis with free intra-abdominal air seen on an X-ray. In some patients, this can be the first manifestation of the diverticulosis.

Recurrent attacks of diverticulitis may lead to stricture of the affected segment and the gradual development of colonic obstruction (**Figure 36.34**). In every case of suspected diverticular colonic stricture or colovesical fistula, underlying malignancy must be ruled out.

## MECHANICAL BOWEL OBSTRUCTION

Intestinal obstruction is the delayed or blocked transport of food, swallowed air and intestinal secretions along the gastrointestinal

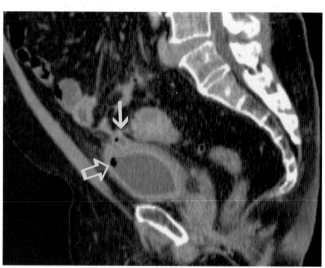

Figure 36.33 A CT scan demonstrating air in the urinary bladder (hollow arrow) in the absence of urinary tract instrumentation and, in this case, a discrete colovesical fistula tract (solid arrow).

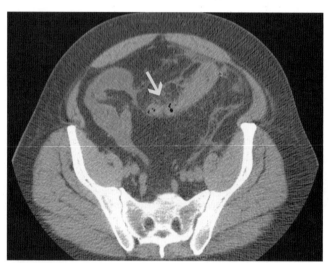

Figure 36.31 Acute uncomplicated sigmoid diverticulitis with thickening of the sigmoid colon and surrounding inflammation (arrow).

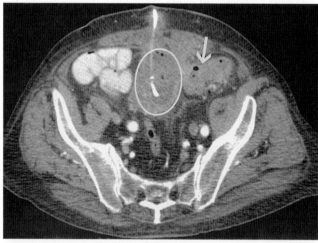

Figure 36.32 Complicated diverticulitis (the arrow marks inflamed sigmoid colon) with a pelvic abscess (outlined). The condition is initially best managed with percutaneous drainage.

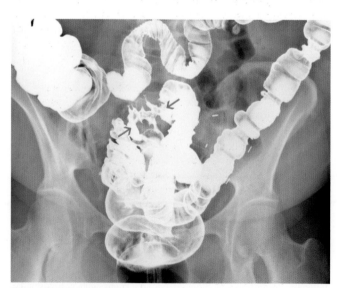

Figure 36.34 A double-contrast barium enema demonstrates a 5 cm long stricture (arrow) in the mid-sigmoid colon, secondary to recurrent diverticulitis.

tract. Mechanical (dynamic) obstruction is caused by obstruction of the lumen (foreign body, faecal impaction, the roundworm *Ascaris lumbricoides*), intrinsic abnormalities of the bowel wall (tumour, stricture) or external compression (such as adhesions, a hernia, an adjacent mass, intussusception or volvulus). Functional (adynamic) obstruction is also called ileus and results from alterations in bowel peristalsis due to electrolyte disturbances, infection, ischaemia and neurogenic causes.

Volvulus is a rotation of the bowel loop around the axis of the mesentery, with a risk of mesenteric blood flow interruption and the formation of a closed loop obstruction. In a closed loop obstruction (from volvulus, hernia or adhesions), the segment of bowel has no outlet for its secretions. Gradually increasing intraluminal pressure leads to overdistension, an interruption of mural venous flow, inflammatory and ischaemic changes and eventually necrosis and perforation. Ischaemic changes are reversible with early correction of the obstruction.

The symptoms and aetiologies of intestinal obstruction vary depending on the level of the intestinal tract affected and the degree of blockage. The hallmark symptoms are colicky abdominal pain, abdominal distension, vomiting and an inability to pass stools and flatus (absolute constipation). The presence of bile in the vomit depends on whether the obstruction is proximal or distal to the ampulla of Vater. If bowel gangrene and perforation occur, peritonitis develops.

With **proximal intestinal obstruction**, the intraluminal contents reflux into the stomach, producing a rapid onset of abdominal pain, with frequent and profuse bilious vomiting. Abdominal distension may be minimal. **Gastric outlet obstruction** represents a very proximal obstruction and results in projectile non-bilious vomiting, dehydration and hypochloraemic metabolic alkalosis. With **distal obstruction** (small or large bowel), the symptoms have a more insidious onset with an eventually pronounced abdominal distension. Intestinal distension is due to the presence of gas (mostly swallowed, but also produced by bacterial fermentation) and intraluminal fluid stasis.

As with other cases of acute abdominal pain, undertake a thorough review of the patient's symptoms, previous operations and medical conditions. Assess and continuously monitor the patient's respiratory and haemodynamic status. It is not uncommon for patients with a poor pulmonary reserve to suffer a deterioration from massive abdominal distension. Prompt nasogastric tube placement may frequently provide relief and prevent aspiration. The hypovolaemic patient should receive appropriate fluid and electrolyte resuscitation.

Examine the abdomen for the presence of surgical scars, and check all the hernial orifices. Assess the function and patency of any ostomy present.

The presence of fever, tachycardia, signs of peritoneal irritation, leukocytosis and lactic acidosis increase the suspicion of bowel ischaemia. The viability of the bowel is the most important issue in a patient with bowel obstruction.

Nasogastric tube decompression is frequently therapeutic in patients with certain types of bowel obstruction. Clear effluent suggests gastric outlet obstruction. A reflux of bile into the stomach indicates obstruction distal to the ampulla of Vater. The heme molecule is metabolized in the liver into the green pigment biliverdin, which is in turn converted to yellow bilirubin. Bilirubin gives a golden yellow colour to bile and a yellowish hue to the succus entericus. In the gastrointestinal tract under the influence of bacterial enzymes bilirubin is converted to colourless urobilinogens. Part of urobilinogens is reabsorbed and the rest is oxidized to brown stercobilin in the colon. During the intestinal flow stagnation, biliverdin forms and the contents of the obstructed bowels turns green. In prolonged obstruction, the stagnant succus becomes particularly dark and foul-smelling (faeculent). A decrease in nasogastric tube output and a change in its colour from green back into a normal light colour indicate the resolution of the bowel obstruction.

An adequate assessment of the abdomen for evidence of obstruction must include both supine and upright radiographs. Assess the pattern of gas, its distribution in the small intestine and colon and any distension on the supine film. Abnormal small bowel gas is generally found in the middle part of the abdomen and is characterized by a 'stack of coins' patterns due to the circumferential plicae circularis.

Colonic gas is expected to be located on the periphery of the abdomen and in the pelvis, and is associated with the haustral folds. Upright radiographs are used to evaluate for free air and to assess the number and size of air–fluid levels, which correlate with the level of obstruction (**Figure 36.35**). An absence of colonic gas indicates complete small bowel obstruction, but this may not be evident until existing stool and gas have been passed. The location of the gas in the colon may similarly indicate the level of colonic obstruction (**Figure 36.36**).

Chronic delayed empting of the small bowel into the colon for any reason may lead to a radiographic appearance of 'small bowel faecalization' due to the change in consistency of the succus entericus (**Figure 36.37**).

Because large quantities of fluid are produced, pass through the gastrointestinal tract daily and are reabsorbed in the small bowel and colon, large losses through vomiting and any intraluminal sequestration of fluid rapidly produce symptoms of dehydration. The more distal the obstruction, the longer it takes for the symptoms of hypervolaemia to become manifest. A proximal obstruction may result in a life-threatening fluid and electrolyte disturbances in 1 or 2 days, whereas in distal ileal obstruction this may take many days.

## Small Bowel Obstruction

Bowel obstruction is the most common surgical disease of the small intestine. In developed countries, the most common cause is adhesions from previous surgery. It may occur within weeks, months or years post-operatively. Depending on nature of the original disease, the operation and patient-related factors, the adhesions may be generalized or limited to a segment of bowel. Thin filmy adhesions are of no significance, whereas dense fibrous bands may compress the bowel or serve as an axis for intestinal volvulus (**Figure 36.38a**). Any abdominal surgery, including the operation to resolve the obstruction, results in the formation of new adhesions, with a risk of further obstruction in the future. Therefore, unless complications develop, bowel obstructions secondary to adhesions are treated non-operatively.

In the absence of previous abdominal surgery, small bowel obstruction is due to an abdominal wall or internal hernia, tumour or bowel ischaemia until proven otherwise. Compression of the third portion of the duodenum is an unusual cause of proximal intestinal obstruction that may develop secondary to significant weight loss in patients with chronic debilitating illnesses (**Figure 36.38b**).

The cardinal symptoms are abdominal pain, vomiting and constipation. The colicky pain is usually felt over the entire abdomen but is worse in the mid-abdomen. It occurs in episodes of a crescendo–decrescendo pattern of variable length. The more

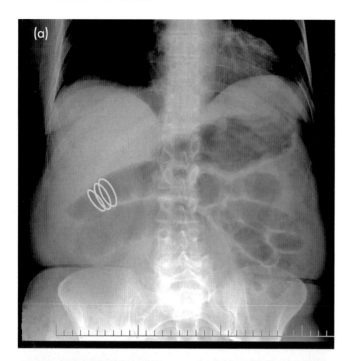

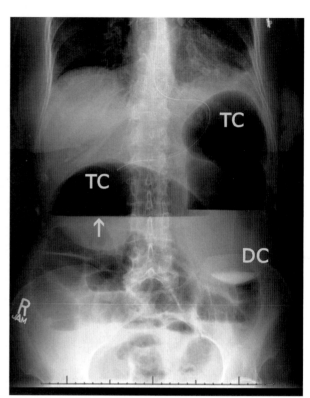

Figure 36.36 Colonic obstruction secondary to a carcinoma at the splenic flexure. Note the distended transverse colon (TC) with a large air–fluid level (arrow), and a collapsed descending colon (DC) distal to the obstruction.

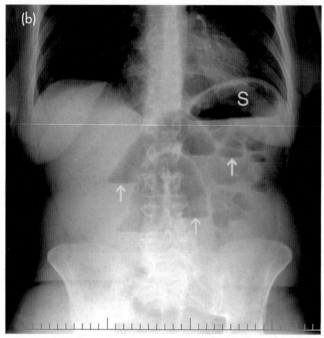

Figure 36.35 (a) A supine abdominal radiograph demonstrates gaseous distension of the stomach (S in part b) and small bowel with characteristic plicae circularis (several being outlined). The upright film (b) demonstrates multiple small bowel air–fluid levels (arrows) consistent with distal obstruction. The lack of colonic gas is consistent with small bowel obstruction.

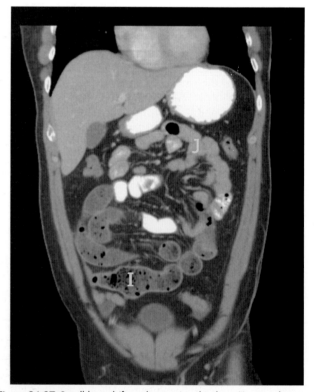

Figure 36.37 Small bowel 'faecalization' in the ilium (I) secondary to a chronic partial small bowel obstruction. Note the normal appearance of the jejunum (J) in the upper abdomen.

proximal the obstruction, the shorter the duration of the attacks and the intervals between them.

Patients vomit undigested food, fluids and gastrointestinal secretions refluxing into the stomach. With distal small bowel and large bowel obstruction due to bacterial overgrowth, the vomit looks and smells faeculent.

Constipation is not a consistent feature of small bowel obstruction. It may take over a day for the colon to empty the gas

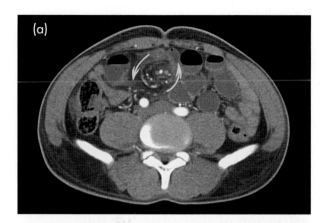

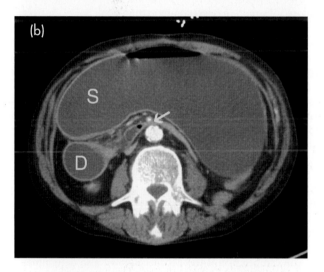

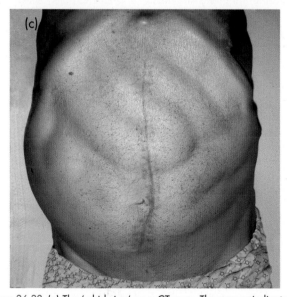

Figure 36.38 (a) The 'whirl sign' on a CT scan. The arrows indicate the volvulus of the small bowel loop around its mesentery (secondary to an adhesive band), creating the whirl of mesenteric vessels. (b) Superior mesenteric artery (SMA) syndrome in a patient with profound malnutrition. Computed tomography demonstrates a distended stomach (S) and duodenum (D), proximal to an area of compression (arrow) between the aorta and SMA. (c) The 'ladder pattern sign' in a patient with a distal small bowel obstruction.

and stool present distal to the level of the obstruction. In cases of a Richter's hernia, the luminal obstruction may be incomplete. If the bowel obstruction is caused by a pelvic abscess, patients may develop diarrhoea secondary to the colonic irritation. In cases of acute mesenteric ischaemia, diarrhoea may be a prominent feature.

During examination, strategically undrape the groins as well as the abdomen so that any inguinal or femoral hernia may be detected. In early obstruction, the abdomen may still be scaphoid. As the condition progresses, the abdomen becomes more distended. In thin individuals, peristalsis may become visible in the late stages. In the so-called 'ladder pattern sign', distended intestinal loops of bowel are visible through the anterior abdominal wall ((Figure 36.38c).

Abdominal auscultation early in the course of the obstruction reveals a characteristic pattern: the low-pitched gurgling sound rapidly changes to a high-pitched tinkling, corresponding to hyperperistalsis. At times, the sounds may be audible even without a stethoscope. Later in the course of the condition, the abdominal sounds may be absent due to overdistension and atony of the bowel. Percussion generally yields a resonant sound and may reveal signs of peritoneal irritation.

Palpation of the abdomen follows the general principles of examination and occasionally reveals the cause of the obstruction, such as a ventral or groin hernia, intussusception or a tumour. Localized tenderness with signs of peritoneal irritation generally indicates the possibility of bowel ischaemia, overdistension threatening the integrity of the bowel and a need for urgent operative intervention before perforation leads to generalized peritonitis. No tests have proven totally reliable for the prediction of bowel ischaemia.

Although rectal examination rarely contributes to the diagnosis, it may reveal gross or occult blood in the stool in the cases of mesenteric ischaemia.

### Gallstone Ileus

Gallstone ileus is an uncommon cause of small bowel obstruction in contemporary practice and generally occurs in the elderly population. Chronic inflammation and a pressure effect may lead to a large gallstone eroding into the stomach or duodenum and causing obstruction at the level of the terminal ileum, pylorus or, if very large, jejunum (Figure 36.39). There is typically a history

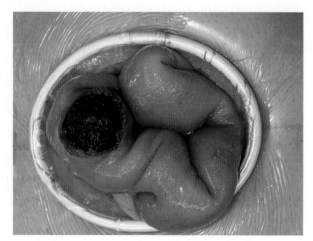

Figure 36.39 A large gallstone causing proximal jejunal obstruction exposed through the intraoperative enterotomy.

of recurrent biliary colic. Physical examination is consistent with a bowel obstruction. Abdominal imaging almost always shows presence of air in the biliary tree (pneumobilia) and occasionally a radio-opaque gallstone.

### Internal Hernias

Internal hernias are an uncommon cause of bowel obstruction. Bowel loops herniate through the defects between the various intra- and retroperitoneal structures. Some of these defects are due to congenital variations in the ligamentous anatomy (paraduodenal, paracaecal, intersigmoid or supravesical hernias) and diaphragmatic defects. Others are post-surgical. They cannot be diagnosed on physical examination. They frequently cause closed loop obstructions and always require surgical correction.

### Intussusception

An intussusception is the telescoping of a segment of bowel (intussusceptum) into a more distal segment (intussuscipiens). Intestinal peristalsis pushes the inner loop further and further down, leading to the intestinal obstruction. Compression of the mesenteric blood vessels between the two loops eventually leads to strangulation.

Intussusception develops secondary to a lead point at the apex of the inverting segment. Intussusceptions are classified as ileocolic, jejuno-jejunal, jejunoileal or colo-colic. Intussusception most commonly occurs in young children (idiopathic intussusception). These cases are commonly associated with minor viral and bacterial infections. They are thought to be due to hyperplasia of the Peyer's patches and are usually ileocolic.

Intussusception causing bowel obstruction is uncommon in children above the age of 5 years and in adults, and is almost always due to a pathological lead point: Meckel's diverticulum, polyp, adhesion or tumour (**Figure 36.40**).

The typical paediatric patient is a 6–24-month-old boy presenting with a sudden onset of severe cramping pain accompanied by inconsolable crying and drawing up of the legs towards the abdomen. Brief bouts of pain are initially separated by

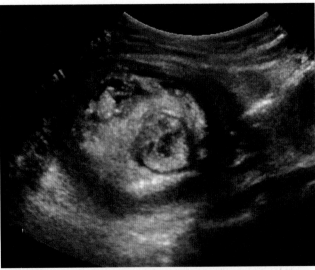

Figure 36.40 Ultrasonography demonstrating a 'bull's eye' or 'target sign' in an adult patient presenting with acute ileocolic intussusception secondary to an adenocarcinoma of the ileocaecal valve: ascending colon (intussuscipiens) and ilium (intussusceptum).

approximately 15–30 minute intervals of almost normal behaviour. The attacks become more frequent and severe as the disease progresses. It may take up to a day for vomiting and abdominal distension to develop. Most children have a containing mixture of mucous and blood. If the child is constipated, rectal examination may provoke a gush of characteristic 'redcurrant jelly'.

In uncomplicated cases, the abdomen is typically soft but may reveal the presence of a sausage-shaped abdominal mass in the upper abdomen with an emptiness in the right iliac fossa (**Dance's sign**). Very rarely, an ileocolic intussusception in children or left colo-colic intussusception in adults may be palpated on rectal examination, resembling a cervix, or progress further and protrude through the anus, mimicking a rectal prolapse.

## Obstruction of the Large Intestine

Colonic obstruction is less common than small bowel obstruction. While most small bowel obstructions secondary to adhesions resolve with non-operative management, colonic obstructions do not resolve, and they require urgent surgical intervention. The most common causes of the large bowel obstruction are colorectal carcinoma, faecal impaction, colonic volvulus, pseudo-obstruction, hernias and compression by an extrinsic mass. A colonic stricture may develop secondary to inflammatory bowel disease, ischaemic colitis and recurrent diverticulitis, and after radiation.

The presentation depends on the aetiology of the obstruction. A history of recent changes in bowel habit, weight loss, anorexia, abdominal discomfort and possibly rectal bleeding (or occult blood), leading to the signs and symptoms of anaemia, should raise a concern about colorectal carcinoma. The acute onset of symptoms and certain demographic characteristics of the patient may point to the diagnosis of a volvulus.

The competence of the ileocaecal valve also determines the presenting symptoms. Normally, a competent ileocaecal valve prevents the reflux of the caecal contents into the terminal ileum. If complete distal colonic obstruction develops, pressure in the caecum rises and may lead to overdistension of the caecum within a few days. Once the intraluminal pressure exceeds the perfusion pressure of the caecal wall, necrosis and possibly perforation ensue. If the retrograde pressure is able to decompress through the valve into the terminal ileum, the symptoms may be less acute and patients may present with symptoms resembling distal small bowel obstruction.

Patients with early colonic obstruction may initially appear less unwell than those with small bowel obstruction. Bouts of colicky pain are less frequent and vomiting is less prominent; the abdomen is distended and tympanitic in the areas where there are distended segments of colon. Pre-existing ascites and hepatomegaly may be sinister signs of metastasis. An obstructing tumour is palpable in only a few advanced cases.

Digital rectal examination is mandatory to rule out faecal impaction and distal rectal cancer. In more proximal colonic obstruction, the rectum is usually empty.

### Caecal Volvulus

Caecal volvulus occurs in individuals with abnormal fixation of the right colon. Its presentation is similar to that of distal small bowel obstruction, with abdominal pain, nausea, vomiting and abdominal distension. Hyperresonance, tenderness and fullness are present on the right and mid-abdomen. On plain radiographs of the abdomen, there is a characteristic bean-shaped mass with a convex aspect pointing towards the left upper quadrant (**Figure 36.41**).

## Volvulus of the Sigmoid Colon

Sigmoid volvulus is most commonly seen in South America, Africa, Scandinavia and Asia. Its exact aetiology is not completely understood. Redundant sigmoid colons with a narrow mesentery and abnormal motility are predisposed to volvulus. The patients are frequently elderly, may be institutionalized and have neuropsychiatric conditions. Large meals after a period of religious fasting or significant rapid changes in altitude may precipitate the disease in predisposed individuals.

Patients usually present with a triad of abdominal pain, distension and constipation. A history of similar attacks may indicate prior, spontaneously resolved volvulus episodes. Abdominal imaging reveals a bean-shaped loop of colon with a convex aspect pointing to the right upper quadrant (**Figure 36.42**), although differentiation from caecal volvulus may occasionally be difficult and require additional imaging.

## Faecal Impaction

Delayed transit through the colon (arbitrarily defined as fewer than three bowel movements per week) may be related to medications (narcotics, anticholinergics), diet (low fibre and fluid intake), immobility and metabolic (diabetes, hypothyroidism, hypercalcaemia) and neuropsychological disturbances. Chronic inadequate evacuation of stool and its build-up may lead to faecal impaction.

Adult and paediatric patients, usually with a history of constipation, may present with acute abdominal pain and signs of colonic obstruction. The abdomen is typically soft but tender, and in severe cases a distended colon of doughy consistency may be palpated through the abdominal wall (**Figure 36.43**). Rectal examination reveals the presence of abundant stool.

Paradoxically, faecal incontinence may develop in some patients, secondary to the leakage of liquid stool around the impaction. Colorectal ulceration, bleeding and rarely perforations (stercoral perforation) are other possible complications.

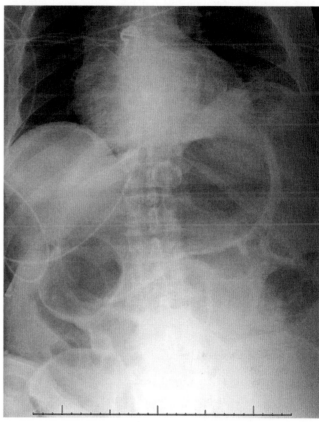

Figure 36.42 Sigmoid volvulus (convex of the distended bowel points to the right upper quadrant).

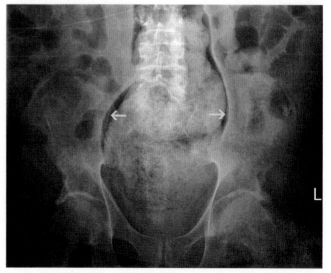

Figure 36.43 Faecal impaction. The patent periphery of the rectal lumen (megarectum) is marked with arrows.

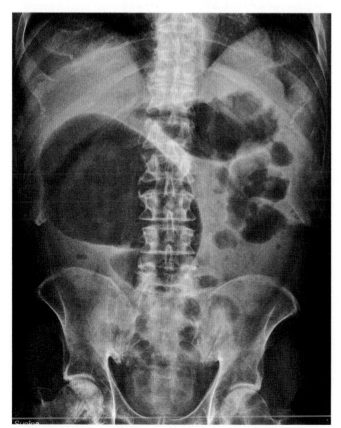

Figure 36.41 Caecal volvulus (convex of the distended bowel points to the left upper quadrant).

## ADYNAMIC OBSTRUCTION

### Paralytic Ileus

Ileus is the dysfunction of normal motor activity of the gastrointestinal tract without mechanical obstruction. The most common cause is a surgical operation. Some degree of ileus follows all abdominal and some non-abdominal operations, but its duration and severity depend on individual patients and the operation performed. It is thought that, after a major uncomplicated abdominal operation, the function of the small intestine recovers within a day, followed by stomach within 2 days and then the colon within 3 days. Electrolyte imbalances (especially hypokalaemia and hypomagnesaemia) and narcotic use are common after major intra-abdominal operations and may further impede the recovery of bowel function.

Symptoms of ileus include anorexia and inability to tolerate an oral intake, nausea and vomiting, abdominal distension and bloating, abdominal discomfort and pain, and an inability to pass flatus and stool. Physical examination reveals various degrees of abdominal distension, tympany, reduction of bowel sounds and mild diffuse tenderness. Bowel sounds are characteristically very diminished or absent. One can only state that the bowel sounds are absent if auscultation is negative when performed in a quite environment for 2–3 minutes in the most sensitive location (just to the right of and below the umbilicus, over the bulk of the small bowel). The symptoms are usually very mild.

An ileus usually resolves with conservative management. It should, however, be differentiated from post-operative bowel obstruction that has a mechanical cause and may progress. This is sometimes difficult. In ileus, abdominal radiographs demonstrate diffuse dilatation of the entire gastrointestinal tract. A paucity of gas in the colon may, however, mimic post-operative small bowel obstruction and vice versa.

Any major trauma, abdominal pathology (e.g. cholecystitis, pancreatitis, pyelonephritis, haemorrhage) or systemic disease (pneumonia, acute renal failure) may result in ileus. Ileus secondary to renal failure may further compromise the recovery of renal function due to hypervolaemia and should be recognized early.

### Acute Colonic Pseudo-obstruction

**Ogilvie's syndrome** is a significant dilatation of the colon (usually to the level of the descending colon) without mechanical obstruction. In most patients, it is associated with an underlying disease: metabolic, neurological, oncological, respiratory failure, renal failure, trauma and others. It may be a part of post-operative ileus.

Most patients appear well, with constipation but minimal nausea and only mild abdominal discomfort despite very significant distension. Severe abdominal distension may occasionally affect respiration. The abdomen is tympanitic, but bowel sounds are frequently present. Tenderness on palpation in early cases is minimal. In certain patients with abnormal motility, colonic pseudo-obstruction can be chronic.

Abdominal films demonstrate colonic distension with no significant small bowel dilatation (**Figure 36.44**). The left colon may be collapsed, with no air present distally. A contrast enema or endoscopy is mandatory to rule out mechanical obstruction of the distal colon prior to making the diagnosis of colonic pseudo-obstruction. Increasing abdominal tenderness or a caecal

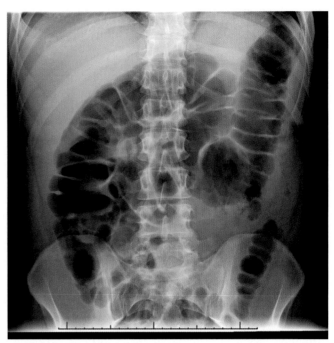

Figure 36.44 Acute colonic pseudo-obstruction in a patient with ascending cholangitis (Ogilivie's syndrome). Note that colonic distention ends at the level of the descending colon.

diameter over 10 cm requires prompt intervention and colonic decompression.

### Toxic Megacolon

Toxic megacolon is a segmental or pancolonic non-obstructive dilatation of the colon and is usually a complication of inflammatory bowel disease (**Figure 36.45a**) or a fulminant *Clostridium difficile* colitis (**Figure 36.45b**). Other causes are *Salmonella*, *Shigella* and *Campylobacter* colitis and, in HIV patients, cytomegalovirus colitis.

Colonic dilatation secondary to impaired motility occurs in variety of other conditions: Hirschsprung's disease, Chagas disease, primary colonic inertia and constipation (**Figure 36.45c**). Toxic megacolon, however, differs from these, manifesting signs of a systemic inflammatory response and being truly life-threatening. Inflammatory changes in the mucosa lead to the release of inflammatory mediators and the translocation of bacterial products. It may be the presenting symptom of inflammatory bowel disease, and the distinction between ulcerative colitis and Crohn's disease may be difficult (**Figure 36.45d**).

The symptoms and signs of colitis (malaise, abdominal distension, pain, diarrhoea) are usually present for several days prior to a severe deterioration. Diarrhoea may be bloody in inflammatory bowel disease and watery in *C. difficile* colitis. Patients have a septic appearance, with fever, tachycardia, hypotension and frequently changes in mental status. The abdomen is distended and tender with or without signs of peritoneal irritation. Imaging demonstrates dilatation of the colon to greater than 6 cm and variable degrees of bowel wall thickening.

Toxic megacolon is life-threatening and requires urgent medical and surgical intervention.

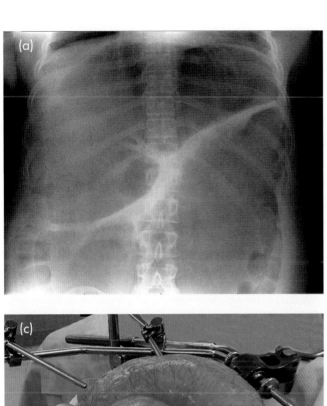

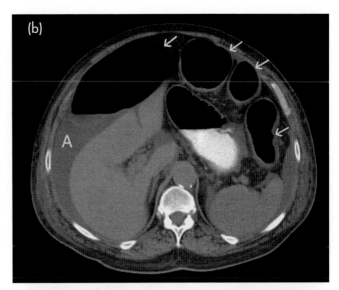

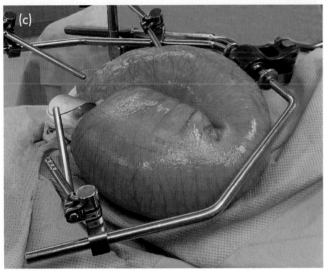

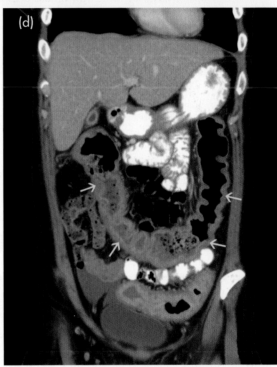

Figure 36.45 (a) Toxic megacolon in a patient with an ulcerative colitis and massive distension of the transverse colon. (b) Computed tomography demonstrating diffuse colonic wall thickening, distension (arrows) and ascites (A) in a patient with fulminant *Clostridium difficile* colitis. (c) Intraoperative photograph of megacolon in a patient with colonic inertia and chronic intractable symptoms of pseudo-obstruction. (d) Fulminant indeterminate colitis in a young patient. Note the non-specific diffuse colonic wall thickening (arrows) with no significant luminal distension.

## ACUTE ISCHAEMIC CONDITIONS

### Mesenteric Ischaemia

Acute mesenteric ischaemia is a life-threatening condition (**Figure 36.46a**). Acute mesenteric arterial occlusion develops due to thrombosis, embolism or vasoconstriction. A dislodged cardiac thrombus is the most common source of embolism and may travel to block the vulnerable segment of the superior mesenteric artery supplying most of the small bowel and proximal colon. Patients with an embolism frequently have a history of atrial fibrillation or recent myocardial infarction.

Patients with severe atherosclerosis of the visceral arteries usually first develop chronic mesenteric occlusion and intestinal angina. In some patients, severe post-prandial pain leads to the avoidance of food and substantial weight loss. Untreated arterial disease can lead to the acute thrombosis of a narrowed major vessel, resulting in an acute presentation.

Non-occlusive ischaemia develops as a result of visceral hypoperfusion and vasospasm in acutely ill patients with cardiac failure, shock and hypervolaemia (**Figure 36.46b**).

Patients complain of a sudden onset of central abdominal pain, initially intermittent but progressing to become extreme and constant. This is followed by vomiting and abdominal distension secondary to a dynamic obstruction of the ischaemic segment.

On examination, the patient looks unwell; some patients have early shock with tachycardia, hypotension and changes in mental status. Abdominal examination may initially be very unimpressive, with a soft but very tender mid-abdomen. The pain is classically 'out of proportion to the degree of abdominal tenderness' and may lead to a delay in diagnosis. Stools testing positive for occult blood or bloody diarrhoea may be present in some patients. When full-thickness gangrene is developing or bowel perforation occurs, signs of peritoneal irritation become manifest.

Mesenteric venous thrombosis occurs in patients with underlying inherited hypercoagulable states or portal hypertension, in women using oral contraception or as a result of intra-abdominal infection. The resistance to venous outflow and developing bowel oedema may lead to a diminished arterial flow. The symptoms are typically less acute than in patients with acute arterial occlusion. Although slower to progress, mesenteric venous occlusion may result in massive necrosis of the small bowel.

An increased lactic acid level, although not specific, and leukocytosis should increase the suspicion of mesenteric ischaemia. Plan radiographs may be unremarkable in the early stages. The presence of gas within the intestinal wall (pneumatosis intestinalis) is sometimes seen in a number of benign conditions. However, pneumatosis encountered in the setting of abdominal pain, leukocytosis or lactic acidosis indicates intestinal ischaemic changes and the breakdown of the mucosal barrier (**Figure 36.47**).

## Ischaemic Colitis

Ischaemic colitis develops secondary to a period of an inadequate flow via the colonic arteries. It is most commonly non-occlusive and occurs in patients with associated medical comorbidities or accompanies the acute illness. The splenic flexure and caecum have a decreased collateral network and hence a poor tolerance to hypoperfusion. Non-occlusive colonic ischaemia occurs during periods of global hypoperfusion: myocardial infarction, cardiopulmonary bypass, haemodialysis and shock. Occlusion of flow may occur with cholesterol emboli and mesenteric thrombosis.

Ischaemia of the left colon is a known complication of aortic surgery and is related to an interruption of the collateral flow. Underlying diabetes and atherosclerosis further predispose to the

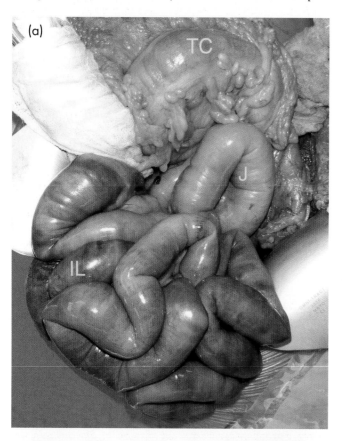

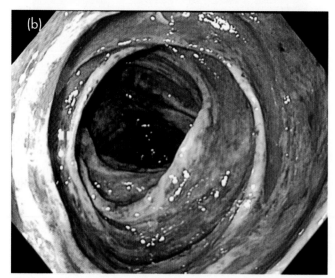

Figure 36.46 (a) Acute mesenteric ischaemia of the ileum (IL) and right colon secondary to arterial embolism in a patient with atrial fibrillation. Note the sparing of the proximal jejunum (J) and distal transverse colon (TC). (b) The endoscopic appearance of non-occlusive mesenteric ischaemia secondary to cardiogenic shock.

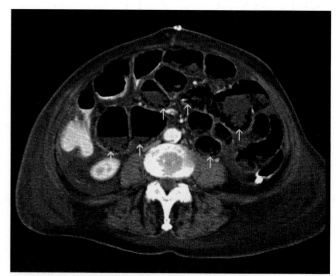

Figure 36.47 Computed tomography demonstrating a gas bubble within the dependent area of the intestinal wall (arrows), consistent with pneumatosis and seen throughout the small bowel secondary to acute mesenteric ischaemia.

poor ability of the vasculature to meet the metabolic demands of the colon. Ischaemic colitis may occur in healthy young individuals as a result of vasospasm due to extreme exercise or illicit drug use (cocaine, amphetamines).

Patients usually present with an acute onset of abdominal pain and anorexia. A small amount of bloody diarrhoea develops within the first day of onset of the pain. The abdominal pain is less severe than in a patient with small bowel ischaemia. Abdominal tenderness is located over the affected segment, usually lateral to the umbilicus.

Most patients recover within a few days with conservative management, normalization of the collateral flow and resolution of the precipitating event. Healing in more severe cases may result in obstructing strictures of the affected areas. In some cases (more commonly in the right colon), acute ischaemia progresses to full-thickness necrosis and subsequent perforation.

## PERITONITIS

Peritonitis is inflammation of the peritoneal cavity. The term implies the presence of a specific disease with various microscopic and macroscopic changes. It should be distinguished from the 'signs of peritoneal irritation', which are not always specific and sensitive, and may be equivocal or present in benign conditions. Peritonitis most commonly results from pathology of the adjacent organs (secondary), as described in the preceding sections, and is only rarely a primary disease.

Peritonitis is classified as infectious (bacterial, fungal, hydatid disease) or non-infectious. Depending on their chemical properties, the leak of sterile fluids (bile, gastric contents, blood, urine, pancreatic fluid, the contents of an ovarian dermoid cyst) into the peritoneal cavity results in inflammation and pain. Talc peritonitis from chemical irritation and fibrosis is now not seen as talc is no longer applied to surgical gloves. A retained foreign object may also lead to an aseptic irritation.

**Secondary bacterial peritonitis** is by far the most common type and usually results from spontaneous, traumatic or iatrogenic perforations of the gastrointestinal tract (the most common aetiologies are discussed individually in this chapter). The severity of the infection depends on the nature of the disease and on patient-related factors.

Depending on the extent of the contamination and the resulting infection, the peritonitis may be focal or diffuse. Contamination and infection stimulate an inflammatory response that in early stages results in fibrin deposition. The resulting adhesions of the greater omentum and adjacent organs, and adhesions from prior operations, may contain the area of spillage and seal the perforation. The greater omentum, 'the policeman of the abdomen', is not very prominent in children and is less efficient for this purpose.

The severity of the disease and its clinical manifestations also depend on the duration of the infection, the nature of the contaminants and the concentration and virulence of the organisms involved. Faecal peritonitis results in a major systemic inflammatory response due to high counts of gram-negative rods and anaerobes. Even initially sterile or nearly sterile peritonitis (bile, pancreatic, gastric) becomes secondarily infected as the time progresses. Spilled solid particles are more difficult for the peritoneal immune system to clear.

The ability to tolerate the acute disease is influenced by the patient's age, nutritional status, medical comorbidities and immune system function. Elderly and immunosuppressed patients are particularly prone to poor outcomes.

Most commonly, **primary peritonitis** results from haematogenous or lymphatic spread or intestinal bacterial translocation in patients with cirrhosis and pre-existing ascites (when it is called spontaneous bacterial peritonitis). Primary peritonitis (usually streptococcal) may also be seen in children with nephrotic syndrome. Tuberculous peritonitis may result from haematogenous spread and may develop in patients who do not have underlying portal hypertension. Tuberculous ascites in these patients develops secondary to the infection.

In women, the fallopian tubes may serve as an entry point for infection of the peritoneal cavity. The alkaline vaginal milieu in prepubertal girls may predispose to pneumococcal spread, and the resulting acute peritonitis may mimic appendicitis. Ascending gonococcal or chlamydial infections in adults result in perihepatitis (Fitz-Hugh–Curtis syndrome), which presents with right upper quadrant pain. Interestingly, in some patients the primary cervicitis and salpingitis may not be clinically prominent. Ascending transfallopian non-specific bacterial infection (pelvic inflammatory disease) may also occur in women using intrauterine devices.

The cardinal sign of peritonitis is somatic abdominal pain. The pain is constant and exacerbated by movement of the abdominal wall, such as in walking and coughing. Patients 'look sick' and tend to lie still to minimize the pain, which gains little relief from analgesics. In diffuse peritonitis, patients reduce the amplitude of their respiratory movements to limit the irritation.

A paralytic ileus invariably follows intra-abdominal infection and is proportional to its severity. Bowel sounds may be diminished and abdominal distension occurs. Signs of peritoneal irritation are present over the areas affected by the peritonitis. The manifestations of the systemic inflammatory response and organ failure progress along with the disease: fever, tachycardia, hypotension, oliguria and changes in mental status.

**Familial Mediterranean fever** is of particular interest. This is an autosomal recessive disorder occurring primarily in the descendants of ethnic groups who originated from the Mediterranean region. The disease manifests by recurrent attacks of fever and inflammation of the serosal surfaces. The first attack occurs in childhood in most patients, and by the end of the teenage years in almost all patients. The frequency of attacks varies from patient to patient, and they typically have no consistent trigger point.

Almost all patients present with abdominal pain and signs of peritoneal irritation, which is the cardinal manifestation of this disease. Some patients develop pleuritis, arthritis and an erysipelas-like erythema of the lower extremities. The symptoms begin with fever, which peaks within 12 hours and resolves without sequelae in 24–48 hours. The signs of an acute abdomen are so convincing that previously undiagnosed patients may be submitted to laparotomy.

## ABDOMINAL AORTIC EMERGENCIES

An abdominal aortic aneurysm (dilatation of the aorta) is associated with atherosclerosis and abnormalities of collagen and elastin metabolism. Aneurysms usually occur in middle-aged men and are commonly asymptomatic. When the aortic diameter reaches 6 cm, the risk of rupture is approximately 20 per cent per year. Acute rupture of the aneurysm results in life-threatening bleeding and is a common cause of sudden death in this population. In two-thirds of patients, acute rupture is the first manifestation of the disease. When an aneurysm is encountered on routine examination as a pulsatile mass or found incidentally on imaging or through screening, it is best repaired electively if it is greater than 6 cm in diameter.

The classic presentation occurs in only half of all patients and consists of severe pain, hypotension and a pulsatile abdominal mass. Some patients complain of nausea. Most have some degree of abdominal distension and a feeling of fainting. Abdominal tenderness is present in most, and 60 per cent of patients have a pulsatile mass in the epigastrium.

The haemodynamic conditions depend on the degree of blood loss the patient has suffered. Most commonly, free rupture occurs into the peritoneal cavity with the rapid development of profound shock. In cases of retroperitoneal rupture, tamponade may occur and hypotension may develop more slowly (Figure 36.48a). Flank, back and groin pain in such cases may initially mimic renal colic and other benign conditions. The term 'symptomatic aneurysm' refers to pain related to expansion of the aneurysm with no evidence from imaging of bleeding on rupture. Such pain and tenderness implies impending rupture and should be promptly addressed.

Aneurysms of the splanchnic arteries (splenic, hepatic, superior mesenteric) are uncommon and are related to atherosclerosis. They are small, non-palpable and generally asymptomatic unless rupture occurs. Patients with rupture present with acute abdominal pain and intra-abdominal bleeding. Splenic artery aneurysms are associated with pregnancy or atherosclerosis (Figure 36.48b).

An acute dissection of the aorta is strongly associated with systemic hypertension. The blood flow dissects a false lumen within the layers of the aortic wall through an intimal tear; this may result in hypoperfusion of its branches with myocardial, cerebral, spinal, limb or visceral ischaemia (Figure 36.48c). Dissection most commonly occurs in the ascending thoracic aorta, presents with excruciating chest and back pain and leads to acute aortic valve insufficiency, occlusion of the coronary arteries or cardiac tamponade. Dissection of the descending aorta may extend into the abdomen, producing back and abdominal pain.

After assessing the vital signs and degree of shock, perform a complete vascular examination. Assess the carotid, brachial, radial, femoral, popliteal and pedal pulses for their presence and symmetry, and note the findings for subsequent comparison. If the pulses are faint due to hypotension or peripheral vascular disease, a hand-held Doppler probe should be used to assess them.

## THE ACUTE ABDOMEN IN WOMEN

Pathology of the internal organs of reproduction is a common cause of abdominal pain in women. A careful history and pelvic examination are essential. Many of these conditions may be treated non-operatively, and an accurate diagnosis may require confirmatory tests. Ultrasonographic examination of the pelvic organs, either transvaginally or transabdominally, is an invaluable tool. Computed tomography should be used only judiciously, since it is associated with significant radiation exposure and other risks.

Some women with certain psychological and social circumstances may not report an accurate sexual history or simply may not be aware of a recent conception. Thus, a pregnancy test is mandatory for women of childbearing age with abdominal pain.

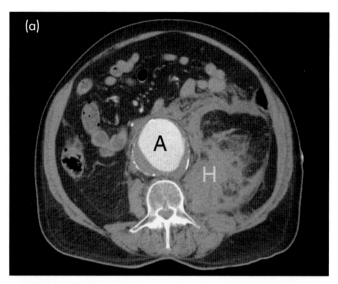

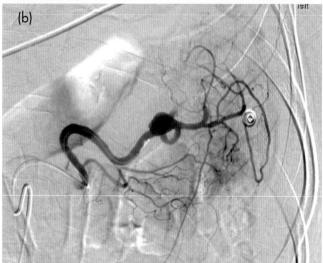

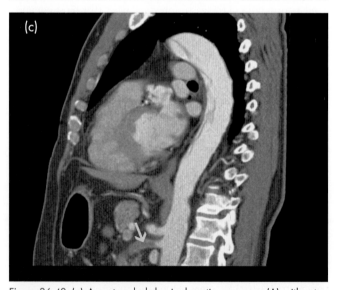

Figure 36.48 (a) A ruptured abdominal aortic aneurysm (A) with retroperitoneal haematoma (H). (b) A symptomatic splenic artery aneurysm in an elderly patient. (c) An ascending aortic dissection (hollow arrow) extending into the abdominal aorta, with complete occlusion of the superior mesenteric artery by thrombus (arrow).

# Ectopic Pregnancy

Implantation of the blastocyst outside the uterus occurs in up to 2 per cent of all pregnancies. Around 95 per cent of all ectopic implantations occur in the segments of the fallopian tube, and the rest may be found in the ovary, peritoneal cavity and cervix. The major risk factors for this condition are a previous ectopic pregnancy, tubal pathology and pelvic surgery. Among other factors are previous genital infections, infertility, assisted reproductive technologies, the use of the intrauterine devices and smoking.

After ectopic implantation, the fertilized ovum initially develops normally, with typical physiology-related symptoms and signs of early pregnancy: morning sickness, breast tenderness and urinary frequency. Amenorrhoea is the cardinal sign of pregnancy and, along with some vaginal spotting or bleeding, is present in the majority of tubal pregnancies. Some patients may not suspect that they are pregnant and may mistake the bleeding for a true menstrual period; in retrospect, however, such bleeding is seen to be different from the normal menses. This bleeding is related to the pathophysiology of ectopic implantation and results from the breakdown of thickened uterine endometrium. Profuse vaginal bleeding is uncommon and generally suggests an incomplete abortion.

Current serum and urine tests for beta-human chorionic gonadotropin are invaluable tools and are positive in 99 per cent of ectopic pregnancies. The tubal pregnancy resolves in two ways: abortion or rupture.

**Tubal abortion** is common in ampullary pregnancy and has a benign course. Placental separation leads to the extrusion of all or parts of the products of conception into the peritoneal cavity. Some blood may accumulate in the cul-de-sac (rectouterine pouch). This manifests with intermittent lower abdominal pain and tenderness of moderate severity that is usually localized to the side of the affected fallopian tube. After all the tubal products have been either extruded or resorbed, the hormone levels return to baseline and the vaginal bleeding stops.

**Tubal rupture** results once the size of the growing trophoblast exceeds the elastic capacity of the lumen where implantation has occurred. It usually occurs spontaneously in the first few weeks, or may follow coitus or pelvic examination. The resulting intra-abdominal bleeding may be life-threatening. There is a development of vasomotor symptoms ranging from feeling faint to occasionally actual syncope. The patient complains of severe sharp or stabbing pain from the blood irritating the peritoneum, which is exacerbated by coughing and movement. Blood in the pelvis produces lower abdominal pain. It may be referred to the rectum, known as a 'toilet sign'. Extensive intra-abdominal bleeding results in diffuse abdominal pain. In the supine position, referred pain from diaphragmatic irritation may cause neck and shoulder pain.

Since these patients are typically young and have good compensatory mechanisms, the pulse and blood pressure may initially be normal even with significant blood loss. Sinus tachycardia and hypotension are the disturbing signs of impending decompensation.

On examination, some abdominal distension may be present. The location of the tenderness is determined by the site of the intraperitoneal blood. Pelvic examination is very uncomfortable, especially with cervical movement. The posterior vaginal fornix may bulge as blood accumulates in the cul-de-sac. A tender boggy mass may be palpable in the area of the involved fallopian tube. Since pelvic examination may exacerbate the bleeding, it should be performed with great care and only by an experienced clinician.

# Pelvic Inflammatory Disease

Pelvic inflammatory disease (PID) describes an acute infection of the uterus, fallopian tubes or ovaries. Extension of the infection may result in peritonitis, perihepatitis and tubo-ovarian abscess. The infection is most often due to sexually transmitted disease, but may also develop as a post-operative or pregnancy-related pelvic infection. *Neisseria gonorrhoeae*, *Chlamydia trachomatis* and normal vaginal flora have been implicated. Infection may also be subclinical or recurrent.

The main symptom is lower abdominal pain of variable severity. The pain, usually bilateral, may initially be mild and progress to being more severe and constant over time. The pain frequently begins after the menstrual period and is aggravated by sexual intercourse and shaking movements. Abnormal uterine bleeding, new vaginal discharge and fever may be associated symptoms.

On physical examination, the lower abdomen is tender, with frequent signs of peritoneal irritation. Right upper quadrant tenderness indicates the presence of perihepatitis. The presence of a purulent cervical discharge, cervical motion tenderness in all directions and adnexal tenderness are the characteristics of PID. A significant lateralization of the tenderness on pelvic examination is uncommon, unlike in appendicitis or diverticulitis. A palpable adnexal mass may represent a tubo-ovarian abscess or other pathology.

# Ovarian Cysts

Ovarian cystic lesions are classified as physiological (follicular and corpus luteum cysts) or pathological – benign, borderline or malignant ovarian tumours. Most cysts are physiological, small and asymptomatic. The complications of ovarian cysts – rupture, bleeding and ovarian torsion – result in acute abdominal pain (see Figure 36.20b). These acute conditions commonly develop during strenuous physical activity or sexual intercourse.

Torsion is twisting of the ovary on its ligaments and vascular pedicle. It presents with non-specific symptoms of an acute onset of sharp, intermittent abdominal pain, frequently associated with nausea and vomiting. The pain may radiate to the back, flank and groins. Fever is uncommon and usually signifies necrosis of the ovary. Signs of peritoneal irritation are rare. A unilateral palpable adnexal mass is detectable on pelvic examination in many patients. Prompt recognition and surgery is necessary to prevent loss of the ovary and the risk to future fertility.

Rupture of an ovarian cyst presents with sudden, severe, unilateral pelvic pain and is not associated with fever or vaginal, gastrointestinal or urinary symptoms. Typically, the rupture precedes the menstrual period. Pain develops via two mechanisms. The bleeding into ovarian tissue may stretch the ovary and cause visceral pain. Bleeding into the abdomen is usually not significant but may produce signs of peritoneal irritation and mimic the signs of an ectopic pregnancy. Serous and mucinous cyst fluid is not very irritating to the peritoneal cavity. In the absence of haemorrhage, it is usually rapidly absorbed and the pain resolves within a few days. Rupture of dermoid cysts are uncommon, but their contents cause chemical peritonitis and significant pain.

Enlargement and rupture of a luteal follicle to release an ovum into the peritoneal cavity occurs in the middle of a normal menstrual cycle. The resulting mid-cycle pain in some women, known as **Mittelschmerz**, is typically unilateral and mild, lasting from a few hours to a few days.

## ABDOMINAL TRAUMA

The abdomen accounts for a large part of the human body surface and is subjected to both penetrating and blunt trauma. The peritoneal cavity extends from the diaphragm to the pelvic floor, the external landmarks being the nipple line anteriorly, the scapular tip posteriorly and the inguinal creases inferiorly. The main results of trauma to various abdominal organs are intra-abdominal bleeding, contamination (faeculent, pancreatobiliary, urinary), disruption of the anatomy (wounds, traumatic ventral and diaphragmatic hernias) and combinations of these.

Blunt abdominal trauma commonly results from motor vehicle accidents. Falls and incidental and direct violence-related impacts account for the rest of the injuries. Powerful blunt forces against the abdominal wall (a seatbelt or foreign object) may crush the organs against the spine and thoracic cage. The 'seatbelt sign' and significant soft tissue trauma are almost always associated with significant underlying injuries to the intra-abdominal organs (**Figure 36.49**). Such abdominal injuries are frequently associated with spine, rib and pelvic fractures.

Sudden deceleration during a high-speed impact creates shearing forces that may result in the laceration and avulsion of both hollow and solid organs from their vascular and ligamentous attachments. A sudden significant rise in intra-abdominal pressure may lead to the rupture of a distended hollow viscus (diaphragm, stomach, bladder). Pre-existing diseases (splenomegaly, cirrhosis, abnormal points of fixation due to postoperative adhesions) may make the intra-abdominal organs more susceptible to injury.

The extent and severity of penetrating injuries from gunshot, stab and impalement wounds vary dramatically depending on the ballistics, trajectory and other characteristics of the traumatizing agent. Surgical repair of the intra-abdominal injuries is required in most cases of gunshot but in only a third of stab wounds.

Injuries to the major abdominal vessels produce massive haemorrhage and are frequently fatal at the scene.

Liver and spleen injuries are common in both blunt and penetrating trauma and may result in various degrees of free intra-abdominal or intraparenchymal bleeding (**Figure 36.50**). Delayed complications are also common. The life-threatening rupture of a subcapsular haematoma of the spleen may sometimes be delayed – even until after the patient's discharge from hospital and seemingly successful non-surgical management. Lacerations of the liver may result in bilious peritonitis several days after the initial trauma. Upper gastrointestinal bleeding presents several weeks after the trauma and is sometimes accompanied by right upper quadrant pain. Jaundice is the result of haemobilia secondary to a traumatic arteriobiliary fistula.

The pancreas and duodenum are highly vascular retroperitoneal structures. Both penetrating and blunt injuries to them produce devastating complications. Blunt injuries may initially produce few abdominal symptoms given the retroperitoneal location of these organs. Pancreatic trauma may result in acute pancreatitis or the delayed development of fistulas and pseudocysts. A child hitting their upper abdomen against a bicycle handlebar is the classic example of pancreaticoduodenal injuries

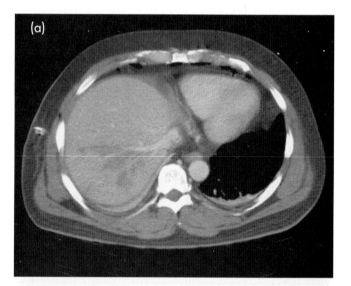

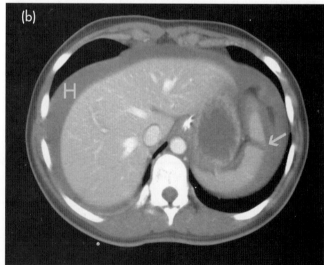

Figure 36.50 (a) Laceration of the liver. (b) Laceration of the spleen (arrow) with haemoperitoneum (H).

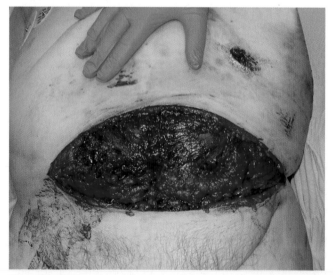

Figure 36.49 Extensive abdominal wall laceration, bruising and abrasions in the victim of a farming accident.

resulting from the compression of these organs against the spine. A duodenal wall haematoma does not produce spillage of the enteric material but may produce symptoms of gastric outlet obstruction (**Figure 36.51**).

The stomach and small and large intestines occupy a significant part of the abdominal cavity. Injury to them occurs more commonly in penetrating trauma and generally results in peritonitis. Blunt trauma (deceleration mechanisms, seatbelt compression) results in rupture, bleeding and ischaemia from mesenteric avulsions and haematomas. Some blunt intestinal injuries may be difficult to diagnose accurately in acute situations without surgery, and require imaging (**Figure 36.52**) and close observation for the development of signs of peritoneal irritation. Significantly damaged or devascularized segments may lead to delayed perforation.

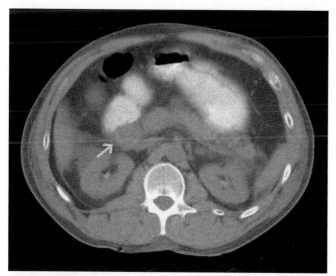

Figure 36.51 A duodenal haematoma (arrow) causing obstruction in a 12-year-old boy after a bicycle handle bar impact.

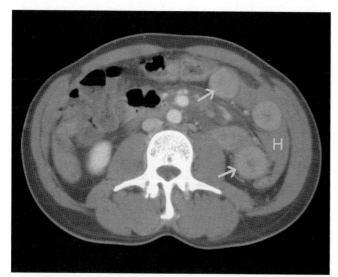

Figure 36.52 Computed tomography scan of mesenteric avulsion with small bowel devascularization in a victim of blunt trauma. Bowel wall thickening (arrows) and haemoperitoneum (H) in the absence of a solid organ injury are consistent with an intestinal injury.

Diaphragmatic injuries may produce acute or chronic herniation of intra-abdominal organs into the chest. They are frequently associated with other injuries. The symptoms depend on the size of the defect and are more common on the left side. Decreased breath sounds, elevation of the hemidiaphragm and the presence of bowel gas in the chest on radiography are diagnostic (**Figure 36.53**).

Most genitourinary injuries occur secondary to blunt trauma, except for ureteral injuries, which are mainly caused by gunshot wounds. Haematuria is the cardinal marker of urinary tract trauma. When it is present, appropriate imaging is needed to determine the level of injury. Bladder and urethral lacerations are frequently associated with pelvic fractures. Urine is very irritating to the peritoneum, and intraperitoneal bladder rupture produces symptoms of peritonitis.

Knowing all the circumstances of the traumatic event is very important to understand its pathophysiological mechanisms and predict the patterns of injury. Many patients, however, have an altered mental status from brain injury, respiratory insufficiency and intoxication, and may not be able to provide details of the trauma. Child abuse and domestic violence need to be ruled out in some cases of abdominal injuries presenting with unclear or unexplainable details of an accident.

Multiple factors, including the patient's agitation, dramatic external deformities and bleeding may distract the attention of the clinician from their priorities in the management of trauma victims. The evaluation of all trauma patients should follow the standard algorithm of primary and secondary surveys (advanced trauma life support) with appropriate immediate interventions when life-threatening abnormalities are encountered:

- **A – Airway.** Assess the patency of the airway and rule out obstruction (troubled speech, stridor).
- **B – Breathing.** Assess the respiratory rate and pattern. Palpate the neck to rule out tracheal deviation. Percuss and

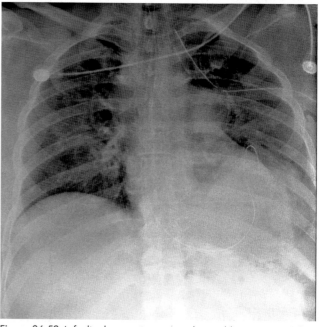

Figure 36.53 Left diaphragmatic rupture due to blunt trauma with a diagnostic elevation of the hemidiaphragm and intrathoracic location of the nasogastric tube for the chest radiography.

PART 8 | ABDOMINAL

auscultate the chest bilaterally to rule out haemothorax and pneumothorax.

- **C – Circulation**. Assess the heart rate, blood pressure and skin colour. Control external sources of bleeding.
- **D – Disability**. Perform a brief neurological examination.

Electrocardiography, blood tests, urinary and gastric catheters, radiographs of the chest and pelvis, and abdominal ultrasonography are adjuncts to the primary survey. Only intra-abdominal bleeding is immediately life-threatening. The presence and degree of the haemorrhagic shock depends on the percentage of blood volume lost:

- *Class I* haemorrhage (up to 15 per cent). This may be associated with an increased pulse pressure but otherwise few symptoms. This is equivalent to the donation of a unit of blood.
- *Class II* (uncomplicated) haemorrhage (15–30 per cent). This leads to an increase in heart rate to above 100 beats per minute and a fall in pulse pressure; orthostatic hypotension may also be noted. Patients may be diaphoretic (show increased sweating) and restless.
- *Class III* (complicated) haemorrhage (30–40 per cent). A progressive tachycardia of greater than 120 beats per minute is now accompanied by supine hypotension. The resulting organ malperfusion manifests with diminished urine output and a decline in mental status. The skin is cool and clammy secondary to peripheral compensatory vasoconstriction.
- *Class IV* haemorrhage (>40 per cent). The tachycardia exceeds 140 beats per minute, profound hypotension is associated with a progression of organ failure, and the condition is immediately life-threatening.

During the secondary survey, the patient is examined from head to toe and their past medical history obtained. Specific attention should be paid to open wounds, bruising, abrasions and deformities of the extremities. Entry and exit points of gunshot wounds are noted to establish an approximate trajectory. The abdomen is assessed for distention, which may be due to a large amount of blood or simply from ileus. Over 1500 mL of blood is required to produce shifting dullness.

Acute gastric dilatation may develop rapidly after trauma, produce significant abdominal distension, especially in children, and impede the examination. This is easily corrected using a gastric tube. The abdomen is evaluated for signs of peritoneal irritation, which may be difficult to evaluate in unconscious patients. Digital rectal examination is indicated to evaluate the presence of blood (although a negative result does not rule out bowel injury) and the position of the prostate, as well as to assess the function of the external anal sphincter in spinal cord trauma.

The main question the clinician needs to answer promptly after assuring a patent airway and adequate ventilation is 'Is the patient actively bleeding?' Frequently, especially with a blunt mechanism, the abdominal trauma is a part of a set of combined multisystem injuries. The haemorrhage from the abdominal injuries should be differentiated from cardiogenic and neurogenic shock and bleeding from other sources (intrathoracic, extremities).

Focused assessment with sonography for trauma (FAST) is a quick, fairly sensitive, non-invasive method to assess the presence of over 300 mL of free intra-abdominal fluid. Four windows are evaluated: pericardial, right and left upper quadrant and pelvis (**Figure 36.54**). In the vast majority of cases, it has replaced diagnostic peritoneal lavage and pericardiocentesis. Ultrasonography

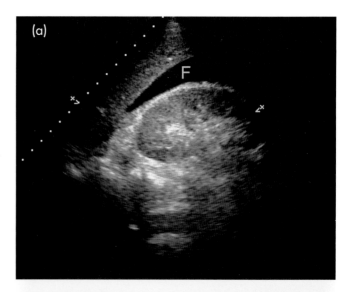

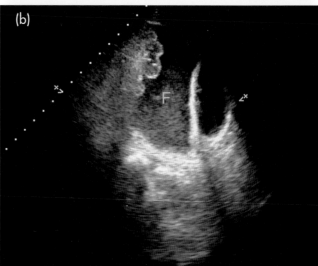

Figure 36.54 Focused assessment with sonography for trauma. (a) Right upper quadrant window positive for fluid (F) between the liver and right kidney. (b) Pelvic window positive for fluid (F) in the rectovesical space. Note the contour of the intestinal loops.

cannot, however, distinguish between blood, urine and ascites. An unstable patient with abdominal trauma and a positive FAST scan is assumed to be bleeding into the abdomen and requires emergency surgery. Advanced imaging, specifically CT scanning, should only be performed on patients with stable vital signs.

## MEDICAL CAUSES OF ACUTE ABDOMINAL PAIN

There are a number of 'medical' ('non-surgical') causes of abdominal pain that can mimic the 'surgical abdomen'. The correct diagnosis can mostly be made with a detailed history and examination. In addition, the clinician must always remember that surgical conditions may occur in a patient with medical disease. If the patient's condition changes, always consider an initial misdiagnosis or the possibility of a surgical complication developing. The cardinal signs of a surgical abdomen are the presence of rebound tenderness and involuntary guarding; these are absent in the conditions described below.

## Ischaemic Heart Disease

Ischaemic heart disease manifests with chest pain that is commonly associated with exercise or stress. The pain is usually described as a tightness, pressure or burning, and or as heartburn, frequently described as central and located behind the sternum. Sharp, stabbing pain, localized to a small area and exacerbated by palpation, movement or swallowing is atypical of a cardiac aetiology.

Cardiac pain is sometimes reported in the C7–T4 dermatomes, typically the epigastrium, shoulders, arms and forearms (often the inner left forearm), neck and lower jaw, and rarely in between the scapulas. Such referred pain is usually described as a diffuse discomfort rather than a focal site. Referred epigastric pain associated with nausea occasionally simulates a peptic ulcer, cholecystitis or pancreatitis. Biliary colic can easily be confused with cardiac pain. An ECG and levels of cardiac enzymes will help in making the correct diagnosis.

## Pleural Inflammation

Pleuritic chest pain is caused by irritation of the nerve endings supplying the parietal pleura. It is often described as stabbing and exacerbated by inspiration, coughing and palpation. Underlying viral and bacterial infections, pleural effusion, pneumothorax and autoimmune conditions (systemic lupus erythematosus, rheumatoid arthritis) may produce pleuritic pain. These conditions are typically accompanied by a cough and dyspnoea.

The lower intercostal nerves supply the abdominal wall, and pleuritic pain may be felt in the abdomen. The classic scenario is right lower lobe pneumonia with an effusion mimicking acute cholecystitis or appendicitis. Auscultation, percussion and palpation of the chest and abdomen, in addition to chest radiography, clarify the aetiology.

## Neurogenic and Musculoskeletal Pain

Radiculopathy of the spinal nerves may be caused by degenerative disease of the spine, injuries, tumours and abscesses. Such nerve root irritations may mimic pain originating within the abdomen. Tenderness may be elicited by paraspinal or intercostal, rather than abdominal, palpation.

A reactivation of latent varicella-zoster virus within the sensory dorsal root ganglia may occur years after the initial infection and results in herpes zoster, or shingles. Herpes zoster manifests with a painful, unilateral vesicular eruptions localized to the area of the affected thoracic or lumbar dermatomes. Acute neuritis with a burning and throbbing pain, and the characteristic hyperaesthesia, may precede the onset of the rash by days or weeks, and may simulate intra-abdominal disease.

Pain related to costochondritis may be confused with upper abdominal pain and may be differentiated by superficial palpation of the costal margins. Acute muscle strain from vigorous physical activity in fit individuals or chronic strain from increased intra-abdominal pressure in obese patients may also present with abdominal pain.

## Diabetic Ketoacidosis

Nearly half of all patients presenting in diabetic ketoacidosis have nausea, vomiting and abdominal pain. The presence of pain is more likely the more severe the acidosis is. Possible aetiologies of the pain include delayed gastric emptying and ileus. The pain typically resolves with resolution of the ketoacidosis, and if the pain persists an additional work-up is needed.

## Lead Colic

The incidence of lead poisoning is decreasing due to the monitoring of work environments and the use of lead-free paints in construction. Chronic exposure leads to cognitive impairments in both adults and children and, with high doses, death.

Acute lead intoxication presents with headache, muscle aches, arthralgias, anorexia and peripheral neuropathy (extensor weakness being common). Colicky abdominal pain (lead colic) and constipation may simulate an acute abdomen. The thin bluish pigmentation ('lead line') along the margin between the gums and the teeth margin may be present in some patients.

## Porphyria

The porphyrias are a group of congenital metabolic disorders of haemoglobin metabolism. Cutaneous porphyrias present with photosensitivity and chronic blistering lesions on sun-exposed areas of skin.

Acute porphyrias (specifically acute intermittent porphyria) present with acute intermittent attacks of non-specific neurovisceral symptoms and no cutaneous manifestations. The usual patient is a young woman. The attacks may be precipitated by smoking, ingestion of alcohol, oestrogens, antiseizure medications or sulphonamides. The neurological symptoms include sensory and motor neuropathy, delirium and seizures.

Persistent diffuse abdominal pain is the most common presenting symptom during acute attacks and is usually associated with ileus and abdominal distension. The attacks may be accompanied by urinary retention or incontinence. Signs of systemic inflammation are minimal. Biochemical urinary tests are diagnostic. Remarkably, the voided urine is of normal colour but turns the colour of red wine after several hours of exposure to light.

## Sickle Cell Disease

Sickle cell disease is a hereditary disorder resulting in an abnormal haemoglobin structure (haemoglobin S). The manifestation and severity of the disease depend on the genotype and on the coexistence of thalassaemia. The disease is most severe in homozygote patients (sickle cell anaemia). The heterozygote condition (sickle cell trait) is associated with milder clinical symptoms and provides some protection against severe malaria infection. This explains the origin and high prevalence of this genetic mutation in Mediterranean, African and Middle Eastern countries. Sickle cell trait is present in 10 per cent of the African-American population.

Abnormal haemoglobin is prone to polymerization on deoxygenation, which causes the red blood cells to lose the normal shape and pliability that are necessary for their normal flow through small vessels. Membrane damage eventually leads to haemolytic anaemia. Chronic haemolytic anaemia produces jaundice, calcium bilirubinate gallstones, splenomegaly and poorly healing pretibial ulcers. The result of the impaired blood flow and complex pathophysiology is vaso-occlusion. This causes recurrent episodes of acute ischaemic pain (sickle cell crises) and leads to a variety of systemic complications and organ failures.

The form of the disease determines the frequency of the episodes, which is approximately once per year. Acute painful episodes, lasting hours to days, may be precipitated by stress, infection, dehydration, the onset of menses, weather fluctuations, smoking or alcohol consumption. Many of the attacks have no definitive cause and are not associated with increased haemolysis.

Patients present with bone and joint pain affecting the back, extremities, chest and head. Acute vascular occlusion may cause strokes and priapism. Severe abdominal pain may be part of an acute crisis or a resulting abdominal complication. The mesenteric vessels may be affected, and ischaemic pain mimics an acute surgical abdomen. Right upper quadrant pain may result from vascular occlusions in the liver or symptomatic pigmented gallstones. An initial splenomegaly in childhood, with repeated splenic infarctions, evolves into autosplenectomy.

## Henoch–Schönlein Purpura

Henoch–Schönlein purpura is an uncommon self-limiting condition associated with IgA immune complexes. It is the most common form of systemic vasculitis in children. The disease is more common in boys, and in half of all cases is preceded by an upper respiratory infection. All patients have purpura, most have arthritis and approximately half have glomerulonephritis and abdominal pain.

The manifestations evolve over a period of days to weeks, usually beginning with development of the diagnostic palpable lower extremity and buttock purpura, or large joint arthritis without effusion. Within a week, this may be followed by gastrointestinal symptoms.

The presentation may vary, with a quarter of patients initially presenting with colicky abdominal pain, nausea, vomiting and frequently bloody stools. The abdominal pain may be very severe, simulating an acute abdomen; however, the pain is often incompatible with the examination findings and is diffuse rather than localized, and signs of peritoneal irritation are generally uncommon. In addition, mucosal oedema and haemorrhage may serve as a lead point and result in small bowel intussusception in some of these patients.

## Malaria

Malaria is a tropical disease caused by *Plasmodium* spp. and transmitted via a mosquito bite. Millions of people living and visiting endemic areas are affected annually, and this diagnosis should be suspected in exposed individuals presenting with a febrile illness. The acute illness manifests with fever, chills, arthralgias and myalgias, vomiting, abdominal pain and diarrhoea. The infected red cells undergo haemolysis or splenic clearance. Splenomegaly may develop after several days of illness in non-immune individuals and may be chronic in individuals living in endemic areas.

## Somatization

Somatization is a broad term used to describe conditions in which a patient's symptoms cannot be reasonably explained after an appropriate work-up and investigations. These conditions are a major public health problem and are associated with variable degrees of psychiatric and social impairment. Conditions are classified in relation to whether the symptoms are produced intentionally and what the individual's motivation is. In a variety of somatoform disorders (pain disorder, hypochondriasis and others), patients do not produce their symptoms consciously or intentionally.

Factitious disorder and malingering should always be considered when patients' complains are not consistent with the findings of a thorough evaluation. However, never ignore any symptoms and risk the well-being of patients presenting with an uncommon manifestation of an unsuspected disease.

Patients demonstrating **malingering** consciously simulate symptoms of illness for the reason of an external incentive: financial gain or the avoidance of criminal prosecution, for example. Malingering is not a mental illness.

In **factitious disorders**, patients also produce symptoms and signs intentionally, but with an unconscious motivation and no objective or response to external incentives. They want to assume a sick role and be a patient. These individuals frequently have some medical knowledge and present with non-healing wounds, self-induced infections, hypoglycaemia, bleeding, gastrointestinal disorders and various other problems.

**Munchausen's syndrome** is an extreme form of a factitious disorder. Such patients persistently submit themselves to surgery and invasive procedures for the condition they simulate. Surgeons most commonly face patients simulating an acute abdomen or bleeding, or manipulating for treatment using the presence of foreign bodies. Such behaviour causes direct bodily harm and also exposes these individuals to the risk of iatrogenic complications. Patients may have previous scars and a long convoluted history of medical care in various institutions. They may be very hostile and even threaten litigation.

The patients present 'the disease' very convincingly and may be very knowledgeable of medical symptoms, terminology and even appropriate management. Careful interviewing, however, reveals some inconsistencies and gaps. Patients may be unwilling to allow contact with family members or previously seen physicians. Examination may be difficult due to the skilled faking of signs of peritoneal irritation. Vital signs, close observation and laboratory tests may help to reveal the discrepancies. All kinds of foreign bodies may be encountered in the gastrointestinal tract or abdominal cavity (**Figure 36.55**).

A very dangerous situation is a **Munchausen's syndrome by proxy**, when a parent exposes a child to unnecessary treatment for a falsified paediatric illness.

### Key Points

- A thorough history and physical examination of the patient are of paramount importance in making the correct diagnosis.
- Imaging (radiography, CT scanning) and laboratory tests are ancillary studies and do **not** replace a careful physical diagnosis.
- The prompt diagnosis of an acute surgical abdomen and the recognition and correction of physiological derangements will save lives.
- The evaluation of any trauma patient should follow the standard ABCD (Airway–Breathing–Circulation–Disability) sequence of advanced trauma life support.

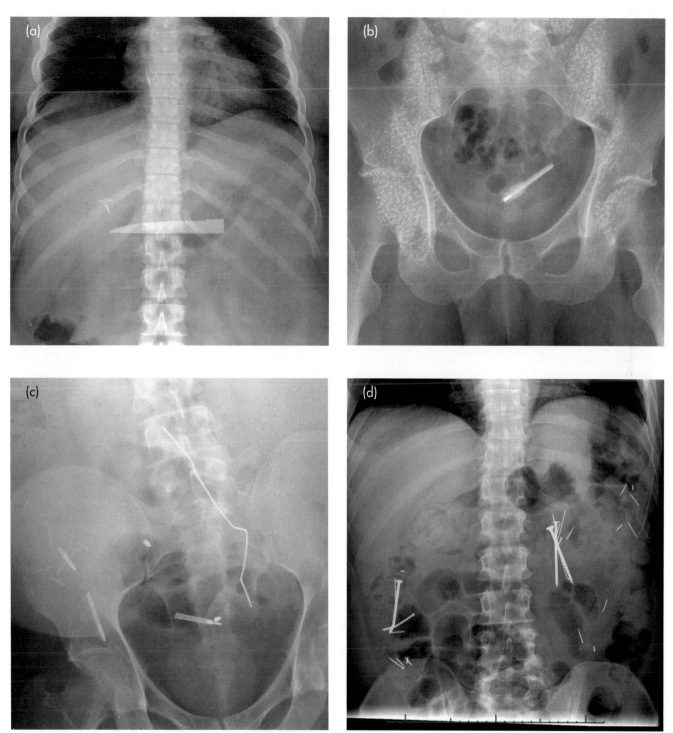

Figure 36.55 (a) A swallowed knife blade located within the stomach. (b) A thermometer introduced into the urinary bladder. (c) Metal wire and other objects introduced into the peritoneal cavity through the fresh laparotomy incision performed for complications of foreign body ingestion. (d) Multiple ingested foreign bodies.

## SBAs

**1. Which statement is not true about colonic obstruction?:**

  **a** Mechanical colonic obstruction can be an emergency surgical condition

  **b** Caecal and sigmoid volvulus may have a similar radiographic appearance

  **c** Colon obstruction is effectively a 'closed loop' obstruction

  **d** Ogilvie's syndrome is caused by intraluminal obstruction

  **e** Adhesions are not the leading cause of large bowel obstruction

**Answer**

**d** *Ogilvie's syndrome is caused by intraluminal obstruction. Acute colonic pseudo-obstruction (Ogilvie's syndrome) is a paralytic dilatation of the colon (usually proximal to the descending colon) that occurs without mechanical obstruction and is associated with a transient loss of normal motility (as a result of severe primary illness, surgery or trauma).*

*Any intestinal obstruction should be approached from the position of whether bowel ischaemia is present or threatened. A threatened blood supply to the bowel is an emergency surgical condition.*

*Due to the competence of the ileocaecal valve (a 'closed loop' mechanism) and the presence of a blood supply with a relatively limited reserve, the colon, even more so than the small bowel, is prone to overdistension, ischaemia and perforation.*

*While the overdistended, bean-shaped loop seen in caecal volvulus characteristically points towards the left upper quadrant, and the one of sigmoid volvulus towards the right upper quadrant, their differentiation may be difficult based on physical examination and plain radiographs alone.*

*Carcinoma is the leading cause of large bowel obstruction. Unlike with small bowel obstruction, post-operative adhesions are a very rare cause of colonic obstruction.*

**2. Which of the following statements is true?:**

  **a** All patients with acute appendicitis have a typical presentation

  **b** In patient with acute appendicitis, the signs and symptoms of peritoneal irritation typically develop within 48–72 hours after the onset of the abdominal pain

  **c** Acute sigmoid diverticulitis causes pain only in the left lower quadrant

  **d** The differential diagnosis of abdominal pain is wider in females

  **e** An acute flare of Crohn's disease can be easily distinguished from acute appendicitis

**Answer**

**d** *The differential diagnosis of abdominal pain is wider in females. Pathology of the internal reproductive organs should always be on the list of differential diagnoses in females with abdominal pain regardless of their age. The 'classic' symptoms and signs of acute appendicitis (nausea followed by abdominal pain, migration of the pain from the epigastrium to the right lower quadrant, and fever) may not be present in many patients with acute appendicitis. The signs and symptoms of acute appendicitis may also vary depending on the anatomical position of the appendix, the patient's age and immune status, and pregnancy. Right lower quadrant guarding and rebound tenderness usually develop within the first day of onset of the symptoms.*

*Acute diverticulitis predominantly affects the sigmoid colon. The sigmoid colon is located in the left lower abdomen and its inflammation typically produces the symptoms and signs of 'left-sided appendicitis'. The sigmoid colon may, however, loop to the right side and the diverticulitis may then mimic acute appendicitis. Acute perforation of the sigmoid colon may cause generalized peritonitis and diffuse abdominal pain.*

An exacerbation of inflammatory bowel disease, gynaecological and urological conditions, and a variety of other conditions causing an acute abdomen may mimic acute appendicitis and may demand observation, additional testing and imaging to make a correct diagnosis.

---

**3.** Which of the following statements is true?
  **a** In the trauma patient presenting with low blood pressure, a diagnosis of intra-abdominal bleeding should be the first priority
  **b** Intra-abdominal bleeding after blunt trauma most commonly originates from lacerated mesenteric vessels
  **c** The presence of the seatbelt sign is worrying in terms of underlying pelvic fracture
  **d** Associated injuries are uncommon in patients with blunt trauma to the abdomen
  **e** The presence of bowel gas and the projection of a gastric tube to within the chest on plain radiographs is characteristic of a diaphragmatic rupture

**Answer**

**e** *The presence of bowel gas and the projection of a gastric tube to within the chest on plain radiographs is characteristic of a diaphragmatic rupture*.
*Visualization of the gastric tube and bowel gas pattern above the diaphragm is pathognomonic for diaphragmatic rupture.*

*Any trauma patient should be evaluated in a systematic manner taking into account the priorities of the primary survey as follows: Airway (patency), Breathing (adequacy of ventilation), Circulation (haemodynamics, hypovolaemia, active visible external bleeding) and Disability (brief neurological examination). Only after the 'ABCD' have been addressed and corrected should the secondary survey (a head to toe examination) and an evaluation of the patient's specific injuries take place.*

*Bowel and mesenteric injuries are more common in penetrating trauma.*

*The seatbelt sign is associated with intra-abdominal injury and should raise a suspicion of underlying solid organ and bowel trauma.*

*Unlike with penetrating injuries (gunshot and stab wounds), multiple system injuries are common in patients presenting after motor vehicle accidents, falls and other blunt trauma. Haemorrhagic shock may result from bleeding external wounds, intra-abdominal and intrathoracic injuries and long bone fractures. The spleen and liver are the most commonly injured intra-abdominal organs in blunt trauma. Bowel injuries are more common in penetrating trauma.*

---

## MCQs

---

**1.** The pathophysiological mechanisms that lead to an acute abdomen include:
  **a** Perforation
  **b** Inflammation
  **c** Gastrointestinal bleeding
  **d** Bowel obstruction
  **e** Ischaemia

**Answers**
*a, b, d, e.* There several pathophysiological mechanisms behind an acute abdomen: perforation, inflammation, bowel obstruction, ischaemia and torsion. Gastrointestinal bleeding typically occurs within the lumen of the bowel and is painless unless it occurs secondary to mesenteric ischaemia.

**2. Which of the following conditions may present with symptoms of bowel obstruction?:**

  a  Crohn's disease
  b  Peptic ulcer disease
  c  Post-operative adhesions
  d  Intra-abdominal malignancy
  e  Acute uncomplicated appendicitis
  f  Incarcerated abdominal wall hernia
  g  Ileocolonic intussusception

**Answers**

*All of the above except **e**. Post-operative adhesions and intra-abdominal malignancy are the most common causes of bowel obstruction. Incarceration of the bowel within the hernia ring or focal oedema of the bowel wall (active Crohn's disease or acute diverticulitis) can be associated with obstructive symptoms. A chronic fibrotic stricture (stricture of the pylorus secondary to peptic ulcer disease, Crohn's disease or a recurrent stricture in diverticulitis) are other possible aetiologies. Ileocolonic intussusception is a common cause of distal intestinal obstruction in children.*
*Uncomplicated acute appendicitis is not associated with symptoms of bowel obstruction.*

# Anorectal and Vaginal Examination

Parth B. Amin and John Byrn

## LEARNING OBJECTIVES

- To be able to describe the gross and histological anatomy of the anal sphincter and anal canal
- To understand the key elements of the anorectal examination, with particular attention to patient positioning

- To be able to describe common and uncommon pathology of the anorectum, and the unique aspects of physical examination that aid in diagnosis

## ANUS AND RECTUM

### Basic Anatomy

The anatomy of the anal sphincter is shown in **Figure 37.1**. The levator ani muscle group forms the pelvic floor. The puborectalis muscle passes between the anal canal (posteriorly) and the urethra and vagina (anteriorly). The puborectalis envelopes the lower rectum on all sides except anteriorly, and is continued interiorly as the external sphincter of the anal canal. This muscle is responsible for the forward angulation of the anorectal junction. It is felt easily in the conscious patient as a posterior ridge, but less easily under anaesthesia. Because of the sling-like arrangement of the puborectalis sling, a shorter length of anal canal is surrounded by striated muscle anteriorly than posteriorly.

The **internal anal sphincter** is a direct continuation of the circular smooth muscle coat of the rectum that has developed specialized properties. The lower edge of the internal sphincter may be easily felt under anaesthesia, with an anal retractor opened in the anal canal, as a tight band that forms the upper border of the anal intermuscular groove. The internal sphincter is crossed by fibroconnective tissue fibres derived from the medial aspect of the conjoined longitudinal muscle as this runs down the intersphincteric

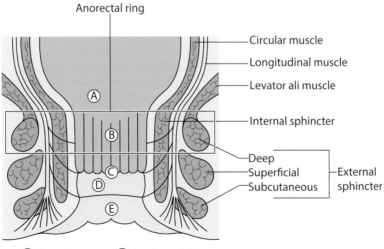

Figure 37.1 Surgical anatomy of the anal sphincter.

Anorectal ring

- Circular muscle
- Longitudinal muscle
- Levator ali muscle
- Internal sphincter
- Deep
- Superficial — External
- Subcutaneous — sphincter

(A) Rectal mucosa  (D) Anal canal skin
(B) Anal mucosa  (E) Anal skin
(C) Dentate line

PART 8 | ABDOMINAL

space; these fibres intermingle with those of the subepithelial space and support the overlying anoderm and mucosa.

These supporting fibres coalesce at the level of the dentate line (see below) to form a structure called the **mucosal suspensory ligament**. This site is important since it separates the vessels of the superior haemorrhoidal plexus (related to internal haemorrhoids) from those of the inferior haemorrhoidal plexus (related to thrombosed external haemorrhoids). It also separates the marginal space from the submucous space.

Between the internal and external sphincters lies the **intersphincteric space**, which is clinically important as it contains the anal glands. Infection of the anal glands is probably responsible for the majority of cases of acute anorectal sepsis. Bacteria pass retrogradely from the crypts at the dentate line and through the anal ducts to create an abscess in the glands in the intersphincteric space. This abscess cannot spontaneously discharge back into the anal lumen because of the normally high resting tone of the internal sphincter. Anal glands may also be found superficial to the internal sphincter, but these are not important clinically since infection in such glands is able to drain and resolve spontaneously.

The skin of the perineum is stratified, squamous, hairy, keratinized epithelium. It contains apocrine glands that may become the site of chronic infection (hidradenitis suppurativa; see below). The distal end of the anal canal is lined by stratified, squamous, non-keratinized epithelium to the level of the dentate line.

The **dentate line** is so called because of its likeness to a row of teeth (or is referred to as 'pectinate' – akin to a comb), the sides of the teeth passing cephalad as the rectal columns of Morgagni. The dentate line may be regarded as the site of fusion of the embryological ectoderm and the hindgut. In practical terms, it is the site of the anal crypts, at which point the anal gland ducts open into the anal lumen, and is the site of the majority of internal openings of cryptoglandular or idiopathic anal fistulas. The dentate line is also a watershed for lymphatic drainage; this drainage – which accompanies the arteries – passes upwards to the inferior mesenteric nodes above the dentate line but downwards to the inguinal nodes below the dentate line.

It is in the region of the line that there is the highest concentration of sensory nerve endings; the sensory component of the anal canal is important, not only in the conscious discrimination of gut contents passing over it, but also in the unconscious reflex in which the internal sphincter relaxes to allow 'sampling' of the rectal contents.

Above the dentate line is the so-called **transitional** zone of the anal canal. This area represents a gradual change from flattened squamous-type cells to the true columnar epithelium of the rectum. Above the dentate line, the epithelium is relatively insensitive, although an appreciation of stretch can be elicited. This pattern of innervation also becomes important when minor procedures are performed in this region.

The arrangement of the muscular and supporting tissues of the anal sphincter complex means that several well-defined anatomical spaces lie in relation to them. As these spaces are important in the spread of sepsis, accurate identification of the site of any sepsis is fundamental to the correct management of the patient.

## Positioning the Patient for Examination or Treatment

Anorectal examination can be made with the patient in one of four positions:

- *The left lateral (Sims') position* (**Figure 37.2a**): The patient is positioned with the left side up and the left lower extremity straightened. This position is useful because it does not require a special table or any particular effort on the part of the patient. The right lower extremity is flexed at the hip, and the leg is flexed at the knee. If the patient is obese, it is essential to have an assistant retract the left buttock and thigh to expose the anus.

- *The knee–elbow (genucubital) position* (**Figure 37.2b**): The patient lies prone with their weight on their knees and the elbows. Examining tables designed for proctology allow the patient to assume this position with far less effort. This provides stable access to the anus. An assistant may be needed to retract the buttocks of an obese individual.

- *The dorsal recumbent position* (**Figure 37.2c**): Use this position when the patient cannot be moved laterally because of a possible spinal injury or when the patient is too ill to turn into the left lateral position. The patient lies semi-recumbent with the knees flexed, and the (right-handed) examiner passes his or her arm under the patient's right thigh to gain access to the anorectum. Digital examination with the dominant hand is used in conjunction with pressure from the other hand upon the lower abdomen, so that pelvic swellings can be assessed bimanually and access to the rectovesical or rectouterine pouches can be made with minimal disturbance of the patient.

- *The lithotomy position* (**Figure 37.2d**): This allows the most thorough examination of the pelvis and allows lesions high in the rectum to be felt, which might not be so in the other positions. This position is usually adopted for examination under anaesthesia (EUA). The buttocks project beyond the end of the operating table, and the hips are flexed beyond the right angle with legs in stirrups outside the poles.

Anorectal examination includes inspection, careful palpation – both within and outside the anal canal – with an adequately lubricated digit, sigmoidoscopy and proctoscopy. If a proper examination cannot be performed, the patient should undergo EUA.

## Examination

### Inspection

Inspection of the perineum is extremely important. Soiling may be a result of incontinence or poor local hygiene. Minor anal seepage from haemorrhoids, a fissure, a fistula, proctitis, a rectal polyp, prolapse or malignancy, from minor incontinence secondary to anal surgery, and from liquid stool from whatever cause may lead to itching, scratching and excoriation of the perianal skin. Excoriation may also result from primary skin disorders that may affect the perineum, fungal, viral and parasitic infections and, not uncommonly, hypersensitivity reactions to washing agents, toilet paper and even those topical agents applied in the hope of relieving the itching.

Inspection of the skin of the perineum may reveal one or more external openings of anal fistulas, openings of multiple sinuses due to underlying hidradenitis, scars from previous infections or surgery, or warts, which may also be present on the external genitalia and inside the anal canal. Look closely at the anal margin itself – look for an olive-shaped subcutaneous perianal haematoma resulting from thrombosis of one of the veins of the external (superficial) haemorrhoidal venous plexus, the external skin components of true haemorrhoids, the sentinel tag of a fissure and simple anal skin tags.

(a)

(b)

(d)

(c)

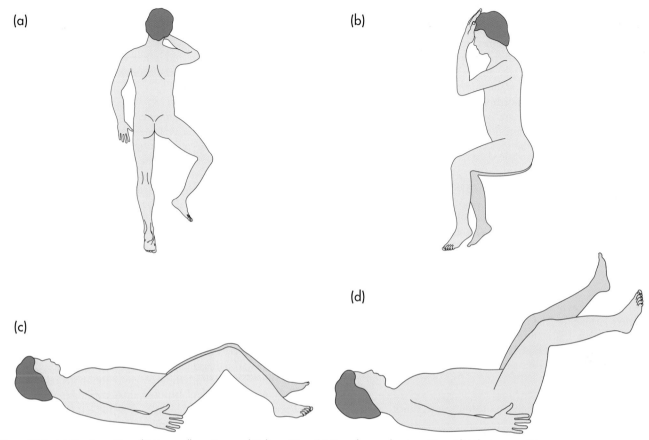

Figure 37.2 (a) Sims' position. (b) Knee–elbow (genucubital) position. (c) Dorsal recumbent position. (d) Lithotomy position.

Look closely at the anus, that is, its position in relation to the ischial tuberosities at rest and on straining – monitoring perineal descent. If there is a history suggestive of prolapse – of piles, a polyp, malignancy or of the rectum itself – and this is not demonstrable by inspection in the left lateral position, observe the anus while the patient is sitting on a lavatory. This is easiest if the patient is crouched forward and the examiner is leaning over to look from behind. This simple manoeuvre can be most informative.

## Palpation

Palpation includes feeling the skin of the perineum as well as actual digital examination of the anorectum itself; tracks leading from the external openings of fistulas may course superficially and may then easily be traced by using a well-lubricated, gloved digit.

Rectal examination, although often embarrassing to the patient, should be a painless process. The left lateral position is adopted. Before proceeding, always warn the patient what you are going to do and what sensations this action may produce. Lay the pulp of the index finger flat upon the anal verge, and slowly introduce the tip of the digit into the anal canal with the pulp facing posteriorly. The patient may be able to assist by bearing down as if having a bowel movement, as this relaxes the sphincter. If an acute fissure is present, the patient will not tolerate digital examination. Abandon the examination and make arrangements for an EUA.

On initial insertion of the finger, feel for the anal intermuscular groove. Make an assessment of the tone of the internal sphincter digitally with the patient at rest, and of the external

sphincter when the patient is asked to squeeze the examining finger. Rotating the pulp of the finger around the circumference of the anal canal and asking the patient to squeeze allows a clinical assessment of the integrity of the external sphincter. This takes much experience, especially the anterior sphincter aspect in women. Feel for induration around the anal canal; above the levators, induration feels bony hard like the sacrum lying posteriorly, and can be best appreciated by comparing one side with the other.

Anteriorly, in men, feel the prostate and assess it for size, consistency and the presence of the median sulcus. A long digit may reach the seminal vesicles, especially if the patient is in the knee–elbow position.

In women, the cervix uteri can be felt projecting through the anterior rectal wall. Assessment of the cervix transanally is difficult for the inexperienced, and occasionally the experienced, examiner because of the variety in its size and shape, and it is not unusual for a normal cervix to be thought a rectal neoplasm. Only practice and experience gives an appreciation of what is clinically normal and what is pathologically valid. Above the prostate or cervix uteri, the rectovesical pouch (in men) and the pouch of Douglas (in women) should be assessed digitally.

## Pathology
### Haemorrhoids

Patients with rectal bleeding may complain of true 'piles', that is, lumps that appear at the anal orifice during defecation and return spontaneously up into the anal canal (second-degree piles), have to be replaced manually (third-degree piles) or lie permanently outside the anus. The term 'first-degree piles' is applied to pain-less rectal bleeding from the potentially prolapsing mucosa. Many so-called fourth-degree piles cannot be reduced because it is the external skin component of the haemorrhoids that represents the irreducible components. These tags arise through intermittent congestion and oedema when the internal components prolapse.

True **strangulated haemorrhoids (Figure 37.3)** usually pre-sent as an emergency. They are associated with severe, constant, unremitting pain. On examination, large pile masses are seen to be protruding from the anal orifice, with gross oedema and later ulceration.

A **perianal haematoma** (thrombosed external haemorrhoid) is a 5–10 mm thrombosed vein in the subcutaneous perianal venous plexus. The lesion is usually of sudden onset and exqui-sitely painful. The lump is blue and tender, and visible at the anal verge. The pain takes 4–5 days to resolve and the lesion slowly fibroses, often leaving a palpable, persistent nodule.

### Acute Perineal Sepsis

Acute anorectal sepsis is common. An understanding of the aeti-ology and anatomy is fundamental to the correct management. Patients with acute anal sepsis present with a story of increasing pain in the region, usually a lump, and occasionally a purulent or bloody discharge and fever. The condition of a high intermuscular abscess is uncommon but must be considered in the differential diagnosis of a patient with fever, vague deep anorectal pain, perhaps difficulty in passing urine and maybe no visible abscess, but in whom digital examination of the anorectum is extremely painful.

For the most part, anorectal sepsis may be divided into sepsis that has nothing to do with the anorectum – for example, simple boils, pilonidal abscess and hidradenitis suppurativa – and sepsis that is intimately related to the anorectum. **Pilonidal disease (Figure 37.4)** and **hidradenitis suppurativa (Figure 37.5)** are usually simple to recognize. **Cutaneous boils** can present as both perianal and ischiorectal abscesses. The key to their distinction from boils associated with anal problems can often be found in the microbiology and the smell of the pus. The incidence of anorectal sepsis due to skin organisms – and nothing to do with fistulas – is equally divided between the sexes, whereas sepsis due to gut organisms is more common in men, reflecting the similar (unexplained) male predominance of the chronic condition, the anal fistula. A history of previous sepsis at the same site is also indicative, but not diagnostic, of a communication with the ano-rectal lumen.

Most cases arise spontaneously and are not associated with underlying diseases, but they are occasionally a presentation of established inflammatory bowel disease and can be associated with underlying diabetes and other immunosuppressed states, which should be revealed by the history and examination.

### Anal Fistula

Anal fistulas represent a communication between the anal canal and the perianal skin. The vast majority of anal fistulas seen in surgical practice are due to persisting infection of the anal glands in the intersphincteric space – the cryptoglandular hypothesis. They may be considered to be the chronic sequel of the par-ent condition, acute anorectal sepsis, although many years may elapse between the two clinical conditions. Anal fistulas are also seen in association with other specific conditions such as inflam-matory bowel disease, tuberculosis, malignancy, actinomycosis, lymphogranuloma venereum, trauma and foreign bodies.

Patients with anal fistulas complain of intermittent anal pain and discharge, either purulent or mixed with blood; the two symptoms are often inversely related, with the pain increasing until it eases off when the pus drains out through the external opening. There is often a history of acute anal sepsis, either treated surgically or that has settled after a spontaneous discharge of pus or insidiously, leaving an opening on the perianal skin.

The surgical management of anal fistulas depends upon an accurate knowledge of both the anatomy of the anorectal sphincter and the course of the fistula through it. According to **Parks' clas-sification**, there are four main types of fistula – trans-sphincteric, intersphincteric, suprasphincteric and extrasphincteric – each of

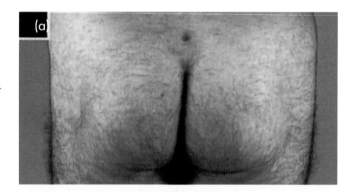

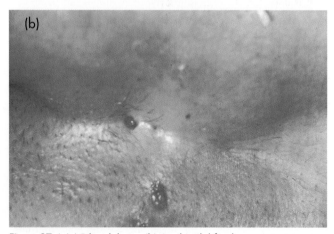

Figure 37.4 (a) Pilonidal pits. (b) A pilonidal fistula.

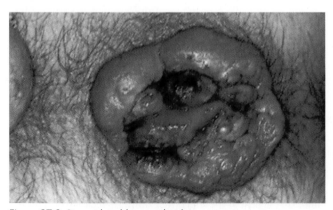

Figure 37.3 Strangulated haemorrhoids.

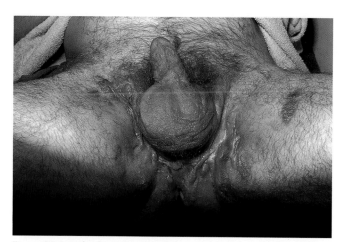

Figure 37.5 Hidradenitis suppurativa.

laid open at a single-stage fistulotomy, would cause significant functional morbidity, and as 'low' the remainder, in which laying open would not cause major incontinence. This does not mean that laying open 'low' fistulas is not associated with functional morbidity, but rather that the incidence and degree of symptoms are less.

The clinical assessment of anal fistulas involves five essential points: the location of the external and internal openings; the

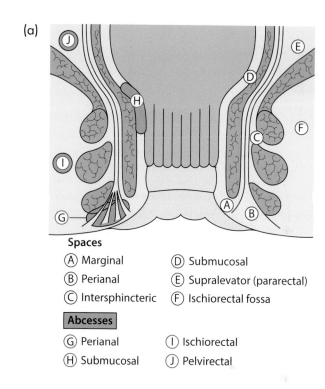

(a)

**Spaces**

Ⓐ Marginal            Ⓓ Submucosal
Ⓑ Perianal            Ⓔ Supralevator (pararectal)
Ⓒ Intersphincteric    Ⓕ Ischiorectal fossa

**Abcesses**

Ⓖ Perianal            Ⓘ Ischiorectal
Ⓗ Submucosal          Ⓙ Pelvirectal

which may be further subdivided according to the presence and course of any secondary tracks (**Figure 37.6**):

- *Trans-sphincteric fistula*: The primary track of this fistula passes through the external sphincter at varying levels into the ischiorectal fossa. Such fistulas may be uncomplicated, consisting only of the primary track opening onto the skin of the buttock, or can have a high blind secondary track that ends either below or above the levator ani muscles.
- *Intersphincteric fistula*: This passes from the anal canal across the internal sphincter, downwards between the internal and external sphincters, and opens onto the perineal skin. Such fistulas are most commonly simple, but others end with a high blind track, have an internal opening into the rectum, have no perineal opening or even have a pelvic extension or arise through pelvic disease.
- *Suprasphincteric fistula*: Suprasphincteric fistulas run up in the intersphincteric plane to loop over the top of the puborectalis muscle and thence to pass down through the levator ani and ischiorectal fossa to reach the skin of the perineum.
- *Extrasphincteric fistula*: This is a fistula that runs without any relation to the sphincters and is classified according to its aetiology. Some are iatrogenic in origin, arising from overzealous probing of the ischiorectal fossa in a patient who presents with an ischiorectal abscess. The underlying fistula in this circumstance is usually trans-sphincteric.

It is important to understand the basic primary tracks of the four recognized types of anal fistula. Superimposed on these primary tracks are extensions or secondary tracks that may be blind or may open onto the perineal skin or back into the anorectal lumen (usually because of injudicious probing). Besides vertical and horizontal spread, sepsis may also spread circumferentially in any of the three tissue planes: intersphincteric (or intermuscular, which implies no restriction to below the anorectal ring), ischiorectal or pararectal.

Parks' classification does not include those low intersphincteric fistulas that result from an anal fissure, and subcutaneous tracks arising from superficial infection, two types that, although relatively minor, are seen much more commonly in local hospitals than tertiary referral centres.

The differentiation of fistulas into 'high' and 'low' is often a point of confusion. A sensible and useful way of implementing such terminology is to describe as 'high' all those fistulas that, if

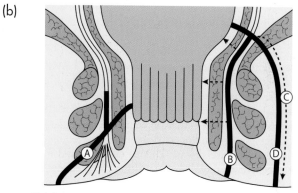

(b)

**Fistulae**
Ⓐ Trans-sphincteric (high or low)   Ⓒ Supersphincteric
Ⓑ Intersphincteric                  Ⓓ Extrasphincteric (supralevator)

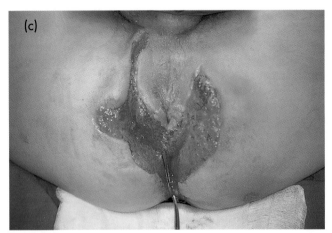

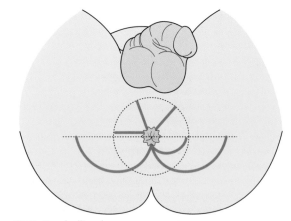

Figure 37.7 Goodsall's rule.

Figure 37.6 (a) Perianal abscesses. (b) Anal fistulas. (c) Surgical laying open of an anal fistula indicating the extent of its various channels.

course of the primary track and any secondary tracks (lateral burrowings); and the presence of other diseases complicating the fistula. The relative positions of the internal and external openings indicate the likely course of the primary track, and the presence of any palpable indurations, especially supralevator, alerts the surgeon to a high secondary track.

The distance between the external opening and the anal verge may assist the differentiation between an intersphincteric and a trans-sphincteric fistula; and the greater the distance, the more the likelihood of a complicated upward extension.

The position of the external opening also gives a clue to the likely site of the internal opening. **Goodsall's rule** (**Figure 37.7**) states that for openings anterior to a transverse mid-anal line, the fistula usually runs radially into the anal canal; for openings posterior to this imaginary line, the track is usually curvilinear to open into the anal lumen in the posterior midline. The exceptions to this rule include anterior openings more than 3 cm from the anal margin, which may be anterior extensions of posterior horseshoe fistulas, fistulas associated with Crohn's disease and those arising from carcinoma of the anal glands.

The internal opening may be felt digitally as an indurated nodule or pit, or may be seen at proctoscopy, aided if necessary by gentle downward retraction of the dentate line, which may expose openings concealed by prominent anal valves. Outpatient assessment must include sigmoidoscopy, but beyond this more information can only safely and comfortably be obtained from EUA or special investigations. Probing fistulas in the clinic is both painful and dangerous. Special investigations are generally reserved for 'difficult' – that is, recurrent or complex – fistulas.

Sigmoidoscopy and/or colonoscopy may be required to exclude inflammatory bowel disease. Endorectal ultrasound and MRI scan are excellent methods for delineating the anatomy of complex fistulas.

### Anal Fissure

An anal fissure (**Figure 37.8**) is a cutaneous tear in the ectodermal portion of the anal canal and is usually found in either the 12 o'clock or the 6 o'clock position around the anal circumference; the orientation of the anus is conventionally described in the lithotomy position, so 12 o'clock is sited anteriorly – towards the scrotum or vagina. Anal fissures commonly occur after a bout of constipation and are very painful. Patients find themselves in

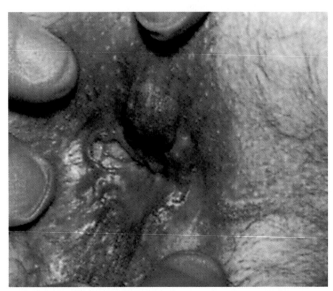

Figure 37.8 An anal fissure.

a vicious circle in which they anticipate that the next bout of defecation will be painful; hence they avoid passing a stool and become progressively more constipated. When the bowel is eventually opened, the tear is made worse. Fresh bleeding is common. This is the most common cause of rectal bleeding in a child.

A diagnostic feature of an anal fissure is anal pain after defecation. In chronic cases, the skin at the lower part of the fissure becomes swollen and can be used as a marker of an anal fissure – the 'sentinel pile'. This may be the only sign of a chronic anal fissure as it is often too painful to examine the patient digitally or proctoscopically.

**Pruritus ani** is an insatiable itch around the perianal region; it may extend to the introitus in women and girls. The skin is usually moist from an anal or vaginal discharge of infected material, mucus or faeces. There is erythema, maceration, excoriation and lichenification (**Figure 37.9**). In females, pruritus vulvae may be associated with pruritus ani. Thrush is common, and urinary leakage may be due to a cystocele or an ectopic ureter.

Every baby develops a nappy (diaper) rash at some point (**Figure 37.10**). This is usually due to prolonged contact with urine or faeces but may be due to a fungal infection or a reaction to an emollient.

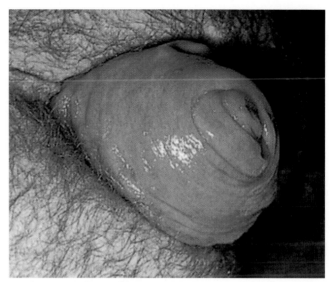

Figure 37.11 Prolapse of the rectum.

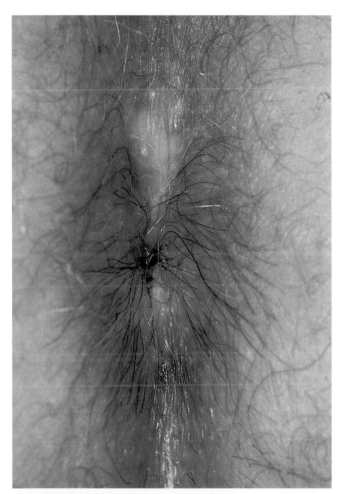

Figure 37.9 Skin changes in pruritus ani.

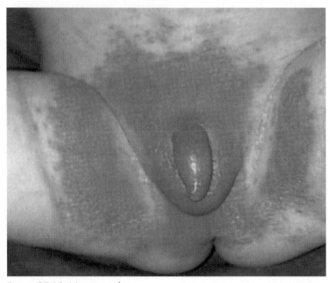

Figure 37.10 Nappy rash.

## Prolapse of the Rectum

This encompasses both prolapse of the rectal mucosa through the anus and full-thickness prolapse of the rectum (**Figure 37.11**). The two can be distinguished by feeling one wall of the prolapse between the index finger and thumb – a full-thickness prolapse feels like a double-layered tube.

A prolapse may be caused by straining excessively at stool, especially if the pelvic floor muscles are weak. Although the young and the elderly are most frequently seen with the condition, any age group can be affected. In children, it may be associated with malnutrition and chronic diarrhoea. If present for a long time, the prolapse may ulcerate and the patient may then present with bleeding and mucus discharge. Occasionally, a prolapse can become ischaemic and present as a surgical emergency.

### Perianal Crohn's Disease

Perianal Crohn's disease (PACD) may be found in up to 75 per cent of patients with Crohn's disease, the incidence relating to the site of gastrointestinal pathology, with higher rates the more distal the disease. It is important to remember, however, that PACD may precede Crohn's disease elsewhere in the gastrointestinal tract by many years.

The spectrum of PACD may be clinically divided into those primary conditions – fissures, ulcerated piles and cavitating ulcers – whose activity reflects that of the intestinal disease, and secondary lesions – either mechanical (skin tags, strictures, epithelialized fistulas) or infective (abscesses, fistulas) – for which local treatment should be determined by local severity. Suspect Crohn's disease when fistulas occur without previous bouts of perirectal sepsis, or when the fistula has a characteristic 'bland' appearance.

### Perianal Warts

The incidence of perianal warts – **condylomata accuminata** (**Figure 37.12**) – caused by the human papillomavirus, is increasing. The highest rates are seen in homosexual men, although heterosexual individuals are certainly not immune, the condition being almost invariably sexually transmitted. For this reason, there is often a history of other sexually transmitted diseases (STDs).

Patients with perianal warts usually complain of itching, bleeding and perianal lumps; there may also be symptoms from warts elsewhere on the genitalia. The appearance of the warts is

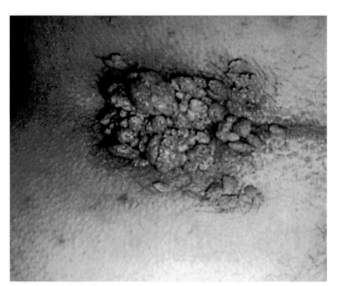

Figure 37.12 Perianal warts.

variable, ranging from one or two discrete excrescences, which may be both within and outside the anal canal itself, to massive cauliflower-like lesions totally obscuring the anal orifice. Warts may occasionally have the appearance of frank malignancy. Excisional biopsy is usually required to exclude squamous carcinoma.

### Pilonidal Disease

A pilonidal sinus (see Figure 37.4) is a chronic inflammatory disorder comprising a midline epithelialized pit between the buttocks that extends, for a variable distance and usually in a cranial direction, as a track lined with granulation tissue, and ends either as a cul-de-sac or at another orifice, and which almost invariably contains a nest of hair. The location is characteristically over the bony sacrum, generally in the midline. The condition is not seen before puberty and rarely seen in patients over the age of 45 years.

The aetiology of the condition is unclear. It is possibly congenital, but a traumatic aetiology is suggested by the fact that the opening is in the natal cleft between the ischial tuberosities at a site of maximum shearing stresses when an individual seated. An attractive hypothesis is that shed hairs 'drill' into congenital midline pits. Such pits are commonly seen as incidental findings on examination and may never be associated with pilonidal disease, which is characteristically seen in hairy truck drivers.

Abscess formation within the sinus leads to the development of secondary lateral tracks since discharge through the midline is prevented by the fibrous septa connecting the skin to the fascia over the sacrum. Such lateral tracks may pass caudally and create an appearance that may resemble hidradenitis suppurativa or fistula-in-ano, both of which may coexist with pilonidal disease.

Patients usually present with an acute abscess or a chronic discharging sinus. The acute abscess usually lies to one side of the midline, although a midline pit is always present.

Rarer versions of the condition are seen on the hands, at the umbilicus and in the axillae. Pilonidal sinuses of the hand are seen in barbers where hair clippings enter the web of the barber's dominant hand between the index and ring fingers. A small black spot is present, as is a palpable lump – a barber's nodule – both of which may become infected. The condition is also reported from wool clippings in sheep shearers.

### Hidradenitis Suppurativa

Hidradenitis suppurativa (see Figure 37.5) is a chronic, recurring suppurative disease of apocrine gland-bearing skin – apocrinitis. It usually affects the axillae but may involve the back of the neck, the areola of the breast, the groins and the perineum. Although it is generally more common in women, those cases involving the perineum – the apocrine circumanal Gay's glands – are more often seen in men. Like pilonidal disease, hidradenitis is not seen before puberty, and most patients present aged 16–40 years.

Its aetiology is unknown, although obesity, acne, poor hygiene and excessive sweating have been suggested as predisposing factors. It may be seen in a variety of endocrine disorders, suggesting that a relative androgen excess or increased target organ androgen sensitivity may be implicated.

Occlusion of the apocrine gland ducts leads to bacterial proliferation within the glands, with rupture and the spread of infection to adjacent glands. Secondary infection causes further local extension, skin damage and fibrosis, eventually leading to multiple communicating subcutaneous fistulas. In the primary stages, it presents with multiple, tender, raised, red lesions around the perianal region, but in its chronic form multiple sinuses are seen, with secondary infection leading to gross fibrosis and scarring. It may rarely extend into the anal canal, but never above the dentate line.

### Sexually Transmitted Diseases of the Rectum and Anus

Anal receptive intercourse is not uncommonly practised by both sexes and may lead to disease that is evident on examination of the anus and rectum. Although drugs are often used to relax the anal sphincters, the anal and rectal mucosa (and underlying muscles) may still tear. This leads to bleeding and problems with continence, and also allows an easier entry of potential pathogens.

**Anorectal Gonorrhoea** – Anorectal gonorrhoea is caused by the gonococcus, a gram-negative coccus that is transmitted sexually. The infection can be asymptomatic or may give rise to constipation, tenesmus and the passage of mucus or pus. Little is likely to be seen on inspection, although the anal and rectal mucosa may look inflamed, congested and covered with discharge.

**Anorectal Syphilis** – Anorectal syphilis gives rise to a chancre that may be confused with a fissure-in-ano but is usually not in the characteristic midline position. It has the appearance of a well-defined indurated ulcer (**Figure 37.13**).

**Herpes Simplex** – Herpes simplex is a viral infection caused by the herpes simplex virus. It gives rise to painful vesicles that may ulcerate. The patient usually presents with pain, especially on defecation, and also constipation and discharge.

**Perianal Disease in the HIV-positive Patient** – The rise in the prevalence of AIDS sufferers has led to a corresponding rise in the associated anorectal lesions. These patients may have any of the STDs seen in the general population – especially those associated with anoreceptive intercourse, for example gonorrhoea, syphilis and chlamydia. Various viral infections and tumours (squamous cell and cloacogenic carcinomas, lymphoma, Kaposi's sarcoma) may also be present.

Anorectal pathology in the HIV-positive or AIDS patient also includes conditions common to all patients, that is, haemorrhoids, fissures and fistulas, as well as those more prevalent in the HIV-positive group, namely herpes simplex virus,

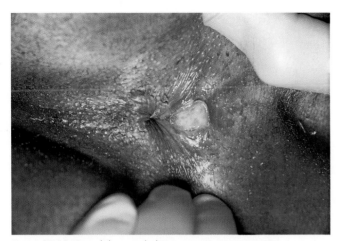

Figure 37.13 A syphilitic anal ulcer.

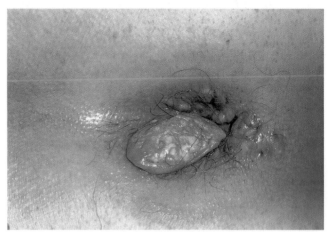

Figure 37.14 An anal squamous cell carcinoma.

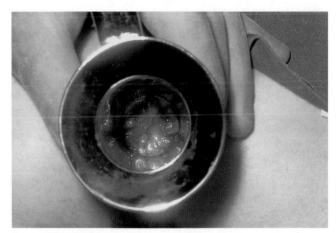

Figure 37.15 Melanoma of the anal canal.

cytomegalovirus, *Mycobacterium avium-intracellulare*, *Candida*, condylomata accuminata and non-specific, primary HIV-positive-induced anal ulcer.

Most HIV-positive patients seen in the surgical clinic are already under the care of a specialist in that disease. A thorough history should include an evaluation of the patient's anorectal symptoms, age, HIV status, Centers for Disease Control classification, previous and current STDs, previous anorectal conditions and treatments, and current medications.

Examination should be carried out with all precautions taken, and specific pathology such as warts, vesicles, ulcers, fissures, fistulas and abscesses looked for. Proctoscopy and sigmoidoscopy should be performed, and intra-anal and intrarectal ulcers biopsied. Biopsies should be sent for routine microscopy, viral cultures (including HIV, herpes simplex virus and cytomegalovirus), acid-fast stain for *Mycobacterium avium-intracellulare* and Indian ink stain for cryptococcus.

Anal condylomas of various viral types are probably the most frequent pathology seen, and there may be a higher incidence of dysplasia and *in situ* neoplasia than in non-HIV-positive homosexuals with warts.

## Tumours of the Rectum and Anus

Adenocarcinoma of the colon and rectum is one of the most common causes of cancer death in the Western world. Most tumours are found in the distal colon and rectum, where they are often detectable by digital and sigmoidoscopic examination.

The presenting complaint is usually one of a change in bowel habit as the obstructing lesion causes constipation or overflow diarrhoea, although other common symptoms are rectal bleeding and tenesmus – the sensation of a desire to empty the rectum caused by a tumour in the rectum mimicking the presence of faeces. Adenomatous tumours are also common and are clinically important as they may give rise to malignant tumours if they grow over a certain size.

Anal tumours are not as common as rectal and colonic tumours, and present as either painful or painless lumps in the anus, usually with bleeding. These arise from squamous epithelium and thus are usually squamous cell carcinomas or melanomas.

On inspection, only the most distal of anal tumours are evident. Anal squamous cell carcinomas (**Figure 37.14**) can appear warty, as an indurated plaque or as an ulcer. Anal basal cell carcinomas have an appearance similar to that of other basal cell carcinomas, that is, a pearly ulcer with a rolled edge. Melanomas are usually wart-like, pigmented tumours (**Figure 37.15**). Spread from anal malignant tumours is commonly to the inguinal lymph nodes, which should therefore be palpated if an anal tumour is suspected.

Digital examination may bring to light the presence of a tumour in the anus or proximal rectum. Colorectal tumours are either sessile, that is, arising without a stalk – in which case they can extend part or all the way round the lumen of the bowel – or polypoid. The benign or malignant nature of the tumour can only be determined with certainty by microscopic examination of the whole tumour.

Benign tumours tend to be more homogeneous with an intact, velvety mucosal surface that can make the tumour quite difficult to feel compared with the heterogeneous consistency and ulcerated surface of a frankly malignant tumour. Invasion through the rectal wall may be determined by the degree of fixity of the tumour to the pelvic wall. Although usually only the distal 10 cm of the rectum can be examined digitally, it may be possible, as with tumours of other pelvic organs, to examine tumours in the sigmoid colon through the rectal wall.

Other tumours of the rectum include lipomas, leiomyomas, leiomyosarcomas and melanomas. Tumours of the colon and rectum usually spread to the liver, and the presence of hepatomegaly should be sought if a malignant tumour of the colon or rectum is suspected.

The **solitary ulcer syndrome** is characterized by an ulcer of the anterior rectum just above the anal canal. The ulcer is usually 2–3 cm across, but there may be just a reddened, oedematous area or even more than one ulcer. The area may be elevated or polypoid, increasing the difficulty of differential diagnosis from Crohn's disease or carcinoma of the rectum.

The syndrome occurs in patients who have difficulty in defecation, with straining and incomplete evacuation, producing an internal intussusception of the rectum or occasionally a prolapse. There is weakness of the pelvic floor muscles, but it is uncertain whether this is primary or secondary to the development of the ulcer. An earlier theory that the ulcer was caused by the trauma of the digital evacuation used to overcome the defecation problem may also be a factor in some instances. The ulcer may bleed, and a good deal of mucus is produced. This, and any associated incontinence, may produce soiling and often pruritus ani.

## VAGINAL EXAMINATION

Although the vagina is mainly the province of the gynaecologist, diseases of the female reproductive organs can mimic conditions that present to general surgeons. Therefore, vaginal examination is invaluable in the evaluation of these diseases. The clinician can gain further access to the pelvis and the organs within it, enabling more information to be gathered about their involvement. For these reasons, all those managing surgical conditions should become skilled in vaginal examination.

The examiner should first wash their hands and put examination gloves on. In the general surgical setting, vaginal examination is carried out before or after rectal examination, so the gloves should be changed in between to avoid cross-contamination. It is usual for the surgeon to use the left lateral position rather than the lithotomy position, which is usually used by gynaecologists.

First, the vulva and introitus are inspected. These are subject to all the lesions that can be found on the penis – primary chancre, the primary lesion of lymphogranuloma inguinale, chancroid, herpes simplex, leukoplakia, cancer and other subcutaneous lesions (**Figure 37.16**). Papillomatous warts can be prolific, and sebaceous and **Bartholin's cysts** (**Figure 37.17**) are also common. A vaginal discharge from these conditions or from uterine abnormalities may give rise to pruritus vulvae, and there may be visible erythema, eczematous changes, excoriation and scratch marks.

A small amount of whitish mucous vaginal discharge is normal, as is a bloodstained discharge due to menstruation. However, bleeding may also be caused by an impending or recent abortion, an ectopic pregnancy or a uterine carcinoma. A profuse whitish or purulent discharge denotes salpingitis, endometritis, cervicitis or, most commonly, vaginitis.

*Trichomonas vaginalis* infection causes a profuse, watery, pale yellow, sometimes frothy discharge with intense pruritis. Thrush – *Candida albicans* infection – leads to a thick yellowish discharge that is particularly excoriating. In gonorrhoea, the discharge is purulent.

At this stage, ask the patient to strain down. This may show a cystocele – descent of the bladder through the anterior vaginal wall – or a rectocele – descent of the rectum through the posterior vaginal musculature. When the pelvic diaphragm and the ligaments supporting the uterus are defective, the cervix appears at the introitus on straining and becomes extruded to a varying degree – **procidentia** (**Figure 37.18**). Ask the patient to cough

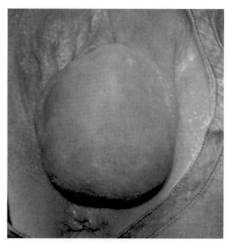

Figure 37.16 A lipoma of the vulva.

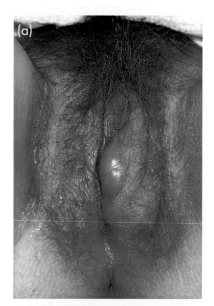

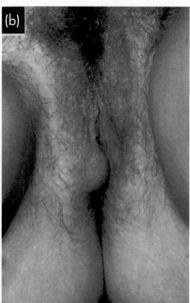

Figure 37.17 (a) A Bartholin's cyst. (b) A Bartholin's abscess due to gonococcal infection.

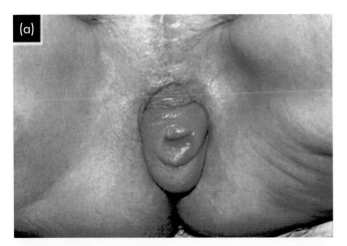

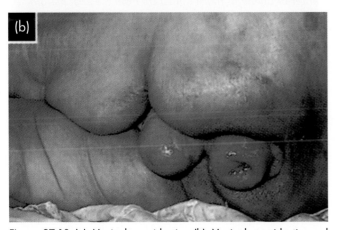

Figure 37.18 (a) Vaginal procidentia. (b) Vaginal procidentia and rectal prolapse.

The size, position and attitude of the corpus of the uterus are noted, and the fornices are examined in turn to palpate the pelvic contents. Abnormalities are then palpated bimanually through both the vagina and the lower abdominal wall. This will establish the relations of any abnormality, especially whether it is fixed to the pelvic wall or other pelvic organs.

The ovaries may be palpable, and the mobility of any ovarian mass should be assessed. The fallopian tubes cannot usually be palpated, but acute salpingitis produces marked tenderness in the lateral fornices and on movement of the cervix. A hydro- or pyosalpinx may be palpated.

In gynaecological practice, a speculum is introduced at this stage, and samples of discharge and secretions are taken for culture and cytology. A cervical smear will also be undertaken for cytological examination.

## Key Points

- The anatomy of the internal and external anal sphincter and the puborectalis is palpable and can aid in the diagnosis of anal sepsis.
- The dentate line marks the end of the hindgut and is the boundary by which internal and external haemorrhoids are differentiated.
- Trans-sphincteric, intersphincteric, suprasphincteric and extrasphincteric fistulas have a clear anatomical basis, and although they are usually related to bacterial infection, they can have an alternate aetiology. Goodsall's rule can help to guide a clinician to the location of a fistula's internal opening.
- Multiple other infectious diseases, Crohn's disease and tumours can also cause pathology in the anorectal region.

several times; this will indicate the competence of the urethral sphincter as urine will leak in cases of stress incontinence.

On palpation, the forefinger and, if the vagina comfortably allows it, the middle finger are introduced into the vagina until the cervix is encountered. The shape, size and surface of the os should be assessed, and irregularities noted for subsequent visualization.

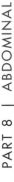

## QUESTIONS

### SBAs

**1. Goodsall's rule describes which of the following?:**
  a Anterior openings follow a curvilinear course to an internal opening, while posterior openings follow a radial course
  b Anterior and posterior external openings follow a curvilinear course towards an internal opening
  c Anterior openings follow a straight course to an internal opening, while posterior openings are curvilinear
  d Anterior and posterior external openings follow a radial straight course towards an internal opening

**Answer**

*c Anterior openings follow a straight course to an internal opening, while posterior openings are curvilinear.* The position of the external opening also gives a clue to the likely site of the internal opening. Goodsall's rule (see Figure 37.8) states that, for openings anterior to a transverse mid-anal line, the fistula usually runs radially into the anal canal; for openings posterior to this imaginary line, the track is usually curvilinear to open into the anal lumen in the posterior midline. The exceptions to this rule include anterior openings more than 3 cm from the anal margin, which may be anterior extensions of posterior horseshoe fistulas, fistulas associated with Crohn's disease and fistulas arising from carcinoma of the anal glands.

**2. The dentate line represents which of the following?:**
  a The watershed area between the superior/middle and inferior rectal artery and vein
  b The watershed area between the superior and middle/inferior rectal artery and vein
  c The watershed area between the internal iliac and inferior mesenteric nodes
  d None of the above

**Answer**

*b The watershed area between the superior and middle/inferior rectal artery and vein.* In practical terms, the site of the anal crypts indicates the point at which the anal gland ducts open into the anal lumen, and is the site of the majority of the internal openings of cryptoglandular or idiopathic anal fistulas. The dentate line is also a watershed for lymphatic drainage; this drainage – which accompanies the arteries – passes upwards to the inferior mesenteric nodes above the dentate line, but downwards to the inguinal nodes below the dentate line.

**3. The most common location for an anal fissure is?:**
  a Posteriorly in the midline
  b Anteriorly in the midline
  c At the 3 o'clock position
  d At the 9 o'clock position

**Answer**

*a Posteriorly in the midline.* An anal fissure is a cutaneous tear in the ectodermal portion of the anal canal and is usually found in either the 12 o'clock or the 6 o'clock position around the anal circumference (the orientation of the anus conventionally being described in the lithotomy position, so that 12 o'clock is thus sited anteriorly – towards the scrotum or vagina).

### EMQs

**1. Match the following fistulas types to the appropriate description given below:**
  1 Trans-sphincteric
  2 Intersphincteric
  3 Suprasphincteric
  4 Extrasphincteric
  a The fistula passes from the anal canal across the internal sphincter, downwards between the internal and external sphincters and opens onto the perineal skin

**Answers**

a 2 *Intersphincteric.*
b 3 *Suprasphincteric.*
c 4 *Extrasphincteric.*
d 1 *Trans-sphincteric.*

**b** Fistulas run up in the intersphincteric plane to loop over the top of the puborectalis muscle thence to pass down through the levator ani and ischiorectal fossa to reach the skin of the perineum.

**c** A fistula that runs without relation to the sphincters and is classified according to aetiology

**d** The fistula passes through the external sphincter at varying levels into the ischiorectal fossa

**2. Match the following positions to the appropriate description given below:**

   **1** Sims' position
   **2** Knee–elbow (genucubital) position
   **3** Dorsal recumbent position
   **4** Lithotomy position

**a** The patient lies semi-recumbent with their knees flexed, and the (right-handed) examiner passes his or her arm under the patient's right thigh to gain access to the anorectum

**b** The patient's buttocks are positioned to project beyond the end of the operating table and their hips are flexed beyond a right angle, with their legs in stirrups outside the poles

**c** The patient is positioned with their left side up and their left lower extremity straightened

**d** The patient is positioned prone with their weight on their knees and the elbows

Answers

**a** 3 *Dorsal recumbent position.*
**b** 4 *Lithotomy position.*
**c** 1 *Sims' position.*
**d** 2 *Knee–elbow (genucubital) position.*

# The alimentary tract and abdomen in children

Andrea Badillo

LEARNING OBJECTIVES

- To understand the key anatomical relationships, the significance of the presenting symptoms and the important physical signs in determining the congenital causes of bowel obstruction in neonates

- To be able to distinguish between the abdominal wall defects gastroschisis and omphalocele
- To become familiar with the typical presentations of common acquired paediatric surgical diseases

## INTRODUCTION

There are a variety of congenital anomalies and acquired disorders of the alimentary tract that have unique presentations in the neonatal period and early childhood. The assessment of infants and children can be difficult because of their inability to articulate specific complaints. A knowledge of embryology, key anatomical relationships and the typical symptom patterns of surgical diseases in neonates and children is an essential tool for arriving at an accurate diagnosis.

## NEONATAL BOWEL OBSTRUCTION

Congenital anomalies of the intestinal tract usually present as intestinal obstruction within the first few days of life and can be grouped under the heading of neonatal bowel obstruction (Figure 38.1). Common symptoms include intolerance of feeding, emesis, abdominal distension and a failure to pass meconium.

The presenting symptoms depend on the level of the obstruction and the relationship to the ampulla of Vater. Obstruction proximal to the ampulla manifests as non-bilious emesis, whereas obstruction distal to the ampulla usually results in bilious emesis. Patients with proximal obstructions tend to develop emesis first with less abdominal distension, while patients with distal obstructions become distended first and develop emesis later. Infants with an obstruction at the colonic level present with abdominal distension and a delay in the passage of meconium.

A differential diagnosis of neonatal bowel obstruction can be narrowed down based on the onset and predominant types of presenting symptoms. In many cases, plain radiographs can confirm the diagnosis.

## Oesophageal Atresia

The trachea and oesophagus develop as a single tube and then separate to form distinct passages between 6 and 7 weeks of gestation. Various patterns of incomplete separation exist, the most common of which is a proximal, blind-ending oesophageal pouch with a fistula tract from the trachea to the distal oesophagus. The second most common variant of oesophageal atresia is a proximal oesophageal pouch without a fistula tract. This variant is known as pure oesophageal atresia and is associated with a significant gap between the proximal and distal portions of the oesophagus.

Neonates with oesophageal atresia are unable to tolerate feeding or even their own oral secretions. Babies exhibit drooling and an inability to swallow their saliva. Feeding attempts are associated with coughing and a risk of developing pneumonia from the passage of oral contents into the lungs. The diagnosis of oesophageal atresia is confirmed by an inability to pass an orogastric tube into the oesophagus. In cases of tracheo-oesophageal fistula, air passes through the fistula, demonstrating air-filled bowel loops on a chest radiograph. In pure oesophageal atresia, a gasless abdomen is present (Figures 38.2 and 38.3).

## Duodenal Stenosis and Atresia

Obstruction at the level of the duodenum can occur as a result of atresia, the presence of a duodenal web or an annular pancreas. The main presenting symptom is emesis with little or no abdominal distension. Emesis is usually non-bilious but can be bilious if the level of obstruction is just distal to the ampulla of Vater. In cases of complete obstruction, emesis and intolerance of feeding are present at birth. When the duodenum is stenotic because of the presence of a web, which allows some passage of contents distally, the presentation can be delayed.

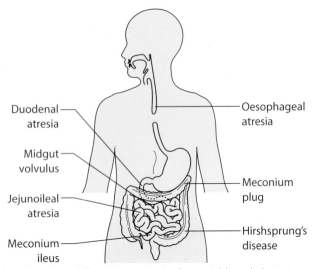

Figure 38.1 The differential diagnosis of neonatal bowel obstruction.

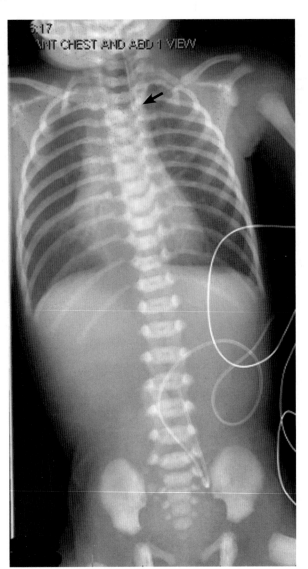

Figure 38.3 X-ray demonstrating the sump tube in the proximal oesophageal pouch (arrow) without distal bowel gas, consistent with pure oesophageal atresia.

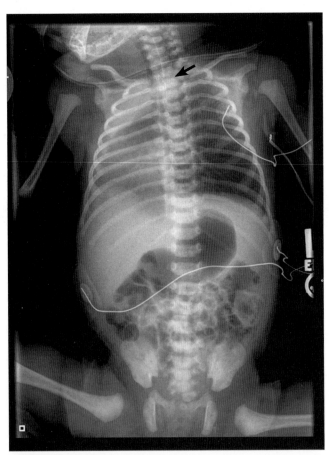

Figure 38.2 X-ray demonstrating the sump tube in the proximal oesophageal pouch (arrow) and the presence of distal bowel gas, indicative of oesophageal atresia with a tracheal fistula.

The diagnosis is often made with an abdominal radiograph showing the classic 'double bubble' sign in which air is present in the stomach and contained by the pylorus, followed by a second

air-filled area representing the obstructed, dilated duodenum (Figure 38.4).

Duodenal atresia is associated with Down syndrome in 30 per cent of cases, and the presence of other physical features of Down syndrome can give a clue to the diagnosis.

## Malrotation and Midgut Volvulus

Disorders of bowel rotation alter the pattern of bowel fixation, leading to a narrow mesenteric base that predisposes the midgut to volvulus upon its vascular pedicle. Bilious emesis in the newborn is a surgical emergency and is considered to be the hallmark presentation of midgut volvulus. The abdomen is rarely distended unless there is also significant bowel oedema and ascites.

Left unidentified, midgut volvulus can lead to necrosis of the entire small bowel and neonatal death. Bilious emesis

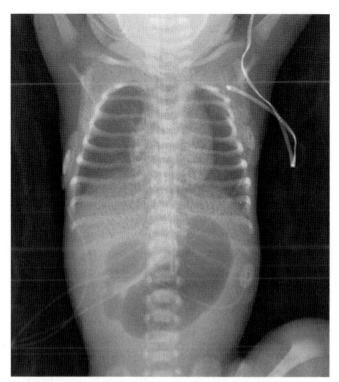

Figure 38.4 The 'double bubble' sign of duodenal atresia.

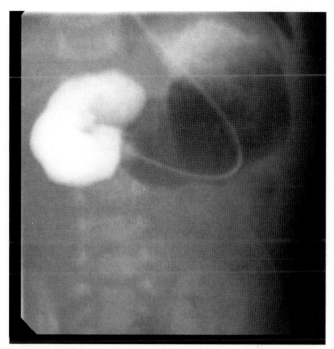

Figure 38.5 Fluoroscopy demonstrating failure of the duodenum to cross the midline and contrast to pass distally, consistent with malrotation with volvulus.

accompanied by infant lethargy is particularly ominous. In stable patients, upper intestinal fluoroscopy can demonstrate malrotation with volvulus (**Figure 38.5**). In unstable patients, immediate surgical exploration is indicated.

## Jejunoileal Atresia

Jejunoileal atresias are due to vascular accidents resulting in some degree of bowel loss, creating an obstruction. These defects usually present with an inability to tolerate feeds and abdominal distension within the first few days of life.

The ability to pass meconium depends on the timing of the initial vascular insult. When the ischaemic insult occurs early in gestation, the colon does not fill with meconium and exists as a microcolon. When the vascular insult occurs late in gestation, a meconium-filled colon already exists, and these neonates may evacuate the meconium distal to the atresia within the first few days of life.

An abdominal radiograph will demonstrate a characteristic pattern of dilated bowel proximal to the atresia. Contrast enema can be used to delineate the distal bowel anatomy, but contrast will fail to reflux into the dilated proximal bowel.

## Meconium Ileus and Meconium Plug Syndrome

An inability to pass meconium within the first few days of life can be indicative of functional obstruction of the distal bowel. These babies tend to be distended, can have bilious emesis and do not tolerate feeds well. Rectal examination with the passage of a rubber catheter is useful to determine the presence of meconium. Rectal irrigations may help to determine the presence of meconium plugs.

**Meconium plug syndrome** is characterized by the presence of white fibrous plugs within the colon that are thick and difficult to pass, thereby causing a functional obstruction. Abdominal radiographs demonstrate a distal obstructive picture. A contrast enema shows filling defects within the colon and a reflux of contrast into the more proximal dilated bowel.

**Meconium ileus** is associated with cystic fibrosis and is characterized by inspissated meconium within the distal small bowel that causes an obstruction. These infants can become quite distended, and the abdomen may have a doughy consistency due to the presence of small bowel loops distended with thick meconium.

Abdominal radiographs may show a 'ground-glass' appearance in the distal ileum consistent with inspissated meconium and grossly dilated small bowel loops. A contrast enema will show a small colon with a reflux of contrast into the area of the terminal ileum, thereby excluding possible atresia. Water-soluble contrast enemas can help with the evacuation of meconium to relieve the obstruction without the need for surgery. Neonates presenting with meconium ileus should be tested for cystic fibrosis.

## Hirshsprung's Disease

Hirshsprung's disease is a functional bowel disorder in which part of the colon lacks ganglion cells. In normal development, neural crest cells migrate in an ordered progression from proximal to distal to innervate the colon. An arrest of migration can occur at any location along the length of the bowel, leaving the bowel length distal to the point of migratory arrest without ganglion cells. This bowel does not have normal motility and produces a functional point of obstruction.

Patients can present within the first few days of life with a delayed passage of meconium, abdominal distension and sometimes bilious emesis. Alternatively, if the segment of aganglionic colon is short, infants may present later in life. Rectal examination can produce a forceful expulsion of liquid stool. In cases of enterocolitis, the stool may appear greyish in colour and unusually foul-smelling. Enterocolitis can result in death and requires prompt treatment with antibiotics, intravenous fluid resuscitation and evacuation of the retained stool with saline rectal irrigations.

A contrast enema may demonstrate a transition point between the proximal, dilated, ganglionated bowel and the distal decompressed, aganglionated bowel. In early presentations, the transition point may not yet be apparent on such studies. The diagnosis is confirmed with a rectal biopsy to look for the presence of ganglion cells.

## ABDOMINAL WALL DEFECTS

Defects of abdominal wall closure are obvious at the time of birth. The two most common abdominal wall defects are gastroschisis and omphalocele. These can be distinguished based on the extrusion of abdominal organs, the presence of a covering membrane and the position of the umbilical cord insertion.

**Gastroschisis** is characterized by exposure of bowel contents without an outer covering (**Figure 38.6**). The defect is usually to the right of the umbilical cord. An **omphalocele** is characterized by extruded abdominal contents covered by a sac composed of amnion. The umbilical cord inserts onto the centre of the sac (**Figure 38.7**). In cases of giant omphaloceles, the sac may contain liver as well as bowel.

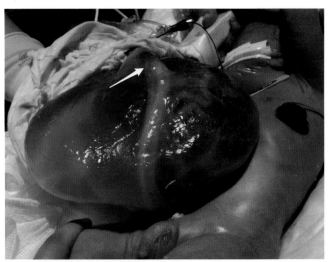

Figure 38.7 Omphalocele. The umbilical cord inserts onto the sac (arrow).

## ANORECTAL MALFORMATIONS

Anorectal malformations or 'imperforate anus' represent a broad spectrum of anatomical defects in which the rectum fails to descend and the anus does not form properly. Physical examination at birth reveals meconium output from a fistula tract located more anteriorly on the perineum and the absence of a well-formed anus in the normal location.

In cases where the rectum is high in the pelvis, the fistula tract may connect with the genitourinary tract instead of the perineal skin. These 'high' defects are associated with a higher incidence of genitourinary anomalies and poorer functional outcomes. In infants with fistulas to the proximal urethra or bladder neck, there is poor development of the perineal musculature and a flat perineum. Infants with features of Down syndrome and an absent anus often have well-formed perineal muscles without a perineal fistula and represent a special category of anorectal malformation.

## ACQUIRED DISORDERS

Some of the most common surgical illnesses present beyond the neonatal period (after 1 month of life) and the age at the time of presentation becomes helpful in distinguishing these entities from one another (Table 38.1).

### Pyloric Stenosis

Pyloric stenosis generally presents between 2 and 8 weeks of life and is characterized by progressive non-bilious emesis. Failure of the stomach to empty because of the hypertrophied pylorus results in an overdistended stomach and retained feedings. Parents often report the forceful projectile emesis of curdled milk of volumes in excess of the volume of their most recent feeding. These infants often appear dehydrated with a sunken fontanelle, and produce less urine.

In the calm infant, the hypertrophied pylorus can be palpated just under the liver edge. Ultrasound is often used to measure the length of the pyloric channel and the thickness of the muscle to confirm the diagnosis.

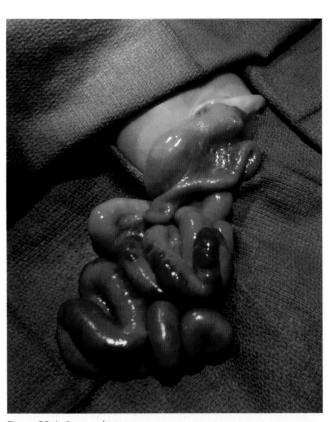

Figure 38.6 Gastroschisis.

Table 38.1 Common acquired paediatric surgical diseases

| | Age of presentation | Physical signs | Tips for interpreting the physical examination |
|---|---|---|---|
| Pyloric stenosis | 2–8 weeks | Right upper quadrant mass | The infant must be calm and the abdominal wall relaxed to palpate the pylorus |
| Intussusception | 3 months – 3 years | Normal examination<br>Blood in the stool | Persistent or recurrent intussusception is sometimes palpable as a right lower quadrant mass |
| Appendicitis | Any age | Right lower quadrant tenderness | Distracting techniques are often necessary to distinguish true tenderness from the child's fear of examination |
| Omphalomesenteric duct remnant (e.g. Meckel's diverticulum) | Any age | Blood in the stool<br>Can mimic appendicitis or bowel obstruction | Physical findings depend on the anatomy of the remnant |

## Intussusception

Ileocolic intussusception generally occurs in toddlers when the proximal bowel 'telescopes' within the adjacent colon. This is frequently associated with a prodrome of gastroenteritis when lymphoid aggregates with the bowel wall hypertrophy and serves as lead points for the intussusception.

The children present with episodic, colic-type abdominal pain. The presence of blood within the stool is indicative of mucosal ischaemia and is a late sign. Abdominal examination is usually unremarkable except in advanced cases in which a perforation has occurred and signs of peritonitis may be present. If the intussusception has progressed distally, the intussusception may be palpated by digital rectal examination. The diagnosis may be confirmed with ultrasound or contrast enema.

## Acute Appendicitis

Acute appendicitis can occur at any age, but the presentation is often delayed in younger children. Young children more often present with perforation and fever. Abdominal examination is characterized by right lower quadrant tenderness but may also demonstrate diffuse tenderness and abdominal wall rigidity characteristic of peritonitis. Physical examination of the abdomen can be difficult due to the child's fear of pain. Distracting techniques such as using a stethoscope or the child's own hand to palpate the abdomen are extremely useful.

## Omphalomesenteric Duct Remnant

The omphalomesenteric duct exists as a connection between the yolk sac and the mesentery during embryological development and is then obliterated by 9 weeks of gestation. Remnants of this *in utero* connection can exist as a diverticulum of the small bowel or Meckel's diverticulum (**Figure 38.8**), a fibrous band from the small bowel to the abdominal wall or more rarely an enterocutaneous fistula from the small bowel to the umbilicus.

The timing of presentation is variable. A Meckel's diverticulum may present with painless intestinal bleeding or diverticulitis with symptoms similar to those of acute appendicitis. In patients without a prior history of abdominal surgery, symptoms of small bowel obstruction should alert the practitioner to the possibility of a fibrous band from an omphalomesenteric duct remnant causing bowel obstruction. Abdominal examination can range from completely benign to signs of peritonitis or emesis and abdominal distension characteristic of small bowel obstruction. The abdominal signs correlate with the anatomy of the variant of duct remnant that is present.

## NECROTIZING ENTEROCOLITIS

Necrotizing enterocolitis is a condition associated with prematurity in which the intestine becomes ischaemic, usually in response to the initiation of enteric feeding. Clinically, this process manifests with abdominal distension, bloody stools and/or emesis. Symptoms often progress rapidly, with neonates exhibiting lethargy, apnoea, bradycardia and hypotension. Abdominal wall erythema can be indicative of perforation. In male neonates with hernias, the scrotum may become discoloured, indicating the presence of free air (bluish) or free meconium (dark) within the abdomen.

Abdominal radiographs may demonstrate pneumatosis within the bowel wall or portal venous gas. In cases of full-thickness ischaemia, free air indicates the presence of a perforation.

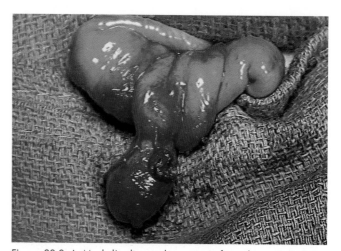

Figure 38.8 A Meckel's diverticulum arising from the antimesenteric surface of the small bowel.

## JAUNDICE IN INFANCY

Jaundice in the newborn period is a common occurrence and reflects the immaturity of the liver. So-called 'physiological jaundice' usually fades within the first week of life as babies begin feeding well and passing stools

Jaundice that persists, is progressive, or is accompanied by symptoms of extrahepatic biliary obstruction (e.g. acholic stools or tea-coloured urine), should raise concern for biliary atresia. On examination, patients have icterus, obvious jaundice and a firm, palpable liver edge. While the precise aetiology of biliary atresia remains unknown, this is a progressive inflammatory process of the biliary architecture, and the outcome is best when the disease is identified and treated before 8 weeks of age.

### Key Points

- The differential diagnosis of neonatal bowel obstruction can be narrowed down based on the onset and type of the presenting symptoms. Most diagnoses are confirmed with plain radiographs.
- Bilious emesis in the neonatal period should prompt immediate concern for malrotation with midgut volvulus and is a paediatric surgical emergency.
- Common paediatric surgical diseases are best distinguished by the age of presentation and the abdominal examination. When examining children, distracting techniques are often needed to differentiate the child's fear of examination from true abdominal tenderness.
- Neonatal jaundice that persists for longer than 2 weeks, is progressive or is associated with acholic stools should prompt evaluation for biliary atresia.

## QUESTIONS

### SBAs

**1.** A 4-week-old infant, feeding well prior to presentation, has a **sudden** onset of bright green emesis without abdominal distension. Which is the most concerning possible diagnosis?:
- **a** Midgut volvulus
- **b** Jejunal atresia
- **c** Pyloric stenosis
- **d** Hirshsprung's disease

**Answer**

**a** *Midgut volvulus. Bilious emesis is the hallmark presentation of midgut volvulus and is a surgical emergency. Infants with jejunal atresia or Hirshsprung's disease can also have bilious emesis, but a baby with atresia would be unable to tolerate feedings at home for 4 weeks. Hirshsprung's disease is a distal obstruction and is associated with abdominal distension. Babies with pyloric stenosis have non-bilious emesis.*

**2.** A newborn baby chokes with initial breastfeeding attempts. The nurse notices that the baby drools and does not tolerate lying down. What is the most likely diagnosis?:
- **a** Duodenal stenosis
- **b** Oesophageal atresia
- **c** Meconium ileus
- **d** Malrotation

**Answer**

**b** *Oesophageal atresia. An inability to tolerate initial feeds is indicative of a proximal obstruction. An inability to handle oral secretions points to obstruction at the oesophageal level. Infants with duodenal obstruction can handle oral secretions but usually have emesis shortly after feeding. Meconium ileus causes bowel obstruction at the level of the terminal ileum and is associated with the development of marked abdominal distension.*

**3.** A 1–month-old premature infant, weighing 750 g, has been tolerating feeds and develops bradycardia, bilious emesis, abdominal distension and abdominal erythema. What is the most likely diagnosis?:
- **a** Midgut volvulus
- **b** Jejunal atresia
- **c** Necrotizing enterocolitis
- **d** Pyloric stenosis

**Answer**

**c** *Necrotizing enterocolitis. Bilious emesis should always prompt concern for midgut volvulus, and this diagnosis must be excluded. However, given the clinical history, necrotizing enterocolitis is the most likely diagnosis. Babies with jejunal atresia may also present with bilious emesis but do so in the first few days of life and would not be able to tolerate feeds for 1 month.*

### EMQs

**1.** Match the characteristics with the appropriate diagnosis given below. Characteristics can be associated with more than one diagnosis:
- **1** Non-bilious emesis
- **2** Bloody stool
- **3** Toddler
- **4** Six-week-old infant
- **5** Fever
- **6** Right upper quadrant mass
- **7** Right lower quadrant mass
- **8** Abdominal cramps
- **9** Right lower quadrant tenderness
- **a** Appendicitis
- **b** Intussusception
- **c** Pyloric stenosis
- **d** Meckel's diverticulum

**Answers**

**a** *5, 7, 9. Appendicitis can present at any age. A perforated appendicitis can be associated with fever and a palpable right lower quadrant inflammatory mass.*

**b** *2, 3, 7, 8. Intussusception occurs in toddlers, and the intussusception can sometimes be palpated in the right lower quadrant. A bloody stool indicates mucosal ischaemia from recurrent or persistent intussusception.*

**c** *1, 4, 6. Pyloric stenosis is characterized by non-bilious emesis in infants aged 2–8 weeks. In the relaxed child, the thickened pyloric muscle is palpable in the right upper quadrant just below the liver edge.*

**d** *2, 5, 7, 8. Meckel's diverticulum can present at any age. If the diverticulum contains gastric mucosa, acid production causes small bowel ulceration and painless bleeding with blood in the stool. When the diverticulum becomes inflamed, the presentation can mimic appendicitis.*

PART 8 | ABDOMINAL

**2. Match the physical findings with the appropriate abdominal wall defect:**

1 Covered defect
2 Herniated liver
3 Herniated bowel
4 Defect to the right of the umbilicus
5 Umbilicus inserts within the defect

a Gastroschisis
b Omphalocele

**Answers**

**a 3, 4.** *Gastroschisis is an abdominal wall defect characterized by herniated bowel that does not have a membranous covering. The defect is seen to the right of the umbilicus.*

**b 1, 2, 3, 5.** *Omphaloceles are covered by a membrane, with the umbilical cord inserting directly onto the membrane. Bowel as well as liver can herniate out of the abdominal domain and into the sac.*

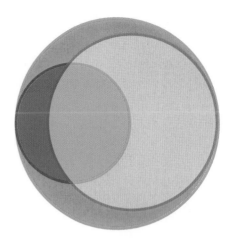

# PART
## 9

# Genitourinary

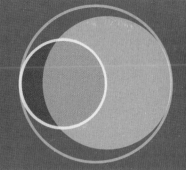

CHAPTER

# 39

# The Genitourinary System and Genitalia

William Cross

## LEARNING OBJECTIVES

- To understand that many urological conditions present with a similar symptom complex
- To elicit an accurate urological diagnosis from a thorough medical history and physical examination
- To understand the importance of routine dipstick urinalysis

- To be able to request appropriate radiological investigations to confirm and further characterize a clinical condition
- To develop skills in identifying the clinical signs of acute urological emergencies that require prompt management to avoid significant morbidity

## INTRODUCTION

The urinary tract is relatively inaccessible to physical examination, and urologists have increasingly become dependent on radiological imaging and laboratory investigations to diagnose urinary tract pathology. Despite advances in diagnostic technology, the cornerstone in the evaluation of the urology patient remains a thorough medical history and physical examination. The application of these basic clinical skills often leads to an accurate diagnosis or, if not, to a differential diagnosis that guides the selection of the most appropriate laboratory and radiological studies.

## URINALYSIS

Examination of the urine is a simple test that should be considered for all urology patients. It is important to assess the colour and odour of the urine, and the presence of blood and sediment. Urine is normally a pale yellow colour as a result of the pigment urochrome, but it can become discoloured from food substances, medications, products of metabolism, blood and infection. The common causes of an abnormal urine colour are listed in **Table 39.1**. Infected urine is characteristically pungent and cloudy.

Further clinical information can obtained from a dipstick urinalysis and a complete urinalysis that includes microscopic examination of the urine. Most dipstick strips test for blood, protein, glucose, ketones, white blood cells, urobilinogen and bilirubin. The correct dipstick urinalysis technique is as follows. **Correct collection of the urine sample is crucial:**

- In the uncircumcized adult man, the foreskin should be retracted and the glans penis cleansed. For a woman, the labia are separated and cleansed from front to back.

Table 39.1 Common causes of an abnormal urine colour

| Colour | Associated condition |
|---|---|
| Clear | Overhydration |
| Milky/cloudy | Pyuria (pus in the urine), chyluria, phosphaturia |
| Red | Haematuria (blood in the urine), haemoglobinuria, myoglobinuria, beetroot and blackberries |
| Green–blue | Amitriptyline, methylene blue |
| Brown | Urobilinogen, porphyria, nitrofurantoin, metronidazole |
| Brown–black | Haemorrhage, methyldopa |

- To avoid contamination of the urine specimen with skin and urethral organisms, the initial stream of urine is discarded into the toilet and a midstream urine sample is collected into a sterile container. The sample is referred to as a midstream clean-catch urine sample.
- If a patient has a catheter *in situ*, a urine sample can be obtained from the catheter or the urine collection bag for analysis (a catheter specimen of urine).
- In babies and toddlers who are not toilet-trained, a sample of urine can be obtained by attaching a small collection bag to the external genital region.
- The urine sample should be analysed as soon as possible after collection, but if this is not possible the sample should be refrigerated.

The dipstick is immersed in the urine specimen and withdrawn against the edge of the container to remove the excess urine. The dipstick should then be held horizontally for the appropriate length of time for reading the reagent pads.

## Haematuria

Haematuria is the presence of red blood cells in the urine, which may be detected by a dipstick test (dipstick haematuria), urine microscopy (microscopic haematuria) or direct visualization of the urine (visible, gross, frank or macroscopic haematuria). Dipstick and microscopic haematuria are often collectively referred to as non-visible haematuria. Urine dipstick tests are highly sensitive for detecting haematuria, but false-positive readings can result from contamination from menstrual blood, recent exercise and dehydration.

The common causes of haematuria are:

- malignancy of the urinary tract;
- urinary tract infection (UTI);
- urolithiasis;
- renal parenchymal disease;
- benign prostatic hyperplasia (BPH);
- prostatitis;
- trauma to the urinary tract.

## Proteinuria

The detection of protein in the urine may be the first sign of renal disease, and persistent proteinuria requires further evaluation by a quantitative and qualitative measurement of urinary protein(s).

## Glucose and Ketones

Very small amounts of glucose are normally excreted in the urine. If the serum glucose concentration rises (e.g. in diabetes mellitus) and the renal threshold for glucose tubular reabsorption is exceeded, glucose will be excreted in the urine and detected on a dipstick test.

Ketones are not normally excreted in the urine, and a positive dipstick test may occur in diabetic ketoacidosis, in pregnancy and following starvation or weight loss.

## Bilirubin and Urobilinogen

Normal urine contains very little urobilinogen and no bilirubin. A positive dipstick test for bilirubin may indicate intrinsic hepatic disease or obstruction of the bile ducts. Increased urinary urobilinogen is associated with haemolysis and hepatocellular disease.

## Leukocyte Esterase and the Nitrite Test

Leukocyte esterase is produced by neutrophils, and a positive dipstick test indicates the presence of white blood cells in the urine. Urine does not normally contain nitrites, but certain bacteria can convert urine nitrates to nitrites. Both tests are used to screen for UTIs.

## Urine Microscopy

Urine is microscopically examined for cells, casts, crystals, bacteria, yeasts and parasites.

### RENAL FAILURE

Renal failure may occur as the result of underlying urinary tract disease, or alternatively a diagnosis of urinary tract disease may bring to light unsuspected renal impairment, together with its associated clinical features.

Intrinsic renal disease as a cause of renal failure is not considered further here, but obstructive renal failure is due to either urinary tract pathology or extrinsic compression of the urinary tract from some other pathological process. It may be acute or chronic in onset, and may result from pathology anywhere along the length of the urinary tract from the kidney to the external urethral meatus. For these reasons, the clinical features of renal failure are considered before those associated with individual urinary tract organs.

Acute or chronic renal failure can be due to pre-renal (renal hypoperfusion), renal (renal parenchymal damage) or post-renal (acute obstruction to renal flow) causes. The predominant cause related to urinary tract disease is the gradual onset of post-renal failure resulting from obstruction to the excretion of urine.

## Acute Renal Failure

Acute renal failure or, as it is more often referred to, acute kidney injury, is defined as an abrupt or rapid decline in renal filtration function. It is often clinically dramatic in onset and, because of the high frequency of associated problems, has a high mortality. It has a tendency to appear in patients with pre-existing renal disease, especially chronic vascular ischaemia. It is a potentially reversible syndrome characterized by a marked rise in the serum creatinine concentration and a retention of nitrogenous waste products. There are many causes but perhaps those most commonly seen are sepsis, drug toxicity and obstruction to urine flow.

### Causes of Acute Renal Failure

Pre-renal causes are:

- fluid loss: haemorrhage, burns, gastrointestinal fluid loss;
- hypotension: myocardial infarction, septicaemic shock, drugs;
- renovascular disease: embolus, dissection, atheroma;
- increased renal vascular resistance: hepatorenal syndrome.

Renal causes include:

- toxins and drugs: for example, aminoglycosides, contrast material, non-steroidal anti-inflammatory agents;
- acute tubular necrosis secondary to ischaemia;
- eclampsia;
- bacterial interstitial nephritis;
- rhabdomyolysis.

Post-renal causes are:

- urethral obstruction: calculus, trauma, posterior valves, phimosis;
- bladder neck obstruction: BPH or prostate cancer, calculus, pelvic tumour;
- ureteric obstruction: trauma, retroperitoneal fibrosis, calculi, pelvic tumour.

The clinical state of patients presenting with acute renal failure ranges from those in whom only a biochemical abnormality has been detected to those who are gravely ill with multiple organ failure. The initial assessment depends on the clinical situation encountered. However, all patients should undergo an assessment of their fluid status by examining their blood pressure, skin turgor and central venous pressure, and by looking for signs of pulmonary, ankle and sacral oedema. It is also useful to review the records of urine output and fluid balance for the preceding hours or days, as well as the recent drug history.

Investigations to document the degree of uraemia, hyperkalaemia and acidosis should be urgently undertaken as early treatment may be imperative.

## Chronic Renal Failure

A chronic failure of renal function results in a number of clinical manifestations that relate to functions of the kidney, namely the failure of body salt and water homoeostasis, a reduction in urea excretion and a failure of normal red blood cell production. The onset is gradual, over many months or years, and the patient typically passes through three clinical stages:

- *Renal insufficiency*: The patient is usually asymptomatic but with mildly abnormal serum and plasma biochemical investigation results, and is at risk of acute renal decompensation.
- *Renal failure*: Persistent malaise and osteomalacia are seen, and nocturia is invariably present.
- *Uraemia*: The patient is unwell, anaemic, acidotic, hypocalcaemic, hypophosphataemic and hyperkalaemic.

A number of clinical features develop during the gradual onset of chronic renal failure. These are all related to the loss of renal function and should each be considered when examining these patients. An obvious cause for the renal failure should also be considered during this examination. Features to assess include:

- signs of chronic uraemia: skin excoriation, brown arcs on the nails, pigmentation, anaemia, neuropathy and pericardial rub, restless legs syndrome;
- acidosis: as demonstrated by rapid shallow breathing – Kussmaul breathing;
- fluid status: skin turgor, venous pressure, peripheral and pulmonary oedema;
- signs of urinary tract obstruction.

If the chronic renal failure persists, the patient ultimately reaches end-stage renal failure and requires some form of renal replacement therapy. The aetiologies of end-stage renal failure in the UK are:

- glomerulonephritis (30 per cent);
- pyelonephritis (reflux) (20 per cent);
- polycystic kidneys (10 per cent)
- hypertension (10 per cent);
- renal vascular disease (10 per cent);
- drugs (10 per cent);
- unknown causes (10 per cent).

## URINARY TRACT INFECTION

Urinary tract infection is a bacterial invasion of the urothelium (the epithelial lining of the urinary tract) resulting in an inflammatory response that usually presents as urinary frequency, urgency, dysuria and associated pyuria and bacteriuria.

Urinary tract infections are among the most prevalent of infectious diseases. It has been estimated that half of all women in the UK will have a UTI at least once in their life, and one out of every 2000 healthy men will develop one each year.

In the majority of cases, the UTI is a simple and isolated infection that responds to short course of an oral antimicrobial agent. However, some patients develop severe symptoms requiring hospitalization and intravenous therapy. In this group, it is important to consider whether the infection is complicated by an underlying structural or functional abnormality of the urinary tract, or by the presence of a condition that can interfere with the host defence mechanisms.

## Acute Pyelonephritis

Acute pyelonephritis is defined as inflammation of the renal parenchyma and renal pelvis. The condition usually presents with loin or abdominal pain, fever and nausea. In the majority of cases, the causative pathogens have ascended from the bladder and the abdominal symptoms are preceded by cystitis.

On examination (Table 39.2), the patient is tender within the loin region, as well as suprapubically if they have coexisting cystitis. Urinalysis usually reveals haematuria, pyuria and occasionally nitrates. Urine and blood cultures are typically positive for enteric gram-negative bacteria.

Pregnant women should be screened for bacteriuria during the first trimester as 20–40 per cent of women with asymptomatic bacteriuria develop pyelonephritis during pregnancy.

## Emphysematous Pyelonephritis

Emphysematous pyelonephritis is a severe necrotizing infection of the renal parenchyma in which gas forms within the collecting system, renal and/or perirenal tissues (Figure 39.1). The condition can be severe and potentially life-threatening, and its diagnosis requires a high index of suspicion as it presents in a similar way to acute pyelonephritis. Although more common in the elderly, it can present at any age. Ninety-five per cent of patients have diabetes, which is often poorly controlled. Physical examination typically reveals flank or abdominal pain and occasionally crepitus in the flank area in advanced cases.

## Xanthogranulomatous Pyelonephritis

Xanthogranulomatous pyelonephritis is a rare condition characterized by focal or diffuse parenchymal destruction and replacement with granulomatous infiltrates containing lipid-laden macrophages. Most cases are associated with urinary tract obstruction (secondary to calculi, pelviureteric junction obstruction or urothelial cell carcinoma), infection and diabetes.

Patients with the condition often present with subacute and non-specific symptoms, including anorexia, weight loss, fever, flank pain and malaise. Xanthogranulomatous pyelonephritis is

Table 39.2 Examination of the kidney

To examine for renal pathology, the patient should lie on their back with their head slightly elevated to relax the abdominal wall. The examiner places one hand beneath the patient's lumbar region and the other on the upper quadrant of the abdomen. If the patient takes deep breaths, the kidney may be palpable between the two examining hands. Although normal kidneys are not usually palpable, the lower pole of the right kidney can occasionally be felt on deep inspiration in thin patients. Typically, an enlarged kidney feels smooth, moves on respiration and is ballotable, that is, it can be 'bounced' back and forth between the examining hands.

An alternative method of examination to palpate the kidney is to turn the patient onto their side with the affected side uppermost and repeat the bimanual examination. A physical sign described is Murphy's 'kidney punch test', which is performed by jabbing under the patient's 12th rib to evoke pain in those with renal inflammation. This physical test is unnecessary as it can cause considerable discomfort and does not elicit any further clinical information than that obtained with gentle palpation.

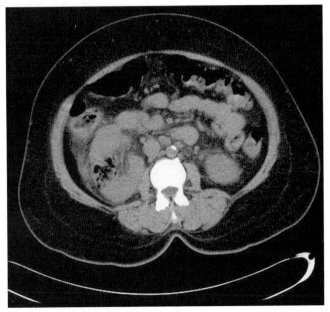

Figure 39.1 Emphysematous pyelonephritis. Note the dark irregular gas shadows in the hilum of the right kidney.

prone to fistula formation, and patients occasionally present with a pyelocutaneous, ureterocutaneous or pyeloenteric fistula.

## Perinephric Abscess

A perinephric abscess is a mass of suppurative material within the perirenal fat, encased within the renal (Gerota's) fascia. It forms either by direct extension secondary to pyelonephritis, by haematogenous seeding from other sites of infection or as a superimposed infection in a perirenal haematoma. Patients who receive haemodialysis for polycystic kidney disease are particularly susceptible to perinephric abscess formation. If a perinephric abscess progresses and ruptures through Gerota's fascia into the pararenal space, it can develop into a paranephric abscess.

Typically, a perinephric abscess presents with symptoms similar to those of acute pyelonephritis, including fever, flank and abdominal pain, weight loss, malaise and gastrointestinal symptoms. In contrast to most patients with an uncomplicated pyelonephritis, those who present with a perinephric abscess have usually been symptomatic for at least a week. Pleuritic pain may be experienced if the abscess is adjacent to the diaphragm.

Physical findings include abdominal tenderness and a flank mass, especially if the abscess is large and located in the region of the inferior pole of the kidney. During movement, the patient may experience pain on flexion of the contralateral thigh and lateral flexion of the spine.

## Pyonephrosis

Pyonephrosis refers to pus in an obstructed collecting system. The condition requires prompt diagnosis and management as any delay can result in sepsis, irreversible renal impairment and death. Patients may present with asymptomatic bacteriuria or, more commonly, infective urinary symptoms, loin pain and a fullness or mass in the flank.

Treatment is with a combination of intravenous antibiotics and decompression of the renal pelvis by placing a percutaneous nephrostomy tube or less frequently an endoscopically inserted ureteric stent.

## Acute Cystitis

Cystitis typically presents with dysuria, urinary frequency and urgency. In most cases, the only abnormality detected on physical examination is suprapubic tenderness. In men, the pathophysiology of cystitis is less well understood than it is in women, and UTIs should be considered to be complicated until proven otherwise. Complicating factors include prostatic enlargement, calculi, urinary tract malignancy, strictures, fistulas and bladder dysfunction. It is therefore important that a thorough urological examination is performed in all men who present with cystitis.

## Prostatitis

Prostatitis is inflammation of the prostate gland that clinically presents as several syndromes with a range of clinical symptoms and investigative findings (Table 39.3).

Prostatitis is a common urological diagnosis, with approximately 50 per cent of men experiencing symptoms of prostatitis during their lifetime. Despite this, acute bacterial prostatitis is relatively unusual in that it accounts for less than 5 per cent of cases of prostatitis. The condition classically presents with fever, chills, pelvic and back pain, urinary frequency, dysuria, urgency and occasionally urinary retention.

If the patient will tolerate it, digital rectal examination (Table 39.4) will reveal a tender, enlarged and warm prostate

Table 39.3 The National Institute of Diabetes and Digestive and Kidney Diseases classification of prostatitis

| Category | Description |
| --- | --- |
| I | Acute bacterial prostatitis |
| II | Chronic bacterial prostatitis |
| III | Chronic abacterial prostatitis – chronic pelvic pain syndrome (CPPS):<br>– IIIa – Inflammatory CPPS (white blood cells in the urine or prostatic secretions)<br>– IIIb – Non-inflammatory CPPS |
| IV | Asymptomatic inflammatory prostatitis (histological prostatitis) |

Table 39.4 Examination of the prostate

The prostate is located beneath the bladder, in front of the rectum. Through the centre of the prostate passes the first part of the urethra (prostatic urethra), into which the prostatic glands drain and the ejaculatory ducts pass to open adjacent to the verumontanum. The prostate is palpable through the rectum.

The examination is commonly performed with the patient in the left lateral position, with the knees and hips flexed so that the buttocks are near the edge of the examining couch or bedside. Using a generous amount of lubricant gel, the gloved index finger is inserted into the rectum and then turned to face the anterior surface, where the lobes of the prostate can be palpated through the rectal mucosa. The seminal vesicles and vasa, neither of which is palpable in the normal individual, lie cranial to the prostate.

The prostate should feel smooth, firm and bilobed with a median sulcus. It is important to assess the size of the prostate, document the maximum transverse distance between the lobes, as well as the consistency, and check for the presence of tenderness, nodules and asymmetry.

gland. If the prostate feels boggy, this suggests the presence of a prostatic abscess, and radiological imaging should be requested. If the patient is systemically unwell, prostatic massage for bacteriology is contraindicated and only the midstream urine is collected for urine culture.

Urinary retention should be managed using a suprapubic catheter to avoid instrumentation of the prostatic urethra. Severe cases of acute bacterial prostatitis require antimicrobial agents first intravenously and then followed by a 3–4 week oral course.

About 5 per cent of cases of acute bacterial prostatitis progress to chronic bacterial prostatitis, which is characterized by recurrent genitourinary and back pain with associated urinary frequency, urgency and dysuria. Other symptoms include urethral discharge, haematospermia and sexual dysfunction. In contrast to acute bacterial prostatitis, the physical findings in chronic bacterial prostatitis are often normal.

The diagnosis is often made by the culture of urine samples taken before and after prostatic massage. The prostatic massage should be performed during the rectal examination and often requires firm palpation to obtain prostatic secretions from the urethral meatus. The ejaculate can also be cultured.

Chronic pelvic pain syndrome (CPPS) is the most common of the prostatitis subgroups. Patients with CPPS often present with a similar symptom complex to those with chronic bacterial prostatitis. The differentiating factor is that CPPS is characterized by an absence of bacteriuria. Examination of the urinary tract in men with CPPS is usually normal. The distinction between inflammatory and non-inflammatory CPPS is academic as the management of the two subgroups is similar.

## Epididymitis and Orchitis

Epididymitis and orchitis are inflammation, usually secondary to infection, of the epididymis and testicle, respectively. Infection of the epididymis that progresses to the adjoining testicle is referred to as epididymo-orchitis.

Both pathologies typically present with scrotal pain and swelling, which develop over a couple of days, in contrast to torsion of the spermatic cord, which presents within hours. Associated symptoms include dysuria, urinary frequency, urgency and occasionally fever and urethral discharge. A common cause of isolated orchitis is mumps, in which testicular pain is usually preceded by fever, malaise and parotiditis.

On examination, orchitis and epididymitis are characterized by swelling and tenderness of the respective tissue with erythematous and oedematous overlying scrotal skin. The discomfort may be relieved by elevating the affected hemiscrotum (Prehn's sign). In advanced cases, a reactive hydrocele may occur, making scrotal examination more difficult.

## Tuberculosis

Tuberculosis (TB) of the genitourinary system is usually caused by haematogenous and/or lymphatic dissemination of mycobacteria from a primary lung infection, or very rarely by direct inoculation during sexual intercourse. Genitourinary TB can affect the whole of the urinary tract from the kidney to the testis, and patients usually present with chronic, intermittent and non-specific symptoms. Often, before a diagnosis of TB is considered, patients will have received multiple courses of antibiotics for suspected recurrent UTIs. The most common presenting features are urinary frequency, nocturia, dysuria, fever, suprapubic pain, flank pain, haematuria and pyuria.

Bacilli can spread into the lower urinary tract from renal granulomas that erode into the calyceal system. Ureteral TB often leads to strictures and upper tract obstruction, or occasionally ureteric dilatation (**Figure 39.2**). Involvement of the bladder usually initially manifests in the region of the ureteric orifices with fibrosis and obstruction or ureteric reflux. Rarely, in severe cases, the bladder wall becomes fibrotic and shrunken. Tuberculosis of the epididymis and vas characteristically causes nodular beading and may result in infertility if there is bilateral obstruction. In severe cases of infection of the scrotal contents, a discharging sinus may form. Prostatic and urethral TB is rare in developed countries.

## Schistosomiasis

It is estimated that over 200 million people worldwide are infected with organisms of the genus *Schistosoma*, with 97 per cent of cases of centred around North and West Africa and the Middle East. Urinary tract schistosomiasis is caused by infestation with a trematode fluke, the most common species being *Schistosoma haematobium*, *S. mansoni* and *S. japonicum*. Travel to endemic areas and swimming, bathing and wading in contaminated water can result in infection.

Schistosomiasis is the result of direct penetration of the skin by free-swimming cercariae released from freshwater snails. The cercariae enter the venous system, traverse the pulmonary circulation and migrate to the perivesical veins. There, each adult female (about 2 cm long) produces 50–300 eggs per day. These migrate into the lumen of the bladder before being shed into the urine. On their way, they induce a granulomatous response leading to ulceration of the mucosa on the release of the eggs into the lumen.

The clinical manifestations depend on the egg load, the patient's immune status and the degree of secondary infection. However, most infected patients exhibit haematuria and, on cystoscopic examination, have typical perioval granulomas visible on the mucosal surface. They later develop ulceration, fibrosis and calcification. Lower ureteric involvement is a feature of heavy or prolonged infection and leads to obstruction and hydronephrosis.

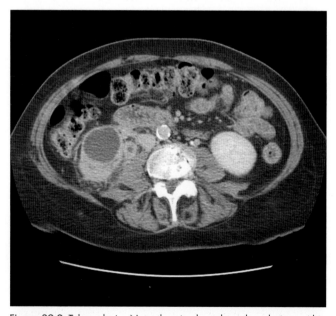

Figure 39.2 Tuberculosis. Note the circular tuberculous lesion within the right kidney.

Chronic infection has also been shown to be a risk factor for the development of bladder cancer, especially squamous cell carcinoma of the bladder, which is an uncommon variant in non-endemic areas.

## Fournier's Gangrene

Fournier's gangrene is a necrotizing infection of the external genitalia that is a urological emergency. Delayed diagnosis and intervention often results in significant morbidity and occasionally death. The typical presentation is with pain, swelling and erythema of the genitalia.

On examination, there may signs of necrosis of the soft tissues (Figure 39.3) and subcutaneous crepitus secondary to gas-forming bacteria. The source of the infection is usually the large bowel, urinary tract or skin of the genitalia. Patients often have multiple comorbidities that compromise the immune system, which precipitates and augments the infection. The mainstay of therapy is broad-spectrum intravenous antimicrobials and surgical debridement of the necrotic tissue (Figure 39.4).

## Sexually Transmitted Infections

### Gonorrhoea

Gonorrhoea is a common infectious condition caused by the bacterium *Neisseria gonorrhoeae*. Approximately 10 per cent of infected men and 50 per cent of infected women are asymptomatic. Men may complain of dysuria and a urethral discharge, which may be clear, yellow or green in colour (Figure 39.5). Infected women may experience vaginal discharge, dysuria and pelvic pain (Figure 39.6).

### Non-gonococcal Urethritis

Infectious urethritis is commonly categorized as either gonococcal urethritis or non-gonococcal urethritis (NGU). The latter is usually caused by infection with *Chlamydia trachomatis*, *Ureaplasma urealyticum*, *Mycoplasma hominis* or *Trichomonas vaginalis*.

Patients with NGU typically develop symptoms 4 days to 2 weeks after contact with an infected individual. Approximately 25 per cent of cases of NGU are asymptomatic and present following partner screening (this can be up to 75 per cent of women with *C. trachomatis* infection). Symptoms include urinary frequency, dysuria and a discharge. The discharge is more watery than that of gonorrhoea (Figure 39.7).

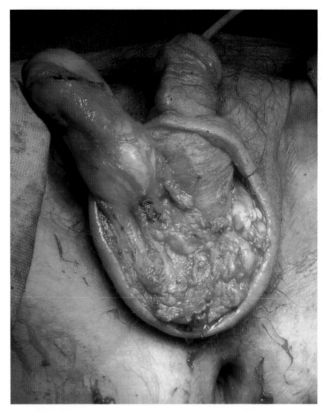

Figure 39.4 Fournier's gangrene – post-surgical excision of gangrenous tissue.

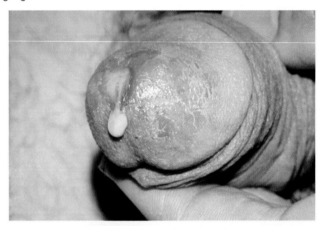

Figure 39.5 Gonorrhoea in a man.

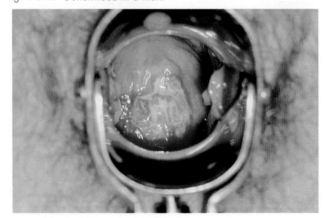

Figure 39.6 Gonorrhoea in a woman.

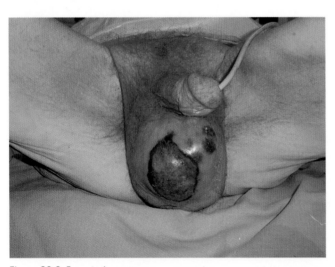

Figure 39.3 Fournier's gangrene – pre-surgery.

## Genital Herpes

Genital herpes can be caused by infections with either herpes simplex virus type 1 or type 2. In primary genital herpes, the patient typically starts to experience constitutional symptoms (fever, headache, malaise) and local symptoms (pain, dysuria, itch, urethral and vaginal discharge) after an incubation period between 1 day and 3 weeks. Herpetic vesicles appear on the external genitalia (Figure 39.8) and progress to encrusted pustules or rupture, resulting in tender ulcers. Recurrent genital herpes is common, occurring in up to 90 per cent of patients within the first 12 months.

## Genital Warts

Genital warts (condylomata acuminata), caused by infection with human papillomavirus (HPV), vary from discrete papules to large exophytic masses. They may appear on the frenulum, glans and shaft of the penis and may extend into the urethra (Figure 39.9). Infection has been associated with changes in the cervical epithelium that may progress to cervical intraepithelial neoplasia and later to invasive carcinoma.

## Syphilis

Syphilis is caused by the spirochaete *Treponema pallidum*. The primary route of infection is through sexual contact, but it may also be transmitted from mother to fetus *in utero* or at birth (congenital syphilis). If not managed appropriately, the condition can progress through four stages: primary, secondary, latent and tertiary.

The **primary stage** usually presents with a single lesion (a chancre) on the glans penis in men (Figure 39.10) and on the vulva or cervix in women. Occasionally, and especially if the patient is co-infected with HIV, multiple lesions may occur. The lesion(s) typically resolves after 4–8 weeks. Non-tender lymphadenopathy frequently occurs in the region of infection.

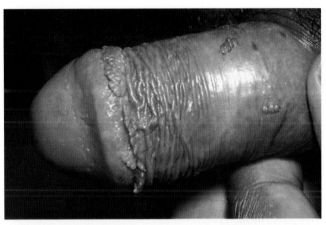
Figure 39.9 Genital warts.

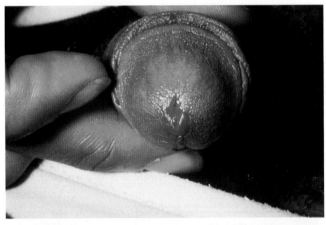
Figure 39.7 Non-gonococcal urethritis caused by *Chlamydia*.

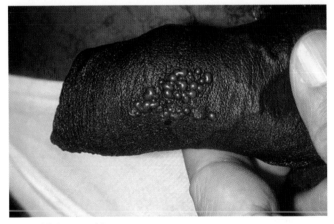
Figure 39.8 Genital herpes.

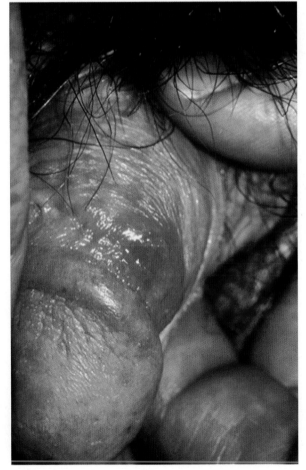
Figure 39.10 Primary syphilis.

**Secondary syphilis** occurs 4–10 weeks after the primary infection and usually manifests as a symmetrical non-pruritic rash on the trunk (Figure 39.11) and extremities, including the palms and soles (Figure 39.12). Other symptoms may include fever, malaise, weight loss, headache and fatigue. The acute symptoms usually resolve after 3–6 weeks.

During the **latent** phase, which may last many years, affected individuals are usually asymptomatic. The manifestations of **tertiary syphilis** include symptoms of neurosyphilis and cardiovascular syphilis.

## URINARY TRACT CALCULI

Urinary tract stone disease is a common condition, with a lifetime risk for stone formation of approximately 20 per cent for men and 10 per cent for women. The highest incidence of urinary tract stones occurs in the 20–50-year-old group, but patients of all ages, including children, can be affected. Risk factors for stone formation include a low urinary volume, metabolic abnormalities, UTI and drug-induced nephrolithiasis.

### Renal and Ureteric Calculi

Clinically, small calculi and even large renal stones (staghorn calculi) may be asymptomatic, and the only abnormality may be dipstick or microscopic haematuria. More commonly, if the stone partially or totally obstructs the upper urinary tract, it induces renal pain, often referred to as a renal colic.

Renal pain is caused by acute distension of the renal capsule, and the discomfort radiates from the flank anteriorly towards the umbilicus. Renal pain may be confused with pain secondary to intraperitoneal pathology. Typically, patients with renal pain usually roll around holding their loin, whereas those with pain due to intraperitoneal disease prefer to lie still to limit irritation of the peritoneum.

Obstruction of the ureter by a calculus induces distension and spasm of the ureter (Figure 39.13). The location of the obstructing stone (Table 39.5) can often be estimated by the location of the referred pain:

- With obstruction of the *mid-ureter on the right side*, the pain is referred to the right lower quadrant of the abdomen and may be misinterpreted as appendicitis.
- *Left mid-ureteric pain* is referred to the left lower quadrant and can present in a similar way to diverticulitis.
- Stones lodged in the *lower ureter*, especially at the vesicoureteric junction, may cause irritative bladder symptoms, such as urinary frequency, urgency and dysuria.

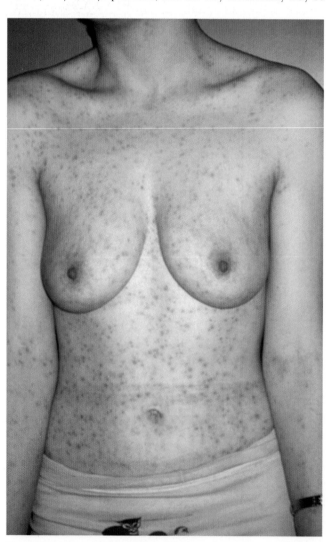

Figure 39.11 Secondary syphilis – lesions on the trunk.

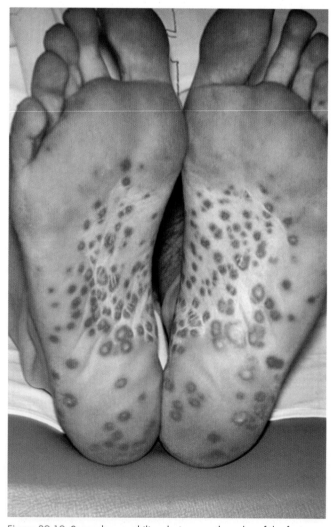

Figure 39.12 Secondary syphilis – lesions on the soles of the feet.

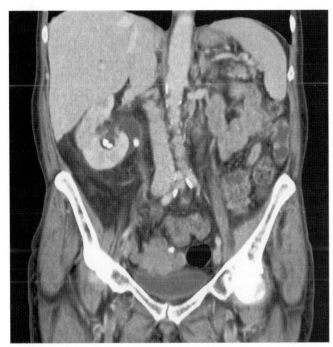

Figure 39.13 Ureteric calculus. Note the two dense white shadows at the same level within the dilated collecting system of the right kidney.

Table 39.5 Examination of the ureter

The ureter descends from the renal pelvis through the retroperitoneum on the psoas muscle, and enters the pelvis in front of the common iliac vessels, anterior to the sacroiliac joint. The ureter then courses downwards and backwards to the level of the ischial spine before turning forwards and medially to enter the posterior wall of the bladder.

The anatomical location of the ureter means that it is impalpable even in diseased states. This means that diagnosis of ureteric pathology usually requires urinary tract imaging and/or direct endoscopic evaluation of the ureter.

Conditions affecting the ureter typically cause obstruction of the lumen, which can cause severe and spasmodic pain, often referred to as ureteric colic. The pain may be referred to cutaneous areas innervated from the same segments of the spinal cord, namely T11–L2. Ureteric colic usually starts at the costovertebral angle and radiates down into the groin and even into the penis or labia majora.

Renal and ureteric colic are often associated with nausea and vomiting because of reflex stimulation of the coeliac ganglion.

## Bladder Calculi

Bladder stones usually result from urinary stasis associated with prostatic enlargement, urethral strictures, bladder diverticula and bladder dysfunction. Patients with static urine who develop a UTI are especially prone to bladder stone formation (**Figure 39.14**). Other predisposing factors include foreign bodies in the bladder, including suture material, ureteral stents, surgical staples and catheters.

The clinical presentation of bladder stones varies from a complete lack of symptoms to suprapubic discomfort, haematuria,

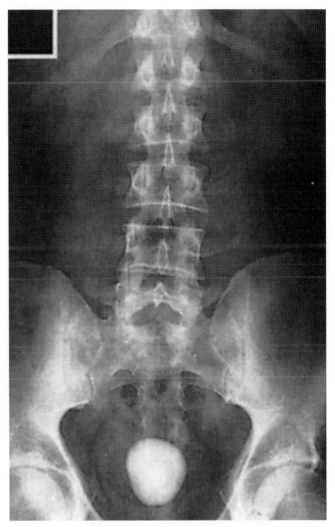

Figure 39.14 Bladder calculi.

dysuria, urinary frequency and an intermittent urinary stream. On examination, the findings may include suprapubic fullness and tenderness, and rarely acute urinary retention if the stone has obstructed the bladder neck or urethra.

## Prostatic Calculi

Prostatic stones are relatively common but are usually of no clinical significance. Occasionally, the calculi form a nidus of infection and lead to chronic UTI. On rectal examination, prostatic calculi in the peripheral aspect of the gland can often be felt as small hard nodules and can be confused with prostatic adenocarcinoma.

### URINARY TRACT MALIGNANCIES

Urological malignancies, specifically cancers of the kidney, bladder, prostate and testis, are very common. Prostate cancer is the most common cancer in men in the UK, with a lifetime risk of 1 in 9 of being diagnosed with the condition. Bladder cancer is the fourth and 11th most common cancer diagnosis in men and women, respectively. This male:female ratio is in part due to the difference in exposure to occupational carcinogens and cigarette smoking.

The risk of prostate and bladder cancer is strongly related to age, with few cases diagnosed below 50 years. In contrast, over 90 per cent of cases of testicular cancer occur in men aged under 55 years, and the condition is the most common cancer in men aged 15–44 years.

## Renal Cancer

Renal cell carcinoma is the eighth most common cancer in the UK and affects more men than women, with nearly two-thirds of patients being over 50 years of age at diagnosis.

Many renal tumours remain asymptomatic until they are advanced. The classic presenting triad of flank pain, gross haematuria and a palpable abdominal mass is rarely seen now as the majority of renal carcinomas are diagnosed at an early stage during abdominal imaging for unrelated and non-specific symptom complexes. These tumours are often referred to as a renal incidentaloma.

Renal carcinoma can give rise to symptoms secondary to local extension, haemorrhage, metastatic spread or paraneoplastic syndromes. Tumour extension into the renal vein can give rise to bilateral peripheral oedema and a varicocele, which supports the role of renal imaging in any man who presents with acute distention of the pampiniform plexus. Other symptoms and signs of advanced disease include weight loss, fever, bone pain, respiratory symptoms and palpable cervical lymphadenopathy.

Approximately 20 per cent of patients with a renal cell carcinoma experience systemic symptoms associated with a diverse range of paraneoplastic syndromes. These include hypertension, hypercalcaemia, hepatic dysfunction (Stauffer's syndrome), anaemia, polycythaemia, neuromyopathy and amyloidosis. These usually improve and return to normal following treatment by radical nephrectomy.

Renal cell carcinoma is associated with von Hippel–Lindau syndrome. Individuals with this rare hereditary cancer syndrome (1 in 36000 births) can develop bilateral, multifocal renal tumours and cysts, haemangioblastomas of the cerebellum and spine, phaeochromocytomas, pancreatic islet cell tumours, retinal haemagiomas and epididymal cystadenomas.

## Wilms' Tumour/Nephroblastoma

Nephroblastoma is the most common solid abdominal tumour of childhood and accounts for more than 90 per cent of malignant renal tumours in children. Typically, the condition presents with a painless abdominal mass in a relatively well child. Pain is unusual but can occur secondary to tumour rupture and haemorrhage following minor abdominal trauma. The symptoms and signs of metastatic spread are rare.

## Renal Pelvis and Ureteric Cancer

Over 90 per cent of tumours that occur in the renal pelvis and ureter arise from the epithelial cell lining of the upper urinary tract, and these are referred to as urothelial or transitional cell carcinomas. Most patients present with microscopic or gross haematuria, less common presentations including flank pain, dysuria or symptoms of advanced disease, including weight loss, anorexia and bone pain. Once suspected, the diagnosis is confirmed with a combination of radiological imaging, urine cytology and ureteroscopy (**Figure 39.15**).

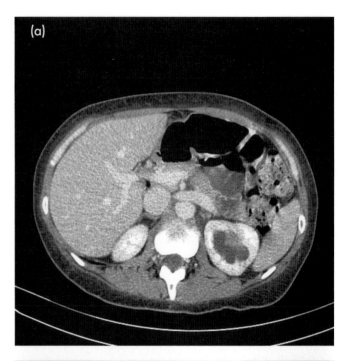

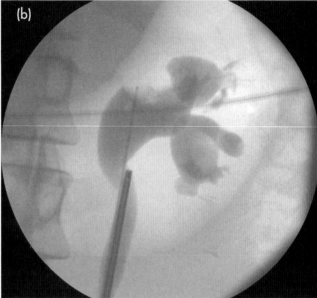

Figure 39.15 (a) A CT scan revealing a left renal pelvic urothelial cell carcinoma. (b) A retrograde pyelogram showing a filling defect consistent with a renal pelvic urothelial cell carcinoma.

## Bladder Cancer

In the UK, urothelial cell carcinoma accounts for over 90 per cent of malignant tumours of the bladder. Less common forms of bladder cancer include squamous cell carcinoma, adenocarcinoma and neuroendocrine tumours. Adenocarcinoma may develop in the bladder as a secondary metastatic lesion from a primary site in the prostate, ovary, endometrium or rectum. Mesenchymal tumours of the bladder are very rare.

Most patients with bladder cancer classically present with painless haematuria, which is gross or microscopic and intermittent in nature. In 20–30 per cent of cases, patients also experience irritative bladder symptoms, including urinary frequency, urgency and dysuria. Bladder cancer should be considered and excluded in all patients with unexplained irritative bladder symptoms, especially if they have had exposure to urothelial carcinogens. Patients with advanced disease may present with weight loss, flank pain secondary to ureteric obstruction, and pelvic and/or bone pain.

Large bladder tumours can cause ureteric obstruction leading to flank pain. Scans reveal large tumours that are capable of causing this degree of upper tract obstruction (Figure 39.16).

At the time of the initial diagnosis, the disease is confined to the superficial bladder wall (Table 39.6) in the majority of patients (75–85 per cent), and they exhibit no signs on physical examination expect for blood in the urine. Patients with muscle-invasive disease may have a palpable bladder mass (Table 39.7).

Examination carried out under anaesthesia allows a more thorough assessment, when the size of the mass and the location and mobility of the tumour can be determined. If the bladder tumour is immobile and the bladder is fixed in position, this suggests that the cancer has invaded the adjacent organs and or the pelvic side wall. Examination should assess for hepatomegaly and lymphadenopathy, both features of metastatic disease.

## Urethral Cancer

Urethral carcinoma is a rare malignancy that is more common in women, with a female to male ratio of 4:1.

The majority of women present with urethral bleeding, urinary frequency and a slow or intermittent urine flow. On examination, the tumour may appear as a papillary growth extending from the meatus, a palpable urethral mass or an ulcerative lesion with induration of the anterior vaginal wall. The tumour may extend into the bladder neck, vagina or vulva, making the clinical diagnosis of the primary lesion difficult. Urethral carcinoma metastasizes to the inguinal lymph nodes, and these must be examined during the clinical assessment (one-third of patients have palpable nodes at presentation).

In men, the condition typically presents in the fifth decade of life and is associated with chronic inflammation secondary to sexually transmitted disease and urethral stricture. The condition

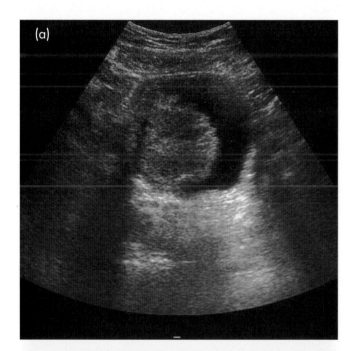

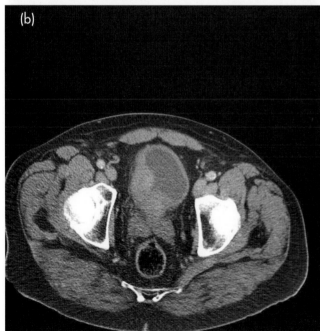

Figure 39.16 Bladder cancer. (a) Ultrasound scan. (b) CT scan.

Table 39.6 Local staging of bladder cancer

| Ta | Tumour confined to the urothelial layer | Superficial/non-muscle-invading bladder cancer |
|---|---|---|
| T1 | Tumour invading the suburothelial layer | |
| T2 | Invasion of the muscle layer | Invasive bladder cancer |
| T3 | Tumour extension into the perivesical fat | |
| T4 | Tumour invasion of adjacent organ and/or the pelvic side wall | |

Table 39.7 Examination of the bladder

The bladder lies in the anterior part of the pelvic cavity, posterior to the pubis. When the bladder fills and distends, it rises above the pubic crest, adopts a spherical shape and comes into contact with the lower anterior abdominal wall. The bladder is extraperitoneal, and surgical access to it can be made without entering the peritoneal cavity.

When significantly distended, the bladder can be felt, especially in thin patients, as a mass in the suprapubic region. It is usually smooth, symmetrical and dull to percussion. In extreme cases, the bladder dome may extend above the umbilicus, and the bladder may also rest on the abdominal aorta, leading to the mistaken diagnosis of an aortic aneurysm due to transmitted pulsations. Other conditions that need to be differentiated from a distended bladder include an ovarian cyst, fibroid uterus and pregnant uterus.

typically presents with urinary symptoms on voiding and, less commonly, urethral discharge, haematospermia and dyspareunia. On examination, the man may have a palpable urethral mass (**Figure 39.17**), urethrocutaneous fistula, periurethral abscess and inguinal lymphadenopathy.

## Prostate Cancer

Prostate cancer accounts for approximately a quarter of all new cases of male cancer in the UK. Although prostate cancer is the second most common cause of cancer death in men, more men die *with* prostate cancer than *because of* the disease.

Most prostate cancers arise in the periphery of the gland and do not cause symptoms in the early stages. It is relatively common for men to be diagnosed with prostate cancer during an investigation of their urinary symptoms secondary to benign prostatic enlargement (BPE) and other pathologies. In this situation, men often falsely believe that their symptoms are a result of the diagnosed prostate cancer.

Men with locally advanced or systemic disease may present with bone pain from skeletal metastases, signs of renal impairment from unilateral or bilateral ureteric obstruction or bowel symptoms from impingement on the rectal canal (despite the close proximity of the gland to the bowel, prostate cancer rarely directly invades the rectal wall).

Spinal metastases can invade or compress the spinal cord, leading to lower limb neurological symptoms and/or autonomic dysfunction, including urinary retention or less frequently bowel or bladder incontinence. Prostate examination is therefore an essential examination in all men presenting with unexplained lower limb neurological symptoms as treatment must be initiated before irreversible damage occurs.

On digital rectal examination (see **Table 39.4**), the clinical signs of prostate cancer include increased firmness of the prostatic tissue, nodularity, loss of symmetry and rarely fixation of the gland due to extension of the cancer into the surrounding pelvic wall.

The prognosis of men presenting with prostate cancer is influenced by multiple factors, especially the stage of the disease (**Table 39.8**). The clinical staging of prostate cancer by palpation can be difficult and requires experience.

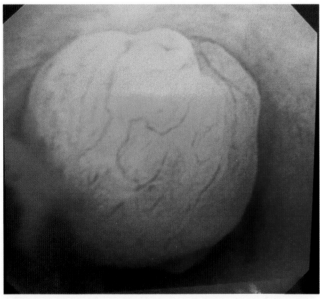

Figure 39.17 A urethral tumour.

## Carcinoma of the Testis

Testicular cancer rarely occurs before puberty. Ninety-five per cent of testicular cancers are germ cell tumours, and 4 per cent are lymphomas, the latter occurring predominantly in men aged over 50 years.

The majority of patients present with a testicular mass that is usually painless or mildly uncomfortable. Rarely, testicular cancer presents with manifestations of metastatic disease, including weight loss, chest symptoms and back pain. Testicular tumours occasionally cause severe scrotal pain secondary to intratumoural haemorrhage.

Examination of the involved testis typically reveals a hard painless mass within the testis, which may extend into the epididymis and spermatic cord (**Table 39.9**). If the tumour has penetrated the tunica albuginea, a secondary hydrocele may be present. General examination can reveal cachexia, enlarged lymph nodes, chest signs, hepatomegaly and gynaecomastia.

Table 39.8 Local staging of prostate cancer

| **T1 – tumour not palpable or visible on imaging** | |
|---|---|
| T1a | Incidental histological finding in <5% of resected tissue (often following transurethral resection of the prostate) |
| T1b | Incidental histological finding in >5% of resected tissue |
| T1c | Positive on prostate needle biopsy |
| **T2 – tumour palpable or visible on imaging and confined to the prostate** | |
| T2a | Involves <50% of one lobe |
| T2b | Involves >50% of one lobe |
| T2c | Involves both lobes |
| **T3 – tumour extends through the prostatic capsule** | |
| T3a | Tumour extends beyond the capsule unilaterally or bilaterally |
| T3b | Tumour invades the seminal vesicle |
| **T4 – tumour extends into adjacent structures other than the seminal vesicles, such as the rectum, levator muscles and/or pelvic wall** | |

Table 39.9 Local staging of testicular tumours

| Tis | Intratubular germ cell neoplasia |
|---|---|
| T1 | Tumour limited to the testis and epididymis without vascular or lymphatic invasion. Tumour may invade the tunica albuginea but not the tunica vaginalis |
| T2 | Tumour limited to the testis and epididymis with vascular or lymphatic invasion, or tumour extends through the tunica albuginea with involvement of the tunica vaginalis |
| T3 | Tumour invades the spermatic cord with or without vascular or lymphatic invasion |
| T4 | Tumour invades the scrotum with or without vascular or lymphatic invasion |

If a testicular tumour is suspected, a scrotal ultrasound (Figure 39.18) and serum tumour markers (alpha-fetoprotein and beta-subunit human chorionic gonadotrophin) should be requested. The prognosis is dependent on the stage of the disease at diagnosis, and treatment should not be delayed as the tumour cell doubling time can be very short. The primary treatment is inguinal orchidectomy unless the patient presents with advanced metastatic disease, in which case urgent referral for primary chemotherapy should be considered.

## Carcinoma of the Penis

Penile cancer is an uncommon malignancy that usually presents at an advanced stage due to delayed medical consultation through fear, embarrassment or self-neglect (Figure 39.19). Delayed diagnosis also occurs as some patients are misdiagnosed and inappropriately managed by their primary care physician.

There are many premalignant penile lesions that, if treated appropriately, can be prevented from progressing to invasive carcinoma. These premalignant lesions can be divided into those related to HPV infection and those that are not HPV-related but are occurring secondary to chronic inflammation (Table 39.10).

Erythroplasia of Queyrat and Bowen's disease are essentially the same condition histologically, differing only in the location of the lesion. Erythroplasia of Queyrat is characterized by smooth, velvety, bright red plaques that occur on the inner prepuce and glans, whereas Bowen's disease produces red, scaly lesions of the skin of the penile shaft.

Bowenoid papulosis predominantly affects young sexually active men and is highly contagious. The lesions are usually multiple, red and velvety, and affect the penile shaft, glans and prepuce.

Condylomata acuminata are exophytic, warty lesions that can affect any part of the anogenital region, especially the coronal sulcus. They occasionally aggregate to produce a giant condyloma acuminatum or Buschke–Löwenstein tumour (Figure 39.20),

Table 39.10 Premalignant penile lesions

| Human papillomavirus-related lesions | Lesions secondary to chronic inflammation |
| --- | --- |
| Erythroplasia of Queyrat | Balanitis xerotica obliterans |
| Bowen's disease | Cutaneous horn |
| Bowenoid papulosis | Leukoplakia |
| Giant condyloma | Pseudoepitheliomatous, keratotic and micaceous balanitis |

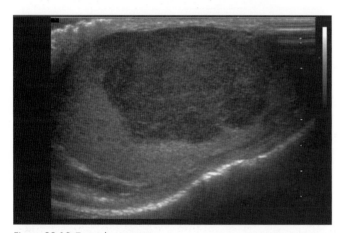

Figure 39.18 Testicular cancer.

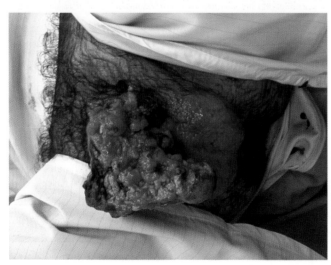

Figure 39.19 Advanced penile cancer

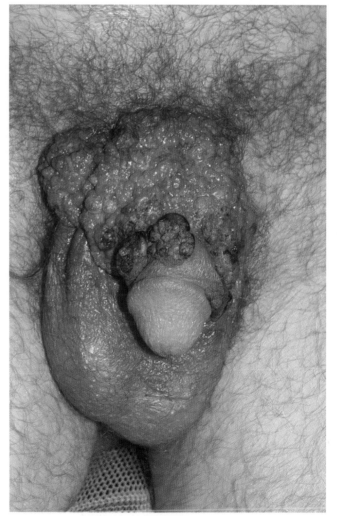

Figure 39.20 A Buschke–Löwenstein tumour.

which can invade adjacent structures in a malignant fashion despite a benign histology.

Balanitis xerotica obliterans (BXO) is a progressive, inflammatory condition of unknown aetiology. It typically presents as pale, atrophic plaques on the glans, prepuce and less commonly the meatus and anterior urethra. In advanced cases, BXO may cause a phimosis and/or meatal stenosis. The association of BXO with invasive carcinoma of the penis remains to be fully established.

A cutaneous penile horn is a rare keratotic lesion that arises secondary to chronic inflammation. Approximately 30 per cent of cases transform into invasive squamous carcinoma.

Leukoplakia is characterized by white plaques that occur on the glans and prepuce. Fewer than 20 per cent of cases reveal dysplastic changes.

At an early stage, penile squamous cell cancer can present in a variety of forms, including a papule, warty growth or ulcerated lesion (Figure 39.21). As most patients are uncircumcised, the lesion may not be discovered until it erodes through the prepuce, becomes infected or bleeds. In advanced cases, the patient may present with a fungating mass involving the metastatic inguinal lymph nodes.

## URINARY INCONTINENCE

Urinary incontinence is defined as the complaint of involuntary loss of urine.

Urinary incontinence is a multifactorial disease process that affects 1 in 4 women and 1 in 9 men at some stage in their lives (Table 39.11). Continence of urine and normal micturition require a complex interplay between the bladder and the urethral sphincter mechanism that is coordinated by the central and peripheral nervous systems. A large number of varied pathologies and conditions can interfere with these mechanisms, resulting in urinary incontinence.

Urinary incontinence is mainly subcategorized based on the symptoms (Table 39.11). **Stress urinary incontinence** usually occurs as a result of urethral sphincter muscle weakness and/or an anatomical defect in the urethral support, leading to insufficient closure pressure in the urethral during physical activity. The urethral sphincter may be weakened after pelvic surgery, neurological injury or pelvic irradiation. Damage to the nerves, muscle and connective tissues of the pelvic floor during childbirth is probably the most common cause of stress incontinence.

**Urge incontinence** may result from detrusor myopathy, neuropathy or a combination of both. If no objective cause can be identified, it is termed idiopathic urge incontinence, whereas neurogenic detrusor incontinence occurs secondary to neurological disease, for example multiple sclerosis, motor neurone lesions and peripheral nerve lesions following pelvic surgery.

**Mixed urinary incontinence** is a combination of stress and urge incontinence. Mixed and urgency incontinence predominate in older women, while stress incontinence is more common in young and middle-aged women.

During the physical examination of patients with urinary incontinence, it is important to check for conditions that may contribute to or exacerbate urinary incontinence or influence management decisions. The abdomen should be examined for masses that may contribute to stress incontinence or may cause bladder outflow obstruction with associated overflow incontinence. The external genitalia and perineum may be erythematous and inflamed secondary to urinary leakage.

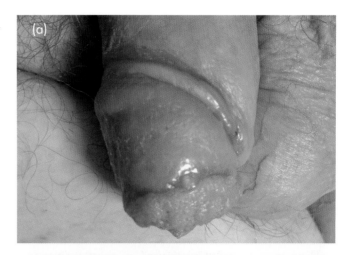

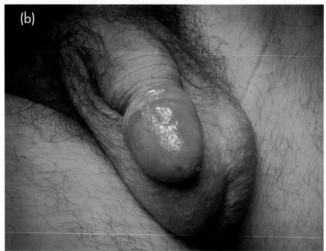

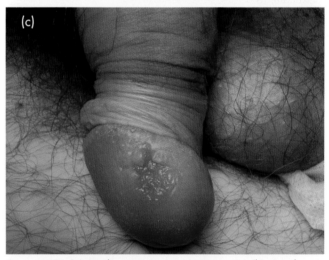

Figure 39.21 (a) Penile cancer – carcinoma-in-situ. (b) An ulcer in penile cancer. (c) Penile cancer.

In women, the tissues of the genitalia may be pale and thin, suggesting oestrogen deficiency (although the role of oestrogen in the continence mechanism remains unclear). The suburethral area and anterior vaginal wall should be inspected for signs of a diverticulum (associated with post-micturition dribbling) or the opening of a fistula tract.

Table 39.11 Types of urinary incontinence

| Type of incontinence | Features |
| --- | --- |
| Stress urinary incontinence | The involuntary leakage of urine on effort, exertion, sneezing or coughing. During these physical activities, the intra-abdominal pressure rises above the urethral resistance, resulting in leakage of urine |
| Urge urinary incontinence | The complaint of involuntary leakage accompanied by or immediately preceded by urinary urgency, urgency being the complaint of a sudden, compelling desire to pass urine that is difficult to defer |
| Mixed urinary incontinence | The complaint of an involuntary leakage of urine associated with urgency and also with exertion, effort, coughing or sneezing |
| Continuous urinary incontinence | The complaint of continuous leakage. This type of incontinence is commonly due to a urinary tract fistula or ectopic ureter |

With the aid of a speculum, a detailed pelvic floor assessment should be performed to look for signs of pelvic organ prolapse, including a cystocele, rectocele, uterine or vaginal prolapse. The patient should be asked to cough and strain to demonstrate stress urinary incontinence by the involuntary leakage of urine from the urethra. A focused neurological examination, concentrating on the sacral segments, should be part of the evaluation to exclude a neurological cause for the incontinence.

## Urinary Tract Fistulas

Urinary tract fistulas are abnormal communications between the urinary tract and the exterior, or with another viscus such as the bowel, uterus or vagina.

Vesicovaginal and ureterovaginal fistulas commonly occur as a complication of gynaecological surgery, pelvic radiation or prolonged and obstructed labour in developing countries. Patients often present with continuous urinary incontinence that may be exacerbated by physical activity, leading to confusion with stress incontinence. Patients who develop a ureterovaginal fistula following pelvic surgery often experience fever, flank pain and gastrointestinal symptoms post-operatively secondary to urinary extravasation. A detailed vaginal examination may reveal an inflamed pinpoint fistula opening.

Enterovesical fistula formation may result from infection, inflammation, neoplasia, trauma or iatrogenic injury. The pathological process is usually intestinal, and diverticulitis accounts for up to 70 per cent of enterovesical fistulas. The symptoms include suprapubic discomfort, debris in the urine, haematuria, pneumaturia and voiding symptoms secondary to UTI. Patients rarely pass urine from their bowel.

## BENIGN UROLOGICAL CONDITIONS

## Kidney

### Renal Cysts

The kidney is one of the most common organs in the body for cysts to occur, and renal cysts are the most common benign renal mass. The incidence of simple renal cysts increases with age, occurring in 20 per cent of individuals by the age of 40 years and approximately 33 per cent after the age of 60 years. Cysts may be single or multiple, and unilateral or bilateral. Typically, they are asymptomatic and diagnosed during abdominal imaging for other clinical conditions. However, they can grow to a considerable size and produce an abdominal mass, discomfort and haematuria secondary to rupture into the upper urinary tract.

Renal cysts that are not simple but contain septations, calcifications, variable margins or suspicious internal areas should be further evaluated by CT or MRI as they may be a manifestation of renal malignancy.

### Renal Angiomyolipoma

A renal angiomyolipoma is a benign renal tumour that consists of adipose cells, smooth muscle and blood vessels. Approximately 20 per cent of cases are associated with tuberous sclerosis syndrome, which is characterized by mental retardation, epilepsy and adenoma sebaceum. Most angiomyolipomas are asymptomatic and found incidentally. Tumours greater than 4 cm in diameter are more likely to cause symptoms, including massive retroperitoneal haemorrhage, which may require selective embolization or total nephrectomy.

## Ureter

### Pelviureteric Junction Obstruction

Obstruction of the flow of urine from the renal pelvis to the proximal ureter can lead to hydronephrosis and progressive renal impairment. Pelviureteric junction obstruction is usually congenital, and multiple aetiologies have been proposed. The condition can present at any age and may be unilateral or bilateral. The patient may experience UTIs, haematuria and flank pain, especially after increased fluid intake.

Clinical examination is usually unremarkable unless the kidney is significantly hydronephrotic, when it may be palpable. It is important to remember that hydronephrosis does not necessarily imply obstruction, and a kidney can be dilated but drain normally. The diagnosis of pelviureteric junction obstruction requires functional assessment, and the investigation of choice is diuresis renography.

### Retroperitoneal Fibrosis

Retroperitoneal fibrosis is characterized by the deposition of fibrotic plaques on the posterior abdominal wall. The fibrosis encases the ureters, causing obstruction, which is secondary to impaired ureteric peristalsis rather than mechanical blockage. Chronic and progressive upper urinary tract obstruction can lead to renal impairment.

The condition usually presents in middle age with nonspecific symptoms, including poorly localized back pain, fever, anorexia, weight loss and malaise. On examination, approximately 50 per cent of patients have hypertension, and there may rarely be peripheral oedema, thrombosis, ascites or a hydrocele. Treatment involves surgical release of the ureters from the fibrosis, or corticosteroids if the fibrosis is secondary to an inflammatory aneurysm.

## Bladder

### Acute Urinary Retention

In an adult man, the finding of a distended bladder associated with an inability to micturate should provoke a search for the possible cause (Figure 39.22). The foreskin and urethral meatus

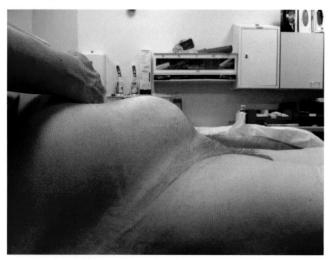

Figure 39.22 Acute urinary retention.

are examined for phimosis and meatal stenosis, and the length of the urethra as far as the bulb can be palpated for a stricture, a periurethral abscess or the presence of a stone or foreign body. The presence of any urethral discharge should be noted. The prostate must be examined as prostatic disease is the most common cause of retention of urine in men.

A full assessment should include examination of the central nervous system to exclude a neurogenic cause for the retention. The bladder sensation and micturition reflex arc can be inhibited or obliterated by central nervous system disease that is localized to the level of the midsacral neural outflow. The physical signs associated with nerve damage at this site are an absent ankle jerk and diminished or absent cutaneous sensation in the perineum and perianal regions. This examination is essential in all younger patients who present with retention of urine and those with any other physical signs of neurological disease.

When retention of urine is due to prostatic enlargement, it is preceded by the typical symptoms of bladder outflow obstruction. If these symptoms are untreated, a proportion of these men develop acute retention, which is the painful inability to micturate. However, in another, albeit smaller, proportion of men, the bladder continues to enlarge as the obstruction increases, and the condition of chronic retention follows.

The **chronic retention** of urine produces similar physical signs but is quite painless for the patient. He may also complain of dribbling 'overflow' incontinence; firm palpation of the enlarged bladder may induce leakage at the urethral meatus. Chronic retention is more likely to produce upper tract hydronephrosis and thus renal impairment – the appropriate physical signs may be present. Why some men with bladder outflow obstruction from prostatic hyperplasia suffer acute retention, while others develop chronic enlargement of the bladder and upper tract dilatation, remains unclear.

In women, retention of urine can also occur. In the younger woman, this is usually neurological in origin and may represent the onset of a more widespread neurological disease such as multiple sclerosis. In the older woman, difficulty with micturition due to obstructed voiding can result from a urethral stenosis. This may develop in the post-menopausal woman as part of atrophic vaginitis due to poor oestrogenization of the vulval tissues.

## Prostate

### Benign Prostatic Hyperplasia

Benign enlargement of the prostate gland is a common finding in elderly men. An enlarged prostate gland on clinical examination is commonly referred to as BPE. Benign prostatic hyperplasia is a histological diagnosis that can only be made on microscopic examination of biopsied or resected prostate tissue. Benign prostatic enlargement is mostly secondary to BPH.

In BPE, the two lateral lobes of the prostate feel smooth and can bulge posteriorly, laterally and superiorly, while retaining the central sulcus. The enlarged prostate is occasionally asymmetrical, and this can be confused with prostatic adenocarcinoma. Benign prostatic enlargement can cause obstruction of the prostatic urethra leading to lower urinary tract symptoms (LUTS) during voiding, including urinary hesitancy, a slow and intermittent stream, prolonged micturition and terminal dribbling. However, it is important to note that not all men with BPE will experience LUTS, and voiding symptoms may be secondary to pathology other than BPH.

Men presenting with bothersome LUTS secondary to BPE are often managed with medical therapy to relax the smooth muscle component of the prostate and/or shrink the prostate. If medical therapy fails, surgical treatment by transurethral endoscopic resection of the prostate is the current gold standard therapy.

## Urethra

### Urethral Stricture

A urethral stricture is a narrowing of the urethra, which can result from a wide variety of conditions, including:

- *congenital*: meatal stricture, bulbar stricture, posterior urethral valves;
- *traumatic*: instrumentation (e.g. catheterization), direct injury, foreign body;
- *inflammatory*: gonococcal and non-gonococcal urethritis, BXO;
- *neoplastic*: urothelial cell carcinoma, squamous cell carcinoma of the penis.

Iatrogenic and traumatic strictures tend to be short and situated in the bulb of the urethra, while infective strictures often involve longer lengths of the anterior urethra. Patients with a urethral stricture often present with similar symptoms to those with prostatic enlargement. They are, however, usually younger and often overcome their poor urinary flow by abdominal straining. They suffer from repeated UTIs and occasionally experience visible haematuria.

Examination and subsequent investigations (urethrography) aim to determine the exact site and length of the stricture as subsequent management is dictated by these two factors (Figure 39.23).

### Caruncle

A urethral caruncle is a benign urethral lesion most commonly diagnosed in post-menopausal women. In the majority of cases, the caruncle is asymptomatic and diagnosed incidentally on pelvic examination. Urethral caruncles can present with discomfort or blood on the underclothes. On examination, they often appear as a red exophytic lesion at the urethral meatus (Figure 39.24).

## Urethral Diverticulum

Urethral diverticula occur in 1–5 per cent of the general female population and classically present with the three Ds (**d**ysuria, post-void **d**ribbling and **d**yspareunia). Diverticula are associated with stones, incontinence and infection, including urethral abscesses. However, many patients have minimal symptoms, and the diverticulum is then diagnosed during the investigation of other symptoms. On physical examination, urethral diverticula can be felt as a mass behind the urethral meatus, which on compression may elicit discomfort and/or a purulent discharge.

## Penis

### Hypospadias

Hypospadias is an abnormal ventral opening of the urethral meatus, which may be positioned anywhere between the ventral aspect of the glans penis and the perineum (Figure 39.25). This anatomical anomaly is associated with a 'hooded' foreskin that is deficient ventrally (Figure 39.26) and a ventrally curved penis (chordee). It is a common congenital abnormality, affecting approximately 1 in 250 male births. Boys with hypospadias should be examined for associated abnormalities including an undescended testis (8–9 per cent) and inguinal hernia and/or hydrocele (9–16 per cent).

### Epispadias

Epispadias is a rare congenital abnormality (1 in 117 000 males) characterized by the urethral meatus opening onto the dorsal aspect of the penis (Figure 39.27). It is classified depending on the position of the urethral opening and varies from a mild form with a glandular defect to the penopubic variety with complete incontinence. Epispadias is associated with bladder exstrophy.

### Phimosis

Phimosis is a condition in which the foreskin cannot be fully retracted over the glans penis (Figure 39.28). In neonates, there is a physiological phimosis because of natural adhesions between the prepuce and the glans. These adhesions are broken down as the penis grows and smegma accumulates under the foreskin. At 3 years of age, 90 per cent of foreskins can be retracted. A pathological phimosis can occur secondary to balanitis (inflammation of the glans) or balanoposthitis (posthitis being inflammation of the foreskin).

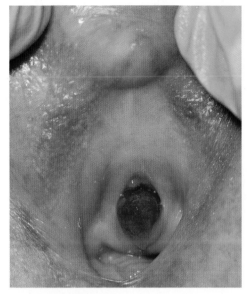

Figure 39.24 A urethral caruncle.

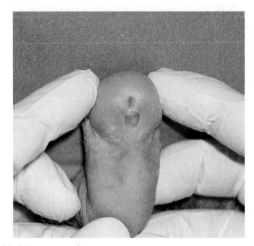

Figure 39.25 Hypospadias.

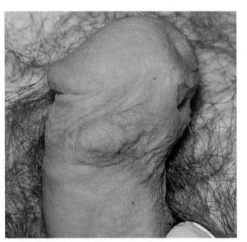

Figure 39.26 Hypospadias, showing the hooded foreskin.

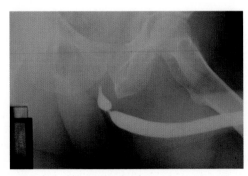

Figure 39.23 A urethrogram showing a bulbar stricture.

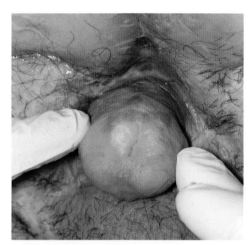

Figure 39.27 Epispadias.

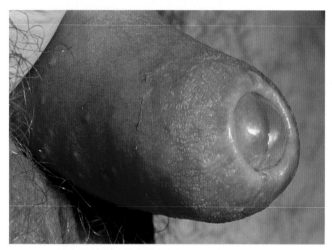

Figure 39.28 Phimosis.

## Paraphimosis

Paraphimosis is a condition in which the foreskin, once retracted back over the glans, cannot be returned to its original position. As a result, the foreskin becomes swollen, oedematous and inflamed. The cause is usually iatrogenic and occurs after failing to replace the foreskin after clinical examination or instrumentation, especially urethral catheterization. The majority of cases can be managed with patient reassurance, local anaesthesia and then manual compression to reduce the oedema, with simultaneous advancement of the foreskin.

## Meatal Stenosis

Meatal stenosis is a narrowing of the urethra at the external meatus. In children, the condition is almost always acquired following circumcision. It has been proposed that meatal stenosis results from ischaemia caused by division of the frenular artery during circumcision and/or inflammation of the glans following removal of the foreskin.

## Inguinoscrotal

### General Examination of the Scrotum

Scrotal examination can reveal a multitude of pathologies, from benign congenital conditions to malignancies and acute surgical emergencies. Coexisting urological conditions are occasionally

present. The scrotum (Figure 39.29) and its contents are readily accessible to physical examination, and an appreciation of the normal anatomy facilitates an accurate diagnosis of most scrotal masses.

It important to always bear in mind that if the patient has a scrotal swelling, it may not be due to pathology of the external genitalia but may instead be a mass that has descended through the inguinal canal into the scrotum (i.e. a hernia; Figure 39.30).

To thoroughly examine the external genitalia, it is important that the patient is warm, comfortable and relaxed. The examination should be performed with the patient both lying and standing. First inspect the genitals for evidence of skin changes.

Any lesion that occurs in the skin, particularly **sebaceous cysts** (Figure 39.31), can affect the skin of the scrotum. These cysts typically present as painless nodules in the dermal layer and are freely mobile over the underlying tissues. Sebaceous cysts are often surgically excised for cosmetic reasons.

**Squamous cell carcinoma** of the scrotum is primarily an occupational illness that has become relatively rare due to reduced exposure to carcinogens (soot, tar, pitch, mineral oil) in the workplace. The condition presents as a raised plaque that enlarges and ulcerates. Primary treatment is wide local excision of the scrotal lesion.

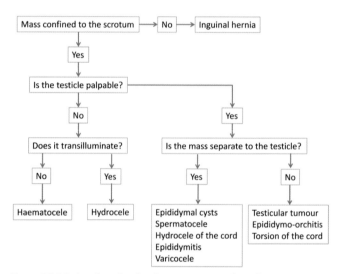

Figure 39.29 An algorithm for diagnosing scrotal swellings.

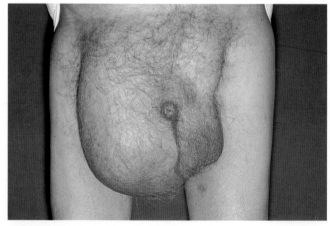

Figure 39.30 A hernia.

- Is the testis palpable?
- Is the mass separate from the testis?
- Does the mass transilluminate?
- Is the mass tender?

## Hydrocele

During normal development, the testis descends into the scrotum from the abdominal cavity and takes with it a projection of peritoneum (the processus vaginalis). The processus vaginalis becomes obliterated, leaving a small potential space between the layers of the tunica vaginalis around the testis. A hydrocele is a collection of fluid within the tunica vaginalis and results from an excess formation or reduced absorption of peritoneal fluid (**Figure 39.32**).

**Congenital hydroceles** occur due to failure of closure of the processus vaginalis (communicating hydroceles). They present at birth or occasionally in later life. Classically, the hydrocele varies in size during the day depending on the patient's posture and level of physical activity. On examination, the fluid within the hydrocele transilluminates and can be compressed and drained back into the abdomen. The differential diagnosis of a congenital hydrocele includes a congenital hernia.

An **infantile hydrocele** occurs when the processus vaginalis closes proximally trapping fluid within the tunica vaginalis (a simple hydrocele). They are often bilateral, large, tense, painless and transilluminate.

A **hydrocele of the cord** occurs when the processus vaginalis closes in a segmental fashion, resulting in a loculated fluid collection anywhere from above the testicle to the inguinal canal. The hydrocele is mobile and may transilluminate depending on its position.

## Haematocele

A haematocele is a collection of blood with the tunica vaginalis and typically results from blunt or sharp trauma to the external genitalia. Haematoceles are often tense and painful, and do not transilluminate. If a haematocele is large or there is a suspicion of testicular rupture, scrotal exploration is recommended.

## The Testes

In the patient who presents with hemiscrotal pathology, it is good clinical practice to first examine the 'normal' side. The testes vary in size between individuals and to a lesser degree within individuals. Palpation of the normal testicle allows, without causing discomfort, an appreciation of the size, shape, firmness and lie of the patient's testicle before moving to the contralateral side.

Testicular Maldescent – In a child, it is important to confirm the presence of two testes. One of the most common congenital anomalies is an undescended testicle (cryptorchidism, or 'hidden testis'), which affects 3 per cent of full-term male newborns and up to 30 per cent of premature infants. Over 70 per cent of cryptorchid testes will spontaneously descend by 3 months, and at 1 year of age the incidence of cryptorchidism is approximately 1 per cent. The testis can also lie in an ectopic position outside the line of normal descent. An ectopic testicle may be located in the suprapubic, femoral or perineal region.

A maldescended testis needs to be differentiated from a 'retractile' testis, which is a testis that is withdrawn out of the scrotum by an active cremasteric reflex (initiated by stroking the skin of the inner aspect of the thigh). A retractile testis can be brought down into the scrotum and remains there after traction

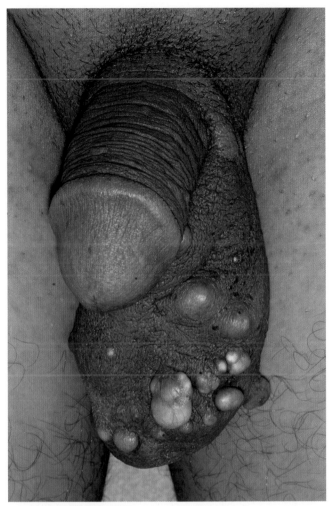

Figure 39.31 Scrotal cysts.

**Scrotal oedema** can affect all ages and is either acute or chronic. Acute oedema occurs secondary to local infection or trauma. Chronic oedema of the scrotum can be caused by a number of conditions such as heart failure, liver failure, peritoneal dialysis, prior surgery and radiotherapy. Lymphoma and penile and pelvic cancers can result in venous compression and/or lymphatic infiltration, leading to lower limb and scrotal oedema.

Idiopathic scrotal oedema is a condition of young boys (usually less than 10 years of age), which typically causes unilateral swelling and erythema, and resolves with conservative therapy over a couple of days. In this group, it is important to exclude acute spermatic cord torsion.

The entire contents of the scrotum, including the testes, epididymides and cord structures, need to be examined individually and assessed for their presence and normality. Any individual component may be absent congenitally, and if a testis and/or vas is absent, the presence of a kidney on that side should be determined by ultrasound as there is an association with renal agenesis.

If a mass is discovered in the scrotum, five key questions should be answered:

- Is it possible to palpate above the mass (i.e. is the mass arising from the scrotum or is it extending into the scrotum from the inguinal canal)?

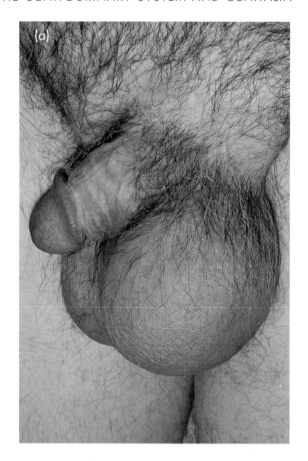

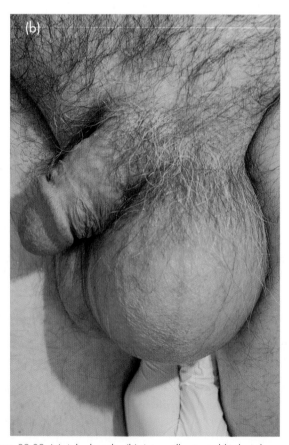

Figure 39.32 (a) A hydrocele. (b) A transilluminated hydrocele.

has been released. Retractile testes typically present between the ages of 3 and 7 years and do not require treatment.

## Torsion of the Spermatic Cord

Torsion of the cord needs to be considered in all patients who present with acute scrotal symptoms. Most episodes of torsion occur during sleep in boys aged between 13 and17 years. Patients typically present with acute and severe testicular pain that radiates to the inguinal region. Testicular swelling is often accompanied by nausea and vomiting. There is usually no history of additional LUTS.

On palpation, the testis may be lying high in the scrotum (Figure 39.33) and have an abnormal transverse orientation due to torsion-induced shortening of the spermatic cord. The scrotal skin overlying the testis may be erythematous and oedematous. The absence of a cremasteric reflex is a good sign of torsion of the cord but is often difficult to assess due to severe pain.

Torsion of the spermatic cord is a surgical emergency and requires immediate scrotal exploration because irreversible ischaemic injury to the testicular tissue occurs (Figure 39.34). The testicular salvage rate for surgical detorsion is 90 per cent if performed within 6 hours of symptom onset, but only 50 per cent after 12 hours and 10 per cent after 24 hours.

Adolescents occasionally present with a history of intermittent episodes of severe scrotal pain that have resolved spontaneously. At the time of the physical examination, the symptoms have

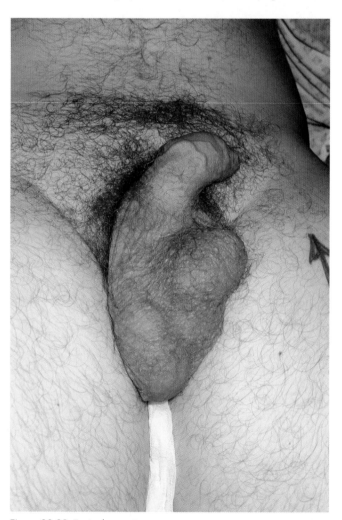

Figure 39.33 Testicular torsion.

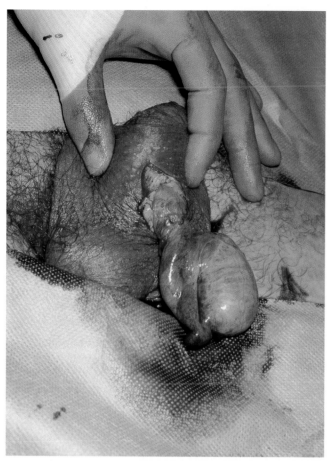

Figure 39.34 Intraoperative view of testicular torsion.

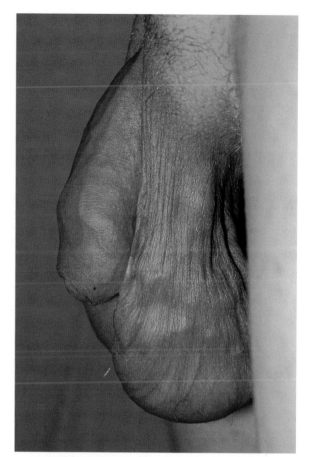

Figure 39.35 Varicocele.

usually settled and no abnormality is detected except for perhaps a bell-clapper deformity. These features are consistent with cord torsion with spontaneous detorsion and are best managed by elective scrotal exploration and bilateral testicular fixation.

## Torsion of the Testicular and Epididymal Appendages

Torsion of the appendix testis and appendix epididymis can present with variable symptoms ranging from mild scrotal discomfort to severe pain indistinguishable from torsion of the cord. In the initial phase, the pain may be localized to the upper pole of the testis or epididymis, where a tender nodule may be palpable. The infarcted appendage is occasionally visible through the skin (the 'blue dot' sign). The testis will be mobile, and the cremasteric reflex should be intact.

Most cases resolve spontaneously with simple analgesia. If scrotal exploration is performed for clinical uncertainty, the torted appendage can be excised.

## The Epididymis and Vas

The epididymis is palpable behind the body of the testis and is continuous with the vas, which passes within the spermatic cord. Examination should be carefully performed to confirm the presence of these structures as congenital absence is not uncommon. Agenesis of the vas is associated with cystic fibrosis and absence of the epididymis and/or the seminal vesicles, as well as with renal anomalies, including renal agenesis.

Epididymal Cyst – Epididymal cysts are commonly found during routine examination. The cysts are typically located in the head of the epididymis and are spherical, smooth and variable in size; they may be multiple and bilateral. They transilluminate and, when small, are easy to differentiate from other scrotal pathologies. Most cysts are asymptomatic, but as they enlarge the patient may complain of discomfort or a feeling of heaviness in the scrotum. Large epididymal cysts can mimic a hydrocele and are often only differentiated on ultrasound examination or during surgery.

A spermatocele is an epididymal cyst that contains sperm and occurs in adults.

## The Pampiniform Plexus

### Varicocele

A varicocele is a dilatation of the veins of the pampiniform plexus within the spermatic cord. It occurs in approximately 15 per cent of male adolescents and up to 30 per cent of men investigated for infertility (it remains controversial whether varicoceles cause oligospermia). Approximately 90 per cent of varicoceles are left-sided, attributable to increased venous pressure in the internal spermatic vein (as the left drains into the left renal vein and the right drains into the vena cava), collateral venous anastomoses and absent or incompetent valves in the veins.

Varicoceles are usually asymptomatic. Occasionally, they present with a dull ache in the scrotum, exacerbated by prolonged standing or physical activity.

Examination should be performed with the patient both standing and supine and with and without a Valsalva manoeuvre. Classically, the veins engorge and feel like a 'bag of worms' (Figure 39.35) when the patient is standing. When he lies down, however, the veins decompress and become less prominent. It is important in boys who present with a varicocele to assess testicular volume, preferably with an orchidometer. Ipsilateral testicular volume loss is an indication to offer surgical ligation or radiological embolization of the varicocele (Figure 39.36).

## GENITOURINARY TRACT TRAUMA

### Renal Injuries

The kidney is the most commonly injured organ in abdominal trauma, occurring in up to 10 per cent of cases. Renal injuries are usually due to blunt trauma sustained in road traffic accidents, sports accidents, falls and assaults. Penetrating injuries can occur with gun shots and stab wounds, and during surgical and percutaneous procedures. Minor injuries to the kidney include contusions and small lacerations, while more significant and potentially life-threatening injuries involve the renal vessels or a shattered kidney. Pre-existing renal abnormalities increase the chance of and complicate the outcome of kidney trauma.

The initial priority in the assessment and management of any trauma patient includes securing the airway, controlling external bleeding and resuscitation of shock. During the stabilization phase, a thorough physical examination should include looking for signs of urogenital injury. The clinical findings may include a penetrating wound in the flank, upper abdomen or lower chest, and if the patient has been shot, there may be an exit as well as an entry wound. It is important not to underestimate the degree of internal injury on the basis of a small penetrating injury wound.

Signs associated with blunt renal injury may include haematuria associated with flank bruising, tenderness and swelling. Blood in the ureter and bladder may clot, producing clot colic, which characteristically occurs 2–5 days after injury.

Although blood in the urine is the most common sign of underlying renal injury, the degree of haematuria, whether it is microscopic or macroscopic, continuous or intermittent, does not always correlate with the severity of the injury. Rarely in major renal injury, the renal pedicle may be avulsed, the pelviureteric junction disrupted or a segmental artery thrombosed, and the patient may not exhibit haematuria.

### Ureteric Injury

The ureter is involved in less than 1 per cent of all genitourinary tract injuries sustained by external trauma. External injury can be penetrating or blunt, with gun shot wounds accounting for over 90 per cent of cases, and stab wounds and blunt trauma together accounting for less than 10 per cent of injuries.

Ureteric trauma more commonly results from iatrogenic injury, specifically abdominopelvic surgery and ureteroscopy. The ureter may be divided, crushed, devascularized, ligated, excised or perforated. The majority of iatrogenic injuries are diagnosed postoperatively and present with flank pain, fever, sepsis, prolonged ileus or occasionally renal failure. On physical examination, there may be a tender flank mass secondary to a urinoma, signs of peritonitis or urine leakage from the wound or vagina.

### Bladder Trauma

The bladder lies in the anterior part of the pelvic cavity behind the pubic bones. The superior surface of the bladder is covered by peritoneum, which in males passes down the posterior surface of bladder before being reflected onto the anterior aspect of the rectum to form the rectovesical pouch. In females, the peritoneum reflects from the posterior bladder wall onto the body of the uterus, forming the vesicouterine pouch.

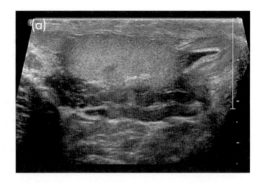

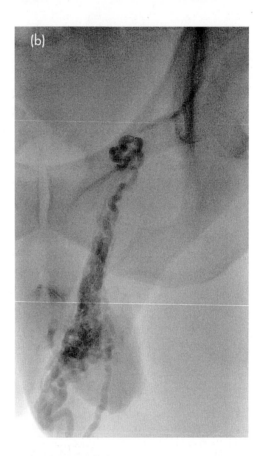

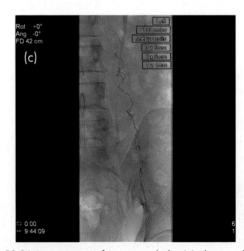

Figure 39.36 Investigation of a varicocele by (a) ultrasound and (b) a venogram. (c) Embolization of a varicocele.

The bladder may be injured by blunt or penetrating injury, and the rupture may be intraperitoneal or extraperitoneal. The risk of bladder injury is related to the degree of bladder distension, a full bladder being more prone to rupture than an empty one.

Traumatic extraperitoneal bladder injuries are usually associated with pelvic fractures, resulting in direct perforation by a bony fragment, a compression burst injury or laceration by shear forces. Pelvic injury can result in simultaneous trauma to the bladder and posterior urethra. Other causes of extraperitoneal injury of the bladder include iatrogenic injury secondary to transurethral resection of the bladder and surgical procedures for urinary stress incontinence (Figure 39.37).

Bladder resection of the dome, the thinnest part of the bladder wall, can also result in an intraperitoneal injury. This is usually diagnosed intraoperatively and requires a laparotomy to close the bladder wall defect. A common cause of intraperitoneal injury due to external trauma is a direct blow to a distended bladder. The classic presentation is an inebriated individual involved in a fight or a person with a car seatbelt injury.

Bladder trauma commonly presents with the classic triad of gross haematuria, suprapubic tenderness and difficulty or inability to void. Extravasation of urine may produce swelling in the scrotum, perineum, abdominal wall and thighs. On physical examination, absent bowel sounds, abdominal distension, guarding and rebound tenderness suggest intraperitoneal injury.

Rectal examination may reveal an elevated or 'high-riding' prostate, suggestive of a posterior urethral injury. If present, this sign is often difficult to elicit due to disruption of the tissue planes by pelvic haematoma.

## Urethral Trauma

Urethral injuries are classified based on the anatomical location of the injury. The urogenital diaphragm divides the male urethra into anterior and posterior sections. The posterior urethra consists of the prostatic and the membranous urethra, and the anterior urethra consists of the bulbar and penile urethra. Only the posterior urethra exists in females.

The classic anterior urethral injury is a straddle injury sustained by a blow to the perineum, usually from a bicycle handlebar or a fence. Other causes include urethral injury associated with penile fracture, and iatrogenic injury during instrumentation and catheterization. Posterior urethral injury is usually secondary to major pelvic trauma and most cases are associated with pelvic fractures.

Physical examination may reveal blood at the urethral meatus, which is present in at least 75 per cent of cases of anterior urethral trauma and more variably with posterior urethral injury. The perineum and genitalia are commonly bruised, the pattern of which reflects the integrity of the fascial boundaries. With anterior urethral injury, a characteristic butterfly-shaped bruise results if Buck's fascial layer is disrupted.

Rectal examination may reveal an elevated or 'high-riding' prostate, suggestive of a posterior urethral injury. If present, this sign is often difficult to elicit due to pelvic haematoma. In cases of significant pelvic trauma, rectal examination is principally performed, not to feel for the prostate gland but to check for a rectal injury. Blood on the examination finger is supportive of a rectal injury and should prompt further investigation.

## Genital Trauma

Genital trauma is relatively common in men due to the exposed nature of the genitalia and a higher level of participation in physical sports. Men who have sustained blunt scrotal trauma classically present with acute, severe pain associated with scrotal bruising and swelling.

Physical examination may reveal a tense haematocele that prevents palpation of the underlying testis. In this situation, it is important to perform an ultrasound of the testis to establish whether the tunica albuginea has been ruptured and whether the parenchyma has sustained injury. If identified, surgical exploration and repair should be performed.

Fracture of the penis (rupture of the cavernosal tunica albuginea) can occur when the erect penis slips out of the vagina and is compressed against the symphysis pubis. Typically, the man usually hears a cracking sound, instantly loses his erection and then develops marked bruising and swelling of the penis (Figure 39.38). The defect in the tunica albuginea can occasionally be palpated, especially if there is minimal associated haematoma.

A penile fracture should be differentiated from a torn superficial blood vessel, which can also occur during intercourse. In contrast to a penile fracture, maintenance of erections is still possible after a vascular injury.

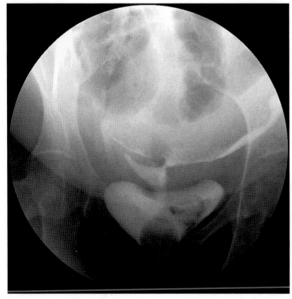

Figure 39.37 Bladder injury.

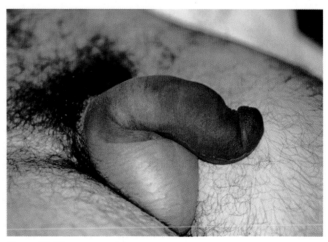

Figure 39.38 Fracture of the penis.

**Key Points**

- Urological conditions often present with a similar symptom complex.
- Laboratory and radiological studies are not a replacement for a thorough medical history and clinical examination.
- Torsion of the spermatic cord and Fournier's gangrene require prompt diagnosis and treatment to avoid or limit potentially significant morbidity.
- Urinalysis should be considered in all patients presenting with urological symptoms.

## QUESTIONS

### SBAs

**1. Which of the following pre-cancerous lesions of the penis is not related to a viral aetiology?:**
- **a** Bowenoid papulosis
- **b** Erythroplasia of Queyrat
- **c** Giant condyloma
- **d** Cutaneous horn
- **e** Bowen's disease

**Answer**

**d** *Cutaneous horn. Bowenoid papulosis, erythroplasia of Queyrat, giant condyloma and Bowen's disease are associated with human papillomavirus infection, whereas a cutaneous horn is thought to predispose to malignant transformation secondary to chronic inflammation.*

**2. In acute bacterial prostatitis, which of the following statements is inaccurate?:**
- **a** The condition typically presents with dysuria, urinary frequency and perineal pain
- **b** Digital rectal examination often reveals a globally tender prostate
- **c** Associated acute urinary retention is ideally managed with the passage of a urethral catheter
- **d** Prostatic secretions obtained by prostatic massage reveal bacteria and inflammatory cells in the initial voided urine specimen
- **e** A prolonged course (3–4 weeks) of antibiotics is required to eradicate the infection

**Answer**

**c** *Associated acute urinary retention is ideally managed with the passage of a urethral catheter. Acute bacterial prostatitis typically presents with a symptom complex of acute febrile illness, infective lower urinary tract symptoms and associated perineal and back pain. If tolerated, palpation of the prostate will reveal a tender, swollen and warm gland. Prostatic massage should be avoided if the patient is too unwell but if performed the culture of prostatic secretions and the voided urine often contain bacteria, especially Escherichia coli. If the patient develops acute urinary retention, it is best managed with a suprapubic catheter, not a urethral catheter, in order to avoid instrumentation of the inflamed prostatic urethra.*

**3. Which of the following is not a common clinical finding in cases of extraperitoneal bladder injury?:**
- **a** Haematuria
- **b** Suprapubic tenderness and fullness
- **c** Difficulty with or inability to void
- **d** Abdominal distension and absent bowel sounds
- **e** Pelvic pain on voiding

**Answer**

**d** *Abdominal distension and absent bowel sounds. Bladder injury with an associated breach of the overlying peritoneum results in leakage of urine into the abdominal cavity. This results in abdominal distension, guarding and rebound tenderness, as well as reduced bowel mobility.*

### EMQs

**1. From each of the descriptions of patients with a urological abnormality, choose the most likely diagnosis from the following options:**
- **1** Wilms' tumour
- **2** Renal angiomyolipoma
- **3** Emphysematous pyelonephritis
- **4** Xanthogranulomatous pyelonephritis
- **5** Pyonephrosis
- **6** Renal tuberculosis
- **7** Renal calculus
- **8** Renal cell carcinoma
- **9** Renal pelvic urothelial cell carcinoma
- **a** A 48-year-old lady presents with a 3 day history of right loin pain that was initially colicky but is now constant. She has a history of recurrent renal calculi. On examination, she is febrile, tachycardic and hypotensive.

**Answers**

**a 5** *Pyonephrosis. The patient's symptoms are consistent with an obstructed and infected upper urinary tract. This is a urological emergency that requires acute management with urinary tract drainage (nephrostomy) and antibiotics.*

**b** A 75-year-old lady with poorly controlled diabetes mellitus presents with a 4 day history of left loin discomfort, rigors and nausea. On examination of the loin region, there is crepitus on superficial palpation and pain on deep palpation.

**c** A 59-year-old man presents with a 2 week history of intermittent painless frank haematuria. He works in the petrochemical industry and smokes 20 cigarettes a day.

**d** A mother notices that her 5-year-old son has recently developed a visible mass in his right loin region. He is otherwise well.

**e** A 35-year-old man with a history of epilepsy and learning difficulties presents with loin pain, tachycardia and hypotension.

**b 3** *Emphysematous pyelonephritis. This condition is more common in older patients with diabetes mellitus and presents with loin pain and crepitus secondary to gas in the soft tissues.*

**c 9** *Renal pelvic urothelial cell carcinoma. Urothelial cell carcinomas are associated with cigarette smoking and occupational chemical carcinogens.*

**d 1** *Wilms' tumour. Nephroblastomas typically present as a painless loin mass in a relatively well child.*

**e 2** *Renal angiomyolipoma. Approximately 1 in 5 cases of angiomyolipma are associated with tuberous sclerosis syndrome, which is characterized by mental retardation, epilepsy and adenoma sebaceum.*

**2. From each of the descriptions of patients with a urological abnormality, choose the most likely diagnosis from the following options:**
   1 Prostatic adenocarcinoma
   2 Prostatic tuberculosis
   3 Urethritis
   4 Chronic pelvic pain syndrome
   5 Urothelial cell carcinoma of the bladder
   6 Acute bacterial prostatitis
   7 Urethral stricture
   8 Torsion of the spermatic cord
   9 Epididymo-orchitis

**a** A 30-year-old man presents with urinary frequency and a slow urine stream. He was treated for a gonorrhoea infection approximately 5 years previously. Dipstick urinalysis is positive for blood.

**b** A 39-year-old man presents with fever, pelvic and back pain, urinary frequency, dysuria and urgency. He is unable to tolerate a digital rectal examination because of the pain.

**c** A 42-year-old man presents with a 12 month history of intermittent perineal and back discomfort, dysuria and reduced libido. Urinalysis is negative.

**d** A 19-year-old man presents with urinary frequency, dysuria and a clear urethral discharge.

**e** A 15-year-old presents with acute right hemiscrotal pain. Dipstick urinalysis is negative.

Answers

**a 7** *Urethral stricture. Voiding urinary symptoms in a young man are often secondary to a urethral stricture, which in this case was induced by a previous gonococcus urethritis.*

**b 6** *Acute bacterial prostatitis. Acute bacterial prostatitis characteristically presents with voiding urinary symptoms, pelvic pain, systemic upset and sexual dysfunction. Treatment requires a prolonged course of antibiotics (e.g. 3–6 weeks of ciprofloxacin or trimethoprim).*

**c 4** *Chronic pelvic pain syndrome. This is often a diagnosis of exclusion. The symptom complex is similar to chronic bacterial prostatitis but the differentiating factor is that chronic pelvic pain syndrome is characterized by the absence of bacteriuria.*

**d 3** *Urethritis. In a young sexually active man with dysuria and a urethral discharge, a sexually transmitted infection is the primary diagnosis until proven otherwise.*

**e 8** *Torsion of the spermatic cord. Acute scrotal pain in a man with no infective symptoms or signs is often due to ischaemic testicular pain. In the acute setting, prompt surgical exploration is required to avoid or limit irreversible loss of testicular function.*

# Index

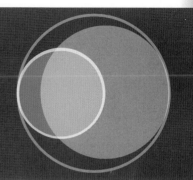

WITHDRAWN FROM LIBRARY
BMA LIBRARY
BRITISH MEDICAL ASSOCIATION